ISBN 978-0-484-07460-5
PIBN 10783903

FB &c Ltd, Dalton House, 60 Windsor Avenue, London, SW19 2RR.
Company number 08720141. Registered in England and Wales.

For support please visit www.forgottenbooks.com

THE

MEDICAL NEWS.

A Weekly Medical Journal.

EDITED BY

J. RIDDLE GOFFE, PH.B., M.D.

VOLUME LXXII.

JANUARY—JUNE, 1898.

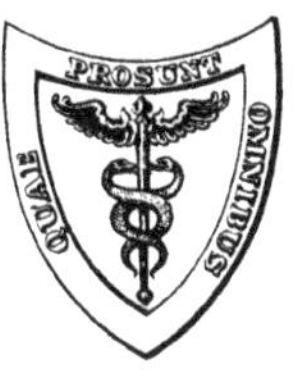

NEW YORK:

LEA BROTHERS & CO.

1898.

ROONEY & OTTEN PRINTING CO.,

NEW YORK.

CONTRIBUTORS

TO

VOLUME SEVENTY-TWO.

R. Abrahams, M.D., of New York.
Albert Abrams, M.D., of San Francisco.
Charles Lewis Allen, M.D., of Washington, D. C.
Royal W. Amidon, M.D., of New York.
Willis S. Anderson, M.D., of Detroit, Mich.
J. A. Bach, M.D., of Milwaukee, Wis.
Gorham Bacon, M.D., of New York.
Wesley B. Bailey, M.D., of Pekin, Ill.
L. Grant Baldwin, M.D., of New York.
G. H. Balleray, M.D., of Newark, N J.
P. V. Ballou, M.D., of Rowena, Ky.
William C. Bane, M.D., of Denver, Col.
L. Bolton Bangs, M.D., of New York.
Carl Beck, M.D., of New York.
A. L. Benedict, M.D., of Buffalo, N. Y.
Herman M. Biggs, M.D., of New York.
Albert E. Blackburn, M.D., of Philadelphia.
I. N. Bloom, M.D., of Louisville, Ky.
Henry P. Bowditch, M.D., of Boston.
Samuel M. Brickner, M.D., of New York.
Harlow Brooks, M.D., of New York.
Everett J. Brown, M.D., of Decatur, Ill.
W. F. Brunner, M.D., of Marine Hospital Service.
Arthur Conklin Brush, M.D., of Brooklyn, N. Y.
E. F. Brush, M.D., of New York.
Joseph D. Bryant, M.D., of New York.
J. N. Buckham, M.D., of Flint, Mich.
J. H. Burch, M.D., of Baldwinsville, N. Y.
James Hawley Burtenshaw, M.D., of New York.
F. C. Busch, M.D., of Buffalo, N. Y.
Glentworth R. Butler, M.D., of Brooklyn, N. Y.
W. K. Butler, M.D., of Washington, D. C.
H. R. Carter, M.D., Marine Hospital Service.
A. Morgan Cartledge, M.D., of Louisville, Ky.
E. C. Chamberlin, M.D., of New York.
George L. Chapman, M.D., of Chicago.
Palmer C. Cole, M.D., of New York.
George L. Cole, M.D., of Los Angeles, Cal.
Henry C. Coe, M.D., of New York.
Joseph Collins, M.D., of New York.
W. L. Coplin, M.D., of Philadelphia.
Edwin B. Cragin, M.D., of New York.
T. D. Crothers, M.D., of Hartford, Conn.
J. C. Da Costa, Jr., M.D., of Philadelphia.
Charles L. Dana, M.D., of New York.
Waller H. Dade, M.D., of Chicago.
E. P. Davis, M.D., of Philadelphia.
D. Bryson Delavan, M.D., of New York.
I. B. Diamond, M.D., of Houston, Tex.
George Dock, M.D., of Ann Arbor, Mich.
Fay M. Dunlap, M.D., of Bloomington, Ill.
Max Einhorn, M.D., of New York.
Henry L. Elsner, M.D., of Syracuse, N. Y.
J. H. Emerson, M.D., of New York.
Rosa Engelmann, M.D., of Chicago.
Henry B. Favill, M.D., of Chicago.
William Flitcroft, M.D., of Paterson, N. J.
Edward M. Foote, M.D., of New York.
George Ryerson Fowler, M.D., of Brooklyn, N.Y.
Melvin M. Franklin, M.D., of New York.
M. Howard Fussell, M.D., of Philadelphia.
A. Ernest Gallant, M.D., of New York.
H. J. Garrigues, M.D., of New York.
C. P. Gildersleeve, M.D., of Brooklyn, N. Y.
Herbert R. Goodrich, M.D., of Philadelphia.
J. Riddle Goffe, M.D., of New York.
M. M. Grady, M.D., of New York.
Egbert H. Grandin, M.D., of New York.
Allen McLane Hamilton, M.D., of New York.
Charles S. Hamilton, M.D., of Columbus, Ohio.
Hobart Amory Hare, M.D., of Philadelphia.
T. A. Harris, M.D., of Parkersburg, W. Va.
George C. Harlan, M.D., of Philadelphia.
Frank Hartley, M.D., of New York.
L. J. Harvey, M.D., of Griggsville, Ill.
Knut Hoegh, M.D., of Minneapolis, Minn.
Charles A. Holder, M.D., of Philadelphia.
George Homan, M.D., of St. Louis.
George T. Howland, M.D., of Washington, D. C.
Arthur M. Jacobus, M.D., of New York.
Jacob R. Johns, M.D., of Philadelphia.

Levi B. Johnson, M.D., of Muscatine, Ia.
Wallace Johnson, of Washington, D. C.
Jas. C. Johnston, M.D., of New York.
Joseph A. Kenefick, M.D., of New York.
H. A. Kilbourne, M.D., of U. S. Army.
Jas. P. Kimball, M.D., of U. S. Army.
Herbert Maxon King, M.D., of Grand Rapids, Mich.
Charles H. Knight, M.D., of New York.
D. L. Lainé, M.D., of Philadelphia.
John A. Lichty, M.D., of Clifton Springs, N. Y.
J. C. Lightfoot, M.D., of Alvaton, Ky.
R. P. Lincoln, M.D., of New York.
Frank E. Lock, M.D., of Buffalo, N. Y.
Eli H. Long, M.D., of Buffalo, N. Y.
M. D. MacDaniel, M.D., of New York.
M. L. Maduro, M.D., of New York.
W. F. Martin, M.D., of Colorado Springs, Col.
Claudius Henry Mastin, M.D., of Mobile, Ala.
Joseph M. Mathews, M.D., of Louisville, Ky.
Emil Mayer, M.D., of New York.
James H. McCall, M.D., of Huntingdon, Tenn.
S. J. McNamara, M.D., of Brooklyn.
A. Dan Morgan, M.D., of Witt's Mills, S. C.
Robert T. Morris, M.D., of New York.
J. B. Nichols, M.D., of Washington, D. C.
F. H. Nicolai, M.D., of Milan, Italy.
N. W. Noble, M.D., of Rochester, N. Y.
W. P. Northrup, M.D., of New York.
F. G. Novy, M.D., of Ann Arbor, Mich.
Seymour Oppenheimer, M.D., of New York.
Lambert Ott, M.D., of Philadelphia.
R. C. M. Page, M.D., of New York.
Thomas D. Parke, M.D., of Birmingham, Ala.
Isaac L. Peebles, M.D., of Hattiesburg, Miss.
Howell T. Pershing, M.D., of Denver, Col.
Frederick Peterson, M.D., of New York.
W. M. Pirt, M.D., of Barrie, Ontario, Canada.
Henry I. Raymond, M.D., of U. S. Army.
R. Harvey Reed, M.D., of Rock Springs, Wyo.
Julius Rosenberg, M.D., of New York.
E. Wood Ruggles, M.D., of Berlin, Germany.
B. Sachs, M.D., of New York.
Robert Sattler, M.D., of Cincinnati, Ohio.
H. A. Sifton, M.D., of Milwaukee, Wis.
W. Kelly Simpson, M.D., of New York.
Ellet Orrin Sisson, M.D., of Keokuk, Ia.
Fred. P. Solly, M.D., of New York.
Raymond Spear, M.D., of U. S. Navy.
W. G. Spiller, M.D., of Philadelphia.
George M. Sternberg, M.D., of U. S. Army.
Charles F. Stokes, M.D., of U. S. Navy.
Heinrich Stern, M.D., of New York.
Dudley Tait, M.D., of San Francisco.
John Madison Taylor, M.D., of Philadelphia.
Jerome B. Thomas, Jr., M.D., of Brooklyn, N. Y.
A. O. Trebeck, M.D., of Charlottesville, Va.
J. S. Triplett, M.D., of Harrisonville, Mo.
Frank Van Fleet, M.D., of New York.
G. Tully Vaughan, M.D., of Washington, D. C.
Victor C. Vaughan, M.D., of Ann Arbor, Mich.
Carl Weidner, M.D., of Louisville, Ky.

THE MEDICAL NEWS.

A WEEKLY JOURNAL OF MEDICAL SCIENCE.

VOL. LXXII. NEW YORK, SATURDAY, JANUARY 1, 1898. NO. 1.

ORIGINAL ARTICLES.

HYSTERIA IN CHILDHOOD AND YOUTH.

BY JOHN MADISON TAYLOR, M.D.,
OF PHILADELPHIA;
PROFESSOR OF DISEASES OF CHILDREN IN THE PHILADELPHIA POLYCLINIC; NEUROLOGIST TO THE HOWARD HOSPITAL; ASSISTANT PHYSICIAN TO THE CHILDRENS' HOSPITAL.

THE tendency during late years has been to make the diagnosis of hysteria much less rashly than of old. The time was, and quite recently, when a large number of puzzling functional affections were called hysteria, and treated as such. Increasing knowledge of the disorder is correcting this unfortunate mistake. True hysteria frequently occurs among children, in whom it is sometimes seen in a very graphic form, in boys as well as in girls, although twice as frequently in the latter. It increases steadily in frequency of occurrence from the third to the thirteenth year, and no age is exempt. The popular idea of this affection is that it is a mere feigning of disease, though hysteria, while simulating many disorders, is never a true imitation of any. It is a psychosis with clearly defined stigmata physical and psychic. Hysteria may be described, then, as a functional disturbance of the nervous system due to no known structural lesion, manifested by paralyses, convulsions, psychic, and sensory disturbances, and impairment of vision. The early recognition of all the neuroses of childhood is peculiarly important. This is epecially true of hysteria, which, if unchecked, seriously modifies character growth and psychic development, as well as obscuring the sequelæ of acute diseases.

In almost no other disorder do we see the influence of remote causes so admirably illustrated as in the hysteria of children. A neurotic ancestry of howsoever wide a variety may be manifested in the child in this form. It is rare, if not impossible, for children to be thus affected unless there is a clear history of neuropathic ancestry, along with debilitating conditions or emotional strain. It readily happens, too, that a powerful example may produce a hysteric outbreak in a well-balanced child. The influence of environment is a most potent factor in the production of hysteria. Exciting causes are: exhausting conditions, depressed health from acute diseases, injuries, abusive treatment at the hands of others, overwrought emotionality, and objectionable education generally, especially in religious matters. A very important study for the general practitioner is to search closely into the hereditary and other causes of all the neuroses in children, and it is also a very essential part of his duty. Whenever there is recognized ancestral alcoholism, insanity, or "marked peculiarities," the children must be doubly watched and guarded.

Hysteric symptoms are frequently seen during convalescence from infectious and other acute diseases. Imitative paralysis, contracture, tremor, and persistent local pain or tenderness are likely to follow various injuries, even very trifling ones. Vexations, disappointments, fright, shame, and, above all, religious excitement, are often potent factors in the production of psychic disturbances. An early encouragement of religious thoughts and training, especially of a kind which cultivates emotional exaltation, is powerful for harm in this direction. Perhaps the very worst influence of all, because more constantly present, is unwise, especially careless, home influences, lacking in systematic and watchful control, encouraging selfishness and minor deceptions deemed necessary by the child to secure what is coveted. Lax regulations as to duty and the higher moral faculties is the atmosphere most congenial to the growth of hysteria and even worse things. However, it must not be inferred that hysteria is solely the outcome of individual blameworthiness, nor is it always the result of lax moral conditions; for, on the other hand, puritanic severity is capable of working a large measure of harm. Disorders of the generative organs, especially those resulting from masturbation, are important causative agents, about which much might be said, especially as parents are singularly unwilling or unable to control habits of the kind mentioned.

By far the most important element in hysteria is the mental phenomena, which are exceedingly varied and complex, and, to a trained observer, capable of clear differentiation, and yet, when superficially studied, appear a mere mass of mental disturbances, imitative procedures, pretense, and deception. It must first be recognized that hysteria is not a simple feature of degeneracy, but a condition which may be acquired by children of unimpeachable parentage and otherwise excellent health. The child subject to hysteria is markedly impressionable, with a great tendency to accept and act upon suggestion. There is a dissociation of the higher mental faculties, as of volition and cerebration, from lower emotional and impulsive states. The actions of a hysteric child during the paroxysm result from morbid concepts of associations of ideas, which permit the organic activities to exhibit characteristic irregularities. The key-note to the whole situation is suggestion, both in the production of the psychosis and the emancipation of the sufferer. Morbid suggestion from without or from within, one or the other, or both, produces the malady and encourages its continuance; and wise, forceful suggestion from without will affect a cure, especially if accompanied by well-chosen auxiliary measures systematically applied.

The paroxysm of hysteria consists of certain definite steps or procedures which continue from prodromal states with regular gradations to a systematic culmination, or they may be checked here or there, producing even more extraordinary features.

The paroxysm or hysteric fit has acquired the reputation of being the most important manifestation of the disorder, because it is the most conspicuous. It may, however, be absent or only rarely observed, or, again, but atypically exhibited. The more severe hysteric paroxysm has received the misleading name of "hystero-epilepsy," and is extremely rare, and when it does occur is difficult to differentiate from an epileptic attack. Nevertheless, it is hysteria, and has nothing in common with epilepsy. A better term, as proposed by Lloyd, is "hysteria-major," just as in epilepsy we distinguish between the larger and lesser epilepsy (or *grand* and *petit mal*).

The hysteric paroxysm usually begins with certain antecedent features, mostly changes in the mental state, a shifting of the mood from its normal plane. There is never absolute unconsciousness. The exciting cause may or may not be apparent; if not, the point of departure of the fit may be some auto-suggestion.

The fit follows close upon an aura, which may be either sensory or motor. It may begin abruptly, or be preceded by alternate laughing or crying. It usually begins with a subjective feeling, as of a lump rising in the throat which is accompanied by a sense of suffocation. Another form of aura consists of loud noises, throbbing or beating sounds in the ears; still another is violent headache, a boring or piercing pain, as of a nail driven into the head (clavus hystericus). At other times there is dimness of vision, or alarming dizziness. Again, there may be sensations connected with the ovaries or testicles. The fit proper is usually divided into periods. The first or convulsive period resembles epilepsy, but is in no sense identical with it. The patient sinks down, or falls prone upon the back, with the limbs extended and rigid, but with the fingers and toes flexed; the eyes are usually rolled slowly from right to left, or crossed; the jaws are firmly clenched; the breathing becomes slow and labored, and later hurried, the face flushed or bluish, the neck turgid; the cardiac action becomes more rapid and forcible, and consciousness is blunted, or even almost, but never entirely, lost. Sensation is much obtunded, and abolished in some portions of the body. Soon clonic movements succeed—a tremor affecting the muscles of the trunk, extremities, and face. This alternates with electric-like startings, during which the patient may fling himself furiously about, or actually out of bed. Presently this stage ends with sighs, and is followed by a short sleep.

The next stage is one of dramatic movements, not so commonly seen here as in Europe. These may appear by themselves, and explain some otherwise puzzling conditions. The most common form is a complete opisthotonos, tonic spasm of the muscles of the back, a bowing of the lumbar curve until the child rests only upon head and heels. This may alternate with, or be replaced by, a variety of quaint attitudes and movements, some of which simulate purposive acts, and others are merely automatic. The final or closing period of the convulsive attack is one of delirium. This is usually an expression of the dominating mental attitude, and likely to be reproduced in each succeeding fit. It usually expresses some condition of fear or sadness, manifested by tears and sobs, and more or less incoherent appealings or pleadings. The attack is not always complete, one period may be exaggerated and the others left out. Especially in children, certain acts may be habitually performed, or changed by suggestion until the combinations are most extraordinary.

A series of apparently purposive movements, or merely automatic acts, may originate in one individual, and be so powerfully suggestive to others that they unconsciously imitate them, and thus a widespread contagion occurs in religious communities and schools, such as gave rise to the dancing manias of the Middle Ages. Somnambulism should be mentioned as having points of contact with the hysteric state. A lethargy, also, sometimes follows the paroxysm. Catalepsy, another psychosis strongly resembling hysteria, may be observed during or after the hysteric fit. The duration of a paroxysm may be but a few minutes, and then, with intervals of rest, be succeeded by others, as many as two hundred attacks having occurred within twenty-four hours in a case recorded by Sachs; or it may last longer, as in a case observed by me, in which the attack continued the greater part of two hours. Those which occur fragmentarily, or present considerable variety in their manifestations, may continue, with almost no intermission, day in and day out, as in the epidemic which occurred in the Church Home of this city while I was on duty there.

The hysteric paroxysm, as has been said, is not the most important symptom of hysteria. The permanent markings (stigmata) of hysteria have to do with changes in sensation, motility, the activities of the viscera, the mind, and nutrition. Alterations in sensibility are nearly always present. Hyperesthesia and local tendernesses are common, as in the well-known hysterogenous zones. These zones and areas of exalted sensation, over which, if pressure be made, pain is produced, and some one or other of the more graphic motor manifestations are elicited; the most common of these are over the ovaries and spine. In boys the testicles are sometimes hypersensitive. Pressure over these zones may give rise to a convulsion, or, again, may cause them to stop. A hysteric pain caused by an old injury may act as a hysterogenous zone, especially in one of the joints, as the hip or knee.

Disturbances or alterations of sensation are characteristic of hysteria. Anesthesia, more or less complete, is nearly always present in the hysteric subject, who may often be ignorant of its presence. Sometimes this is only of one side of the body, divided with great exactness in the middle line from head to heel (hemianesthesia); and sometimes occurs in irregularly distributed areas (disseminated anesthesia); or, again, is distinctly localized in one arm or one leg (segmental anesthesia). This last may be accompanied by motor impairment (palsy) of the part. The areas of anesthesia, when pricked, do not readily bleed (ischemia). The organs of special sense are often disturbed in hemianesthesia, and always upon the affected side. Of these the most important are the eyes; there may be a concentric narrowing of the visual field, or an alteration in the color fields (amblyopia or color-scotoma). There may be deafness of one side, or impairment of smell or taste. The changes in the color field (when characteristic) are one of the most certain points for differential diagnosis.

The disturbances of motility in hysteria are either loss of function (paralysis), or perversion of function (contraction and tremor). These symptoms are very apt to appear by themselves. The paralyses of hysteria simulate those due to central nervous disease in their distribution, but not in their clinical history. They may be named in the order of frequency with which they occur in children, *viz.:* paraplegia, monoplegia, and hemiplegia. The paralysis of motion is commonly, but not always, accompanied by paralysis of sensation. The onset is usually sudden, and in form may be flaccid or spastic. The immediate cause is usually some emotional perturbation, which may be psychic or traumatic. The contractures in hysteria may be either partial or complete, a local stiffening, or a spasm. These contractures may persist for years, though not always constant, and sometimes returning upon slight excitation; they may remain in the same place, or pass from one part to another. Tremor is rare in children; loss of voice is not common, neither is increased rapidity of respiration. Hysteric vomiting, also rare in the young, is a very serious matter when it does occur, imperiling health, or even life. Its character is *sui generis*, a mere regurgitation, due to a spasm of the esophagus. The intestine is sometimes paralyzed in hysteria, producing an immense bloating, with noisy belching, which is usually concomitant with a condition of emotional excitement.

Hysteria is a psychosis, a profound disorder of functional activities, of almost universal distribution, but due to no known demonstrable lesion. By some change in mechanism, an entire half of the brain is temporarily invalided, which alone can explain the complete hemianesthesia. The possibility of transferring this anesthesia from one side to the other would show the two halves of the brain to be in sympathy, one with the other. The cortical inhibition is lessened, leaving the lower centers unchecked. Recent views upon the mobility of the neuron points the way to a clearer understanding of hysteric states, but as yet scarcely explains the accompanying phenomena. The hysteric child evidences a marked vulnerability to certain perturbing influences, is always susceptible to psychic changes and functional disturbance. The manifestations of the disease may disappear during many years and yet readily recur under the influence of slight morbid agencies or changes in condition, or emotional irritation.

The treatment of hysteria in children or in adults is always complicated by the fact that the causes which produce it have so much to do with environment. It is difficult, almost impossible, to effect a cure unless the unfavorable environment be changed. It is easy to point out how a case may be benefited or cured, but not so easy to enforce the measures with sufficient thoroughness to produce a satisfactory result. The most important point in treatment, to be always insisted upon, is a complete separation of the child from its parents or previous caretakers during a considerable period of time. The physician finds himself in a very difficult situation, and will usually be compelled to compromise. Indeed, it may sometimes be wiser to do this, and then gradually lead up to other measures more and more efficient and complete. The first part of the treatment should consist of the systematic application of measures directed to the improvement of general health, which may not seem obviously much impaired. An essential factor in the production of a cure is a properly qualified nurse, or (in rare instances), a wise and patient member of the family who can be taught to exercise the necessary control. The next most important element in the treatment is moral training, a complete remodeling of the point of view of duties to self and others.

It is of the greatest importance for physicians to realize that drugs are of no value whatsoever in the treatment of the psychosis known as hysteria. Judicious reasoning, frank conversation of an educational kind, and vigorous suggestions, with sometimes the added pomp and circumstance of the proper place and conditions, are powerful agents for good. Thus, a steady repetition of suggestion, with judicious and thorough detail, by a nurse or attendant trained to this end, is of great efficacy. As soon as the more severe symptoms are overcome and the child restored to uniform good health, proper educational measures must be steadily pursued. Remedial measures, directed to the removal of functional disturbances, for instance, hydrotherapy, electricity, especially the static form, massage, and regulated exercises, are of direct value. Strong faradic applications help to overcome hysteric paralyses, particularly in conjunction with encouraging words. The manner assumed by the physician exerts the utmost influence for good or evil. A frank, candid exposition of the patient's need should be clearly given. The medical man should be recognized by the patient as most kindly disposed, encouraging, and yet relentlessly firm.

For the sensory disturbances, the cold douche, or alternate use of hot and cold water, or the employment of some of the more picturesque devices, such as metalotherapy, may prove beneficial. Hypnosis will control a certain proportion of phenomena, and is rather easy to produce in children who, at best, are very impressionable, but is little better than repeated, direct suggestion at the hands of a physician whom the child has learned to respect and esteem. To overcome a paroxysm or convulsion the following measure may prove efficient: ice water dashed repeatedly over the face or back, or trickled steadily upon one point, as from a small hose or watering-pot; pieces of ice rubbed here or there on the back or chest, and lastly, inhalations of ammonia or nitrite of amyl.

THE OPERATIVE TREATMENT OF PTOSIS.[1]

BY FRANK VAN FLEET, M.D.,
OF NEW YORK.

PTOSIS is a condition characterized by a drooping of the upper lid. It may be unilateral or bilateral, partial or complete, congenital or acquired. The congenital variety is generally bilateral, although it may be of varying degree on either side. In one of the cases in which I operated ptosis was apparent only on one side, but when corrected the contrast made it evident that the same condition, in lesser degree, existed in the other eye.

It is supposed that congenital ptosis is due to a lack of development of the levator palpebræ superioris muscle, although it is possible that it is the result of a malposition of the muscle, or to an anomalous distribution of the nerves. It causes a most characteristic appearance on the part of the affected individual. The drooping upper lid narrows the palpebral orifice in varying degree, depending upon the amount of ptosis present. The head is thrown back, and the eyeball rotated downward so as to bring the pupil on a line with the narrowed opening between the upper and the lower lids. While the downward rotation of the eye is generally due to this cause, it may result from a faulty development, or maladjustment of the superior recti muscles, a not unusual accompaniment, and one which must receive consideration in operative procedures directed to the correction of the ptosis.

In the three cases of congenital ptosis in which I have operated this complication was not present. In this affection there is also a wrinkling of the forehead due to the efforts of the occipitofrontalis muscle to assist in the elevation of the upper lids.

Acquired ptosis may result from syphilis (or any constitutional trouble which produces paralysis of the third nerve), traumatism, or diseases of the conjunctiva. A cause I had never heard of until it was mentioned by the first patient upon whom I operated for this affection was the use of the Davy lamp in coal-mining. It may have been only a coincidence, but the patient himself was firmly convinced that it was the cause of his eye trouble, and furthermore he said that it was not an uncommon occurrence among miners in the Welsh collieries who use the Davy lamp. The case of this patient is as follows:

J. H. P., aged forty-six years, formerly a miner in South Wales, presented himself for treatment in July, 1896. He had marked ptosis in both eyes. Until his eighteenth year he had never observed anything peculiar about his eyes, but at that time noticed that his upper lids drooped. In the mine in which

[1] Presented before the New York Medico-Surgical Society, October 4, 1897, and the Section on Ophthalmology of the New York Academy of Medicine, November, 1897.

the patient was employed there were about 1000 men, and the occurrence of ptosis, he said, was not uncommon. In the bituminous mines, where the naked lamps were used, this affection did not occur. When the disease manifested itself, the only remedy was to seek other employment, or at least to stop using the Davy lamp. However, the patient continued to work until the ptosis was so nearly complete that to see straight ahead it became necessary to raise the eyelids with the fingers. Fig. 1 shows the condition some time before he was compelled to give up his work, and is an enlarged copy of a photograph taken in England many years ago. Fig. 2, a copy of a photograph taken by Dr. E. S. Thomson, formerly house surgeon at the Manhattan Eye and Ear Hospital, shows the appearance of the same patient about thirteen months after the operation.

FIG. 1.

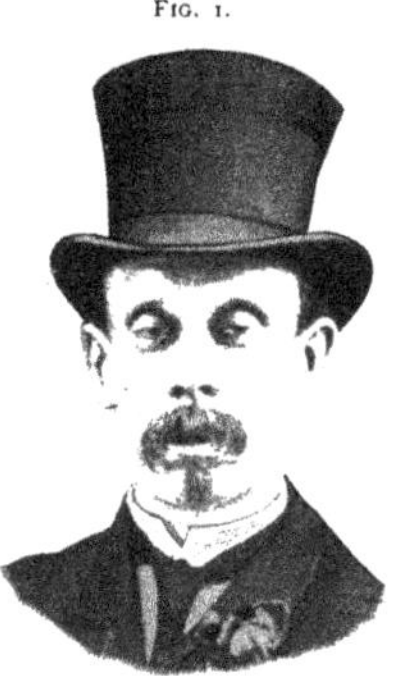

Showing appearance of patient with ptosis.

I would like to remark that the cause, as given by my patient, is not recorded as one of the known causes of ptosis so far as I have been able to ascertain, and may have been imaginary on his part.

The treatment of ptosis due to affections of the third nerve, is generally satisfactory when directed toward the cause, whether it be syphilitic or traumatic. When the result of trachoma, or any congenital condition, in which the drooping of the lid remains after the causative disease is cured, the deformity may often be remedied by simply removing an elliptic piece of skin from the upper lid and stitching the edges together. When this does not suffice, and also when the ptosis is the result of deficient muscular development, more extensive operative procedures have been unsatisfactory until recently. The levator palpebræ superioris muscle, having its origin in the orbit, is attached to the lid at about the convex margin of the tarsal cartilage, and its action draws the lid not only upward but backward as well. In the absence of this muscle, operators have endeavored to make the occipitofrontalis, the anterior portion of which is intimately adherent to the skin, take its place. The results produced by the devices of Pagenstecher, DeWecker, and others are satisfactory for the time being, but the objection has been that they are not lasting. We have, however, in the operation devised by Panas, a method which is generally satisfactory as to results, both immediate and remote. To this operation there is but one objection, *viz.*, it is complicated and difficult to understand. In fact, I know of no other operation the description of which is so confusing as this. An excellent description of this procedure may be found in De Schweinitz's work, "Diseases of the Eye," and a somewhat shorter one in Roosa's book, "Treatise on the Diseases of the Eye." There are many modifications of this operation, and I have taken the liberty of adding another. Possibly my operation is a copy of one which is already in existence, but be that as it may, I have employed it in five cases in which the immediate and remote results have been entirely satisfactory. My operation (Fig. 3), as I have taken the liberty of calling it for the time being, differs from that of Panas (Fig. 4), inasmuch as the lines of incision

FIG. 2.

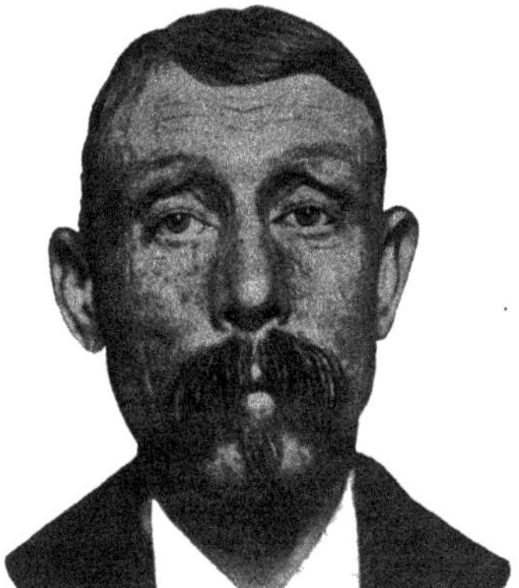

Showing the appearance of the same patient thirteen months after operation.

are straight and extend only through the integument. There is no danger of wounding deeper structures, and the flap, uniting by first intention to the upper edge of the incision in the brow, becomes a part of the skin controlled by the occipitofrontalis muscle quite as much as it would had the incision extended down to the periosteum. A short description of this procedure is as follows:

The patient being anesthetized and the brow shaved, the face and forehead should be cleansed with a mercuric bichlorid wash. An assistant then inserts an ordinary horn shield under the lid, and with his free hand steadies the skin of the brow as directed by Panas. The operator makes an incision into the upper lid somewhat above the superior margin of the tarsal cartilage, commencing at the inner side and including the middle third of the lid. From the inner extremity of this incision another is made extending down to the ciliary border, and a third incision is made in like manner from the outer extremity of the first. The integument enclosed by these three incisions is dissected from the underlying tissues down to the ciliary border, and constitutes the flap. A final incision is made in the brow parallel with the first, but slightly longer. The integument between the two is then undermined and forms the bridge. The parts are again carefully cleansed, the flap passed up under the bridge, and its upper margin stitched to the upper edge of the incision in the brow by means of five sutures. The outer and inner extremities of the final incision, *i.e.*, external and internal to the flap, are sutured, the wound dusted with iodoform, covered with bichlorid gauze, and bandaged. The latter is left in place two days, after which it is removed and daily reapplied during a week; when the stitches should be removed and the dressings discontinued. The epithelium of the flap becomes macerated and exfoliates, and the true skin unites with the under surface of the bridge, of which it becomes a part, or, perhaps disappears.

FIG. 3.

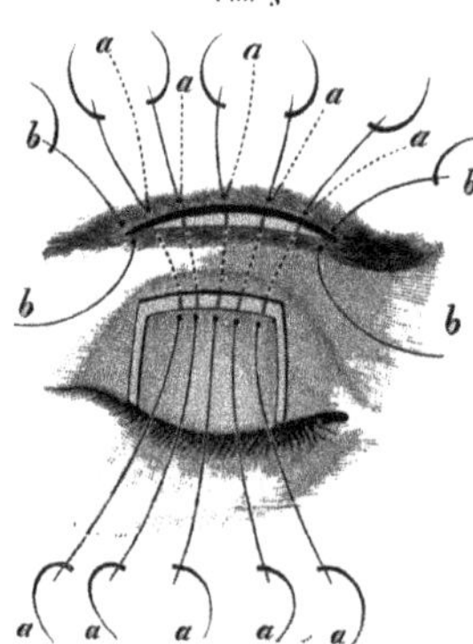

Van Fleet's modification of Panas' operation for ptosis.
a, *a*, sutures uniting flap to integument of brow.
b, *b*, sutures closing extremities of incision in brow.

I believe it is well not to make the flap too narrow, but better, perhaps, to include even more than one-third of the lid. Its length should vary with the degree of ptosis to be overcome, always bearing in mind that it is better to have too great, rather than too little, resulting elevation of the lid, as the subsequent stretching of the skin tends to counteract the primary results.

I performed this operation upon a child, two years of age, for a physician in Brooklyn, who, after the operation, was alarmed because when the child slept the eye remained partly open. This continued a long time, perhaps six months, and the doctor feared the occurrence of keratitis, which we find following the inability to close the eye in facial palsy. In regard to such an accident the danger is nil; the patient may close the eye, and does so when occasion requires.

FIG. 4.

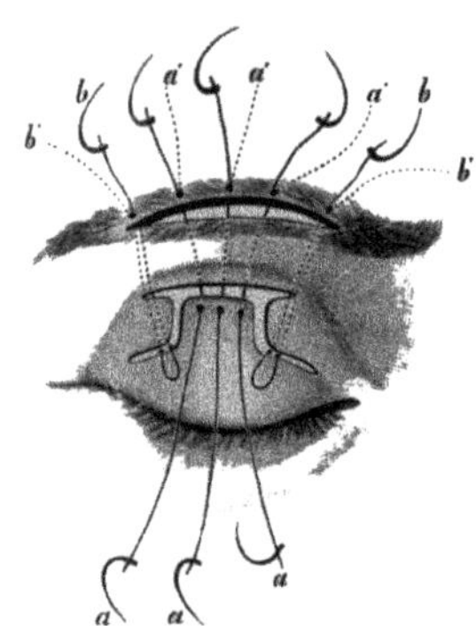

Panas' operation for ptosis (after de Schweinitz).
a, *a*, sutures uniting flap to integument of brow.
b, *b*, sutures advised by Panas to prevent possibility of ectropion resulting.

Another point to be remembered is that the shrinking of the bridge may cause a deformity, as shown in the left eye (Fig. 2) of the patient, to whose case I have previously referred. This has occurred in three of my five cases, and was easily remedied by freshening the edges of the wound and again stitching them together.

The two lateral sutures advised by Panas (Fig. 4, *b*, *b*,) I have not employed, but think that it may, perhaps, be well to do so in future cases; not because of the possibility of resulting ectropion, for in this I do not believe, but because the two sutures mentioned serve to prevent stretching of the flap and consequent lessening of the good effect. Another question to be decided is whether the stitches which unite the flap to the upper margin of the incision in the brow should include the upper edge of the bridge. This latter has a tendency to curl, and if the upper edge be fixed, the tendency to cicatricial distortion will be lessened. There may be other points to be considered which will be suggested by individual operators.

NOTE.—Since writing the above I have been informed that Dr. J. Ascroft Tansley, of this city, has devised a similar operation. He has very kindly forwarded to me a reprint of an article describing his operation.[1] There is little similarity in these two operations except that they are both modifications of Panas', at least mine is, and I should imagine Dr. Tansley's to be so likewise.

[1] *American Medical and Surgical Bulletin*, February 8, 1896.

EXPERIENCES WITH RETAINED INTUBATION TUBES AND ANTISTREPTOCOCCIC SERUM.

BY ROSA ENGELMANN, M.D.,
OF CHICAGO;
PROFESSOR OF PEDIATRICS IN THE POST-GRADUATE MEDICAL SCHOOL OF CHICAGO; CLINICAL INSTRUCTOR OF PEDIATRICS IN THE MEDICAL DEPARTMENT OF THE UNIVERSITY OF ILLINOIS; CONSULTANT PHYSICIAN TO THE MARY THOMPSON HOSPITAL FOR WOMEN AND CHILDREN.

A MOST trying case of laryngeal diphtheria in which I performed intubation nineteen times within twenty-five days first called my attention to retained tubes as a complication of this procedure. Had O'Dwyer's brilliant and helpful article upon this subject then been published two lives might have been saved. Moreover, I would not have blamed myself for failing to do an early tracheotomy in the one case, although this operation proved futile in the second. At that time I had no knowledge of the short O'Dwyer tubes with larger head and lower, broader swell, nor of the tubes with built-up heads designed for cases of this kind.

The course of the disease and the *post-mortem* demonstration of subglottic ulcers, according to O'Dwyer, contraindicates tracheotomy. He says: "If extensive subglottic ulceration exists at the time the trachea is opened, the rapid healing which follows is very likely to produce a close cicatricial stricture, if not complete occlusion of this narrow portion of the larynx. Slow healing around a properly fitting tube is much less likely to be followed by contraction, and is the only safe method in these cases." His ingenious method of local astringent application by means of a medicated gelatinized intubation-tube might have been as efficacious in my cases as in his.

CASE I.—James L., Italian, 2½ years old. I saw him for the first time on December 17, 1896, and the following history was elicited: Previous health good; father syphilitic, as learned from the family physician; child robust and well-developed; had been ill one day; primary laryngeal involvement; severe stenosis; temperature, 101° F.; pulse strong and full. At 5 A.M. I injected 5 c.c. of No. 6 antitoxin. At 11 A.M., No. 1 tube was inserted; it was expelled, after three-hours' retention, at 2 P.M., and we thought it to be too small. At 4 P.M., reintubated with No. 2 O'Dwyer tube; culture showed the presence of Löffler bacillus and staphylococcus pyogenes.

December 18th: Injected 5 c.c. of No. 6 antitoxin and 5 c.c. of antistreptococcic serum. After every antitoxin injection the temperature rose 2½° F., dropping the same number of degrees within eighteen hours. At 4 P.M. the tube was coughed up, with membrane, having remained in place twenty-four hours; 5 P.M., reintubated.

December 19th: At 9 A.M., seventeen hours later, tube expelled; 9.30 A.M., reintubated; 8.30 P.M., 11½ hours later, tube again coughed up; 9.30 P.M., reintubated.

December 20th: At 5.30 P.M., tube expelled, retained twenty hours; reintubated at 8 P.M.; pulse, 150; temperature, 102.8° F.; administered 5 c.c. No. 5 antitoxin.

December 21st: At 3 A.M. child suddenly became dyspneic, cyanosed, and convulsed in its effort to expel tube; some membrane appeared with the tube, the boy being strong enough to cough up the tube with, and ahead of, the membrane which doubtless had been occluding it; tube retained but 9½ hours; 4.30 A.M., replaced tube; retained eighteen hours; 10.30 P.M., tube expelled; retained 5½ hours.

December 22d: At 5 A.M., inserted a No. 3 tube, thinking that the edema had subsided to some extent and that pressure would hasten its disappearance. Five c.c. No. 4 antitoxin was given, 6500 units having been injected within six days. Later experience taught me that the antitoxin should have been more heroically and rapidly administered.

The diphtheria bacillus and staphylococcus were now associated with the streptococcus. Albumin appeared in the urine, remaining until the eleventh day of the disease, when it finally vanished. The No. 3 tube now remained *in situ* four days and five hours, then, on December 27th at 10 A.M., I removed it for cleansing, it having been worn ten days. It seemed to me about time for its permanent removal, but the boy was comfortable without it only three or four hours, respiratory difficulty increasing until twenty-one hours after its removal its reinsertion became imperative; temperature, 100.8° F.; pulse, 95; child taking nourishment well.

December 30th: At 3 P.M., or three days and five hours later, I extubated, fearing loss of resiliency and ulceration of the laryngeal walls; 6 P.M., reintubated for what seemed to be laryngeal and bronchial spasm. Whistling râles were heard over the entire chest;

temperature, 100.4° F.; pulse, 90; respirations embarrassed. A culture was taken which revealed the presence of the bacillus lanceolatus. To my mind this threatened pneumonia, for in quite a number of my cases this bacterial report had been significant.

December 31st: Temperature, 101.6° F.; pulse, 120 and irregular; physical examination revealed a bronchopneumonia.

January 1, 1897: Pallor; cyanosis; cold extremities; pulse 120, and regular; temperature, 100.8° F.

January 4th: At 3 A.M. the tube was again expelled; it had remained in place four days, 9½ hours; 4.30 A.M., tube replaced; 8.30 A.M., four hours later, it was again expelled; temperature, 99.2° F.; lungs clearing; 11 A.M., intubated; tube retained four hours, and was again coughed up; 4 P.M., reintubated; retained only three hours, and at 7 P.M. was again expelled. A No. 4 tube was now easily inserted, meeting absolutely no resistance. I was well aware of the danger of so large a tube, but apnea was threatened after each expulsion, and the father so dreaded this occurrence that he had learned to press back the tube which now rose with every expulsive effort.

January 5th: At 4.30 P.M. the boy strangled, and was so nearly asphyxiated that the father pulled out the tube. From its large size it was probably being impacted in the post-pharyngeal space. The larynx was undoubtedly so lacerated that it had become intolerant of the foreign body.

January 6th: At 12.30 A.M., ten hours later, reintubated with a No. 3 tube, although from the stretching of the parts I feared it might slip down into the trachea. A culture from the tube showed Löffler bacillus and staphylococcus; temperature, 100.4° F.; pulse, 120.

January 8th: At 12 M. the lungs appeared to be normal; temperature, 101° F.; pulse, 120; removed the tube after a retention of three days, 7½ hours; 2 P.M., replaced the tube as asphyxiation was imminent; no albumin in the urine; tracheotomy was advised, but refused by the parents.

January 9th: At 4.30 P.M., 5 c.c. of No. 4 antitoxin was injected. Up to this time 7500 units had been administered, but, as I now believe, not nearly enough, since upon this, the twenty-third day of the disease, the diphtheria bacillus still remained. The child had readily learned to drink inverted, but at each and every draught almost suffocated.

January 10th: Child playing.

January 11th: At 10.20 A.M., removed the tube to cleanse it; 10.25, gasping for breath; 10.30, dead before I could replace the tube or open the trachea.

Having gained the consent of the father, and in order to explain the cause of sudden death, we removed the larynx entire. Upon looking down past the vocal cords we could see absolute approximation of the subglottic walls, due to ulceration and loss of substance of the subglottic space. Another ulcer was seen in the right vestibule and still another on the posterior laryngeal wall. The laryngeal side of the epiglottis was about destroyed. Unfortunately the specimen was lost. Thus were the symptoms and unfortunate termination accounted for.

The futility of tracheotomy was proved in the following case:

CASE II.—Libbie M., aged two years and three months. She was a healthy, well-nourished girl, whom I had been treating for urticaria and some slight gastro-intestinal disturbance.

April 2, 1897: She had been ill thirty hours. Respiratory embarrassment was so rapidly progressive that intubation was at once performed. Before my arrival the child had received an unknown dose of antitoxin to which I added 5 c.c. of No. 6. The first culture showed staphylococcus; second culture, April 4th, showed the Löffler bacillus and the streptococcus pyogenes. Five c.c. of antitoxin and 10 c.c. of antistreptoccic serum were injected. The urine was normal; pulse, 120; temperature, 101.8° F.

April 5th: Morning temperature, 99.5° F.; pulse, 96; evening temperature, 98.2° F.; pulse, 100; respiration, 30, and unembarrassed; 11.30 P.M. Coughed up the No. 2 tube with some membrane; very cyanotic, and collapsed at 12.15 A.M., April 6th, when the tube was replaced.

Antitoxin administration doubtless caused local turgescence which, until its subsidence, was an added source of danger in the absence of a tube. Rapid membrane exfoliation obstructing the tube caused its expulsion at this most critical time. There were some peculiar erythematous patches around the site of the first injection.

April 6th: At 10 A.M. the temperature was 100.4° F.; pulse, 114; 5 c.c. of No. 4 antitoxin was injected.

April 7th: At 6.30 A.M. she coughed up the tube, which was completely filled with a semi-gelatinous, non-tenacious substance, probably dissolved membrane, for no shreds appeared later. At 7 A.M., when the tube was replaced, the child was almost asphyxiated and cold; rapid reaction; temperature, 101.8° F.; pulse, 150. At 6.30 P.M. the temperature was 103.6° F.; pulse, 150.

April 8th: 2 A.M. Giant urticaria involving entire body; face and eyelids enormously swollen; neck swollen even with angles of the jaw, so seriously affecting respiration that the tube was not fulfilling its purpose; there was doubtless pressure and edema above and below it. Dr. A. M. Thorpe, who had given me great assistance in the previous case, saw this child at my request, and reported no immediate danger. I did not see her until 11 A.M., when she was found delirious, scarlet, swollen beyond all recognition, and panting for breath; pulse and respiration too rapid to count; temperature, per rectum, 107° F. She was packed in sheets which were continually flooded with cold water, rubbed with ice, and ice applied to the head. Iced colonic flushings were likewise given. She sucked voraciously at the ice pellets placed in her mouth. Nitroglycerin, strychnin, and brandy were hypodermically administered.

Within twenty minutes the temperature was reduced to 101.2° F., and the pulse to 100. True, the respiration was still sighing and the body blue, but at 2 P.M. the thermometer registered 100° F., the respirations were 48, and the pulse 180, but regular. Such absolute loss of respiratory and circulatory control I hope never to see repeated. Infected antitoxin was unquestionably the cause of this trouble, for neither previous nor later doses had any such deleterious effect, profound toxemia evidently affecting the respiratory, thermogenic, and cardio-inhibitory centers. It seems clear that idiosyncrasy may be excluded.

April 9th: At 5 P.M. she coughed up the tube; great dyspnea and depression; 6 P.M., reintubated; general edema and urticaria disappearing.

April 10th: At 1 P.M., tube expelled with glairy mucus; no membrane; 3 P.M., intubated with No. 3 tube.

April 11th: 11 A.M., coughed this large tube into postnasal space, from whence it was extracted with difficulty by a neighboring physician who refused to reinsert it. The child was almost moribund when I arrived at 1 P.M. I temporarily inserted a No. 4 tube, wishing to reduce the laryngeal edema by pressure as well as by the length of the tube, in order to get above and below the edematous tissues which were interfering with respiration. When reaction was established, within two hours, tracheotomy *for the edema, not membrane,* was performed by Dr. Bayard Holmes; no membrane to be seen; some mucopurulent discharge from the tracheotomy tube. A culture made therefrom showed streptococcus, staphylococcus, and Löffler bacillus. The tracheotomy tube was clear most of the time, and the breathing comfortable.

April 12th: Sent to Cook County Hospital, where she died shortly afterward from sepsis and bronchopneumonia.

The next case may be classed with the above, but in one sense only. After what was supposed to be a final extubation and recovery there seems to have been a reinfection ten days later, necessitating another intubation.

CASE III.—Jennie B., two years old; ill three days; tonsils and larynx involved; temperature, 100.2° F.; stenosis.

January 16th: Intubation. Given 5 c.c. No. 6 and 2 c.c. No. 5 antitoxin, and 5 c.c. antistreptococcic serum.

January 18th: Extubated in order to convince myself that the period of wearing the tube could be shortened; for in a series of six of my cases it had been worn respectively two and one-half days, three days, three days and three hours, four days, five days, and six days. That it could not be effected in this instance was conclusively demonstrated, since a reintubation was performed within half an hour; culture showed diphtheria bacillus.

January 19th: 10 A.M., temperature, 100° F.; breathing more labored than at the time of the first intubation, due to a complicating bronchitis; temporary anuria, but no albumin.

January 20th: Final removal of tube.

January 22nd: Father reports that the child is well; culture; Löffler bacillus.

January 24th: Culture showed Löffler bacillus, but very few and not characteristic.

January 26th: Child hoarse again and coughing.

January 27th: Bacillus lanceolatus was found, but no Löffler bacilli.

January 28th: Bronchopneumonia, and patches of membrane on the tonsils.

January 29th: Streptococcus and staphylococcus; severe stenosis requiring intubation; gave 5 c.c. No. 6 antitoxin.

February 1st: Sent to isolation hospital of Dr. F. W. Gillespie, to whom I am indebted for the subsequent detailed report.

Löffler bacillus again found, and 1500 units of antitoxin was injected. On February 2d, when the tube was removed, having been worn five days, pulse, temperature, and respiration were normal. The child was discharged on February 11th, having made an uninterrupted recovery.

Antistreptococcic serum was tentatively used in the previous and following cases, but because of the small dosage and the character of the infection, *viz.*, a mixed one, no conclusion can be adduced, nor would an expression of opinion be in order after so few observations. Nevertheless, the citation of a few cases in this connection will not lack interest:

CASE IV.—Mary S.; thirty years old; no history of previous throat trouble; a strong, robust individual; ill twenty-four hours before coming under observation.

January 8, 1897: Pulse, 100; temperature, 101.8° F.; tonsils, soft palate, and uvula swollen, almost occluding interpalatal space, a typical picture of peritonsillar abscess. There were gray adherent patches on the tonsils; severe adenitis. A culture demonstrated the presence of the streptococcus and staphylococcus. Gave 10 c.c. antistreptococcic serum; urine negative before and after the injection; the temperature fell 2° F. within twenty-four hours. She was also given a bichlorid of mercury and iron mixture, and a gargle consisting of a twenty-per-cent. peroxid-of-hydrogen solution. Twenty-four hours after the injection there was the most remarkable subsidence of the local edema, redness, and some disappearance of the membrane. Within twenty-four hours, however, the swelling again appeared and there was so much distress that I lanced the tonsil, but did not find a clean staphylococcic abscess. There was much burrowing and many very small pockets of pus which no knife could reach. This condition was nuquestionably of streptococcic origin. Another dose of 10 c.c. of antistreptococcic serum was injected. Results were as rapid and satisfactory as with the previous injection; cervical glandular enlargement also disappeared. Had I used a larger primary and secondary dose I believe lancing would have been obviated. I gave a third and final injection on the fifth day of the disease, when again some turgescence had taken place. Within one week the patient was discharged cured, a very rapid recovery from what would have become a large peritonsillar abscess, ordinarily running a course of from two to three weeks.

The following is a case of scarlatina in which antistreptococcic serum was employed. The first throat culture showed the presence of the staphylococcus, the second, both staphylococcus and streptococcus.

CASE V.—Morris McK., six years old, excessively emaciated and asthenic; ill thirteen days with what had been called diphtheria. The tonsils, palate, and uvula were still covered with gray, adherent, foul smelling membrane. An adenitis was present; no albuminuria. The hands and feet were desquamating. Erythematous patches were located upon different parts of the trunk.

March 30, 1897: Twenty c.c. of antistreptococcic serum was injected. Temperature, 103.4° F.; pulse, 158; some bronchitis.

April 1st: Pulse, 156; temperature, 103.8° F. Only slight rise of temperature after the injection. Some inflammatory reaction and erythema at the point of injection which subsided within three days following the use of an ice bag, and a little later, application of ichthyol ointment.

April 2d: Patches exfoliating; adenitis decreasing; temperature, 101.2° F.; pulse, 120; bronchitis.

April 3d: Temperature, 102.6° F.; pulse, 120; bronchitis improving.

April 4th: Temperature, 101.8° F.; pulse, 120; injected 10 c.c. antistreptococcic serum; urine negative.

April 5th: Temperature, 98.2° F.; pulse, 100; patches disappearing; rapid desquamation. Tonics were administered, and the child now regained strength and flesh, and made what the parents called a marvelous recovery.

The following is a brief history of a coincident scarlatina and diphtheritic infection. The sudden typical onset of fever and rash was evidenced, but overlooking this the attending physician called the case one of diphtheria; I pronounced it scarlet fever. The report from the culture was Löffler bacillus and staphylococcus. Thus, we were both right and both wrong:

CASE VI.—Bessie S., eleven months old; tonsils, nares, and larynx involved; ill four days previous to observation. Culture showed staphylococcus and diphtheria bacillus. Gave 5 c.c. No. 6 antitoxin, and two doses of 20 c.c. antistreptococcic serum on alternate days. The attending physician reported a very rapid recovery from both diseases without complications. To prevent the latter might be a sufficient reason for the use of antistreptococcic serum in scarlet fever.

The difficulty of differentiating a simple streptococcic, scarlatinal, not necessarily streptococcic or diphtheritic throat, except by taking both clinical and cultural findings into consideration, is thus illustrated. In my first series of 100 cases of true diphtheria I was inclined to believe that the density and color of the membrane, excessive turgescence of the parts, even in the absence of membrane and low temperature, were characteristics of diphtheria. On the other hand, I have seen many cases with these peculiar attributes in which only staphylococci and streptococci could be demonstrated. Again, the infective agent of scarlatina has been supposed to be a variety of streptococcus, and many clinicians have asserted that the tonsils are its point of entrance into the body. In an article on "Scarlatina and the Streptococcus Infection," written in 1895, I suggested other infective atria, such as the gastro intestinal tract and skin. It is a curious fact that all throat cultures taken by me in cases of scarlatina during the past six months, and in five recent cases of scarlatina, show no other germ than the staphylococcus; whereas, I had expected in each and all of these cases to find the streptococcus. Much yet remains to be learned in regard to the genesis of throat lesions and their associated complications.

CLINICAL MEMORANDA.

A CASE OF HODGKIN'S DISEASE ASSOCIATED WITH MULTIPLE NEURITIS.

BY R. ABRAHAMS, M.D.,
OF NEW YORK;
DISTRICT PHYSICIAN TO MOUNT SINAI HOSPITAL.

M. L., Russian, male, single, aged thirty-five years. Family history unknown. During childhood he had smallpox as well as all the diseases peculiar to this period. His boyhood and youth were spent in idleness, both of mind and body. At the age of twenty, probably sooner, he began to masturbate. This habit continued until he was thirty years of age. About this time his fancy turned to thoughts of matrimony, but he soon relinquished the idea, as "by trial" he found himself incapable of performing the sexual act. His genital organs, however, were well developed. His second bad habit was the excessive use of alcoholic beverages. During six years he drank heavily and promiscuously—anything that was alcoholic. At the end of this time he began to experience pain in the lower extremities. The pain was dull, and at times shooting or lancinating, but always present. Some time after slight ataxia supervened, when he sought refuge in a hospital. At this institution he received both medicinal and electric treatment nearly a year, with neither real nor apparent amelioration of his symptoms. During his stay in the hospital alcohol was absolutely withheld.

At this time a small "fleshy lump" made its appearance on the right side of the head, joining the neck. The lump slowly but steadily increased in size. A few weeks after a second tumor appeared on the same side of the head. When the second swelling attained the size of a horse-chestnut it stopped growing, while the first continued to increase until it reached the size of a small orange.

He consulted me during March, 1897. On examination the patient was found to be of medium size, with a mild lateral curvature of the spine (Fig. 2). Otherwise

FIG. 1.

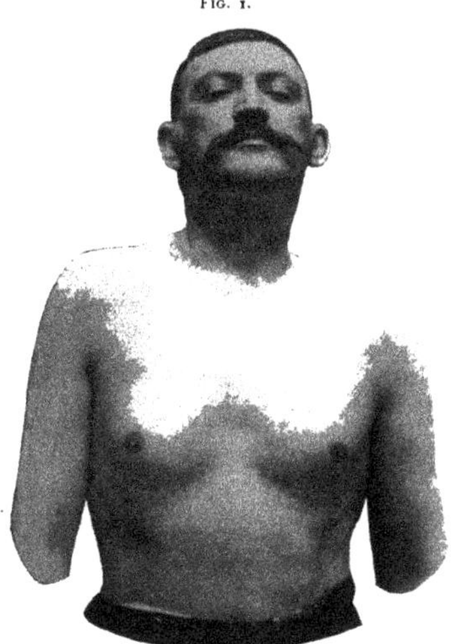

Showing appearance of patient with Hodgkin's disease.

he was well built and well nourished. The heart, lungs, liver, spleen, and kidneys seemed to be normal. He had dyspepsia of moderate degree. He stoutly denied alcoholism, but admitted masturbation; never had any venereal disease. He complained of constant shooting and burning pain in the lower extremities. The pain was aggravated by pressure. Mild ataxia was present; total absence of patelar reflex on both sides; staggering on walking with closed eyes; feeling as if walking on sand, and, *upon suggestion*, he owned to the girdle sensation. It must be mentioned that the Argyll-Robertson pupil was absent; the sphincters were normal, and electric tests yielded negative results. The clinical picture, therefore, was suggestive of locomotor ataxia.

The man had scarcely been two weeks under observation when new features developed. The glands of the neck showed an appreciable increase in size. At the same time two glandular enlargements became visibly apparent at the upper borders of the parotid glands. In the course of two weeks more the axillary and mammary glands gave optical evidence of abnormal growth. A glandular, movable mass appeared over the sternal notch. It was also noticed that while these glands were increasing in size the abdomen also was growing larger, although repeated and careful examination did not reveal any alteration in the size of the internal organs. The rapidity with which the glands enlarged was very remarkable. Within six weeks the cervical glands presented one continuous mass, hanging down like a double chin; the mammary glands attained the size of large oranges. The two old enlargements on the back of the head shared in the general hypertrophy, so that they became double the original size. The accompanying figures fairly illustrate the condition.

The only subcutaneous lymphatic glands which escaped enlargement were the epitrochlear and inguinal. The constitutional disturbances accompanying the glandular phenomena were slow but progressive anemia and loss of appetite and muscular strength. At this stage, with a clinical diagnosis of leucocythemia, the blood was examined. Dr. F. S. Mandelbaum, Pathologist to Mt. Sinai Hospital, to whom I am indebted for the examination, reported May 19th as follows: "Your patient's blood shows 2,900,000 red and 4500 colorless corpuscles per c. m. The ratio, therefore, is 1 to 644, which comes within the normal limit. The percentage of hemoglobin is 60 per cent. (Fleischl.) The dried and stained preparations showed that the majority of white corpuscles were of the

FIG. 2.

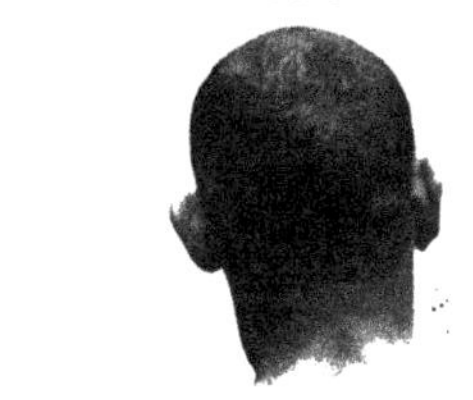

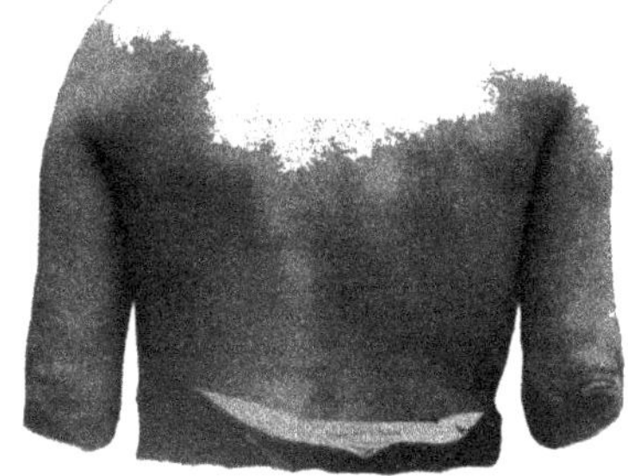

Back View of same patient, showing to some extent the glandular enlargement.

ordinary neutrophile, polynuclear type. A few mononuclear forms were seen, but no lymphocytes or eosinophile cells were present. There was a moderate degree of poikilocytosis, but no nucleated red corpuscles were found."

About the first of June the patient began to complain of marked weakness in his forearms and legs. This terminated, within a day or two, in complete motor-paralysis of the extensor muscles of the forearms and legs. Sensation was undisturbed, and there was pain on pressure along the nerves. Within a few days the muscles grew flabby, showing a tendency to rapid degeneration. At the same time a mild delirium tremens developed, accompanied by a reluctant confession to a history of prolonged and profound alcoholism. The delirium was quite active during the night. During the day the patient's intellect was comparatively clear, although he never ceased picking snakes around his bed and bedding. Slight jaundice and bronchitis, difficult breathing, and loss of control over the bladder developed. Intestinal hemorrhages were frequent and marked after the patient took to bed. On the 10th of June he died of acute edema of the lungs; no autopsy.

The treatment was carried out with system and regularity. It consisted of the internal administration of strychnin, $\frac{1}{60}$-grain doses, gradually increasing to $\frac{1}{10}$-grain three times daily, and also increasing doses of the arseniate of soda. Alcohol was absolutely forbidden. Nourishing food and every obtainable comfort were secured for him, but all were of no avail.

Besides the interesting combination of multiple neuritis and Hodgkin's disease presented by this patient, the case emphasizes a valuable lesson in diagnosis. Strümpel and others regard the differential diagnosis between chronic alcoholic-neuritis and tabes dorsalis as not only important but quite difficult. The resemblance of this case to one of locomotor ataxia was only intensified by the absolute denial of a history of alcoholism, which was steadfastly maintained almost to the end. Other interesting features of the case are the utter failure of treatment and the rapid and fatal termination, justifying, indeed, the name given to Hodgkin's disease, namely, malignant lymphoma.

A CASE OF PURPURA RHEUMATICA.[1]

By WALLACE JOHNSON, M.D.,
OF WASHINGTON, D. C.

W. L., male, aged twelve years. The patient was anemic, not well developed, and complained of pain in the back and abdomen, and also in the left elbow and right knee. The joints were found to be slightly swollen, red, and painful on motion. The thermometer indicated a slight rise of temperature. The patient's mother stated that during the few days preceding the examination he had had pain in various joints and also abdominal pain, particularly at night. At night, when the pain was most severe, vomiting occurred. Sodium salicylate in 10-grain doses was ordered to be given every three hours.

The next day, October 1st, the location of the pain had changed from the joints previously affected to the opposite elbow and left ankle. The severe abdominal pain at night continued; temperature, 101° F.

October 6th: During the first few days of this month the location of the pain frequently changed from one joint to another, and at present has entirely disappeared. The abdominal pain previously referred to persisted, though only at night, and was still accompanied by vomiting. There was no rise of temperature after October 2d; the bowels acted daily. During the morning there was present a slight tenderness over the upper abdomen, which by evening disappeared. Owing to the regularly recurring attacks of colic, the blood was examined for malarial parasites, but none were found.

October 8th: A dose of calomel emptied the bowels of a large quantity of feces, which was examined for the presence of any intestinal parasite that might be the cause of the colic. A few eggs of the tricocephalus dispar were found; but as all authorities agree that this parasite has no clinical significance, its presence was not considered a causative factor of the colic.

October 9th: Patient felt well and did not have colic the previous night.

October 12th: Three days before, after unusual exertion, the patient's feet swelled, became painful, and that night another attack of vomiting and colic occurred. At the time the mother noticed an eruption, "like that of scarlet fever," over his hips, ankle, and knee-joints. This eruption soon faded, and left only a few purpuric spots over the joints mentioned; colic and vomiting persisted at night.

October 27th: The joint-pain was entirely overshadowed by the severity of the colic and vomiting; temperature normal.

October 28th: After the administration of calomel and castor-oil the patient had a large movement of the bowels in which some blood was observed; no colic on the preceding night.

November 1st: No colic since October 27th; profuse purpuric eruption was present over both legs and extended as high as the waist; a few spots over wrists and elbows; none on the upper part of the trunk.

November 8th: The pain did not recur until the night of November 6th; it lasted a few hours and was not accompanied by vomiting. The next day the ankles were swollen and painful, but this condition disappeared within twenty-four hours.

November 10th: Slight abdominal pain on the preceding night; a few new purpuric spots had appeared.

November 15th: A new outbreak of purpura was present over both legs. A careful examination of the heart by Dr. J. D. Thomas did not reveal the presence of any abnormality. During the last two attacks of colic a rise of temperature did not occur.

The course of the disease was characterized by an apparent division into three successive periods, separated by intervals of eight to ten days of comparative health. Each exacerbation was marked by attacks of colic accompanied or preceded by rheumatic pains in the joints and followed by a purpuric eruption. The three prominent symptoms apparently had some relation one to the other, and were evidently not affected by treatment. During the first attack the relief of the colic was coincident with active purgation; in the second, relief preceded purgation; and in the third, a carthartic was not given. Under

[1] A disease resembling a form of purpura observed by Henoch of Berlin, and sometimes called Henoch's disease.

these circumstances it seems likely that the end of an attack and the action of the calomel were but coincident, not interdependent. After the first each subsequent attack was seemingly due to over-exertion.

NEW INSTRUMENT.

A NEW LABORATORY DISH.

BY W. L. COPLIN, M.D.,
OF PHILADELPHIA;
PROFESSOR OF PATHOLOGY AND BACTERIOLOGY IN THE JEFFERSON MEDICAL COLLEGE, PHILADELPHIA.

IN the laboratory of the Jefferson Medical College we almost exclusively use for routine work the paraffin method of embedding. The blocks of tissue are infiltrated in the usual manner, and the sections cut with the Ryder, or Minot microtome. The student cuts his sections and fastens them on the slide by means of Ohlmacher's combined water-albumen method, in combination with certain improvements of the methods of Gaule and Mayer. These are then kept from twelve to twenty-four hours in the drying-oven at a temperature of 37° C., until all the water is evaporated, the paraffin and section having, during the evaporation of the water, straightened out perfectly. The slide is now gently warmed until the paraffin, which has a melting-point of 45° C., begins to melt when it is thrust into kerosene, which in ten minutes completes the removal of the paraffin. The excess of kerosene is wiped off, the slide washed with a few drops of alcohol and then placed in a dish of alcohol; from this dish of alcohol the staining is conducted as usual. If the tissue has been hardened in corrosive sublimate, it is necessary to carry the cemented section through diluted tincture of iodin to remove the mercuric salt; this is followed by washing in alcohol when the section is ready for staining. The stains are conveniently kept in large salt-mouthed bottles into which the slides are placed for staining, mordanting, dehydrating and clearing.

FIG. 1.

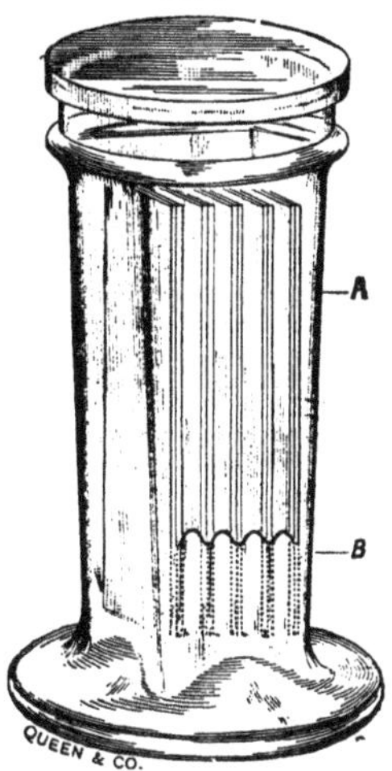

This cut is about two-thirds of the exact size of the dish. At *A* can be seen ten slides, placed back to back, and passing down between the ribs at *B*. Since this figure was drawn the width of the base has been increased, so that the base is now the width indicated in Fig. 2.

It is usual for the student to take from five to ten slides through the various solutions at one time, and in so doing he not uncommonly scratches the section off one slide by rubbing it against another. This difficulty arises no matter whether the method of Gaule, Suchannek's modification of Gaule's method, Gulland's modification of Gaule's method, or what is better, Heidenhain's water method be used. Even employing any of the collodion methods does not permit us to escape this danger. In order to overcome this, the writer sought very carefully through the dishes which have been designed by various workers, but failed to find anything which was ideally available. True, Ranvier has designed a rack upon which a number of slides may be supported, but this is entirely too cumbersome for general laboratory use, and besides involves a large amount of fluid, which makes it an expensive luxury. With these points in view, I have devised a dish which is expected to overcome some of the above difficulties.

FIG. 2.

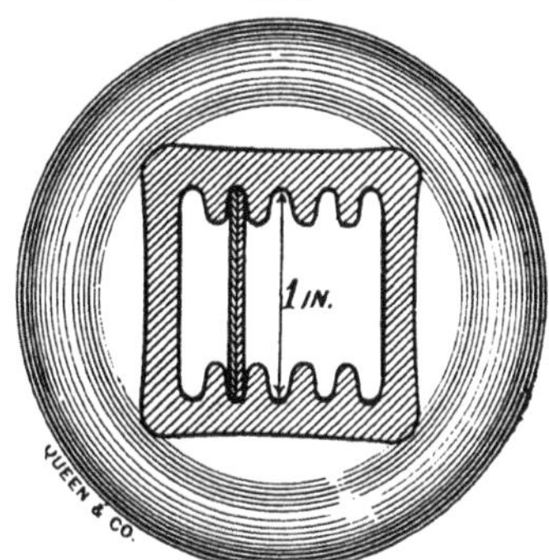

This represents a transverse section of the dish at the point marked *B* in Fig. 1, viewed from above and showing the ribs and intervening grooves. The two arrows mark the position occupied by a slide one inch in width. Just to the left of the arrow is shown a transverse section of two slides placed back to back, as is usually done for staining.

The inside measurements of the dish are 3⅛ inches in height, 1 inch square at the bottom, 1⅜ inches square 3 inches from the bottom, and 1¾ inches in diameter at the top which is round, and closed by means of a ground, grooved, Stender cover which when in place makes the dish air-tight. In order to render the dish stable, the base is the broadest and heaviest part, measuring nearly 2½ inches in diameter. Extending upward from the bottom on the inside and on two opposite sides, are eight ribs, four on each side, forming between them three grooves sufficiently wide to admit in each groove two slides of ordinary thickness. Two slides can also be placed in the outside groove, between the outside ribs on either side and the inside of the dish. This gives the dish for ordinary purposes convenient and not crowded accommodation for eight slides standing on end, or if the sections are small, and the slides thin, four slides may be placed outside of the ribs, two on each side, back to back, making ten in all.

An ordinary Stender dish requires about 120 cubic centimeters of fluid to immerse a slide sufficiently to cover a section cemented to its center. The above dish requires less than one-third of that amount to secure an equivalent degree of immersion. Of course, these dishes vary slightly in their capacity, as all pressed glassware will; such a variation, however, does not amount to more than from ten to fifteen cubic centimeters.

Where, for reasons of economy, or otherwise, it may be desirable to close the top of the dish by means of a cork or rubber stopper, the expense may be materially reduced. Wheh closed by means of a glass cover, as described above, and shown in the illustration, the cover and the dish will each bear the same number cut in the glass, so that the student working at his desk, may easily avoid mixing the covers which would not only be detrimental by mixing incompatible fluids, but as each lid can be ground only to fit the dish which accompanies it, exchanged lids would not fit tightly.

In order to facilitate cleaning and to avoid inaccessible corners, all the angles are rounded.

The advantages claimed for the dish are: (1) Convenience; a number of slides can be safely handled at one time. (2) Great economy in the use of reagents; not only is the amount used less than is required with the Stender dishes, but in case, as will not uncommonly occur with students, anything happens which ruins the contained fluid the loss will be materially less. (3) No other dish of the same height and the same capacity possesses equal solidity. (4) Contained fluids are prevented from evaporating by the tight-fitting top. This is not secured in the Naples dish.

I desire to express my appreciation of the assistance rendered by Messrs. Queen & Co. in securing working drawings from which the above cuts have been made, and the final successful production of the dish.

THERAPEUTIC NOTES.

Gelatin as a Hemostatic.—CARNOT (*Ther. Wochenschr.*, September 26, 1897) finds that of all the agents used to induce coagulation of the blood none equals gelatin. Its power of coagulability was shown by experiment some years ago, and even in small doses this is evident in hemorrhage from an exposed surface, such as the nose or the skin, where the temperature is below that of the melting-point of gelatin. In the organization of a blood-clot, the influence of the contained gelatin is for good, as it has a favorable nutritive effect upon the forming granulation-tissue.

Gelatin may be used in a five-to-ten-per-cent. solution in water, or, better, in normal salt solution. This preparation should be sterilized, on two successive days, at 100° C. during fifteen minutes. In several cases in which children were brought into the hospital bleeding from the nose, of several day's duration, Carnot was able to stop the hemorrhage at once by the injection into the nasal cavities of an ounce or two of this mixture, and the insertion into the nose of a tampon soaked in the same fluid.

The fluid must not be above the body temperature when brought into contact with the bleeding surface. In hemorrhage from the stomach or intestine, the remedy is useless, as the digestive action of the stomach destroys its virtue. In metrorrhagia, it is of incalculable value, if injected into the cavity of the uterus under aseptic precautions. Similar treatment serves to stop persistent rectal bleeding.

In surgical operations in situations in which hemorrhage is not easily controlled, the application of swabs of cotton soaked in the gelatin solution will stop the bleeding almost instantly. This is especially valuable in operations on the liver, kidney, etc.

To further coagulability of the blood in general, the gelatin solution may be introduced into the rectum, or injected subcutaneously. By the latter method a hemophiliac may be saved from a long hemorrhage and a beginning purpura hemorrhagica may be cut short.

The Hypodermic Administration of Quinin in Malaria.—DUNHAM (*Vir. Med. Semi-monthly*, November 12, 1897), who has had a great deal of experience with malaria, is an advocate of its treatment by means of the subcutaneous administration of quinin. It is recognized that the segmentation of the plasmodia occurs just before or at the time of the chill. A much smaller dose of quinin than is ordinarily required, if administered at this time, will quickly control the attack. It is in the case of patients who do not well tolerate the drug, or when it is desirable to cut short an attack, that the hypodermic method is especially valuable. The hydrochlorosulphate is the best salt for injection, as it has the strength of the sulphate, and its use in the manner indicated is not painful. In many cases, a 5-grain dose of this salt injected four hours before the expected paroxysm and the same quantity injected four hours after its occurrence, will at once check the disease, and completely cure it within four or five days. In some instances larger doses will be required. In cases of the estivo-autumnal form, it is advisable to begin treatment at once and to push it relentlessly, at the same giving the patient the benefit of the best hygienic surroundings. A relapse is even then likely to occur, and the cure must not be considered perfect until several weeks have passed without a recurrence of the disease.

THE MEDICAL NEWS.

A WEEKLY JOURNAL
OF MEDICAL SCIENCE.

COMMUNICATIONS are invited from all parts of the world. Original articles contributed *exclusively* to THE MEDICAL NEWS will after publication be liberally paid for (accounts being rendered quarterly), or 250 reprints will be furnished in place of other remuneration. When necessary to elucidate the text, illustrations will be engraved from drawings or photographs furnished by the author. Manuscripts should be typewritten.

Address the Editor: J. RIDDLE GOFFE, M.D.,
No. 111 FIFTH AVENUE (corner of 18th St.), NEW YORK.

Subscription Price, including postage in U. S. and Canada.

PER ANNUM IN ADVANCE	$4.00
SINGLE COPIES	.10
WITH THE AMERICAN JOURNAL OF THE MEDICAL SCIENCES, PER ANNUM	7.50

Subscriptions may begin at any date. The safest mode of remittance is by bank check or postal money order, drawn to the order of the undersigned. When neither is accessible, remittances may be made, at the risk of the publishers, by forwarding in *registered* letters.

LEA BROTHERS & CO.,
No. 111 FIFTH AVENUE (corner of 18th St.), NEW YORK,
AND NOS. 706, 708 & 710 SANSOM ST., PHILADELPHIA.

SATURDAY, JANUARY 1, 1898.

THE DISPENSARY BILL.

THE text of the "Dispensary Bill" which it is proposed to introduce in the State Legislature this winter will be found on another page of this issue, incorporated in the final report of the Committee on Charity Abuses as presented to the Medical Society of the County of New York at its last monthly meeting. This measure is the result of mature and careful deliberation, and has the endorsement of the principal medical societies of the State through their representatives in joint committee.

The bill as presented differs materially from the one which passed the Legislature last winter but failed to receive the Governor's signature. The great improvement—for this measure is vastly better than the former—lies in the fact that too much "reform" is not attempted. It avoids the fatal mistake of the now famous Raines' law, inasmuch as impossibilities are not contemplated—no effort is made to define a "poor person," which was an organic error in the former bill.

The primary essential object that will be accomplished by the enactment of this law is the placing of the dispensary question upon the statute books, giving it, as it were, a legal status. Practical experience in its application will suggest from time to time such amendments as the exigencies of the future may necessitate. The admirable feature of the measure lies in its conservatism, which cannot fail to insure for it a united effort on the part of the profession to place it among the laws of the State.

The State Board of Charities, which is given power to grant and revoke licenses under which dispensaries are to be conducted, will be responsible for the administration of the law. It will not be necessary for the medical profession to do police duty as has been the case in the enforcement of the general medical law of the State—a law successful only through the efforts of the profession. The members of this Board will no longer be able to say "we lack power," for, possessing authority to make rules and regulations governing the conduct of dispensaries, and armed with the power to revoke licenses in aggravated cases, the members of the Board will have it in their hands to elevate the present defective dispensary system to a constructive instead of a destructive charity.

THE MEDICAL NEWS bespeaks for the bill the prompt and favorable consideration, not only of the Legislature but also of the Governor, and foresees in the wise administration of such a law prompt relief from a great social abuse.

THE FAITH-CURE AGAIN.

DURING the last two weeks two deaths have occurred, the immediate result of the nefarious practice known as the "faith cure." The child of a man in Camden, N. J., died of what we understand to have been diphtheria. Later the father and a certain "faith-cure" professor were summoned before the court on the ground that they had caused the death of the child. There is no necessity to go into the details of the hearing and the hopeless ignorance and superstition displayed, but it is gratifying to know that the jury, after being out a few minutes, returned a verdict that "the child came to her death through the criminal negligence of her father, the aforesaid professor being an accessory." Something of the same kind occurred at Baltimore, the particulars of which we do not happen to have at hand. It is mentioned in order to emphasize the pressing need of legislation against such preposterous, indeed, criminal practices.

From Pennsylvania comes the report that Christian Science has received a set-back in that State from which it will find it most difficult, if not impossible, to recover. Through a judicial ruling recently made by Judge Pennypacker, permission for the incorporation of the creed which substitutes "metaphysical healing," as it is termed, for rational diagnosis and therapeutics, has been denied, and the practice of this ridiculously fatuous belief, if it may be called a belief, has been uncompromisingly declared as "against the law of the State."

Some of the points brought to light in this legal investigation as to the claims of the Christian Scientists appear both absurd and dangerous; absurd, because of the revelation they bring of the queer medieval mental perceptions prevalent among this sect; dangerous, on account of the immense risk to human life their application involves. Their teachings declare, for example, that "metaphysical healing" extends to such serious and fatal diseases as rheumatism, scrofula, cancer, smallpox, and consumption; in the latter disease, the *naïve* advice is given to "take up the leading points included, according to the individual's belief in the disease, show that it is not inherited, that inflammation, tubercles, hemorrhage, and decomposition are only beliefs, and these ills will disappear." Regarding luxations, they are equally hopeful, and in all seriousness "authenticated records" of the cure "through mental surgery alone of dislocated joints and spinal vertebræ" are offered for the Court's inspection. In the case of infants and children too young to understand the wonderful intricacies of the Christian Scientist's mind, the mental receptivity of the little one's elders transfers the cure through them to the child! The technic point of law upon which the ruling of the Court was based was obviously that which relates to the practice of medicine in Pennsylvania; and coming as it does so soon after the two lamentable instances of loss of life above referred to, the decision must be considered a timely piece of judicial action.

TREPHINING FOR HEMIPLEGIA AND NEWSPAPER NOTORIETY.

IN THE NEWS of last week we commented editorially on the Public Press and the Academy of Medicine anent the question of allowing reporters of the daily papers to be present at the meetings of the Academy and its Sections, and to make such report of the proceedings as they decided would startle or interest their readers. The fact that much surreptitious advertising, evading the letter of the code of ethics, while violating its spirit, is indulged in, is patent to the most unobservant. But the transgressor who thus attempts to bring his wares to the uncritical eye and gullible mind of the laity, is in nowise to be compared, in the matter of depravity, with him who gets the ear of the reporter in private and fills it with glowing statements of his own revolutionizing discoveries and brilliant achievements.

Such a flagrant example of the latter kind of advertising, not to speak of other reprehensibilities, has recently been perpetrated by a surgeon of this city, that we are constrained to call attention to it. As it involves not alone the ethical side of the question, but concerns as well, probably, a mistaken diagnosis and possibly an unwarranted procedure in the treatment of the patient, we shall content ourselves at this juncture with a recitation of the case, leaving for a future time, until the surgeon in question has had an opportunity to deny and disprove the report of statements attributed to him, a more personal consideration.

The facts of the case, so far as we have been able to learn them, are as follows: A man, fifty-six years old, was seized suddenly, without particular premonitory symptoms, save that of headache of several days' duration, with a sensation of numbness and unwieldiness of the right leg, and within a few minutes with a similar condition of the right upper extremity of the same side. The right half of the body rapidly became hemiplegic, and within a quarter of an hour the patient was comatose. He was seen immediately by a physician, who called a surgeon in consultation. The latter, on seeing him, advised that he be removed to a hospital and trepanned. And within four hours from the occurrence of the apoplexy the patient was trepanned over the left parietal region. With what object in view it seems difficult to conjecture.

Nothing abnormal was discovered, although an exploratory needle was carried into the brain in different areas, the lateral ventricle among them. A considerable quantity of cerebrospinal fluid, including that of the lateral ventricle, escaped. No blood, fluid or clotted, save that spilled in the operation, was found. The patient rallied, and after three or four days began to recover consciousness in a way exactly parallelizing a goodly number of apoplectic patients whose lesion is a thrombosis or moderate rupture of the middle cerebral artery, even when they are not bled or given vasomotor equalizers and absolute rest, the sequelæ of the attack symptomatically being right hemoplegia and total aphasia. Then comes the startling information through the medium of the secular press that a new treatment, "Trephining for Apolexy," had been vouchsafed to afflicted humanity at the hands of a surgeon to —— Hospital. The symptoms of the patient's illness are given in detail, and then the surgeon is quoted as saying to the reporter, his remarks being in quotation marks as they are here: "I have given much thought to the subject for a long time." Alas, that such things should be! "And I had been waiting for just such a chance as this to put my theory into practice. I have proved now that ordinary apoplexy may be cured by trephining." The *naïvete* of this concluding remark, the hope that it holds out to sorrowing ones who see those immeasurably dear to them stricken with this alarming condition, is to them like the Balm of Gilead, and the genesis of the hopeful statement may have been founded on the belief that the hand which applied the balm so skilfully and efficaciously in this case might be asked to do it in another; yes, even in scores of others, until his megalomaniac claims shall be shown by sad experience to be an air bubble. But, to continue the reputed words of the surgeon, "I believe that this is the first time that trephining for an ordinary case of apoplexy has been resorted to." We concur in this belief, and we gratefully thank the surgeons, past and present, for their concurrence in establishing this most praiseworthy status. And if prayer or supplication is of avail to keep this so, we humbly offer it. That any man should be so bereft of the faculties constituting common sense or judgment as to believe for one moment that he can reach the seat of lesion without sacrificing the patient in a case whose features mirror absolutely the most typical case of cerebral apoplexy due to occlusion or rupture of the middle cerebral artery, surpasses human understanding.

"Any literature that I have read upon this subject does not refer to the treating of ordinary apoplexy in this manner, and I believe that I am a pioneer in this direction." And again we concur! No, a thousand times no. There is no literature on the subject, and so long as the rank and file of physicians are recruited from men and women endowed with sufficient gray matter to comprehend the rudiments of anatomy and physiology, and the underlying principles of pathology, so long as the geniuses of our profession do not outrage their endowments and the unknowing do not violate their trust, there never will be such a literature. He is a pioneer indeed; the pioneer who prepares the holocanst and brings grief to many. We are desirous of doing no man an injustice. We contend for the rights of the individual, and we believe in the supremacy of personal opinion. If the surgeon in this instance believed that he had to do with a supracortical hemorrhage, then operative interference was justified. But in a man fifty-six years old, whose urine was shown on examination to contain casts and albumin, who develops the symptoms of cerebral apoplexy without preceding trauma or evidences of local contagious disease, supracortical hemorrhage is so extremely rare that, in truth, careful deliberation on the part of those to whom his fate is entrusted and the counsel of those whose experience has been great along the lines of such disease is the smallest consideration that should be granted him.

We refrain from further comment on this matter for the time being, for we would gladly learn and convey to our readers that the words of the daily papers, apparently coming directly from the surgeon, were false, and that the case is one that must be ascribed to misplaced zeal or mistaken diagnosis.

ECHOES AND NEWS.

Medical Faculty of Paris.—The theses for the degree of Doctor of Medicine presented to the medical faculty of Paris during the year 1896-97 numbered 640.

A Statue to Pasteur.—A statue to the memory of Pasteur has been erected at Melun by the agriculturists and the veterinary surgeons of the Departments of Seine and Marne.

The Sale of Serum.—The authorities of Paris have discovered that, although there is a law which forbids it, certain chemists have been manufacturing and selling preparations of serum. It has not yet been ascertained whether, as in the case of tuberculin, any of these preparations are fraudulent.

A Healthy Locality.—Friendsville, a little village in the Pennsylvania mountains, is remarkable for the longevity of its inhabitants. The town contains 135 inhabitants, of whom 27 have passed the age of ninety.

Medical Men and Preliminary Imprisonment.—The Obstetrical and Gynecological Society of Paris has appointed a committee to draw up a proposition to modify the law concerning preliminary imprisonment of medical men in cases of malpractice.

X-rays in Military Surgery.—The Röntgen rays are being employed with great success in cases of gunshot wound among the British troops in India in locating splinters of lead which would otherwise escape detection, as well as fractures and splinters of bone.

Typhus Fever at Skye.—A number of cases of typhus are reported at Skye, a small hamlet near Portree, Scotland. The inhabitants did not know the nature of the disease, and consequently children from infected houses were permitted to go to school. As a result, several members of the teacher's family have been stricken with the disease.

Vaccination or Prison.—A young woman of Atlanta, Ga., was recently fined $25.75 by Recorder Calhoun of that place for refusing to be vaccinated. She was unable to pay the amount and was ordered to serve twenty-five days in the city prison. After having been locked up for three hours she decided to be vaccinated, and was subsequently released after this had been done by her family physician.

The Stringencies of New York Quarantine.—A case of smallpox was discovered on board the Steamship "Edam," which arrived in New York Harbor on December 19th from Amsterdam with 277 steerage passengers. The health officer ordered all on board vaccinated and their detention at Hoffman Island for fourteen days. The vessel was thoroughly fumigated before being permitted to proceed to her dock.

Cattle-fever Quarantine.—The Department of Agriculture has issued a circular to railroads and transportation companies notifying them in regard to a contagious and infectious disease known as splenic or Southern fever which exists in certain parts of the country, and forbidding them to transport any cattle from below a certain line to any portion of the United States, except by rail or boat for immediate slaughter, from January 15th to November 15th of each year.

The Blood of the Buzzard as a Source of Antitoxin.—Dr. Eugene Street of Fall Creek, North Carolina, writes to ask if the blood of the buzzard has ever been tested for antitoxic properties. He suggests that the buzzard seems immune to disease ptomains and toxins, and that it may be within the range of possibility that a principle of more or less antitoxic powers could be obtained from it. Here is an original field of investigation for the ambitious serum-therapeutist.

Another Bogus Dentist Fined.—In New York General Sessions a man was recently fined $500 for practising dentistry under an assumed name, that of a man who was a graduate of a Western dental college and is now dead. The officers of the New York State Dental Society are reported as declaring that in many instances men are practising dentistry under the names of dead persons who held regular diplomas, and, moreover, that there is a regular traffic in dentists' diplomas.

Approval and Disapproval in Georgia of the Marine Hospital Service.—A joint resolution was recently adopted in the Georgia Legislature providing that all quarantine matters be entrusted to the United States Marine Hospital Service, and memorializing Congress to embody this resolution in a National Quarantine Law. The Governor of the State signified his disapproval of it by refusing to append his signature, on the plea that such action was contrary to the doctrine of State rights. Comment is unnecessary.

Explosive Hair-combs.—The explosion of a quantity of celluloid hair-combs which recently occurred on an elevated-railroad train in New York City, draws attention to the dangerously inflammable nature of this substance. In referring to this subject, the *British Medical Journal* mentions the case of a young girl who, while wearing one of these celluloid combs, bent over a lighted candle, with the result that, although the comb had not touched the flame, it exploded from the heat, and the girl was badly burned about the face and eyes.

Smallpox in a Dog.—In the smallpox hospital at Atlanta, Ga., there is a small hairless Mexican terrier which is suffering from the disease. Two weeks ago the dog's master was attacked with smallpox, and was removed from his home to the hospital by the Health Department. Three days later the little dog, which had been in the habit of sleeping with his owner, developed the typical smallpox eruption, and the matter was reported to the health authorities. The dog is now at the hospital with his master, and is being well cared for.

Obituary.—The death is announced of Dr. Joseph Lewi of Albany, N. Y., on December 19th. Dr. Lewi was born in Radnitz, Austria, August 17, 1820. He received his medical education at the University of Vienna, and came to this country soon after his graduation. He was at one time President of the Albany County Medical Society, and at the time of his death was the senior member of the Board of Censors of the New York State Medical Society. For twelve years he served as a member of the State Board of Public Instruction, and refused re-election after four terms of service.

Dangerous Lay-Press Prescriptions.—The *British Medical Journal* comments upon the appearance of a dangerous prescription which recently appeared in the "Answers to Correspondents" column of an English paper called *The Hearth and Home.* The prescription is as follows: "℞ Potass. bromidi, grains 10; Liq. strych., ♏. 5; Tinct. cinch. co., ℥ ½; aq., ℥ ss. Misce. Ft. haustus, 6 ter die." The fact is pointed out that strychnin and bromid of potassium are pharmacologically antagonistic and chemically incompatible, and also that in the above mixture they form a combination of a most dangerous character.

The Antivivisection Bill Again in Congress.—Senator Gallinger is reported in the *Congressional Record* of December 15, 1897, as saying: "Upon solicitation from several Senators saying that they were receiving letters from constituents protesting against the passage of the bill, I allowed it to drift along. On the 13th day of May the bill was again reported and is on the calendar. At an early day I shall move to take up that bill, which is *Senate Bill 1063, Calendar No. 136.* I trust that when I ask the consideration of the bill it may not be objected to, but that that matter which to my mind is extremely important—and a controverted matter, I will say, on the part of physicians, scientists, and humanitarians—may have a fair discussion, and that we may have a vote of the Senate deciding whether or not that bill shall pass this body."

Requirements of the Various States Regarding the License to Practise Medicine.—To obtain a license to practise medicine it is necessary to pass an examination in the following States: Alabama, Delaware, District of Columbia, Florida, Georgia, Idaho, Louisiana, Maine, Maryland, Massachusetts, Minnesota, Mississippi, Montana, New Hampshire, New Jersey, New York, North Carolina, North Dakota, Oregon, Pennsylvania, South Carolina, Utah, Virginia, Washington, and West Virginia. Examination is required although certain diplomas are recognized as an equivalent in the following States: Arkansas, Colorado, Connecticut, Illinois, Indiana, Iowa, Missouri, Oklahoma, Rhode Island, Tennessee, Vermont, Wisconsin, New Mexico. A diploma only is required in the following States: California, Kentucky, Nebraska, Ohio, South Dakota, Texas (practically). The law practically imposes no restriction in the following: Alaska, Arizona, Kansas, Michigan, Nevada, Wyoming. Dr. D. C. Newman of Seattle, Wash., writes us that the law requiring a license to practise medicine in that State is practically a dead letter, for it is never enforced, and adds that fully one-fourth of the practising physicians of that State have never complied with it.

Hospital and Dispensary Abuse in Boston.—The Boston Medical Society, at its meeting December 18th, 1897, adopted the following resolutions: "*Whereas*, the unrestricted abuses of medical charity in the great hospitals and dispensaries of Boston is being seriously complained of by a large number of general practitioners; and *whereas*, the State has granted charters to these hospitals and dispensaries for the definite purpose of giving medical and surgical care and treatment to indigent persons within the city and commonwealth; and *whereas*, the Boston Medical Society, individually and collectively, recognize, with every feeling of sympathy, the rights and just claims of some of our citizens to the benefits of public and private charity, and will not be found wanting in generosity in whatever may tend to foster the moral, social, and physical well-being of the sick, the poor, the destitute, the lowly, the worthy, and the unfortunate; and *whereas*, large numbers of persons, of both sexes, frequently, daily, and repeatedly receive medical and surgical advice and treatment gratuitously for numerous cases of minor surgery and ordinary illness who are believed to be financially competent to pay moderate fees; and *whereas*, the time, facilities, and attention at the dispensaries being necessarily limited, that which is received by the well-to-do and the undeserving is, in that proportion, withheld from those who, by the chartered rules of these institutions, are justly entitled to their benefits; and *whereas*, the practitioners of medicine and surgery of any community, who have duly graduated from accredited medical colleges, and have incurred the expense of locating in such communities, naturally and justly feel that their present and prospective rights and privileges are wrongly encroached upon by the abuses now in practice in connection with medical charities. Therefore, *resolved*, that it is the opinion of this society that some means can be found to check or modify this formidable evil; and, *resolved*, that an urgent call be made upon all such members of the profession who are in sympathy with the movement, and have at heart the best interests of the medical profession, to render such moral assistance and financial support in the adoption of such measures as will tend to eradicate and prevent these evils, abuses, and practices; and *resolved*, that an open meeting be held in the near future, and the profession at large be invited to be present; and *resolved*, that a copy of these resolutions be sent to the *Boston Medical and Surgical Journal, Journal of the American Medical Association, Medical Record, New York Medical Journal*, and THE MEDICAL NEWS for publication. Signed for the Society, M. GERSTEIN, M.D., Secretary, 1038 Washington street."

SPECIAL ARTICLE.

FINAL REPORT TO THE MEDICAL SOCIETY OF THE COUNTY OF NEW YORK OF ITS COMMITTEE ON THE ABUSES OF MEDICAL CHARITY.

(Transmitted December 27, 1897.)

MR. PRESIDENT AND GENTLEMEN: Report has already been made of the work done by your Committee on the Abuses of Medical Charity since its appointment one year ago. In its final report, here presented, the committee offers for your consideration and approval the text of a Dispensary Bill which it is proposed to have introduced in the Legislature during the early days of the approaching session. This bill, which has been prepared by the Joint-Committee on Medical Charity Abuse, has received the endorsement of the several committees appointed, with power, by the New York State Medical Association, New York County Medical Association, New York Medical League, New York Society for Advancing the Practice of Medicine, Kings County Medical Society, Kings County Medical Association, Brooklyn Medical Society, Brooklyn Medical Association, and the Long Island Medical Society.

The text of the bill is as follows:

SECTION 1. By and for the purpose of this act, a dispensary is declared to be any person, corporation, institution, society, association, or agent, whose purpose it is, either independently or in connection with any other purpose, to furnish, at any place or places, to persons non-resident therein, either gratuitously or for a compensation determined without reference to the value of the thing furnished, medical, or surgical advice, or treatment, medicine or apparatus; provided, however, that the moneys used by and for the purposes of said dispensary shall be derived wholly or in part from trust funds, public moneys, or sources other than the individuals constituting said dispensary, and the persons actually engaged in the distribution of the charities of said dispensary.

SEC. 2. Six months after the passage of this act it shall not be lawful for any dispensary to enter upon the execution, or continue the prosecution of its purpose unless duly licensed by the State Board of Charities as hereinafter provided.

SEC. 3. Upon the filing with the State Board of Charities of an application and statements in such form and of such substance as shall be prescribed by said Board, said Board may issue a license in such form as it shall prescribe to any dispensary, if in the judgment of said Board the statements filed and the evidence submitted therewith indicate that the operations of said dispensary will be for the public good.

SEC. 4. The State Board of Charities is hereby empowered to make rules and regulations, and to alter or amend the same, in accordance with which all dispensaries shall furnish, and applicants obtain, medical or surgical relief, advice or treatment, medicine or apparatus, but nothing in this act contained shall be construed to mean that said Board shall have power to determine the particular school of medicine in accordance with which any dispensary shall manage or conduct its work, or to determine the kind of medical or surgical treatment provided by any dispensary.

SEC. 5. When it shall appear to the satisfaction of the State Board of Charities that any dispensary licensed by it under the provisions of this act has violated any of the provisions of this act, or any of the rules and regulations made by the said Board under authority of this act, then, and in that event, the said Board is hereby empowered, due notice and an opportunity for a hearing having been given to said dispensary, to suspend or revoke the license of said dispensary.

SEC. 6. Six months after the passage of this act no dispensary shall make use of any place commonly known as a drug-store, or any place or building defined by law or by an ordinance of a Board of Health as a tenement-house.

SEC. 7. Six months after the passage of this act it shall not be lawful to display or cause to be displayed in any manner whatsoever anything which could directly, or by suggestion, make public the existence of the equivalent, in purpose and effect, of a dispensary.

SEC. 8. Any person who violates any of the provisions of this act, or any of the rules and regulations made and published under the authority of this act, shall be guilty of a misdemeanor, and, on conviction thereof, shall be punished by a fine of not less than ten dollars, and not more than $250.

SEC. 9. Nothing in this act contained shall in any wise be construed to abridge any of the powers of the said State Board of Charities, or of any of the members or officers thereof, or inspectors duly appointed by it, now existing under and by virtue of Chapter 546 of the Laws of 1896, known as the State Charities Law.

SEC. 10. This act shall take effect immediately.

As will be seen, this bill differs essentially from that with which the first report of your committee had to deal, the most important feature being that each and every dispensary must obtain a license from the State Board of Charities, by virtue of which its operations shall be conducted; and that, in case the law, or the rules and regulations framed by the Board be not complied with, said Board is empowered to revoke the license of the dispensary so offending. The vested rights of corporations will in no wise be interfered with, and the effort to correct the crying abuses now so widely prevalent will not result in injury to those institutions which are, and will be, properly and conscientiously conducted. This bill, as now presented, embodies the result of much paintaking and earnest consideration, and it is hoped that it will receive the hearty and unqualified support of those who have the subject of the correction of medical charity abuse nearest at heart. The State Commissioners of Charity have already been informally consulted regarding its provisions, and a copy is about to be sent, together with other literature, which has been prepared, to every legally constituted medical society in the State for indorsement.

It is not the idea of your committee that the universal abuse of dispensary privileges can either be done away with or even adequately controlled all at once, but the enactment of a law, such as provided for in the accompanying bill, will, in its opinion, mark an era in the effort which, during the past twenty years, has been made by so many earnest workers toward this end. Experience has shown that without a law on the statute books, just and equitable alike to the laity and the members of the medical profession, absolutely nothing can be accomplished in the direction of bettering existing conditions, and, therefore, it is with the full confidence that the Medical Society of the County of New York will heartily indorse the action of its committee, and will attach its seal of approval to this amended Joint-Committee Dispensary Bill that this report is submitted.

(Signed) JAMES HAWLEY BURTENSHAW, Chairman.

A. BRAYTON BALL,	ALEXANDER HADDEN,
H. J. BOLDT,	WILLIAM M. POLK,
E. S. BULLOCK,	W. WASHBURN,
HENRY DWIGHT CHAPIN,	W. H. WESTON,
CARTER S. COLE,	FREDERICK H. WIGGINS.

For the Relief of Migraine.—Excellent results are reported by ESHNER from the administration in this affection of the fluid extracts of gelsemium and cannabis Indica. The dose is 3 to 5 drops of each, given three times daily, until physiologic action becomes apparent.

CORRESPONDENCE.

AN ANSWER TO DR. MUNDE.

To the Editor of THE MEDICAL NEWS.

DEAR SIR: I have noticed in the issue of your journal of November 27th a letter from Dr. Paul F. Mundé in which he offers several criticisms of my article on "The Treatment of Abortion," which appeared in THE MEDICAL NEWS of November 6th,

With reference to Dr. Mundé's criticism of the name applied to the large, blunt curette, I beg to say that I have seen the one I use offered for sale in one shop as Mundé's, and in another as Lusk's. So far as I know, it was Dr. T. G. Thomas who introduced the dull, wire curette for scraping the inside of the uterus, and in my opinion an instrument does not become a new one by being made larger and stronger, and used for a kindred purpose. I take, therefore, all intra-uterine dull wire curettes to be essentially Thomas' dull curettes as opposed to Sims' sharp curette, and, if Dr. Mundé is the first who described their use in obstetrics, which I can neither affirm nor deny, his merit in this regard consists in extending the principle of Thomas' curette from gynecologic to obstetric surgery.

As to the other three criticisms, they only prove that Dr. Mundé, on the points in question, does not agree with me, in which he has the same right as anybody else.

H. J. GARRIGUES, M.D.

NEW YORK, December 14, 1897.

CONSTANTINOPLE LETTER.[1]

FROM GEO. R. FOWLER, M.D.,
OF BROOKLYN, N. Y.

MASSING THE TURKISH TROOPS AT THE "SELAMLIK"—THE YILDIZ HOSPITAL—DJEMIL PASHA—TRANSPORTATION EQUIPMENT—THE GERMAN RED CROSS SOCIETY'S WORK—ASEPSIS IN TURKEY—CONSERVATISM OF THE TURKISH SURGEON—THE GRAS RIFLE—THE HAIDA PASHA HOSPITAL—FLORENCE NIGHTINGALE—TURKISH CEMETERIES—EDUCATION OF MILITARY MEDICAL OFFICERS—MILITARY CADETS—THE HOSPITAL CORPS—THE RED CRESENT—THE X-RAYS IN TURKEY.

CONSTANTINOPLE, August 4, 1897.

IN response to a request through our efficient *chargé d'affaires* here, Mr. Riddle, Muchir Theoket Pasha, the commander of the Second Turkish Brigade, in whose district the *Yildiz Hospital*, the largest military hospital in Constantinople, is situated, detailed an adjutant to conduct me to the latter institution. While waiting for the horses to be saddled the Pasha invited me, with true Turkish hospitality, into the beautiful garden adjoining his headquarters, from which point an extensive view of the Bosphorus, with Scutari in the distance, is obtained. There I partook of a refreshing ice and a delightful cup of coffee. By the aid of German, of which the Pasha possessed some knowledge, and the Turkish and English of our dragoman, I endeavored to obtain some information as to the number of Turkish troops, as well as the losses sustained during the recent Greco-Turkish war. With characteristic Turkish caution, however, the Pasha was not disposed to talk very freely upon this subject, but from other sources it was learned that, of the 750,000 men which constitute the war footing of Turkey, less than one-fifth were sent to the front. Certainly there are not less than 10,000 soldiers in Constantinople at the present time, as I had opportunity of estimating upon witnessing the ceremony known as the *Selamlik*, or visit of the Sultan to the mosque, which takes place every Friday afternoon. At this ceremony the troops in Constantinople and vicinity are massed about the palace and mosque, which are only about 500 yards apart, the opportunity being thus afforded for the Sultan to come face to face with his troops upon this, the only occasion upon which the descendant of the Prophet and Ruler of the Nation leaves the palace grounds.

Arriving at the hospital I was greeted most courteously by the Turkish medical officers. These, for the most part, have had the advantage of a training in France or Germany, and I had no difficulty in obtaining information as to the hospital buildings and their capacity.

The *Yildiz Hospital* is beautifully located upon an eminence overlooking the city, and is not far from the Sultan's palace of the same name. It consists of twenty-two pavilions, built of wood, and lined with heavy sheathing-paper. These pavilions or barracks are placed in regular order upon an extensive plateau, with wide streets between, and were erected in less than a month to meet the emergency caused by the war.

We were shortly joined by Djemil Pasha, who, although but twenty-seven years of age, is the surgeon-in-chief of this large hospital. It is currently reported that this young man owes his exalted position to the fact that he is the son-in-law of a prominent and influential individual at the Sublime Porte.[1]

We learned that the hospital has ample accommodations for 1000 patients. At the present time it contains between 800 and 900. We were informed that in the neighborhood of 3000 soldiers have been treated here for injuries alone since the commencement of the war. With the natural desire to lessen the importance of their losses this may be taken as a low estimate, as this is the hospital in which was received the majority of those who survived the somewhat crude means of transportation frequently employed (donkeys and rough carts). The equipment for transportation purposes at the disposition of the Medical Corps consists of eight ambulances and two hundred litters for the entire Turkish army. Many of the wounded were strapped upon the backs of donkeys and mules, and conveyed in this manner miles to the nearest railroad.

A tour of the grounds, including a well-shaded garden for advanced convalescents, was first made, escorted by

[1] This letter was lost in transit, and only recently came to light. It is considered of sufficient importance and interest to warrant its publication even at this date.—ED.

[1] From what I saw of his work in Constantinople, as well as the impression which he produced at Moscow, where he appeared as the representative of the Turkish Army Medical Department at the International Congress, I am convinced that whatever influences were at work to secure his rapid promotion he is largely deserving of the confidence that is reposed in him.

the Surgeon-in-Chief and his staff, after which the pavilions were inspected in detail, and many interesting cases shown.

Two of the pavilions, until a few days ago, were under the care of Dr. Nasse, assistant to Bergmann, and a corps of surgeons and nurses of the German branch of the Red Cross Society. Upon the eve of their departure to return to their own country, they were entertained at dinner in the Yildiz Palace, at the close of which they received at the hands of the Sultan the gold medal and green military decoration, conferred upon those who have distinguished themselves in the performance of some especially valuable service to the Turkish Government. In the hospital mentioned there are two operating-rooms, provided in a special operating pavilion, one at each end of the building. One of these is used for aseptic cases, while the other is for septic cases. To the fact that the majority of the Turkish military surgeons receive an additional training in France or Germany is to be attributed the care exercised in respect to wound treatment. While this was not always ideal, yet such as it was it excited my surprise. There seemed to be an earnest desire, and in some instances an enthusiastic and well-directed effort, to comply with the requirements of modern aseptic work.

While the Turkish surgeons are strikingly conservative, sometimes to a fault, and energetic and ambitious operative attacks are not encouraged, yet this conservatism is not the result of timidity on the part of the operators. Djemil Pasha has twice sutured the axillary artery, after Murphy's suggestion, for injury of that vessel occurring in the course of the removal of secondary carcinomatous glandular masses in the armpit—a procedure requiring surgical courage and skill decidedly above the average. Almost all of the operations performed at the *Yildiz Hospital* were done by the native Turkish surgeons, a fact to which they called attention with pride.

Here, as at Athens, I was shown a large number of gunshot wounds of joints, particularly of the shoulder and elbow. Singular to say, these occurred, in the vast majority of cases, upon the right side. In many of the instances of joint injury secondary resection had been done, some of which were typical. Cases of amputation were conspicuous by their absence. The Turk is violently opposed to noticeable mutilation, and to this is to be attributed his abhorrence of losing a member. Of the twenty-two cases of traumatic destruction of the eye, enucleation had been positively refused in the larger number. Up to the present time none of these have developed sympathetic ophthalmia. In those in which the globe was removed in connection with operations upon the orbit, the authorities had at once supplied an artificial eye, of which the wearer was childishly proud.

The Turkish wounded were rather more severely injured, as a rule, than the Greeks. This is probably due to the fact that the latter were armed with the Gras rifle, which carries a large lead projectile. These were obtained from a supply representing the discarded weapons of the French army, and, in many instances, the pieces were shortened by sawing off the barrel after being purchased by the Greek Government. When employed at short range, however, they are capable of considerable execution. That so many Turks were wounded at short range, and in the head and the upper portion of the trunk, rather serves to contradict the stories of want of coolness, if not actual cowardice, of the Greek soldier, which are current. In justice to the Turk it should also be stated that in no instance was a case observed in which the wound was received from behind. This was likewise true of the Greeks.

A visit was made to the *Haida Pasha Hospital*, in Scutari, upon the Asiatic side of the Bosphorus. This is the hospital made famous as the scene of the labors of Florence Nightingale during the Crimean War. The Turkish authorities in charge seemed to evince some interest when reference was made to the work of this noble and self-sacrificing woman: although her labors were of inestimable value, not even a tablet commemorates her services. This is not to be wondered at, however, when one considers some of the peculiarities of the Turkish character. The average Turk lives only in the present. He puts the past behind him as soon and as far as he may, and devotes but very little thought to the future. Only a short walk from the spot where Florence Nightingale won the love and admiration of the civilized world is to be found the largest Turkish cemetery about Constantinople, where lie the remains of many of the highest dignitaries, as well as warriors and statesmen, that Turkey has ever produced; for the soil of Scutari is considered sacred ground. Here the Ottoman dynasty was founded, and from here Islamism spread itself in Europe. Many illustrious men, therefore, have been buried here. The condition of the place would disgrace the potter's field of the meanest hamlet in Christendom. The tombstones, many of which are painted green to indicate the grave of a descendant of Mahomet, are to be seen leaning in all directions in a shiftless, tumbled-down manner, and many have fallen and are half buried beneath the *débris* of broken-down branches of the Oriental cyprus, the invariable accompaniment of a Turkish burial-place. There is no railing about the place, and the dogs, idlers, and cattle rove about its three-mile area at will. That this was not due to the fact that it is no longer used as a cemetery was attested by the presence of a newly made grave, the freshly painted green tombstone of which, surrounded by a carved turban in many folds, proclaimed the importance during life of its occupant.

I could not help contrasting this with the well-kept English cemetery within sight of the spot where I stood, in which lie buried many of the English officers who died here during the Crimean War.

The *Haida Pasha Hospital* is now only occupied by convalescents, these being principally medical cases. Typhoid fever formerly prevailed here to a considerable extent; but, since the water-supply has been changed and water has been brought in casks from the mountains, it has been greatly lessened.

I was somewhat surprised to find that both Armenians and Greeks are serving at the present time in the Turkish Army Medical Corps. It is a fact that only the faithful followers of the Prophet are allowed to fight under his banner, and to join its actual combatant rank and file.

The Turkish military medical officer has a special training, and this at the expense of the government. Upon passing his examination and receiving his commission he pledges himself to serve the government twenty-six years, at the end of which time he may be pensioned. If for any reason other than actual physical disability this obligation is not fulfilled, he is forced to refund to the government the amount expended by the latter upon his education.

About one-fourth of the classes at the University of Constantinople are entered as medical students, or about 500 yearly. While at first glance this seems like a large class, yet it should be remembered in this connection that this is the only school in which medicine is taught in Turkey. There is a special department of military medicine, which, together with the regular course, covers six years. In the case of those intending to practice in civil life the examinations are conducted by a civil board, but those designed for the army or navy must pass an examination at the hands of a board of military surgeons.

A surgeon and an assistant surgeon are assigned to each battalion. In addition to these, *medical cadets*, who have attended two or more courses of lectures and demonstrations, are placed under the orders of the medical officers. These are selected from among those who have but a limited preliminary education, and who are not deemed of sufficiently promising material to do credit to the service in the higher grades. The medical cadet may, however, aspire to the latter, and occasionally succeeds in obtaining a commission. Usually, however, he spends his life in performing the most menial duties of the medical service, these including cupping, bleeding, tooth-drawing, and such services as were demanded of the old-time barber-surgeon of the European armies.

The hospital corps consists of non-combatants enlisted for the purpose. Upon occasions of ceremony they parade as a separate organization. This corps corresponds in some respects to the ambulance corps of our National Guard. It is much below the latter in efficiency; for the reason that its members are not trained in rendering first aid to the injured. The brassard is a *red crescent*. The natural aversion of the Turk to anything in the shape of a cross forbids the adoption of the insignia of the Geneva convention. The corps flag is a green field with a red crescent. The corps numbers 3000 for the entire army, including hospital stewards, who must be regular graduates in pharmacy, and pass a special examination before admission. The hospital corps is especially trained in the transportation of the wounded and care of the sick, but its members are not expected to render first aid, save of the simplest character.

The discovery of Röntgen has found its way into Turkey and has been utilized by the medical department of its army. Several cases were shown in which missiles have been located by the aid of the X-rays, and their removal successfully accomplished. The erratic course of the missiles and their inaccessibility rendered their localization impossible by any other means.

OUR PHILADELPHIA LETTER.

[From our Special Correspondent.]

PATHOLOGICAL SOCIETY OF PHILADELPHIA—PHILADELPHIA COUNTY MEDICAL SOCIETY—SOME COMMENTS APROPOS OF THE RECENT OUTBREAK OF DIPHTHERIA AND ENTERIC FEVER.

PHILADELPHIA, December 25, 1897.

AT the last stated meeting of the Pathological Society of Philadelphia, held on December 23d, Dr. Joseph Sailer read a paper on "Results of Laceration of the Brain Substance," based upon the following experiment: A cat having been anesthetized, a trephine opening was made in the skull large enough to expose a rather large area of brain substance, into which a hot platinum needle was then plunged, and moved to and fro in order to lacerate the organ; the wound was then dressed aseptically, and the animal placed under observation. At the end of seventy-two hours the animal died, the brain was removed, and sections were cut from areas near and remote to the site of the lesion and stained by appropriate methods. Microscopic examination of these sections showed that in the vicinity of the clot which resulted from the hot needle, the neuroglia cells had proliferated and were noticeably increased in size, and that extensive degenerated changes in the neighboring ganglion cells had ensued; karyokinetic figures were not observed. Away from the immediate site of the lesion no abnormalities were apparent. Dr. W. E. Hughes reported two interesting cases of Weil's disease occurring in men of middle age. The first case, after a vague history of malarial infection some months before, suddenly developed acute jaundice, hematuria, irregular chills, and hyperpyrexia, followed by rapid collapse and death; *post-mortem* findings showed an enlarged spleen, kidneys, and Pyer's patches, with advanced fatty degeneration of both suprarenal capsules. In the second case, sepsis resulting from an urethral stricture for which perineal urethrotomy was performed, preceded anuria, jaundice, signs of acute hepatic and renal congestion, and obstruction to the venous return flow. In both cases extensive small round-cell infiltration of the capsule of Glisson, and acute parenchymatous degeneration of the liver were found after death. Dr. Joseph McFarland and Dr. J. M. Anders reported a case of pneumothorax in which the site of the perforation had been discovered, this joint-paper including a careful *résumé* of the literature of the lesion, and its discussion from a pathologic standpoint.

At the last stated meeting of the Philadelphia County Medical Society, held on December 22d, Dr. Joseph Price read a paper on "Operative Detail in Appendicitis," in which he advocated a radical operation in cases demanding operative interference at all, and in which many minor details of the procedure were elaborated; he described, among these, a method by which sutures are introduced before final severence of the appendix, thus obviating to a large extent, the speaker claimed, the risk of infection through the wound. Dr. Williams F. Arnold gave a most interesting account of "Some Personal Observations on the Bubonic Plague," which he made in Hong Kong and its environs in 1894. Speaking of the specific cause of this disease, Dr. Arnold said that he had been unable to convince himself of the specificity of Kitasato's plague bacillus, and that he thought rather that Yersin's bacillus was the true cause of the disease. He seemed to be favorably impressed with the results of Yersin's serum-treatment of the plague, by the use of which he had seen the mortality fall from 80 or 90 to 50 per cent. in severe cases, and from 50 to 10 per cent. in mild cases. Dr. Milton B. Hartzell reported an unusual instance of epithelioma occurring in a boy of fourteen years; the growth was situated at the left ala of the nose, with slight secondary involvement of a small area around the outer canthus of the left eye. It was removed by the local use of pyrogallic acid, healthy cicatrization following this treatment. Dr. Edward Jackson reported a case of ivory exostosis about the size of an almond, growing from the lateral aspect of the nasal side of the orbit, the removal of which he accomplished without difficulty. The speaker also referred to two other cases of a like character, and showed a specimen of the growth. Dr. J. B. Learned read a paper on "The Induction of Sleep by Means of Producing Muscular Fatigue in the Patient," an original feature of which was his advocacy of slow breathing, instead of rapid respiratory movements, as usually recommended for hypnotic effects.

The resources of the Philadelphia health authorities have been greatly taxed during the recent outbreaks of diphtheria and typhoid fever—taxed, it would appear, to an extent which left them completely distanced in the race between health and disease, for the infection spread merrily on, involving whom it chose in what would have been called an epidemic, had the nature of the infection been, for instance, some imported tropical fever, or smallpox. But being only diphtheria and typhoid, to which tuberculosis is, of course, a necessary adjunct to every respectable community—particularly communities with Health Boards—the outbreak had to sink its identity in the official obscurity of "a prevalence in certain sections" of the diseases in question. The epidemic, for such it certainly was, has now subsided, some say because of the intervention of the Board of Health; others, less charitably inclined, say it was because it ran its course. At all events, it has subsided, but at the cost of many lives, and leaving in its wake an unsavory odor of general public mistrust in our methods of municipal hygiene. And is the public, after all, so far wrong in its judgment? What, with foul water, inadequate food-inspection, and a whole host of relics of municipal insanitation of a past era still flourishing here, is the public to infer? Is it not natural for it to place greater confidence in personal immunity and prophylaxis rather than upon the labors in its behalf made by its health and legislative bodies? The time has come for this city to possess a modern water-supply, to abolish with a firm hand nuisances which would not be tolerated for a moment in many centers, to equip its medical-inspection officers with every facility for the intelligent pursuance of their work, and, finally, to legislate so that for such necessities as these she will not be dependent upon the humor of a clique of politicians whose ideas of sanitation and public health are distinctly subservient to the machinations of practical politics, and to the pecuniary plums with which other forms of legislation fill their councilmanic pockets. Councils must be importuned for every improvement needed by the Board of Health, and with the approval of this body only may the present inadequate equipment for coping with epidemics be made effective. The question, therefore, can be solved only by the entire cooperation of both bodies, or by the complete divorce of the one's dependence upon the other. The former seems futile of accomplishment; the latter is palpably impossible. And thus the situation remains, to the detriment of the health of the city at large, and as a tremendous handicap to the efforts of the Board of Health in dealing with these outbreaks of endemic infections, such as the two which have just terminated.

OUR BERLIN LETTER.

[From our Special Correspondent.]

A NEW OPINION ON THE THYROID QUESTION—THE IMPORTANCE OF MIXED INFECTION IN TUBERCULOSIS—AMYLOID DISEASE DUE TO STAPHYLOCOCCIC, BUT NOT OTHER BACTERIAL PRODUCTS—LONG INCUBATION OF GONORRHEA AND ITS SIGNIFICANCE—PROFESSOR MOMMSEN'S EIGHTIETH BIRTHDAY.

BERLIN, December 18, 1897.

PROFESSOR HERMANN MUNK'S article on the "Thyroid Gland" which appeared in the last number of *Virchow's Archives* has naturally attracted a great deal of attention. The Professor of Physiology at the University of Berlin and the successor to the chair of Du Bois Reymond would be deferentially listened to in any case, but besides, Professor Munk's own work in physiology has given him a place among the greatest living workers in this line. It is a little startling to find that he does not agree with the generally accepted theories as to the thyroid gland in animals being essential to life, or that its function is necessary for the proper performance of the processes of nutrition. For years he has been known to hold such opinions, but his reassertion of them now, after a long series of careful experiments in the face of the supposed acquisitions to physiology and therapeutics which prevailing opinions involve, has appeared somewhat in the light of a medical sensation. He states very definitely what are considered to be the cardinal points of the present physiology of the thyroid gland: (1) That animals cannot exist without it. (2) That where death is not immediate a cachexia develops resembling myxedema in the human species, or the so-called cachexia strumipriva after surgical removal of the gland. (3) That the implantation of the thyroid or its internal administration will obviate the symptoms caused by its removal. He then categorically denies each one of these principles and also the doctrine as a whole.

As to animals dying sooner or later as a consequence of the removal of the gland, while in his experiments of ten years ago all animals perished after the operation, now fifty per cent. of the apes and rabbits, and twenty-five per cent. of the dogs and cats are not affected at all by removal of the thyroid. The difference in the results of the operations performed with the antisepsis of 1887 and the asepsis of 1896 and 1897 is a very suggestive series of experiments for the modern surgeon to study. The completeness of the experiments seems to eliminate any chance of error. That the thyroid was thoroughly removed was made positive from the results of autopsies in a number of cases where the animals were killed after months and sections made to decide this point. Nor did any organ develop to replace the supposedly necessary function of the gland. The parathyroids played no such rôle, as they were always carefully sought and removed, except in one instance in which they were left and the animal subsequently died, but the *post-mortem* did not reveal any tendency to compensatory hypertrophy. The hypophysis was very carefully examined in a number of cases to be sure that it did not develop a compensatory function, but no evidence of any change was ever found, and no thymus nodules took on regressive activity to replace the romoved thyroid.

As to the myxedematous cachexia so often described, he has never observed it. He has frequently seen animals die some months after the operation from a progressive wasting, seemingly without cause, but the changes present could never be described as myxedematous. The lesions usually (*post-mortem*) found were those of a chronic gastro-intestinal affection. This was probably due to the well-known tendency of animals to die during captivity from nutritional disturbances because of the unsuitable food and insufficient exercise. By no means all the experimental animals died, but on the contrary, many of them grew fat after the operation. Professor Munk especially criticizes Horsley's two series of experiments on apes. The first is the basis of all the claims which have been made for the development of myxedema in apes. In it, all the apes that did not succumb to the operation became myxedematous within from four to seven weeks. During the last year or two Professor Munk has had thirteen out of seventeen apes live from one to nine months after the complete removal of the thyroid gland, but has observed the development of nothing like myxedema. Some of the comments on Horsely's work and his failure to answer Professor Munk's request to be shown a myxedematous ape or a photograph of one are rather caustic.

As to the question of implanted or ingested thyroids preventing the accidents remote or proximate which follow thyroidectomy, Munk has never observed any such effect. It certainly does not prevent the immediate accidents. The cachexia which so often develops after the operation as the result of captivity, etc., is not influenced by thyroid medication, Professor Munk quotes, in this regard, the work of a number of others who have reached similar conclusions; for instance, one set of observations are detailed in which a fair percentage of thyroidectomized animals survived without thyroid feeding or implantation, while eleven out of twelve, the thyroids of which had been extirpated, and to which thyroid extract had been given as food, died within a few weeks.

Tetany has sometimes been observed after the removal of the thyroid, but it is very irregular in its manifestations, sometimes occurring immediately, sometimes not for some time, and is often interrupted by irregular intervals, during which no spasms occur. All these irregular phenomena point to other conditions for their origin besides the extirpation of the thyroid, which, of course, was a constant factor in the observations. The course of the tetany does not seem to be modified by thyroid medication.

The important question in the study of tuberculosis throughout the German medical world just now, apart from the erection of institutions for its treatment, is the influence of mixed infection on its course and fatality. Some time ago Dr. Michaelis, working in Professor Leyden's clinic, was able to demonstrate staphylococci in the blood of eight out of ten tuberculous patients. Some recent work from Professor Stadelman's clinic more or less confirms the studies of Michaelis, though the percentage of cases in which the staphylococci could be demonstrated was not so high.

A special feature of the work in Professor Stadelman's clinic was the determination by inoculation experiments that the staphylococci found were not especially virulent, but, on the contrary, seemed to have lost their virulency owing to unfavorable circumstances for their growth in the organism. Petruschky, some time ago, observed the same lack of virulency in the streptococci which he had found in the blood of tuberculous patients. The explanation of this would seem to be either Spengler's theory that bacterial growth in the non-succulent cicatricial tissue of tuberculous cavities, in an unfavorable medium, leads to the loss of certain vital properties, or that the comparatively slow growth and the consequent gradual absorption of toxins leads to the formation of certain antitoxic and immunizing agents in the blood which react unfavorably upon the vitality of the streptococcus.

An interesting commentary on the whole subject is the very thorough review of amyloid degeneration which appeared in a recent number of *Virchow's Archives*. Dr. Davidsohn, of Virchow's laboratory, at the suggestion of his chief, has reviewed the literature of this subject, and confirmed by a series of careful personal investigations the results of those observers who claim to have experimentally produced amyloid disease in animals. With the immense material of the Pathological Institute in the Charité to draw from for comparative studies in amyloid disease in man, his conclusions may be accepted as absolutely final.

Dr. Davidsohn has been able to experimentally induce amyloid disease only with injections of staphylococci and their products. Streptococci, though carefully experimented with, did not lead to amyloid degeneration, neither did carefully graduated doses of more virulent bacteria, nor the injection of putrefactive material. The work of others with tubercle bacilli he considers amply sufficient to prove that they alone never produce amyloid degeneration, which somehow seems to be the specific effect of the staphylococcus.

Dr. F. Bruck, in the last number of the *Allgemeine Medicinische Central-Zeitung*, reports a case of gonorrheal infection in which all the circumstances seem to point to an incubation-period of thirty days. The case was carefully studied, and there seems no reason to doubt the facts or the conclusions drawn from them. Such cases are not so rare as they used to be, and generally are not received with the air of incredulity which was formerly customary. Lesser, here in Berlin, and Finger in Vienna, consider that the possibility of a gonorrheal infection running a very subacute course so that no symptoms are to be noted and yet later lighting up into an acute process cannot be entirely excluded. It is the same principle as that involved in the question of chronic gonorrhea, which may continue years with practically no symptoms. Acute exacerbations, which were once regarded as reinfections, are now considered to be cases of self-infection from an old persistent focus. There are some interesting possibilities in the medico-legal aspects of these cases of gonococcus infection with very long incubation periods, which seem to make the subject worthy of more than passing attention.

TRANSACTIONS OF FOREIGN SOCIETIES

Vienna.

EFFECT OF DIET IN DISEASES OF THE LIVER—EXPANSION OF THE STOMACH WITH AIR—PERONIN AS A SUBSTITUTE FOR MORPHIN—THE IMPORTANCE OF SKIAGRAPHY IN THE DIAGNOSIS OF CALCULI—PHYSIOLOGY OF THE URINARY BLADDER—UNRELIABILITY OF THE HEMOGLOBINOMETER.

AT the session of the Medical Club of November 3d, KOLISCH read a paper upon the *prognosis and treatment of diseases of the liver*, in which he showed as a result of reasoning as well as from experiments upon animals, it is indisputable that in all cases of severe liver disease life may be greatly prolonged by the restriction of the amount of albumin in the food. If too much of this substance is taken at once, NH_3 remains in the blood, and poisons the individual. To facilitate the removal of toxic products, diuretics should be given, calomel being the best of all. Drugs which produce increased metamorphosis of albumens, such as salicylic acid, are distinctly contraindicated. Preparations of bile or its salts are the best cholagogues.

At the session of November 10th, HERZ described a case of *hysteric expansion of the stomach with air*. The patient was a male aged nineteen years, who, after a period of overwork, suffered so greatly from difficulty in breathing and palpitation of the heart, that he was obliged to remain eight weeks in bed. Later the curious symptom developed that with each inspiration the stomach filled with air, emptying again on expiration. The chemic and motor conditions of the organ remained normal and there was no sign of pyloric stenosis.

OSER has observed several such cases, some of which seemed to be due to intestinal disturbances following the abuse of cathartics. In other cases, the swallowing of air apparently resulted from the alternate action of the constricting and dilating nerves of the stomach.

STAMPFL recommended the use of *peronin as a substitute for morphin*, especially in cases of laryngeal and pulmonary disease accompanied by an irritating cough. By the use of this remedy the cough is made less severe and painless, expectoration facilitated, and reflex vomiting ceases. This drug is also valuable in mild neuralgias. Patients do not quickly become accustomed to its use. As peronin frequently produces itching of the skin and increases diaphoresis, it must not be given to phthisical patients with night-sweats, and cannot be used as a laryngeal insufflation. It has no bad effect upon the heart, and does not constipate.

At the session of November 17th, BUXBAUM spoke of the *importance of radiography in the diagnosis of calculi*. Contrary to the opinion which has sometimes been expressed, he found that all varieties of urinary calculi including those composed of uric acid, cystin, or cholesterin, are impermeable to the X-rays. However, he has had so many failures in his attempts to demonstrate biliary and nephritic calculi in the living, that he is still in doubt as to the true value of this method of diagnosis.

At the session of the Imperial Royal Society of Physicians, November 12th, SCHLESINGER narrated two cases which have a bearing upon the *physiology of the urinary bladder*. A woman, aged sixty-one years, suffered some time with symptoms of paralysis of the sphincter and detrusor urinæ muscles and also with complete anesthesia of the perineum, vulva, and mucous membrane of the bladder, followed later by motor and sensory paralysis of the rectum. At autopsy, it was found that a carcinomatous nodule had almost completely destroyed the fourth sacral segment by means of the pressure it exerted. In another patient, a glioma which was found at autopsy to be situated in the third and fourth sacral segment of one side, produced motor disturbances of the bladder without any loss of sensibility. These cases show that the spinal nerves to these organs are bilateral, and, furthermore, that the controlling center for the rectum is not identical with that of the bladder, but it is situated somewhat lower down.

At the session of November 19th, JELLINEK showed by clinical evidence that there is, even in healthy individuals, *no constant relation between the color of the blood and its percentage of iron*. In pathologic conditions this is even more striking than in the normal. Thus, in anemias the color of the blood is changed much more than the percentage of iron is diminished, while in purpura hemorrhagica the reverse is true. This proves the hemoglobinometer to be an unreliable instrument.

SOCIETY PROCEEDINGS.

HARVARD MEDICAL SOCIETY OF NEW YORK.

Stated Meeting, Held November 27, 1897.

THE President, JOHN WINTERS BRANNAN, M.D., in the Chair.

DR. JOHN H. HUDDLESTON read the paper of the evening, entitled

VACCINE.

The paper consisted of a collection of interesting notes upon the following subjects: (1) Vaccination in Europe; (2) a good vaccine laboratory; (3) tetanus following vaccination; (4) generalized vaccinia, and (5) vaccinal immunity. The author described the various methods of preparation of vaccine virus employed in Europe, and stated that vaccination with calf-lymph is generally practised on the Continent, while it is rarely used in England, where human virus is preferred. Vaccine laboratories in Germany are under Government control. The percentage of successful vaccination in Berlin is 96.84; in Hamburg, 94.85. The best laboratory, in buildings and equipments, is that of Cologne, which the author described at length. A case of tetanus following vaccination was referred to, also forty-five cases of generalized vaccinia in patients varying in age from three days to sixty-two years. Twelve of these were vaccinated with bovine virus, either direct from the animal or preserved; 18 with humanized virus; 1 with cow-pox, and 1 with horse-pox by accidental inoculation. The source of the virus in the other cases was not stated. Nine out of the 45 cases were not vaccinated in the usual way; 8 were inoculated with virus from the vaccine vesicle of another person, and the ninth ate vaccine crusts given accidentally with the food. Seven of the cases terminated fatally as a result of some complication. In regard to vaccinal immunity, the author said that little or no immunity is given the fetus by vaccination of the mother, as shown by Wolf and Gast, who vaccinated respectively sixteen and seventeen women in various stages of pregnancy and subsequently vaccinated the children with complete success. Natural immunity is so rare that those who have seen the largest number of vaccinations are least inclined to admit the possibility of its existence. Immunity is acquired slowly through the medium of vaccination. Repeated experiments have been made by vaccinating a person daily until the vaccinations failed to take, and it has been found that immunity is usually secured within from seven to ten days. The duration of the immunity when obtained is extremely variable; in some cases it apparently lasts a lifetime. Allbutt has reported the case of a woman who was successfully vaccinated three times, and who had smallpox three times. At North Brother's Island, New York, where patients are vaccinated on arrival, it has happened that persons repeatedly sent there have, on each occasion, been successfully vaccinated, revaccination having followed within six months of the first inoculation. Buchanan has reported a series of cases occurring in prisoners in which successful revaccination followed the first inoculation within a very short time—in 4 cases within less than a month; in 9 within two months or less; in 3 within three months or less, and in 12 within six months or less.

DISCUSSION.

DR. FRANK H. DANIELS: I have at present a child under observation whom I have unsuccessfully vaccinated three times. The mother tells me that she has never been vaccinated with success, although several attempts have been made. I used fresh vaccine, and I am going to try again, but it has occurred to me that this may be a case in which there is an inherited immunity.

THE PRESIDENT: I remember seeing a case some years ago at North Brother's Island in which a man was vaccinated and the pustule formed; in spite of this smallpox was contracted, and the two processes went on at the same time. The patient had a most malignant form of the disease, and died of it while the vaccinia was still going on. It would be interesting to know whether many such cases have been reported.

At a recent meeting of this society I spoke of a fluid vaccine which I employed in vaccinating six adults; it was successful in every case, but in all there was a good deal of trouble while the process continued, several patients developing abscesses in spite of the fact that I took antiseptic precautions before using the vaccine. I am not now so enthusiastic about fluid vaccine as I was at that time, and would like to ask if the unpleasant effects in these cases were due to the preparation employed.

DR. HUDDLESTON: The President's question immediately brings to mind what is known concerning "germ-free" lymph. It is at present impossible to collect vaccine virus without germs. But two different, and partially successful, methods of sterilizing virus have been discovered; one consists of the centrifugalization of virus which has been diluted with water, and the second, of mixing the virus with varying proportions of glycerin. The former method reduces the number of bacteria present, but does not entirely remove them; the latter is much more effective, and by means of it the number of germs in lymph, as tested by making cultures on agar, can always be materially reduced within a period which varies from a few days to a few weeks. Sometimes this does not secure sterility, but when old glycerinated virus is not sterile the inference simply is that the germs present are such as resist the action of glycerin; the bacillus subtilis, for instance, which is non-pathogenic, is unaffected by glycerin. It may then be fairly stated that lymph practically, although not absolutely "germ-free," can be secured with considerable certainty. The results from the use of this so-called "germ-free" lymph, whether absolutely sterile or nearly sterile, have not, however, secured freedom from the inflammatory complications of vaccine. On the contrary, it is the general testimony given by those who have experimented at length with such lymph that inflammatory reactions occur in about the same proportion of cases as before this lymph was introduced, and also that not merely inflammatory complications are present, but occasionally vaccinal eruptions as well. At Hamburg vaccination of 1700 primaries with "germ-free" lymph gave eight cases of skin eruptions. The Imperial Berlin Commission recently reported that in its judgment inflammatory appearances are due, first to the condition of the person vaccinated, second to the greater or less amount of effective lymph in the material applied, and, third, to the technic employed in the inoculation. The commission stated that inflammatory complications are especially frequent if the incisions made in the inoculations are numerous, long, deep, and close together. It is a familar fact that inflammation is more frequent in secondary than in primary vaccination. It is also unfortunately the case that a number of German reports state that quite thorough disinfection of the arm by means of sublimate solution and ether before vaccination does not prevent all inflammatory complications, but in some cases has actually seemed to increase them. Nevertheless, it has been a great advantage to vaccine production that practically germ-free lymph may be obtained; because the germs present, while, as a rule, non-poisonous, are, it is thought, injurious to the vaccine organism, and it is a fact, that by employing "germ-free" lymph, the so-called "purulence" in the producing animals, one of the former bugbears of the vaccine laboratory, has practically disappeared.

Finally, it should be added that while every brand of vaccine has its own bacterial flora, the few germs which are common to almost all are very clearly non-pathogenic to men or animals. Repeated inoculations of germ-bearing lymph have been made in guinea-pigs, rabbits, and other test animals, and almost invariably without any pathogenic results.

DR. REYNOLD W. WILCOX then read a brief paper, entitled

BOERHAAVE ON THE CANINE MADNESS.

Before reading his paper, Dr. Wilcox said he wished to correct some inaccuracies which appeared in the report of the last meeting as published in a recent number of THE MEDICAL NEWS. In speaking of Pasteur Institutes, he did not refer especially to any one. Nor did he mean to convey the idea that all patients died who received antirabitic treatment at such institutions. What he said was, that those patients who did die after receiving the treatment, died at about the same length of time after the inoculations. Again, in speaking of the symptoms described by Dr. Cabot as occurring in animals inoculated with rabies as similar to those which took place in guinea-pigs which he had inoculated with cod-liver oil for experimental purposes, he referred to the so-called alkaloids of cod-liver oil.

The author first spoke of the variations in the period of incubation of hydrophobia in the human being, as given in the old books, in which it is variously stated as being from twenty-four hours to as long a period as forty years, and repeated his statement made at the last meeting that there is no known infectious disease with such an indefinite incubation period as the one under consideration. He then read extracts from Van Swieten's Commentaries on Boerhaave "On the Canine Madness," published in 1776. He further said that, in carefully looking over the literature of the subject, he had been surprised to find that since 1776 all authors, in writing of hydrophobia, have copied Van Swieten's description of the disease, and that even the most modern writers have copied from each other the self-same description. In a work published as late as 1875 the maximum length of the incubation period is given as three years. To show that inoculation against rabies, with attenuated virus as an immunizing agent, is not an entirely new idea, he read a passage from Van Swieten's book, in which it is recommended that "the burnt liver of a mad dog" be eaten by the person bitten in order to ward off hydrophobia.

DISCUSSION.

DR. WILCOX: I have studied the *post-mortem* findings in persons alleged to have died of hydrophobia, and have learned that it is distinctly stated in the later books that the blood-vessels of the pons and cortex are enlarged and congested, that the perivascular spaces are infiltrated with round cells, and that small hemorrhages are also found; whereas, in the old books special mention is made of "dry brain" being present in such cases. I have been trying to recall some of the patients I have seen who were supposed to have suffered from hydrophobia, and I think I have seen twelve, of whom three died. Of those who survived there can be no reasonable doubt but that four were hysterics; one had tic convulsif, and another tetanus; the remainder suffered from fear of hydrophobia. In the three who died the usual *post-mortem* signs of septicemia were found. I repeat that I do not believe there is a definite disease hydrophobia, although I am willing to be convinced of its existence. I do not want to convey the impression that I do not appreciate the work which is being done by Dr. Cabot and others; but as long as no lesion can be demonstrated after death, and not one of the dicta for the determination of an infectious disease, as Koch has set forth, is found, I cannot believe in the existence of hydrophobia.

DR. FOLLEN CABOT: In regard to Wilcox's last remarks I want to say that such criticism is rather stimulating than depressing, for it makes me all the more determined to prove what I believe to be the truth. I am convinced of the existence of a disease which produces certain definite symptoms by inoculations from one animal to another. For instance, the virus which is used in the laboratory of the Board of Health has probably been inoculated into 2000 rabbits here and in Baltimore, and was used many years in Paris. The virus is now a "fixed virus," that is, it produces the same symptoms with death following on about the same day in each consecutive inoculated animal. The rabbit is subdurally inoculated with an emulsion made from the medulla of a rabbit dead from rabies. The animal is apparently perfectly well during six days following the inoculation, then a beginning tremor is noticed, most marked in the hind legs, and combined with weakness; on the seventh day the animal is markedly paralyzed; may be excited, and froth at the mouth; on the eighth day complete paralysis supervenes, and the animal dies any time from the tenth to twelfth day. These animals do not attempt to bite, but open and close the jaws, and have an increased flow of saliva from the mouth. Toward the last the bladder is paralyzed. Guinea-pigs have the furious form of the disease after an incubation period of from five to six days; they then become excited; run around furiously, biting at everything, showing some paralysis of the throat, and an abundant flow of saliva. Paralysis soon begins in the hind legs, and death occurs on about the seventh day.

I have here to-night a guinea-pig and a rabbit which have been inoculated with virus from an animal dead with rabies. The rabbit was inoculated eight days ago and is nearly wholly paralyzed which has been made more marked by transportation and exposure. The guinea-pig is just at the beginning of the stage of excitement of rabies. The animals are not what I intended to show as typical, but I wish any gentleman here, particularly Dr. Wilcox, would come to the laboratory and see many of the animals in the condition I have described. All cultures made from the emulsion, prepared by mixing a small piece of medulla from a rabid animal and a little water, are sterile to all tests in different media, if not so the animal inoculated will die in different media, if not so the animal inoculated will die of septicemia, always traceable to some impurity which has entered the material during the autopsy or in the process of emulsifying.

DR. SCHRAM reported a case of

CONJUGAL DIABETES.

The patient, a woman, first came under observation seven years ago, at which time she was sixty-nine years of age, and had been married forty-eight years. Sugar was constantly found in the urine in amounts varying from less than one to four per cent. She refused to submit to rigorous diet and died in July, 1897, in diabetic coma. Thirst and pruritus had been the most troublesome symptoms. An extensive ischiorectal abscess developed two weeks before death. One week later the husband's urine was found to contain three per cent. of sugar. Symptoms of the disease sufficient to attract his attention antedated his wife's death by about two weeks. Sugar is now found in his urine in abundance, but disappears for a time under diet and opium. He is now seventy-six years of age and apparently contracted the disease seven years after it was first discovered in the wife and after nearly fifty-three years of married life. The couple had eleven children, seven of whom are alive and well.

In a series of 5000 cases Boisumeau found 1.8 per cent. of conjugal diabetes. Most investigators agree that the development of the disease in both husband and wife is not accidental, but that an etiologic relation exists. The facts thus far published do not shed much light on the two theories of causation now held, *viz.;* (1) that the ordinarily accepted causes of diabetes are active in both husband and wife, and (2) that the disease is contagious. Cases have been reported with almost conclusive evidence of contagion, but the nature of the contagium and how it is conveyed are mysteries.

DISCUSSION.

DR. DANIELS: I should doubt whether it is a question of contagion or infection in such a case as the one reported. The disease could have existed undiscovered a long time. These people had lived together fifty years, and were exposed to identical conditions; therefore, whatever conditions favorable to the prodution of the disease were present in the case of the wife might also have been present in that of the husband. I would rather attribute it to this fact than to contagion or infection, especially as it did not appear in the man until seven years after its onset in the woman.

DR. SCHRAM: In regard to the doubt which has been expressed as to contagion in diabetes, I would ilke to mention some recently reported cases in which laundresses apparently contracted the disease by washing the clothing of diabetics. However, the question is still an open one. The authorities differ very much, but the French school is inclined to believe that diabetes is contagious.

DR. DANIELS: Some time ago I reported the case of a man, forty years of age, in whose urine sugar was found. He soon contracted syphilis during the early stage of which the sugar disappeared to reappear later on.

DR. J. P. MCGOWAN: I have a patient, a man thirty-nine years old, who has been under observation four years, and who during years has had more or less sugar in his urine, the amount depending upon his habits, which are not always what they should be. About two years ago he contracted syphilis, and a strict diet and the usual treatment were administered. Sugar entirely disappeared from his urine two months after the occurrence of the secondary symptoms. He was under observation the ten months subsequent to the manifestations of syphilis, during which time frequent examination of the urine failed to reveal any sugar; this fact, I think, was due more to the regulation of his habits than to any special effect of the syphilitic poison.

DR. ROBERT H. GREENE: It is a well-known fact, I think, that sugar often disappears from the urine in diabetics who have been attacked by syphilis, although, so far as I know, no explanation has been given as to why this is so. There are some writers who claim that diabetes proper is always the result of syphilis.

NEW YORK NEUROLOGICAL SOCIETY.

Stated Meeting, Held November 2, 1897.

THE President, DR. C. A. HERTER, in the Chair.

DR. GEORGE W. JACOBY exhibited a patient with a typical case of Thompson's disease. He is a young man who had been referred to him by Dr. Schwinn of West Virginia, with a correct diagnosis. The patient is twenty-eight years of age, and has lived in this country since 1884. There is nothing in the family history especially bearing upon the condition, except that a distant cousin is said to have walked stiffly and in a peculiar manner for fifteen years. The patient himself has always been delicate, but has been as active as other boys. He had typhoid fever in 1889, and on recovering from this first noticed a cramp in the legs. After a little it was found that he could not execute movements as quickly as before. In 1893, he first sought treatment. During the past year or two his arms and hands have also been affected. The condition varies considerably at different times, but is apparently not influenced by meteorologic conditions. The examination showed quick reaction of the eye muscles, with spasm of the external rectus; cramp of the masseter muscles on bringing the jaws together forcibly; no involvement of the pterygoids. All the muscles of the upper extremity and of the thorax are involved—indeed, nearly all the muscles of the body. The contraction of the muscles is decidedly tetanic, and at first was very marked, but, on repeated tests, it gradually subsided. The electric examination showed marked myotonic reaction, and also a wave-like appearance, but Dr. Jacoby could not make up his mind that this latter phenomenon consisted of a series of waves, such as are observed in water. A piece of muscle had been excised from the biceps, and also from the quadriceps, but they had not yet been minutely examined. The case is quite characteristic on account of the marked variations occurring from time to time. The speaker said that in an article published by him ten or more years ago he had taken the stand that these cases are probably of myopathic origin, due to some congenital defect in development, but in the light of modern investigation he is now disposed to believe that some central cause is operative—that there is a functional hereditary derangement of the central nervous system—a condition of lessened resistance in the cells. This does not seem to him a strange assumption, when one considers the well-known idiosyncrasies exhibited to various toxic influences. On the theory that some kind of toxemia is the foundation of this disease, he thought the observed phenomena could be explained—at least in this direction seemed to lie the possibility of solving the pathogenesis of this variety of disease. This patient had not been affected by the trouble until he was eighteen years of age; hence, there is no propriety in calling such a case "myotonia congenita." He divides these cases into three classes as follows: (1) myotonia congenita; (2) myotonia acquisita; and (3) myotonia transitoria.

DR. FREDERICK PETERSON asked, why a theory of causation might not be founded upon chemic changes in the muscles? Changes in the structure of the muscles, he said, are known to arise—for instance, in connection with typhoid fever.

DR. HERTER thought that we must look to toxic agents as furnishing at least a clue to the causation of such conditions. The peculiar susceptibility to certain types of poisons, seen, for instance, in epilepsy, must be referred to peculiarities of the central nervous system. He would agree with Dr. Peterson that these cases do not seem to be of central origin, and that it is more probable that they arise from chemic changes in the muscles. To study this subject successfully, it would be necessary to inquire into the condition of the secretions and excretions at the time of the onset of the disease, and not after it had become chronic.

PACHYMENINGITIS HEMORRHAGIA INTERNA IN CHILDREN

was the title of a paper by DR. C. A. HERTER, in which he said that internal hemorrhagic pachymeningitis is usually considered to be a very rare condition in children, yet one German observer has found it in about seventeen per cent. of his autopsies. The following cases were reported:

CASE I.—A female child, five and one-half months of age, was admitted to the Babies' Hospital, May 15, 1897, with an entirely negative family history. The illness had begun one month previously with persistent vomiting. The head was of normal shape, and the fontanels were not bulging. There was a soft spot over one parietal bone. The child had no teeth. On the fifth day after admission tremor and nystagmus developed. Four days later there was a general convulsion, in which the mouth deviated to the left. Cyanosis was a feature of the convulsion. A second attack occurred within ten hours. After these seizures the fontanels were sunken. The child now became semi-comatose, and died after a few days. The autopsy showed the presence of hemorrhagic pachymeningitis, fibrinopurulent pleurisy, pulmonary congestion, fatty liver, and nephritis. Along the superior longitudinal fissure, over the entire base and over the island of Reil on both sides was a membrane covering the pia. The ventricles were normal in size, and contained about one dram of hemorrhagic fluid. There was fluid blood in all the sinuses. The cervical cord showed the same conditions. Under the microscope the right occipital region showed the pia attached to the cortex in many places, and there was a splitting up of the membrane overlying the cortex into two or more layers. The inner layer was infiltrated with small round-cells. The outer membranous layers consisted of the same cells, fibroblasts, and connective-tissue fibers. The island of Reil showed the same condition, but much more marked, as was also the case over the cerebellum. In the spinal cord there were only slight traces of hemorrhage.

CASE II.—Female infant, colored, twenty-two months old. The child had been nursed seven months. It had never walked or stood alone, and was very rachitic. The first two months in the hospital were marked by slight loss in weight and considerable prostration. In October, 1897, the child was readmitted, with the statement that she had been well up to three days before, at which time she had had four convulsions followed by three more the next day. The general condition was very bad. The hands and feet were in a position of persistent flexor contraction, characteristic of tetany. The knee-jerks were unobtainable; the fontanels were bulging. There was slight, but varying rigidity of the muscles at the back of the neck. Bloody mucus diarrhea was present, and the child died comatose. The autopsy showed pachymeningitis hemorrhagica interna, bronchopneumonia, and acute and chronic ulcerative colitis. Over the right side of the brain was a recent blood-clot covering the entire hemisphere, and also the left occipital lobe. The inner surface of the dura was covered with a membrane extending from the superior longitudinal fissure on either side. The pia was congested. The ventricles and brain substance were apparently normal. All the sinuses were filled with recent clots. The microscopic examination showed thickening of the pia over the right temporosphenoidal lobe, and the vessels of the pia were thickened. There was also a thick membrane splitting up into layers, as in the other case. There were numerous small blood-vessels, and hemorrhages had occurred into the meshes of the membrane. In places, there were aggregations of small round-cells undergoing fragmentation. They were chiefly found in the superficial layers of the membrane. In the dura the fibers were separated from each other by serous infiltration, and the dura was covered with a membrane similar to that already described. In places, there was very extensive pachymeningitis.

It is at about the age of five months, the speaker said, that this disease is especially frequent. The majority of these infants are badly nourished, many of them being subjects of rachitis or of chronic colitis. The new membrane must be regarded as originating from proliferation of the dural endothelial cells. In some cases there is little inclination to hemorrhage. The membrane is very variable in thickness; sometimes it reaches a thickness of two or three lines. There seems no good reason for thinking that the locality of the pigmentation indicates that the layer of blood originates from the inner surface of the dura. On the other hand, there is no conclusive proof of the old notion that the disease is of inflammatory origin. It is so common to find severe intoxications without such lesions that the intoxication theory does not seem tenable. It is apparently impossible to recognize the condition until the hemorrhage has occurred, and even then it is extremely difficult to make a positive diagnosis. Slight cerebral symptoms are probably masked in these very young and usually marantic children. The hemorrhage is probably more often unilateral, and the usual symptoms present are rigidity, hemorrhage, and coma. Paralysis is rarely noted. The pyrexia is usually less than in meningitis, but these cases are so commonly complicated with other diseases that the range of temperature is variable. The speaker did not think there is any symptom or combination of symptoms in hemorrhagic internal pachymeningitis which might not be encountered in any acute infection without any cerebral affection being present; but whenever unilateral rigidity and convulsions with deepening stupor are present in a cachectic or rachitic child under one year of age, we should think of such a diagnosis. It is probable that relatively slight traumatisms to the head may occasion rupture of the vessels in the highly vascular membrane. This gives these cases a certain medico-legal importance.

DR. PETERSON remarked that the condition is interesting to him because of the possibility of its being occasionally found in infantile cerebral palsy.

DR. HERTER said that he was inclined to think that these membranes are considerably more frequent than one would suppose from the literature. It is quite possible to overlook the presence of the membrane if it is not decidedly vascular.

A paper, entitled

THE PATHOLOGY AND MORBID ANATOMY OF HUNTINGTON'S CHOREA, WITH REMARKS ON THE DEVELOPMENT AND TREATMENT OF THE DISEASE,

was read by DR. JOSEPH COLLINS, who said that the neurologist frequently encounters knotty problems, and among these none had the secret of its genesis more carefully concealed than the hereditary degenerative diseases. The pathogenesis of the acute inflammatory diseases of the nervous system is an open book, but the degenerative diseases are discouragingly slow in yielding the mystery of their being. This is especially true of such degenerative affections as the hereditary ataxias, choreas, and dystrophies. The status of the original lesion cannot always be inferred from a consideration of the lesion found at the time of death, and this is particularly true if the disease has existed a great number of years. No one could do much laboratory work on the central nervous system of individuals who had succumbed to degenerative nervous diseases of long duration without having forced upon him the fact that there are certain abnormalities of the circulatory system—varying degrees of degeneration of vessels, changes in the size of the lymph spaces, and relative disproportion of connective tissue to the parenchyma —which occur in all degenerative diseases, considered entirely apart from their causation. He is convinced that such changes are very often secondary, and have no other significance than as evidences of protracted disturbance of nutrition, and that this nutritional depravity is the result of the existence of the original lesion. There is nothing more certain than the occurrence of glia proliferation in all slowly progressing, destructive lesions of the nervous system, but nothing can be more misleading than to consider this glia overgrowth to be primary, and the changes in the parenchyma secondary.

Huntington's chorea, Dr. Collins said, is a comparatively rare disease, and of rather recent recognition; hence, the reports made upon its pathology have not been uniform. The discrepancies are apparently the result of the varying points of view of different observers. In studying the nervous system in cases of Huntington's chorea it is scarcely justifiable to maintain that all the morbid conditions are inherent to the disease; for, as had been said, many of them might be the consequence of prolonged interference with nutrition. Although the present study of the pathology of the disease is upon an individual who has had the disease a considerable time, it is compared with a case of much shorter duration reported by Dr. C. L. Dana. A study of these two cases, he felt confident, would go far toward establishing the morbid anatomy and hinting at the pathogenesis. His patient was a man, fifty-five years of age, who had married in early manhood, and who was the father of three children—all of them giving evidence of neuropathic inheritance. The known duration of the disease in his case was ten years. In the beginning the hands only were affected, but in the last years the lower extremities were also involved. The mind remained in fairly good condition up to about three years before his death, when he began to have suspicions about his relatives and friends, and became forgetful and suicidal. His speech was so imperfect that during the last years of life he was understood with difficulty. Dr. Collins had seen him for the first time a few days before his death. He then had a temperature of 105° F., and it remained at about this point until the end. The movements were very severe and incessant, except during sound sleep, although even then they frequently wakened him. He was was quite conscious, but made no response to questions. The cause of death seemed to be exhaustion and high temperature. The disease was traceable to the maternal grandfather, an Irishman, who had three children, two of whom were similarly affected. One of these was the mother of this patient, and of her seven children, five were so afflicted. The other daughter had two children, one of whom became choreic. In three generations there had been no less than nine affected individuals, and when it was considered that many of these children died in infancy, the number of cases that had developed was surprisingly great.

At the autopsy, on opening the skull, the dura was quite adherent, the diploe dense, and the Pacchionian depressions marked. The brain had a wet appearance, as did also the cord. The pia was not adherent to the brain. The convolutions of the anterior pole of the brain were very small, and the entire encephalon weighed forty-two and one-half ounces. The dura was intimately adherent to the spinal column. The principal fissures were somewhat wider, more shallow, and shorter than in the normal brain, but there was nothing pointing to defective convolutions. The average thickness of the gray matter was uniformly less than the normal, but this thinness could not be attributed to age. An examination of the pons and medulla oblongata did not show any marked variation from the normal, but the changes were more noticeable lower down. Microscopic changes were not confined exclusively to the Rolandic region, but the process here was more advanced. The specimens were stained by various methods, and carefully examined. The macroscopic changes were briefly as follows: (1) thinness and atrophy of the cortex; (2) the mottled, streaked appearance and cribriform state on cross-section of the brain, due to diminution in number and in health of the ganglion cells, and to the increased perivascular and pericellular spaces and increased patency of the blood-vessels. The microscopic changes were: (1) a decay or slowly progressive degeneration of the ganglion cells of the cortex throughout the brain, especially of the two deepest layers, the layers of large pyramids and polymorphous cells. This cell death was particularly evident in the Rolandic region, very much less so in the anterior pole of the brain, and incomparably less in the posterior pole; (2) increase of glia tissue, but not sufficiently prominent to constitute sclerosis, the conspicuous increase being about the blood-vessels and ganglion cells; (3) enlargement and distention of the pericellular spaces; (4) slightly diseased blood-vessels, consisting principally of a proliferation of the nuclei of the adventitia and a thickening of the intima. This involvement of the vessels was not regular or symmetric, but showed itself only in certain sections of vessels; (5) relative paucity of the medullated fibers of the cortex. In short, it might be said, that the lesion was a chronic parenchymatous degeneration of the cortex, with consecutive and secondary changes in the interstices, the brunt of the disease having been borne by the motor regions. There was, in consequence, a degeneration of the pyramidal tracts in the spinal cord. In Dr. Dana's case the central convolutions suffered most, and the process occurred in patches throughout the affected cortex. There was nothing to justify the opinion, that it was an inflammation—the process was evidently one of degeneration.

In connection with the treatment, Dr. Collins said, that he desired to emphasize the necessity for delaying the advent of the disease in those who had a hereditary tendency to it, and also to emphasize the folly of tenotomy of the eye muscles—a method of treatment now being carried out upon one of these unfortunate individuals in this city, with a promise of a cure. If we wished to influence the course of hereditary chorea after it had once become manifest, it would be necessary to administer whatever drug was selected in the largest possible doses consistent with life, and to maintain this medication for a long time.

DR. ONUF said that he had been present at the autopsy on the case reported in the paper, and had been especially impressed with the general narrowing of the gyri—a general atrophy. On section, the mottled condition of the cortex had been most striking, but the cribriform appearance produced by the enlargement of the perivascular spaces was also worthy of note. The general appearance of the brain resembled very closely that of general paresis. The microscope confirmed the macroscopic findings, although the changes were not as marked as one would have expected from the gross appearance. The cell changes were of the atrophic order. The characteristic feature was the accumulation of neuroglia cells in the pericellular and perivascular spaces. His impression was, that this accumulation is due to a secondary process following atrophy of the cells. The disease is evidently a degenerative one, originating in the parenchyma of the brain, and not in the interstitial tissue.

THERAPEUTIC HINTS.

The Tonic Effects of Zincohemol.—This remedy is said to be very efficient in increasing the quantity of hemoglobin in the blood, and maintaining the percentage attained. It is recommended by CERVELLO and SAVOCA in the following combinations:

For anemia and chlorosis:

℞ Zincohemol
Ext. gentianæ } aa . . . gr. lxxx.

M. Ft. pil. No. LXXX. Sig. Two to four pills three times daily.

For chronic diarrhea:

℞ Zincohemol
Ext. hæmotox. } aa . . . ʒ iss
Glycerini
Aq. dest. } aa . . . . q. s.

M. Ft. pil. No. LXXX. Sig. Two to four pills four times daily.

As a sedative nervine in chorea and hysteria:

℞ Zincohemol
Ext. valerianæ } aa . . . . gr. lxxx.

M. Ft. pil. No. LXXX. Sig. Two or three pills three times daily.

Suppositories for Bleeding Hemorrhoids.—

℞ Ferri subsulph. . . . . . gr. iii
Plumbi acetat. . . . . . gr. i
Mass. hydrarg. . . . . . gr. ss
Ol. theobrom. . . . . . q. s.

M. Ft. suppos. No. 1. Sig. Insert one suppository morning and evening.

For Catarrhal Jaundice.—

℞ Ammon. iodi. . . . . . ʒ i
Liq. potass. arsenit. . . . ʒ ss
Tinct. calumbæ . . . . ℥ ss
Aq. dest. . . . . . . ℥ iss.

M. Sig. One teaspoonful three times daily before meals.

THE MEDICAL NEWS.

A WEEKLY JOURNAL OF MEDICAL SCIENCE.

VOL. LXXII. NEW YORK, SATURDAY, JANUARY 8, 1898. NO. 2.

ORIGINAL ARTICLES.

SOME OF THE VAGARIES OF CROUPOUS PNEUMONIA.[1]

BY HENRY L. ELSNER, M.D.,
OF SYRACUSE, N. Y.;
PROFESSOR OF THE SCIENCE AND ART OF MEDICINE AND CLINICAL MEDICINE IN THE SYRACUSE MEDICAL COLLEGE.

THE deductions presented in this paper are the result of a careful consideration of 150 cases of pneumonia observed in private, consultation, and hospital practice. It occurred to the writer as he examined the records of these cases that it might be of interest to the profession to learn something of the peculiarities of croupous pneumonia as seen in Central New York.

I was surprised to find many cases in which, at some time during the course of the disease, unusual features presented, frequently making a positive diagnosis impossible, and at other times obscuring the diagnosis of pneumonia which had already been made.

The pneumonia of Central New York may be considered the most typical disease of an infectious nature which the physician is called upon to treat. In eighty per cent. of our cases the characteristic chill and fever and all of the other usual symptoms followed each other in regular order, the disease running a typical course within from six to eleven days. In twenty per cent. of our cases, however, there were vagaries which occasionally masked the diagnosis. In these, careful and acute diagnosticians were puzzled during the period which preceded the appearance of characteristic objective and subjective signs.

The 150 cases may be tabulated as follows:

TABLE I.

Age.	Number of Cases.
Between 1 and 5 years	2
" 6 " 10 "	2
" 11 " 15 "	3
" 16 " 20 "	31
" 21 " 25 "	29
" 26 " 30 "	18
" 31 " 35 "	15
" 36 " 40 "	13
" 41 " 45 "	12
" 46 " 50 "	11
" 51 " 55 "	4
" 56 " 60 "	2
" 61 " 65 "	3
" 66 " 70 "	2
" 71 " 75 "	1
Over 75 "	2

[1] Read at the last meeting of the American Climatological Association.

The right lung was involved in sixty per cent. of the cases; the left lung in twenty-four per cent.; both lungs in sixteen per cent. The localization of the disease in the various parts of the lungs corresponded very closely with that given by Jurgensen, Grisolle, Busse, and other voluminous writers on this disease. There were twelve cases in which the apex was involved; in seven of these the right apex was diseased; in five, the left.

It may be remarked in connection with *apex-pneumonia* as we see it in Central New York, that, as a rule, it is not associated with active cerebral symptoms which would justify us in speaking of it as synonymous with cerebral pneumonia. Indeed, the majority of these cases presented less delirium than was true when other parts of the lung were involved, and most of them were marked by a typical course, terminating by crisis without further complication. Those forms of mixed infection in which active pneumonia attacks a tuberculous apex are not included; attention will be directed to them in another place. One of the apex cases was a traumatic pneumonia in a boy eleven years of age, who had sustained a fracture of the skull three days before the onset of the disease; his mind was at all times clear, and he made a full recovery.

In fourteen per cent. of the cases in adults the initial chill was absent. This was commonly observed in cases of pneumonia occurring in alcoholics or in aged and enfeebled subjects, and in most of the severer forms of the disease occurring in children. It is rare to find evidence of the occurrence of a chill in the subjects of croupous pneumonia previous to the tenth year of life. The disease is more frequent in early life than it was formerly supposed to be. In a number of our cases of secondary croupous pneumonia, particularly that associated with or following other infectious disease, the chill was absent, the first evidence of the disease being a marked increase of the already existing fever, with an increasing frequency of respiration. In such cases positive physical signs were absent for from one to three days; the symptoms of the primary infection were intensified, there being present a true typhoid condition and characteristic sputum, while the objective symptoms followed on the third or fourth day of the pulmonic affection.

In thirty per cent of the *influenza-pneumonias* of the croupous variety the disease developed gradually after a period of malaise accompanied by the usual symptoms of the primary affection. Seventy per cent. of the influenza-pneumonias were ushered in with a well-defined chill, severe but characteristic of the ordinary form of the disease. When this occurred we found that the pneumonia was of much shorter duration than in those cases in which the chill was absent; that it was associated with a more sthenic condition of the patient, and gave a decidedly better prognosis. In a few cases of this type we were surprised to find large areas of consolidated lung tissue, sometimes remnants of recent pneumonias, without marked subjective symptoms, but with positive physical signs, in which the condition had not been suspected. Many of these cases dragged along during a number of weeks with but little sputum, although, at times, there was marked rusty sputum during a day or two. During the later weeks, the sputum usually became mucopurulent, nummular, and finally disappeared as gradually as did the physical signs. Most of these patients made a full recovery. Microscopic examination of the sputum showed the presence of the pneumococci of Fränkel and Friedlander and frequently streptococci in abundance. It may be readily understood that these cases aroused a suspicion of existing tuberculosis. The microscope served to differentiate this latent form of pneumonia from the tuberculous infection which we have learned to fear as a complication or sequel of *grippe*.

No cases were more difficult to diagnose than were those of *central pneumonia without chill* occurring in children, occasionally in adults, with marked gastric symptoms, slight jaundice, abdominal distress and pain. In many of these there was but little cough during the first twenty-four hours, hurried respiration and a continuously high temperature being the only accompanying symptoms. The physician who has had much to do with croupous pneumonia occurring during early life, has learned from his experience to be suspicious of its presence when persistently rapid respiration and elevation of temperature are present, even though other marked pulmonary symptoms of a subjective or objective character are not manifested. Abdominal pain misled a number of physicians with whom I saw these cases, and when this was associated with slight jaundice, central pneumonia was not suspected. In the case of a child five years old, with the symptoms just mentioned, we found tympanitic resonance over the lower lobe of the left lung persisting for two days without other physical signs, save bronchophony over a small area. Gradually it became evident that a central pneumonia was spreading toward the surface; bronchial breathing with crepitant râles became clear, and the child died after a three-weeks' illness with every portion of both lungs consolidated.

The method of Leube, in which, in such cases, he searches at an early stage for an area of bronchophony, and in which after twenty-four or thirty-six hours he has found confirmatory signs of the disease, such as bronchial breathing and crepitant râles, has often proved an important aid, but it, too, has occasionally failed. It may be safely concluded that the cases of pneumonia characterized by absence of chill were, as a rule, of the asthenic variety; that they ran a protracted course, rarely terminating before the eleventh or thirteenth day, usually by lysis, and in a large number there was an alarming typhoid condition which developed during the fourth or sixth day and was evidenced by profound nervous symptoms, muttering delirium, considerable albuminuria, feeble and rapid pulse, death usually ending the scene with less evidence of carbonic-acid poisoning than was present in the equally serious sthenic cases of the disease.

Among the noteworthy pathologic features presented in this asthenic type of pneumonia may be mentioned an ultimate though diffuse infiltration of the lung. Several foci were usually found, and the inflammation was prone to attack both lungs. The stage of red hepatization was short, the lung tissue was soft, tore easily, and there was a great tendency to puriform infiltration. The spleen was enlarged. In a number of these cases pleurisy appeared at an early stage, usually serous, sometimes purulent, but it was not at all uncommon to observe the occurrence of empyema after serous pleurisy. Among the other complications, kidney involvement was common, and in a few cases endocarditis, pericarditis, or meningitis, were the final concomitants. There can be no doubt that these forms of asthenic pneumonia without chills are increasing, and that the greater mortality of pneumonia in many sections of this and other countries is very largely due to this fact.

Another variety of pneumonia to which I wish to call attention, and which is among the more difficult forms of the disease to diagnose, is the one presenting *the symptom complex of an acute meningitis*. In such instances there was not a single physical sign or subjective symptom to call attention to the lungs, but there was present a clear picture of meningitis, often without respiratory embarrassment. In these cases the deep involvement of the brain is due to pneumococcic toxins. In some of these we found *post-mortem* a limited area of lung tissue involved, usually central, without a single lesion or change in the brain to account for the symptoms during life. These cases are not uncommon.

Three instances of *afebrile pneumonia* were observed in patients aged respectively sixty-five, sixty-seven, and seventy-four years. The first example of this type occurred without any prodromata or initial chill, but all the characteristic physical signs of the disease were presented, the lower lobe of the right lung being involved; there was rusty sputum. This patient had suffered many years from interstitial nephritis accompanied by polyuria, a moderate amount of albuminuria, tense pulse, and arteriosclerosis. The disease terminated favorably by crisis on the sixth day, although the crisis was followed by an alarming condition of the patient, which continued, with profuse perspiration, almost twenty-four hours; the patient ultimately rallied, living six or seven years after his recovery and finally dying of uremia.

The subject of the second case was also an albuminuric, with less marked arteriosclerosis, but with evidences of secondary contracted kidney. The patient died on the fifth day of the disease. The diagnosis was confirmed by autopsy. One-half of the left lung was found to be completely consolidated, and there was positive evidence of the presence of the second stage of croupous pneumonia. The heart was hypertrophied in all directions, and the kidneys had undergone secondary contraction.

The third patient had been previously healthy, had no evidences of renal or cardiac disease, but had been subject to great nervous strain and was in a very much reduced mental and physical condition during the two or three weeks preceding the onset of the disease. The case terminated favorably by lysis.

All of these patients were well nursed, carefully watched by trained attendants, and the temperature taken four times daily. In none did the latter at any time go above 100.1° F.

There seems to be an antagonism between the pneumococcic toxins and blood which is surcharged with urea, or changed as the result of chronic nephritis. This fact has been observed by a number of writers, and we are at the present time carrying on experiments to determine whether this conclusion is justifiable. It may be still further asserted that in all of the cases of afebrile pneumonia which the writer has observed there has been great nervous depression. In several cases there was an afebrile period, varying from one to three days, during which there was progression of pneumonic infiltration without preceding chill. On the third or fourth day the temperature began to rise gradually, reaching its maximum about the sixth day, the disease ultimately becoming asthenic. Death followed in the majority of these cases between the tenth and fourteenth days, with rapid pulse, but without evidences of carbonic-acid poisoning. In these we did not find preceding albuminuria, but the patients were much reduced in strength and nerve force before the advent of the fatal affection.

Hyperpyrexia was frequently found in the sthenic forms of the disease. We observed it more frequently in hospital than in private practice. In fifteen hospital cases the temperature rose above 105° F. in five. In one of these the temperature reached 107.5° F., remaining there almost twenty-four hours before death occurred. In two in which recovery occurred, the temperature reached 106.2° F.; in private practice, in 135 cases, the temperature rose above 105.5° F. in only ten, seven of which occurred in children. With corresponding involvement of lung tissue, it may be assumed that the temperature in children ranges from one and one-half to two degrees higher than in adults.

Among the unique clinical manifestations observed was a condition to which the writer gave the name "*post-pyrexial* delirium" a number of years ago. Since reporting my first case with this characteristic I have noticed a number in medical literature, all presenting about the same features. Four such cases are included in the collection. In all the disease had been of sthenic variety. The febrile period averaged six days, during which the patients were unusually clear-headed. *Following the crisis* in from three to ten days, these patients became the subjects of active and wild delirium during which they were restrained with difficulty—a true "delirium-ferox," without the slightest increase of body heat. In three such cases the period of delirium continued between seven and twelve days, in the other, the patient was wildly delirious during two weeks, then merged into an irresponsible condition in which she was easily controlled, making a final recovery after the fifth week. The writer does not include in these cases of post-pyrexial delirium those forms of insanity and nerve depression which sometimes follow influenza, for in the majority of such cases there usually was more delirium during the active period of the disease than during the period of convalescence, and finally, the train of nervous symptoms which persisted weeks and months, at times leading to permanent insanity.

Among the vagaries of pneumonia, a peculiar behavior of the pulse in the subjects of *arteriosclerosis*, with or without manifest renal complication, has occasionally been noted. During a period varying from two to four days, the pulse remained tense and slow, rarely being above eighty per minute. After this period, the tension became suddenly lowered, the pulse rapid, irregular, and intermittent, and the patient died with all of the evidences of cardiac asthenia on the fifth or sixth day of the disease. Experience has taught that this period of calm and slow pulse in the subjects of arteriosclerosis, is something to be feared, for it almost invariably leads to a fatal termination, preceded by a sudden lowering of arterial tone and almost immediate cardiac failure.

Ambulatory pneumonia is rarely observed in Central New York. In the cases reported there was only one in which the diagnosis was made positive by *post-mortem* examination. This case occurred in a man forty-two years of age in whom the disease existed four days, during which time he was up and about. He died within twenty-four hours after his admission to the hospital. The *post-mortem* showed the right lung to be entirely solidified, well advanced in the second stage of the disease, and marked edema of the left lung; the right half of the heart dilated with a large thrombus extending into the pulmonary artery.

Among the cases of *malignant pneumonia* are three which occurred in one family within one week of each other. All resulted fatally before the sixth day of the disease. The toxemia seemed over-powering, the local disturbances being subsidiary.

Traumatic pneumonias are comparatively frequent, particularly after serious head injuries, and it has been the writer's experience to find the larger number during early life. In children this type is almost always fatal.

Aspiration, or the "*Schlück pneumonia*" of the Germans, was observed three times. Two cases resulted in recovery. The disease was protracted, and complications, particularly edema of the lungs, were not unusual. The only case of pneumonia which followed the inhalation of ether was that of a woman whose breast had been amputated for cancer. The disease was of sthenic variety; there was a chill within twenty-four hours after the operation; the disease was severe, but ended favorably by crisis without interfering with the primary union of the wound.

An annoying complication of *senile pneumonia* was the blocking of the bronchial tubes with retained mucus, with ultimate collapse of air-cells, all of which masked the physical signs of pulmonary infiltration.

In spite of the fact that several cases were seen in which there was a characteristic intermittent fever, with at the same time advancing lung involvement, there were no data, microscopic or clinical, which justified the assumption that there was present an added malarial infection. The administration of quinin in these cases failed to influence the fever in any way.

In three cases there was sudden and unexpected death; once during the period of convalescence; twice after crisis, when a favorable prognosis had been given. These deaths were in all probability due to the effects of the specific toxins upon the heart, and the accompanying acute myocardial degeneration. I do not include those cases in which there had been preceding nephritis, or organic heart disease. In this connection it may be added that the toxemia is by far the most important element to be taken into account in considering the treatment and prognosis of pneumonia, and it is certain that in the majority of cases it stands in no relation to the extent of lung tissue involved. Limited areas of disease have often been associated with more profound evidences of infection than was the case with far-reaching consolidation.

Eighty-five and one-half per cent. of the cases terminated by crisis, and 14.5 per cent. by lysis; the crisis occurred in the majority between the fifth and eighth day of the disease; in one it occurred on the thirteenth. The longest-deferred crisis was noted on the fifteenth day. It was not uncommon to have the fever continue with but slight change until the eighth or tenth day, when crisis occurred. The old notion of the ominous uneven days is not justified. Persistence of fever after the eighth day without positive evidence of fresh involvement of lung tissue or other discoverable complications must lead to the suspicion of tuberculous disease. A sharp rise of temperature during the twenty-four hours preceding the crisis was not uncommon. A decided rise of temperature following crisis, sometimes three or four exacerbations, alarmed many physicians who were not warned of the possibility of such an occurrence. In twenty-four cases there were pseudo-crises. These occurred, as a rule, between the fourth and sixth days; the earliest was observed on the third, the latest on the twelfth day. After the crisis, and during the period of convalescence, it was not uncommon to observe one or two sharp rises of temperature without accompanying leucocytosis, or other demonstrable complication.

The majority of cases of croupus pneumonia showed a *marked increase of the polynuclear leucocytes* during the febrile period, with a reduction as the temperature declined. In thirty cases in which we made blood counts there were evidences of leucocytosis in twenty-two. The greatest number of white corpuscles were found immediately before the crisis. In all cases examined within thirty-six hours after crisis there was no further evidence of leucocytosis. As a rule, there was no reduction during pseudo-crisis; in two cases an increase of leucocytes was observed. The occurrence and intensity of leucocytosis may be said to depend almost entirely upon the virulence of the pathogenic micro-organism causing the disease. This clinical fact is emphasized by the result of animal experimentation. It was impossible to demonstrate satisfactorily any relation between the extent of the disease and the existing leucocytosis. The malignant forms of pneumonia with far-reaching and rapid infiltration, also asthenic cases with or without extensive consolidation, particularly in those subjects who were poorly nourished, gave low average blood-counts. For differential purposes it may be concluded that the presence of leucocytosis in acute febrile disease favors the diagnosis of pneumonia; that its absence favors the diagnosis of typhoid fever or of a severe form of lung inflammation; that marked leucocytosis favors the diagnosis of croupous pneumonia against purulent pleurisy; that the presence of leucocytosis is a favorable, but by no means certain, prognostic sign.

From the cases here considered I conclude that the *fully developed physical signs* which justify a *positive diagnosis of pneumonia are rarely present before the end of the second day of the disease*, and it is not infrequent to see the third day pass without the development of the characteristic breathing and râles. I have notes of several cases in which, with fully developed physical signs, there was no expectoration. The expectoration was typical in the majority of cases, but it, too, was often atypical in color, consistency, and quantity.

It would draw this paper to too great length if all the complications observed were considered. Without going into detail it may be said that following heart weakness, edema of the lungs was one of the most serious disasters. The various serous and purulent effusions were usually successfully treated. In one case the disease was complicated with abscess of the lung, and the pus was finally located after seven unsuccessful explorations with the hypodermic needle. The abscess was opened and drained, and the patient made a perfect recovery. Albuminuria was present at some time during the course of the disease in over ninety per cent. of the cases; in ten per cent. of these there were evidences of nephritis.

In considering the clinical material, those forms of mixed infection which have been brought to light by the bacteriologic study of the cases cannot be ignored. Under this head are included those cases of tuberculosis which were accompanied by inflammatory processes in the lung caused by the concurrence of two or more infecting agents, one of which was the tubercle bacillus. The fact has been repeatedly demontrated, experimentally and clinically, that the tubercle bacillus alone, without the presence of other infecting agents, has the power of causing changes in the lung which simulate very closely the various forms of acute and non-tuberculous pneumonia. Clinically, such cases are necessarily differentiated with great difficulty, and require repeated microscopic examination of the sputum (the centrifuge aiding materially) before a positive diagnosis can be made. It is possible to have two pathologic processes in many cases of pulmonary tuberculosis; one leading to the formation of tubercle, the other giving rise to pneumonic infiltration.

These cases I have classified as follows:

1. Cases of acute fibrinous pneumonia, in which the disease attacks an area of lung tissue, the greater part of which is the seat of infiltrating, but latent, tuberculosis. The previous history includes disease in a distant organ, from which pulmonary tuberculosis took its origin, or with which it was coincident. The latent pulmonary deposit, as a rule, did not give rise to subjective symptoms before the advent of the acute pneumonia.

2. (*a*) Cases in which there is an acute croupous or catarrhal pneumonia in the immediate vicinity of tuberculous areas, the latter previously recognized, with changes in the infiltrated areas, usually at the apex, the fibrinous disease running its course and terminating by crisis or lysis. This type is not associated with hemoptysis as a prodromal or initial symptom. (*b*) Cases of chronic or subacute pulmonary tuberculosis in which acute catarrhal or croupous pneumonia attacks distant areas of the diseased or opposite lung, in which there is no early hemoptysis, but in which the tuberculous process is actively progressive, with physical signs of beginning or already completed disorganization.

3. Cases which may be called streptococcus-pneumonia, in which the disease is added either to a latent or an active pulmonary tuberculosis. Hemoptysis is present, usually, during the early stage of the acute exacerbation, or immediately precedes the pneumonia. Here the complication depends largely upon the aspiration of infecting agents from the seat of the original infiltration and ultimate disorganization.

4. Cases of acute catarrhal, occasionally fibrinous, pneumonia with concurrent infection, when, as a result of lowered vitality, resulting usually from child-bearing, alcoholism, or unfavorable environment, there is, in a comparatively short time, rapid disorganization of lung tissue, ultimate cheesy infiltration, with the clinical evidences of coagulation-necrosis, hectic fever, and finally death.

The most unique and at the same time surprising cases of mixed infection which have come to my notice, are those in which there has been no suspicion of existing pulmonary tuberculosis antedating the accompanying pneumonia. There were no lung symptoms until the violent outbreak of croupous disease, and in no case which I have seen had the physician been consulted to prescribe for or examine the patient. The general appearance had, in many cases, been so good that during the early days of the acute pneumonia no suspicion of the true state of affairs was entertained, and not until it became plain that the pneumonia was not following a typical course and bacteriologic examinations were made, were the facts established which made it positive that a mixed infection was present. In the majority of these cases the added element gave rise to a croupous pneumonia which involved the area of latent disease and the tissues immediately adjacent to it.

While there are in many of these cases no subjective complaints, or objective symptoms of pulmonary tuberculosis before the appearance of pneumonia, careful inquiry and a thorough search reveal the fact that there have been foci in distant organs, from which pulmonary tuberculosis proceeded, or with which it was originally closely related. Many of these patients present good family histories, while their personal record strengthens the conclusion that lung tuberculosis may be present, but dormant, awaiting the advent of some depressing agent or added pulmonary disturbance. In other words, lower by the addition of the second germ the resisting power of the patient who has an unsuspected tuberculosis, and, as a rule, the result will be tissue disorganization and consequent progression of the original disease. I know that this conclusion is contrary to the belief of many who attribute to mixed infection little influence on latent tuberculosis, and who prognosticate favorably in cases of this class, but I give it as being in accord with my own clinical experience.

SCHOOL HYGIENE: LIGHTING OF SCHOOLROOMS AND ITS RELATIONS TO ANOMALIES OF REFRACTION.

BY J. A. BACH, M.D.,
OF MILWAUKEE, WIS.

IT is a well-known fact among oculists that nearly all eyes at birth are far-sighted. As the general development of the body proceeds, the eyes approach nearer and near to the normal, and under certain conditions the relative length of the anteroposterior axis of the eyeball may, by the stretching following abnormally rapid growth, go beyond the normal and produce near-sightedness. Unequal curvatures in the different meridians of the eye, especially of the cornea, produce astigmatism. This condition, with a few exceptions, is always congenital.

Persons whose occupations do not necessitate close vision, such, for instance, as may be found among the Indians, rarely lose all their far-sightedness during development, and as a class are a far-sighted people. On the other hand, it is the oculist's daily observation that persons who apply themselves to close work from childhood, as a rule, not only lose their far-sightedness, but a very large percentage of them become near-sighted in varying degrees. Especially is this true when the conditions are such as to necessitate a close approximation to the work under unfavorable surroundings. This tendency to the development of near-sightedness is most marked during the years of active growth, when the tissues are soft and unresisting. Any influences which produce an abnormal congestion of the eye with a consequent poor circulation in this organ, tend to favor the development of anomalies of refraction by lowering the resistance of the coats of the eye and increasing the intra-ocular tension. The result is that the organ will gradually yield at its weakest point—the posterior part—producing elongation of the eyeball, a condition constituting myopia.

Persistent use of the eyes in near work, thus strongly exercising the accommodation and convergence, is beyond doubt the chief immediate cause of the development of myopia. The lateral compression of the eyeball by its muscles, together with the congestion of the eye, resulting partially from the effort and partially from the stooped posture which is generally assumed during close vision, are responsible for a great deal of injury to the eyes. Close approximation to work and the consequent unfavorable conditions referred to can only be avoided by having proper and sufficient light, which becomes a source of the greatest relief to the eye already burdened with the effort to overcome any mechanical defect which may be present; the demand upon accommodation and convergence will be much lessened, as it enables the holding of work at a greater distance from the eyes. With proper light the retinal image becomes brighter and more clearly defined, and the ocular irritation resulting from the efforts for greater distinctness is distinctly lessened.

Light reaches the eyes in three different ways, as follows: (1) Direct light, or that which strikes the eye directly from its source. (2) Reflected light, or that which strikes the eye after it has been thrown back by one or more surfaces sufficiently smooth to reflect a considerable number of rays in the same general direction. (3) Diffused light, or that which reaches the eye after it has been reflected from all possible surfaces round about. In diffused light the air is crowded, as it were, with silent lines of light. Back and forth they pass in all directions, every surface receiving light, every little grain and fiber acting as a reflector to send it out again. Thoroughly diffused light does not cast shadows, all surfaces participating in reflection and re-reflection.

The most favorable light, as to quantity and quality, to work by is the diffused white sunlight from a northern sky. Using this as a basis, we must further consider the direction from which this light is admitted for use, so as to avoid annoying reflections and other disturbing elements. It will be seen that the question of light may be considered under three heads, *viz.*, quality, quantity, and direction.

Quality.—White sunlight is the normal stimulant of the retina, and any light which does not at least nearly correspond in composition with sunlight is defective by just so much, and may become a source of fatigue. Many schoolrooms through the entire day, and nearly all rooms for a portion of it, have no direct sunlight, and all the light they receive is entirely by reflection. Of this the portion coming from surfaces on the earth, etc., is a very considerable part. Light-colored surfaces are the most valuable reflectors, as they least disturb the composition of sunlight, and, at the same time, reflect the largest number of rays. It becomes, therefore, a matter of no little importance to see that the surroundings of school buildings be as free as possible from colored reflecting surfaces. Each substance has its effect upon the light which it reflects; some of the light is absorbed and that which is reflected carries with it the effect of color characteristic of the reflecting object. Again, surfaces may be illuminated by colored light depending upon nearby surfaces. Thus, conditions occur when there will be very noticeable flushes cast over the pages of the books of school children and which may be easily traced to the predominating influence of some one of the reflecting surfaces.

Concerning the function of light when it finally reaches a room, it may be said that that which passes directly from the window to the eye is of no benefit, except as it enables one to see the outside view. After the light passes into the schoolroom it is reflected back and forth between walls, floor, furniture, and occupants. The light which these various surfaces reflect gives impressions of form and color by which we appreciate objects. To preserve the light as pure as it entered, it will be readily seen that colored surfaces in a schoolroom should be avoided. A neutral gray, or such a shade of gray as may be necessary to modify the light in a room, should be used on the walls, curtains, and other reflecting surfaces. This, containing all the elements of white light, does not disturb the composition of light, and yet enables a variation of the amount of light by varying the degree of the color of the window-shade.

Quantity.—The darkest place occupied by any pupil should have at least sufficient light so that he may, without special effort, on account of insufficiency of light, read diamond type at a distance of at least twelve inches from the eye. By diamond type I mean the smallest type used by printers. The size of this type approximately subtends an angle of five degrees at a distance of twelve inches from the eye, and represents about the limit of distinct vision. This test is sufficiently accurate for practical purposes. The diffused white sunlight from the northern sky, in general terms, is a close approximation to the desired amount. It is more usual to err on the side of insufficiency of light than on the side of excess. Therefore, it is safe to allow as much desirable light as possible to enter the schoolroom. To facilitate this the school building should have full and free exposure to the sun in order that the most perfect source of light may be fully utilized, either directly or indirectly. Such buildings should, if possible, stand upon elevated ground of sufficient area to prevent any adjoining building or trees from casting interfering shadows. The windows should be large and should be equal to about one-fifth the area of the floor. As little space as possible should be occupied by divisions in the windows. The windows should reach to the ceiling, and no obstructing ornamental projections, either outside or inside, should exist. The best effect is obtained with square-topped windows, the Gothic style being objectionable. The regulation of the amount of light, especially in those rooms of a school which are exposed to the direct rays of the sun, is of great importance. Blinds and curtains are used for this purpose. The essential qualities which these light-regulators should possess are as follows: (1) They should intercept the direct rays of the sun. (2) They should not dazzle. (3) They should transmit a maximum amount of white light. It is, indeed, difficult to find material which perfectly meets all these indications, but this can be approximated by such material as will not interfere with the quality, nor yet too much with the quantity of light.

This we find in combining the extremes, black, or the absence of all light, and white, giving such a shade of gray as may be desired to meet the indications. Blackboards, although not disturbing the quality, absorb a considerable portion of light, and, if the general amount is not plentiful in a given room, these should not cover too much surface; such rooms, as well, should have the walls colored white or nearly so. The ceilings of all rooms should be white, as by this is gained a valuable diffuser and reflector of light. Glass dulled on one side by sand-blowing, and gray cathedral glass, make desirable substances for shading, but being too costly, are hardly practicable. Colored materials of whatever shade, except gray, should never be employed. Shades should roll at the bottom of the window; this will allow the more advantageous light to enter, besides making it easier to lower the upper window for other purposes.

No artificial light can ever equal diffused sunlight, and, therefore, it is very desirable that children should be required to do their studying during the day if possible. However, when required, artificial light should be made to correspond as nearly as possible to natural light. It should be ample in quantity, good in quality, and come from a suitable direction. It should, furthermore, be steady, otherwise it will be dazzling and fatiguing. Experiments have been carried on by means of concave mirrors throwing the light to the white ceiling, thus diffusing it equally through the whole room, while the source of light remained hidden. The results are said to have been perfect. The electric light possesses an additional advantage over other artificial light, in that it does not vitiate the air—a very important consideration when large classes are confined to one room during a long period of time.

Direction.—The most favorable direction in which light can enter a schoolroom is probably from above. The photographer well knows the excellent service of diffused skylight. Unfortunately, however, school buildings are more than one story high, making this impracticable, excepting for the upper floor. All light that is not reflected directly from the work can only be a source of annoyance. If it is direct light which strikes the eye, the retina becomes unduly irritated, and cannot properly perform its function. Reflected light, as well, irritates the retina excessively, and often causes a confusion of the letters on the printed page with the images of other objects from which it may be reflected. For this reason blackboards should not be placed beween windows, as the direct light from the windows will be a source of the greatest danger to the eyes of the pupil using them. The surface of the blackboards must not be glossy, but rather a dull black to prevent strong reflections. Light coming from below the level of the work or the head of the child is often worse than useless.

It will be readily seen that light should enter from such a direction that it strikes the work from above and from the left side. Light from the right side is, as a rule, objectionable, because it casts shadows, and for the same reason light from behind is not desirable, shadows of head and shoulders being cast over the work, either reading or writing. To increase the general lighting effect, partially diffused light from behind, but from as high a level as possible, may be permissible. If the rooms are properly arranged, sufficient light from the left side may be admitted without resorting to other sources. It will be noted that the light as it comes from the left strikes the page, and most of it is reflected from the page at the same angle that it originally touched it. This light does not pass on as so much useless light, but as it passes from surface to surface, lighting the room from millions of reflections and re-reflections until finally becoming thoroughly diffused throughout the room, each nook and crevice is equally well illuminated with the general light in the room. This light being so strongly diffused does not cast shadows, is sufficient in quantity, and, if the reflecting surfaces are free from color, non-irritating in quality. It is the ideal light, and it has been amply proven that many, if not all the aggravating eye-strains and their varied consequences, so prevalent in our schools, could be avoided by close attention to this subject.

Bearing directly upon the well-being and health of the child's eyes as well as of his body is the position assumed during study. The seating of school children, therefore, becomes a subject of almost as great importance as the provision of proper light. A bad posture is not only injurious to the health of the eye, but is a fruitful source of curvature of the spine. Eulenberg says that ninety per cent. of curvatures of the spine, not induced by local disease, are developed during school life, and are directly traceable to improper seating. The improvement in American school-desks, as all know, has been great during the last few years, yet in many particulars we are far from perfection in this respect. As a rule, insufficient attention is being given to the size of the desks relative to the size of the children, and in many schools may be found desks all of the same size. As has already been pointed out under the subject of light, the great object in view is the prevention of undue approximation of the pupil to the work, and to avoid stooping. Desks should, therefore, correspond relatively in size to the size of the pupil. A back rest is necessary, but in nearly all desks this is too high, and interferes with the free movements of the body, besides encouraging a sliding down of the body. A good and substantial support to the pelvis and lower part of the back is sufficient and decidedly the least fatiguing. Furthermore, a child should rest the feet on a foot-board or the floor to sit easily. Non-support of the feet while sitting produces great fatigue and restlessness in children. The height of the seat, the height of the desk, and its slope are all very important. The slope for reading should be about 40°, and for writing 20°. The edge of the desk should at least come up to or slightly overlap the edge of the seat. This is an important consideration, and assists much in preventing the habit of stooping. It must, however, be borne in mind that, however important and necessary a proper school desk may be, it is equally essential that the habit of correct sitting be acquired, and the teacher should dwell on this point at the beginning of the school year. Cramped and awkward positions are not likely to be assumed by an occupant of a properly fitting desk, except in writing and drawing, yet the habit of bad positions of sitting for all work may be acquired by the pupils unless properly instructed. Pupils should never approach their work closer than twelve inches.

It remains an undisputed fact among oculists that the constant stooping forward of the head and the close approximation to the page, is the most effective factor in the causation of myopia, save possibly constitutional predisposition. Eyes under these conditions are working in a state of tension, as it were, which, if long continued, produces a deep intra-ocular pressure, softening and stretching of the coats of the eyeball, and results, in milder forms, in a slight elongation of the eyeball characteristic of myopia. It has been noted with a great deal of satisfaction that whenever radical improvements in the lighting and seating of schools have been carried into effect, the reduction in the prevalence of myopia has been so great that its ultimate absolute prevention would seem a probability.

It must be observed, however, that not only must pupils be properly protected while in school, but the parents as well must cooperate, and the close application of the scholars at home under unfavorable conditions must be discouraged. After the child has attained its full growth, its tissues become more resisting, and injury to the eyes in the manner above stated, becomes less frequent.

CLINICAL MEMORANDA.

EXCISION OF THE RIGHT CLAVICLE FOR OSTEOSARCOMA.

BY GEORGE TULLY VAUGHAN, M.D.,
OF WASHINGTON, D. C.;
PASSED-ASSISTANT SURGEON, U. S. M. H. S.; PROFESSOR OF PRINCIPLES AND PRACTICE OF SURGERY IN GEORGETOWN UNIVERSITY.

W. S., American, aged twenty-eight years, was admitted to the marine ward of the German Hospital, Philadelphia, October 15, 1895. His family history was negative, and he denied all venereal diseases and rheumatism. During March, seven months before admission, he began to complain of pain situated in the right clavicle. Shortly afterward enlargement of the bone became apparent. The pain was of a dull aching character, often radiating to the chest and mastoid process on the right side, and was aggravated by use of the arm. On examination, the inner two-thirds of the clavicle was found to consist of a hard, spindle-shaped tumor, extending to within 2½ cm. of the joint. The right external jugular vein was distended.

October 22d, under ether anesthesia, the entire right clavicle, with the tumor, was removed by an incision extending along the bone from one end to the other, disjointing the acromial end first, dissecting the tumor loose from the surrounding parts, and last, disarticulating at the sternoclavicular articulation. The tumor was broken through while using the bone as a lever in separating its sternal attachments. To control the hemorrhage, it was necessary to apply over twenty ligatures. To prevent dropping of the shoulder, the detached portions of the trapezius and sternocleidomastoid muscles above were carefully sutured to corresponding portions of the deltoid and pectoralis major muscles below. The wound was closed with catgut sutures, leaving an opening in the middle for a gauze drain, and the dressing was applied, with the arm in the Velpeau position.

Subsequent to the operation, the highest temperature was 102.2° F., which continued for one day only.

FIG. 1.

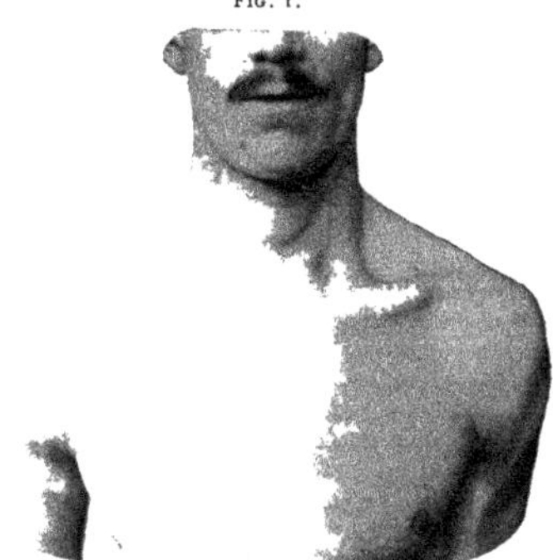

Showing site of operation and resulting deformity after excision of the clavicle.

Fourteen days after the operation the patient was out of bed. The wound healed by primary union, except at two points, one in the middle and one at the outer end, which healed by granulation. Forty-one days after the operation the patient was discharged. There was no deformity and no interference with the function of the arm. The tumor measured 11.25 c.cm. in circumference, and, on microscopic examination, was pronounced a mixed-cell sarcoma. The accompanying illustration shows the condition of the parts one year subsequent to the operation, and it will be seen that there is absolutely no deformity except the absence of the clavicular prominence on the right side. During the interval he had been performing his accustomed work as fireman on a steamboat, and stated that he felt no inconvenience from the loss of the clavicle, his arm being free from pain and as strong as ever. With his clothes on there was no evidence of dropping of the shoulder, and after stripping it was barely perceptible—not more than one centimeter—which is no more than is often observed in the normal individual.

Excision of the entire clavicle seems to be a rare operation, though partial excision is comparatively common. Professor Ashhurst up to 1893, had been able to collect but 36 cases of the complete operation at one sitting, following which there were 7 deaths, a mortality of nearly 20 per cent. It seems that Dr. Charles McCreary did the first complete excision in 1813, removing the right clavicle from a boy of fourteen, with scrofulous caries; that of Remmer in 1732, given by Gross as the first operation, having been, according to Ashhurst, a partial excision. The same author gives the mortality from partial excision, or excision *a deux temps*, in 76 cases as a little over 14 per cent. The celebrated operation of Dr. Mott,[1] performed during 1828, for sarcoma of the left clavicle, which required nearly four hours for its performance, and in which forty ligatures were employed, was a case of partial excision, though from the size of the tumor and the part of the clavicle removed—the inner end—was really a more formidable operation than the majority of cases of complete excision. Dr. Mott referred to it as his "Waterloo operation," and said that it was without a precedent, and far surpassed in tediousness, difficulty, and danger anything he had ever witnessed or performed.

A CASE OF SEVERE TOXEMIA; RECOVERY AFTER TREATMENT WITH COLD BATHS.

By KNUT HOEGH, M.D.,
OF MINNEAPOLIS.

THE patient, Mrs. G., thirty-two years of age, entered St. Barnabas' Hospital on September 2, 1897. A diagnosis of multiocular cyst of the left ovary having been made, the usual preparatory treatment for operation, consisting of bathing, scrubbing, shaving, evacuation of the bowels, and restricted diet, was carried out according to routine practice. On the morning of the operation breakfast was not allowed. An enema was given, and at eight o'clock a hypodermic injection of 1/6-grain of sulphate of morphia was administered. At nine o'clock the patient was etherized and oophorectomy performed. The hands of the operator and assistants had previously been thoroughly scrubbed, the operating-gowns, caps, and dressing material sterilized in Schimmelbusch's steam sterilizer, the instruments boiled fifteen minutes in a ten-per-cent. solution of sal soda, and the silk suture material, an hour in a five-per-cent. solution of carbolic acid. Böckmann's catgut was also used.

The sterilization was accomplished under the personal supervision of the operator. The operation was as easy as an oophorectomy can be, and no mishap occurred, except that a knuckle of bowel, about four inches long, was twice forced out of the wound by the vomiting and retching of the patient, and was immediately replaced by the fingers covered with gauze wrung out of sterilized hot water. In puncturing the cyst, a very small quantity of its contents, of an apparently bland nature, escaped along the trocar. There was no bleeding and the emptying of the cyst largely occurred outside of the abdominal cavity. Nothing but the operator's hands was introduced into the cavity; sponging or flushing was not employed, and the peritoneum was not interfered with in any way. Including the insertion of sutures in separate layers and the application of the dressing, the operation occupied exactly thirty minutes, and at its completion a most hopeful outlook was presented.

Some hours after the operation five ounces of urine was withdrawn by catheter, and for the first few days the secretion of urine was normal. On the evening of the first day the temperature rose to 100.4° F. and the pulse to 84; the patient complained of abdominal pain; no flatus was passed; nothing but hot water was given by mouth and drugs were not administered. On the following day the morning temperature was 100.6° F., the evening 100.8° F., and the pulse varied from 90 to 98. The patient complained of severe abdominal pain and slept but little. The urine was withdrawn by catheter, and while scanty was as much as could be expected considering the small quantity of hot water taken. Food was not given during the thirty hours following the operation. At the end of this time a small quantity of broth and a little dry toast was allowed. Nothing more was given that day, as nausea was provoked. The patient passed a restless night, having short snatches of sleep interrupted by pain in the back. Forty-six hours after the operation she vomited a dark-green fluid. The temperature remained very much the same as on the previous day—100° F. to 100.8° F., and the pulse, 88 to 92. During the day she repeatedly vomited a little dark-green fluid. She rested but little during the night, and the next morning vomited a somewhat larger quantity of similar appearance.

Sixty-six hours after the operation the temperature was 99.9° F., the pulse had risen a little, and the patient had a somewhat collapsed appearance. She had urinated spontaneously, but neither fecal matter nor flatus had passed. The wound looked healthy, the abdomen was slightly distended, but no ascitic fluid could be discovered. Hourly doses of 1/4-grain of calomel were administered, but the vomiting continued and no signs of intestinal peristalsis appeared. On the afternoon of the fourth day, eighty hours after the operation, the temperature began to rise; at 4 P.M. it was 102.6° F., pulse, 112; at 8.45 it was 103.2° F. and the pulse, 118; the vomiting continued. The administration of two enemas of salines and turpentine resulted in a fairly large movement of the bowels. The vomiting, however, continued during the night and the next morning; it must have been feculent, as it was described as offensive, although still green. The patient appeared slightly delirious. The matter next vomited was brown in color. The calomel was continued and small doses of strained barley-water were given. The following morning, at the end of the fourth day, the stomach was emptied by means of a flexible tube, a large quantity of distinctly fecal matter being evacuated. The calomel was then stopped and citrate of magnesia given. The patient was very feeble and decidedly delirious, but answered questions rationally.

During the forenoon of the fifth day the temperature remained 102.6° F., while the pulse increased in frequency and lost in volume and strength. An enema at noon produced a loose dark-brown evacuation. As the vomiting con-

[1] *American Journal of the Medical Sciences*, January, 1883.

tinued it was deemed advisable to use the stomach tube again, and about a quart of yellowish-brown fluid of fecal odor was removed. She was more delirious and restless than before, the pupils were dilated, the lips dusky, and a clammy perspiration covered the upper part of the body; temperature, 103.6° F., pulse, 148. It seemed as if the end were approaching, an event the more deplorable as the operation had appeared one of unusual simplicity and freedom from complications. As a last resort, she was carefully lifted from her bed and placed in a portable bath-tub filled with water at a temperature of 90° F. A towel rung out of ice water was placed upon her head, and the temperature of the bath reduced to 70° F. by adding ice to the water. She was kept in the bath ten minutes, during which time the body and limbs were briskly rubbed. She enjoyed the bath very much, spoke intelligently on being taken out, and went to sleep immediately after. An hour and a half later the temperature was 100.3° F., while the pulse still remained 148. A hypodermic injection of 1/30 of a grain of strychnia was administered.

A little less than three hours after the first, a second bath was given, the temperature of which was lowered to 75° F. After this bath the patient's temperature was 102° F., pulse, 134, and a slight amount of flatus was passed, which was observed both by the patient, who had become more rational, and by the nurse. After a short time she became restless and vomited again, whereupon the stomach tube was used, and another hypodermic of strychnia given. At midnight, another tub bath reduced the temperature to 101.8° F., after which the patient became more quiet, and the pulse, which had remained 138, became perceptibly stronger. As she had not passed any urine since seven o'clock the previous morning, the catheter was used, and an ounce and a half withdrawn.

At two o'clock on the morning of the fifth day, that is before the one hundred and twentieth hour was completed, a fourth tub bath was given which calmed the restlessness and brought down the temperature to 100.8° F. and the pulse to 128. At four o'clock another hypodermic of strychnia was given, and at five, she was given a fifth bath which had the usual quieting effect. The temperature was then 100° F. in the rectum, and the pulse 124. The stomach was again emptied by means of the tube. At six o'clock hot water and whiskey, three ounces of each, were given per rectum, whereupon she went into a somewhat restless sleep. During the forenoon of this, the fifth day, two more tub baths were given and the stomach again emptied. The fluid removed was now green and did not smell so badly. In the afternoon, another tub bath was given, although the temperature had not risen above 100.6° F., but the patient wanted it, and, as it seemed to have a good effect upon the pulse which had dropped to 120 and finally to 110, it was deemed advisable. She was then given some barley-water which was retained an hour or more. At eleven o'clock at night the stomach was again washed out, and for the first time the contents were not feculent; there had been a slight natural movement a short time previously. The catheter had been used several times during the day, and altogether about seven ounces of urine obtained.

From the morning of the sixth day there was a steady improvement. The pulse went down to 104, occasionally rising to 110, the temperature ranged between 98° F. and 99.6° F., and there was a corresponding improvement in the general condition which continued until recovery was complete. It would be tedious to dwell upon the successive steps of her convalescence; it is only necessary to mention that she received in all ten tub baths and that the stomach tube was not used after the end of the seventh day. Her recovery was slow owing to extreme weakness, and was complicated by the appearance of a number of carbuncles on the back, which were satisfactorily treated by parenchymatous injections of a six-per-cent. solution of carbolic acid and applications of permanent wet antiseptic dressings. October 10th she returned to her home perfectly well.

In trying to account for the condition which came so near being fatal (and at one time was hourly expected to be so) it seems reasonable to assume that it was due to an absorption of toxins. The case did not impress the physicians as one of septic peritonitis, for there was no fluid or other effusion or exudation discoverable in the abdominal cavity, nor was there marked tympanites, at least not enough to correspond to the gravity of the constitutional symptoms, nor was there pronounced abdominal tenderness. At the end of the sixth day, when the crisis was over, the abdomen was absolutely flat and entirely free from pain upon pressure. It seems to me that the best explanation of the condition is the assumption of absorption through the edematous mucous membrane of toxic products from the paralyzed intestinal tract.

Why was the intestinal tract paralyzed? Could it have been the result of the administration of morphia before the operation? Was it due to the ether narcosis or to the compression of the knuckle of bowel by the rather violent vomiting and retching during the operation? Is it possible that the escape of, at the very utmost, two teaspoonfuls of the apparently bland cyst contents could have produced it? And if so, should we not rather have expected peritonitis, and not this paretic condition of the intestinal tract?

The patient was of large frame, looked strong and robust, and had always been healthy; but her mother and a brother are said to have died after surgical operations. Does this point to the possibility of a congenital lack of resistance and power of reaction? Is such a paralysis of the intestinal tract to be classed with the anuria which sometimes follows abdominal operations, to be looked upon as an effect or evidence of shock?

It seems to me, and it appeared so to other physicians who saw the patient, that she would not have survived but for the cold baths. It is certain that they were very grateful to her at the time, although after her recovery she could not remember the first ones. That they were beneficial was evidenced by the lowering of the temperature, the strengthening of the heart's action, and the mental clearness which followed their administration. I was led to use them in this case because of the good effect which usually accompanies their employment in typhoid fever when the toxin poisoning is often the main cause of a fatal issue.

AN ADDRESS.

SANITARY SCIENCE, THE MEDICAL PROFESSION, AND THE PUBLIC.[1]

BY HERMANN M. BIGGS, M.D.,
OF NEW YORK;
PROFESSOR OF THERAPEUTICS AND CLINICAL MEDICINE AND ADJUNCT PROFESSOR OF THE PRINCIPLES AND PRACTICE OF MEDICINE IN THE BELLEVUE HOSPITAL MEDICAL COLLEGE; PATHOLOGIST AND DIRECTOR OF THE BACTERIOLOGICAL LABORATORY OF THE NEW YORK CITY HEALTH DEPARTMENT.

IN an address on public medicine delivered before the British Medical Association some years ago, Sir Charles Cameron referred to a writer in the *Scotsman* who objected to the appointment of medical men engaged in practice as officers of health, on the ground that "no sane body of men can bring themselves to believe that medical practitioners, whose livelihood depends upon sickness, are likely to exert themselves in exterminating it." Dr. Holmes once humorously said, "Physicians desire for their patients great longevity with frequent illness." To such an audience as this arguments or proofs are not necessary to refute these suggestions.

The history of sanitary science is indissolubly related to the history of medicine, and its achievements may almost be written in the recital of the work, investigations, and discoveries of medical men. It may perhaps be justly said, that no class or profession has contributed as much as the medical profession to the advance of civilization, to the prosperity of nations, and to the preservation and prolongation of human life, all of which are closely related to the vast contributions to the progress of civilization which have been made by sanitary science. Sanitary science aims to prevent disease. In former times at least four-fifths of all deaths were due to preventable causes, and even now, when the death-rate has been reduced to a quarter of what it once was, still one-third of the deaths occurring in our large cities are due to distinctly preventable diseases.

During a discussion in the British Parliament of a bill for the protection of the public health, one of the greatest English ministers, Disraeli, pronounced these memorable words, "The public health is the foundation on which repose the happiness of the people and the power of a country. The care of the public health is the first duty of a statesman." England has long and justly been regarded as the birth-place and home of sanitary science. English methods in sanitation have been the models for the world. No other country has had in modern times so high a standard of public health and such low death-rates. These conditions have, without doubt, largely contributed in placing the British nation foremost in civilization, and have assisted much in laying the foundation of, and in building up, the British empire, in which is included to-day nearly one-quarter of the world's population. Such results are, in fact, the logical and far-reaching consequences of broad statesmanship in sanitary matters.

[1] The anniversary discourse delivered before the New York Academy of Medicine, October 21, 1897.

So complex are the relations, that it is impossible, even after the most careful consideration, to gain an adequate conception of the vast influence which the health of a nation has upon its material prosperity and its standard of morality. We realize more fully how close is the relation of the public health to the material prosperity of a community, when we recall the deadening influence on business and commerce produced in 1892 by the appearance in New York harbor of several ships, each with a few cases of Asiatic cholera on board, and the occurrence of a dozen cases in New York City itself. Almost a panic was created among the more fearful of the inhabitants. All the Southern, Central, South American and Mediterranean ports were quarantined against New York, and but for the short duration of the outbreak a most serious interference with commerce would have resulted.

The appearance at that time of cholera in Europe and in New York was the result of sanitary neglect. We realize how dearly this was paid for, when it is remembered what the epidemic of cholera in 1892 cost the city of Hamburg. Can one by any stretch of the imagination conceive of the terrible results which would follow the extension of such an epidemic to a number of the large cities of Europe and the United States, or over the whole continent of Europe, as occurred in the great epidemics of earlier times? Consider the results which only this year followed the introduction, at the end of the season too, of yellow fever into some of the Southern cities. The material loss has been enormous, although the actual number of deaths comparatively insignificant. The expenditure, on sanitary and quarantine improvements, of one-tenth of the loss involved in this insignificant epidemic would render another introduction of yellow fever well-nigh impossible. With the numerous close and rapid lines of communication which now exist between all parts of the civilized world, the rapidity of extension of one of the medieval epidemics would be frightful to contemplate, should sanitary conditions and lack of sanitary knowledge rendered such an epidemic possible. In temperate climates we have no longer reason to fear the occurrence of epidemics of any diseases more terrifying than scarlet fever, measles, typhoid fever, and diphtheria, and the occurrence of an epidemic of any one of these is to be chargeable to remediable sanitary defects.

The public health bears quite as close a relation to public morality as to general material prosperity. Sickness brings in its trail, especially among the poor, uncleanliness, poverty, misery, wretchedness, destitution, and death. The physical and the moral man are interdependent. That which degrades one, degrades the other; individual exceptions to the rule do not invalidate its force.

The most casual review of history shows in a striking manner the extraordinary improvement which has taken place in the public health in modern times. The plague and the other great epidemic diseases of the Middle Ages, which decimated and sometimes well-nigh exterminated the human race, are vanquished; smallpox, typhus fever, epidemic dysentery, and cholera have been restricted to the narrowest limits. The prevalence, in temperate climates and under favorable sanitary conditions, of yellow and typhoid fever has been diminished to a small fraction of what it formerly was. Diphtheria and hydrophobia are now absolutely preventable, and even the less alarming, because more familiar, but hardly less fatal diseases, measles, scarlet fever, whooping-cough, and summer diarrhea—a formidable array of preventable affections—have been confined by the energies of the sanitary authorities within much narrower boundaries. The great plague of modern civilization, tuberculosis, shows a steady and continuous decline in its death-rate, and the most gratifying improvement in the percentage of recoveries from it, as the result of improved general and personal hygiene. Smallpox, in former times with all its terrors, before the discovery of vaccination, was scarcely more to be dreaded than tuberculosis is even now. Smallpox then caused a relatively smaller proportion of deaths than tuberculosis does to-day. We are all familiar with pulmonary tuberculosis. It is seen everywhere; it occurs among all classes of the population. It is insidious, and extends slowly; it is not dramatic in the manner of its appearance or course. As it is so familiar to everyone, we do not fear it. We neglect it; and many would deny proper sanitary supervision and refuse to provide special hospitals for the care of the poor suffering from it. Therefore, its ravages still continue, and it causes nearly one-seventh of all deaths, and nearly one-fourth of all deaths among the adult population, although, be it remembered, no disease is better understood or more preventable; none more amenable to simple and easily applied measures of cleanliness and disinfection. A consumptive may be absolutely free from danger to his immediate family and to his most intimate associates, provided only simple precautions be observed.

But at last we may hope that light is breaking upon sanitary authorities, the medical profession, and the people. Rational measures of prevention are taking the place of insane fear, or helpless, hopeless, ignorance and neglect, and before another generation has passed away the death-rate from tuberculosis in cities under the best sanitary control will, I believe, be less than one-third what it is in New York to-day. I do not wish this statement to be received as the opinion of an enthusiast; but as the deliberate conviction, reached after most careful and prolonged consideration and study, of one who has had considerable experience in sanitary matters and exceptional opportunities for the investigation of this dread disease.

The diminution in the number of deaths occurring from all causes in proportion to the population is shown in the most striking way when we compare the present with previous conditions. The healthfulness of a community or locality is to be judged by the statistics of the number of cases of sickness and death considered in relation to their causes. The condition of the public health should be studied, not simply with relation to the number of deaths or number of cases of sickness in proportion to the population, but also with relation to the nature and preventability of the diseases which cause the morbidity and mortality. The mortality is usually expressed by stating how many persons die each year to each thousand of the population. In the Seventeenth and Eighteenth Centuries the average annual death-rate per thousand living, throughout the civilized world, probably varied from 50 to 80, that is, of every thousand persons in the population 50 to 80 died each year. The average duration of life of each person born was not more than fifteen to eighteen years. From 1628 to 1635, in London—these years being free from pestilence—the average death-rate was 50 per thousand, and the absolute annual mortality for twenty-four years, from 1620 to 1643, inclusive, was nearly 80 per thousand. With what incredulity would the prediction have been received two hundred years ago that the then average annual death-rate of 80 per thousand in England would be reduced at the present time to 17. The mortality during 1894 in London was only 17 and a fraction, or less than one-quarter of that of two hundred years ago. The mean expectation of life at birth one hundred years ago in London was only about nineteen years, the annual death-rate being 51 or 52 per thousand. At the end of the first half of this century it had already diminished more than one-third, to an estimated 30 or 35 per thousand, and as the century draws to an end it has diminished again to only 17 or 18, and the average duration of life has increased to more than 40 years, or more than doubled during the century. From 1770 to 1780 smallpox alone caused a higher annual death-rate in London than diphtheria, croup, consumption and all other tuberculous diseases, measles, smallpox, scarlet fever, and typhoid fever together caused in New York last year. Fever at the same time caused an even greater death-rate, and in the Sixteenth-Century plague, cholera and dysentery, diseases which are now practically extinct, annually destroyed nearly twice as many of each thousand of the population as now die from all causes added together. More than 40,000 people died in Paris during one epidemic of smallpox in the last century, and a third of the population of Iceland in another. Ten per cent. of the population of a city or country were often destroyed during one epidemic.

It is perhaps desirable to define more specifically what is meant by infectious, contagious, and communicable disease. Infectious diseases are those caused by some simple form of animal or plant life, which possesses, under favorable conditions, unlimited powers of reproduction. The contagious diseases include those infectious diseases which are transmitted by contact or proximity to the infected individual or infected material. For convenience we refer to another class of the infectious diseases as communicable, in distinction from the contagious, because the susceptibility is far less general and the means by which they are transmitted are well understood.

In the communicable diseases the observation of simple measures of prevention almost entirely robs them of danger to others. This is not true of the contagious class, which includes smallpox, scarlet fever, measles, chickenpox, whooping-cough, and typhus fever. The communicable diseases include diphtheria, typhoid fever, tuberculosis, cholera, and some others of less importance, in all of which it is possible to reduce to a minimum the danger of transmission by the observation of simple measures. In diphtheria the germs causing the disease are contained solely in the discharges from the nose and mouth; in typhoid fever and cholera they are contained only in the discharges from the stomach or intestines; in pulmonary tuberculosis, or consumption, only in the expectorations. It at once becomes evident that very different measures of prevention are to be adopted in these different diseases. In the contagious class, it should be said, we are as yet unable to adopt any measures which will protect an exposed and susceptible individual.

The most serious array of preventable diseases with which we have at present to contend are those which are highly contagious, such as measles, scarlet fever, and whooping-cough, and a group of infectious diseases, partly communicable, such as diphtheria, typhoid fever, summer diarrhea, pneumonia, influenza, and some other affections of the respiratory tract. In all the diseases of this list there has been a constant decrease in frequency of occurrence, excepting diphtheria, pneumonia, and the epidemics of influenza. Diphtheria has been gradually increasing for a number of years in all of the larger cities until the discovery of the diphtheria antitoxin in 1894. With the extensive use of this remedy it commenced to diminish rapidly, and in Berlin and Paris the death-rate from this disease has been reduced to almost one-quarter of what it previously was. Much has also been accomplished in New York, a diminution of forty per cent. having taken place; but as yet the field is by no means exhausted. The constant increase of diphtheria in the large towns was a remarkable and inexplicable fact, until the observations first made on a large scale by the New York City Health Department showed how it was disseminated through the diphtheria bacilli present in the throat during convalescence and in health.

In the control of whooping-cough, measles, and scarlet fever, exceptional difficulties must be contended with, especially in the great tenement-house population of New York. These diseases possess many features in common. In no one of them is the cause known, and, therefore, the difficulties in their control are greatly increased. These difficulties arise in part from the great crowding in our tenement-house districts, and in part from the fact that they are regarded by the ignorant as only children's diseases, and consequently inevitable. They are, therefore, neglected, and, as a result, being excessively contagious, are prevalent and familiar, and unnecessarily destroy many hundred lives in this city every year—more than ten times as many as smallpox and cholera together; yet there is more dread of the latter two diseases than of all other zymotics combined.

I believe that much could be done to reduce the death-rate from the diseases under consideration if they were managed in an efficient and intelligent manner and with a genuine determination to restrict and prevent them. Probably a satisfactory result will only be attained by the education of the masses, so that they will be able to estimate the actual danger attending these diseases. This opinion as to the possibility of their prevention is justified, as has been shown by Dr. Hill, Medical Officer of Health to Birmingham, by the success which has attended the measures taken in that city with regard to scarlet fever. In Birmingham the annual average death-rate during three periods—1875 to 1878, 1878 to 1882, and 1883 to 1889—has been reduced from 425 per 100,000 to 235 and to 72 during the last period, the number of deaths being only about one-sixth as many as during the first. This reduction has been ascribed to the compulsory reporting of cases and to the hospital accommodations which have been provided for the care of patients with this disease. During 1875 only 20 cases of scarlet fever were admitted to the hospital. In 1889 this number increased to 3759. During the intervening period the decrease in the prevalence of the disease was coincident with the knowledge obtained of the occurrence of cases, and the extent to which the public availed themselves of the advantages of hospital care.

It is said by Dr. Hill that "the prejudice against hospital treatment, which was general at first, has mostly disappeared, and the public now appreciates the advantages to health and life of an institution which enables patients to be removed from unhealthy rooms and other unfavorable conditions to a properly equipped hospital, where better air, suitable food, superior medical treatment, careful nursing, and all those appliances are at hand which a hospital affords, but which are wanting in the homes of the poor." The mortality of the disease in the hospitals varies from five to six per cent. It is noted also that "the social and professional objections to the act controlling the notification of infectious diseases have been proved to have had no foundations whatever. The distrust and friction between the practitioner and the medical officer of health, which were predicted, have not appeared, the concealment of disease which was to have followed has not occurred; the sacred confidence between patient and doctor, which was to have been destroyed with most disastrous results, remains inviolate. And so every theoretic objection which timidity, selfishness, or ignorance could find or invent has been refuted by practical experience.

"One of the objections put forward in this matter, and which deserves special comment, was that notification would be useless in the absence of isolation-hospitals. Without seeking to refute this assertion, which, however, would not be difficult, it may be said that to make compulsory the notification to the sanitary authorities of cases of infectious disease which ought to be isolated constitutes one of the strongest inducements to provide hospitals for their care. These follow as a natural sequence. Every town should provide at least one bed in such a hospital to every thousand of its population.

"The past triumphs of preventive medicine have been achieved in relation to the majority of the scourges afflicting mankind through cleanliness. Malarial fever, smallpox, and hydrophobia have yielded to different and special influences, but the plague and the medieval epidemics have been banished by cleanliness. Typhus and cholera, which formerly wrought such terrible havoc where filthy conditions prevailed, have disappeared through the influence of cleanliness. Typhoid fever is becoming less common through the improved cleanliness and better water-supply of our cities; and while filthy conditions do not seem to give rise to measles, whooping-cough, scarlet fever, and diphtheria, yet there can be no doubt that they seriously aggravate their severity. Nevertheless, the old lesson of thousands of years ago is still unlearned. The sanitarian must still go forth and try to teach that without cleanliness health is impossible."

A Royal Commission, appointed to inquire into the sanitary condition of the British army in India in 1859, found that during a long period the annual average death-rate had remained 69 per thousand. The inquiry resulted in extensive improvements in the housing, clothing, food, and occupation of the soldiers. After these were carried into effect there was a steady decline in the death-rate, the rates for 1886, '87, and '88 vary between 14 and 15.2 per thousand, or less than one-fourth of that previously prevailing; in some years the rate has been even lower.

The impetus to modern sanitary progress may be said to have commenced in England with the passage of the Public Health Act of 1875. Since that time there has been a diminution of twenty per cent. in the death-rate for the whole of England and Wales, while in certain individual communities the fall has equaled thirty per cent., and in Maidstone the unusual figure of forty per cent. has been reached. In New York City, in more recent years, an equally great reduction in the death-rate has been obtained in a shorter period. The average annual death-rate for the ten years ending in 1893 was about 26 per thousand of the population, while the present year will show a death-rate of only 19 and a fraction—a reduction equaling about twenty-five per cent. since 1893. The improvement in New York is especially notable, because it has not been the result of, or associated with, any single great public work or improvement, such as the introduction of a purer water-supply or a better system of sewerage, but is the result of a gradual improvement in every respect in the general sanitary conditions—the improvement in the character of the housing of the poor, the condemnation of rear tenements, the prevention of overcrowding and the habitation of basements and cellars; the improvement in the character of the pavements, and in the cleaning of the streets; the improved character of the water-supply, through a better control of the watershed; a closer supervision of foods, attained by a rigid inspection of meat, fish, and fruit, and the precise control of the milk-supply; the inspection and supervision of offensive trades; the application of modern scientific discoveries in the supervision and control of infectious diseases, and the education of the people in all matters connected with general and personal hygiene.

While the splendid results which have been obtained may well serve for congratulation, it is not to be supposed for a moment that the limit of the improvement has been reached, or that the resources of preventive medicine have been exhausted. On the contrary, the reverse is true, and while we cannot rationally hope for as rapid a reduction of the death-rate in the future as has been the case in the past, because the limit placed by the natural duration of human life is being more nearly reached with each advance, yet it may be said that almost as much remains to be done as has been accomplished in the immediate past. Notwithstanding the increased strain which is associated with the complexity of modern civilized life, there is no inherent reason why the death-rate, even in such a densely populated city as New York, should not be reduced to 14 or 15 per thousand, or even less, and the average duration of human life increased to fifty years or more.

In speaking of sanitary authorities in relation to the medical profession I desire to refer more especially to the Board of Health of New York City and its relation to those who practice medicine it this city. I would not be understood as speaking for the Health Department, but wish to give only my personal impressions as one of its officials.

The attitude of the Board of Health of New York City toward the medical profession has been in many respects more advanced than that of any other sanitary body in the world. The broad position has been taken that it is the function of the Health Department to furnish to physicians all such specific and general information and assistance in relation to the infectious diseases as can be afforded by thoroughly equipped bacteriologic laboratories, in which the work is fully abreast of the most recent observations in scientific medicine. The sanitary authorities of New York City were the first in the world to assume this position, and while their example has been widely followed in the great cities of this country and Greater Britain, yet nowhere else has this position been frankly taken and consistently followed to the extent that it has been here. It has been the attempt of the Health Board to introduce new measures or to adapt existing measures to the new requirements of every additional observation with regard to any of the infectious diseases which had a practical bearing on prophylaxis or therapeutics. Two considerations, as I interpret the action of the Department, have mainly influenced the Board in the adoption of this position: (1) The desire to extend as rapidly as possible the knowledge of the most recent discoveries in regard to the infectious diseases and the means for their restriction, prevention, and cure. (2) The desire to afford the general practitioner of medicine, without charge, such expert assistance and special information as may be useful to him in clinical work, which could not be otherwise obtained, excepting at greatly increased trouble and considerable expense.

It has been the hope of the Board of Health that such a course would materially aid in establishing more cordial and mutually confidential relations between the members of the medical profession of this city and the Health Department, and thus facilitate the work of the Department; and it was thought that the information thus offered would be, in a sense, received in lieu of the money compensation given to private physicians in some countries for reports of births, deaths, and cases of contagious disease. In this country no such compensation is offered; the position assumed being that it is the duty of the physician to make such reports, and that no payment should be received for the discharge of such a duty. Whether this attitude is a proper one or not does not concern us now. My own belief is that the welfare of the community and the rights of the medical profession would be better conserved by the payment of money for reports of the occurrence of births, deaths, marriages, and contagious diseases.

In considering the relations of the sanitary authorities to the medical profession the fact must be kept in mind that the points of view of the Health Department and of the profession are widely separated. The interests of the community, as guarded by the sanitary authorities, and of the individual practitioner of medicine, are apparently divergent, but the real interests of the practitioner, who is at the same time a citizen, are quite in line with those of the community, and it cannot be for one moment assumed that the conscientious, intelligent, and broad-minded physician will view the situation from any point other than that of the community as a whole. Whether the practising physician then arrives at the same conclusion as the Health Board as to the proper course to be pursued by the sanitary authorities will be a question of opinion; there will be harmony of purpose, and, at most, only a difference of opinion as to the methods to be adopted to secure a common object. Considering the apparently diverging interests of the physician and the community, it is not strange that the action of the Health Board and the position adopted by it in relation to some of the infectious diseases should be the subject of criticism by members of the profession.

But physicians apparently often think that radical measures are adopted by the Board of Health after too little consideration and without a full knowledge of all the facts bearing upon the situation—a much fuller knowledge than, from the nature of the conditions, the members of the medical profession can possibly possess. Consequently, the Health Department is severely and often very unjustly criticised for a course which is the only logical one, and one wholly justified when all of the facts are taken into consideration. The medical profession sometimes forgets that the Health Board legislates and acts for the whole city, not for special sections or for individuals; that many measures which are not demanded or necessary in the best portions of the city are required for the well-being of the inhabitants of the tenement-house districts, and also that special legislation is generally objectionable, must be very carefully restricted, and only resorted to when it has an absolutely special application.

Great discretion has always been exercised in enforcing sanitary measures and the provisions of the Sanitary Code in New York City, and much greater liberty is allowed in private houses than in tenement-houses, because of the lessened danger to the public as a whole. It has never been the policy of the Health Department to interfere in any way in the management of cases of contagious disease occurring in private houses as long as there is no exposure of persons outside of the patient's family. The Department requires that such precautions shall be taken as will protect persons outside from possible infection, but in the family the Department does not interfere. This has always been the policy and the course pursued; but it does not seem to have been fully understood by many of the members of the medical profession.

Physicians occasionally criticise the Health Department for indiscretion or want of judgment on the part of its employees. These criticisms are often justifiable, but unfortunately, they are not, as a rule, made directly to the Health Board, so that the facts may be determined and any wrongs or defects remedied; often they are facts made known through the medical journals or through discussions in the medical societies, and thus, only long after the occurrence the Board becomes aware, indirectly, of the cause of the complaint. There are over two hundred physicians in the employ of the Department, all appointed after passing a civil-service examination. Their instructions are always definite, specific, and detailed as regards duties, and all employees of the department are strictly held to account for their actions. Judgment and discretion cannot be furnished to its employees by the Health Board, or by any other body. Every possible precaution is taken to prevent any just cause for complaint, and each and every one is most carefully investigated, and, so far as is possible, the cause removed and the errors corrected. The Board, however, cannot remedy defects which are not brought to its knowledge. Investigation has also shown in many cases in which complaints have been directly made to the Board that the physicians have been misled by the statements of the patient or family, or by lack of knowledge of all of the facts in the case. The greatest cause for misunderstanding and complaint arises from the fact that only with rare exceptions can physicians be induced to read the circulars of information issued by the Department in regard to its work and the methods pursued. Most of the unsatisfactory results in the work of the bacteriologic laboratories are due to the failure on the part of physicians to follow specifically the directions given. It is impossible where examinations are made from several hundred cases each day, as frequently occurs, to attain anything like a reliable service unless the specific and definite directions given are accurately followed. Still, I think it may be fairly said, that as a whole the work of the Health Department of New York City during recent years has deserved and received the commendation of the large majority of the medical profession of this city.

The duties and reponsibilities of the sanitary authorities with relation to the general public are numerous and comprehensive. To a very great extent the general welfare of the community is in their hands. Everything which is detrimental to health or dangerous to life, most broadly interpreted, is properly regarded as coming within their province, and so wide should be the construction of the law that everything which improperly or unnecessarily interferes with the comfort or enjoyment of life, as well as those things which are detrimental to health or dangerous to life, should become the subject of consideration and action. Sanitary authorities must protect the community from the individual, "the greatest good to the greatest number" furnishing the first rule of action. They must ensure the safety of the community as a whole, and, so far as possible, of each person in it, by protection of the community from its component parts, and then again from each other. The interests of the individual and of the community are often divergent, or apparently divergent; for example, in factories and noxious trades, the observation of such sanitary precautions as are necessary for the protection of the health of employees often involves serious expenditures which fall upon the owners. Again, the welfare of the individual frequently requires such changes in the physical condition of property—tenement-houses for example—as the tenants would not themselves demand. In cases of contagious disease it may sometimes be to the interest of the individual to be left in his own home, while the good of the community urgently requires his removal to an isolation hospital. It becomes at once evident, in all such instances and many similar ones, that it is the plain duty of the sanitary authorities to exercise judiciously, but firmly, the autocratic powers given to them by law. They should not interfere in regulating individual action, at least only to a very limited degree, unless such action involves danger or detriment to the community.

A glance at the functions performed by sanitary authorities shows how broad is their scope: Primarily, sanitary science aims to insure to a community and to each individual an abundant and pure supply of air, light, water, and wholesome food. In the great aggregations of population found in our large cities the preservation of the purity of the air and insurance of an abundance of light and good ventilation involves most comprehensive measures relating to the character of the habitations—their cleanliness and the cleanliness of their surroundings, including the streets; the provision of efficient plumbing; good sewerage; sufficient air-space to the individual, that is, the prevention of overcrowding; protection against noxious vapors or odors arising from offensive trades, slaughter-houses, gas-houses, decomposing animal and vegetable matter, and the purity of the atmosphere, so far as suspended solid particles are concerned.

These functions of the sanitary authorities are performed through official inspections made by inspectors of plumbing, ventilation, overcrowding, nuisances, noxious trades, and by the general sanitary inspectors. An abundant and pure water-supply is one of the first and most essential factors in insuring healthfulness in a large community. Without this, cleanliness, in a broad sense, is impossible; and, of course, cleanliness is the first consideration in all sanitary work. Further, the purity of the water-supply is a most important factor in the prevention of many forms of water-borne disease. New York City is particularly fortunate in this respect; no great city of the world has a more abundant or purer water-supply. In this connection we must not confuse what is unpalatable to the taste or appearance with actual purity. At certain seasons of the year the Croton water is unattractive in appearance and has a disagreeable odor and taste, due to suspended vegetable matter. There is no evidence, however, to show that this is really detrimental to health.

It is also incumbent upon the sanitary authorities to prevent adulteration and to guarantee the wholesome quality of food. This is attained through specially trained inspectors of meat, milk, fish, fruit, and general foods. The purity and quality of various drinks must be inquired into, and the relative food values of different articles of diet determined. Not only must an abundant supply of light, pure air, and water be insured in the homes of the individuals of the community, but the same must be found where they are engaged in their daily occupation, in factories, mercantile establishments, etc.; all the sanitary conditions surrounding these must be supervised.

The general sanitary inspections include inspections relating to street excavations, wells, privies, stables, the conditions surrounding the removal of garbage and dead animals; conditions in public places and places of assembly; the manner and place of burial, etc.

A special feature of the work relates to the restriction and prevention of infectious diseases. Personal and general cleanliness is to be regarded as a most important and almost universally valuable safeguard against all forms of infection, yet the most ingeniously devised systems of plumbing, drainage, and street-cleaning cannot avail to protect the individual from direct contagion. The greatest value of the system of notification of the existence of contagious disease is due to the fact that it enables the authorities to adopt intelligent and scientific measures to prevent the direct transmission of contagion. Their energies are not then wasted in ill-conceived and inefficient measures. It should be clearly understood that the reporting of the occurrence of infectious diseases is most useful only when the direct causes of the diseases reported and the methods of their transmission are accurately known and amenable to control. The public, and even the medical profession, have not yet fully learned the lesson, though it seems almost axiomatic, that different diseases require to be controlled by different methods, and the more accurate and extensive our knowledge of the nature and causes of the different infectious diseases the more unlike become the intelligent measures devised for their prevention.

The condition of the general sanitary administration in this country now much resembles that existing in Great Britain twenty-five years ago, previous to the enactment of the Public Health Act of 1872. There is everywhere lacking the presence of intelligent, thoroughly trained sanitary officers, because there are no provisions in this country for the education of men in matters of public health. The knowledge required for the intelligent discharge of the duties of medical officers of health is broad, comprehensive, and entirely unlike that required for a medical adviser. There is, so far as I am aware, no place in this country where the complete training required can be obtained. Consequently, outside of the large cities the medical officers are generally physicians without special knowledge, experience, or ability in the performance of the work required. Unfortunately, too, the compensation is insufficient and the tenure of office insecure, frequently depending upon local political influences. It, therefore, becomes almost impossible that such officers should act in the prompt, firm, and fearless manner often required, and especially is this true when the interests of persons prominent in the community are jeopardized by their action. The community, in other words, must suffer because the interests of its prominent members are different from those of the people at large. In regard to even the larger towns and cities all this may be said with almost equal force.

There are no men to be found anywhere in this country with a broad knowledge of public medicine. In the great cities there are officers in the service of the health departments who, from practical experience and long training, have acquired the special knowledge requisite for the efficient discharge of duties in a narrow sphere of work. But even in the large cities none are to be found whose knowledge covers the whole sphere of public medicine. The great sanitary need of the time is for the establishment of training-schools in public health (similar to those existing in Great Britain), the education of physicians in the special knowledge required, and the enactment in the various States of laws requiring that medical officers of health should have diplomas in public health, such diplomas representing the requisite sanitary knowledge; and those not possessing such credentials should not be eligible for public-health appointments. The compensation for sanitary work should be larger, the tenure of office more secure, and the appointments made by State or National authorities, rather than dependent upon local influences.

As the country grows older and more densely populated, the cities larger and more crowded, the demand for intelligence in the administration of sanitary affairs will become more urgent. In addition to the improvement in local conditions, there should be added a National supervision exercised through a properly constituted National Bureau or Department of Health. With the fulfilment of these two requirements in the future, we may hope finally to attain more nearly ideal sanitary conditions throughout the whole land.

MEDICAL PROGRESS.

A Case of Tetanus.—J. RUDIS-JICINSKY (*N. Y. Med. Jour.*, Nov. 13, 1897) describes a case of tetanus following a bite in the thigh produced by a boar. Five hours later there had already developed stiffness of the muscles of the neck and jaws and tonic spasms of the diaphragm. The temperature in the axilla was 99° F. The wound was thoroughly curetted and irrigated with a strong solution of potassium permanganate, followed by hydrozone, and was then dressed with iodoform gauze and equal parts of iodoform and calomel. Forty grains of bromid of potassium and large doses of morphin were given every two hours, while chloroform was administered during the spasms. Twenty-four hours later treatment with antitoxin was commenced, about 40 c.c. being given every day for five days. Up to the time of the first injection the spasms had recurred with unpleasant regularity. From that time on they became lighter, and the intervals between them longer. The patient recovered.

The Best Gauze for Drainage.—HALL (*Boston Med. and Surg. Jour.*, Nov. 18, 1897), who has been testing the capilliary power of different gauzes, finds that wicking or cordine has a decided advantage over ordinary gauze wicking as it contains in a small compass a maximum number of longitudinal threads. In ordinary gauze each transverse thread proves a little obstacle to the upward progress of fluids. "A study lamp," says the writer, "which burns a pint of oil during an evening may teach a lesson in drainage. In most lamp-wicks the threads all run as nearly longitudinally as is consistent with stability of the fabric. Steps have already been taken toward securing the manufacture of an absorbent tape on the principle of the selvage. Such a tape, it is hoped, will supplant the faulty gauze drain."

Omental Grafts.—JORDAN (*Lancet*, October 30, 1897) used omental grafts in sixteen cases of intestinal resection in dogs. In every case their application worked disadvantageously. In dogs killed a short time after operation the omental graft was found to be thickened and adherent to surrounding coils of intestines. Later, it was changed into a dense fibrous ring which either constricted the lumen of the bowel or, contracting longitudinally, produced a sharp angle in the intestine, or threw the mucous membrane into folds, or by extensive adhesions with other coils of intestines so matted them together as to make their separation difficult or even impossible. Such conditions, even if they are not followed by obstruction of the bowel, cause so much disability and pain, that the practice of covering intestinal sutures with omental grafts should never be resorted to.

A Case of Combined Intra- and Extra-uterine Pregnancy at Term.—ROYSTER (*Amer. Jour. Obstet.*, December, 1897) reports that a negress, aged thirty-four years, was delivered by a midwife of a healthy male child. Forty-eight hours afterward, inasmuch as the midwife felt in the abdomen another child which she was unable to deliver, she sent for a physician, who, by introducing his hand into the uterus, made out that a living fetus at term was outside of this organ. He advised operation, which was refused. The fetus lived more than a week, and then movements ceased. One week later, as the woman's temperature had begun to rise and death seemed imminent, she consented to operation. Celiotomy was performed, and a female child weighing four and one-half pounds was successfully removed. The placenta with its membranes was attached to the anterior abdominal wall, and it would not have been necessary to open the peritoneal cavity in order to remove the whole. This was done, however, accidentally. The patient recovered. The history in this case reveals the fact that during the third month of pregnancy, while squatting down to pass urine, the patient had had a sharp pain in the right side which caused her to call for help. She fell, half-fainting, and was carried into the house and put to bed, but recovered within a few hours. There was no external loss of blood.

A Curved Hypodermic Needle.—LEGRAND (*Bull. Gen. de Therapeut.*, Nov. 8, 1897) suggests that the use of a long curved hypodermic needle will enable the operator to more perfectly anesthetize with cocain those surfaces of the body which are difficult of access, especially the anal region. Such a needle has been tried by several European surgeons with the greatest satisfaction.

THE MEDICAL NEWS.

A WEEKLY JOURNAL

OF MEDICAL SCIENCE.

COMMUNICATIONS are invited from all parts of the world. Original articles contributed *exclusively* to THE MEDICAL NEWS will after publication be liberally paid for (accounts being rendered quarterly), or 250 reprints will be furnished in place of other remuneration. When necessary to elucidate the text, illustrations will be engraved from drawings or photographs furnished by the author. Manuscripts should be typewritten.

Address the Editor: J. RIDDLE GOFFE, M.D.,
No. 111 FIFTH AVENUE (corner of 18th St.), NEW YORK.

Subscription Price, including postage in U. S. and Canada.

PER ANNUM IN ADVANCE	\$4.00
SINGLE COPIES	.10
WITH THE AMERICAN JOURNAL OF THE MEDICAL SCIENCES, PER ANNUM	7.50

Subscriptions may begin at any date. The safest mode of remittance is by bank check or postal money order, drawn to the order of the undersigned. When neither is accessible, remittances may be made, at the risk of the publishers, by forwarding in *registered* letters.

LEA BROTHERS & CO.,
No. 111 FIFTH AVENUE (corner of 18th St.), NEW YORK, AND NOS. 706, 708 & 710 SANSOM ST., PHILADELPHIA.

SATURDAY, JANUARY 8, 1898.

RECENT TYPHOID-FEVER EPIDEMICS.

THE serious outbreak of typhoid fever at Paterson, N. J., and in its neighborhood, caused as it was by a tainted milk-supply requires no comment on that account, but it brings into glaring light a most astonishing lack of proper dairy and milk inspection here at our very doors. First, the dairyman's three sons were ill with what had been carelessly diagnosticated "remittent fever," but which in reality was typhoid, and were allowed to continue their work in the dairy for a month. Secondly, the dairy inspection has been so outrageously lax that a large dairy supplying Paterson, Arlington, Dover, Newark, Morristown, the Oranges, Jersey City, and New York, was allowed to draw its water for all purposes, washing the utensils, cans, etc., *from a small stream, taking its water through a pipe only twelve feet below the outlet of the drain-pipe from the dairyman's privy.* Thirdly, the criminal carelessness of the proprietor who used water which he must have known was in imminent danger of being infected at any moment. Fourthly, the entire absence of any law in New Jersey requiring physicians in the country districts to report cases of infectious and contagious disease. To point out these salient points ought to be sufficient to bring speedy reform. Comment is unnecessary.

Even typhoid epidemics have their humorous side. A large number of the typhoid cases in Paterson were traced to ice cream which had been prepared from milk from the above-mentioned dairy, and which had been eaten at a "pure-food show" inaugurated by the good denizens of the town to show what they could do in that line. They did it.

The second epidemic to which we desire to call attention is that at Maidstone, England, in which up to date there have been nearly 2000 cases. As is usual in large epidemics, this was spread by water, the lake from which the water was drawn for the larger part of the town having been infected, through a camp of hop pickers. The percentage of cases is based upon the population of the entire town, but if the number of inhabitants of the central district, which was not supplied with the contaminated water, was known, it would show that in the parts of the town where the infected Farleigh water was drunk the percentage of cases was very much higher. The curious thing in connection with this epidemic is the significant immunity enjoyed by that part of the town which contained 17,000 persons, or nearly one-third of the entire population, there having been in this district up to date but thirty-five cases. To be sure, this particular section of the city was not supplied with the Farleigh water, but there was probably not a single inhabitant of the central district who had not relatives, friends, or business connections living in one or more of the districts which did use the Farleigh water, and they must have consumed a great deal of it at one time or another in going about their daily avocations, and yet there were only thirty-five cases in this district, as opposed to 1073 in the districts immediately surrounding. It does, therefore, seem as if the inhabitants of this locality were for some reason or other less susceptible, and in the course of his investigation the *Lancet's* commissioner made a special study of this point, and found that the epidemic was not only limited to those districts supplied with the Farleigh water, but established the curious fact that the greater number of cases occurred in the *higher parts* of those districts which were higher than the rest of the town, and this was particularly the case at the commencement of the epidemic. The second characteristic fact noted was that the epidemic did not coincide with the distribution of the Farleigh water-supply only, but also with the higher altitudes.

It seems curious that while it is generally considered more healthy to live on high ground, the reverse seems to have been proven in the epidemic under consideration. This fact, however, has been noted before, as in Paris, where much typhoid fever has been noticed in such high districts as Belleville, Montmartre, and Les Batignolles, while the low-lying quarters near the Seine were comparatively free from the disease. This fact was explained by the Paris authorities on the ground that the sewer air traveled upward and that a greater volume of sewer air forced itself into the mains draining into the upper extremities of the sewer, and this would also seem to explain the fact that the Maidstone epidemic was almost exclusively confined to the higher parts of the city.

The *Lancet's* commissioner, however, finds that the manner in which the sewers of Maidstone are built and laid does not confirm this theory, and he calls attention to the fact that the great majority of sewers in Maidstone are pipe, that is to say, very small sewers, whereas, in Paris, the sewers are usually very large with proportionately less water, and hence, the downward flow does not prevent an upward current of air, whereas, when the sewer is small and the pipe nearly full of water, there is sufficient friction caused by the downward rush of the water to attract the air of the sewer-gases. It, therefore, would follow the flow of the water, and go down instead of up. While this is true, it seems that in Maidstone the sewer-pipes, though small, are poorly flushed, and the discharge of sewage is irregular, and though the air would probably travel downward in the morning when the sewers are full, it would scarcely be the case at night when the pipes are empty. And hence there would unquestionably be a steady flow of sewer-gas drawn by the warm air upward and into the houses, more especially at night, in houses in the higher portion of the town. It is at night that sewer air, as we know, produces the most deadly results, for there is naturally less free ventilation and the power of resistance of the sleeper is probably not so great as that of the person awake. Add to these considerations the fact that the domestic drainage of Maidstone is in anything but a good condition and that there are many closets without any flushing apparatus, and there are produced the favorable circumstances which weakened the resistance to typhoid infection when introduced by the medium of the contaminated water-supply in those who lived in houses in the higher parts of the city.

It also appears from the work of the commissioner that the sewers of Maidstone are so laid that they are much more likely to act as ventilators for the main sewers which flow through the lower part of the city, than those which flow through the central or non-infected district. The conclusion to which he comes is that under the conditions, it was most essential that the investigations, whether concerning the epidemic at Maidstone or elsewhere, should not be limited to the water-supply, for while, naturally, it is first necessary to discover what is the primary cause of the epidemic, so that practical measures may be taken during the emergency to do away with the same, it would be folly to imagine that having done this much no further measures need be adopted, for a town, like a patient, is composed of individual parts which together form the collective whole. Some are strong and wholesome, others are weak and susceptible to disease, and, as the *Lancet* writer says, the duty of sanitary science is to discover and remove the cause of this condition.

The Farleigh water-supply of Maidstone is in the hands of a private company. The fact occurs to us that the terrible epidemic in Duluth, Minn., occurred at a time when the water-supply was in the hands of a private company, and the officers of the company denied that their water-supply was the cause of the infection and refused to move in the matter. In this case it was known that the intake-pipe was not at a very great distance from the emptying sewer-pipe in the lake, although it extended out a much greater distance. The officers insisted that it was sufficiently far away to be perfectly safe. As the epidemic increased, the citizens took the matter in hand and investigated it for themselves, and lo and behold, they found a break in the intake pipe close to the shore, and at very little distance from the emptying sewer-pipe. There was naturally a political upheaval about it, and the city of Duluth now has its water-supply in its own hands and under the direction of its Health Commissioners.

While there was apparently no such criminal carelessness on the part of the Farleigh water-supply company, at the same time the occurrence should lead us to ask whether the water-supply of all cities should not be operated by the city, under the direction of proper health-officers.

THE PHILADELPHIA MEDICAL JOURNAL.

THE first number of the *Philadelphia Medical Journal* is at hand. Its appearance is pleasing, and its contents varied and interesting. The one new feature which is quite distinctive in a medical weekly is the method of abstracting articles from other journals. Instead of selecting leading articles, certain journals are chosen and brief abstracts of their entire contents are presented, after the now familiar method of the *Medical Review of Reviews*.

In its Announcement the declaration is made that "the Company is to be its own publisher, so that by sins neither of omission nor of commission can commercial interests influence a line of the reading columns. By the advice of experts of national reputation the *Journal* will seek to draw the line against all nostrums in our advertisement columns, in order that from cover to cover the best scientific and ethical standards shall be safeguarded."

This is, indeed, most commendable, and it will be interesting not only to medical editors, but also to the profession at large, to observe how this "band of experts" discriminate between "nostrums" and numerous proprietary preparations, some of which have already found a place in their advertising columus, and have thus received the stamp of their approval. In these iconoclastic days the birth of an ethical arbiter, such as the *Philadelphia Medical Journal* evidently aims to be, marks an epoch in the history of medicine.

THE MEDICAL NEWS cordially welcomes the new journal to the sisterhood of medical weeklies, and predicts for it the meed of success which its enterprise merits and its unquestionable excellence will command.

ECHOES AND NEWS.

Bubonic Plague in Bombay.—Despatches from Bombay report a recrudescence of the plague in the vicinity of that city. Many new cases are daily reported, and many deaths have occurred. Up to date 14,257 cases and 11,882 deaths have been reported in Bombay alone.

Higher Salary Desired.—The subordinate staff of the Paris Medical Faculty have sent to the Deputies and Senators a petition signed by sixty-four medical men asking for an increase of salary.

Bequests to Charity.—By the will of the late Charles H. Contoit, who recently died in New York City, the bulk of his estate, estimated to be worth over $1,000,000, is left to New York charitable institutions.

Pneumonia Transmitted by Parrots.—According to the Paris correspondent of the *British Medical Journal*, seventy cases of psittacosis (pneumonia transmitted by parrots) have occurred in that city and its environs since 1892.

A New Editor for the Columbus Medical Journal.—Dr. H. Harvey Reed has tended his resignation as president, editor, and manager of the Columbus Medical Publishing Company, and Dr. J. E. Brown has been elected editor and manager.

Chinese Medical Maxims.—"The physician who is sure of his diagnosis says little; he who is not sure talks much without being understood." "The greatest enemy to the health of men is woman; the worst enemy to the health of women is man."

Medical Colleges Must Give Bond.—In the State of Pennsylvania all medical colleges are required to give a bond of $1000 as a guarantee that no human bodies will be dissected except those which come to them through the regularly appointed legal channels.

Bequest to the Philadelphia Hospitals.—Mrs. Henrietta R. Fales Baker, whose will was recently probated in Philadelphia, left an estate worth $2,000,000. Should her son and daughter die without issue the whole estate will revert to the University of Pennsylvania and the Pennsylvania Hospital.

Dr. Reed's Appointment.—Dr. Harvey Reed has accepted the position of superintendent and surgeon in charge of the Wyoming General Hospital located at Rock Springs, Wyoming. This hospital is a State institution, and the building, when completed, will have accommodations for eighty patients.

Loomis Sanitarium for Consumptives.—The Building Department recently refused to approve plans for this hospital, soon to be erected in New York City, on the ground that they did not call for a fire-proof building. A writ of mandamus has been applied for to compel the department to approve the plans.

Polhemus Memorial Clinic.—The opening of this institution, which is situated on the southwest corner of Henry and Amity streets, Brooklyn, N. Y., took place on December 30th. The building provides luxurious accommodations for clinic patients, and lecture-rooms and an amphitheater for the use of the Long Island College Hospital.

Obituary.—Dr. Henry Parke Wilson recently died at his home at Baltimore, Md. Dr. Wilson was born in Workington, Md., in 1827. He was graduated from Princeton College, and studied medicine in the University of Virginia and the University of Maryland. He settled in Baltimore in 1851, and practised medicine there until the time of his death.

Sanitary Inspection of Barber-shops.—The Metropolitan Barbers' Association of the State and City of New York have prepared a bill which will be presented to the Legislature in the near future. Among other things the bill provides for a sanitary inspection of all barber-shops and for the appointment of a board of inspectors, to be selected from the ranks of the Association.

A Question of Pronunciation.—A correspondent writes to *The Lancet* (London) pointing out the fact that the usual pronunciation of the word "angina" (an-jai'na) is incorrect. Etymology and metrical usage make it "an-ge'na," with the penult short. The editor of *The Lancet* adds that the 1886 edition of Smith's Small Latin-English Dictionary gives the latter pronunciation of the word.

Preventive Inoculation and Plague.—From the joint report of the recent epidemic plague in Portuguese India, presented by M. Haffkine and Surgeon-Major Lyons, the president of the Bubonic Plague Research Committee, it is seen that the preventive serum was employed with good effect, both as regards limiting the number of persons attacked and in decreasing the mortality. Especially good results were obtained when strong lymph was used.

Dr. O'Dwyer Ill.—The medical profession throughout the world will be pained to learn of the serious illness of Dr. Joseph O'Dwyer of New York, who has contributed so much to diminish the death-rate in laryngeal diphtheria by the invention of his now famous laryngeal tubes. Dr. O'Dwyer has been suffering from what he himself diagnosticates as tuberculous meningitis. His diagnosis has been concurred in by numerous professional brethren who have been called in. Dr. O'Dwyer himself admits the fatal nature of his illness.

A Naval Hospital Corps.—A movement is under way toward the organization of a naval hospital corps similar to that of the army. It is proposed that the corps consist of twenty pharmacists at $75 per month, five at $100; sixty-five hospital stewards at $60; thirty-five first-class hospital apprentices at $24; sixty hospital apprentices at $18; and that naval hospitals be established at Portsmouth, N. H., Chelsea, Mass., Newport, R. I., New York City, Philadelphia, Washington, D. C., Norfolk, Va., Pensacola, Fla., Mare Island, Cal., and Yokohama, Japan.

Dr. Roswell Park.—Our readers will be gratified to learn that Dr. Roswell Park of Buffalo, who has been abroad during his convalescence from a serious septic infection, has returned to his field of labor. While passing through New York City, he called at the editorial office of THE MEDICAL NEWS, and we can, therefore, assure his many friends from personal observation that although the doctor does not present the satisfactory picture of perfect vigor which characterized his former appearance, he gives evidence of being on the way to complete restoration of health.

New Hospital for Contagious Diseases.—The opening of the New York Hospital for Scarlet Fever and Diphtheria, at the foot of East Sixteenth street, took place December 30th. The hospital consists of two pavilions, forming the letter "U," each two stories in height, and built of pressed brick. The laundry and fumigating apparatus are in the center. A special feature is the solarium for the use of convalescent patients. It is situated on the south side of the building and has a wall of heavy plate-glass. There is also a roof-garden. The beds are of iron, the chairs and tables of agate, and the shelves of glass. The hospital was open for patients on the first of January. There are no free beds.

Dr. Sherow a Victim to Cocain Poisoning.—Dr. E. J. Sherow of New York died at his home New-Year's morning from the effects of an overdose of cocain. Dr. Sherow graduated from the College of Physicians and Surgeons of New York in 1890, and supplemented his medical education by hospital experience at the New York, and Nursery and Child's Hospitals. Four years ago the Doctor began treating himself with cocain for the relief of annoying nasal catarrh. Steadily the insidious habit grew upon him, and he became a victim of cocain. Aside from this, it is said his professional prospects were bright. The probabilities are that he took the fatal dose of the drug by mistake.

St. Louis Laryngological and Otological Society.—On December 27th the St. Louis Laryngological and Otological Society was formed, composed of those physicians of St. Louis who limit their practice to the treatment of diseases of the nose, throat, and ear. Dr. J. C. Mulhall was elected president; Dr. J. B. Shapleigh, vice-president; Dr. F. M. Rumboldt, secretary, and Dr. A. S. Barnes, Jr., treasurer, for the year 1898. Meetings will be held monthly, and it is expected that the scientific programs furnished will be highly interesting and instructive. While the membership is limited, the privilege of inviting professional friends is reserved to each member.

Filtration of Milk.—In several European cities, sand filtration of milk is employed at a central depot after its arrival from the country. The filters consist of large cylindrical vessels, divided by horizontal perforated diaphragms into five superposed compartments, of which the middle three are filled with fine clean sand, sifted into three sizes, the coarsest being placed in the lowest, and the finest in the topmost of the three compartments. The milk enters the lowest compartment through a pipe under gravitation pressure, and after having traversed the layers of sand from below upward, is carried by an overflow to a cooler fed with ice water, whence it passes into a cistern from which it is drawn direct into the locked cans for distribution. Milk thus filtered is not only freed from dirt, but the number of bacteria is reduced to about one-third. In new milk the loss of fat is said to be very slight, but the quantity of mucus and slimy matter retained in the sand is surprising. The sand is renewed each time the filter is used.

SPECIAL ARTICLE.

EXAMINATION OF APPLICANTS FOR POSITIONS IN THE MARINE HOSPITAL SERVICE.

A BOARD of officers will be convened at Washington, D. C., January 25, 1898, for the purpose of examining applicants, for admission to the grade of Assistant Surgeon in the United States Marine Hospital Service.

Candidates must be between twenty-one and thirty years of age, graduates of a respectable medical college, and must furnish testimonials from responsible persons as to character.

The following is the usual order of the examination: 1. Physical. 2. Written. 3. Oral. 4. Clinical.

In addition to the physical examination candidates are required to certify that they believe themselves free from any ailment which would disqualify for service in any climate.

The examinations are chiefly in writing, and begin with a short autobiography by the candidate. The remainder of the written exercise consists in examination on the various branches of medicine, surgery, and hygiene.

The oral examination includes subjects of preliminary education, history, literature, and natural sciences.

The clinical examination is conducted at a hospital, and when practicable candidates are required to perform surgical operations upon the cadaver.

Successful candidates will be numbered according to their attainments on examination, and will be commissioned in the same order as vacancies occur.

Upon appointment the young officers are as a rule first assigned to duty at one of the large marine hospitals, as at Boston, New York, New Orleans, Chicago, or San Francisco.

After five-years' service Assistant Surgeons are entitled to examinations for promotion to the grade of Passed-Assistant Surgeon.

Promotion to the grade of surgeon is made according to seniority, and after due examination as vacancies occur in that grade. Assistant surgeons receive $1600. Passed-assistant surgeons, $2000, and surgeons, $2500 a year. When quarters are not provided, commutation at the rate of thirty, forty, or fifty dollars a month, according to grade, is allowed.

All grades above that of assistant surgeon receive longevity pay, *i. e.*, ten percentum in addition to the regular salary for every five-years' service up to forty percentum after twenty-years' service.

The tenure of office is permanent. Officers traveling under orders are allowed actual expenses. For further information, or for invitation to appear before the board of examiners, address Walter Wyman, Supervising Surgeon-General, United States Marine Hospital Service, Washington, D. C.

CORRESPONDENCE.

ANSWER TO DR. WILLY MEYER.

To the Editor of THE MEDICAL NEWS.

DEAR SIR: Please grant me sufficient space in your worthy paper to mention that I reaffirm my statement made in my article on "A New Method of General Anesthesia" regarding the doses in the administration of the Schleich mixture. My claims are based on personal experience which, although not very large, is sufficient to convince me of the correctness of my observations, and to prove that the use of such large amounts of the anesthetic as Dr. Willy Meyer states he uses is wholly unnecessary. Details of my observations will be presented at a later date. Yours very truly,

M. L. MADURO, M.D.

NEW YORK, December 24, 1897.

PRE-COLUMBIAN LEPROSY IN AMERICA.

To the Editor of THE MEDICAL NEWS.

DEAR SIR: I read in your report of the recent Lepra Conference at Berlin that, "He (Virchow) considers that the mutilations observed in certain ornamental figures found on what evidently is Pre-Columbian pottery, point to the existence of leprosy on the American Continent before the Spanish discoveries. There is no other disease which could have produced the mutilations of the feet observed in the figures. The nasal mutilations point to lupus rather than to leprosy, but Professor Virchow called attention to certain faces in Professor Lassar's collection of wax models of Norwegian lepers which very closely resemble those found on the potteries."

This discussion was on my paper: "The Question of Pre-Columbian Leprosy in America." Your reporter, however, fails to give what Dr. Carrasquilla of Colombia had to say on the subject. This South-American doctor, who knows a great deal about South-American history and customs, very probably far more than Professor Virchow, as soon as he saw the photographs which accompanied my paper, said: "The clear cut of the nose and upper lip shown in the pottery faces, and the amputated feet represent punishment inflicted by the Incas for certain crimes." I think that this settles the matter. As Professor Virchow said, "No other disease could have produced the mutilations observed in the feet;" but the sharp sword of an executioner could.

Other mutilations I am inclined to consider as evidences of lupus and syphilis; yet, it is natural to think if the amputated nose and lip are the result of punishment, that the amputated feet are so, too. But then there are marks which point to disease, such as the prognathous jaws, the spinal curvature, the side of the face eaten away, etc., which appear in the amputated-feet images, at least in some of them.

Perhaps this will make Dr. Carrasquilla pause; but, if these signs lead us to suspect disease, they just as naturally make us reject the idea of this disease being leprosy. It may have been facial lupus, tuberculosis of the vertebræ, or syphilis. If leprosy had eaten off the feet, as

Professor Virchow thinks, it would at the same time have mutilated the hands. Now, the hands in all the images are perfect.

I will conclude in a few words: The mutilations shown by my photographs may represent punishment, and some of them lupus, etc., but, Professor Virchow to the contrary notwithstanding, *not leprosy*.

ALBERT S. ASHMEAD, M.D.

NEW YORK, December 26, 1897.

OUR PHILADELPHIA LETTER.

[From our Special Correspondent.]

THE ISOLATION OF THE CRIMINAL INSANE—AGAINST THE ESTABLISHMENT OF A FOUNDLING ASYLUM—PHILADELPHIA NEUROLOGICAL SOCIETY—LARGE CONTINGENT BEQUESTS TO PHILADELPHIA HOSPITALS—DR. F. P. HENRY FOR HEALTH-OFFICER—DR. G. S. WOODWARD APPOINTED A MEMBER OF THE BOARD OF HEALTH—IN MEMORY OF DR. HARRISON ALLEN AND DR. GEORGE H. HORN.

PHILADELPHIA, January 1, 1898.

THE State Board of Charities of Pennsylvania is making a determined effort to establish in this State, by an act of Legislature, a hospital exclusively for the treatment of insane convicts and the criminal insane, there being at the present time 118 of the former, and 158 of the latter class confined, under wholly unfavorable surroundings, in the various State penitentiaries. Between the insane convict and the criminal insane there seems to be a decided difference, according to the general sentiment of the public, which holds that the one is a person who, while insane, commits a criminal offense, while to the other is attached the stigma of criminality prior to the development of insanity. This fine point which is shared by the State law-makers, as well as by the laity at large has been in the past the stumbling-block which has thwarted the efforts of the Board and of others in favor of their project; and their attention at present is directed against this prejudice, in many quarters, of placing these two classes of lunatics in the same category, and in the same institution. The intention is to establish a moderate-sized hospital on the grounds of some one of the State penitentiaries, and to there carry out the efficient plan of caring for the "detained," we will say, insane, which has been so long in vogue at the New York State Hospital for the criminal insane, first at Auburn, and later at the present site at Matteawan.

A unanimous opinion against the advisibility of establishing a foundling asylum in this city was expressed last week at a meeting of several prominent citizens, held to consider this subject, about which considerable agitation is going on in other quarters. Physicians, the law, the clergy, and the laity were represented at this meeting, and declared the founding of such an institution inexpedient, lowering to the general moral standard of the community, and entirely to be deprecated. It remains, however, to see what effect, if indeed any, this protest will have upon the growth of the project. Could the helpless babes abandoned on the vacant lots, or heartlessly consigned to some one else's doorstep have a voice in the matter, which would they prefer, a childhood passed in the precincts of the city almshouse, or the training and care and comforts of an institution devoted to their welfare? And under which of the two surroundings will the name, bastard, be sooner lost ?

At the last meeting of the Philadelphia Neurological Society, held December 20th, Dr. James Hendrie Lloyd exhibited a case of astasia-abasia, occurring in a hysterical woman, who had recently undergone a gynecologic operation. The patient had been confined to bed under the delusion that she was paralyzed, but had improved under suggestive therapeusis, to such an extent that she is now able to walk without support, although incoordination of gait and station was still present. Dr. D. L. Edsall reported, by invitation, a case of dissociation of sensation of the syringomyelic type in Pott's disease. The patient, a boy, in early adolescence, suffered from caries of the second, third, and fourth cervical vertebræ, together with the manifestations of analgesia, thermo-anesthesia, and the preservation of tactile sensation—the dissociation of sensation generally believed to be a characteristic symptom of syringomyelia. The speaker expressed his belief that the lesion causing these symptoms was an intraspinal tumor, probably associated intraspinal tubercle. Dr. W. E. Hughes exhibited, by invitation, a tumor of the pituitary body, and also described a similar case. One of these neoplasms proved to be a small lymphosarcoma; the other a large carcinoma. It is of interest to note that symptoms of acromegaly were absent in both cases. Dr. A. A. Eshner further discussed an interesting case of meningitis which had been presented before the Society at a previous meeting, provoking at the time considerable discussion of the question of the differential diagnosis between basilar meningitis and posterior sclerosis. In the case in question *post-mortem* examination showed that death was due to cerebellar hemorrhage, following a diffuse meningo-encephalitis. Dr. H. M. Schreiner reported an instance of arsenic neuritis, in a choreic girl ten years of age, who, after the administration of moderate amounts of the drug, developed widespread paralysis.

A contingent bequest of the late Henrietta R. Fales Baker bequeaths, in event of the death of her son and daughter without issue, the sum of $2,000,000 to the Pennsylvania Hospital, to erect and maintain a hospital to be known as the Fales Hospital for Surgical and Infirmary for Chronic Diseases. The University Hospital is to receive, under the same terms, $200,000, and the University of Pennsylvania $300,000 to endow professorships in the medical and scientific departments.

Dr. Frederick P. Henry, Professor of Practice of Medicine in the Woman's Medical College of Pennsylvania, is being urged for the position of Health-Officer of this port by those interested in the elimination of this important office from city politics, and it is hoped that Goveruor Hastings will act favorably on the recommendations being made in favor of Dr. Henry's appointment. The resignation of the former incumbent of the office, Theodore B. Stulb, has been "accepted" by the Governor.

Dr. George S. Woodward has been appointed by the Mayor to fill the vacancy in the Philadelphia Board of Health, caused by the death of Dr. William H. Ford.

A special meeting commemorative of the late Doctors Harrison Allen and George H. Horn, the two distinguished scientists, was held by the Academy of the Natural Sciences on December 31st. Addresses were made by Doctors Daniel G. Brinton, Edward S. Nolan, Professor John B. Smith of Rutgers College, and others.

The total number of deaths occurring in this city for the week ending December 25, 1897, was 396, of which 106 were in children under five years of age. Deaths from diphtheria numbered 24; from scarlet fever, 2; and from enteric fever, 15. The general health of the city is fair, and the number of new cases of zymotic diseases is on the decline, as compared to previous weeks reported.

The annual report of the Registration Division of the Bureau of Health for the year 1897 shows that the total number of deaths in Philadelphia last year was 22,735, or a ratio of 18.72 per thousand inhabitants. This proves to be the lowest annual death-rate recorded here since 1879, when the ratio was 17.37 per thousand. During the past year there were 1231 deaths from diphtheria, or an increase of 369 fatal cases over 1896; 282 deaths from scarlet fever, an increase of 221 over 1896; and 401 fatal cases of enteric fever. Pulmonary tuberculosis caused the death of 2388 persons, while the victims of influenza, which was not considered to have been especially prevalent during the last twelve months, numbered 160. The past year, among other things, witnessed 20 homicides and 143 suicides within the city limits.

OUR BERLIN LETTER.

[From our Special Correspondent.]

LECTURES TO THE UNIVERSITY STUDENTS OF ALL DEPARTMENTS ON "THE SIGNIFICANCE AND PROPHYLAXIS OF VENEREAL DISEASES"—THE THERAPEUTIC INFLUENCE OF CONGESTION AND INFLAMMATION—UNCOOKED FISH AND PARASITIC AND MICROBIC DISEASES—NOMENCLATURE OF BACILLI AFTER VARIOUS DISCOVERERS.

BERLIN, December 31, 1897.

PROFESSOR LASSAR is at present delivering the best-attended lectures at the University of Berlin. Nearly a thousand students of all faculties, mainly, however, non-medical men, will be found in the largest lecture-room of the principal University building any Tuesday evening, listening with every appearance of the greatest interest. The subject is "The Significance and Prophylaxis of Venereal Diseases." These lectures have now been given during the past three years, and the opposition manifested toward them in certain university circles before their institution and during the first months, when they were on probation, has faded away before the evident beneficial effect of accurate knowledge on subjects of such immense practical importance.

There is no danger, in the present state of our knowledge of venereal diseases, that "familiarity will breed contempt." Additions to our knowledge during the past fifteen years have practically revolutionized opinions as to the results of venereal infection of whatever kind. The significance of venereal diseases has become much more comprehensive, and the idea that they are a passing event in the life of mortals, that, like the diseases of childhood and colds in the head which nearly every one must go through and which almost never have any serious consequences, is now entertained only by those who are not abreast of the times.

No better sermon could be preached to the ordinary young man thrown for the first time on his own responsibility amid the temptations of a great city, for universities, fortunately or unfortunately, are, in our day, situated in large cities, than the inculcation of a clear, succinct idea of the present state of medical knowledge with regard to venereal diseases and their immediate and remote consequences. It would almost seem to be the duty of university authorities to furnish the opportunity for the acquirement of such knowledge as a safeguard of health quite as much as the encouragement of athletics.

Here university responsibility in the matter has been squarely faced and met by the establishment of a special lectureship, supported by an extraordinary government provision for the purpose. The matter is excellently placed in Professor Lassar's hands. The interest has never waned, and there is always, as previously mentioned, a large and appreciative audience at the lectures.

No exaggeration is required to make the fearful cousequences of venereal disease clear, and there has been, on the other hand, no mincing of matters in the lecturer's descriptions. The lectures are illustrated by stereoscopic pictures, and in the first lecture of the course, for example, after the diplococcus of Neisser, as found in a recent case of gonorrhea, had been exhibited, the same organism from a case some fifteen years old, where its existence was absolutely unsuspected by the patient, was shown. The conjugal infection that had followed all unwittingly, and the consequent innocent suffering involved was dwelt upon. Some of the statistics of serious diseases of the female pelvic organs which have been traced to such infections were given. The personal experience of even the youngest of the men was appealed to as furnishing examples of young and healthy women falling victims to insidious disease shortly after marriage, the root of the trouble, not being some obscure woman's ailment, insidiously developing no one knew how, but, in reality, an infectious remnant of a husband's gonorrhea, existing very often without his knowledge.

To most young men such information comes as a distinct surprise. Information of the most varied kind, from quacks and mountebanks, from advertisements, and so-called medical books he has had, but the evident purpose to exploit his failings has led him to distrust it all. Plain talk from a man thoroughly conversant with the subject, utterly trustworthy and disinterestedly solicitous, he heartily welcomes.

It is an interesting study to watch the students' faces while they hear such home truths as that a gonorrheal infection may continue many years, or may finally end fatally in involvement of important membranes, or that most of the so-called women's diseases, with their necessitated mutilating therapeutics, and 80 to 90 per cent. of the blindness in the world, is the result of innocently acquired gonorrheal infection. Such information puts in a new light a host of things which before seemed trivial, and shows their real importance. When to all this is added the fearful significance of syphilis in the development of the hopelessly incurable nervous diseases, from the apoplexies to paresis in middle life to tabes and the varied results of arterial degeneration in later years, a wonderful lesson is taught. A lesson, too, that under present circumstances is owed to every young man; for the unknown dangers of life, with their inevitable cousequences, are plentiful enough already without leaving him in the dark on a subject like this, where definite knowledge is ready at hand and prophylaxis a comparatively simple matter.

Such a course of lectures would be eminently suitable for our large American universities. That they would be well attended no one would think of doubting. That they would do great good seems just as indubitable. The candid admission, however, of the imminence of the danger to young men is not in accord with Anglo-Saxon principles generally in such matters, and so, it may be supposed, the suggestion of such a thing to most university faculties would be met by prompt discouragement. Some time, however, in the near future the wisdom of such a course of action will dawn upon educators who are sincerely interested in the student's welfare, and then young America, too, will have the chance to learn these important truths.

Dr. Hamburger has just published some very interesting investigations of the influence of congestion and inflammation on bacterial life (*Deutsche Med. Wochenschrift*). He starts with the observation, which has now been confirmed upon all sides, that patients with mitral stenosis very seldom acquire tuberculosis of the lungs; while, on the contrary, those affected by congenital pulmonary stenosis almost invariably are ultimately carried off by this disease. He finds that, while jugular serum—*i. e.*, the serum of blood drawn from the jugular vein—is much more bactericidal than ordinary serum taken from blood-vessels at the periphery of the body, carotid serum (from the internal carotid) is much less bactericidal in character.

He has found, too, that when CO_2 is added to ordinary serum its bactericidal properties are much increased. This procedure adds, of course, to the alkalescence of the serum. He calls attention to the fact, which Behring and Cantani and other distinguished serum-therapeutists have already pointed out, that increase of alkalescence in animal serum increases its protective power.

Dr. Hamburger thinks that there is here the explanation of certain phenomena of inflammatory processes, and points out that the congestion incident to these is perhaps a protective reaction on the part of Nature which may well deserve imitation in local infections. He finds, too, that in such processes there are changes in both red and white blood-cells, notably a swelling and irregularity of outline which is accompanied by the giving off of CO_2, which is obviously, to his mind, only another phase of this natural protective process.

Among the varieties of food which have been the subject of investigation, fish has not had as important a place as some others. The epidemics of typhoid fever which have occurred during recent years have called attention to the fact that shell-fish constitutes almost the only animal article of diet which is now consumed uncooked. The necessity for extreme caution and the advisability of eating this variety of food only when cooked, unless one knows the origin, just as with water, is being insisted upon.

Attention has also been called to the fact that there are certain forms of smoked fish often consumed uncooked which are equally liable to be infected with the morbid element of various infections and communicable diseases, and that the process of smoking does not destroy the vitality of the unwelcome additions to the fish. Certain of the Baltic provinces of Germany have had quite a few cases of fish tapeworm, bothriocephalus latus, and some scattered cases throughout the Empire have been observed as the result of the more careful diagnostic methods of recent years. A note of warning has recently been sounded, and it would seem as though fish will soon come in for as careful government investigation, here in Germany at least, as do other animal foods.

The nomenclature of bacilli does not grow more satisfactory as time goes on and the field widens. More than one bacteriologist has lately been outspoken in the hope that a botanic classification of bacteria may soon replace the personal nomenclature which is so utterly unscientific and so varying under different circumstances. It is really the general practitioner and the specialist in other lines who have just cause for complaint. It is they who find it more than annoying, for it is often positively confusing. The calling the bacillus of tuberculosis Koch's bacillus may seem unpardonable enough to those who know better, but it has been known to occur even here. In a recent work on laryngology the bacillus of typhoid fever is called Gaffky's bacillus, with never a word of Eberth. The honor of having their names attached to the microbes of diphtheria and pneumonia is divided among four men, while the world knows that there are least four others, one of them an American, who equally deserve the honor. This faulty method will continue, it may be persumed, until, as in anatomy, an organized effort at systematization will have to be made, and then the adopted nomenclature will be as slow in finding its way into general use as have the results of the very meritorious effort of the anatomic committee in the same direction. Here, meantime, every step toward a purely scientific classification and nomenclature from the botanic standpoint is receiving deservedly widespread encouragement.

TRANSACTIONS OF FOREIGN SOCIETIES.

London.

IMMEDIATE REDUCTION OF ANGULAR DEFORMITY OF THE SPINE—PREVENTION OF ENTERIC FEVER—PNEUMOTHORAX OF SOME MONTHS' DURATION CURED BY FREE INCISION—MECHANOTHERAPY OF MOVABLE KIDNEY—HERNIA OF THE ABDOMINAL CICATRIX AND THE OPERATIONS FOR ITS CURE—EMPYEMA OF THE ANTRUM OF HIGHMORE.

THE Clinical Society at its meeting of November 26th continued the discussion of CALOT'S paper on *immediate reduction of angular deformity of the spine.* Those members who expressed themselves as opposed to this operation base their objections chiefly on theoretic grounds, and besides, claim that the good results reported are of too short a duration, to enable the deduction of safe conclusions. CLARKE insisted that it is bad policy to keep a patient in a plaster jacket, as Calot's plan necessitates. Those who advocated the operation pointed to the success which Calot has had in more than 600 cases. THOMAS said that the theoretic objections that such treatment might produce (1) paraplegia, or (2) abscesses, or (3) dissemination of tubercle have all been proved to be groundless. Only one objection remains, *viz.*, that Nature cannot fill the "gap" with new bone; but as she is quite able to accomplish this in other bones in which surgeons have caused a solution of continuity, there seems no reason to doubt her ability to do the same in the spine.

At a meeting of the Royal Medical and Chirurgical Society, November 23d, POORE opened a discussion upon he *prevention of enteric fever*, by stating that the contagion of enteric fever is contained in excreta, and may gain access to the bodies of the healthy by means of drink, food, or inspired air. Records were given of forty-six instances, occurring during the last thirty years, in which epidemics followed contamination of public water-supplies. Attention was called to the possibility of pollution, often facilitated by the bad practice of laying water- and sewer-pipes side by side, neither being open to inspection. Pollution at the periphery is liable to occur whenever a tap is left turned on, and a vacuum thus produced in the supply-pipe by intermission of the supply, so that gas, or water, or even solids, may be drawn back into the house-pipe, Thus, in one house the water-pipe at certain times yielded blood, which was sucked into an open tap in a slaughter-house next door. It must be remembered that in big towns there are many foul places other than water-closets over which there may be open taps. A few of the practical remedies suggested were: the maintenance by water companies, just as by large dairies, of a staff of chemists and bacteriologists; the separation of water- and sewer-pipes, and the location of them as far as possible in subways; cremation of excreta in country places, or the scattering of this material upon suitable soils, when, under the influence of sun and rain, aided by frequent light plowing, such material soon becomes harmless. As enteric fever is preeminently a water-borne disease, the excreta from patients having it should never be mixed with water, as the property of water is to return to its source. There can be no purity of soil without tillage, and organic filth must be placed upon the humus to increase the food-supply, and not beneath it to endanger the water-supply. At present our population is silently taught that the only decent way to treat feces is to mix them with water to brew sewer-gas, and thus insure the aerial, as well as the aquatic, convection of enteric fever.

THORNE did not admit that the conclusions of Poore in regard to the danger of the present systems of water and sewage are correct, and in support of his position he quoted statistics to prove that the death-rate from typhoid fever is less than half of what it was under the old systems of wells and privies. No doubt the spreading of normal stools upon frequently tilled fresh soil in a short time destroys all enteric bacilli; but it has not been shown that this is a safe practice to follow in disposing of infected sewage. Experiments have shown that though typhoid bacilli will grow only a few days in sterilized virgin soil, they will grow 200 days in sewage-soaked soil which has not been similarly sterilized.

BOYCE made a plea for more thorough bacteriologic examination, which he regards as the real safeguard of a community from epidemics of enteric fever.

At a meeting of the Medical Society, November 22d, WEST read a paper on a *case of pyopneumothorax of some months' duration cured by free incision.* About four pints of seropurulent fluid were removed, and the patient rapidly improved, though a tube was kept *in situ* seven months. As a rule such cases are left alone from a belief that the lung is bound down by adhesions. The reader cited several cases to show that this view is by no means always correct. Another false notion is that pneumothorax is generally associated with tuberculosis of the lung, and that the pressure of the air or fluid in the pleural cavity will arrest the development of tubercle, a view absolutely without foundation, though it was once held in regard to serous or purulent collections in the chest. In short, the presence of air does not effect the principles of treatment in case of fluid in the pleural cavity.

BOWLES said that the position of the patient with the sound side upward is of great importance during anesthesia in pyopneumothorax. Two cases have been recently recorded, in each of which death followed the turning of the sound side of the patient upward to facilitate operative procedures, death being due to a flow of pus into the bronchial tubes of the sound lung.

ECCLES read a paper on the *mechanotherapy of movable kidney.* Sixteen patients were treated by means of "rest," with especial attention to abdominal massage and exercise during periods varying from two to eight weeks. Seven of these patients disappeared from observation; in one instance the treatment was a complete failure, but the remaining patients almost immediately improved, and five of them were greatly, and to all appearances, permanently benefited by abdominal massage, exercises, and the application of a pad and belt. It is of importance that the displaced kidney be replaced as early as possible and kept in its normal position. Replacement is best secured when the patient lies upon the sound side, flexes the thigh of the affected side acutely on the abdomen, and extends the arm of that side well above the head.

DORAN read a paper before the Harveian Society, November 18th, on *hernia of the abdominal cicatrix and operations for its cure*, in which he took the ground that such conditions may be most satisfactorily relieved by suture of the abdominal wall in layers, avoiding a too deep suture in the peritoneum, in which case this membrane may be everted and an actual hernial pouch produced. The edge of the rectus muscle should be included in the aponeurotic suture.

ROUGHTON read a paper on *empyema of the antrum*

of Highmore. The essentials of treatment were stated to be: (*a*) a removal of the cause by dealing with nasal or dental disease; (*b*) evacuation and drainage of pus; (*c*) antiseptic irrigation, and (*d*) removal of morbid tissue (when present) from the antrum. He advocated that an alveolar tube be fitted in every case. The points which SPICER regards as essential to the success of a radical operation are: (1) a large opening through the canine fossa; (2) thorough curettement of the diseased antral mucosa; (3) very free counter-opening from the nose into the antrum, and (4) no drainage apparatus (the air-blast sufficing to clear the antrum of pus until the mucosa is healthy). No bad results, certainly no sinking of the cheek, had occurred in any of his cases.

Berlin.

ADVANTAGES OF CELLULOID-TRICOT-CORSETS.

At the session of the Medical Society, on November 10th, JACQUES spoke of *the advantages of the celluloid-tricot-corset.* Celluloid has ordinarily been employed upon wide strips of mull in order to make a stiff corset, but there is danger, especially in the case of women having a large bust and small waist, that there will be parts of the corset which contain air-spaces. This can be avoided by using a very light tricot in the following manner: The cloth is first cut in squares large enough to reach conveniently around the patient. One such piece is stretched tightly about her, an easy process owing to the elasticity of the tricot, and carefully rubbed full of celluloid-gelatin. Another layer is applied and this again filled with celluloid-gelatin, and so on until the corset is sufficiently thick. After two days it is cut off and prepared with laces. If applied in this way the corset will be both elegant and durable.

At the session of November 24th, PLACZEK described a *case of uncomplicated paralysis of the serratus magnus.* The only history obtainable from the patient was that some months previously he had fallen from a ladder, jerking his right arm above his head. Soon after he had had pain in the right suprascapular region, which was ultimately followed by the paralysis. If the patient attempted to bring his arm from a horizontal position forward, the scapula fell away from the thorax like a flail. If an attempt was made to raise the arm to a vertical position it failed, unless the lower angle of the scapula was drawn outward, thus making good the deficient action of the serratus muscle.

PLACZEK also showed a patient who suffered from spasm of the masseter muscle. This patient was a locomotive fireman, and by reason of his occupation was subjected to sudden changes of temperature, increased by the habit of leaning out of the window. The patient suffered from neuralgia of the third branch of the fifth nerve, and with the attacks of pain. There usually was a contraction of the masseter muscles of both sides, the spasm ending with the mouth wide open. The attacks occurred about every five minutes.

At the session of the Union for Internal Medicine, November 22d, LOWENTHAL spoke of disinfection of the intestines. There are two methods of determining the efficacy of an intestinal antiseptic, one being the bacteriologic examination of the stools. This has proved absolutely unreliable. The other method is the chemic examination of the urine in order to determine quantitatively the presence of those substances which are due to intestinal putrefaction. Using this method as a test, Lowenthal made experiments with amyloform, a substance which yields formaldehyd if introduced into the alimentary tract. In the test cases the dose was gradually increased until formaldehyd could be demonstrated in the urine. The quantity of the products of intestinal fermentation in the urine were distinctly decreased by this means in spite of the somewhat constipating effect of the drug.

STRAUSS has made similar experiments with steriform, and BLUMENTHAL with itrol. Both of these observers reported inconstant results.

ZIEGELROTH spoke of the prophylactic value of periodic sweats. Recently, numerous investigations have proved that sweat contains pathogenic microbes. The speaker himself, by a comparison of the bacteriologic condition of water, before and after a patient had bathed in it, found that the water contained three times as many microbes after a sweat bath as after an ordinary bath. The advantages of such a bath before an operation are therefore plain, and serves an even greater purpose in stimulating cellular oxidation. Such baths are contraindicated in diseases of the heart and circulatory apparatus. They act as a specific in rheumatism, and while they may increase the symptoms of an attack of gout they improve the general condition of the patient. The specific gravity of the blood is the same before and after a bath, so that the blood is not changed by it. Two points should be carefully observed: first, the duration of the bath should not exceed fifteen to thirty minutes, and second, care should be taken to at once replace the fluid which has been lost by the sweating by copious draughts of water.

SOCIETY PROCEEDINGS.

THE NEW YORK CLINICAL SOCIETY.

Stated Meeting, Held November 26, 1897.

THE President, DR. FRANK W. JACKSON, in the Chair.

DR. B. FARQUHAR CURTIS read a paper, entitled

SOME EXPERIENCE WITH URETHROTOMY FOR STRICTURE.

The author said that in speaking only of urethrotomy he did not wish to be understood as believing in this operation to the exclusion of dilatation. The paper was devoted to a discussion of the results of operations performed with certain definite ideas in view as to treatment. The cases, though few in number, were much alike, and were all observed in hospital practice. The list included nearly twice as many external as internal operations, owing to the severity of the class of cases seen in St. Luke's Hospital. The operator had aimed to make the urethra of sufficient caliber to admit a No. 30 (French) sound measured with a bulbous bougie, which, as is well known, usually is two sizes smaller than a steel sound of the same number. The usual aseptic precautions were observed in all instrumentations and operations. Steel and soft rubber instruments were boiled. For the urethra, Thiersch's solution was employed, except in a few very foul cases, in which a 1-to-10,000 or even a 1-to-5000 solution of bichlorid of mercury had been used. As a rule it was necessary to incise the meatus, the incision usually being made on the floor of the urethra, although the roof and the sides were nicked when necessary. About half of the patients were operated upon under cocain anesthesia. Ill effects from the use of this drug were not observed, although the delay and the nervous excitement incident to the employment of local anesthesia prevented its use in many instances; it is necessary to retain the cocain solution in the urethra four or five minutes, and to wait as long again before beginning the operation. Failures with this method of anesthetization may generally be explained by too great haste. Cocain intoxication is the result of allowing the solution to remain in the urethra. Nitrous oxid gas is also a useful anesthetic agent in these cases.

The two dangers of internal urethrotomy are hemorrhage and sepsis. In none of the cases was hemorrhage alarming. When it had been free, he had employed a strip of muslin, one foot long, and as wide as the penis was long, torn at each end so as to make a many-tailed bandage. A couple of layers of gauze were wrapped around the penis and then bass-wood splints were applied, and finally, over them, the many-tailed bandage. It is, of course, necessary to loosen the dressing during urination. The foreskin must always be retracted before applying the dressing, else it will certainly swell badly. In only one or two cases had the severity of the hemorrhage made it necessary to insert a catheter into the urethra, and then bandage the penis. The perineal crutch had only been employed in one or two cases. Sometimes an ice-bag or a hot urethral injection of alum solution had been of value. The immunity from hemorrhage was doubtless due to the fact that the operation of internal urethrotomy had been restricted to the anterior five and one-half inches of the canal, and in a large proportion of the cases the wound extended only to a depth of three inches from the meatus. In those few cases in which chill and rise of temperature occurred, the administration of 10 or 15 grains of quinin two hours before the passage of a sound, prevented the chill and fever, so that it was not probable that very serious sepsis was present.

In one case, a fatal result, probably from auto-infection, occurred—the only death from internal urethrotomy in the speaker's experience. The case was that of an Italian, twenty-eight years of age, who was admitted to St. Luke's Hospital, December 8, 1891. He had had one attack of gonorrhea eleven years previously. No instrument larger than a No. 10 (French) sound passed down the whole length of the urethra. The urine did not contain albumin or sugar. After urethral irrigation for four days, internal urethrotomy was performed on December 12th. Bulbous bougie, No. 20, entered the meatus; No. 18 passed one-eighth of an inch; No. 12, five-eighths, and No. 10, five and three-eighths inches. The meatus was incised on the floor and roof, and the Otis urethrotome could then be passed four inches and a half. It was screwed up and withdrawn, and then bulbous bougie No. 26 passed. The urethrotome was again employed, and after this cutting, a No. 34 (French) sound passed into the bladder. A foul discharge then escaped. The operation continued twenty-five minutes, during which time eight ounces of ether was consumed. The patient rallied well, and the next morning appeared comfortable and in good condition. At 1.30 P.M. he passed eight ounces of urine with some bleeding and pain. This was followed by a rise of temperature from 99° to 102° F. He was at once given 8 grains of quinin, and at 4 P.M. his temperature was again 99° F. That evening he had severe pain in the region of the kidney after urinating, and then another chill, with a rise of temperature to 102° F. He passed seventeen ounces of urine mixed with blood during the twenty-four hours subsequent to the operation. The next morning he appeared flushed and restless, but without definite complaint. On the right leg, near the ankle, an emphysematous crackling was detected along the course of the veins. There was no redness, edema, or swelling at that time, and this was the only point of crepitation. Lead and opium applications were made to the part. The urethra was being regularly irrigated with Thiersch's solution. The temperature remained high, and sixty-three hours after the operation the man died. There was no redness, swelling, or unusual tenderness in the penis or groin. The autopsy showed nothing unusual in the urethra, but gas was found in the veins of nearly all the organs of the body. The kidneys were healthy. It seemed improbable that the infection took place at the operation, because the same technic and instruments were employed in another case on the same day without any untoward result. Considering the foul discharge behind the stricture, the theory of auto-infection of the wound seemed the most plausible. The speaker believed if the urethra had been opened through the perineum the man might have been saved, and this had been his principle of practice in similar cases since then. It was interesting to note that the strictures were situated in the anterior three and a quarter inches of the canal, where operations are generally considered trifling.

In regard to external urethrotomy, the principal objections to this procedure are as follows: The danger of hemorrhage, and the possibility of a troublesome fistula and the resulting confinement to bed. By the external operation at the present time is understood a short perineal incision made for the purpose of draining the urethra and bladder behind the stricture, but it is generally admitted that the strictures themselves are rarely situated in the region opened by this wound—namely, six or seven inches below the meatus. The perineal opening must be made when it is impossible to introduce instruments through the meatus to the bladder. It is also generally employed when the stricture is deeper than five and one-half inches, because of the danger of hemorrhage in such a deep-seated internal wound, and also on account of the danger of retention of the discharge and consequent sepsis. When cystitis is present the advantage of draining the bladder during a few days is obvious, and constitutes another indication for the external operation. Again, if there is a foul discharge behind a narrow stricture, even though this is within two inches of the meatus, the perineal section should be employed. The longer confinement to bed is not a weighty objection to the operation. No matter how small and shallow the wound in the urethra may be, it is a wound which we are largely obliged to leave to itself during recovery, and hence the patient is safer in bed during a few days, even in the simpler cases. Moreover, the perineal section is chiefly advised for a class of cases which should be confined to bed because of the gravity of the lesion. The perineal operation is only difficult when performed without a guide, and in such cases internal urethrotomy is manifestly impossible. The difficulty arises only when no other operation is possible. The most serious objection is the possibility of a permanent or slowly healing perineal fistula. In a certain number of cases this is unavoidable, but they generally occur when drainage has been maintained a long time on account of a coexisting cystitis. Dr. Curtis endeavors to avoid fistulæ by very early removal of the tube when cystitis is not present. The external incision is generally indicated when it is necessary to divide a deep stricture, to find the urethra behind an impassable stricture, or to drain the posterior urethra. The tube should, therefore, be removed within a day or two, and the perineal wound lightly packed with gauze. If chill or rise of temperature does not follow the next urination the tube is no longer required. If fever occurs, the tube should be reinserted, and another attempt made within a few days to discontinue its use. The speaker had observed, in some instances, such rapid healing of the perineal wound that there was no leakage after the first week. Not infrequently cases are seen in which the perineal wound must be rather extensive in order to deal successfully with strictures, fistulæ, false passages, or other lesions. Such a wound may be almost closed with sutures, leaving, of course, a small opening posteriorly. The speaker has succeeded in closing permanent sinuses by means of the double-flap operation, although as a rule several attempts were required before success was achieved. The most serious difficulty in cases of impassable stricture is the location of the urethra without a guide—still one of the most difficult operations in surgery. The difficulty in passing these strictures is often due to the existence of false passages. In two cases observed by Dr. Curtis there had been extravasations of urine with complete sloughing of the perineal urethra. In one case there were many sinuses through which the patient urinated as from a watering-pot.

He has been able to subsequently observe only a few of his cases. Of those patients upon whom internal urethrotomy had been performed, twelve had been kept under observation, in four of whom relapse had occurred. Two had frequently used the sound during a period of two years and one-half, and a year and one-half respectively. The remaining six presented symptomatic cures. One patient who had had a stricture equaling in size a No. 16 (French) sound remained well without instrumentation two years, and finally died of phthisis. Another patient, on leaving the hospital, could pass sound No. 30 (French), and the same instrument could be passed two years later, although dilatation had been practised only during the six months after the operation. Still another patient, in whom there had been a stricture of No. 14 (French), could pass sound No. 30 (French) four years after the operation. One patient could pass a No. 28 (French) five years after the operation, although treatment had not been continued. Another, with an original stricture of No. 14 (French), could pass a No. 22 (French) sound eight years after operation, although there had been no subsequent treatment. Another, who had had a stricture of No. 22 (French), could pass a No. 26 (French) sound ten years after operation, dilatation having been practised three years. This patient had had two attacks of gonorrhea in the interval.

Dr. Curtis said that he had been able to follow the subsequent history of thirteen patients upon whom urethrotomy had been performed. It was found that in one relapse had occurred, and that in eight there had been symptomatic cure, but examinations of these patients were not made. Of those examined, one could pass a No. 32 (French) sound one year after operation; another a No. 26 at the end of two years, no sound having been passed for six months. Another patient passed steel sound No. 26 (French) to the ligament and No. 18 to the bladder six years after operation. Considering the severity of the cases and the common neglect of after-treatment, he thought these results were quite satisfactory. Of course, regular dilatation subsequent to operation would probably have produced still better results.

DISCUSSION.

DR. F. TILDEN BROWN said that the plan of controlling hemorrhage from the anterior urethra described in the paper was new to him, and he thought it a valuable suggestion. He fully endorsed the reasons given for making perineal section, yet, personally, he was inclined to resort to this operation more frequently, even in the more anterior strictures. The object is to secure perineal drainage for a *brief* time. It was his practice to wait until the first sound had been passed, usually on the third or fourth day, before deciding upon the removal of the drainage-tube. If the passage of the sound does not cause a disturbance, he withdraws the tube and carefully dresses the wound so as to secure healing of the deeper parts first. He has not had trouble with perineal fistulæ except in one case—a broken-down patient who had a suprapubic fistula of two-years' duration, a tuberculous testicle, and foul urine. Perineal drainage was maintained for some time, and a good deal of broken-down material was discharged through the fistula. A very simple operation was eventually sufficient to completely close the fistula.

The speaker referred to a patient who had worn a silver catheter continuously twenty-eight years, because of a traumatic stricture and severance of the urethra. The wound had at first been sutured, and subsequently a perineal operation performed, but the man had finally been advised to wear a catheter permanently. The stricture was found to be at four and a half inches, but owing to the small size of the penis it was deeper than would have been the case in an ordinary adult man. A perineal incision was made, long posteriorly, for drainage. The anterior part of the incision opened the way to the stricture, which was very short. The mucous membrane over the stricture was cut transversely and laid back anteriorly and posteriorly. The dense layer was next dissected out from one edge of the longitudinal incision to the other, and the mucous membrane sutured together. A drainage-tube was inserted posteriorly, and kept in place eight or ten days. The man made an excellent recovery, and is now passing sound No. 32 (French) upon himself.

Regarding the occurrence of chill and fever in these urinary cases, Dr. Brown said that he believed that some cases of this kind cannot be explained on the theory of sepsis; they seem to be due rather to a nervous reflex. One great advantage of the perineal operation is that it admits of treating a contracted condition of the posterior urethra, not uncommonly found in old men.

DR. L. BOLTON BANGS said that he was quite in accord with the reasons presented in the paper for the performance of external urethrotomy. In his own practice he rudely grouped strictures into those of small caliber, those of large caliber, and traumatic strictures. Unless there is some emergency requiring it, he does not perform any cutting operation upon a urethra from which there is a discharge, no matter whether it is gonorrheal or due to some mixed infection. He agreed with the reader of the paper regarding the treatment of strictures of small caliber, but he makes it a rule to paint the posterior urethra, from the bulbomembranous junction back to the neck of the bladder, with a solution of nitrate of silver. This coats the urethra with an albuminous substance, prevents infection, and renders the urethra less sensitive for a number of days.

Regarding the treatment of strictures of large caliber, Dr. Bangs said that he believed there were many of these cases in which an operation is not required. In every case the mucous membrane is diseased, and, irrespective of stricture, one would have to first treat the affected mucous membrane. It is his rule to measure the urethra at intervals of a few months, meanwhile treating the lesions of the mucous membrane. In this way he determines the necessity for operation by the degree of contraction. If this plan were followed, it would be found that fewer strictures of this variety require operation. Dr. Bangs exhibited an endoscopic picture of the urethra of an old man who had not had urethritis since his boyhood, and who had been operated upon most zealously by a skilful surgeon, but without relief. Two or three distinct ulcers were revealed by the endoscope, and then it became an easy matter to apply successful treatment.

DR. MURRAY said that he personally resorts more and more to external urethrotomy, never trusting to internal urethrotomy when the stricture is below four or four and one-half inches from the meatus. If it is fairly tight, he always does an external urethrotomy. In the removal of the tube he is governed entirely by the condition of the bladder, but believes in as speedy removal as possible. Regarding the fatal case cited in the paper, he doubted very much if it were an example of auto-infection, and in this connection he agreed thoroughly with the criticism made by Dr. Curtis himself regarding the better result that would probably have followed perineal drainage.

DR. CURTIS, in closing the discussion, said that he usually passes a sound twenty-four or thirty-six hours after the operation, and then not again for a week. After this they are passed at intervals of a week. It seemed necessary to him to pass the first sound before the wounded surfaces have a chance to unite. He has had no case of tight stricture which seemed suitable for resection, nor any of large caliber, except the one case in which a No. 22 (French) sound could be passed. This patient, however, had strictures extending from the meatus to a point five inches backward. It seemed to him impracticable in a hospital service to postpone operative work until the mucous membrane behind the stricture has been put in a healthy condition, for the patient would often have to be kept under constant observation many months. Of course, if there is a profuse purulent discharge, the operation would have to be postponed for a time, but even then it is difficult to treat the condition until the stricture has been divided.

APPENDICITIS AND PERITONITIS WITH LOW TEMPERATURE.

DR. A. J. MCCOSH referred to a case, seen that afternoon—a young man who had had rather severe abdominal pain for about eight days, and had frequently vomited. The temperature had not been below 98° or above 99° F. He had been able to take a short walk the day before. He had been freely purged. When seen by the speaker at 3 P.M. the patient seemed to be seriously ill. A diagnosis of general peritonitis due to appendicitis was made. The belly was quite tense; the temperature was 98° F., and the pulse 110. The patient had been very carefully watched by a good physician and nurse, yet he had not been considered a sick man, because he had not had fever. He was operated upon at 5 P.M. About ten separate pockets of pus were found, holding, in the aggregate, three or four pints of thin, watery, and very offensive pus.

THE PRESIDENT asked if the surgeons could furnish any points which would aid in the early diagnosis of these serious cases.

DR. MCCOSH replied that vomiting and regurgitation of gas whenever pressure was made upon the abdomen, together with the general appearance, are perhaps the signs of most value.

DR. FRANK HARTLEY said that the increasingly rapid pulse, rigidity of the recti muscles, and a general cyanotic appearance are fairly reliable indications of the gravity of the condition. Many cases run a serious course without any marked rise of temperature. Many laborers work in the streets up to the day before coming to hospital, and yet the appendix is found to be gangrenous. The rise of temperature seems to depend chiefly upon the amount of absorption of septic material.

CASES OF REMARKABLE SUBNORMAL TEMPERATURE.

DR. A. ALEXANDER SMITH said that during the night of November 22d a patient had been admitted to Bellevue Hospital with a temperature of 91.4° F. There was some doubt about the accuracy of this record, so it was taken with four thermometers. The only complaint made by the patient was that he thought he was freezing to death. He had a very disseminated pulmonary tuberculosis, and also nephritis. He was placed in an improvized incubator, and his temperature gradually rose until, at the end of twelve hours, it reached 102° F. and his pulse 84. His pulse on admission had been 64. At no time was the pulse over 100. When the temperature reached 98° F. he became very bright, and expressed himself as feeling well. After reaching 102° F., it gradually dropped back to 96° F. He lived twenty-nine hours and forty-five minutes. An hour and a half before death the temperature was 98° and the pulse 72. The autopsy confirmed the diagnosis.

A few weeks ago a patient had been admitted during the night to the same hospital with a temperature of 90° F., as determined by three thermometers. He made the same complaint as the other man, and under the same treatment his temperature gradually rose. He also had pulmonary tuberculosis and nephritis, but the autopsy showed, in addition, a small cancerous deposit in the head of the pancreas. Both patients, of course, had been living under the most unfavorable conditions, particularly as regards nutrition.

DR. WALTER MENDELSON said that while an hospital interne he had seen a man who was admitted during the summer with a temperature of 90.5° F. The patient was rather dazed, but seemed otherwise healthy. It was ascertained that he had had nothing to eat for a week. Food soon restored his normal temperature, although during the week after entering the hospital there was a tendency for the temperature to fall to 97° or 98° F. As the patient recovered, it was observed that his mental condition was not normal, although possibly this had existed previous to the illness in question.

REVIEWS.

A TEXT-BOOK OF PRACTICAL THERAPEUTICS, with Especial Reference to the Application of Remedial Measures to Disease and Their Employment upon a Rational Basis. By HOBART AMORY HARE, M.D., Professor of Therapeutics and Materia Medica in the Jefferson Medical College, Philadelphia, etc. With special chapters by DRS. GEORGE E. DE SCHWEINITZ, EDWARD MARTIN, and BARTON C. HIRST. Sixth edition, thoroughly revised and largely rewritten. Philadelphia and New York: Lea Brothers & Co., 1897.

THE eminent success of Dr. Hare's book on therapeutics is evidenced by the appearance of the sixth edition within seven years. This is to be attributed somewhat to the excellent arrangement of the subject-matter, the first part of the work dealing with therapeutic agents of recognized worth, the second containing the principal diseases, with a brief description of their pathology and symptomatology and their treatment in full. The present edition has been brought fully up to date and includes a full discussion of diphtheria antitoxin and of the newer remedies whose usefulness has been proven. Therapeutic measures of a non-medicinal nature are fully considered, and include cold, heat, mineral springs, and diet-lists.

The present edition will undoubtedly meet the same kindly fate as its predecessors, for the work is one of the few books which are really of value to the physician in his daily work.

THE CARE AND FEEDING OF CHILDREN. A Catechism for the Use of Mothers and Children's Nurses. By L. EMMETT HOLT, M.D., Professor of Diseases of Children in the New York Polyclinic, etc. Second edition, revised and enlarged. Flexible cloth; 104 pp. New York: D. Appleton & Co.

IN the second edition of this practical little work the author has preserved the form of question and answer of the first edition. While this makes the book much less readable, clearness and simplicity are gained thereby, and it has the further advantage of making it easy to find quickly any given point to which reference is desired. If put in the hands of the mothers of young children, this book will serve not to take the place of the doctor, but to make his visits and advice pleasanter and more profitable for both parties.

THERAPEUTIC HINTS.

For Whooping-cough tussol is recommended in doses of 1/6-grain, for an infant one month old, to 8 grains for a child of five years. It may be administered in raspberry syrup one to three times daily.

For Tabetic Neuralgia.—

℞ Malacini . . . . . ʒ iss
Sod. bicarb. . . . . grs. xlviii.

M. F. Chart No. xii. Sig. One powder two to four times daily.—*Kutky*.

To Remove Warts painlessly and with avoidance of scars apply a supersaturated solution of bichromate of potassium once daily.

Destruction of Small Vulvar Vegetations may be accomplished by the repeated application of the following powder after the parts have been bathed and well dried:

℞ Pulv. sabinæ }
Iodoformi } aa . . . . ℥ ss.
Ac. salicylic. }

M. Sig. External use.

Ichthyol Applied to Anal Fissures, in conjunction with dilatation of the sphincter muscle under cocain anesthesia, is said to act efficaciously, not more than ten treatments being requisite to effect a cure in recent cases.

For the Bites of Poisonous Insects it is recommended to paint the wound with pure ichthyol, or in case swelling and inflammation have occurred, apply ichthyol plaster, and adminster the drug internally in 10-drop doses in spirits of ether.

THE MEDICAL NEWS.

A WEEKLY JOURNAL OF MEDICAL SCIENCE.

VOL. LXXII. NEW YORK, SATURDAY, JANUARY 15, 1898. No. 3.

ORIGINAL ARTICLES.

COUGH DUE TO LESIONS OF THE NOSE AND THROAT.

BY WILLIS S. ANDERSON, M.D.,

OF DETROIT, MICH.;

LARYNGOLOGIST TO HARPER HOSPITAL POLYCLINIC; ASSISTANT TO THE CHAIR OF LARYNGOLOGY IN THE DETROIT COLLEGE OF MEDICINE.

THE physician is frequently called upon to treat the symptom cough, and to do so intelligently an accurate idea of the many different lesions capable of producing this disagreeable symptom is necessary. In diagnosis, cough is too often associated with diseases of the chest, and we are prone to forget that it may be dependent upon a lesion remote from the lungs. It is the unusual causes of cough, especially those dependent upon pathologic changes in the nose and pharynx, to which I wish to call attention. If the usual explanation be accepted, irritation of the branches of the vagus nerve must be regarded as the principal factor in the production of cough. When the general distribution of the branches of this nerve and their frequent communications with others are recalled, it may be readily understood how lesions of many different organs may give rise to reflex cough. Those who are accustomed to examining the nose, throat, and ear will have noticed how frequently a reflex cough is excited by the examination *per se.*; the introduction of an aural speculum is often sufficient to excite it. The explanation of this phenomenon is simple, when it is remembered that the auricular branches of the vagus are distributed to a portion of the auditory canal. Sprays and applications to the nares frequently provoke a cough, which varies in character in different individuals. We are indebted to John Mackenzie for calling attention to the fact that irritation of the nasal chambers is one of its causes. He found that certain areas in the nose, when irritated, gave rise to the symptom in question. These areas are the inferior and middle turbinate bodies and that portion of the septum opposite the posterior end of the inferior turbinate. So commonly are lesions of these areas the cause of the cough that they may be considered the nasal areas of reflex cough. In like manner, examination of the pharynx frequently produces the same result.

If it is true that the mere touching of these various surfaces causes this symptom, then it should certainly be expected as a regular accompaniment of lesions in this portion of the respiratory tract, and so it is found that it is frequently caused by hypertrophic rhinitis, and can only be relieved by curing the nasal affection. It is not usually a concomitant of a recent hypertrophy of the anterior portion of the inferior turbinate, but is frequently caused by the same pathologic lesion of the posterior end of the same structure. This condition may be permanently relieved by removal of the hypertrophic tissue or by its destruction with the galvanocautery. Hypertrophy of the middle turbinate is often the cause of the same symptom. The trouble may be due to hypertrophy of the mucous membrane alone, or to a thickening of the bone itself. If the enlargement, in either case, is sufficient to press against the septum, or nearly to occlude the nares, a train of disagreeable symptoms, of which cough is one, will be manifested. In many cases this condition is a troublesome one to relieve. When simple hypertrophy exists the symptoms may often be removed by cleansing and astringent sprays, followed by the application of menthol, grains v-x to ℥i of albolene. In true hypertrophy, the galvanocautery may be carefully employed with good results, or in case the original lesion has undergone polypoid degeneration the cold snare will be found to be of special service. When the bone is thickened it is often necessary to saw off a portion. This is often a very difficult operation, especially when the space in which the operation is to be performed is small and the field of operation very sensitive. In spite of the use of cocain the pain is usually severe, and hemorrhage interferes with the view. Care should be taken not to destroy more of the mucous membrane than is actually necessary, as the resulting cicatrix is sometimes a source of irritation, occasionally leading to symptoms almost as disagreeable as those on account of which the operation was performed.

Various observers have reported many cases of persistent cough due to fibrous and mucous polypi. The etiology of these growths is not well understood. These have been carefully studied by Zuckerkandl, who, in his admirable work, "Normal and Pathological Anatomy of the Nasal Cavities," gives a number of plates showing them to orginate, in a large majority of cases, around the ostium maxillare, under the middle turbinate. They push out from the middle meatus and fill the greater portion of the nares, and may even hang down into the nasopharynx. They may be single, more frequently multiple, and may involve the accessory sinuses of the nose. Asthma and hay fever, with their accompanying coughs, are frequently dependent upon polypoids. There is but one treatment, and that is the removal of the growths. After this has been accomplished the stumps should be cauterized to lessen the danger of recurrence. The results of this treatment are often very gratifying, yet prognosis must be cautious, as in some cases there is an underlying neurotic element which resists all treatment. It has been the experience of the writer that in but few cases of asthma and hay fever of long standing can a permanent cure be obtained by treating the nasal cavities alone; but in the large majority a marked improvement follows, and in some, a complete cure. Of the other lesions of the nose which may cause cough, spurs and deviations of the septum are probably the most important. Deviations of the septum are estimated to be present in ninety per cent. of all adults, and spurs are commonly found. When these conditions present, the rhinologist must decide as to the advisability of operative interference. It seems to the writer that too many of these operations have been performed during recent years. There are many cases in which a moderate deviation of the septum or a small spur does not give rise to any symptoms. There are other cases with an S-shaped deviation causing an apparent stenosis, but on more careful examination one can satisfy himself that in spite of the irregular and tortuous channel the patient has a fair breathing space. In other cases there is present such a marked deviation of the septum as to occlude one side, and yet, in spite of the exaggerated lesion, there is no complaint from the patient. In any of these types cough may or may not be presented as a symptom. One ought not to be too hasty in attempting operative interference for the relief of cough, or, in fact, for the relief of any other symptom, unless there is an evident connection between the local disease and the symptom.

The surgical treatment of these lesions is one requiring judgment and careful study of all the factors of each individual case. If operations upon the septum were never followed by a disagreeable train of symptoms it would be a different matter, but the practical fact is, that the condition often returns, or a train of annoying symptoms follow, due, in some cases, to a resulting perforation, or to the cicatrix which forms at the site of operation, or, as may possibly happen, to the formation of adhesions between the septum and the outer wall of the nose. I do not wish to take the position that operative treatment is never indicated, but feel that a careful study of all cases and a consideration of the probable condition after the lapse of a few years will reduce the number in which an operation is apparently justifiable.

Lymphoid hypertrophies of the nasopharynx are a very frequent cause of cough, especially in children; and although a very common affection, its importance does not seem to be appreciated. One frequently observes children going about with open mouths, broad and flattened noses, and dull, vacant expressions, all indicating the obstruction to nasal breathing usually due to lymphoid hypertrophy. The oft-repeated phrase, "They will outgrow it," accounts for many cases of chronic coughs and permanent deafness, as well as impaired mental and physical vigor. These children do not outgrow the affection. The cough which often accompanies this condition is a persistent symptom, increasing in damp weather and lessening in warm, dry weather. The treatment is largely surgical. It is true that in recent cases, if mild, marked improvement follows spraying of the nose and nasopharynx with iodin, grains ii to ℥ i of water, and the internal administration of syrupus ferri iodid; but in most cases a permanent cure is not possible without more radical treatment. Ablation of the growths and the application of the galvanocautery are the only surgical methods which commend themselves to a surgeon. The galvanocautery is the more tedious method, usually requiring more than one sitting, and each application is followed by as much or even more reaction than excision of the growths. It seems to the writer that cauterization should be employed only when some special indication exists. The removal of the growths by the post-nasal cutting forceps or the curette is a very satisfactory procedure. The pain and annoyance following the operation are usually slight, and the disappearance of the symptoms is very gratifying, both to patient and operator. A general anesthetic is necessary in very young or nervous patients, but in older children cocain anesthesia is usually sufficient. The use of a general anesthetic adds danger to the operation, partly because the patient is unable to freely expel the blood from the throat. The danger from this cause is lessened by careful administration of the anesthetic and maintenance of the head on a level lower than the body.

There are many morbid conditions of the pharynx capable of giving rise to cough. All of the acute and chronic diseases of the mucous membrane of this region may be accompanied by this symptom in greater or less degree. The accumulation of mucus in the pharynx will often excite a reflex cough, which is relieved by the removal of the offending substance.

Hypertrophy of one or both tonsils is a frequent source of cough. There does not seem to be any special relation between the severity of the latter and the size of the former. Some patients having large tonsils have little or no cough, while others, in whom the hypertrophy is moderate, have a very persistent cough which disappears only when the hypertrophy is removed. An accumulation of a white, cheesy matter in the crypts of the tonsils will often keep up an irritating cough, which will promptly disappear upon the removal of the accumulation with a curette. Elongation of the uvula is a common cause of an irritable, hacking or a spasmodic cough. Many cases of months' or even years' duration, in which a diagnosis of consumption has been made, have been cured within a few days by amputating the tip of the uvula. One ought to be careful not to remove too much of this organ. It is usually not necessary to remove any of the muscular substance, but simply the relaxed, edematous tip.

Cough is frequently a result of hypertrophy of the follicles in the posterior wall of the pharynx. The writer has found the best treatment for this condition to consist in the application to each follicle of the galvanocautery point. More than three or four applications should not be made at one sitting, as there is sometimes considerable reaction. Cleansing applications should also be employed to remove the accumulations of mucous, and if there be atrophy of the membrane between the follicles, stimulating applications are indicated.

Hypertrophy of the lymphoid tissue at the base of the tongue may be responsible for an irritating cough. One can easily detect this condition with a laryngeal mirror, and an application of the cautery will bring speedy relief, or if the follicles are numerous, or very much enlarged, they may be curetted or removed with a cutting-forceps.

Hypertrophy of the lymphoid tissue in the lateral wall of the pharynx frequently causes a hacking cough. This chronic lateral hypertrophy is often overlooked as a cause of this symptom. Objectively, the posterior wall of the pharynx may be found to be normal, or the seat of follicular hypertrophy, and along the lateral wall of the pharynx, behind the posterior pillar of the fauces and parallel with it, may often be seen an intensely congested and thickened ridge. This ridge of hypertrophied tissue is sometimes nearly covered by the posterior pillar, and may be best observed when the patient phonates or gags. Schmidt calls attention to the frequency of this condition in singers. The treatment is very satisfactory. Mild cases rapidly improve by applying nitrate of silver, grains xv to ℥ i of water. Two or three applications are sufficient to relieve the cough in some cases; but more permanent benefit may be obtained by applying the galvanocautery.

There are, no doubt, many other lesions of the nose and throat which may give rise to cough, but those mentioned by the writer have, in his experience, been frequently overlooked.

The following brief histories may be of interest in this connection:

CASE I.—Female, aged seventeen years. The symptoms were: cough for one year, with no expectoration, pharynx dry, frontal headache. Examination of the chest was negative. The pharynx showed commencing atrophy of the posterior wall, with injection of the vessels and accumulation of mucus. Treatment consisted of applications of ichthyol, grains x to ℥ i of water, after thoroughly cleansing the mucous membrane. Under this treatment the cough entirely disappeared.

CASE II.—Male, aged twenty-one years. He complained of a sore, irritable throat which was worse in the morning. Cough for four years, with some mucus expectoration, occasionally tinged with blood. There was also nocturnal nasal obstruction. Examination: Chest, negative; nose, hypertrophy of both inferior turbinates; pharynx, very much congested and irritable; uvula, elongated and relaxed. Treatment: Astringent sprays were used in the pharynx for about a week with some improvement. The uvula was then amputated, with entire relief of the cough.

CASE III.—Male, aged twenty-nine years. He had had trouble with his throat for over five years, causing him to cough and to hawk up mucus, and he complained of a sensation as of a lump in his throat. Examination revealed moderate hypertrophy of the anterior portions of both inferior turbinates; the vessels of the posterior wall of the pharynx were injected, with commencing atrophy of the mucous membrane, and an accumulation of mucus; the larynx was somewhat congested, though otherwise normal. On examining the lymphoid tissue at the base of the tongue, one follicle was found to be very much enlarged. After cleansing the mucous membrane of the nose and throat, an application of a fifty-per-cent. solution of oleum picis in albolene was made. The galvanocautery was applied to the enlarged follicle at the base of the tongue, with the result that the symptoms entirely disappeared. About three weeks later the cough and sensations as of a lump in the throat returned, with the addition of a constant, bitter, metallic taste in the mouth. I found on examination that the same follicle was again enlarged, and its thorough cauterization resulted in permanent relief of the symptoms, but there remained an ulcer at the site of the cauterization which would not heal under local applications. I suspected specific trouble, and on carefully questioning the patient, found that he had had syphilis many years before. Ten grains of iodid of potash was administered three times daily, and in about a week the ulcer was entirely healed.

CASE IV.—Female, aged thirty-five years. She complained of a dry, hacking cough which she had had two months, so severe at night as to prevent sleep. She also had a sensation as of a foreign body in the throat. She was in good health up to the time of the commencement of the cough; since then her appetite had been poor and her nutrition had suffered. Examination of the nose was negative. The pharanyx was congested, there being lymphoid hypertrophy behind and parallel to the posterior pillar. There were several good-sized hypertrophied follicles in the posterior wall, with commencing atrophy between them. The upper portion of the larynx was congested. The tongue was covered with a white coating. After cleansing the pharynx, a solution of nitrate of silver was applied, grains x to ℥ i of water. Codein, ¼-grain, was administered for two nights to control the cough. The galvano-cautery point was applied to the hypertrophied follicles, several sittings being necessary. The cough had almost ceased in less than a week, and in another week and a half she was entirely free from it. She was obliged to leave town before all the follicles had disappeared, but when last seen the cough had not returned.

CASE V.—Male, aged twenty-six years. In regard to asthma or nervous diseases the family history was negative. He had had asthma since an attack of whooping-cough which occurred when he was a child. Three years before coming under observation he gave up farming because of dyspnea and general ill-health. He had noticed marked nasal obstruction in the right side for several months. He had asthma all this time, but it was worse during wet weather. Cough, which was most annoying during the early morning hours, pain in the left side of the chest, and constant dyspnea were the principal symptoms noted. Examination of the lungs showed the sibilant breathing, prolonged expiration, and an abundance of coarse mucous râles. The right side of the nose was obstructed by polypi. The use of drugs gave but temporary relief. The polypi were removed with a snare, and their bases cauterized. The patient experienced prompt relief, and when last seen he was much better than he had been at any time for many years.

A CASE OF INFANTILE SCURVY, WITH COMMENTS ON INFANT-FOODS AND FEEDING.[1]

By ARTHUR M. JACOBUS, M.D.,
OF NEW YORK.

THE health and family history of the parents of the girl baby whose case is herein reported has always been good, excepting that from overwork in looking after a large household, the mother's physical condition was not up to par during the early part of the pregnancy which resulted in the birth of the patient. The mother had previously given birth to four children, two girls and two boys, all of whom have enjoyed excellent health, excepting that the fourth child, a boy, was inclined to mild attacks of eczema during the latter part of the nursing period, when he was also given artificial food. The parents and all of the children are of the auburn-blonde type. Three months before the fifth baby was born, the one whose case is here reported, the mother and family, who had been under my care at different times during three or more years, removed to a mountainous country home, having an elevation of nearly 1400 feet above sea-level, with most healthful surroundings, and it was at this place that the baby was reared.

The patient was born July 13, 1896, the labor being normal in every respect. The child, a small one, was not weighed at birth. The family history has been purposely mentioned to show that it could not have been an element in the case. The mother's version of the baby's illness is so significant and excellent that it is given in full, as follows:

"I nursed the baby, and apparently had enough milk for her, but she did not seem to grow as rapidly as she ought, and when I spoke to the doctor about it, he said he thought the quality of my milk was probably not good and I had better wean her. I was very well at this time, had a good appetite, but was growing quite stout. I weighed 146 pounds, and my usual weight is only about 127 to 130. I thought that what I ate seemed to make flesh rather than produce milk, and the doctor seemed to think so too. I never gave her any other food as long as she had breast-milk, and after she was weaned, which was when she was just five months old, she had —— [mentioning the name of a well-known baby-food] and nothing else, until I went to New York in the spring, when I told you [Dr. Jacobus] about her wetting so much, and you advised me to try more solid food, and also to give two or three teaspoonfuls of cream with each feeding, which I did. We could not make her eat anything like eggs, or solid food in any form. . . . I do not remember the weight at different ages, but I know that just before we took her away in the middle of September, 1897, when fourteen months old, she weighed 14¼ pounds. She has never been sick until the present illness, excepting a slight attack of measles, which she had at the same time she was cutting her first teeth, which she did when she was seven months of age. Her food seemed to agree with her, was well digested, and her bowels were in good condition. She never had more than two or three loose passages at a time, and those usually just preceding the appearance of a tooth. The doctor here never said anything about her, although I told him that she did not seem to grow like the others. He only said, 'She's taking it easy.' She had a faint color, and her lips were red, until September 15, 1897, when she suddenly seemed to droop, refused her food (the proprietary food) and in a week's time became so emaciated that to handle her caused pain, and so we carried her on a pillow.

"During this time she passed very little water, sometimes going as long as seven hours without doing so. She had a little fever, but not much. During this week she cut four teeth, the anterior molars, making twelve between the ages of seven and four-

[1] Read before the Northwestern Medical and Surgical Society of New York, November 17, 1897.

teen months, and her bowels became distended, the stools being curdy and green. The doctor here attributed this to the fact that we had given her two doses of cod-liver oil, but they continued in the same condition until after we had changed her food as you directed when we consulted you some time later. In the middle of September the doctor here advised a change of air to the seashore, in order to save her life, which seemed rapidly passing away. We took her to Seabright, N. J., after calling at your office and finding you out of the city, and the doctor there said at once that her trouble was scurvy, and ordered orange juice for her, also meat juice. But he told us to let it get cold and take the grease off and then heat it. This she took for a few days, but soon got so she could not keep it down. She did not begin to gain until after we saw you in New York two weeks later and changed her food. That was the 27th of September, and she still weighed only 14¼ pounds. We brought her home October 1st, and the next day noticed a slight swelling of her hands and feet. It did not seem to extend further than her wrists and ankles, was at its worst on October 4th, began to decrease by that time, and had entirely disappeared in about a week. Her urine was examined at that time, and found to be normal. During the week her color began to improve, although so slightly as to be scarcely perceptible. She gained a pound that week, a quarter the next, and seven ounces last week. She now (October 25, 1897) weighs sixteen pounds, and is as rosy a baby as you would wish to see, but is still very thin in the legs and arms. The skin on her limbs is dry and scaly. We have been rubbing her with cod-liver oil, and I hope it will soon be better. Lately we have been giving her oatmeal in her milk and cream mixture, in place of the barley, and her constipation seems better.

"I met the doctor on the street this morning, and he asked me if I was still giving the baby meat and orange juice, and advised me to discontinue it, saying the necessity for it was past. I have not done so, nor do I intend to unless by your advice. A week previous he had also told me to skim the milk and not give the baby any cream, as it was too rich for her. Baby never had any rash or blood spots."

This ends the mother's intelligent history, as she observed the baby's illness, and, to my mind, depicts a typical case of scurvy. I have given it in full for the purpose of showing that her physician, a skilled surgeon with a large general practice, had evidently failed to make a diagnosis of the real condition, or to suggest the proper remedy—a change of food. When I saw the baby for the first time it was in New York on September 27th last, on its return from Seabright, N. J. The child lay on a pillow, was profoundly emaciated, with lips and face bloodless, pulse so weak and rapid that it was almost imperceptible, and apparently the baby had but a few hours to live. I had, a short time previously, on hearing the mother's story, made a diagnosis of scurvy without seeing the baby, and then the mother told me the Seabright doctor had said the same thing, but had not changed the food, excepting to order meat and orange juice. The mother said that the child's gums, which were a dark red and swollen, were somewhat better, but otherwise it had continued to fail, had a slight cough and fever, and had not improved by the trip to the seashore. The legs at this time were puffy, and movements seemed to cause pain, but there was no real edema. The baby, then fourteen and a half months old, had been fed almost wholly on the proprietary food since weaning, at the age of five months, and though the mother was not going home for several days, where the best milk from her own select herd of cows could be obtained, she was directed to stop entirely the food referred to and to give the following instead:

Robinson's prepared barley, well cooked with water, and as thick as rich milk, and the best cow's milk that she could obtain in the city, *unsterilized* or raw, in equal parts, with two teaspoonfuls of pure cream, two teaspoonfuls of lime water, and one-half to one teaspoonful of the best granulated sugar at each feeding. It was directed that the child be fed about once in two to three hours, depending upon the quantity she could take and retain at each feeding. At first she could only take about three ounces at a feeding, but by the end of the second week she took as much as five or six ounces, and later, eight to ten ounces. After the second week the proportion of milk was increased to two-thirds, and barley or oatmeal water and the rest of the mixture together making one-third. From the first she was also given the juice of two medium-sized choice sweet oranges each day in teaspoonful doses, with sugar, and as much water then and between feedings as she desired. The mother was told that she could give the baby the diluted sweetened juice of one lemon each day if at any time unable to obtain good oranges. The child was also given beef juice prepared as follows: I had heard from some teacher that beef juice should never be allowed to become cold from the preparation to the feeding, otherwise there would be a chemic change injurious to the juice, so that the mother was told to take a small piece of "top sirloin," sear it quickly, first on one and then on the other side, and then to broil it over a bed of live coals until the juice began to run, when she was to score it with a hot knife, squeeze it with a hot lemon-squeezer into a hot saucer, and add a pinch of salt and serve with a hot spoon as it cooled down sufficiently to be fed to the baby without burning its mouth. The baby was fed from two to four teaspoonfuls of beef juice freshly prepared in this manner twice each day. This was the entire treatment. No medicine whatever was given either for the cough, fever, profound anemia, indigestion, constipation, edema, scanty urine, sore gums, or anything else. The result has been sure and rapid, as might have been expected by any one with previous experience with this dread and often unrecognized condition. I should add that at first, as usual in scurvy, the baby rebelled against taking the beef juice, but subsequently it was taken with relish. It should also be recalled that though the physician in Seabright recognized the condition and ordered beef and orange juice, which was given, the baby continued to fail, and it was not until the food was changed that she began to improve. A recent report is that the baby is steadily gaining in appearance, weight, and strength, and in fact is apparently well in every respect.[1]

Had this baby been under my immediate care, as were the other children, the mother would never have continued to give the proprietary food so long as she did, with my consent, but as the mixture had apparently agreed with the next older child who, however, was also given other food, she continued it with this one, especially as her local physician had made no comment that the child's illness was due to improper food.

Scurvy is generally considered to be a disease of malnutrition, and customarily attributed to a lack of vegetables, but the latter cause is certainly very doubtful in the case of children. Dr. W. Gilman Thompson, in his work on "Dietetics," says that it is a disease due to omission and not to consumption of certain foods, and that it depends rather upon the quality than quantity of food. He also says, in opposition to the theory that the want of fresh vegetables acts as a cause of scurvy in man, that the fact is stated by Lieutenant Greely that among the Danish Eskimos, who have a population of ten thousand, not a pound of vegetables, nor a dozen pounds of bread per man are eaten annually, and yet they are practically free from this disease, and the same statement is made in regard to the most Northern tribes of Eskimos of pure blood, who were studied by Lieutenant Peary, and also in regard to the natives of the Alaskan Archipelago and some tribes of North American Indians who do not include either vegetable or bread in their food. Scurvy in infants is said to occur as early as the fourth month, but most frequently between the ages of nine and eighteen months, or about the time the mother's milk begins to fail and artificial foods are resorted to. In looking over the literature of scurvy, it is found that the disease in children, in nearly every instance, is reported to have occurred where the infants had been fed almost exclusively on some one of the following foods: Proprietary preserved foods, condensed milk, peptonized milk, sterilized milk, and even barley water is mentioned as a cause. Northrup, according to Thompson, does not state it any too strongly when he says: "It is a significant fact that the country which furnishes most of the literature of scorbutus in children is the same which is posted from end to end with advertisements of proprietary foods." It may be inferred, therefore, that preserved, cooked, or sterilized foods lack something essential to the infant's healthful development. The remedy, then, lies in raw milk or simple mixed foods.

In the Addenda of Dr. A. Jacobi's valuable book on "The Therapeutics of Infancy and Childhood" may be found a number of lines which, perhaps unintentionally on his part, confirm the inferences just made in regard to the causes of scurvy. He says, for instance, that "*sterilized* milk, if the only nutriment, as in many instances it will be found to have been, must be combined with cereal decoctions, and meat broths should be added as a regular food." And yet, though he lauds sterilized and pasteurized cow's milk, chiefly in intestinal disorders, he admits, "There can scarcely be a doubt that if raw milk could always be had unadulterated. fresh, and untainted, it would not require boiling; it would even contraindicate it, for high temperatures at once destroy the bacteria whose action is desirable for normal digestion." He admits also that "boiling or sterilization is not a safe protection under all circumstances," that it takes hours of sterilization to destroy certain bacteria, and that such protracted sterilization, besides being far from certain in its effects, is a clumsy procedure, and one not calculated to benefit the milk, and that it has been claimed to have been no unmixed boon because of its changing the chemic constitution of milk. Again Jacobi states, "But what I have said a hundred times is still true, and borne out by facts, *viz.*, that no matter how beneficial boiling, sterilization, or Pasteurization may be, it cannot transform cow's milk into woman's milk, and that it is a mistake to believe that the former, by mere sterilization, is a full substitute for the latter. Further, that the substitution of cow's milk or of sterilized cow's milk for woman's milk, as the *exclusive infant* food, is a mistake. Also that experience teaches that digestive disorders, such as constipation or diarrhea, and constitutional derangements, such as rachitis, are frequently produced by its persistent use, and it appears to be more than an occasional (at least cooperative) cause of scurvy."

If all this is true, and certainly Dr. Jacobi ought to know whereof he speaks, what is the use of going to all the trouble to sterilize milk, thereby injuring its nutritious and healthful qualities, and in the end run the risk of causing infantile scurvy, rickets, and kindred disorders? Why not absolutely discard all artificial proprietary foods, sterilized and peptonized milk, excepting the latter two as a temporary diet in acute intestinal disorders, and in the absence of *good* human milk give pure, fresh, filtered cow's milk properly modified and diluted to conform to human milk, and which now, owing to the rigid inspection of dairies can be readily obtained in most cities?

[1] Examination of the baby, December 26, 1897, showed her to be in excellent health.

Jacobi,[1] Soxhlet, Caillé, Seibert, and others, deserve great credit for their work in calling attention to the deleterious influences and dangers of impure milk, and in advocating so thoroughly sterilization and the best methods of performing the same, but excepting as a temporary diet in intestinal disorders, or where it is absolutely impossible to obtain pure milk, I believe time will show that it, like proprietary foods, condensed milk, etc., when relied upon as the main diet, will prove detrimental to the health of infants, and particularly that it is a causative factor in scurvy.

In my opinion, scurvy is mainly a constitutional disorder due to slow or chronic starvation, resulting in profound anemia and other morbid processes in the animal economy, and due to a lack of foods in proper variety, suitable to the digestive powers and requirements of the individual. In other words, that preserved or proprietary foods and condensed and sterilized milk, lack certain natural chemic acids and substances necessary to the health of a child, and which cooking and sterilization seems to destroy and which we are not yet in a position to isolate.

Seibert has shown in a series of experiments that sterilization as usually performed, and even by himself, does not eliminate all bacteria, or at least, that bacteria develop in previously unfiltered sterilized milk much quicker than in milk which has been filtered before sterilization according to the method described by him. I believe that in filtered milk lies the solution of the difficulty. That is, first, in the absence of good human milk obtain the purest rich cow's milk which can be obtained; carefully filter it, as directed by Seibert, dilute it freely, and modify it, as described by Jacobi, Rotch, and others, by the addition of water, cane-sugar, and barley, rice, or oatmeal, and lime-water, according to the necessities of each particular case, and a food is obtained which will be perfectly satisfactory. In addition, after the age of six months, there being no special contraindication, and certainly, if the infant is failing on a restricted patent or milk diet, other simple foods, such as baked potatoes (which Watson, in his celebrated work on "Practice," proved over fifty years ago is a specific equal to lemon juice in scurvy), beef juice, fresh fruit juices, vegetables, crackers, etc., should be carefully given as extra diet.

In my experience, the infants most affected with malnutrition, anemia, scurvy, etc., are those of the well-to-do classes who can afford to purchase artificial foods, and who give them because some friend's child apparently did well under such circumstances. On the other hand, the children of the tenement population, as I recall them, as a rule suffer less from these disorders because they sit at the table and are fed on everything that the parents eat, such as tomatoes, potatoes, fruit, meat, crusts of bread, rice, etc., and even beer. Unfortunately, in hot weather, owing to the heat and foul air of the crowded tenement-houses and the exposed and infected groceryman's milk and other infected foods, the infants suffer and frequently die of acute intestinal disorders.

In selecting cow's milk as a portion of the diet, we should be careful to exclude all milk from cows fed on beer grains, as the latter increases the amount of water, acids, etc., in the milk and diminishes the cream. The one cow's milk also, should not necessarily be used, unless its quality has been determined by analysis. I recall a case in which an infant was suffering from dyspepsia and malnutrition following the use of very poor milk from one cow; I suggested an investigation, which resulted, as I expected, in finding that the one cow from which the milk was derived was housed in a filthy stable, and was fed on beer grains and sour, decaying garbage and swill. A change of milk at once effected a cure. We must also, when possible, exclude milk when the morning and evening milkings are mixed together. Milk of different ages, like wine, should be kept separate.

Owing to the length of this paper, but little will be said on the modification of cows' milk to make it correspond as nearly as may be to average good human milk. In the writings of authorities already alluded to and, in fact, in any of the recent well-known text-books on diseases of children, will be found a full discussion of this subject, and I have nothing new to report. It is only necessary to remember that in the "artificial feeding of infants no routine mixture will in all cases prove successful," and that "slight changes in the three elements of milk of which we have the most accurate knowledge, namely, fat, sugar, and albuminoids, are of real practical value in managing the digestion and nutrition of the infant. Cows' milk must be well diluted with water, containing by preference a cereal; in order to diminish the excess of proteids or albuminoids, and in doing this we must make up the loss, in proportion, of the fats and sugars." Dr. Jacobi is a great believer in high or extreme dilution of milk with water, and since I have adopted his advice in that respect my success in feeding cows' milk to children has correspondingly increased. Infants are often sick and famished for the want of water, even during the nursing period. Lime-water or bicarbonate of soda must, of course, be added to cows' milk to diminish the occasional excess of natural acidity, and for

[1] Jacobi claims to have practised sterilization of milk forty years, and to have taught it thirty-five years.

its effects in breaking up the casein into small, easily digestible flakes. Holt advises it in the proportion of one part of lime-water to twenty of milk, or one grain of soda to one ounce of milk. Finally, to again quote from Jacobi, who says: "I am pleased to state that Auerbach agrees with me on another subject. The sugar he adds to the milk-food of infants is not milk-sugar, but cane-sugar, of which he gives twenty grams daily, and also, according to my old teaching, more during constipation. He undoubtedly prefers cane-sugar for the reasons which guided me in my recommendations, though it is true that milk-sugar is being stripped of its dangers in the same degree as boiling, sterilization, or Pasteurization is carefully practised." I will add that since adopting the foregoing suggestion in regard to cane-sugar, it, too, like the extreme dilution previously referred to, has given me the happiest results.

Summary.—The causes of scurvy are many—chiefly poor human or cows' milk, improperly modified good cows' milk, proprietary foods, condensed and sterilized milk, the three latter being relatively unsuitable in the order named, and, finally, a lack of cereals and raw foods, meat, fruit juices, etc., in variety and quantity suitable to the age of the infant.

The treatment, fortunately, is generally simple. First, we must absolutely prohibit the use of patent and proprietary foods, and next supply a food, in the absence of good mother's milk, such as has been suggested. As Thompson says, and Osler, too, in nearly the same words, "the treatment of scurvy in children consists first in throwing away all proprietary foods, condensed milk, etc.," and sterilized milk also, it might be added; and then, if the disease has not progressed too far, improvement and cure rapidly follow change to a normal diet, including expressed beef juice, and a little fresh orange, lemon, or peach juice.

TUBERCULOSIS OF THE TONSIL.[1]

BY SEYMOUR OPPENHEIMER, M.D.,
OF NEW YORK;
ATTENDING LARYNGOLOGIST TO THE OUT-DOOR DEPARTMENT OF BELLEVUE HOSPITAL; ATTENDING LARYNGOLOGIST AND OTOLOGIST TO YORKVILLE HOSPITAL AND DISPENSARY; SENIOR ASSISTANT TO THE CHAIR OF LARYNGOLOGY, UNIVERSITY MEDICAL COLLEGE.

IN the study of tuberculosis of the tonsil it becomes necessary to divide the disease into two classes, the primary and the secondary. The primary form is very rare, but few cases having been reported from time to time, and even the authenticity of these admits of considerable doubt. Störck submitted twenty tonsils, removed *post-mortem*, to minute microscopic examination, and found two presenting tuberculous changes. That tubercle bacilli are present in a considerable proportion of apparently normal tonsils and especially in the hypertrophic form of tonsillitis, has been demonstrated by several Continental pathologists and laryngologists, experimental inoculations being performed upon guinea-pigs and rabbits. In all these experiments the tonsils were removed from the ordinary class of patients seen in a throat clinic, and though hypertrophy was present in all, no evidence of either local or general tuberculosis could be detected. Shenker and Kruchmann, in an extensive consideration of the pathology of this disease, establish the causal relation between primary infection of the tonsillar tissues with the tubercle bacilli and tuberculosis of the cervical lymph-glands.

Primary infection may occur from the use of contaminated instruments (and especially the laryngoscope, which is very difficult to keep surgically clean), from the inhalation of air containing the tubercle bacilli, or from the ingestion of tuberculous food. In dispensary practice, where the number of patients treated within a limited space of time is very large, it is almost marvelous that more cases of tuberculous infection do not occur. The necessary instruments are often not properly cleansed previous to use with each patient, frequently being merely wiped off with a towel or napkin which has sufficed in perhaps ten or twenty similar instances. There is no doubt that tubercle bacilli are frequently transmitted from one patient to another in this way, but on account of the natural resistance of the parts, infection does not result. The dust in the majority of dwellings, especially those occupied by the poorer classes, contains a considerable number of tubercle bacilli, and, as the subjects of the ordinary hyperplasia of the tonsil sleep and usually live with the mouth open, using the nose but seldom as the primary respiratory organ, it is very apparent why the bacilli should be found in the tonsillar crypts. It is hardly necessary to say anything in regard to the ingestion of tuberculons food as a cause of local infection; for, with the exception of milk, the majority of food-stuffs are free from this contagion.

On examination of the tonsils suspected to be the seat of primary tuberculosis, we will not be able to discover anything indicating the character of the affection; they may appear normal, or, as is usually the case, hypertrophied. If a small piece of tonsillar tissue be removed for diagnostic purposes and subjected to staining with hemotoxylin-eosin, the lymph-cells will be colored bluish-red, while the tubercle bacilli will assume the peculiar shade known as eosin-red. Occasionally the diagnosis must be

[1] Read at the Fourteenth Annual Meeting of the New York State Medical Association, October 13, 1897.

based upon this staining method alone, but usually giant-cells and tubercles, more rarely caseation, may be found. Primary tuberculosis, although rare, is probably present more frequently than we suspect, and possibly many cases of pulmonary tuberculosis find their origin in infection through the tonsils.

When the tonsil is the seat of a tuberculous process, distinctly localized in this gland, one of two results follow: either the disease remains local, not affecting the patient in any way and only discovered after removing the tonsil for other causes, or pulmonary tuberculosis develops from infection through the lymphatic system. The treatment of this primary form is very simple, and, if the disease is localized in the tonsil, is absolutely curable by removing the infected tissues. Tuberculosis of the tonsils consecutive to the pulmonary form is of quite frequent occurrence. If you consider, according to reliable statistics, that about every seventh human being dies from pulmonary tuberculosis, while *post-mortem* records of various large hospitals prove that certainly not less than eighteen per cent. of all patients dying from tuberculosis of the lungs have some pharyngeal or laryngeal complication, you will see that, broadly speaking, every thirty-fifth patient dying in the practice of a general practitioner, is afflicted with the ravaging disease under consideration. Strassman found the tonsil involved in thirteen out of twenty-one fatal cases of tuberculosis.

On examination of fauces, the seat of the tuberculous changes, we find the tonsils hypertrophied with no distinctive lesions, or, ulceration may be present on the tonsil, soft palate, or pharynx. The ulcers on the external surface of the tonsil are uneven or ovoid in shape, pale in color at their circumference, but having a red, slightly granular base. Anemia of the surrounding mucous membrane is usually well marked. The ulceration is very superficial, extending laterally rather than deeply, the surface being covered with a dirty, yellowish-gray secretion. The soft palate and uvula are usually thickened with a semi-solid infiltration peculiar to this disease, and known as submucous infiltration in contradistinction to deep infiltration as observed in syphilis. Frequently the tissues are thinned from atrophy or lack of nutrition and the epithelium covering the tonsil is thinned in patches from submucous swelling or from the pressure exerted by a distended crypt. The mucous membrane of the pharyngeal cavity and soft palate is markedly anemic, often in strange contrast to the apparently normal complexion of the patient. The anemia shows itself in the form of either a general pallor of the soft palate and pharynx, or in the form of what at first sight appears to be congestion, but which, on close inspection, is seen to be an injection of the capillary vessels, so marked that even the smallest branches may be distinguished on the intensely anemic mucous membrane. In the neighborhood of the ulcers are small elevations or tubercles, varying in color from deep red to yellow. Schnitzler made the diagnosis of tuberculosis, in one case even before there were signs of the disease in the lungs, by excising one of these small granulomata and finding tubercle bacilli present.

The local symptoms are principally pain and dysphagia. The pain is intense, but is usually confined to the diseased region. Frequently the suffering is so severe that it is impossible for the patient to swallow without the use of an anodyne, and in this connection it is interesting to note that liquids are generally more badly borne than solids or semi-solids. The pain is especially severe if the posterior pharyngeal wall and larynx is involved. The extreme disphagia will often necessitate the use of nutrient enemata, especially as the fatal termination draws near. The voice, as a rule, is not impaired unless the larynx is involved; but if the disease is far advanced, and especially if the tonsils are hypertrophied or ulcerated, the voice is changed in quality, and its use is extremely painful. The mere swallowing of the saliva causes excruciating pain, and the patient goes without food to avoid the agony accompanying the act of swallowing. Taste and smell may both be impaired, or even abolished, and the breath has a peculiar, offensive odor, which is more or less characteristic of the disease in this locality.

The diagnosis of tuberculosis of the tonsil in the majority of cases may readily be made, especially if there is marked concomitant pulmonary changes. The characteristic ulcers on the tonsils and soft palate, the intense pain, and the emaciation with hectic fever, are all readily recognized. A study of the temperature affords considerable evidence in favor of the disease, if the tonsillar lesions are not well marked.

There are three diseases to some extent resembling tonsillar tuberculosis: *viz.*: lupus, syphilis, and cancer. Lupus of the tonsils and pharynx is very rare, and the coexistence of a cutaneous lesion will assist in clearing the case. Cancer may usually be distinguished by the ulcerations, which are deep and angry-looking; its course is very rapid, and the cachexia is generally present. In the early stages of carcinoma, before ulceration is present, resource to the microscope and the finding of the characteristic epithelial elements readily solves the question of diagnosis.

As to syphilis, its differential diagnosis may occasionally present greater difficulties, the more so as the possibility of a double infection being present in one and the same patient must be borne in mind; the tonsillar lesion may be syphilitic, while the pulmonary is tuberculous. Resort to the therapeutic test with mercury and iodid of potassium in sufficient dosage will assist in establishing the diagnosis. In the more ordinary cases, however, tuberculous infections may be distinguished by the pallor of the affected parts, the syphilitic lesions being more of a decidedly inflammatory character. The development of the tuberculous ulcer is slow, that of the syphilitic rapid.

The general diagnostic features of syphilis, the absence of fever, the history of a primary sore, and the post-cervical glandular enlargements are not present in tuberculous affections. The characteristic pathologic changes in tuberculosis of the tonsil are not different in any respect from those seen in other portions of the body, the locality of the disease alone giving rise to its definite local symptomatology. Before the ulcers form tubercle must be present; these may occur as part of the morbid changes of other diseases, for example, syphilis; but the tubercle of tuberculosis is characteristic of the affection, and occurs in no other disease. Briefly, it may be described as consisting of an enlargement of connective tissue, translucent, grayish in color, and about the size of a millet-seed. The cellular elements are lymphoid and round cells, varying in size. The nuclei are generally small and homogeneous. Between the cells are found fibrous tissue, which is not very vascular. The vessels are never newly formed, but have existed in the tonsillar tissue before the development of the tubercle, the latter growing around them. The blood-supply is at all times very deficient. The nodules may be isolated or joined together in a mass from inflammatory changes, imperfect granulation tissue resulting. As the nodule grows older caseation begins in the center, the degenerating process progressing until the nodule is a mass of granular *débris*.

The prognosis is, as a rule, very unfavorable. If the tonsil alone is affected, removal, or prompt and radical medication, offers some hope, but if ulceration is present, and the larynx and pharynx are involved, little can be accomplished, except such palliative measures as will prolong life and make the patient as comfortable as possible.

Lenox Brown outlines the treatment as follows: "Counteract the general tuberculous tendencies; give as much functional rest to the diseased parts as possible; relieve the pain in swallowing; administer suitable nourishment, and attempt to heal the ulceration."

The constitutional treatment must always be enforced, as success cannot be hoped for unless strict attention is paid to the condition of the general health. The administration of cod-liver oil, the hypophosphites, nutritive tonics, proper feeding, etc., should be carried out as if the case were pulmonary in character. Functional rest of the parts is extremely important, as every time the patient swallows or talks the movements of the muscles concerned in phonation or deglutition keep up the irritation. If the ulcerations are extensive, speaking must be prohibited, and food administered by means of the esophageal or rectal tube. Relief of the pain in swallowing will necessitate a careful consideration of the food. The nutriment should be of a semi-solid consistency, such as jelly, eggs, poached, soft, or boiled, scraped meat juice, etc. Heat is usually very painful, while cold is grateful; so ice may be given in small pieces.

Of the drugs used to relieve the pain, cocain is undoubtedly the best. I have lately been employing a pastil composed of morphin, cocain, and antipyrin, which the patient allows to dissolve in the mouth. The treatment of the ulcers is very unsatisfactory. In my experience but one method of treatment has proved to be at all efficacious, *viz.*: that of curetting the ulcer with a sharp spoon, and then cauterizing with lactic acid. We owe the application of this drug to the therapeusis of tonsillar tuberculosis to Krause of Berlin. Moorhoff of Vienna had extolled its merits in the treatment of tuberculous disease of the joints, and Krause utilized the suggestion in the treatment of the same disease in the larynx. In the majority of cases this method gives the best results, cocain being used before the application of the acid. Of the internal remedies recommended at various times for the treatment of pulmonary tuberculosis I now, in most cases, employ but one, *viz.*: creosote in large doses. The use of this drug, combined with lactic-acid applications, has yielded the best results in my hands. In conclusion, quoting Semon, "I can only recommend you, as long as we have nothing better, to adopt this method of treatment, and I hope your endeavors may be crowned with successful results."

THE ANATOMY AND SURGERY OF THE MIDDLE MENINGEAL ARTERY.

By H. A. SIFTON, M.D.,
OF MILWAUKEE, WIS.;
PROFESSOR OF ANATOMY IN THE WISCONSIN COLLEGE OF PHYSICIANS AND SURGEONS.

IN order to investigate the origin, relations, course, distribution, anastomoses, and size of the middle meningeal artery, sixty dissections were made upon thirty-four subjects. The origin was from the internal maxillary artery in fifty-seven of the sixty cases; in one it was from the external carotid; in one from the internal carotid, and in one from the ophthalmic. The anomalies were all observed on the left side. The point of origin was very constant, always being between 11 and 13 mm. from the division of the external carotid; in five instances the division into branches occurred before the skull was entered. In the fourteen cases in which the artery was injected it was found to anastomose freely with other meningeal arteries and with the corresponding artery of the opposite side. Its size was noted in forty cases in which a plug of the injecting material was squeezed out and measured, and the vessel was found to vary between 1 and 2 mm. in diameter. The anterior branch was from ¾ to 1 mm. in diameter, and the posterior branch less than 1 mm.

The location of the artery in question is not between the dura mater and the bone, but in the substance of the dura mater, surrounded by a fibrous process of that membrane. A rupture may occur without a fracture of the skull; and in case of injury the rupture of the artery may be some distance from the point of traumatism, or even on the opposite side of the head. The symptoms caused by a rupture of the artery are those resulting from the pressure of the extravasated blood. It has been estimated that the force exerted by an extravasation 10 mm. in diameter, with a tension of 10 mm. of mercury in the arteriole, is about three atmospheres, a pressure sufficient to destroy any portion of the brain.

The symptoms following rupture are as follows: An interval of consciousness after the injury, followed by coma with spastic movements, ending in paralysis. The condition of the pupils and the character of the pulse vary with the degree of pressure. The respirations are irregular; coma comes on slowly or rapidly, according to the rapidity with which the blood is poured out. The only rational treatment consists in an immediate opening in the skull, turning out of the clot, and arrest of the hemorrhage.

The following cases will serve to illustrate the symptoms and treatment:

CASE I.—John D., a farmer's boy, aged ten years, was sent to turn a horse loose in a pasture, the latter being about a quarter of a mile from his home, at 11 A.M. in the forenoon, and as he did not return to dinner, search was made for him. He was found near the house lying on the ground in an unconscious condition with blood oozing from a small cut over the left temple. A physician was sent for who diagnosed a fractured skull. On my arrival, about three hours after the accident, the boy was in an unconscious condition with slow pulse, cold extremities, and irregular breathing. He was so profoundly comatose that it was impossible to get any response from pinching.

The doctor stated that at the time he first saw him, two hours earlier, he responded to pinching on the left side, but gave no response on the right, although there was marked twitching of the right side of the face, shoulder, and arm. The wound of the left temple was 1½ inches posterior to the external angular process, and one inch above the zygoma. It was about an inch long, and had evidently been inflicted by the cork of a horseshoe, as the outline of the flat part of the shoe could be seen extending backward from the wound. On exploring the opening with the finger a fracture of the skull was found, although no marked depression could be detected.

The boy must have walked a quarter of a mile after being struck, as the horse was found in the pasture with the gate shut. This was conclusive evidence that he did not at once become unconscious, or if he did, he had recovered from the first blow for a sufficient time to allow him to walk the quarter of a mile. The unconscious condition had gradually grown more profound, progressively involving the various groups of muscles of the right side from the face downward, showing that the pressure was increasing and extending. A diagnosis of probable injury to the middle meningeal artery was made.

The external wound was enlarged by a curved incision which disclosed a slightly depressed area with a fissure extending backward. A trephine was applied, and a button of bone removed, including a part of the depression. On taking out the button of bone a dark clot was exposed. The opening was enlarged with the bone-forceps and the clot broken up and turned out. It was large, extending in every direction, and was an inch in thickness opposite the opening. As soon as the clot was broken up, free arterial hemorrhage occurred, which after much difficulty, owing to the depth of the wound and the limited size of the opening, was arrested by passing a ligature under the bleeding-point and tying. This controlled the hemorrhage, and we were able to clear out the clotted blood as far as it could be reached. The artery from which the hemorrhage came could then be distinctly seen pulsating on the surface of the dura mater directly beneath the opening. It was the anterior branch of the middle meningeal, and seemed to have been torn completely across. The dura mater was apparently not injured. The brain did not expand and fill up the space left by the clot, so the cavity was loosely packed and the wound closed. No anesthetic was used, the patient manifesting no sense of pain.

On removal of the clot the breathing immediately become regular and the patient's condition improved, but he did not become conscious until twenty-four hours had passed. He was markedly dull during the following three or four days, and manifested some twitching of the right side of the face, shoulder, and arm, which were partially paralyzed. He did not fully recover for five weeks.

The gauze was removed on the third day, the wound healing by first intention. One year after the injury the opening in the skull had closed, and he was in perfect health.

CASE II.—J. M., aged twelve years, a healthy boy, while plaguing an Italian fruit-vender was struck upon the head by a broomstick. He was apparently not much hurt. A few minutes later, feeling sick, he walked home, a distance of four blocks, telling his mother that the vender had struck him, and complained of headache. As there was nothing but a slight bruise to be seen she thought little of it, and had the boy lie down. About an hour later he was noticed to be breathing hard an attempt was made to rouse him, but was unsuccessful.

I found him in a partly comatose condition, with slow pulse, irregular breathing, cold extremities, and subnormal temperature. He was restless, throwing himself from side to side, muttering and crying out if touched. It was apparent that he could not use his right hand with as much freedom as the left. After a few minutes, he lost all control of the arm and leg. Both eyes were rotated outward, with the pupil of the left dilated and immobile. An examination of the head revealed a slight bruise over the left temple, extending from the external angular process backward, and showing as a faint swelling on the line where the stick had struck him. It was evident that he was suffering from cerebral pressure, and that it was gradually increasing and extending. A diagnosis was made of intercranial hemorrhage, probably from the left middle meningeal artery.

He was removed to a hospital and prepared as quickly as possible for an operation. All the pressure symptoms had markedly increased so that by this time he was in a profoundly comatose condition. A curved incision was made over the left temporal region, the center of which was 1½ inches posterior to the external angular process and 1¼ inches above the zygoma. On turning back the flap no evidence of any injury to the skull could be found.

As a trephine could not be obtained, I opened the skull without difficulty with a metacarpal saw, taking out a piece of bone about 1¼ inches square, the center of which was located at a point over the anterior branch of the middle meningeal artery. On removing the bone, which was easily accomplished as it was quite thin, a large clot of blood protruded through the opening. This was broken up and removed. There was considerable oozing which seemed to come from the lower angle of the opening. After chipping away considerable bone, and being still unable to locate the bleeding-point, the wound was loosely packed with gauze, which finally controlled the hemorrhage. On removal of the clot the brain immediately expanded so that the dura mater came well up to the opening in the skull, and the breathing at once became regular. All the symptoms improved, and at the end of four hours the patient regained consciousness, although there was still some loss of power over the right hand and leg which did not pass off for two or three days. The gauze was gradually withdrawn until by the fourth day it was entirely removed. At the end of ten days the wound had healed, and the boy left the hospital in apparent good health.

Two weeks later he returned showing a small opening at one end of the scar which was discharging a serous fluid. A probe disclosed roughened bone at the edge of the opening. As there were no symptoms an antiseptic dressing was applied. After five weeks, during which time there was a very scanty discharge, I was able to detect with the probe that a shell of bone had separated, and without much difficulty it was removed. The death of this piece of bone is of interest in showing how the stripping off of the dura mater may determine the life of the overlying bone which receives its nourishment from it. Especially is this so in the young subject in which the dura mater is much more firmly adherent to the bone than in the adult.

It is conceded that had the wound been aseptic the piece of bone would not have exfoliated, but would have acted as a bone chip. Had the nourishment of the bone not been impaired, Nature would have overcome the shortcomings in the technic of the operator, and the wound would have remained closed after it had once healed. After the removal of the dead bone, the wound at once closed. Six months later there was still a small opening in the skull through which the pulsation of the brain could be felt. At the end of a year this had disappeared, and no evidence of the large opening remained other than a slight roughening of the bone beneath the scar.

CLINICAL MEMORANDUM.

A PERSONAL EXPERIENCE IN RENAL SURGERY.

BY ROBERT F. WEIR, M.D.,
OF NEW YORK;
PROFESSOR OF SURGERY IN THE COLLEGE OF PHYSICIANS AND SURGEONS, AND SURGEON TO THE NEW YORK HOSPITAL;
WITH THE COLLABORATION OF
EDWARD M. FOOTE, M.D.,
OF NEW YORK;
SURGEON TO THE RANDALL'S ISLAND HOSPITALS.

THE kidney was long the undisputed domain of internal medicine, but little by little surgery disputed this territory until now the only affections of these organs which may be considered strictly "medical," are acute and chronic, bilateral, non-pyogenic inflammations, and even the former of these have lately been made the subject of surgical interference by Harrison of London. This rapid advance in the surgical treatment of diseases of the kidney has been brought about not only by the daring of aseptic surgery, but by the improved methods of establishing an exact diagnosis, and this latter result is very largely due to the introduction of the cystoscope and ureteral catheterization. With this improvement in diagnosis and a corresponding increase in knowledge of the course of diseases of the kidney, treatment of affections of the ureter itself came into being, and the "surgery of the ureter" now occupies a well-recognized place in our art. In publishing the succeeding cases, based upon a personal experience, brevity is of necessity observed, and only such comments as are of practical import are presented, with the addition of such condensed formation as bears directly upon the points developed by the histories. For convenience, rather than for pathologic or surgical reasons, all the cases in which operation was performed have been arranged in the following order:

TABLE I.

No.	Diseases.	Number of cases.
1	Nephralgia	5
2	Movable kidney	5
3	Renal calculus	7
4	Renal abscess	4
5	Hydronephrosis	3
6	Renal tuberculosis	9
7	Cysts of kidney	2
8	Neoplasms of kidney	3
	Total	38

Or stated differently the following operations were performed:

TABLE II.

Operations.	Number of Operations.	Recoveries.	Deaths.	Mortality per cent.
Nephrorrhaphy	9	9	0	0
Nephrotomy	10	9	1	10
Nephrolithotomy	7	6	1	14
Nephrectomy	25	18	7	28
Exploratory exposure	1	1	0	0

The table gives a total of fifty-two operations upon thirty-eight patients. In order to make the list complete, of necessity, several previously published cases have been included.

The mortality from nephrectomy, if divided according to cause, is as follows:

TABLE III.

Diseases.	Cases.	Deaths.	Mortality per cent.
Calculi	5	0	0
Abscess	6	2	33
Hydronephrosis	2	0	0
Tuberculosis	6	2	33
Cysts	3	1	33
Neoplasms	3	2	67

Most of the fatalities occurred in the earlier years of kidney surgery. During 1896-7 I performed ten nephrectomies with but one death, and the last six patients all recovered.

NEPHRALGIA—EXPLORATORY NEPHROTOMY.

The principal symptoms of kidney disease which admit of such varied interpretation as to beget obscurity in diagnosis are pain and renal enlargement. With these present, or sometimes with the association of other urinary and renal disturbances, such as hemorrhage, etc., we are compelled, in order to make a satisfactory solution of the diagnostic mystery, to resort to an exploratory incision. Of the various conditions which lead to this action none are more interesting, because none are more puzzling, than those placed under the ample cloak of nephralgia.

The benefit obtained from these indefinite and exploratory operations and in those of like nature performed elsewhere in the body, notably in the abdomen, has been attributed by some surgeons to the operation *per se;* but this explanation needs itself to be explained. Since a renal incision in certain instances relieves, as Harrison reports, the congestion due to ordinary nephritis, it is more than probable that in nephralgia a similar relief follows incision. This, however, does not explain the few cases where relief has been obtained by the simple splitting of the fat envelope and mere palpation without incision of the kidney. Some have thought that the improvement in such cases might result from the division of nerves encountered in the wound area; but in the few instances reported more light is required.[1] The mechanical handling or palpation of a kidney during its exploration may also aid in dislodging minute calculi, and thus relief be afforded. One of the following cases (Case I.) seemed to admit of this explanation.

Of course, when there is intermittence in the attacks of pain or enlargement, the influence of a loose kidney, its production of temporary hydronephrosis, which is often overlooked at the time of an operation, is to be kept in mind, particularly as this is a condition likely to be benefited by the fixation induced by an exploratory operation.

It is, however, known to all that the apparent absence of a calculus, the commonest cause of persistent pain, does not prove that it is not present. Morris has recorded a typical example of this condition, when, even after the removal of the kidney, a stone the size of a marble could not be localized by palpation. In Case III. a nephrotomy and exploration of the pelvis and ureter by a flexible metallic bougie, and also by the finger introduced into the cavity of the organ, while counter pressure and palpation were carefully made by the opposing finger (bidigital examination), failed to detect any lesion, yet a recurrence of the pain led me subsequently to extirpate the organ. Three tense hemorrhagic cysts were found which had caused the patient's trouble.

CASE I. *Renal Colic—Hysteria (?)—Exploratory Exposure—Recovery.*—Mrs. P., aged thirty-five years, was referred to me by Dr. H. C. Coe. During 1884 she had an attack diagnosed as renal colic, and in June, 1886, she suffered from occipital neuralgia and showed a marked hysteric tendency. She then continued in excellent health until January 1, 1887, when she was awakened one night with a severe darting pain in the left lumbar region. The pain radiated to the left groin and was spasmodic in character. During the intervals between the spasms, there was a steady aching pain in the loin. There was vomiting from the onset. For a few days previous to the attack the urine had contained considerable "brick-dust" sediment, but after its beginning very little urine was passed; it was of high specific gravity, contained numerous uric-acid crystals and quantities of urates, but no albumin, blood, or casts. This condition lasted a week, the spasms recurring at irregular intervals. Scarcely any liquid was retained, and sleep did not average more than two to three hours daily. From sixteen to twenty ounces

[1] Tuffier, *La Semaine Med.*, 1893, p. 481.

of urine was passed in twenty-four hours. The temperature was at no time above 100° F.

I first saw the patient on January 6th. She had not had a spasm for a couple of hours, and appeared comfortable. With the first deep pressure into the left side of the abdomen such a spasm of pain was produced that it was necessary to induce profound anesthesia before proceeding with the examination. Its results were negative, but the patient slept four hours after the ether narcosis and seemed easier. Then the vomiting recurred, and as the pulse became weaker and the condition of the patient indicated impending exhaustion, nephrotomy was decided upon and performed January 8, 1887.

The left kidney was exposed by a vertical lumbar incision and freely separated from its fatty sheath. Nothing was detected by thorough palpation of the anterior and posterior surfaces of its pelvis and of the ureter as far as it could be followed. An aspirating-needle was thrust into the kidney in several places, but nothing but blood was found. As the kidney had been so well separated from its fatty sheath, two tubes were placed, one above and one below the organ, for drainage, and the wound was elsewhere closed by deep and superficial sutures. At the close of the operation the patient was in a critical condition, having a thready pulse of 160 or more. The condition gradually improved under the administration of stimulants subcutaneously and *per rectum*. Vomiting was persistent, and nutrient enemata were continued more or less regularly during the following week. The wound healed promptly, and the condition of the urine improved. From the moment the patient recovered from the ether narcosis the attacks of pain vanished.

The hysteric element came out strongly during couvalescence, and on several occasions the patient convinced herself, her family, and her attending physician that she was about to die. Sixteen days after the operation, when the wound was almost healed and the urine had been normal some days, and the patient was in good spirits and eating and sleeping well, and sitting up each day, she was suddenly seized in the middle of the night with a pain in the right side exactly like that which she had had on the left. Much to her disgust, she was immediately etherized, and the pain disappeared and did not recur. The patient died during 1890 of pneumonia, having been in good health up to the time of the last illness.

CASE II. *Nephralgia—Supposed Calculus—Movable Kidney — Nephrotomy — Nephrorrhaphy—Recovery.*— Mrs. R., aged thirty-five years, and the mother of four children, the youngest being thirteen years of age, noticed, during the spring of 1891, a soreness in the right side of the abdomen near the navel. During the summer of that year the amount of urine was unusually small. She never passed any gravel. About February, 1892, she began to have severe pain in the right lumbar region, extending into the right groin. The urine was much diminished in quantity, and contained mucus and some pus, but no blood. When I saw her, March 1, 1892, with Doctors H. C. Coe and H. F. Walker, the tenderness was exquisite and paroxysmal, any change in position or any starting of the abdominal muscles sufficing to bring it on. The greatest pain was felt over the edge of the right quadratus muscle, near the ribs, and also about the middle of the right rectus. Under ether, neither the kidney nor the ureter could be felt. The uterus and appendages were normal. The conclusion was drawn that a calculus was impacted either in the kidney or ureter.

Before examination the temperature was normal and the pulse 118; during the twenty-four hours following examination the patient was free from pain, and the urine increased to a total quantity of twenty ounces. The pain then returned, and the urine greatly decreased in quantity.

Operation being finally agreed upon, March 10th, by means of vertical lumbar incision, the kidney was exposed. It was enlarged to one and a half times the normal size. It was probed with a steel hat pin, but the presence of a stone was not detected. Traction showed it to be abnormally movable. It was slightly deeper in color than a normal kidney. An incision was, therefore, made into the kidney pelvis through the lower part of the cortex, and, by means of the finger and a sound, the pelvis and all of its calices were systematically examined.

The ureter was next investigated. After passing a large floss silk thread through the kidney for the purpose of traction, the angle between the wound into the pelvis and the uterer could be so far obliterated as to admit of the passage of a curved steel sound. [Traction by means of a thread passed through the lower portion of the kidney answers the same purpose in probing the ureter as does putting the head well back in esophageal instrumentation.] A solid instrument could in this way be passed six inches

FIG. 1.

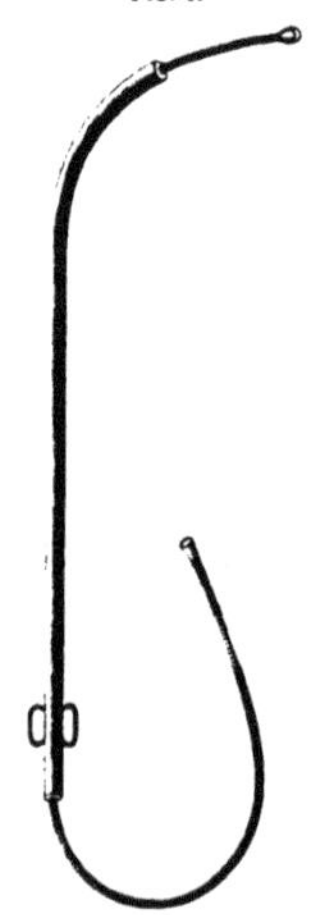

Open-end catheter and flexible metallic ureteral probe.

down the ureter. A flexible probe thirteen inches long, made by winding a narrow, flat steel strip spirally upon itself (Fig. 1), was passed its full length without detecting a stone. A catheter in the bladder detected nothing, but drew off some blood, thus establishing the pervious condition of the ureter. There was, therefore, a perfect demonstration that the trouble was due to a movable kidney, and a kinking of the ureter, thus probably obstructing its lumen. The wound in the kidney was closed by catgut sutures, and a strip of its capsule an inch broad was removed from the whole posterior surface, and the organ stitched with silk to the muscular and fascial edges of the wound. The wound was left open, and stuffed with iodoform gauze.

The patient's condition progressed satisfactorily. Further clots and blood were drawn by catheter the evening following the operation. The urine constantly increased in quantity, being 28 ounces in the first twenty-four hours. The paroxysms of pain were greatly lessened, and by the third day were altogether absent, while the urine had already risen to 40 ounces daily. April 27, 1897, the patient's physician, Dr. Coe, wrote that there had been no recurrence of the paroxysms of pain, but that a more or less constant pain in the lumbar region had been present, which varied in intensity at different times. The urine was occasionally reduced from 20 to 24 ounces (her normal amount) to 12 to 16 ounces. A strong current of electricity through the loin promptly relieved the pain and "ischuria." The general health continued excellent.

CASE III. *Renal Colic—Hemorrhagic Cysts—Nephrotomy—Subsequent Nephrectomy—Recovery.*—Thos. B., aged thirty-two years, suffered during six years with sharp attacks of lumbar pain, growing more frequent and more severe. Upon entrance to the hospital, February 21, 1893, nothing could be ascertained by physical examination except tenderness on pressure over the left lumbar region. The urine contained a little blood and pus.

March 1, 1893, the left kidney was exposed by the incision recommended by König, passing along the edge of the quadratus lumborum muscle to just above the ilium, and then forward along the crest of this bone nearly to the anterior superior spine. The presence of stone could not be determined by means of needle punctures or the finger. The cortex was incised, and the pelvis and eight inches of the ureter exposed without other result than a profuse renal hemorrhage, which cut short further investigation. This was so severe that it was necessary to partially fill the wound in the kidney with gauze. Seven days later, under ether narcosis, the kidney and ureter were again exposed, but nothing was found. The sinus rapidly closed, and until the patient's discharge from the hospital, five weeks after the first operation, there was no recurrence of the painful attacks.

He was again seen during December, 1896, when he reported at the Vanderbilt Clinic, complaining of a recurrence of pain, which showed itself soon after the wound had healed. March 1, 1897, acute pain like the puncture of a needle was still felt on pressure under the twelfth rib near the line of the quadratus lumborum muscle. There was no enlargement of the kidney, and the urine was clear, although at times it was said to be slightly bloody. There was a slight hernial bulging in the cicatrix on coughing and expulsive effort.

The pains increased, radiating from the loin to the breast, groin, and testes, and accompanied with chills and nausea, so that nephrectomy was performed March 25, 1897. König's curved incision was employed. The kidney was so firmly adherent that the peritoneum was twice torn through in the attempt to separate and remove the organ. These openings were at once sutured. The pedicle of the kidney was tied *en masse* with silk, the ligature including the loop of a cautery-point (Cleveland's method), so that the silk could be subsequently divided by simply passing an electric current through the cautery-point. The wound was partly closed with deep sutures of kangaroo-tendon and skin sutures of silkworm-gut and silk. The Mikulicz packing was removed on the third day. The ligature was divided and removed on the seventh day.

Examination of the extirpated kidney showed that it contained three hemorrhagic cysts, each the size of a large marble, and also that it was somewhat inflamed. There was no evidence of tuberculosis.

The patient recovered well from the operation, and resumed his work. He suddenly died, August 9, 1897, the cause of death being heart failure, according to the report of the coroner.

CASE IV. *Renal Colic—Exploratory Nephrotomy—Recovery.*—Samuel J., aged thirty-six years, entered the hospital, November 12, 1897, with the following history:

He had had three attacks of gonorrhea, occurring respectively 9 years, 2 years, and 6 months previously, and recovery always ensued without complications. One month before coming under observation there had been a sudden attack of severe pain in the right lumbar region, followed by vesical irritation, chill, fever, and sweating. Subsequently there had been two such attacks. The urine contained ten per cent. by volume of pus and albumin. Pressure over the right loin was painful.

König's curved lumbar incision was made, as in Case III., and, the kidney being exposed, an incision was made into its pelvis, but nothing abnormal was found. The ureter was also exposed for a short distance and explored by the flexible probe with a negative result. The wound was closed over gauze drains. The effect of the operation was slight. There was blood in the urine at first, and the albumin and pus were diminished for a time, but later increased again, up to eight per cent. by volume, and there was considerable purulent sediment. The wound was superficial at the time of the patient's discharge, and he has since passed from observation.

CASE V. *Renal Pain—Nephrotomy—Nephrorrhaphy—Recovery.*—Ellen W., aged twenty-two years, suffered during five years from attacks of pain and tenderness in the right lumbar and iliac regions, which were not relieved by removal of the appendix, performed at Roosevelt Hospital. The seat of tenderness and pain was along a tract running from the right kidney to the bladder. Examination, with and without an anesthetic, revealed nothing further. The urine was pale, acid, clear, with a specific gravity of 1020, and contained neither albumin nor sugar, and no pathologic sediment.

October 16, 1896, the right kidney was exposed, probed by needles, incised, and examined. A probe was passed seventeen inches into the ureter, and it was palpated as far as possible. Nothing abnormal was found. The renal wound was sutured, and the kidney itself anchored in the incision in the loin by means of catgut sutures. The lumbar wound was closed by sutures. The patient made a good recovery, and during some months was free from pain; but when seen in March, 1897, she complained of pain in the old situation and down the front of the thigh, though she was not prevented from following her occupation as a silk-weaver, standing on her feet ten hours daily. The kidney was in place.

December 10, 1897, she again returned to the hospital, still complaining of pain over the right kidney, which on examination seemed to be enlarged and tender. There was no elevation of temperature and no abnormal deposits in the urine.

MOVABLE KIDNEY—NEPHRORRHAPHY.

At a time when the kidney was still *terra incognita* to most surgeons, the attempt to relieve the pain caused by a wandering kidney by anchoring it in the loin excited a widespread interest. Like other diseases to which general attention has been directed, this condition has proved to be of frequent occurrence,[1][2] and the operation for its relief has become almost a routine performance. During 1883 an

[1] Glénard, *La Presse Méd.*, Belge, xli, p. 65, 1889, says that sixty per cent. of 215 women had movable kidney.

[2] Mathieu, *Ann. des Malad. des Org. Gen.-Urin.*, xii, p. 70, 1894,

account[1] of one of the first successful attempts of this character was published (Case VI.). Although over fourteen years have passed since this operation was performed in the case referred to, there has been no recurrence of the difficulty, and the patient is reported to be in good health. In this, as in Case VII., the capsule of the kidney was simply stitched to the wound, while in the cases operated upon more recently a strip of the capsule has first been peeled off, in order to give a wider band of adhesion.

CASE VI. *Movable Kidney—Nephrorrhaphy—Recovery.*—Eliza I., aged thirty-three years, the mother of several children, entered New York Hospital during December, 1882, for relief from constantly recurring attacks of pain and nausea. She attributed her trouble to a concussion of the abdomen, received five years previously, when she was caught between two slowly moving cars. At that time she was confined to her bed for a brief period, and then resumed her work. Five weeks later she began to have pains in the right abdomen, running up the side and down the thigh, and soon after a tumor was observed in the right lumbar region, the manipulation of which increased the pain. Occasionally an attack of pain was followed by hematuria or uterine hemorrhage, and attacks of nausea and vomiting coincidently occurred. By crowding inward the lower ribs the kidney was easily displaced and palpated at the level of the umbilicus, with its hilum upward and its long diameter transverse. Several examinations of the urine showed it to be normal.

November 18, 1882, the patient was turned upon her face and a vertical incision made from the twelfth rib to the crest of the ilium, about three inches to the right of the spinous processes. The overlying tissues were divided and the kidney exposed, seized, and crowded into the wound. The mobility upward and downward was nearly four inches. Its capsule was stitched to the wound by means of seven carbolized catgut sutures, and the wound left open to granulate. Healing was complete within five weeks, and the patient's condition was much improved. May 12, 1897 (fourteen years later), the patient was reported to be in good health and free from her former affection.

CASE VII. *Movable Kidney—Nephrorrhaphy—Recovery.*—Augusta K., aged thirty-four years, suffered with paroxysms of pain in the right side of the abdomen during sixteen years, growing more frequent and more severe. Two years before admission to the hospital an ovariotomy was performed, but without relief. Examination showed the presence of a smooth, movable, and tender kidney. The urine was normal.

December 14, 1889, an incision extending obliquely forward and downward was made in the right loin, and the kidney exposed. After removal of part of the fat capsule, the kidney was sutured in an elevated position with strong catgut to the muscle and fascia of either edge of the wound; the incision was partly closed. After the operation the patient complained of great pain, similar to that which had characterized previous attacks. In time this somewhat subsided, but was still present at the time the patient was discharged, five weeks after operation. An abscess subsequently presented itself in the lower part of the cicatrix, and after the discharge of its contents the pain disappeared. February 27, 1897, the patient reported that she had had no further symptoms referable to the kidney.

CASE VIII. *Movable Kidney—Nephrorrhaphy—Recovery.*—Frances S., aged thirty years, referred to me by Dr. E. Cushier, entered the Woman's Infirmary with a history of general disturbance during one year, with occasional sharp attacks of epigastric pain. A movable kidney was found which was not benefited by compress and bandage, and an operation was performed May 8, 1894. An incision was made along the outer border of the quadratus muscle, and the kidney exposed. A strip of its capsule, 1.5 inches wide was removed from the posterior surface of the organ, and the kidney was sutured in the abdominal wound with chromicized catgut. The external wound was closed over gauze drains, and it promptly united. Recovery, according to a report from her physician two years afterward, was satisfactory and permanent.

CASE IX. *Movable Kidney—Nephrorrhaphy—Recovery.*—Margaret H., aged forty-two years, was troubled during two years with intermittent pain in the right hypochondriac region, disappearing on lying down. She had noticed a movable body in the right side of the abdomen. Examination showed that she had a characteristic movable kidney on the right side, which could be grasped and pulled upon, thereby causing the same pain which she described as having suffered spontaneously; the urine was normal.

January 5, 1895, the right kidney was exposed, and a strip of its capsule 4 x 1.5 inches was peeled off and six kangaroo-tendon sutures were passed through the substance of the kidney, fastening it into the wound. The end sutures were passed through the skin as well as the kidney, thus partly closing the wound, which was elsewhere filled with iodoform gauze. Recovery was uneventful. The gauze was removed on the fourth day, and the wound rapidly healed by granulation. The patient has passed from observation.

CASE X. *Movable Kidney—Nephrorrhaphy—Oophorectomy.*—Mrs. S., aged twenty-eight years, was referred to me by Drs. Roberts and Nammack, with a history of attacks of pain radiating from the right kidney all over the right side, and sufficiently severe to confine her to bed several days at a time. The assumption of the recumbent posture did not give relief. During March, 1896, she had such a severe attack, characterized by such marked symptoms referable to the right iliac fossa, that two able physicians agreed that the trouble was appendical in origin, one advising operation and the other being against interference.

When seen by me, during May of the same year, examination of the right iliac fossa was negative, but she undoubtedly had a floating kidney and also a painful ovary, prolapsed into Douglas' cul-de-sac. There was no abdominal distension characteristic of enteroptosis. In June, 1896, the kidney was replaced and stitched into position after Tuffier's method, and an enlarged and cystic right ovary removed at the same time. The patient made a prompt recovery, and when seen fifteen months later, the kidney was in good position, but the paroxysms had recurred in a somewhat abated form. In the absence of a definite lesion I was obliged to lean upon her description of the attacks. I advised an exploratory operation for the examination of the previously suspected appendix. This was recently done by another surgeon, and the appendix was removed.

CASE XI. *Movable Kidney—Nephrorrhaphy—Recovery.*—Helena L., aged thirty-six years, had complained for years of gastric indigestion and pain in the stomach and bowels, recently increasing, and especially severe after exertion, or when standing for any length of time. There was at times difficulty in micturition, and the amount of urine daily passed greatly varied. During the six months previous to examination the patient had observed a tumor

found that of 306 women, 85, or twenty-eight per cent., had movable kidney.

[1] Weir, *New York Med. Jour.*, February 17, 1883.

in the right side of the abdomen. Both kidneys could be felt as low down as the iliac fossæ.

June 9, 1896, an incision was made along the outer border of the left quadratus lumborum muscle. A rent into the peritoneal cavity exposed the spleen. This opening was closed by catgut, as was another in the pleural cavity which occurred when the incision was extended upward. The left kidney was then freed from its surroundings, dislocated into the wound, and a portion of its capsule, ¾x2 inches, was removed. The kidney was sutured to the muscles with kangaroo tendon, and the wound partially closed with silk. A similar operation was performed on the right side, and the right lobe of the liver was found to be enlarged three or four inches in a downward direction. Both wounds healed promptly, and recovery was uneventful.

March 8, 1897, the patient reported that she had no pain in the right side, but a great deal in the left, and especially a pulling sensation on stooping.

These six patients, with seven operations (*i.e.*, in one a double nephrorrhaphy), all recovered In no instance, so far as can be ascertained, did recurrence take place, and the elapsed time varies from one to fourteen years. One patient upon whom double nephrorrhaphy was performed suffered from pain in one side following the operation; in others, the pains continued though the kidney remained fixed. These results are no better than the careful surgeon should expect, but they are somewhat better than the average. Thus, according to Neumann, who published a dissertation on this subject at Berlin in 1892; out of 274 nephrorrhaphies, 5 patients or 1.8 per cent. died; while 222 patients, the histories of whom were followed for a time, 65.3 per cent. were cured, 10.3 per cent. were improved, and 22 per cent. were not improved. McCosh[1] found 3 deaths from operation in 117 reported cases of nephrorrhaphy. Of the 62 patients of whom a record was given after a lapse of three months or more, 55 per cent. were cured, 25 per cent. improved, and 20 per cent. not improved. Albarran collected 374 cases with only 4 deaths; Küster had 1 death in 50 cases, and secured 60 per cent. of cures. The latter figures are probably more reliable than those collected from many sources, since fatal cases are apt to be omitted. The mortality from this operation has usually been due to septic peritonitis, this occurring either when the transperitoneal route was selected, or when an accidental opening was made into the peritoneal or pleural cavities.

Relapses may be frequently expected, since the renal ptosis is but one symptom of the general enteroptosis so clearly described by Glénard, and of which the distended stomach or overloaded colon, are usually prime factors. It may also be stated that in none of my cases did bandages or pads give any relief; indeed, I have never observed a good result follow the application of external support.

Numerous operative procedures have been advocated for the relief of a movable kidney. Their number and slight variation, one from the other, show that something more than anchoring the kidney is often required for the relief of the dyspeptic, neurasthenic, and painful symptoms which characterize this affection. The pain may be most easily removed, but the neurasthenia is often unchanged.

[1] McCosh, *New York Med. Jour.*, 1890, vol. 51, p. 281.

As an instance of the remarkable operative feats which have been attempted in this connection, it is sufficient to mention that Riedel[1] is said to have several times stitched the kidney to the diaphragm and quadratus lumborum muscle. Others have imitated him in dislocating the kidney and suturing it to tissues, muscular and otherwise, distinct from the proper renal bed. The secret of success in operating, however, seems to lie in two points, *viz.*: careful stitching of the organ into the depths of the lumbar wound by material which will maintain its integrity a considerable length of time; and allowing a portion, if not the whole wound, to heal by granulation, in order to secure a broad cicatricial support.

In about three-fourths (78 per cent.) of the cases reported by Albarran, the kidney was sutured without the decortication suggested by Tuffier, and he protests strongly against this stripping off of the capsule, as likely to produce a considerable degree of renal sclerosis. Guyon is of the same opinion, contenting himself with the passage of the supporting sutures through the kidney substance. These sutures are usually placed, three or four in number, transversely through the organ; but lately it has been advised to make two of them longitudinal stitches, to be fastened to the muscles on either side of the incision. In my later cases I have employed the decortication already described, and have not found, in several of the patients examined at remote periods, any albumin in the urine or any other indication of renal disease. If such should occur it would as likely as not be due to the suture as to the decortication. But the latter can, in my judgment, be omitted, provided the wound be kept fairly open so that the granulations make a broad band of adhesion.

To illustrate what should not be done, however, attention is directed to the procedure of Küster who, in twelve cases, sutured the lower end of the kidney to the twelfth rib with silver wire. The result was good in ten cases, but five times he opened the pleural cavity during operation, although, thanks to his skill, no bad results followed this accident. Holl long ago called the attention of surgeons to the possibility of this mishap in work in this region, on account of the low attachments of the pleural sac. As far as possible, the fat capsule should be dissected away. A point of importance is a prolonged and, at first, quite rigid rest in the recumbent posture. This, I insist, should continue at least four weeks.

The patients upon whom I have operated have all been females. It is rare, indeed, that a man seeks relief for a wandering kidney.

If a movable kidney cannot be felt in the recumbent or lateral position, it is well to adopt a method of examination which has given me good results for many years. This consists in placing the patient in an erect position with the hips steadied against a solid table, and the head and trunk inclined forward with the hands resting on the back of a chair, or on the shoulders of the surgeon who sits or kneels in front of the person examined. This will relax the abdominal wall and allow of its free palpation, and particularly of the parts overhung by the ribs.

(To be continued.)

[1] Reineboth, "Inaug. Diss.," Jena, 1892.

MEDICAL PROGRESS.

Relation between the Testicle and Prostate.—FLODERUS (*Deut. Zeit. für Chir.*, vol. 45, p. 110, 1897) says that as extirpation of a single testicle is often followed by atrophy of the corresponding side of the prostate gland, it must be due to some nerve relation between the two rather than to any altered internal secretion. Removal of both testicles before maturity interferes with the full development of the prostate. That castration after full maturity will reduce a normal prostate is in dispute. If it does so, it reduces the volume and elasticity of the organ, and increases its consistency. The effect of complete castration in beginning, or fully developed hypertrophies, is irregular, and often not demonstrable. The reduction in volume is sometimes confined to the upper part of the prostate, and is accompanied by a loss of elasticity, while in others a shortening of the urethra is noticeable. Tuberculous processes in the gland may be brought to a standstill, or even cured, by castration.

Unilateral castration sometimes produces in the corresponding side of the normal adult prostate such changes as have been above described. It will not prevent future hypertrophy. Its effect on existing hypertrophy is slow, and consists in a shrinkage of the corresponding side, especially in the upper portion of the gland. It may cause healing of tuberculous lesions. Unilateral castration is not followed by a demonstrable reduction in size of the opposite lobe of the prostate. There usually results atrophy of the seminal vesicles, with compensatory hypertrophy of the other testicle (and prostatic lobe?). The advantages of double over unilateral castration are, therefore, plain.

Periostitis Following Muscular Exertion.—DENT (*The Practitioner*, October, 1897) calls attention to the complex of symptoms which may follow the unfair use of a single muscle, or particular group of muscles. Under such circumstances it is not the muscle itself nor its tendon which suffers, but the investing fascial plane, or the periostial attachments. The constant use of muscles attached to bones produces a vascular condition of the periosteum, and a formation of extra bone. In this manner are built up the bony prominencies which are observable in the long bones of muscular individuals. The abuse of a single muscle may cause a degree of vascularity which in time may amount to inflammation in the region of the bony attachment of the muscle or its tendon. Examples of this condition are seen in persons who make long descents from mountains, or who kick violently in football games, without being used to such exertions. Dent, in speaking of a patient presenting this affection, said that "In all probability the boy had become accustomed to a bad style of play. It is curious to note that in all athletic exercises and games the most efficient play is secured by the most scientific use of the muscles; this means the adroit combination and concerted action of many muscles rather than the undue use of one or a few. Whether using a bat, a tennis-racket, a fishing-rod, or other implement of sport, it is of profound importance to adopt what is called a good style. Teachers of games rightly, and very strongly, insist upon this point. They do so in order to get the best possible results. For example, to make a good cast with a long fishing-line, or to put on what tennis-players call a "heavy cut,' necessitates a good style. The teacher is satisfied with the result if the stroke is made effectively, or the cast is a dexterous one. He may not be aware how truly scientific his instruction is, and how, by insisting upon combined action of numerous muscles, and by using leverage in the most effective possible manner, he diminishes the strain of any one particular group of muscles, or any single muscle, and distributes it over a larger number, thus most effectively preventing such disorders as form the subject of this paper."

Other instances of the occurrence of periostitis which may be cited, are that of the housemaid, who by sweeping irritates the attachment of the pectoralis major to the humerus; that of the man who by pumping inflames the attachment of the biceps to the scapula, etc. Such continued irritation may cause an osteitis. Paget mentions a case of necrosis of the humerus, and suppuration of the elbow- and shoulder-joints, following violent exertion in a university boat-race.

Complete Inversion of the Uterus.—WOOTON (*Vir. Med. Semi-Monthly*, Nov. 26, 1897) reports a case of complete inversion of the uterus occurring in a white primipara. The placenta was adherent, and the attending midwife caused the woman to stand upon her feet while she pulled upon the cord. In this way the placenta was in great part removed. Six hours later the patient was found by the physician in a state of shock, and the uterus was inverted and entirely outside of the body. Under chloroform, and after two-hours' effort, the uterus was replaced, but the woman died the following day.

THERAPEUTIC NOTES.

Therapeutic Value of Salophen.—LEHMANN (*Ther. Wochenschr.*, September 26, 1897) finds that salophen has a most favorable influence upon psoriasis. He treated the left leg of one patient with ten per cent. chrysarobin-tramaticin, and the right one with ten-per-cent. salophen salve. The better result was obtained with the latter method.

BAQUE found that salophen has an indisputable action upon acute and subacute rheumatism. Although it does not have as powerful an effect as sodium salicylate, it possesses the great advantage of not producing unpleasant symptoms, such as headache, dizziness, ringing in the ears, etc. It disintegrates in the intestine, and cannot, therefore, upset the stomach. It does not seem to have any better effect in chronic rheumatism than the numerous other remedies proposed. It has a powerful analgesic action, comparable to that of antypyrin or phenacetin. It appears to be of benefit in skin affections, especially those accompanied by itching. It is without disagreeable taste or smell. A medium dose is 60 grains daily, given in divided doses.

THE MEDICAL NEWS.

A WEEKLY JOURNAL

OF MEDICAL SCIENCE.

COMMUNICATIONS are invited from all parts of the world. Original articles contributed *exclusively* to THE MEDICAL NEWS will after publication be liberally paid for (accounts being rendered quarterly), or 250 reprints will be furnished in place of other remuneration. When necessary to elucidate the text, illustrations will be engraved from drawings or photographs furnished by the author. Manuscripts should be typewritten.

Address the Editor: J. RIDDLE GOFFE, M.D., No. 111 FIFTH AVENUE (corner of 18th St.), NEW YORK.

Subscription Price, including postage in U. S. and Canada.

PER ANNUM IN ADVANCE	$4.00
SINGLE COPIES	.10
WITH THE AMERICAN JOURNAL OF THE MEDICAL SCIENCES, PER ANNUM	7.50

Subscriptions may begin at any date. The safest mode of remittance is by bank check or postal money order, drawn to the order of the undersigned. When neither is accessible, remittances may be made, at the risk of the publishers, by forwarding in *registered* letters.

LEA BROTHERS & CO.,
No. 111 FIFTH AVENUE (corner of 18th St.), NEW YORK, AND NOS. 706, 708 & 710 SANSOM ST., PHILADELPHIA.

SATURDAY, JANUARY 15, 1898.

TEACHING THE SIGNIFICANCE AND PROPHYLAXIS OF VENEREAL DISEASES TO NON-MEDICAL STUDENTS.

IN a recent letter our Berlin correspondent comments favorably upon the lectures on "The Significance and Prophylaxis of Venereal Diseases," which, during the past three years, have been given at the University of Berlin to non-medical students. We take pleasure in referring those who may be especially interested in the matter to the letter itself (MEDICAL NEWS, January 8, 1898), as it would be difficult to give a more able presentation of the subject, or a more entertaining description of Professor Lassar's lectures.

It has become the fashion during late years to look to Germany for much that is good, and not a little that is best, but the present innovation, from a standpoint of radicalism, is apparently more consonant with American or English institutions than with Continental. We can almost hear the caustic criticism from across the water which would in all probability have followed the announcement that an American college had been the first to add to its general curriculum a course on the prevention and significance of venereal diseases—another Yankee notion!

Individual opinions are frequently a century in advance of general practices, and the establishment of such a course, not only in the university but in all higher institutions of learning, from the high-school to the college, has not lacked advocates; but, as our correspondent aptly remarks: "The candid admission, however, of the imminence of the danger to young men is not in accord with Anglo-Saxon principles generally in such matters, and so, it may be supposed, the suggestion of such a thing to most university faculties would be met by prompt discouragement." In common with our English cousins we prefer to remain only semi-cognizant of the existance of immoral practices—a frank exposition of the question might shock some one's venerable idea of modesty.

While teaching our young men and women many useful things, we neglect, for no substantial reason, to inculcate the fearful lesson of venereal diseases—the most preventable of all; fail to teach them how to avoid paresis, tabes dorsalis, stricture, sterility, and all the fell host that surely follow indiscriminate venery; how to avoid the species of homicide, conceived in the womb of ignorance, which unwittingly sacrifices wife and children; and last, though none the less true, that the most careful therapeusis is not infrequently absolutely inefficacious in preventing the remote consequences of venereal infection.

We flee the presence of the leper, but allow the syphilitic freedom to menace us, each and every one—to drink from the same cup, eat from the same dish, occupy the same chair in the barber-shop. The physician and the health-officer are in an altercation about the disposition of a case of measles; the syphilitic slips between the legs of both.

The data of venereal diseases are so familiar to physicians that we, as a class, fail to read their real meaning—that the least we can do in order to avoid culpability in the possible wreck of a fellow being is to energetically assist in the furtherance of the teaching that every young man and woman should be sent out into the world free to choose, knowing all the facts in the case, whether or not the path will be followed that leads to suffering, invalidism, the hospital, or the insane asylum. Then, at least, we would not have to bear with equanimity the reproach: "Had I but known all." Innocence that implies ignorance of the principles of correct ethics is never admirable, but rather always lamentable, and the peculiar attitude of the human mind that leaves one's sexual environment to be imagined had best be eradicated, and this almost herculean task no profession is better able to handle than ours.

The positive isolation of the cause of syphilis will no doubt be intensely interesting medically, but it is hardly necessary to a system of rational prophylaxis of *lues venerea*.

We forestall reference to the proverbial moral laxity of medical students, a laxity seemingly paradoxic when considered in relation to the knowledge they are supposed to possess but which, our observation justifies, grows every year less obtrusive; in fact, it may be said that progress in medical-student morality goes hand in hand with a constantly higher standard of qualification for entrance to the medical college. In this connection we may utilize the truism that constant familiarity with danger begets carelessness in its presence. This may in a measure explain the medical student's fearlessness in exposing himself to venereal infection in spite of an evident knowledge of the subject.

However, we can hardly expect to educate the "Old Adam" entirely out of existence; what we may do, and what it is our plain duty to do, is to teach the significance of venereal diseases, that it may not be said that as a profession we stand idly by and watch the mechanism of the trap in which youth is caught without once trying to injure its evil perfection; content, as it were, to sit in the curule chair without exercising the perogative—the duty of him who occupies it.

THE JUSTIFICATION OF THE PEDIATRIST'S EXISTENCE.

OUR Berlin correspondent remarked in one of his recent letters that the specialty of pediatrics has contributed nothing to the enrichment of medical science, particularly of therapeutics, during its existence now approaching a half century. This may appear on first sight to be a gross exaggeration, nearing falsehood, yet when the matter is carefully considered its truthfulness seems to be in keeping with its candor.

There are undoubtedly many physicians well versed in the ailments of childhood who do not wish to be regarded as specialists, and who maintain that pediatrics can in no wise be considered a specialty. Nevertheless, the existence of a constantly increasing number of physicians who devote their time exclusively to the treatment of diseases of children and to teaching their art to others shows that many are not adverse to the garb and cult of specialism.

Moreover, those who devote themselves enthusiastically to diseases of children are continually bewailing the fact in public that too little attention is given to their department in the undergraduate medical schools, while they point with pride and in terms of general exaltation to the benefit which has accrued the "assumption of the dignity by pediatrics as a special department in colleges." To quote further from a recent writer in *Pediatrics*, as a result of establishing special professorships of pediatrics in medical schools, he says, "A field of inquiry has been opened by those who have given this subject earnest attention which has been fruitful in its results and which must inevitably reclaim thousands from an untimely grave." That there is a general air of conviction in such swinging statements no one can deny. But what is the justification for them, one is led to ask? Can such a writer as the one whom we have just quoted descend from generalizations and enumerate specifically some of the measures now utilized in the handling of the infant which reclaim thousands from an untimely grave and which we owe to pediatrists or their teachings? Or must they admit, with our correspondent, that their existence has been more barren of results than that of any other specialty? Have they by their own efforts altered in any way the mortality statistics of diseases peculiar to children? Have they contributed one diagnostic help in the recognition of the more obscure conditions sometimes afflicting children? Have they unraveled any of the mysteries obscuring the pathogenesis of such a common disease as Sydenham's chorea, or such an obscure condition as diabetes in children? True it is that they may point with pride to the present status of the treatment of diphtheria, but they will scarcely contend that they did more in bringing about this fortunate condition than to follow the road pointed out to them by one working in an entirely different field. They may suggest that the different forms of meningitis and other intracranial and intraspinal conditions may be differentiated early, and thus the proper measures employed for their relief. With this every one must agree but Quincke, Fürbinger, Freyhan, and the others to whom we owe our knowledge of the efficaciousness of such measures and who are not particularly interested in pediatrics.

The subject of infant-feeding demands consideration. Until one examines the proceedings of pediatric societies and the files of pediatric journals he has no idea of the amount of time and energy which is consumed every year in learning and teaching how to feed babies. No one will deny that we are more adept because of this desirable possession than we were a few decades ago, yet it would be a mistake to flatter ourselves that a satisfactory stage has yet been reached. Within the memory of almost the youngest of the present generation three or four quite individualized waves have swept across the pediatric sea in reference to infant-feeding. There was a time, and that not long removed, that artificial infant-foods came in for unmerited, but considerable praise. Later, modified milk seemed to be the thing, but it was succeeded after an interval of mingled satisfaction and distrust by the cry for sterilized milk; while to-day the contest for supremacy of this form of milk and Pasteurized milk goes on apace, with the odds very decidedly in favor of the latter. It would verily seem that Pasteurization of milk is the most fitting process to which it may be subjected at the present day to make it more nearly the ideal food which we are told Nature intended it to be. But what of PASTEUR?

Taking it altogether perhaps our correspondent has given pediatrists food for reflection; they may cease drawing the long bow and concentrate their attention on centering their arrows.

ECHOES AND NEWS.

Trephining for Apoplexy Followed by Death.—The patient recently referred to editorially in the MEDICAL NEWS as having been trephined for apoplexy, is dead. The fatal issue occurred a short time after the operation, and the autopsy revealed the presence of a blood-clot in the internal capsule—a condition forever beyond the reach of the surgeon's knife.

The Brooklyn Neurological Society.—At the annual meeting of the Brooklyn Neurological Society, Dr. A. C. Brush was elected president, and Dr. W. H. Haynes, secretary, for the ensuing year.

Doctors Ill with Diphtheria.—Dr. Frank C. Bunn of East Orange, N. J., and Dr. Harriet K. Burnet of Newark, N. J., are suffering from diphtheria as a result of infection while performing tracheotomy upon a child suffering from that disease.

Death of Dr. O'Dwyer.—Dr. Joseph O'Dwyer died at his home in New York City on the 7th inst. of tuberculous meningitis. Dr. O'Dwyer was fifty-five years of age, and was graduated from the New York College of Physicians and Surgeons in 1866.

First Medical College Lectures in America.—According to Dr. Roswell Park the first lectures on anatomy given in America were those of Giles Firman, delivered some time before 1649 in Harvard College which had been established ten years previously.

A Jewish Hospital for the Borough of Brooklyn.—The Hebrew Hospital Fund Society of Brooklyn have made application to the State Board of Charities for a certificate of incorporation for their proposed new hospital and dispensary for the use of their poorer brethren.

United Hebrew Charities of New York City.—An anonymous donor has purchased the valuable property on the southeast corner of Second avenue and Twenty-first street for the purpose of erecting there a large building for the use of the "Charities" as a headquarters, for their various industrial and training-schools.

Death from Lead Poisoning.—Four deaths from lead poisoning have recently occurred in England among enamel workers in earthenware and china factories. The enamel contains from fifteen to twenty per cent. of lead. One of the deaths was that of a young girl who not long ago was fined for not wearing the respirator provided by the firm.

The Seney Hospital, Borough of Brooklyn.—A handsome bequest has been made to charity under the will of the late George Barlow. The sum of $28,000 is thus devised for the endowment of beds and for other funds of the Seney Hospital. In addition to this there are bequests to various societies, homes, and colleges amounting to nearly $100,000.

The Hoagland Laboratory, Borough of Brooklyn.—Dr. C. N. Hoagland has again made a donation to the above-named institution, by way of a New-Year's gift, by the conveyance of a security valued at $24,000. Dr. Hoagland's benefactions to the cause of scientific research are said to have reached a figure considerably in excess of a quarter of a million of dollars during the last ten years.

Importance of Haste in Dispensary Legislation.—Authoritative information has been received from Albany that the session of the Legislature this winter will be very short. An effort is being made to fix the date of adjournment at February 15th. Under these circumstances no bill introduced later than January 20th will receive any consideration. Who is responsible for the County Society Dispensary Bill? And why has it not been introduced?

Randall's Island Hospital Alumni.—A meeting will be held at the New York Academy of Medicine, at 8.30 P.M., on the 18th inst., for the purpose of forming an Association of the Alumni of Randall's Island Hospital. All who have at any time served on the staff are requested to be present. Dr. David T. Marshall, No. 205 West 106th Street, New York City, is the Secretary.

Murder of Professor Rogers.—Dr. S. A. Rogers, Professor of Anatomy at the Memphis (Tenn.) Medical College and at one time president of the Memphis Board of Health, was shot in the back by a woman on the 7th inst., and was taken in a dying condition to St. Joseph's Hospital. Immediately after shooting Dr. Rogers, the woman sent a bullet into her own heart and died instantly. There were no witnesses to the tragedy and its cause is a mystery.

Boston Medical Society.—At a meeting of this Society, held on January 1, 1898, the following officers were elected for the ensuing year: President, Dr. S. Goodman; first vice-president, Dr. R. K. Noyes; second-vice-president, Dr. F. J. Kelleker; secretary, Dr. M. Gerstein; treasurer, Dr. V. Bychower. The subject of Medical Abuse was discussed by Doctors S. Goodman, F. F. Whittier, N. M. Goodman, G. Liebman, M. Gerstein, F. J. Kelleker, and P. Losnowsky.

Colonel Bache Appointed Professor of Military Medicine.—Colonel Dallas Bache, Assistant Surgeon-General, will be relieved from duty as Chief Surgeon, Department of the Platte on January 20, 1898, and will repair to Washington, D. C., and report in person to the Surgeon-General of the Army to assume charge of the Museum and Library Division of his office, and also to enter upon duty April 10, 1898, as Professor of Military Medicine in the Army Medical School, to which he is assigned accordingly.

Medical Requirements in Tennessee.—In a recent issue of the MEDICAL NEWS we published a note in regard to the laws of the various States regarding license to practice medicine. Dr. John M. Bass of Nashville, Tenn., writes us that Tennessee is no longer among those States which accept certain diplomas in place of an examination. A new law making an examination obligatory in order to practice medicine was passed last year, and is being vigorously enforced by the State Board of Medical Examiners.

Department of Health of the Borough of Brooklyn.—This branch of the city's service has been reposed in the hands of Dr. R. A. Black, whose title is Assistant Sanitary Superintendent. Dr. Black is reported as saying that he intends to move slowly in the matter of recommending the removal of medical inspectors, it being his wish not to see the efficiency of the department impaired by hasty action. The fact that the great Borough of Brooklyn has no medical representation in the Board of Health has led to the report that legislation will be sought at Albany to the end that a medical man may become eligible to the position of president, that one of the medical commissioners will be made the successor of the Hon. Nathan Straus in that office, and that in this roundabout way the Borough of Brooklyn will come in for an adequate representation. Dr. Black was formerly connected with the Sanitary Committee of the Department of Public Instruction of Brooklyn.

Druggist Glogau Sued.—Druggist Conrad Glogau of Jersey City, N. J., is defendant in a suit brought against him by Scott and Bowne, the manufacturers of Scott's Emulsion. Some months ago *The Western Druggist*, published in Chicago, printed an article in which it was stated that the preparation put up by Scott and Bowne was found on an analysis ordered by the Food and Dairy Commissioners of the State of Ohio to contain one-tenth of a grain of morphin to every ounce. The article in question went on to say that the presence of morphin in such a quantity rendered the emulsion prejudicial to health. Mr. Glogau read the article and cutting it out exposed it in one of the show cases in his store, so that his customers could read it. It is alleged that whenever Scott's Emulsion was asked for, he would first refer the purchaser to the *Western Druggist* story. It is further alleged that Mr. Glogau explained his conduct by saying that he wished to be on the safe side in case the services of a coroner should ever be required. Scott and Bowne claim that Mr. Glogau by his action has slandered their firm and demand $25,000 damages. They deny that morphin in any dangerous quantity is present in their emulsion.—*Jersey City Evening Journal.*

Consolidation of Chicago Medical Colleges.—At its meeting of December 29th, the trustees of the University of Chicago, in response to a petition from the trustees of Rush Medical College, voted to enter into affiliation with that college. The date proposed for the consummation of the relationship is June 1, 1898, but it is specifically stipulated that the affiliation shall be dependent upon three conditions, as follows: The first is that the board of trustees of Rush Medical College shall be reorganized. At the present time a great majority of the trustees are physicians who are at the same time members of the faculty. This is acknowledged to be an unfortunate arrangement. The new trustees will be representative business men of the City of Chicago, who have no pecuniary interest in the college. The second condition provides that the requirements for admission to the college shall gradually be increased, until, in the autumn of 1902, only those who have completed the freshman and sophomore years of regular college work shall be admitted. This proposition, which had already been adopted by the present trustees of Rush Medical College, is a most significant step in the history of medical education. The third condition relates to the present debt of the college, which amounts to $71,000. It is provided that affiliation shall not take place until the debt has been paid. The trustees of the University of Chicago assume no financial responsibility in connection with Rush Medical College. Affiliation does not mean organic union. The degrees will be the degrees of Rush Medical College, not those of the University of Chicago.

A Quarantine Convention.—The recent epidemic of yellow fever in the Southern States has led to the proposition

Dr. W. H. Sanders of the Alabama State Board of Health that a quarantine convention be held, at which the South Atlantic and Gulf States shall be represented by delegates in every business and profession, with a view to making a scientific and exhaustive study of both the theory and practice of quarantine. The following preliminary program has been submitted by Dr. Sanders: 1. Quarantine with reference to international rights and interest. 2. Federal and State powers as to quarantine. 3. State and National quarantine as affecting commerce. 4. Quarantine as it affects personal rights. 5. Sanitary inspectors of foreign ports; what is being and can be done in this direction; sanitary conditions of foreign ports which menace us most, and what can be done to improve them. 6. Policing the sea along the South Atlantic and Gulf Coast to prevent the introduction of contagious and infectious diseases; what is being and can be done. 7. National disinfecting-stations for ships; where located; how operated; under what rules; with what results, and whether others are needed. 8. State maritime disinfecting-stations; how many; where located; how operated; under what rules, and with what results. 9. Medical inspectors of South Atlantic and Gulf seaports and coast towns to discover first case or cases of infectious or contagious diseases; how best to provide for. 10. What steps should be taken in dealing with first case or cases of infectious or contagious diseases which may reach our shores? 11. State and local quarantines; how best to adjust their relations. 12. Depopulation of infected cities; how to be accomplished, and to what points may refugees go. 13. Quarantine diseases; what are they, and how should they be dealt with? 14. Infection; how conveyed, and periods of incubation of infectious diseases. Disinfection; when needed, and how applied. 15. The mails and quarantine; how to deal with them practically when proper authority has declared that they should be disinfected. 16. Management of railroad trains during an epidemic of yellow fever from a railroad standpoint. 17. Classification of freights as to their liability of conveying infection. 18. What may be done to check the spread of and to exterminate yellow fever after it has become prevalent in a city? 19. Boards of health; of whom should they be composed, and how should they be appointed? To whom should the practical administration of quarantine be committed? 20. Practical difficulties in diagnosing yellow fever. 21. Interstate quarantine from a constitutional, commercial, and sanitary point of view. 22. Experiences of a quarantine officer in the recent epidemic. 23. National quarantine. 24. A National Bureau of Public Health. 25. The relation of the press to epidemics and quarantine. 26. Quarantine from a moral standpoint. 27. Sins and absurdities committed in the name of quarantine during the recent epidemic. 28. Introduction of yellow fever into the country in the past; from what places introduced and how.

A-Naphthol as an Intestinal Antiseptic.—For this purpose Maximowitsch considers α naphthol superior to β naphthol. It has three times the antiseptic power of the latter, and exhibits only one-third its toxic properties.

OBITUARY.

MR. ERNEST HART OF LONDON, ENGLAND.

MR. ERNEST HART, late Editor of the *British Medical Journal*, died at London, England, January 7th. Mr. Hart was born in the year 1836. He was educated at the City of London School and the School of Medicine attached to St. George's Hospital. In addition to his editorial connection with the *British Medical Journal* he was during some years co-editor of the *Lancet*. At one time he was ophthalmic surgeon and lecturer on ophthalmology at St. Mary's Hospital. Mr. Hart's great reputation however, does not depend so much upon his work along strictly professional lines as in the departments of hygiene and sanitation. Indeed, he might be called the great high-priest and indefatigable preacher of hygienic morality. He interested himself early in this work, and rendered great service in exposing defective arrangements for the sick poor in the workhouses of England, his efforts leading to the passage of an act of Parliament creating the Metropolitan Asylums Board. He carefully investigated during 1868 the practice of criminal baby-farming in London, and his report on the subject was the most effective argument in securing the passage of the Infant Life Protection Act. He also gave his powerful aid to the movement which resulted in the establishment some twenty years ago of the so-called "coffee-taverns" in London.

Not content with introducing these improved sanitary and economic measures at home, he carried the war into India and, as was said in these columns at the time, endeavored to hammer into the Mohammedan ears and understanding the great lesson of sanitation and preventive medicine upon which not only the health of the Orient but that of the Occident depends. His work in India was directed more especially against the spread of cholera through Mecca pilgrimages. His persistent advocacy of disinfection and quarantine was the most potent factor in the establishment of the international system of quarantine applied to these pilgrims. For his tireless efforts in such noble work Mr. Hart has placed the whole world under a deep debt of gratitude. Mr. Hart's more recent work is the report of the Parliamentary Bills Committee of the British Medical Association upon water-borne typhoid. In this report was presented a summary of the various outbreaks of typhoid fever in Great Britain and Ireland from 1858 to 1893. Upon this the MEDICAL NEWS commented editorially in the issue of November 27, 1897.

Mr. Hart was Honorary Chairman of the National Health Society of England and President of the Medical Sickness, Annuity, and Life Assurance Society. He was appointed editor of the *British Medical Journal* in 1866, which position he filled up to the time of his death. For several years he was also responsible for the editorial management of the *Sanitary Record* and the *London Medical Record*. To record the death of one whose contributions to the cause of advancing civilization have been as great as those of the subject of this obituary is indeed a lamentable necessity, and in closing it may be said that to this man is largely due the preeminence of England in matters of public sanitation.

CORRESPONDENCE.

TREPHINING FOR HEMIPLEGIA AND NEWSPAPER NOTORIETY.

To the Editor of the MEDICAL NEWS.

DEAR SIR: The editorial comments upon the subject of "Trephining for Newspaper Notoriety," which appear in the MEDICAL NEWS for January 1, 1898, are quite in accord with my own views on such matters—in cases to which such strictures are applicable.

Here is my brief rejoinder: It is a difficult matter to operate constantly in the presence of fifty or one hundred men without occasionally presenting something which interests them and which causes discussion outside of the class-room. I depend entirely upon the members of the medical profession for my livelihood, and whenever any of my cases are reported in the lay press it costs me hundreds or thousands of dollars. It does not disturb any of the physicians who know me personally, but it irritates physicians who do not know me, and who delight in reading such brightly caustic diction as that which appeared in your editorial.

I have several times received attention by the lay press, as has nearly every surgeon in New York City. The only case that ever came to me directly or indirectly, as far as I know, as a result of such "advertising" was a case in which I did not receive any fee for my work, but was threatened with a suit for malpractice. Other surgeons who have been placed in my position must be amused indeed at the idea of lay-press notices being classified under the head of "advertising."

The apoplexy case has not been correctly reported in the lay press or in the MEDICAL NEWS. A proper report upon the case will be forthcoming at the proper time. Meanwhile it may be well if speculation upon its character be allowed to rest. The editorial in the MEDICAL NEWS on the subject of "Trephining for Newspaper Notoriety" would do me great injury if it were not for the fact that I have so many good friends among the medical editors of the country. Although the editor of the MEDICAL NEWS does not know about me, or about my work, I assume that he would not intentionally do harm to any one, and I will be quite satisfied if he will take the trouble to address letters to the editors of the various newspapers of this city asking if their reporters obtained their information about the apoplexy case from me or from any of my assistants, or if it came from outside parties, and if he will publish the answers received.

All of the newspapers in New York City made news out of the case in question. A great many reporters came to ask about it. Out of the number I had to say something to three only. The reporter for the *World* kindly published the reasons which I gave him for physicians not being allowed to talk about their cases. The reporters for the *Times* and for the *Herald* did not mention my name, but they did publish the questions which they had put to me, and in such a way as to make it appear that I had volunteered the information. This was unintentional on their part as they were evidently gentlemen, and appreciated the reasons why I could not give them information. The "news" about the case did not come from me or from any of my assistants, as all of my friends know very well.

ROBERT T. MORRIS.

NEW YORK, January 8, 1898.

OUR PHILADELPHIA LETTER.

[From our Special Correspondent.]

HYGIENE OF THE SCHOOLROOM—FIRE AT THE UNIVERSITY HOSPITAL—ANNUAL ELECTION OF OFFICERS BY THE COLLEGE OF PHYSICIANS OF PHILADELPHIA, OBSTETRICAL SOCIETY OF PHILADELPHIA, AND PHILADELPHIA ACADEMY OF SURGERY—PRESENTATION OF A PORTRAIT OF THE LATE DR. KIRKBRIDE TO THE COLLEGE OF PHYSICIANS—DR. CHAS. E. SAJOUS—DR. TYSON'S RECEPTION TO THE PHILADELPHIA COUNTY MEDICAL SOCIETY—THE LATEST VERSION OF DR. EVANS' WILL—BACTERIOLOGIC INVESTIGATION OF THE WATER-SUPPLY.

JANUARY 8, 1898.

THE wave of reform which has of late swept over the health authorities of this city has extended to those having school matters in charge. Prodded on by the official hints from the former as to the need of radical improvements in the hygiene of the schoolroom, the latter officials having decided to further school sanitation by furnishing each pupil with an individual drinking-cup, by providing separate receptacles, which may be antisepticized, for each student's pencils and other paraphernalia, by prohibiting the decoration of rooms occupied by classes with potted plants and vines, and by directing that the schools in infected districts be scrubbed out weekly with carbolic-acid solutions. These details, while essential and valuable prophylactic measures, to be really effective must be supplemented by a thorough attention to school lavatories and drains, and to energetic instruction tending to impress upon the pupils (and their parents) the value of personal cleanliness and hygiene. Until the latter is done, no amount of antisepticizing and inspecting will prevent contagious diseases spreading from pupil to pupil.

A fire which for a time threatened the destruction of the hospital of the University of Pennsylvania originated in the dispensary of the hospital on January 4th, but owing to the prompt action of the hospital employees the flames were prevented from communicating to the wards. The fire originated in the basement, immediately under the men's surgical ward, and was due to the explosion of a gas stove. Dr. Schaeffer, the pharmacist, was severely burned in attempting to keep the flames from reaching the adjoining room, where a large quantity of alcohol and benzine was stored. No unusual excitement among the patients occurred, all of whom, it is said, were ignorant of the danger. The loss is estimated at over $2000.

At the last stated meeting of the College of Physicians of Philadelphia, held on January 5th, Dr. John B. Deaver read a paper on "The Necessity for Prompt Surgical Interference in Typhoid Perforation and Appendicitis Complicating Typhoid Fever." The speaker urgently recommended immediate operation in these complications o enteric fever, citing a number of instances from his service at the German Hospital which illustrated the advisability of this plan of treatment; many of the cases quoted were transferred to him from the medical ward of the hospital, operated upon, and then transferred back again to the medical ward, where the bath treatment was resumed, with a gratifyingly low mortality, considering the desperate character of the cases. Dr. James C. Wilson, who opened the discussion of Dr. Deaver's paper, approved in decided terms of surgical intervention in such cases, and held that a moribund condition of the patient was the only contraindication to its employment. Dr. M. B. Hartzell read a paper, entitled "Infectious Multiple Gangrene of the Skin; Report of a Case, with Illustrations." At the close of the scientific business of the evening, a portrait of the late Dr. Thomas Story Kirkbride was presented to the College by members of his family. Dr. John B. Chapin, the successor to Dr. Kirkbride as Superintendent of the Insane Department of the Pennsylvania Hospital, made the presentation address, paying the highest tribute to his predecessor's high attainments and to the advances in the treatment of the insane which he had inaugurated at the Pennsylvania Hospital. The President, Dr. J. M. DaCosta, made a speech of acceptance of the portrait on behalf of the College. At the annual election of officers which then took place, Dr. John Ashhurst, Jr., was elected president, and Dr. W. W. Keen, vice-president. On the recommendation of the Council the following were elected to Fellowship: Drs. George M. Stiles, Stricker Coles, Russell H. Johnson, and George G. Ross.

At the last meeting of the Obstetrical Society of Philadelphia, held on January 6th, Dr. Charles P. Noble read a paper on "Some of the Disadvantages of Vaginal Drainage." He quoted a group of six cases of pelvic cellulitis and abscess, in none of which had the vaginal route secured proper drainage; in two of these cases, moreover, a secondary abdominal section was necessitated in order to evacuate the purulent collections. At the annual election of officers, which followed the speaker's paper, the following were elected officers of the Society for the ensuing year: President, Dr. Charles P. Noble; vice-presidents, Drs. J. M. Fisher and George M. Boyd; secretary, Dr. Frank W. Talley; treasurer, Dr. George I. McKelway.

At the annual business meeting of the Philadelphia Academy of Surgery, held on January 3d., the following officers were elected for the ensuing year: President, Dr. J. Ewing Mears; vice-presidents, Drs. W. W. Keen and John Ashhurst, Jr.; secretary, Dr. William J. Taylor; treasurer, Dr. William G. Porter; recorder, Dr. L. W. Steinbach; council, Drs. Henry R. Wharton and Thomson R. Neilson; business committee, Drs. Richard H. Harte and DeForrest Willard.

Dr. Charles E. Sojous has resigned the deanship of the Medico-Chirurgical College, to take effect immediately. The resignation has been accepted by the trustees of the college, who elected Dr. Seneca Egbert, formerly vice-dean, his successor. Dr. Sajous' resignation was prompted by his desire to devote more time to scientific work and private practice than such an onerous position allowed him.

Dr. James Tyson, the President of the Philadelphia County Medical Society, gave a large reception on the evening of January 8th to the members of the Society. The reception was held in the banquet-room of the Hotel Bellevue, and was attended by over 500 guests.

The latest version of the will of the late Dr. Thomas W. Evans, leaves the sum of 20,000,000 francs to found and maintain a museum in this city, and to erect to the donor a statue (in one of the public squares to cost between 1,000,000 and 2,000,000 francs). The news comes from the Paris *Figaro*, and is not disbelieved by the late doctor's relatives in this city.

The Board of Health has instructed the Bacteriological Department of the Health Bureau to undertake on a large scale bacteriological examinations of water from hydrants of all houses in which there are at present cases of enteric fever. The continued large number of typhoid cases is very generally thought to be due to the polluted water-supply, and these instructions were ordered to determine, if possible, the cause of the epidemic. Diphtheria is still active, and scarlet fever and typhoid are on the increase again, as shown by the following statement of returns of contagious diseases for the week ending January 8th: New cases of diphtheria, 119, or 2 more than last week, with 25 deaths; new cases of scarlet fever, 62, or 16 more than last week, with 6 deaths; new cases of enteric fever, 165, or 68 more than last week, with 15 deaths—a total increase in contagious diseases of 86 cases over the preceding week. The whole number of deaths from all causes for the week was 475, an increase of 14 over the week before, and a decrease of 38 from the corresponding week of last year. Of the total number, 161 occurred in children under 5 years of age.

OUR BERLIN LETTER.

[From our Special Correspondent.]

THE PROPOSED LAW TO PREVENT THE EMPLOYMENT OF MARRIED WOMEN IN FACTORIES—ITS PROBABLE EFFECTS UPON INCREASE OF THE POPULATION—THORACIC ANEURISM AND PULMONARY TUBERCULOSIS—AN UNUSUAL CASE OF MECHANICAL OBSTRUCTION OF THE PYLORUS—DETECTION OF SEMINAL STAINS AFTER A LONG LAPSE OF TIME.

BERLIN, January 7, 1898.

THE German Government is nothing if not paternal, and scarcely a session of the Reichstag passes without the enactment of laws which are expressive of this tender sentiment. All interest in the Reichstag proceedings just now centers around the appropriations for the navy, but still there is occasional attention given to some of the ethical measures which it is proposed to make laws. One of these, involving the question of forbidding married women to work in factories, has attracted a good deal of attention from medical men.

The discussion has taken on a rather typically German aspect, but still presents features which seem of universal interest. It is urged that the absence of mothers from home necessitated by factory work frequently involves the early artificial feeding of children, careless bringing up, and neglected training. From the first comes the high infant mortality which it is the effort of sanitarians the world over to lessen; from the second and third result defective physical and moral training. Deformities are acquired from accident and from increased morbidity, and constitutions congenitally healthy are undermined. The lack of the mother's constant influence is the root of much more of the weaknesses of character, of acquired bad habits, of tendencies to evil, kleptomania, dipsomania, and the like, than all the innate hereditary moral defects which have of late occupied so much attention. Besides, it is urged, excessive competition has already ruined wages. The number of those seeking employment is so great that employers can obtain ordinary hands for what are really not living wages. The gradual entrance of woman into the labor circle has only resulted in obtaining for husband and wife together what the husband alone formerly received, and the family is, of course, no better off. The exclusion of married women from factory work would lesson some of the ruinous labor competition which now exists, and lead in course of time to a better state of affairs.

The German law for the absolute exclusion of children from factories enacted in 1893 has produced excellent results, and those in favor of the new law look with confidence for corresponding results from its enactment. Germans, anyhow, have much more confidence in the reform of social conditions by lawmaking than have most other peoples, and the paternal features of their government are by no means the most unpopular ones. The proposal will, however, meet with considerable opposition, and from points of view which would be utterly unlooked for with us, but which, owing to the national circumstances over here, will throw sidelights upon the question which will probably prevent action at present.

It is argued that the modern woman's duties in the household are much overestimated. She still has the housework to do it is true, but she no longer has the spinning and making of the wearing-apparel for all the various members of the family, which once constituted the principal part of her occupation. Her duties in the care and education of her children are now transferred to schools, which, in the form of kindergartens, are begun while the child is still very young.

All this is supposed to plead for the privilege of the woman working for hire outside of her house, but the real argument of the question, the one which carries weight with the Germans, comes last. If the wife is not allowed to work then the prospective husband will be brought face to face with the fact that he must support the family alone, and with wages as they are, most workmen can scarcely afford to do this. Then he will follow the example of so many of his betters and be content to remain single, in which case Germany's at present rapidly increasing population, as has happened in France, though for other reasons, will come to a standstill. This would mean the lessening within twenty years of the available military force, and that must not happen at any cost. Everything here is arranged with a single eye to the prevention of any such catastrophe as that. So, while those interested in the health of the nation have discovered a source of danger and suggested the remedy, the projected reform is apt to fail of accomplishment.

Professor Fränkel, of the throat and nose clinic at the Charité, called attention some time ago to the frequency with which pulmonary tuberculosis develops in cases of aneurism of the aorta. He attributed this to the fact that a bronchus is probably pressed upon, air circulation and the proper aeration of blood interfered with, and the resistant vitality of the lungs thus lowered. His explanation was not accepted as readily as the facts he reported. Further observation showed the truth of his statement as to the liability to tuberculosis in aneurism, but two other explanations of the fact were presented. One was that the pulmonary artery is pressed upon, and the blood-supply to the lung being thus interfered with its tissues are predisposed to infection. Traube's observation as to the frequency of tuberculosis in cases of pulmonary stenosis, for similar reasons, has been very generally accepted. Still another explanation is that pressure on the vagus causes trophic changes in the lungs, and thus vitality is lowered. This last theory has been confirmed so often in experiments upon animals, when interference with the vagus is almost invariably followed by pulmonary disease, that it was considered very plausible.

At the last meeting of the Society for Internal Medicine, however, Professor Fränkel showed the specimens from a case which would seem to prove his theory. The aneurism was of one of the pulmonary arteries, and by pressure it had narrowed the corresponding bronchus to a considerable extent. Primary tuberculosis of the lungs existed only in the lobe to which this bronchus was distributed, while whatever disturbance of the circulation there was from the aneurism *per se* should have affected much more of the lung parenchyma.

A favorite object of curiosity and of general interest here used to be an elderly hippopotamus in the Zoological Garden. His favorite occupation, when conscious of the presence of an interested audience, used to be a series of playful antics with a rubber ball, his ungainliness making up for his lack of agility—to the amusement of the crowd. One day the ball disappeared, and shortly after the animal showed signs of not being himself. He had evidently something on his heart or his stomach. It was thought that either his failure to attract the admiration of the crowd by his playful antics weighed upon his sensitive spirit, or that the lack of exercise consequent upon the absence of incentive to effort disturbed his metabolic equilibrium and reacted upon his digestion.

Like other elaborate diagnostic theories when patients higher in the scale of evolution have been concerned, these opinions did not lead to any therapeutic result. Another ball was supplied, and every encouragement and opportunity for the resumption of his old-time activity and playfulness were furnished him, but all was of no avail. After a while he absolutely refused all food, and death from inanition closed the scene. The *post-mortem* revealed that he had swallowed the rubber ball, and that this, by peristaltic action of the stomach, had become firmly wedged at the pylorus, absolutely preventing the passage of all food from the stomach to the intestines. The stuffed hide with the story of his tragic fate adorns a pedestal in the Zoological Museum. The accident is an extremely unusual one, but the possibility of such a thing happening in children is not entirely out of the question, so that the story seems not without interest for the medical man.

Of late a good deal of attention has been paid in Germany and Austria to the claim of a new method of detecting spermatic stains, if necessary, years after their original occurrence. Further investigation seems to show that while it is not the ready infallible method that was at first claimed it will prove of great help in such examinations. To a small amount of material scraped from the surface of the supposed seminal stain is added a little saturated Lugol's solution. If spermatic particles are present rather large, brown rhomboid crystals may be discovered with ordinary microscopic magnification. These crystals, while not absolutely characteristic of spermatic substance, as has been shown at the morgue here and elsewhere, always occur if spermatic fluid has been present. If they cannot be demonstrated after careful trials, then it is useless to go on with the often long and patient microscopic search for spermatozoids which used to be necessary. The crystals described are not a chemic combination of spermin, as at first thought, for they have been demonstrated by adding Lugol's solution to mucus from an infantile vagina, but represent a degenerate stage of certain albuminous products. Where a seminal stain exists, however, there they will always be found.

TRANSACTIONS OF FOREIGN SOCIETIES.

Paris.

SYPHILITIC CHANCRES OF THE FOREARM DUE TO TATTOOING—CHOLEDOCHOTOMY—A CASE OF SUBPHRENIC ABSCESS ASSOCIATED WITH THE PRESENCE OF GAS—REMOVAL OF TUMOR OF THE LIVER—ANTAGONISM BETWEEN THE POISONS OF HORNETS AND VIPERS.

AT the meeting of the Society for Dermatology and Syphilography of November 11th, FOURNIER presented a patient who had two typical *syphilitic chancres on the middle region of the forearm due to tattooing*. BESNIER referred to a question to which as yet no satisfactory answer has been given, *viz.*, how long does an instrument infected by the syphilitic contagium retain its virulent properties? It is probably only for a short time, as the instances of its transmission upon surgical instruments, caustics, etc., are comparatively rare, and in almost all of the reported cases the transfer of the virus from one patient to another has been an immediate one. It appears, therefore, that the syphilitic virus loses its power within a short time outside the human organism, and that it requires frequent transmission from person to person in order to remain active.

At a meeting of the Surgical Society, December 1st, QUENU spoke of *choledochotomy*, basing his conclusions upon six cases of his own and ninety-five others which he has been able to collect from medical literature. In four of his personal cases, the common duct was sutured. One of these patients died, and in the other three it was necessary to remove the sutures on account of biliary intoxication. Two of these patients recovered without permanent fistulæ. Two patients, in whom no suture was attempted, also recovered without fistulæ. From his experience in these six cases Quenu is convinced that the ductus choledochus should not be sutured after choledochotomy.

At the session of December 8th, LEJARS described a *case of subphrenic abscess associated with gas* and originating in a perforation of the anterioı wall of the stomach. The patient, a woman aged thirty-two years, had suffered a long time from gastric troubles with symptoms simulating intestinal obstruction. Medium laparotomy was performed, allowing a great quantity of pus and considerable gas to escape from a huge pocket in the right hyperchondrium. The patient died on the fourth day, and at autopsy it was discovered that there was a second smaller abscess also containing gas and pus, situated between the stomach and spleen, and resulting from a second perforation, this one being in the posterior gastric wall. This abscess was overlooked at the operation, and from its situation it seemed doubtful whether it could have been relieved had it been discovered.

TERRIER reported the *successful removal of an epithelial tumor from the middle of the anterior border of the liver*. He made use of the method advocated by Kousnetzoff and Pensky, consisting of a system of chain ligatures, and divided the tissue of the liver with a thermocautery. Hemorrhage was in this way almost entirely avoided. The abdominal wound was left open and it rapidly granulated. POIRIER, in a similar manner, removed a nodule of cancer the size of a large nut from the surface of the liver. Hemorrhage was controlled by cross sutures, and the patient recovered readily from the operation, but died of cancer six months later.

PHISALIX, at a session of the Biological Society, December 4th, stated that the venom of wasps and that of the common honey bee produce symptoms very similar to those seen in viper poisoning. He has examined the *relationship existing between the venom of a hornet and that of a viper*, with the purpose of ascertaining whether the former does not possess immunizing properties in respect to the latter. This appears indeed to be the case, as hornet poison introduced in small doses into guinea-pigs, confers on them marked immunity to viper poison. The true nature of the virus is still to be determined.

HALLION stated that *sea-water may be employed with advantage for hypodermoclysis*, instead of a 0.7 per cent. saline solution, as has already been shown by Quinton. Diluted sea-water is better borne than salt water, for it may be administered in larger doses and injected much more rapidly. It is consequently less toxic than the solutions of salt water usually employed. It is to be noted, moreover, that sea-water reduces the temperature, where ordinary salt water raises it. QUINTON and JULIA have experimented upon dogs of all ages and under varying conditions to determinine the relative value of sea-water and artificial serum, and in every case the results have shown the superiority of the former for subcutaneous injections. Under the influence of the injections of sea-water the renal action is better, both quantitatively and qualitatively.

MERCIER found in the urine of women in a state of eclampsia, a large quantity of albumin, which was soluble, entirely or in part, in the presence of a very small amount of acetic acid. This albumin, therefore, differs from that usually found in albuminuric subjects, more particularly from the presence of serin.

WIDAL reported to the Medical Society of the Hospitals, December 3d, a case of *idiopathic pyopneumothorax which terminated fatally*. The symptoms had existed ten days. The pleura was distended with an extremely fetid fluid, containing a great variety of micrococci and bacilli, both aerobic and anaerobic. No focus of gangrene, pneumonia, bronchopneumonia, or tuberculosis could be detected in the lung. Nor was there any trace of gangrene or perforation in the pleura. Examination of these organs, therefore, gave no clue to the origin of the infection.

GUINON, at the session of December 10th, reported that *three cases of typhoid fever had developed almost simultaneously in a certain hospital ward*. The patients were boys, aged five, six, and twelve years, who were under treatment, respectively, for acute poliomyelitis, purpura, and bronchitis. There were at the time in this ward several cases of typhoid fever. The mode of infection was not evident.

Vienna.

RESULTS OF SUBCUTANEOUS FRACTURE OF THE SKULL IN THE FIRST YEAR OF LIFE—TAMPONS INCLOSED IN GELATIN FOR USE IN THE VAGINA—HEADACHE AND ITS TREATMENT.

At the session of the Imperial Royal Society of Physicians, December 3d, WEINLECHNER spoke of the *results of subcutaneous fracture of the skull in the first year of life*. These results may be twofold in character. Either there may be a defect in the skull with attachment of the brain, or defects of the skull with false meningocele. Both forms develop from fissures. In the first form the edges of the bones are raised and thickened, and pulsation of the brain is easily detected, although with the most powerful expiratory effort there is no protrusion of the brain itself. Such defects in the skull of themselves do not produce symptoms, but they are of importance because they leave the brain exposed to all sorts of injuries. False meningocele may be emptied by pressure, which sometimes does not produce symptoms of pressure upon the brain. When so emptied, it is possible to feel a distinct wall of the cavity, as in case of a hematoma. The contents are connected with either the subdural or subarachnoid space. Both forms may be combined.

With reference to treatment, it was formerly the custom to apply pressure to such false meningoceles. This was without lasting benefit. The effects of puncture are usually transitory unless the meningocele is of very recent origin. Injections of tincture of iodin are too dangerous. The best treatment consists in splitting up the cyst and allowing it to heal by granulation. Later t defect in the bone may be remedied by an osteoplastic ope tion. In some cases Weinlechner said that he had us plates of celluloid with good result. One of the most i teresting of these cases was one of neuralgia of the th branch of the the trigeminal nerve, in which resection w performed and a celluloid plate introduced to preve union of the divided ends of the nerve.

At the session of the Medical Club, of December 1 FISCHER showed *tampons inclosed in gelatin for use the vagina*. The tampons may be saturated with a desired drug, and after their introduction the gela melts and the tampon comes into contact with the muc membrane.

At the session of the College of Doctors of Medici November 29th, BENEDIKT spoke at length upon *hea ache and its treatment*. He recommended for essent headache, the iodids, electricity, and the actual caute the wounds made by the latter being kept open by an irrit ing ointment. In symptomatic headache (occurring in c nection with constitutional maladies such as enemia, c gestion, nephritis, etc.) treatment should be direc toward the disease itself. In hemicrania, Benedikt a recommended the iodids and faradization. Natural these measures will relieve, and not cure, the trouble, migrain is a congenital constitutional affection. He e ploys iodids and mercurials for headache produced tumors of the brain, as he finds these remedies hav favorable influence upon the symptoms, even when tumor is not syphilitic. Before applying the cautery head must be shaved. According to his view the h is too frequently trephined for pain in connection w cerebral tumors. Such treatment rests upon a misc ceived idea that pressure in such cases is the cause of headache.

SOCIETY PROCEEDINGS.

NORTHWESTERN MEDICAL AND SURGIC SOCIETY OF NEW YORK.

Stated Meeting, Held November 17, 1897.

THE President, DR. CHARLES L. DANA, in the Ch

DR. ROBERT MILBANK presented a case of cyclo gia. The patient was a man, thirty-five years of age, contracted syphilis eight years ago. He was put u antisyphilitic treatment, which was continued three y without bad effect, and during this period he faith carried out all directions. While under treatment he an attack of syphilitic iritis in the *right* eye, from w he finally recovered. When the treatment was dis tinued he was in perfect health. In 1894, four years the appearance of the primary lesion, he suddenly dis ered that there was slight interference with the visio the left eye. An ophthalmologic examination reve dilatation of the left pupil, with no change in the retir optic nerve. The pupil reacts under eserin and piloca and at such times vision is perfect. The eye trouble not increased since its sudden onset. The man ha disorder of speech. He is strong and muscular and erwise in perfect health. The case is reported because of the sudden appearance of the eye symptom after two years of good health preceded by three years of careful antisyphilitic treatment.

DISCUSSION.

DR. FREDERICK PETERSON: I understand that this patient has been examined only by an ophthalmologist, whereas, to my mind, the case of this man is one for the neurologist. Such a condition is often preliminary to neuritis and locomotor ataxia, and is also a manifestation of cerebral syphilis. It is frequently observed during the course of syphilis, and may come on five, ten, fifteen, or even twenty years after the other lesions. I consider it an indication for specific treatment.

DR. JOSEPH COLLINS: This condition of the pupil is so suggestive of locomotor ataxia that it is impossible to think of anything else. There is nothing remarkable in the fact that it appeared several years after other manifestations of syphilis, nor that it has neither progressed nor retrogressed since its occurrence. These symptoms often develop late and in spite even of heroic treatment. Some years ago I analyzed a hundred cases in which syphilis was a prominent element. Those patients who were treated in the most approved manner developed nervous lesions a little sooner and with more severity than those who had not been so well treated, so one cannot place much dependence upon the treatment of syphilis to cause delay in the appearance of nervous symptoms. The case in question should be carefully watched, thus anticipating the occurrence of serious brain lesions. The eye symptoms are certainly an indication for treatment by means of mercury and hydrotherapy.

DR. PETERSON: The patient is still young—only thirty-five—and the manifestations of locomotor ataxia usually come on later than this. Perhaps within three or four years from now they will develop, or he may have general paresis. I agree with Dr. Collins as to the necessity for specific treatment, especially if the eye symptoms are an indication of cerebral syphilis.

DR. MILBANK: Can it be possible that a capillary hemorrhage has occurred along the optic nerve and produced this condition? It came on so suddenly, and he tells me that his father died of cerebral hemorrhage, and had several attacks previous to the one which proved fatal.

DR. COLLINS: The visual disturbance may have gradually come on, although the patient may have suddenly discovered it. Patients often think these eye symptoms come on all at once, when in reality they have continued some time before being noticed. This is explained by the fact that they have unconsciously become accustomed to monocular vision. The condition under discussion is not an uncommon pretabitic symptom. I have had patients who complained of it during as long a period as eight years before other symptoms developed,

DR. A. M. JACOBUS presented a child, nine months old, with an extensive subdermal growth or induration of of the vulvoperineal region. The child was apparently healthy at birth, was delivered by the speaker with forceps after a somewhat tedious labor, and without injury. The growth was first noticed by the mother when the baby was two and a quarter months old, but it was not until nearly seven months later that she consulted him about the disease. According to the mother, it first made its appearance between the right labia majora and the anus, and gradually extended upward to the anterior superior spine of the ilium and backward to the coccyx. The glands of both inguinal regions were very much indurated and enlarged. A few small glands could be detected in the right cervical and axillary regions. The child seemed to be in good health otherwise, Since first seen, about three weeks ago, the disease has steadily extended. Drs. Adami, Piffard, Vissman, LeFevre, and others, had very kindly examined the case at the speaker's invitation. Various diagnoses have been made, such as granuloma (originally, perhaps), scrofulosis, epithelioma, sarcoma, and tuberculous infection of the glands. A very doubtful specific history was elicited from the father, who confessed to having had a venereal lesion, probably a chancroid, some four or five years before marriage. At that time he was seen by several physicians in a large dispensary, who said the trouble was a chancroid; while a physician in private practice had declared it to be a chancre, and had given him suitable internal treatment. So far as the father knew there had been no subsequent symptoms or trouble. The disease in the child is increasing rapidly, but, except to interfere with natural defecation, does not appear to affect it. It appears to have commenced in the vulvar glands and not in the skin. There has never been any tendency toward suppuration or ulceration. I am of the opinion that the growth is malignant, either adenoma or sarcoma, No tissue has as yet been removed for a microscopic examination. In the way of treatment the baby has been given arsenious acid, $\frac{1}{100}$-grain, three times daily, and chlorid of gold, $\frac{1}{80}$-grain, once a day.

DISCUSSION.

DR. S. H. DESSAU: If this child presents a malignant disease which has been developing ever since the child was a little over two months old, it seems to me that the baby would not be in such apparent good health. I cannot pretend to say what it is. It may be specific, although the history does not point especially to that, nor does the appearance of the lesion, for in a child of this age there would be some ulceration of the skin. I am inclined to believe, however, that it is tuberculous.

DR. J. H. FRUITNIGHT: It seems to me that an accurate diagnosis is impossible without a microscopic examination of the growth. I am inclined to think that it is an epithelioma; it certainly has the appearance of malignancy.

DR. R. C. M. PAGE: I would like to suggest the possibility of it being Hodgkin's disease, which is characterized by a widespread involvement of the glands. I once saw a case occurring in a boy nine years of age. He was also seen by the late Dr. Henry B. Sands, who refused to operate because the glandular involvement was so extensive and because of the proximity of so many important blood-vessels. I would suggest that the child's spleen be examined, for in Hodgkin's disease there is usually enlargement of this organ; there is also not only a deficiency in the number of red blood-corpuscles, but, in time, an increase in the white. The disease remains stationary during a long period, and will all at once be characterized by rapid changes.

DR. BULKLEY; I have never seen malignant disease in a child so young, and I do not think it is epithelioma or carcinoma. It strikes me as a local infective process. There are present many of the features we observe in sluggish conditions, which we now recognize as tuberculous.

DR. A. M. JACOBUS then read the paper of the evening, entitled

A CASE OF INFANTILE SCURVY, WITH COMMENTS ON INFANT FOODS AND INFANT-FEEDING.

(See page 68.)

DISCUSSION.

DR. S. BARUCH: I have seldom heard a paper which has stirred me as much as this one, but there are three points to which I would like to refer. In the first place, the case presented is very interesting, and certainly demonstrates the author's skill in making the diagnosis and treating the condition. I have seen but one such case. The second point is the condemnation of all prepared foods, in which I fully agree with the author. However, I entirely disagree with him in regard to a third point—that of deprecating the value of Pasteurized and sterilized milk because scurvy may be produced. This is a dangerous doctrine, I think, and I would like to hear the point discussed. Up to 1894 there have been reported but seventy cases of scurvy in infants, and when we recall the fact that many babies are fed on sterilized milk, we ought not to admit this as a cause of scurvy. Looking back over an experience of thirty-five years, part of which was spent in the country, where good milk is to be had, and seeing many children, I can say that there is nothing, not even hydrotherapy, which has given me more satisfaction than the introduction of sterilized milk. Twenty-five years ago, I remember making a record in my mind as to how many babies among my clientele would die of summer complaint during the coming hot weather; and I could find no preventative, because we did not then know that the cause of summer diarrhea is the bacterium lactis. We know now what it is and how to destroy it—by boiling the milk. In regard to the modification of milk, my views are these—that it does not make so much difference how you modify it, it will agree with the child if you destroy the bacterium lactis. In order to prove this fact, Eserich some ten years ago gave a baby four weeks old a quart of sterilized milk; he then examined the feces, and found that nearly all the nitrogen had been utilized. This proves that infants are capable of digesting ordinary milk without modification. The great point in infant-feeding is to make cow's milk like mother's milk. The latter is superior because it is always *sterile* and is received in the child's mouth direct from the mother's nipple; therefore, cow's milk must be made sterile. Good milk should be obtained from cows which are kept in a clean stable, where every precaution is taken to keep the milk pure, and it should be sent to the laboratory to be made perfectly sterile before it is used. The grade of the milk is not of so much importance if only it be *sterile*.

DR. J. H. FRUITNIGHT: In 1894 I wrote a paper on scurvy, and at that time was able to find but seventy recorded cases of the disease occurring in infants. Up to the present time I have seen but ten such cases, and in all but one the child had been fed on prepared foods. In the one exception the mother's milk had evidently not been sufficiently nutritious, and the baby was put on modified milk and antiscorbutic treatment. One of the cases occurred in a baby two or three months old, whose mother had phthisis and had been obliged to wean it. It was given several of the prepared foods and soon developed scurvy. It presented a terrible appearance; it was covered with ecchymotic spots, the knee-joints were swollen, the gums spongy, and the whole body so sensitive that the slightest touch gave pain, and it was necessary to carry it about on a pillow. It recovered under the treatment detailed by the author. This case is one of the most severe ever recorded and was clearly due to artificial food. A microscopic examination of the blood showed marked leucocytosis. The diagnosis in these cases generally lies between scorbutis and acute rheumatism, for which it is frequently mistaken. The condition was formerly called acute rickets, and is due to faulty nutrition, which leads to a deviation from the normal composition of the blood. Occasionally, a case is reported due to sterilized milk, but the latter should not be condemed for that reason. Prepared foods are much more apt to be the cause. Pasteurized is to be preferred to sterilized milk because it is not raised to so high a temperature as is necessary in the preparation of the latter. The prognosis is nearly always favorable under proper treatment, and if this is faithfully carried out the mortality will be reduced to nil.

In regard to infant-feeding in general, all men who do much work among children condemn the proprietary foods and agree that mother's milk is the best food. Cow's milk is next best. Pasteurized milk has saved many children, and it will be a retrograde step if we discard it. Mere sterilization, however, is not sufficient; it must be *modified* to suit the cases—some babies require more fat, others more casein, and so on. As it requires some thought to prescribe the proper formula for modified milk, artificial foods are often ordered because it is easier to do so.

DR. DESSAU: I have seen but two cases of scurvy and both occurred in children fed on proprietary foods, but it is a question whether this food *per se* was a factor in causing the disease. In regard to the feeding of healthy children, I agree with those who recommend Pasteurized milk for summer feeding. I have used other elements added to the milk, and have come to the conclusion that the best food for infants, rich and poor, is a kind of Pasteurized milk which anybody can prepare. In the first place, good, clean milk must be obtained. This is not always easy, for I am told that since separators have come into general use in dairies, milk from which the cream has been thus separated is sold, and a great deal of it used by the condensed-milk companies, and, of course, such milk contains hardly any fat. Having obtained a good milk, dilute it one-quarter with water (more or less if the child does not thrive), add a little cane sugar and a pinch of salt, and place this mixture in a double boiler, allowing it to cook ten minutes after the water in the lower vessel has begun to boil. A double boiler can be bought for 35 cents, and is within the reach of even poor people. Children generally thrive on this **mixture.**

DR. H. LING TAYLOR: I saw one of the cases referred to by the last speaker; that of a child brought up on a certain brand of condensed milk. It is interesting to note that two other children in the same house were fed on this same kind of condensed milk and developed the same symptoms as the child first mentioned, and one of them finally died. A third child living in the neighborhood, also fed on the same food, was affected in the same way as the others. The reason why scurvy in infants is not more often recognized is because there are no stomach or bowel symptoms. This fact leads the physician astray. In my case the diet was changed to Pasteurized milk, and the child recovered. It was also given beef- and orange-juice. There has been of late a decided reaction against sterilized milk. If good milk can be obtained, give it to the child raw, except in hot weather, when some kind of sterilization must be resorted to. Another thing in connection with scurvy is that the child may appear to be perfectly healthy, and even robust, while it is beginning to develop this condition. The infant foods are only indicated when starvation diet is necessary.

DR. ROBERT A. MURRAY: The different expressions of opinion by the members are rather confusing. I consider that Dr. Dessau, by his method, does Pasteurize the milk. In regard to modified milk, it is a fact that mother's milk a few days after delivery is practically the same as it is at the end of lactation. The essential point seems to me is to make a milk as nearly like mother's milk as possible, and to keep it free from germs. Milk must be sterilized, and, whatever method we employ, the same thing is accomplished in the end—it is modified by adding water, salt, and sugar.

DR. JACOBUS: In the first place, I wish to say that, as stated in the paper, I referred to scurvy and not to infant-feeding in summer diarrhea. I limited my remarks to feeding in scurvy and in healthy children. In regard to the statement made by a previous speaker that there are recorded but seventy cases of scurvy in infants, I would like to ask how many thousand cases of this disorder have occurred unrecognized, and progressed, in many instances, to a fatal termination. I also wish to take exception to the statement that mother's milk is always sterile. Laboratory tests show that this is not the case. During the nursing period, a woman's nipple, by reason of the saliva, dirt, and sour milk which collect there, is often a perfect hot-bed of bacteria. Of course, this can be remedied by cleanliness. I have even seen a case of scurvy in a baby which was breast-fed, and in which the disease was due to the poor quality of the milk. In closing, I can only say that for infant-feeding I prefer *raw*, pure, rich milk, the best to be had, which has been filtered after the method of Seibert and modified as suggested in the paper. In addition to this, after the fourth to sixth month, the artificially fed infant should be given beef- and fruit-juice, baked ripe potatoes, with milk, butter and salt, crackers, and other suitable, easily digested foods in small portions at least twice daily.

ANNOUNCEMENT.

MEDICAL SOCIETY OF THE STATE OF NEW YORK; PRELIMINARY PROGRAM, NINETY-SECOND ANNUAL MEETING.

Albany, January 25, 26, and 27, 1898.

TUESDAY MORNING SESSION, 9.15 O'CLOCK.

PRESIDENT'S inaugural address. Reports of officers and committees. Executive business.

PAPERS.

1. "Throat and Nose Affections and Their Relations to General Medicine." Walter F. Chappell, New York.

2. "Ear Manifestations in General Disease." Wendell C. Phillips, New York.

3. "Cases of Acute Non-diphtheritic Inflammation of the Larynx, Requiring the Prolonged Retention of the Intubation Tube." John O. Roe, Rochester.

4. "The Report of a Case of Unusual Contraction of the Visual Field and Disorder of the Color Sense Following an Injury." T. F. C. Van Allen, Albany.

5. "The Railway Surgeon and His Work." C. B. Herrick, Troy.

6. "What Shall the State and County Do for the Consumptive?" John H. Pryor, Buffalo.

7. "The Advantages of State Control in Medicine, with Results Observed." William Warren Potter, Buffalo.

Election, by districts, of members of the Committee of Nomination at close of morning session.

TUESDAY AFTERNOON SESSION, 2.15 O'CLOCK.

8. "A Contribution to the Study of Melancholia, with a Report of the Examination of the Blood in Fifty-seven Cases." B. C. Loveland, Clifton Springs.

9. "The Cold-water Treatment of Typhoid Fever in Private Practice." John T. Wheeler, Chatham.

10. "Anemia." R. C. M. Page, New York.

11. "On the Vagaries and Wanderings of Gall-stones, with Clinical Reports." Henry L. Elsner, Syracuse.

12. "The Treatment of Delirium." Joseph Collins, New York.

13. "Paralysis; Prognosis and Treatment." Edward D. Fisher, New York.

14. "The Relation of Bacteria to the Normal Alimentary Canal." Herbert U. Williams, Buffalo.

15. "The Rivals of the Physician in Practice." Reynold W. Wilcox, New York.

16. "The Hygienic Management of Dairies." E. F. Brush, Mt. Vernon.

17. "The Municipal Control of Milk-supply in Cities and Villages, with Report of Health Regulation." T. B. Carpenter, Buffalo.

18. "The Present Status of Expert Medical Testimony." Evarts M. Morrell, Yonkers.

19. "Expert Testimony." J. B. Ransom, Dannemora.

TUESDAY EVENING SESSION, 7.15 O'CLOCK.

"Practical Exposition of the X-ray in Medicine and Surgery." Exhibition in charge of Arthur L. Fisk of New York. (*a*) "Technic and Apparatus." Samuel Lloyd, New York. (*b*) "The X-ray in Medicine." Dr. Williams, Boston. (*c*) "The X-ray in Surgery." Arthur L. Fisk, New York. (*d*) "The X-ray; Clinical Experiences." Wm. Hailes, Jr., Albany.

WEDNESDAY MORNING SESSION, 9.15 O'CLOCK.

20. "Some Points in the Technic of the Alexander Operation." Herman E. Hayd, Buffalo.

21. "The Present Status of Vaginal Operations for Diseases of the Pelvic Organs." Edward B. Cragin, New York.

22. "Remote Consequences of Excessive Uterine Hemorrhage." W. E. Ford, Utica.

23. "Gauze Drainage in Laparotomy." Henry C. Coe, New York.

24. "The Anatomy and Function of the Female Perineum and the Operation for Its Repair When Lacerated." J. Riddle Goffe, New York.

25. "Traumatic Injuries of the Brain." J. H. Glass, Utica.

26. "Formaldehyd Disinfection." E. H. Wilson, Brooklyn. Discussed by Alvah H. Doty and Herman M. Biggs.

27. "The Past, Present, and Prospective Methods of Treatment of Insanity in the State of New York." P. M. Wise, Albany.

WEDNESDAY AFTERNOON SESSION, 2.15 O'CLOCK.

28. "A Year's Work in Appendicitis." Herman Mynter, Buffalo.

29. "The Management of Undescended Testicle in Hernia Operations." William B. DeGarmo, New York.

30. "Investigation and Exploration of the Other Kidney in Contemplated Nephrectomy." Geo. M. Edebohls, New York.

31. "Congenital Dislocation of the Shoulder Backward, with a Report of Seven Cases and an Operation for Its Relief." A. M. Phelps, New York.

32. Discussion—"The Management of Hypertrophy of the Prostate Gland and Its Complications." (*a*) "General Consideration and Catheter Life." L. Bolton Bangs, New York. (*b*) "Prostatectomy and Prostatotomy, Suprapubic and Perineal." Samuel Alexander, New York. (*c*) "Bottini's Galvanocaustic Radical Treatment, and the Palliative Treatment for Hypertrophy of the Prostate." Willy Meyer, New York. (*d*) "Castration for the Relief of Hypertrophied Prostate." L. S. Pilcher, New York. (*e*) "Stone, Associated with Hypertrophy of the Prostate." E. L. Keyes, New York.

33. "Excision of the Fibula for Sarcoma." Samuel Lloyd, New York.

34. "The Treatment of the Fracture of the Femur in Children." Theodore Dunham, New York.

WEDNESDAY EVENING SESSION.

In the Senate Chamber at 7.45 o'clock. Anniversary address by the President. Reception by the President to the members, delegates, and invited guests at the Albany Club at 9.30 o'clock.

THURSDAY MORNING SESSION, 9.30 O'CLOCK.

Business session and reports of committees.

35. "Treatment of 'Deficient Excretion from Kidneys not Organically Diseased, and Some of the Diseases Peculiar to Women,' and Diseases of the Skin." L. Duncan Bulkley, New York.

36. "The Relations of the Physician to the Practice of Midwifery." C. F. Timmerman, Amsterdam.

37. "The Conservative Surgery of the Fibroid Tumor." A. H. Goelet, New York.

38. "Report of a Case of Osteotomy of Both Tibiæ and Fibulæ for Symmetrical Anteroposterior Angular Deformity." F. H. Peck, Utica.

39. "Intratracheal Injections for Diseases of the Bronchial Tubes and Lungs." H. S. Drayton, New York.

SENECA D. POWELL, New York, President,
LUCIEN HOWE, Buffalo, Vice-President,
FREDERIC C. CURTIS, Albany, Secretary,
CHARLES H. PORTER, Albany, Treasurer.

THERAPEUTIC HINTS.

To Remove Silver Nitrate Stains.—

℞ Hydrarg. bichlor. } aa . . . ʒ i
Ammon. chlorid. }
Aq. dest. . . . . . . ℥ i.

M. Sig. Apply by means of a cloth and friction.

In Infantile Colic.—

℞ Tr. lobeliæ . . . . . . gtt. i
Aq. dest. . . . . . . ℥ i.

M. Sig. One-half teaspoonful when indicated.

For Baldness of Parasitic Origin.—

℞ Pilocarpini . . . . . Parts iv
Sulphuris præcip. . . . . Parts x
Balsam. Peru. . . . . . Parts xx
Beef marrow . . . . . Parts c.

M. Sig. External use.—*Sabauraud.*

For Fetid Diarrhea in the Initial Stage of Scarlatina.—

℞ Mag. sulph. } aa . . . . ʒ ss
Ac. sulph. dil. }
Syr. simpl. . . . . . . ℥ ss
Aq. dest. . . . . . . ℥ iii.

M. Sig. One teaspoonful to one tablespoonful every hour according to the age of the child.

For Scabies.—

℞ β naphthol . . . . . . gr. xl
Sulph. præcip. . . . . . gr. lxxx
Styracis } aa . . . ℥ ss
Pulv. rad. pyrethri }
Adipis . . . . . . ℥ iss.

M. Ft. Ungt. Sig. Rub into affected areas once daily for three days. Woolen undergarments should be worn during the treatment.

THE MEDICAL NEWS.

A WEEKLY JOURNAL OF MEDICAL SCIENCE.

VOL. LXXII. NEW YORK, SATURDAY, JANUARY 22, 1898. NO. 4.

ORIGINAL ARTICLES.

NIL NOCERE, IN OBSTETRICS.

BY JULIUS ROSENBERG, M.D.,
OF NEW YORK.

IN consideration of the fact that ninety-five per cent. of all confinements terminate normally and never require medical aid, this axiom, *nil nocere*, is of special significance in the practice of obstetrics. Labor is, as a rule, a physiologic act, and yet this normal phenomenon is not infrequently transformed into a pathologic process by excessive zeal and a desire to do something.

Puerperal infection stands foremost among the complications of childbirth which are artificially produced. Although the mortality from this dread affection has been much decreased, still we observe its clinical manifestations all too frequently. It is my belief that puerperal infection is an absolutely avoidable sequel of labor, and that women need not die or suffer from it, regardless of their immediate environment.

Previous to 1847 the mortality from puerperal infection in the Vienna General Hospital was more than ten per cent. In May, 1847, Semmelweiss established the rule that students, before taking charge of a labor, should wash their hands in chlorin water; he also restricted the number of digital examinations. The result was an immediate fall in the death-rate. Within six months it dropped from 10 to 3 per cent., and in the second year of the new régime it did not exceed 1.5 per cent. To my mind this brief recapitulation of Semmelweiss' work absolutely indicates the etiology of puerperal infection. A woman is practically aseptic until contaminated by the infected examining finger. The simple washing of the hands in chlorin water reduced the mortality from 10 to a little over 1 per cent., and it is but rational to conclude that if the hands had been thoroughly cleansed the death-rate from this affection would have been reduced to nil. Unfortunately for womankind this conclusion has not been universally accepted; thus, many consider the disinfection of the obstetrician's hands without a more or less thorough vaginal douching insufficient antisepsis. This idea originated through the fact that even after disinfection of the hands women continued to die from puerperal infection; but instead of tracing this to imperfection in the preparation of the hands, the vagina was accused of containing the disease-germs.

It cannot be denied that the vagina of every woman contains numerous micro-organisms, but these are, as a rule, non-pathogenic and not responsible for infection, and, what is more, they prevent subsequent sepsis; and by removing them and the normal vaginal secretions we are inviting instead of guarding against infection.

König[1] demonstrated that not only is the normal vaginal secretion free from pathogenic germs, but he has shown that it has a distinct germicidal power. Experiments were made by introducing different germs into the vaginæ of a great number of pregnant women. It was found that all pathogenic bacteria were destroyed within two days after introduction. He further proved that syringing the vagina with antiseptic solutions has the effect of reducing or completely destroying its germicidal power. Hence, he concluded that prophylactic syringing should be abandoned.

During 1894 Menge published an account of researches as to the bactericidal properties of the vaginal secretion, and his results are identical with those of König. Further investigation of the mechanism of this germicidal action shows that it depends mainly upon the antagonism between the normal bacilli of the vagina and the pathogenic micro-organisms (the presence of which is accidental), and upon the acid reaction of the vaginal secretions. These theoretic deductions and investigations are well substantiated by practical results:

In 1893 Leopold and Goldberg published the statistics of several thousand confinements with and without the employment of vaginal disinfection. Their tables show the best results when vaginal douches were omitted. Fischel, in 880 births at the Prague Maternity Hospital, lost nine women from puerperal sepsis with the employment of preliminary disinfection. After stopping the irrigations he delivered 521 women without a death. Neumann reports 700 cases without the employment of vaginal douches and without a single death from sepsis. Frommel reports 500 cases in which vaginal douching with a solution of bichlorid of mercury was employed, with two deaths from sepsis.

I have delivered during the past four years a fair number of women living under the most varying

[1] *Deutsche med. Wochensch.*, No. 43, 1894.

conditions; I never employ vaginal douches except under strict indications, and every one of my cases have recovered without any complications. I have also, during the same period, seen quite a few cases of puerperal fever, and, though it may have been only incidental, in the virulent types a history of prophylactic vaginal and uterine douching was presented. The restriction of vaginal examinations, thorough disinfection of the external genitals of the parturient woman, and an aseptic condition of the examiner's hands are, to my mind, the only essential requirements for the successful management of a normal labor; whatever is added constitutes an unnecessary interference.

The second subject to which I desire to direct attention is the complication of pregnancy and labor by uterine fibroids. I have observed during the last four years six cases of fibroid of the pregnant uterus; four are reported in detail in the *American Journal of Obstetrics*, May, 1895. In five of these cases pregnancy and labor terminated without serious complications; one woman aborted during the fourth month. The growths ranged in size from that of a lemon to colossal tumors. I record ***six living mothers*** and ***five living children***. These statistics are far superior to those offered by the advocates of operative interference. Leopold[1] collected thirty-one myomectomies during pregnancy, with a maternal mortality of twenty-three per cent., while forty-five per cent. of the children perished. Such varying results should lead one to ask whether myomectomy during pregnancy is ever indicated. As for myself, I consider it entirely unjustifiable, and, with but few exceptions, these cases should be left alone until labor has commenced.

The few cases which I have observed prove that even large tumors may cause but slight complications, and I find not a small number of cases reported in which seemingly insurmountable obstacles disappeared during labor and did not interfere with a normal delivery. Some operators justify operative interference by the plea that the operation relieves the woman of the tumor. Against this I have to reply that the structure of fibromyomata closely resembles that of the uterus, and that they partake in the evolution and involution of this organ. Growths which may be of alarming size during pregnancy become, *post-partum*, utterly insignificant, and may never cause the woman any discomfort. If they should do so, then it is time enough to resort to operative procedures.

Fortunately, the current opinion seems to be against operating in these cases. Hofmeier advises strongly against operative interference. His conclusions are that "the presence of myomata durin[g] pregnancy, labor, and the puerperium is rarely th[e] cause of serious consequences, and the dangers ma[y] be essentially diminished by patience, proper judg[-]ment, and an antiseptic management of the case.

[1] *Am. Journal of Obstetr.*, May, 1895.

Dr. Bantock has observed a large number of case[s] of pregnancy associated with uterine fibroids, an[d] never had any of the accidents usually ascribed t[o] this condition. He quotes the case of a large fi[-]broid occupying the pregnant uterus in which hi[s] opinion was requested as to the advisability of sur[-]gical interference. He advised non-interference, i[n] the belief, founded upon experience, that as preg[-]nancy advanced the tumor would rise out of the pel[-]vis and allow the passage of the child; and this wa[s] just what occurred. He was present at the delivery and the labor proceeded perfectly normally. H[e] examined the woman *post-partum*, and had he no[t] known that she had a fibroid, he would have believe[d] the uterus to be normal.

Armstrong has recorded the case of a woman wh[o] had a large fibroid. She became pregnant, and wa[s] strongly pressed to have an abortion induced, bu[t] declined. She had an easy labor. He examined the woman some time later, and found that ever[y] trace of the tumor had disappeared.

Routh relates the case of a woman who, when si[x] months pregnant, was admitted to the hospital. [A] fibroid the size of a fetal head occupied the lowe[r] portion of the uterus, and delivery *per vias natural[es]* appeared impossible. It was decided to let th[e] woman go to term and then perform Cæsarian se[c-]tion; but one day the tumor rose out of the pelvi[s,] the head descended, and a living child was delivere[d] without difficulty.

To represent the other side of the argument, I sha[ll] briefly relate the history of a case, reported by Ban[tock] (*Am. Journal of Obstetrics*, April, 1894). A sing[le] woman, thirty-six years old, who had always be[en] regular, missed four menstrual periods, and consult[ed] the doctor to ascertain why she was growing so larg[e;] she suspected pregnancy. Upon examination, h[is] diagnosis of pregnancy was confirmed; it was al[so] found that the lower portion of the uterus contain[ed] several small fibromata. She was told that she w[as] pregnant and that she had a tumor, which, if l[eft] until the end of pregnancy, might put her life [in] danger. Operation for the removal of the tumor, [if] possible, with preservation of the uterus, was advise[d.] She consented to the operation, uterus and tum[or] being removed. The patient died of sepsis on t[he] fifth day.

It is a deplorable fact that obstetric text-boo[ks] preserve a too great reverence for old dicta hand[ed] down from book to book. Because some one h witnessed a few fatal results in confinement cases in which myomata were present, although the tumor was generally not the cause of death, we are advised to operate if the tumor gives rise of symptoms. Many operations are reported in which the tumor was the sole indication. But should a procedure which has a mortality of twenty-five per cent. be undertaken except under most pressing indications?

After a most exhaustive study of the literature, and from my own experience, I cannot verify the statement that fibroid tumors occurring during gestation are the cause of so many alarming complications. The reported deaths have mostly been due to sepsis, and to interfering operations.

Clean hands constitute the best prophylaxis for the former, and a regard for the axiom "*nil nocere*" will make the latter less frequent.

EDIBLE AND POISONOUS FUNGI.

By J. N. BUCKHAM, M.D.,
OF FLINT, MICH.

THE increasing use of fungi as food has led me to investigate their botanic structure, their value as an article of diet, and last and most important, to determine the marks of distinction between the noxious and wholesome varieties.

The fungi are next to the lowest order of plants, and are between the algæ and the lichens. The higher forms of fungi and lichens are now grouped together under the name—fungales. Lichens are a fungous growth parasitic on an algal base. Fungals are thallogens; that is, they are nourished through a thallus, mycelium, or spawn. They are parasitic, and absorb the products of decomposing animal or vegetable matter, and generally grow underground. The edible fungi are known as mushrooms, lichens, puff-balls, and truffles.

The fungi consist of a volva, which is the membrane enveloping the fructifying part of the embryo, a stalk, and of a receptacle or expanded cup, to the under surface of which the cortina or veil is attached, covering the hymenophore or conceptacle. The principal appendages are the gills or lamellæ, and their shape, appearance, color, and changes of color, are all important in determining species.

The lichens consist of a thallus and the reproductive organs borne upon it. The *Cenomyce rangiferina*, or reindeer-lichen of Lapland and other Northern countries, furnishes pasturage for the deer in winter. With *Cetraria Islandica*, or Iceland moss, we are all familiar. The *Umbilicaria vellea*, or rock-tripe, is eaten by hunters in the Arctic regions. *Lecanora esculenta*, a lichen of Asia Minor, is supposed to have been the manna of the Exodus.

The commonest form of edible mushroom is the *Agaricus campestris*, or meadow mushroom. The *Agaricus arvensis*, another but coarser variety, grows wherever cattle graze. The *Agaricus cretaceosus* is an excellent table variety. Other wholesome species are *Agaricus ægeritæ* and *avellanus*, *Lipiota procera*, and *Amanita cæsarea*. Puff-balls should not be picked, but a slice cut off when wanted.

Tuber melanospermum, *Tuber cibarius*, and *Tuber moschata* are varieties of truffle found in France, Italy, and other European countries. Truffles grow underground and give off a peculiar odor, which leads to their detection by dogs and pigs trained to hunt for them. Among the noxious species are *Amanita muscaria*, or fly agaric; this is used in this country and in Europe as a fly poison. It is sometimes eaten by the inhabitants of Northern Asia for its intoxicating effect.

In many parts of the world mushrooms form a very large portion of the food of the inhabitants, and in many countries of Europe and Asia they are cultivated on a large scale. In Terra del Fuego they are the chief food of the natives. In France, Italy, New Zealand, Tahiti, and Japan they are an important article of export, and are under government control and inspection. Rollrausch and Ziegel state that they deserve to be placed with meat as sources of nitrogenous nutriment. One man in Thuringia is said by Dr. Gautier to have lived upon nothing but mushrooms for thirty years, and died a centenarian. Dried morel has been found to contain thirty-five per cent. of protein, and *Hellvella esculenta* twenty-six per cent. Different foods contain the following averages of protein substances: bread, eight per cent.; oatmeal, ten per cent.; barley meal, six per cent.; potatoes, five per cent.; beans and peas, twenty-seven per cent., and mushrooms thirty-three per cent.

Many popular fallacies exist concerning certain tests for determining the noxious or wholesome qualities of fungals. One old one is that poisonous varieties will discolor a silver spoon or white onions during cooking. All kinds are liable to liberate H_2S in process of cooking or of decay, and this, of course, will discolor silver, brass, lead, or onions. Another is that all varieties which turn black on being sprinkled with salt are poisonous, and those which do not are wholesome. Other tests are, that all which change color when cut, or have vivid colors or viscid caps are poisonous. These distinctions are not to be depended upon, nor are the contrary hypotheses. It is best to avoid all fungi growing in filthy places, those with an unpleasant odor, those which produce a biting or burning sensation in the mouth, those which yield a white milk, or turn blue or greenish when broken, or those in which the flesh is soft, deliquescent, spongy, hard, corky, or maggoty. The amanitas are nearly all dangerous, and some are *very* poisonous, their active principle being amanitine which acts like morphin; eating them does not produce any symptom for six or eight hours, and then the patient is usually beyond help unless sulphate of atropia, $\frac{1}{60}$-grain, is at once administered. All of these have cups, and all fungi with cups had best be avoided.

In edible varieties the flesh is usually firm, but tender, and the odor and taste pleasant and agreeable, resembling fresh meal or hazelnuts. Many of the wholesome kinds are dangerous when old or over-mature, and some of the noxious ones become wholesome when properly cooked. Cases have occurred in which unpleasant or serious results have followed from eating well-known esculent fungi; such may have been due to idiosyncrasies of the victim or simply to overeating. I have thought it possible that ptomains might be developed under favorable conditions; this and the comparative indigestibility of fungi should be investigated more fully than has been done. The only *sure* test of wholesomeness is the hackneyed one of eating them first and letting the result be determined by your own after-consciousness, or appear in your obituary.

THE GOUTY AND RHEUMATIC AFFECTIONS OF THE UVEAL TRACT.

By ROBERT SATTLER, M.D.,
OF CINCINNATI, O.

Affections of the eye are among the earliest recorded facts in the history of gout. Long before the gouty or rheumatic origin of other ocular lesions was inferred or established affections of the iris were among the recognized complications of gout and rheumatism, being formerly described under the general term "ophthalmia arthritica." More recently, however, the careful study of clinical histories in typical cases has conclusively demonstrated that, not only in iritic disturbances, but also in certain other lesions of the uveal tract, gout and rheumatism must be considered as among the principal etiologic factors (relapsing cyclitis, iridochoroiditis, etc.). These ocular diseases are, in most instances, associate manifestations of the maladies in question, and start as such in one or the other part of the uveal tract; less commonly, they appear as complications of pathologic expressions due to the same causes (episcleritis, scleritis migrans, sclerotitis, neuritis optica, neuroretinitis, etc.).

Clinically, both gout and rheumatism are thoroughly understood. But, however unmistakable the expression of local and general gout as well as of rheumatism may be, it must be admitted that the obscure nature of both these maladies, as well as the complete absence of a distinct morbid anatomy, are equally incontrovertible facts. If this holds good of gout and rheumatism as a whole, it applies with especial force to the local manifestations of the general disturbance observed in ocular lesions. At the very outset, in disorders of the uveal tract presumedly of gouty or rheumatic origin, every observer of the clinical phenomena is confronted with the ever vexing questions, "Are gout and rheumatism independent diseases, or are they, as Haig and others assume, different utterances of one and the same malady, or is there such a blending of the two that their *common identity* must be upheld?" Are we to believe with Hutchinson that "gout is but rarely of pure breed and often a complication of rheumatism?" How shall we classify that chronic affection of the joints which, in clinical manifestations at least, strikingly resembles both rheumatism and gout, *viz.*, arthritis deformans? These and other equally perplexing questions suggest themselves to the specialist from time to time.

On the other hand, there are certain facts derived from his own observation, the literature of the subject, and the known experience of fellow-physicians, which serve to guide him in his endeavors to analyze the ocular symptoms and establish their dependence upon and association with the general disease. These personal deductions may not add much that is new, but they may tend to confirm or supplement some of the many points in the history of gouty and rheumatic disturbances of the eye, concerning which imperfect conclusions are entertained.

Can gout or rheumatism be considered the principal etiologic factors in those cases of iritis in which a searching examination fails to disclose that the disturbances of the joints are dependent upon syphilis, gonorrhea, chronic lead intoxication, malaria, anemia, and other alleged or actual constitutional causes?

This has long been admitted. The older literature refers to these lesions of the uveal tract as ophthalmia arthritica, iritis varicosa, arthritica, rheumatica, etc. Von Ammon, von Walther, von Beer, Himly, and others are among the earliest German observers to refer to the frequency and severity of this special variety of iritis, and assign its cause to gout or to rheumatoid arthritis. In England, although rheumatic iritis and its causal relationship with rheumatism is recognized, Mackenzie[1] and others hesitatingly refer to iritis of gouty or arthritic

[1] Mackenzie mentions the fact that in Germany chronic arthritis and gouty affections are common among the poorer classes, especially in wine-growing districts. Before the advent of reliable mydriatics these affections, characterized by insidious onset, were fraught with great risk, one acute attack being almost invariably followed by recurrent fatal complications with loss of sight, etc.

origin, even though it is mentioned, admitted, and described in the text books.

Recently, in Germany and on the Continent, less stress is laid upon these causes as etiologic factors; this is evidenced by the scarcity of the literature on the subject and by the infrequent reference and even the complete absence in most of the text-books of the designation "gouty," arthritic, or rheumatic iritis. On the contrary, in England where formerly much doubt was expressed, especially concerning the gouty or rheumatic origin of certain forms of iritis and choroiditis, opinion has gradually changed. Jonathan Hutchinson was the first to accumulate, by painstaking labor and observation, such a mass of clinical evidence that the gouty and rheumatic origin for these and other affections of the eye can no longer be questioned. Since then it has been known that many cases which were formerly described by the vague term "idiopathic" or were indiscriminately classified as being of rheumatic origin are really expressions of the uric-acid diathesis and belong to the stage of goutiness (a variable period which precedes acute local paroxysms), or again, are evidences of the rheumatoid stage with its common and uncommon manifestations, including many neurasthenic and neuropathic symptoms, oxaluria, intestinal indigestion, eruptive and herpetic lesions of the faucial and other mucous and cutaneous surfaces, and finally terminating in an acute invasion of the larger joints.

If, as it is claimed, 60 to 75 per cent., or even a higher percentage of iritic, ciliary, and choroidal disease is dependent upon constitutional syphilis, acquired or inherited, 5 to 10 per cent. upon toxic and septic causes (lead-intoxication, gonorrhea, etc.), and the remaining portion—15 to 30 per cent.—upon gout and rheumatism, what share of this is assignable to gout, what proportion to rheumatism, and lastly, what portion to the manifestation of disease which is a blending of both and is designated as rheumatic gout?[1]

Mr. Hutchinson assigns an important share to gout as an etiologic factor, but a major share to what has been termed by him and others rheumatic gout. "The more purely a case is one of rheumatism the less is the possibility that iritis will occur. When iritis is present, the complications are almost invariably those which suggest what we call rheumatic gout, rather than rheumatism pure and simple." In this country, with its diverse and changeable climate, mixed population living amid every condition of favorable and unfavorable hygienic surroundings, rheumatic affections are not rare, and it is not uncommon to meet with iritis and other choroidal complications which, on account of their unmistakable resemblance to rheumatism, must be classed with "rheumatic affections."

Under all circumstances it is evident that in a certain number of cases the ocular disturbances mentioned represent a part of the group of symptoms which are an advanced expression of one and the same diathesis; on the one hand, in gout, the presence of uric acid in the blood and deposits of biurate of soda around the small joints constitute the main pathologic alterations; while, on the other hand, in rheumatism—in its acute or chronic form—the characteristic inflammatory invasions of the larger joints are found. Among other deleterious agents, the same morbid product (uric acid) is present, but undergoes different transformation after accumulation in excessive quantities. As a necessary sequence, in both cases, there are enacted peculiar changes which interfere with and pervert the metabolic processes, especially of the connective tissues and lymphatic channels. It follows from this that we may expect iritic and other ocular complications in both of these maladies, and also in that form which is a fusion in both, the so-called rheumatic gout.

At what period are iritic and other lesions of the uveal tract apt to occur? Are they more common during the acute outbreaks of local gout and rheumatism or during the latent periods of these affections?

As a rule, ocular complications appear during the early manifestations of the uric-acid diathesis, or during the stage which precedes for a longer or shorter period acute outbreaks of either gout or rheumatism, or during the intervals of acute or sub-acute recurrent attacks.

In one of my cases a violent rheumatic seizure affecting the larger joints persisted more than a year and finally disappeared without tophaceous deposits or stiffening of the joints. Recently, five years after the first and only attack, the patient developed acute iritis of the right eye after walking over damp grass. After violent suffering and typical objective symptoms the attack rapidly subsided. It was preceded during several months by neurasthenic disturbances, malaise, migraine, etc. In another case, coincident with the clinical picture of so-called serous iridochoroiditis and unmistakable evidences of a uric-acid diathesis, a most persistent disturbance with frequent and violent relapses occurred. Seven years afterward, inflammatory invasions of the joints followed and continued more than a year. During this period the ocular symptoms were quiescent, but after the subsidence of the joint disturbance they recurred with violence. The patient came to me about this

[1] Unquestionably, cases of iritis have been added to this category which occur in the course of that chronic affection of the joints known as arthritis deformans or crippling rheumatism. This disease, on account of its symmetric deformities, etc., is looked upon as a trophoneurosis (allied to the chronic arthropathies met with in chronic affections of the spinal cord), and should not be considered in this classification.

time, and an iridectomy was at once advised and performed, with temporary arrest of the inflammatory activity. Since then repeated recurrences have taken place, and have resulted in a low grade of chronic iridochoroiditis with dense precipitates on the posterior surface of the cornea, but no tendency on the part of the coloboma to become occluded. The ultimate fate of this eye will most probably be its removal to avert uncontrollable inflammatory disturbance and suffering.

The question whether in exceptional cases iritis and choroiditis may be simultaneous expressions and prominent among the other clinical phenomena during an acute outbreak of either gout or rheumatism, has generally been negatively answered, and no reliable clinical data are to be found among the mass of recorded cases in the literature of gout or rheumatism. In fact, it is safe to state that the ocular attack is never simultaneous, although, in exceptional instances, it may be a concomitant expression. If such processes are lighted up during an acute attack, they must rather be considered a coincidence than otherwise. The following observation is interesting because it bears upon this point: A woman, aged fifty years, complained of a persistent burning sensation about the eyelids. Her eyes had the typical "hot eye" appearance so often seen in gouty subjects. A simple collyrium was advised. The following day I was sent for, and found that a violent rheumatic seizure, affecting the shoulders and hips, had occurred with severe pain in both eyes. Examination disclosed marked episcleral injection, aqueous humor discolored, and dusky irides. The interesting feature was that rapid subsidence of the attack followed the administration of salicylates and the application of the usual local treatment.

Do the ocular disturbances, and in particular the lesion under consideration, offer any confirmatory evidences to any one of the many theories advanced to explain the morbid changes which affect the joints, tendons, and fibrous tissues in gout and rheumatism?

It must be at once admitted that there is nothing distinctive in the pathologic appearance of an iritis or iridochoroiditis by which it may be invariably recognized and connected with these constitutional maladies. A part of the entire category of symptoms of the uric-acid diathesis, or the unmistakable gouty or rheumatic cachexiæ, must be present before the ocular lesion can with reasonable certainty be assigned to these causes. Nevertheless, there are certain local features which strongly suggest this origin, even though there may be a lack of evidence as far as the general symptoms are concerned. So far as offering a positive deduction concerning the morbid anatomy of gout, the pathologic process appears to attack principally the lymphatic circulation and the delicate connective-tissue fabric, thus resembling the great connective-tissue disease—syphilis.

As to the question whether it is possible to differentiate between gout and rheumatic affections at any time during the progress of these maladies, and whether the greater share, as an etiologic factor in iritis and other uveal lesions, may be assigned to gout or rheumatism, it may be stated that during the prodromic stages or after a blending (local and general) of the symptoms occurs it is impossible to do so. But during the early stages, before the characteristic alterations have occurred in the joints,—either as the typical gouty or rheumatic affection—as specialists we can establish a more rational etiology in assuming one or the other or both of the general diseases in question as the cause of the lesions affecting the eye.

1. During the stage before gouty or rheumatic invasions of the joints occur, we can scarcely speak of either of these affections as gout or rheumatism *per se*, but they must be regarded as goutiness, so-called, or a rheumatic or rheumatoid tendency.

2. After the malady is declared it may happen that the pure characteristics are preserved a long time, or even become permanent, so that the patient, on the one hand, presents only the typical gouty manifestations, or on the other, only the typical rheumatic evidences, as far as the joints and other general symptoms are concerned.

3. In other cases again, as both progress or develop, one affection partakes more or less of the characteristics of the other, until such an intimate fusion takes place that by common consent the term rheumatic gout has been selected.

The Gouty Affections of the Uveal Tract.—During the stage of goutiness or latent gout, before its declaration as an acute disturbance of the smaller joints, especially of the foot and hand, we meet with annoying complaints, chiefly referable to the constant presence of muscæ volitantes. In most cases, careful examination discloses a normal fundus oculi, with unimpaired sight and function. In addition there may be found a passive congestion of the vessels of the sclera and episcleral region, the typical "hot eye" of the English. The ocular may only be part of other neurasthenic disturbances, or of an overwrought state of the nervous system; but not infrequently the muscæ volitantes have a pathologic importance and are prodromic of exudative choroiditis. A definite pathologic expression of iritis is rare. It is more frequently observed as a complication of scleritis, episcleritis, and disseminated sclerochoroiditis, as the following cases show:

CASE I. *Sclerotitis or Sclerocyclitis Migrans, Complicated with Iritis.*—Miss B., aged twenty years, a large, over-developed young woman, weighing about 200 pounds. Tophaceous deposits in the hands. Has had several violent attacks (3) in left eye, always accompanied by iritis. During the early stages of relapse activity seems to be concentrated in the sclera and episcleral tissues. Typical "hot-eye" appearance is also present. The last attack occurred in January, 1897; the new feature was an infiltration around the insertion of the internal rectus muscle, with severe complaint when an attempt was made to move the eye to the right. The attack lasted longer than the former ones, but recovery finally occurred.

A far more frequent lesion is an insidious variety of exudative choroiditis (Case II.) which appears under the clinical picture of so-called serous iritis or iridochoroiditis, usually occuring during the initial stage of gout or during the intervals between acute attacks.

CASE II. *Serous Iridochoroiditis and Exudative Choroiditis.*—The disease of the choroid began when the patient was nineteen years old. At the age of thirty-four years complicating cataract, preceded by increasing vitreous opacities, hemorrhages into the choroid, etc., with total abolition of function resulted. Seven or eight years after the ocular lesion manifested itself, evidences of goutiness appeared, and since then he has had repeated typical expressions of local gout. The family history in this case conclusively suggests gout, the father had rheumatic gout, and of a family of four, two, both sons, have had declared gout, a daughter has had goutiness, and the oldest son has also had gouty manifestations in the eyes in the form of persistent muscæ volitantes with unimpaired function.

Of all the obscure ocular lesions caused by an outbreak of gout this is the most treacherous. Muscæ volitantes, functional disturbances of vision, subjective "glimmering," luminous appearances, etc., are present for months, when the so-called "iritis serosa" is added. The disease causes seroplastic exudation into the anterior chamber and on the surface of the iris, posterior synechia, floating opacities in the vitreous humor, especially in the anterior portion, and deposits on the posterior lens-capsule. Progressive failure of vision and most annoying subjective disturbances are usually present. In rare cases, the ocular tension may be reduced; far more frequently it is increased, finally terminating in secondary glaucoma.

The local treatment requires the utmost care and discrimination. Mydriatics and myotics are dangerous, and cocain is useless. Benefit may result from the application of moist heat or hot irrigation to the closed lids. Paracentesis of the anterior chamber, repeated daily according to indications, is in many cases a beneficial measure. If in spite of this the tension remains increased, an iridectomy or a sclerotomy may become necessary. Active internal medication by means of colchicum, salicylates, etc., hot baths, together with local application of moist heat, supplemented by paracentesis corneæ, and the cautious use of either myotics or mydriatics in weak solutions, according to indications, may alone avert enucleation. Nevertheless, in many cases removal of the eye finally becomes the only measure of expediency to rid the patient of an interminable and incurable affection. In the more favorable cases recovery ensues with impairment of vision; in others, one or several scotomata are left, especially if the goutiness develops into declared gout. This is almost the rule, and if a persistent, chronic, degenerative process affecting the entire uveal tract is excited, the disease terminates with atresia pupillæ, cataracta complicata, etc.

This lesion of the uveal tract is, in my experience, the most frequent expression of the gouty diathesis. It is as obscure as the nature of gout itself. It manifests itself as a serous or seroplastic inflammation of low grade, accompanied by chemic changes in the composition and quality of the aqueous humor. The alterations in the anterior chamber and iris only mask the real lesion, which consists of single or multiple exudates into the choroid near the equator, or in the anterior part of the choroid and ciliary body.

Another less frequent lesion is iritis, associated with zona ophthalmica, or herpes zoster of the eye. This may occur in gouty subjects, especially males with inherited gout, or as an expression of advanced "goutiness," or during the intervals of declared gout. It is important to differentiate between iritis which is primary and that which is secondary to the eruption of herpetic vesicles on the cornea, and along the course of the frontal divisions of the ophthalmic branches of the trigeminus. Two of the cases reported below illustrate the more infrequent primary iritis, and the third shows the more frequent form in which the iritis is secondary to the primarily affected cornea.

CASE III. *Zona Ophthalmica—Iritis Plastica.*—E. S., aged sixty-nine years, family history unmistakably gouty. He has two brothers, one of whom had rheumatic gout, the other rheumatism. Patient has tophaceous deposits and gives a history of subacute gouty disturbances. Coincident with the herpetic eruption (brow), violent iritis plastica occurred, but no herpes vesicles on the cornea or conjunctiva. Subsidence of attack took place after six weeks. Disturbance of vision and floating opacities first noticed February, 1896. There was a recurrence of the choroidal trouble, and greater impairment of vision. January, 1897, a more violent attack occurred, accompanied for the first time by severe pain and hemorrhagic iritis. Repeated paracentesis of the anterior chamber was resorted to, in conjunction with absolute rest, use of hot applications, and the internal administration of colchicum, salicylates, etc. There was little or no improvement in vision, no synechiæ, but gouty manifestations continued.

CASE IV. *Zona Ophthalmica—Irits Plastica.*—A. K., aged sixty-seven years, had a neuralgic seizure and typical eruption of herpes following the course of the frontal and lachrymal branches of the right trigeminus. Iritis commenced when this subsided; the suffering returned, but was not as violent as that accompanying the herpes vesicles. He is at present under treatment. No adhesions, but deep and typical herpes scars in skin of brow and scalp.

CASE V. *Zoster Ophthalmicum—Kerato-iritis.*—Mrs McC., presented typical local and constitutional symptoms of herpes zoster; eye trouble was coincident with eruptive stage; suffering intense. Family history conclusively demonstrated a gouty tendency. Patient has tophi and unmistakable evidences of goutiness, but has never had declared gout.

Another rare expression of the gouty diathesis appears under the guise of a low grade of iritis, or of the iridochoroiditis referred to, the process being secondary to degenerative changes which affect the retina, and finally resulting in glaucoma. Iridectomy, in such cases, although indicated, is fraught with danger.

CASE VI. *Chronic Iridochoroiditis Plastica—Synechiæ Posteriores.*—Mrs. H., had rheumatism twenty-two years ago. Insidious chronic iritis commenced ten years ago; numerous exacerbations. In spite of local and general treatment, double iridectomy, etc., the degenerative process continued. Recently, patient has had fresh exudative choroiditis in best (right) eye, attended by all the local symptoms of the so-called "serous" affection.

Equally rare are those cases, also unquestionably of gouty origin, manifesting themselves during the later periods of chronic glaucoma (frequently unilateral), in which the most experienced surgeons as a measure of rational empiricism would first propose an iridectomy rather than immediate enucleation. The inevitable prognosis in such complicated lesions may be inferred from the brief history of the two cases which follow. Severe hemorrhage from the retinal and choroidal arteries, followed by the almost instantaneous extrusion of the contents of the globe, is rather a depressing experience, but one that many have encountered, and which has been reported in some instances, and perhaps left unrecorded in a larger number:

CASE VII. *Chronic Inflammatory Glaucoma.*—Mrs. G., aged sixty-nine years; vision gradually lost after repeated subacute inflammatory exacerbations of glaucoma. T : : No. I. General appearance of eye, with the exception of the glaucomatous changes, favorable. Patient being adverse to enucleation, an iridectomy was substitued, and instantaneously followed by complete extrusion of the contents of the globe through the incision; incision closed by sutures, and globe at once enucleated. The patient was a gouty subject, as tophi and history disclosed.

CASE VIII. *Chronic Glaucoma.*—H. B., aged seventy years, presented evidence of rheumatic gout. Left eye has been blind and painful several months. Although the eye's appearance did not suggest degenerated blood-vessels, enucleation was nevertheless advised as the safest plan. The patient being adverse to this, decided to have iridectomy performed first. This was done, and was immediately followed by hemorrhage and extrusion of the vitreous humor, of course, necessitating enucleation.

I also wish to refer to the gouty diathesis as one of the causes of glaucoma. The subject is of such interest, and requires such extensive consideration, that it is impossible to make more than a passing reference here to the fact that among the alleged causes of glaucoma, the source and origin is placed in the iris angle and lymphatic spaces of this locality. In this connection the condensed history of two cases is given, both women, with double non-inflammatory glaucoma:

CASE IX.—An iridectomy, with large, key-hole-shaped opening, was performed on both eyes. For months before the operation the disease was kept under control by the use of eserine, and on account of the controlling effect of the myotic and the favorable appearance of the external structures an operation for permanent relief was undertaken. Operative interference resulted disastrously, a chronic iritis or iridochoroiditis, doubtless due to miliary hemorrhages in the retina and choroid, hopelessly destroyed the sight of both eyes.

CASE X.—Patient is at present under observation A double iridectomy, clean and smooth, was followed within eight weeks by a low grade of iridochoroiditis in both eyes, resulting in complete abolition of sight in the right eye and with a fragment of vision remaining in the left.

I believe that in both these cases a gouty origin was responsible for the glaucoma, and directly for the disastrous complication, although no general manifestations of gout were present, either immediately before or after the operation. I believe that these cases are identical with those unfortunate experiences (fortunately rare) which some oculists have had after an operation for the extraction of mature cataract, which, from all external indications, functional tests, etc., promised favorable results, and which, regarding the operation as such, was smooth and uncomplicated. During the operation or immediately afterward successive hemorrhages occur in the retina, choroid, and vitreous, without exciting any active disturbance. The healing of the wound is uncomplicated, and there is no visible unfavorable reaction, but when finally the sight i tested, vision is found to be nil. Several years ago an experience like this happened to me in a case of "rheumatic gout." Uncomplicated extraction of cataract was followed by uneventful healing. Eight days later, after insisting that the patient must be able to count fingers, an assertion which she persistently denied, I was at last convinced of the truth of her statements when ophthalmoscopic examination disclosed the vitreous full of hemorrhages, and retina and choroid detached.

In concluding this part of the subject, the history of a case is given which, as far as my experience is concerned, is exceptional:

CASE XI.—Mrs. McM., aged forty-seven years, was attacked during the night with excruciating pain in the left eye. This continued several hours, attended by profuse weeping, photophobia, but especially great suffering when she attempted to move the eye.

I saw the patient on the following day in consultation. I learned that she had just passed the menopause amid great strain and suffering. She was a confirmed neuralgic; had had herpes zoster, eczema, and migraine. In fact, she showed every evidence of the so-called uric-acid diathesis, but no frankly declared gout or rheumatic disturbance. The history of a former eye trouble was absent, and from her account my first impression was that she had acute glaucoma.

The examination, however, revealed a different state of affairs. The lids were glossy and tense. The ocular conjunctiva was intensely congested and chemotic; the sclera, bluish gray, aqueous, discolored; the pupil, contracted and sluggish; iris, dull; globe, exophthalmic, with an appearance resembling incipient panophthalmitis; motion of the globe visibly constricted in every direction and excessively painful. She complained of nausea on attempting to open the eye; tension, unchanged; moderate dilatation of pupil after a drop of atropin solution. Ophthalmoscopic examination disclosed precipitates on anterior capsule of lens and posterior surface of cornea, and exceptionally pronounced optic neuritis, with enormous swelling and edematous infiltration of the adjacent retina.

During the following days, amid recurrences of suffering which in character resembled gout, on account of the exquisite sensitiveness of the lids and the attendant constitutional symptoms, the globe became almost immobile and moderate proptosis continued several days.

By the use of anodynes, absolute rest, leeches, and atropin, the iritis and swelling of the external parts subsided within eight or ten days, but any atttempt to move the globe was attended by pain during many weeks. The optic neuritis slowly subsided, and complete restoration of sight finally resulted. The patient was recently seen, and has had no recurrence.

It may be asked was this an attack of acute iritis in a gouty subject with optic neuritis—a complication which is not uncommon? Was it angioneurotic, or a sudden vasomotor paralysis of the tissues of the orbit? Was it a sudden obstruction in the lymph-channels in the cavernous sinus, or was it a local expression of gout?

Gout is infrequent among women, even though "goutiness" is not. It is admitted that these disturbances are more frequently met with after the menopause.

The Rheumatic Affections of the Uveal Tract.—We not infrequently observe lesions of the uveal tract in regard to which a distinct history is obtained which suggests either a rheumatic tendency without acute disturbances of the joints, or positive inference that one or several paroxysms of declared rheumatic seizures preceded the ocular disturbance. Such manifestations, in character resembling those seen during the stage of goutiness, may precede or follow the active local rheumatic invasions of the larger joints, and we are almost constrained to admit their rheumatic origin.

If such active paroxysms assume all the other characteristics which force us to assign them to the rheumatic group *per se* before a blending with gout or a rheumatoid arthritis has occurred, we can furthermore determine that it is during the period of unknown duration which precedes the acute local attacks, or during the intervals between recurrent attacks, that lesions of the iris, ciliary body, and choroid are apt to be manifested; just as in gout, ocular disturbances of rheumatic origin rarely or never happen during an acute or subacute rheumatic invasion of the joints.

The designation "rheumatic" has always been a vague one, for evident reasons. There is no marked morbid anatomy; therefore, all conclusions concerning its real nature are based upon speculative knowledge, supported, it is true, by a mass of clinical facts. In the search for a rational etiology for these lesions of the iris, when all other known causes have been excluded, it must be assumed, in the absence of more positive proof, that there exists a so-called "rheumatic tendency." Although we do not know exactly what the rheumatic tendency is, we do know, with much more certainty, what it is not.

Goutiness possesses a more or less definite expression. The rheumatic tendency has no end of expressions, because it includes almost every known clinical manifestation. The well-known etiologic dependence of rheumatic seizures upon syphilis, gonorrhea, septic and toxic disturbances, malaria, anemia, etc., demands of every specialist a most stringent examination into the real cause. In this rheumatism differs from gout; with the latter struma, phthisis, herpes zoster, and glycosuria are known to be only occasionally correlated; however, the former, besides its own clinical peculiarities, is very often the conspicuous local expression of a number of constitutional diseases.

Among the early manifestations of the rheumatic diathesis may be found affections of the uveal tract, and functional derangements of the ciliary muscles, or distressing asthenopic disturbances are observed. The most frequent inflammatory affection of the uveal tract due to this cause is iritis, acute and chronic. In its acute plastic form it may be insidious, and in some cases it is only the most conspicuous expression of a general iridochoroiditis; and in others, less commonly, its onset is sudden, its course more rapid, and its symptoms more violent.

CASE XII. *Acute Plastic Iritis.*—Mr. C., married. Iritis came on after overheating and over-exertion; severe pains in muscles of lower limbs, with stiffness of joints, developed within six hours. Iritis, coincidently developed in both eyes.

Upon the administration of salicylates, and the use of rest, leeches, and atropin, the attack subsided, without synechiæ, and without implication of the choroid.

CASE XIII. *Acute Plastic Iritis.*—Mrs. R., aged twenty-six years, was a strong, healthy woman. She was suddenly attacked with pain in the eye and severe neuralgia. In spite of the most rational treatment, suffering persisted. When I first saw her objective symptoms of iritis were pronounced. Absolute rest in bed, large doses of salicylate of sodium, and vapor baths were resorted to, recovery, without synechiæ, resulting.

CASE XIV. *Iritis Plastica.*—F. S., aged sixty years, had had rheumatic manifestations many years, never acute, but frequently disabling him weeks at a time; no tophaceous deposits. Mental worry was an element in the case. A residence along the river bank predisposed him to these attacks, which have occurred with especial frequency during the fall of the year. Both eyes have been affected, but never at the same time.

Another more accentuated expression of plastic iritis is occasionally observed. The onset is sudden, the course stormy, and the suffering intense. Amid local symptoms so violent that at first a parenchymatous or a suppurating variety is suggested, an acute plastic process occurs, and assumes exceptional characteristics. The anterior chamber becomes completely filled with an opalescent grayish-yellow exudate of plastic lymph. As the inflammatory symptoms disappear this yellowish exudate subsides, and generally may be noticed to contract around a central point, which appears agglutinated to the anterior capsule in the middle of the moderately dilated pupil. Another feature of interest is that synechiæ are not as common as one would be led to infer from the apparent severity of the attack.

The following cases are typical of this variety « rheumatic iritis:

CASE XV. *Acute Plastic Iritis in Both Eyes.*—Dr. P., after a violent acute catarrhal or rheumati attack, follicular sore throat, muscular soreness, an lumbago, had, after subsidence of these symptoms, sudden and violent inflammation of both eyes.

The diagnosis was unmistakable, the sympton being so violent that Dr. S. C. Ayres of Cincinna saw the case in consultation with me. The usu remedies were resorted to, and paracentesis was als performed. The exudate, however, was tenaciou and the aqueous humor so completely absorbed th nothing escaped. The opalescent mass, throug which the pupil could be seen, gradually contracte around a central point at or near the middle of th pupil. The periphery cleared up first, and perfe vision was finally restored.

CASE XVI. *Acute Plastic Iritis.*—A. P., age forty-two years. An exudate into the anteri chamber completely filled it. In addition, the were numerous hemorrhages on the surface of th iris, resulting in a vivid, straw-colored appearanc This contracted around a central point near th middle of the pupil, and disappeared completel No recurrence has taken place.

The chronic variety either as an expression general iridochoroiditis or as the result of an acu process, beginning and confining itself to the an terior portion of the uveal tract, is, with all its un fortunate consequences, one of the most dreadf of the lesions of the eye. The following case lustrates the gravity and hopelessness of such di turbances:

CASE XVII.—Miss A. B., presented an indefini family history pointing to a predisposition to rhe matism. During girlhood she had a rheumatic kne joint followed by permanent deformity; no pain disturbance since. Two years ago she had plastric iri which merged into the chronic form, and result in atresia pupillæ of both eyes. When she co sulted me she refused operation, and when s returned, six months later, the prospects were ho less, and the operation failed to bring about i provement in vision.

Cyclitis is not uncommon. It is most commo observed in young girls or during early womanho It is generally associated with sclerotitis, or milder equivalent, episcleritis migrans. The pat logic process of exudative choroiditis, which beg in the choroid and assumes the picture of so-cal iridochoroiditis and serous iritis, is not o destructive to vision, but, because a chronic iri choroiditis is excited with especial liability to he orrhagic extravisations into these structures, enucl tion is frequently rendered necessary, as shown the following case:

CASE XVIII. *Relapsing Cyclitis—Exudative C roiditis, and Later, Iritis.*—Sister B., aged twen five years. The patient, a delicate woman, had subjective symptoms suggesting exudative choroiditis. This was confirmed by ophthalmoscopic examination. In spite of tonics, alteratives, etc., it became necessary, because of exquisite suffering and hopeless degeneration, to enucleate the eye. Rheumatic disturbances affecting the muscles and the larger joints were persistent and frequent.

Affections of the Uveal Tract Associated with Rheumatic Gout.—It must be held that in this group, which is a blending of gout and rheumatism, lesions of the uveal tract, and iritis in particular, may occur. The iritis does not possess distinctive local characteristics, but because of the typical changes in the joints, the diagnosis of the ocular lesion is almost suggested by the appearance of the patient. My own observations have familiarized me with several typical instances conclusively proving iritis to be one of the complications of this general affection; cyclitis and choroiditis are not so common. Of four cases of which I have preserved brief notes two are mentioned because they all have in common stiffening, tophaceous deposits, and other deformities of the smaller and larger joints, and also hereditary tendency to affections of the joints.

CASE XIX. *Chronic Iritis Plastica.*—A. R., aged sixty-eight years, had exceptionally severe attacks of rheumatic gout affecting the knees and ankles, during which he never had eye trouble. It was during the intervals between the attacks of the general affection that several different times he was led to the office for treatment of the eye trouble. Finally atresia pupillæ resulted, but vision remained exceptionally good. Operative interference was refused.

CASE XX. *Plastic Iritis.*—A. F., aged thirty-six years. Had frequent relapsing attacks during intervals of joint-disturbances; great distortion of articular surfaces.

CLINICAL MEMORANDA.

NOTES ON CASES OF SYPHILIS.

By JAMES C. JOHNSTON, M.D.,
OF NEW YORK;
DERMATOLOGIST TO THE NEW YORK LYING-IN HOSPITAL; PHYSICIAN TO THE CLASS OF SKIN AND GENITO-URINARY DISEASES IN THE OUT-DOOR DEPARTMENT OF THE PRESBYTERIAN HOSPITAL.

Precocious Gummatous Syphilide. — The patient, a woman aged thirty-five years, acquired her disease, maritally and genitally, during June, 1897. When she presented herself for treatment in September her face was disfigured by the lesions of syphilis. According to her statement, the gummata developed gradually without intermission from the early secondary outbreak. In addition to the face, the tumors were dotted over the upper and lower extremities. They were rounded, almost hemispheric, not scaling nor crusted, and varied in diameter from a quarter to one inch. They projected considerably above the surrounding skin level. As a rule, the color was a deep, purplish-red, shading through stages of regression to pink. They were freely movable over the fascia, and in the case of the newer lesions, under the integument, thus proving their origin in the subcutaneous tissue. No other symptoms of the early period were present with the exception of nocturnal headache and multiple adenopathy.

Ulceration did not occur since involution began shortly after the institution of treatment, which, in order to secure a swift and sure constitutional result, consisted of inunctions with blue ointment. An ounce of the latter was divided into ten equal parts, one of which was vigorously rubbed into the skin ten to fifteen minutes each night. The residue was washed off in the morning. In order to prevent an outbreak of mercurial dermatitis, the site of inunction was rotated as follows: first the right and left chest, then the abdomen, and finally the inside of the thighs. After three weeks of nightly rubbing, a change to every other night was ordered. This routine was continued without a break. At the present writing (December, 1897) only a few scaling spots remain to mark the sites of the gummata.

In using inunctions, care should be taken to select non-hairy parts. It is singular that as a rule women raise so little objection to the application of the ointment, dirty as it undoubtedly is. Whether a haunting fear of the disease or the relief from the mental burden of pill-taking is responsible for this complaisance, is hard to say. In private practice, Dietrich's ointment is preferable to the officinal unguentum hydrargyri, as it has a soap base, seems more readily absorbable, and is certainly more easily removed. Iodid of potassium, in 20-grain doses, three times daily, relieved the headache within a week.

Nephritis During Early Syphilis.—The patient is the husband of the woman whose case has just been described. He is an engineer on an ocean steamship, exposed to much hardship and temptation in the way of dissipation. He was sent to me by his wife September 20, 1897, five months after infection—according to his statement. No trace of cutaneous eruption could be found; a slight scar remained at the site of inoculation, but a diagnosis of active syphilis could be made from the mucous patches in the mouth. His health was completely broken down. A pronounced anemia was present, the hue of the skin resembling that of chlorosis. He complained of headache, cardiac palpitation, and shortness of breath to such an extent as precluded sustained effort. His lower extremities were edematous, and his urine scanty and high-colored. On examination the urine showed a specific gravity of 1028, albumin, and a few epithelial casts. He was placed on a milk diet and mercurial treatment (inunction, as in the case of his wife), but grew worse and, attempting another trip, was invalided home from Havana.

Three weeks from the date of his first visit his powers of assimilation seemed to have failed. In consequence, his appetite was enormous—the bulimia syphilitica described by Fournier. Specific medication was stopped, the milk diet was continued, and a tonic, consisting of the syrup of the iodid of iron with cod-liver oil and hypophosphites, was administered. A month later, the condition was much improved; the symptoms of nephritis had almost disappeared, and a more liberal diet was permitted. The use of mercurials will be resumed when the general condition warrants specific medication. Fordyce (*Jour. of Cutan. and Genito-Urin. Diseases*, April, 1897), Mauriac, and others have reported similar cases.

Syphilitic Myositis.—The two cases of this manifestation of syphilis of which I have notes possessed almost exactly similar characteristics. Both occurred in young men under thirty years of age, in the early stage of the disease, and in otherwise apparently good health. In both, the middle third of the sternocleidomastoid muscle of the left side was affected. The symptoms were a diffuse swelling in the body of the muscle, stiffness, and slight pain on movement. The myositis is easily differentiated from swelling of underlying lymph-nodes, from rheumatism, by the involvement of a single muscle, the brawny character of the swelling, the presence of other signs of syphilis, and the reaction to medication. It is rather unusual to find syphilitic myositis before the end of the second year of the general disease; both of these cases occurred earlier, and both patients recovered following local and general inunction of gray ointment, used as in the first instance mentioned.

Quite a number of such cases have been reported, and from a study of them it has been determined that the relative order of frequency is (one muscle being usually affected), the gastrocnemius, biceps, sphincter ani, masseter, sternomastoid, and others only exceptionally. Syphilitic muscle inflammation is of two kinds, interstitial and gummatous. Occasionally, a mixed form is observed. In the first, the inflammation spreads diffusely through the endomysium; in the second, there is usually a single node. In either case, a degeneration and absorption of the muscular fibers may result if the process is allowed to continue, the place of the fibers being taken by new connective tissue. In this event, permanent shortening and deformity is, of course, to be expected. Prognosis is good with proper treatment.

A PERSONAL EXPERIENCE IN RENAL SURGERY.

BY ROBERT F. WEIR, M.D.,
OF NEW YORK;
PROFESSOR OF SURGERY IN THE COLLEGE OF PHYSICIANS AND SURGEONS, AND SURGEON TO THE NEW YORK HOSPITAL;
WITH THE COLLABORATION OF
EDWARD M. FOOTE, M.D.,
OF NEW YORK;
SURGEON TO THE RANDALL'S ISLAND HOSPITALS.

(Continued from page 81.)

RENAL CALCULUS.

Renal Calculus—Nephrolithotomy.—Under this heading are embraced seven cases, all resulting in recovery, although in three the renal damage was so great that nephrectomy was necessary. In five of the seven cases there was an associated abscess in the pelvis of the kidney (pyonephrosis) or in the cortical tissue (pyelonephrosis). The calculi removed were principally composed of calcium oxalate or of phosphates. Only once was a stone composed of uric acid found. The largest calculus weighed 510 grains; the greatest number found in any one case was forty-one.

The Röntgen ray was employed in but one instance, a recent case, with a negative result—an experience which has occurred to many in the early employment of the X-rays. This is partly due to the fact that the calculi composed of uric acid and the urates are easily penetrated by the rays, while the only ones which give a good shadow are those of oxalate of lime, and, to a less degree, the phosphatic calculi. With the later improvements in the tubes and plates better results have recently been obtained, and to this end additional benefit may be derived from the advice given by Myles,[1] based upon anatomic experiments, that the light should pass through the kidney from a point backward and outward, as this prevents the obscuration by the liver. A further suggestion has been made by Fenwick[2] that in exploring the kidney, the viscus should, as is often possible, be brought well into or out of the wound. It may then be examined by the aid of the Röntgen rays with more chance of success than when it is *in situ*, and that thereby, as he has shown, calculi small enough to escape detection by puncture or palpation may be recognized and treated.

Occasionally it may occur, as in Case XIII., that the absence of pus or other urinary signs will obscure the diagnosis, especially if there be no decided enlargement of the kidney. In Case XVIII. there existed, it is true, a tumor, but nothing pointing toward the presence of a calculus. It was not only of interest as showing the effect of an untreated calculus when no complications occur, but also from the unusual surgical concomitant which happened during the operation of nephrectomy. The patient was the sister of a skilled physician, who had watched and treated her for many years, making numerous examinations of the urine and finding nothing abnormal except the occasional presence of albumin. During the year preceding the operation a diagnosis of tumor of the kidney was made. Cystocopic examination, though difficult, showed some purulent urine, but it was only at the operation that the real state of affairs became known.

The principal accident which complicated the operation was the tearing of the vena cava. The resulting hemorrhage was successfully controlled by immediate suture of the vein, and the accident did not interefere with rapid recovery. No better evidence could be given of the advantage of the large incision used than the ease with which this vein was sutured. Fortunately no edema or other symptom of thrombosis followed, and the vessel without doubt remained pervious. A similar experience has been recorded by Enderlen.[3] During extirpation of the kidney the vena cava was torn by him and immediately sutured. Death occurred forty-five hours later. The cause of death is not stated, but it was preceded by coma

[1] *Edin. Med. Journal*, September, 1897.
[2] Fenwick, *Brit. Med. Jour.*, October 16, 1897.
[3] *Deut. Zeitschr. f. Chir.*, vol. 41, p. 217, 1895.

and almost complete suppression of urine. There was some suppuration about the suture, but the closure was perfect, and from within, the lumen was seen to be scarcely narrowed. A thrombus the size of a pea was situated upon the inner side of the suture. Thornton[1] also encountered this mishap during a nephrotomy for renal calculus and pyonephrosis. A curved clamp was temporarily applied to the renal vessels. On its removal after extirpation of the kidney and ligature of the vessels in the pedicle, alarming hemorrhage occurred. The tip of the clamp had opened the vena cava. Death ensued before the bleeding-point was secured. I have also knowlledge of yet another accident of this kind which occurred in this city in a similar manner during a nephrectomy and likewise terminated fatally.

CASE XII. *Renal Calculus—Suppurative Pyelitis—Nephrotomy — Subsequent Nephrectomy — Recovery.*—James W., aged thirty-seven years, suffered four weeks before entrance to the hospital with pain in the right loin and frequent micturition, followed two weeks later by chills and fever, and a swelling in the region of the kidney. A needle inserted in the distinct tumor disclosed the presence of thick greenish pus. The urine, which was alkalin, and of a specific gravity of 1030, contained a trace of albumin and a few pus-cells. January 8, 1897, a three-inch incision was made downward and forward from the twelfth right rib, and the kidney exposed and incised. Over a pint of foul, greenish pus escaped. The reticulated cavity was washed out as thoroughly as possible, and drained. Exploration did not detect the presence of a calculus. Under irrigation and drainage, the wound was reduced to a sinus, which showed no signs of closing. The patient left the hospital April 28th at his own request, but returned within two weeks for further treatment. At the site of the previous operation the sinus admitted a probe to a depth of five inches, and at the bottom, on probing, a distinct click was obtained. May 17th the patient was again etherized, and the sinus opened. A stone composed of calcium oxalate, one-half inch in diameter, and weighing 6 grams (90 grains) was extracted with the aid of a vesical scoop. Rubber and iodoform gauze drains were used. There was considerable hemorrhage during the next two days. The tube was removed at the end of six weeks, and the sinus closed soon afterward. This was not a permanent closure, however, and on its recurrence and persistence, about six months later, nephrectomy was performed by one of the other surgeons of the hospital, but no other calculus was found in the removed organ. Seven years later the patient was in good health.

CASE XIII. *Renal Calculi—Nephrolithotomy—Recovery.*—Thos. M., aged fifty-six years, entered New York Hospital, January 12, 1892. For ten years previously he had attacks of renal colic on the right side with passage of gravel and sharp-pointed calculi. These attacks increased in frequency, and during two years there was almost constant lumbar pain. The patient appeared to be healthy, but of a "gouty diathesis." Several examinations did not reveal anything abnormal in the urine. It was alkalin, and presented a specific gravity of 1010.

January 6, 1892, a vertical incision was made from the last rib to the ilium, along the border of the quadratus lumborum muscle, and from its middle a horizontal incision, running forward a distance of three inches, was made. The kidney was freed and explored with a hat-pin. A stone was promptly detected. A longitudinal incision was, therefore, made through the cortex of the kidney posteriorly into the pelvis, and one large stone and about forty small ones were removed. The wound in the kidney was closed by a single catgut suture and the external wound partially sutured and drained with gauze. Blood disappeared from the urine within ten days, and the wound in the loin was superficial within three weeks, at which time the patient left the hospital. The large calculus removed measured 1-inch by ¾-inch, and weighed 7½ grams (112 grains), and the small ones varied in size from that of bird-shot to a buckshot. Their total weight was 9 grams (135 grains). They were composed of calcium oxalate and phosphate. Now, six years later, the patient is in excellent health, having had no urinary symptoms since leaving the hospital.

CASE XIV. *Renal Calculus—Nephrolithotomy—Recovery.*—William S., aged twenty-three years, presented a history of renal colic of some months' duration, with constant lumbar pain, and slight fever. The right lumbar region was tender, but no tumor could be detected. The urine was acid and contained albumin, red blood-cells, and casts. May 3, 1893, the right kidney was exposed by König's curved incision; it was enlarged and lobulated, and a hard mass could be felt in its pelvis. The cortex was incised and a triangular calculus removed. It measured 1.8 cm. (½-inch), 1.8 cm. (½-inch), .8 cm. (¼-inch), and weighed 4.3 grams (65 grains). The wound in the kidney was sutured with catgut, and a strip of gauze placed in front and behind the organ, and the wound elsewhere sutured; it healed readily, and relief of all symptoms followed. The patient has since passed from observation.

CASE XV. *Renal Calculus—Pyonephrosis—Double Nephrotomy — Death.* — Harriet S., aged thirty-eight years, suffered four years from attacks of pain on the left side, usually followed by a chill and fever, and the painful voiding of dark scanty urine, though the general health was fairly well maintained. At the time of entrance to the hospital, to which place she had been sent for operation by Dr. Skinner of Greenpoint, L. I., March 14, 1894, a large smooth tumor occupied the left lumbar region, extending nearly to the iliac crest, and it was not affected by respiration. The urine was alkalin, of a specific gravity of 1012, and nearly half pus. March 21st, the left kidney was exposed by the usual curved lumbar incision, and explored by means of punctures. The presence of a stone was at once detected. The kidney was incised along its convex border, letting out a large quantity of thick foul pus. A large friable phosphatic calculus was then extracted and the kidney flushed with hot water and filled with gauze. The wound was partially sutured. The operation was followed by a temperature of from 101° to 102° F., but it was noted that the urine did not contain any blood.

Two weeks after the operation the patient had a chill which was followed by a temperature of 104° F., and pain in the *right* lumbar region. These symptoms were repeated several times during the following weeks, and the right kidney became so large as to be easily palpable, while the condition of the patient became more and more septic. No increasing tenderness was experienced in the left renal area. Operation was determined upon as giving a slight chance of relief, and the right kidney was exposed May 16th. The presence of pus or stone could not be detected by a needle, though the kidney was very large and soft. An incision was followed by profuse hemorrhage, though no pus was found. The action of the heart failed rapidly, and the patient died within fifteen hours. Though an autopsy was not permitted, yet the inference was plain, after the exploration of the right kidney, that the sepsis was due to another abscess or ab-

[1] *Med. Chir. Transactions*, vol. 72, p. 29.

scesses in the first kidney operated upon. The surgical error made was in not exploring at the last operation the left kidney thoroughly before invading the right one, even though the symptoms pointed so decidedly to the latter organ.

CASE XVI. *Pyonephrosis from Renal Calculus—Nephrolithotomy—Recovery.*—Mrs. E., aged thirty-six years, suffered during ten years with attacks of renal pain, chiefly upon the left side. She was admitted to New York Hospital, October 10, 1894. Eighteen months previously she had passed a number of stones, and more recently the urine constantly contained pus. Her general health was good. By physical examination the right kidney was found to be enlarged and tender. The left kidney was not enlarged, but pressure upon its ureter at the brim of the pelvis was painful. By cystoscopic examination, it was further observed that both ureteral openings were congested, and that the water flowing from the right ureter was purulent, while that from the left appeared to be clear.

By means of König's incision the right kidney was exposed. It was much enlarged, and an aspirating-needle thrust into it disclosed the presence of pus. A two-inch incision was made into its pelvis through the cortex, and two ounces of pus and a large, soft, phosphatic calculus and several small fragments were removed. After irrigation the kidney was filled with iodoform gauze. The transverse part of the lumbar wound was sutured. Operation was followed by a moderate fever. The gauze was removed on the seventh day. Though suppurating freely, the wound granulated well with a constant flow of urine through it. The urine from the bladder also contained a little pus. Within four weeks the patient left the hospital with a small lumbar sinus. Cystoscopic examination showed that purulent urine flowed from the right ureter, and a slightly turbid urine from the left. The water from the bladder was acid, and contained a sediment of pus equal to twelve per cent. of the volume of the specimen.

The calculus with its fragments weighed 35 grams; 1¼ ounces when dry.

In response to an inquiry concerning her health, the patient wrote, March 10, 1897, as follows: "My general health is very good; good appetite; good color; I am able to exercise freely, and weigh 165 pounds. The fistulous opening in my back still discharges, so that I am obliged to wear constantly a small gauze pad over it, and my urine still contains pus, but never any blood. I have no acute pain in the region of the right kidney, but there is a sensation of weight and fulness there which extends to near the groin on that side, and which is more troublesome on some days than on others. Two or three times within the last six months I have had sharp pain on the left side, lasting from one to five minutes. I feel that I have been very much benefited by the operation."

It may be fairly inferred from the above that there is, perhaps, another calculus in the affected kidney.

CASE XVII. *Multiple Calculi — Pyelonephritis — Nephrectomy — Recovery.* — Mrs. K., aged forty-nine years, was attacked at the age of thirty-seven years with a sudden pain in the left lumbar region. Hematuria followed, and this and the pain continued ten or twelve days. There have since been occasional attacks of pain without fever. Five years ago the urine was found to contain pus. Her physician, Dr. Whittemore of New Haven, who placed her under my care, reported that during the summer of 1895 there was blood in the urine from time to time, but he never found any calculi. When I first saw the patient, during September of that year, there was found, on bimanual examination of the left loin, an enlarged kidney reaching half way to the iliac crest. It was tender on pressure, and yielded when compressed, a grating, rubbing sensation. This was the first time I had been able to elicit this symptom in a case of this kind, for it meant, of course, the presence of more than one stone. The patient had occasional elevations of temperature, but was in good condition.

October 4, 1895, the kidney was exposed by the usual König incision, its distended pelvis opened, and over a dozen calculi extracted, each nearly one-half an inch in diameter, rough and irregular, facetted, and composed of uric acid, covered by phosphates. The finger in the thin renal mass detected many other embedded stones, which in turn were released by breaking down tissue or by incision until the kidney had been split throughout nearly its whole extent. Each separate calculus now extracted was either deep in between a calyx or in the true tissue of the kidney, and was surrounded by a suppurating zone. Under such circumstances, it became impracticable to surely remove all the calculi, and therefore the kidney was extirpated; and its examination afterward confirmed the

FIG. 2.

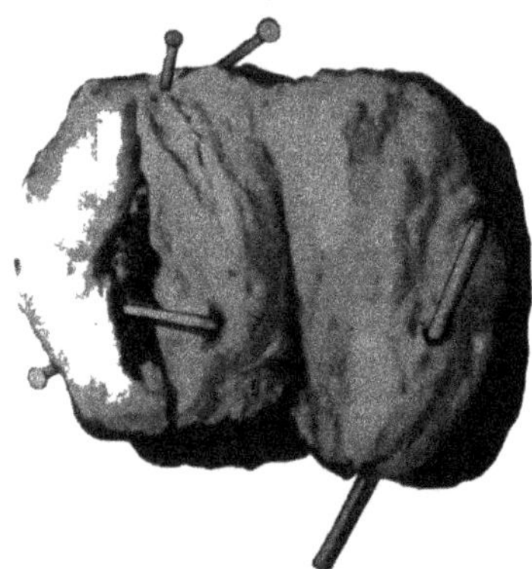

Showing renal calculus *in situ*; atrophy of the kidney; much thickened perirenal fat, which has been split; patency of ureter shown by catheters passed through it to the calculus.

fitness of the proceeding, as, in all, twenty-seven stones were found, many so small as to permit them to escape detection by the eye or finger. The patient made an uninterrupted recovery, and when seen two years later was in excellent health.

CASE XVIII. *Renal Calculus—Complete Atrophy of Kidney—Nephrectomy—Wound of Vena Cava—Suture—Recovery.*—Mrs. T., aged fifty-two years, enjoyed excellent health until she was forty years of age, when, from no apparent cause, she become very anemic, and lost flesh. The urine was then found to contain a large amount of albumin, but no casts. Under tonic treatment and the free ingestion of milk the health improved and the albumin disappeared from the urine. Subsequent examinations, made from time to time, usually showed traces of albumin, though at times the amount was large. At no time did the urine contain pus.

During the past year the patient had had sharp attacks of pain in the right lumbar region and along the course of the right ureter, followed by tenderness and fulness in this region and a vesical irritation lasting some days. During November, 1896, an unusually severe attack occurred, and the pain continued several hours. The urine was then turbid with pus, and contained a large amount of albumin. Within ten days it was again perfectly normal. Palpation at this time first revealed the presence of a hard tumor in the right lumbar region, projecting nearly to the level of the umbilicus. Through the aid of cystoscopic examinations, conducted by Dr. Meyer, it was determined with difficulty and after a number of trials that the left ureteral orifice was normal, and excreted clear urine, while the right was surrounded by granulations, and at the time of examination excreted no urine at all.

March 10, 1897, the right kidney was exposed by the usual König incision. The fat capsule of the kidney was readily exposed, but it was adherent on all sides, especially toward the peritoneum, and not to be separated from the kidney beneath. The incision in the abdominal wall was prolonged to the anterior superior spine of the ilium to permit the dissection of the mass which occupied the site of the kidney, and in so doing a rent about an inch long was made in the vena cava. The flow of blood was readily checked by a finger placed above and below the rent, which was stretched out and held taut and immediately sutured with fine catgut, one continuous suture being sufficient to stop the bleeding without invasion of the edges of the rent. An opening into the peritoneal cavity was closed in like manner. The kidney, with its fat capsule thickened and changed by chronic inflammation, was then removed, and the ureter tied with catgut and cauterized, the renal vessels being ligated separately with catgut. When the specimen was cut open, no trace of the kidney other than its ureter and pelvis could be found. The pelvis contained a Y-shaped phosphatic calculus about 1½x1 inches in size. (Fig. 2.) The rest of the mass, the size of a fist, was composed of fatty and fibrous tissue of inflammatory origin. The patient made a perfect recovery, and has since remained in good health.

(To be continued.)

MEDICAL PROGRESS.

Differential Diagnosis of Inflammations and Tumors of the Ileocecal Region —SONNENBURG read a paper upon the above subject which is reported in the *Berliner Klinische Wochenschrift*, September 15, 1897. According to this writer not only inflammations and diseases of the pelvic organs of women may simulate appendicitis, but also affections of the gall-bladder, liver, kidneys, and, under certain circumstances, even the pancreas may confuse the surgeon. It should first be noticed that a perityphlitic exudate is usually immovable; therefore, if a swelling is movable, it is probably not such an exudate. The reverse of this statement is not true, for a carcinoma, for instance, may be immovable. In such cases injection of the intestine with air will assist in clearing up the diagnosis, for if there is present a new growth of the intestine the wall of the latter will be so stiffened that the injected air cannot cause dilation.

Tuberculosis of the ileocecal region may cause infiltration, and thus may resemble either an old perityphlitic focus or a carcinoma, but here the history of the case, which often includes the symptoms of stenosis and completely fails to reveal characteristic attacks of recurrent appendicitis, will usually suffice to establish the diagnosis. Naturally, if the appendix itself is the seat of tuberculosis the characteristic attacks may be present and the differential diagnosis, at least in the early stages, be well nigh impossible.

Of the rarer conditions which may lead to error may be mentioned sarcomata, myomata, dermoid cyst, etc. Various forms of intestinal obstruction, especially invagination, may also give rise to difficulties. In the latter case, the tenesmus and the presence in the stools of bloody mucus, ought to suggest to the observer the correct diagnosis. If there is complete obstruction of the bowels without passage of fecal matter or even of gas, the case is probably not one of appendicitis, as in this trouble intestinal obstruction comes on more gradually.

Abscesses, either from the psoas muscle or from the vertebral column, lie behind the iliac fascia, and are, therefore, flat and not projecting. Moreover, the pain, in acute cases, extends more toward the right extremity and the genital organs; the right thigh is flexed and rotated inward, and peritonitic symptoms are wanting.

The differential diagnosis between appendicitis and diseases of the gall-bladder and liver is peculiarly difficult in those cases in which the perityphlitic exudate is situated high up. Here there are present chills, fever, tenderness, and resistance in both cases. A carefully taken history will still determine the diagnosis in many instances. In colic originating in the gall-bladder or liver the pain usually shoots toward the shoulder, while in appendicitis it extends toward the navel, the most painful point being in the ileocecal region. The most painful point in hepatic affections is close to the border of the ribs. In appendicitis vomiting is not so persistent as in diseases of the liver. In inflammatory or calculous disease of the gall-bladder the high position of the exudate, the relatively slight disturbance of the general system, and the extension of dulness in immediate relation with the normal liver dulness are characteristic points. In perityphlitis a tympanitic zone exits between the abscess and the liver. In both cases there may be jaundice. It must be confessed that empyema of the gall-bladder is often difficult to differentiate from appendicitis. Dilation of the gall-bladder due to obstruction by gall-stones may simulate a chronic form of appendicitis.

The relations of appendicitis to diseases of the female pelvic organs are most important. It has often been remarked that men suffer from appendicitis more frequently than women. The relative frequency is expressed by the figures 60 and 40. It is interesting in this connection to note that the appendix in women has an especial blood-supply which is not found in men, and which is contained in a ligament extending from the right ovary to the appendix. The pelvic diseases which may be confounded with appendicitis are pelvic peritonitis, acute perimetritis, perisalpingitis, and peri-oophoritis. The gynecologists know how often a careless examination may result in a wrong diagnosis, one of the above affections being mistaken for appendicitis, or the reverse. The relation of the suspected tumor to the uterus may usually be made out toward the median line, and, furthermore, the lack of disturbance of intestinal action will point toward a pelvic trouble. Here again the position of the exudate is of the utmost importance; in appendicitis it is higher up and can seldom be reached from the vaginal vault. In those cases in which the appendix extends into the pelvis and becomes attached to some of the pelvic organs, the position of the tumor is of little assistance in determining the diagnosis.

A pelvic peritonitic exudate usually forms in Douglas' pouch, pressing the uterus against the anterior abdominal wall. Such an exudate is fluctuating in its early stages. On account of congestion the mucous membrane of the rectum is swollen and secretes an abnormal quantity of mucus, and bits of membrane are exfoliated. To these pathologic features may be added several that are clinical. Acute diseases of the adnexa usually begin with vomiting and hiccough, but the seat of the trouble is located from the very beginning in the vicinity of Poupart's ligament. If there is also trouble on the left side, the diagnosis is, of course, clear. In pelvic troubles the pains extend toward the genitals rather than toward the epigastrium; the general condition is less affected; the signs of diffuse peritonitis are wanting. It doubtful cases it may be laid down as a rule that a higher position of the tumor and a localization of the pain on the right side point to an affection of the appendix. In chronic pelvic disease there may be acute recurrences just as in chronic appendicitis, but in the former the symptoms are almost always markedly increased at the menstrual periods, and in chronic cases, moreover, repeated examination will almost always establish a correct diagnosis.

The writer mentioned the fact that he had operated three times in cases of appendicitis which were sent to him with a diagnosis of parametritis. Twice a supposed appendicitis turned out to be an abscess extending upward from the genital organs; in six cases there was combined inflammation of the appendix, and adnexa, and in four cases inflammation of the adnexa followed an operation for appendicitis. He had seen one case in which tubal pregnancy was complicated by appendicitis.

The Mortality of Tetanus with and without Antitoxin.—OWENS and PORTER (*Jour. Amer. Med. Assoc.*, November 13, 1897) report three cases of tetanus, one treated symptomatically, and two with tetanus antitoxin. All proved fatal. A study of the published cases shows two facts, *viz.*, that mortality rates have been but little influenced by the treatment with antitoxin, and that the relation of the period of incubation to the mortality is practically the same whether the antitoxic serum is or is not employed. The writers have analyzed 26 cases in which the serum had been used, and found 12 recoveries, and 14 deaths, giving a mortality of 53.8 per cent. Of those patients who recovered, the shortest period of incubation was six days; of those who died the longest period was twelve days. They are, therefore, of the opinion that those cases in which symptoms appear before the sixth day will die in spite of any antitoxin treatment, and that those in which the development of symptoms is delayed beyond the second week will invariably recover. The Medical Bureau of the Columbian Exposition treated 202 cases in which nail-punctures had been received during the erection of the buildings, in most cases the puncture being made by a rusty nail. Their treatment was as follows: (1) Thorough cleansing of the part with a solution of bichlorid of mercury, 1–1000. (2) Trimming the edges of the wound. (3) Swabbing out the wound with a probe lightly covered with cotton, and dipped in a ninety-five-per-cent. solution of carbolic acid. (4) Drainage. (5) Antiseptic dressing. (6) Rest. Tetanus did not develop in a single case. This shows the value of the preventive treatment which ought to be followed rather than to place dependence upon any possible good effect of serum administered after tetanus has developed.

THERAPEUTIC NOTES.

Treatment of Anemia.—A writer in *Archives of Pediatrics*, October, 1897, recommends the following method as one of the most efficient for the treatment of anemia or chlorosis:

℞ Ferratin . . . . . gram. xv
Natr. bicarb. . . . . gram. ix
Sacchar. alb. . . . . gram. xv.

M. et. div. in chart. No. XXX. Sig. One powder three times daily in a glass of sweetened water.

This is designed for children over fifteen years of age. The dose for children between five and fifteen years is one-half this amount, and one-fourth the amount for children five years of age. An overdose will not do any harm, as about twenty per cent. of ferratin is absorbed without deranging the stomach or causing constipation.

Anemia Treated by Ferratin.—ROLER (*Chic. Med. Rec.*, November, 1897) gives an abstract of three cases, in which treatment by means of ferratin alone, in 3-grain doses, three or four times a day, was efficiently employed. A girl of twelve years, suffering from simple anemia of a marked degree, was practically cured within a month. The number of red blood-corpuscles increased during the administration of ferratin from 2,000,000 to 3,800,000 per c.cm. The appetite improved, constipation disappeared, the cheeks and mucous surfaces were tinged with a healthy red color, and the sensation of fatigue disappeared. Another girl, aged eighteen, suffered three years from anemia and constipation. Ferratin was given, as in the first case, but no marked improvement was manifest until the end of the third week. At the end of the seventh week all symptoms had disappeared. A young man, aged seventeen, suffering with insomnia, anorexia, headache, and fatigue, which latter prevented his engaging in sports, was given 2 grains of ferratin four times daily. Within a month the symptoms had greatly improved, and the blood count showed that the red corpuscles had increased from 2,800,000 to 3,400,000 per c.cm.

For Syphilitic Impetigo.—

℞ Hydrarg. oxid. rubr. } aa . . gr. xxiv
Zinci oxid. }
Resorcini . . . . . gr. x
Vaselini . . . . . . ℥ i.

M. Ft. Ungt. Sig. For external use.

THE MEDICAL NEWS.

A WEEKLY JOURNAL

OF MEDICAL SCIENCE.

COMMUNICATIONS are invited from all parts of the world. Original articles contributed *exclusively* to THE MEDICAL NEWS will after publication be liberally paid for (accounts being rendered quarterly), or 250 reprints will be furnished in place of other remuneration. When necessary to elucidate the text, illustrations will be engraved from drawings or photographs furnished by the author. Manuscripts should be typewritten.

Address the Editor: J. RIDDLE GOFFE, M.D.,
No. 111 FIFTH AVENUE (corner of 18th St.), NEW YORK.

Subscription Price, including postage in U. S. and Canada.

PER ANNUM IN ADVANCE	$4.00
SINGLE COPIES	.10
WITH THE AMERICAN JOURNAL OF THE MEDICAL SCIENCES, PER ANNUM	7.50

Subscriptions may begin at any date. The safest mode of remittance is by bank check or postal money order, drawn to the order of the undersigned. When neither is accessible, remittances may be made, at the risk of the publishers, by forwarding in *registered* letters.

LEA BROTHERS & CO.,
No. 111 FIFTH AVENUE (corner of 18th St.), NEW YORK,
AND Nos. 706, 708 & 710 SANSOM ST., PHILADELPHIA.

SATURDAY, JANUARY 22, 1898.

A PLEA FOR CHLOROFORM ANESTHESIA.

THE recent introduction to the profession of this country of the Schleich mixtures for anesthetic purposes by Maduro in the MEDICAL NEWS of November 27, 1897, and later by Willy Meyer has led to quite general experimentation with it in the hospitals of New York. Its general use, however, does not confirm that confidence in its absolute safety which the report of Schleich's experience inspired. Its extreme volatility or some other as yet undefined quality seems to unexpectedly overwhelm the patient with a depressing influence, producing great pallor and enfeeblement of the pulse. In one or two instances it has seemed prudent to stop its use and substitute ether.

In view of this experience it would seem to be only a wise prudence on the part of those experimenting with this new agent to constantly bear in mind that its use is still in the realm of experimentation and to watch its effects carefully at every stage. The death-rate from chloroform anesthesia is about 1 in 500, and from ether about 1 in 5000. It will, therefore, require a very extensive experience to establish the merits of the Schleich mixture as compared with chloroform or ether.

In an article in *The Practitioner* for December, 1897, Pringle disputes the assertion which was recently made, "that even in Edinburgh, the birthplace and home of chloroform, medical men and teachers are becoming afraid of its use." The reverse, he says, is nearer the truth.

It may be instructive to consider the conditions of its administration in that city. In the first place there are no especial anesthetists, the anesthetic being given by the various house-surgeons or junior house-surgeons, or by a student. It is usually the rule that two persons must superintend its administration. Chloroform is given by the open or Symes' method, and students are taught to watch the breathing and not to "give chloroform with the finger on the pulse." An ordinary, smooth, hospital towel is folded into a cone, leaving a space at the apex large enough to admit two fingers. The anesthetist holds the lower jaw forward with the fingers of the left hand, keeping the thumb over the mouth to feel the breathing. The chloroform is dropped on the upper part of the inside of the cone and the patient thus receives a sufficient quantity of air mingled with the chloroform.

Pringle kept a careful record of 500 anesthesias. Aside from alcoholic cases, 22 of these patients took chloroform badly, but only 2 of them gave cause for alarm, and this was only momentary. And in both instances, drawing out the tongue and clearing the throat were sufficient to restore respiration.

By reference to reports of twenty-one deaths from chloroform occurring during the past few years, it appears that the operation was usually of a trivial character, such as extraction of teeth, tonsillotomy, circumcision, etc. In sixteen cases a mask, inhaler, or lint was used. Pringle looks upon an inhaler as dangerous. "All apparatus for giving chloroform," he says, "are an abomination." Besides the danger of asphyxiation when an inhaler is used, the patient is obliged to inhale the germs of previous patient's exhalations, for there is no doubt that the air-bag of a frequently used Clover's inhaler contains a great variety of bacteria. In a patient with weak lungs this is a serious responsibility to assume.

The point in the article, however, to which attention is especially called is that it is the imperative duty of medical schools to see that the administration of chloroform is thoroughly taught. If the schools continue to teach their students simply how to administer ether, putting aside chloroform except in occasional cases, on the ground that it is dangerous, just so long will there be a high death-rate to report from the use of this anesthetic. For as long as chloroform continues to be the pleasantest and the most convenient anesthetic known, just so long will it continue to be used. It is absolutely necessary, therefore, from the point of view of this writer, that every student should have individual clinical instruction and that he should be compelled, before receiving his diploma, to produce a certificate stating that he has personally administered chloroform in a certain number of cases. When this is done deaths from chloroform will be less frequent; for all observers are agreed that many of the deaths which now occur are due to an overdose of the anesthetic.

NEW YORK STATE AND THE AMERICAN MEDICAL ASSOCIATION.

THE annual banquet of the Harlem Medical Association of New York City was held January 15th at the Harlem Casino. There was an unusual attendance both of members and invited guests; one hundred covers were laid. Among the speakers were Surgeon-General Sternberg, president of the American Medical Association; Dr. J. E. Janvrin, president of the New York County Medical Association, and Dr. A. M. Jacobus, president of the Medical Society of the County of New York. A striking feature of the evening's entertainment was the strong and universal sentiment which prevailed in favor of abolishing all differences in reference to codes of ethics, and of uniting, regardless of previous sentiment, in a strong rally in favor of membership in the American Medical Association. The remarks of the three speakers above mentioned abounded in this sentiment.

Many members of the profession in New York State are members of both the State and County Societies, as well as of the State and County Associations. The time seems ripe for the obliteration of all differences and the acceptance by the national association of all who seek its affiliation. In joining the national organization each member pledges himself to abide by its code. This should be a sufficient requirement, and the condition formerly insisted upon, "that a member of the State or County Society should first join the State or County Association," should no longer be required.

No one who did not participate in the discussions which took place at the time New York State was excluded from the national association can realize the bitterness of feeling which then prevailed and the strong prejudices then formed. These smoldering embers may be kept alive if constantly fanned, but will quickly die if ignored. It is sometimes difficult for two contending parties to settle their differences by a mutual conference without the mediation of a third. The American Medical Association has the opportunity of acting in the capacity of peacemaker in a way which will obliterate all lines of distinction in the profession of New York and unite both parties in one organization which shall be loyal to the national association.

The growth of the American Medical Association during the year 1897 was something phenomenal in its history. With the strong prevailing sentiment in the profession of New York in favor of harmony and consolidation, there would seem to be no reason why the increase in membership in 1898 should not equal or exceed that of 1897. The assurance of a cordial welcome at the hands of the American Medical Association is undoubtedly all that is necessary to ensure this end.

FURTHER EFFORTS TO RESTRAIN THE "FAITH-CURE."

WE recently had occasion to refer with satisfaction to the legal treatment which had been awarded the parties responsible for a death which occurred at Camden, N. J., the immediate result of the neglect involved in the application of the "faith-cure." The father of the child and the "faith-cure professor" were promptly arrested and held in custody. We are now enabled to record the fact that this notorious faith-curist, W. F. Randall of Philadelphia, under whose "treatment" the child died of diphtheria, has been indicted by the Grand Jury, and will immediately be placed on trial for responsibility in causing its death. The father of the child, for his failure to provide proper medical treatment, is to be tried on the charges of neglect and cruelty.

This trial promises to be a most important one in that it will be the means of determining in Camden County, N. J., where faith-cure is said to be rampant, whether this practice will continue to be winked at by the authorities or brought up with a round turn. The Christian Scientists, immediately interested, announce that they are prepared to bitterly contest their rights, and have engaged expert legal counsel to fight the case in the courts. It is sincerely hoped that the New Jersey judges will follow the example of Judge Pennypacker of Philadelphia, who recently refused to recognize the cult of faith-curism as worthy of incorporation, on the ground that the practice of this ridiculously fatuous belief was contrary to public policy and to the laws of the State. By this trial is furnished an opportunity to administer full punishment to those responsible for this latest homicide, and to crush out with an iron hand the iniquitous trifling with human life which, under the guise of a religious belief, the faith-curists practice.

ECHOES AND NEWS.

Plague in Bombay.—During the week ending January 13th, there were 450 deaths from plague in Bombay.

Medical Men in England.—The English Medical Directory for 1898 shows that there are 6081 practitioners of medicine in London, and 15,400 in England in addition to those in London.

Death of Dr. Braymer.—Dr. O. W. Braymer of Camden, N. J., died on the 9th inst. of blood-poisoning, which he contracted while operating upon a septic case at the Cooper Hospital in that city.

Death in Raccoon Hide.—A taxidermist of Reading, Pa., recently died of malignant diphtheria, contracted, it is said, from a raccoon which he had mounted some days previously and which had apparently died of that disease.

Acetylene in England.—Acetylene can be neither manufactured nor sold in Great Britain now save by express permission of the Home Secretary, the prohibition being made in a recent order in Council.—*Scientific American.*

Professor Koch in Africa.—Professor Koch has been invited by the Indian Government to return to India and study the plague, but has declined, for the reason that Germany has engaged his services to study the rinderpest in German East Africa.

Typhus Fever at Glasgow.—The continued spread of typhus fever at Glasgow, Scotland, is attributed to the unsanitary condition of congested parts of that city and to lack of enterprise in destroying the strongholds of the disease.

New Hospital for Pittsburg.—A new hospital, to be called St. Margaret Hospital, will be dedicated by Bishop Whitehead during May next. The hospital is a bequest from John H. Shoenberger, a steel manufacturer of that city, as a memorial of his wife.

Death of Dr. William H. Robb.—The death is announced of Dr. William H. Robb at Selma, Ala. Dr. Robb was a resident of Amsterdam, N. Y. He was fifty-four years of age, and a prominent member of the New York State Medical Society and the American Medical Association.

Yellow-Fever Serum.—Surgeon-General Wyman, of the Marine Hospital Service, and Dr. A. H. Doty, Health Officer of the Port of New York, recently received some of Sanarelli's yellow-fever serum, which was forwarded to them by him from the experimental laboratory at Montevideo.

A Correction.—The strength of the carbolic-acid solution recommended in the article by Dr. Charles E. Lockwood of New York (MEDICAL NEWS, December 25, 1897), for irrigation of the pleural cavity in empyema, should have been given as 1 to 100 (a one-per-cent. solution) instead of 1 to 1000.

Legislation against Hypnotism.—A bill intended to limit the lawful use of hypnotism to licensed physicians will soon be introduced into the New York Legislature, on the ground that its use by irresponsible persons is dangerous and opposed to the public good. The bill should receive the support of all medical men.

Sloane Maternity Hospital Alumni.—The alumni of the Sloane Maternity Hospital have organized a society, and the following officers have been elected: President, Dr. E. A. Tucker; vice-president, Dr. Samuel M. Brickner; secretary, Dr. Ernest A. Gallant; treasurer, Dr. George L. Brodhead. The association will be scientific and social in character.

Post-mortuary Parturition.—In German literature, says the *Lancet*, is to be found a term for which there appears to be no English equivalent, namely, "sarggeburt," or coffin-birth. That is to say, a pregnant woman dies and the body is placed in a coffin and then, before or after burial, an expulsion of the fetus occurs. A few cases of this kind are on record.

Damages for a Broken Jaw.—A woman recently obtained a verdict of $10,000 in a suit for damages which she brought against a New York dentist for injuries to her jaw caused by his unskilful extraction of a tooth. A certificate asserting the fact that the defendant had been convicted by the Court of Special Sessions for practising dentistry without a license, was submitted as a part of the testimony.

Bananas as a Food in Typhoid.—According to Dr. Ussery of St. Louis, Mo., the banana is an excellent food in typhoid fever. This he explains by stating that the banana, although a solid food containing 95 per cent. of nutritive properties, is almost completely absorbed in the stomach, and does not possess sufficient waste to irritate the intensely inflamed and engorged lining membrane of the small intestine.

New Hospital for Berlin.—A new hospital of 1600 beds is to be constructed in Berlin by the municipal authorities. In addition to medical and surgical departments there will be special wards for diseases of women and for venereal diseases, and also a lying-in ward. The institution of special departments is a new feature in municipal hospitals in Berlin, for heretofore they have been divided into medical and surgical departments only.

The Functions of a Medical Society.—In his presidential address to the Glasgow Southern Medical Society, Dr. James Allan summarized the functions of a medical society as the cultivation of good will and the advancement of science. He closed with the sensible statement that "the public will respect and have faith in the profession in proportion as it sees the members of the profession respecting and reposing faith in each other."

Delegates to the New York State Medical Society Instructed.—The Medical Society of the County of New York has instructed its delegates to the State Society to attend the next meeting of that society: to present its dispensary bill to that society for indorsement; to cast their votes in favor of such indorsement, and to vote only for those candidates for offices of the society who individually pledge themselves to indorse the passage of this bill by the Legislature, and to vote against any and all candidates for office who may be opposed to said bill or to any similar bill or legislation.

The Practice of Medicine in Arizona.— The tabulated statement which recently appeared in the MEDICAL NEWS giving the requirements for the practice of medicine in the various States was based upon conditions which obtained in February, 1897. Since that date, *viz.*, on March 18, 1897, Arizona has passed a law stipulating that all applicants for a license to practise medicine in that Territory must not only possess a degree from a reputable medical school, but must also pass an examination before the Territorial Board of Medical Examiners.

Complementary to Dr. Biggs' Address on Sanitation.—The following may be taken as complementary yet antithetic to the opening paragraph of Dr. Hermann M. Biggs' admirable paper, published in the MEDICAL NEWS for January 8th: "Once upon a time when General Sherman was ailing and under the care of a medical friend of ours for quite a long time, he said, 'Doctor, I do not seem to be getting any better for all your medicines.' 'Well, General,' was the reply, 'perhaps you had better take Macbeth's advice and throw physic to the dogs.' 'I would like to do so, Doctor, but there are a number of valuable dogs in this neighborhood.'"

Kings County Effluvium Producers.—Governor Black, following in the footsteps of his two predecessors, Hill and Morton, has issued a precept condemning the offal and garbage works upon Barren Island. The report of the State Board of Health was made October 25, 1897, while the Governor's action bears date of January 7th. We notice that the garbage reduction-plant is in the same group of offensive businesses, or trades, as the notorious fish factory, and the five various condemned plants are alike called upon to apply to the State Board of Health for a permit to conduct their operations in a manner conformable to the regulations of that Board.

Charity and the Queen's Jubilee.—*The Charity Record and Hospital Times* (England) has published its usual annual review of the chief charitable bequests and donations made during the year, and comments upon the fact that the year 1897 has not proved so prosperous for London charities as was hoped and expected. It attributes this in a great measure to the multitudinous appeals made for all sorts of objects in celebration of the Diamond Jubilee. Another object which probably diverted considerable sums from hospitals and other established charities was the Mansion House Fund for the Relief of the Indian Famine, which led to the raising of nearly a million and a half.—*British Medical Journal.*

Health Board Appointments.—At a meeting of the Board of Health of New York City held January 11th, the following appointments were made: Dr. O. L. Lusk of Rockaway Beach, Assistant Sanitary Superintendent for the Borough of Queens; Dr. E. P. Roberts, colored, who has yet to pass the civil service examination, vaccinator for the Borough of Manhattan; Dr. H. D. Goetchius, medical inspector for the Borough of Manhattan. The Board dispensed with the services of Dr. R. M. Wyckoff, deputy commissioner of health of the Borough of Brooklyn. It was also decided to do away with the Brooklyn Department of Bacteriology. Dr. R. B. Randolph of this department was transferred to that of the Borough of Manhattan. E. H. Wilson and J. B. Thomas were removed.

Bill to Enlarge the Board of Health.—A bill has been introduced into the Legislature at Albany enlarging the Board of Health of New York City to four commissioners instead of three, and shortening the term of service from six years to four. A clause in this bill declares that the birth of every child must be reported in writing to the board within ten days of its occurrence by the physician, midwife, nurse, or next of kin assisting at the birth. A fine of $100 dollars is imposed for neglect to comply with this law. The latter clause seems most objectionable. The division of responsibility is a weak point in the bill, and the penalty of $100 is certainly unfair. No physician should be obliged to perform this duty without compensation. The law in England grants a fee of $1 for every such report.

Alcohol and the Russian Death-rate.—An official inquiry into the comparatively larger increase among the Tartar population of the city and government of Kazan has, according to the *British Medical Journal*, brought out some remarkable facts as to the effect of alcoholic indulgence on the death-rate. The Kazan Tartars, numbering about 640,000 souls, have a rate of mortality of only 21 in the 1000, while the mortality among the Russians is 40 per 1000. The general conditions among Orthodox Russians and Mohammedan Tartars are practically the same, except in so far as personal habits are concerned. The medical investigation leaves no room for doubt that the lesser mortality of the Mohammedan Tartars is directly due to their abstinence from spirituous liquors, in which the Russians indulge freely.

Sailors' Snug Harbor.—The investigation recently made into the affairs of the Sailors' Snug Harbor, Staten Island, N. Y., resulted in the resignation of the governor, Captain Trask. Dr. H. D. Joy, the surgeon of the institution, was temporarily placed in charge pending the appointment of a new governor. The Board of Trustees have finally elected Lieut.-Commander Daniel Delahanty, U. S. N., to be governor. The tenure of office is at the pleasure of the Board of Trustees, and the salary is $5000 a year. Lieut.-Commander Delahanty, who was chosen from more than seventy-five applicants, is at present detailed as executive officer of the United States Battle-ship Texas, but the Navy Department has granted to him a year's leave of absence. He was formerly Supervisor of the Harbor of New York, and is the inventor of the self-dumping garbage scow used by the city.

Pension Examining Surgeons.—The United States Civil Service Commission announces that on March 5, 1898, an examination will be held at Washington and at other places throughout the United States for the position of Pension Examining Surgeon. As the result of this examination vacancies will be filled at Bridgeport, Conn., Lynn, Mass., Washington, Ind., and Vicksburg, Miss. Applicants must be graduates of reputable medical colleges, and not barred by State or other laws. The subjects of the examination are as follows: thesis, anatomy and physiology, physical diagnosis, general and special pathology, and surgery. The subject of the thesis will be upon some common medical theme, and each competitor will be required to write not less than 250 nor more than 500 words. Persons who are legal residents of the places where the vacancies exist will be given preference in appointment. Persons desiring to enter this examination should at once write to the United States Civil Service Commission at Washington for application-blanks, forms 304 and 375, which should be properly executed and promptly filed with the Commission at Washington. No applications will be accepted after the hour of closing business on Friday, February 25th.

Voluntary Determination of Sex.—Attention has been called anew by Professor Schenk to the possibility of determining at will the sex of human progeny. George Maccloskie, Professor of Biology at Princeton University, in discussing this subject says: "Sex selection has already been accomplished in the plant world and in some forms of animal life. It has been found that hemp when grown in rich soil produces the female plant, while in scant soil it produces the male. Working bees will, when fed upon very rich food, become queens, and salamanders, when fed upon the fragments of their brothers and sisters will produce almost twice the percentage of females as when they are fed upon ordinary foods. On the other hand, the starving of caterpillars has been found to result in the production of a large percentage of males. Modern biology has established the fact that there is no fundamental difference between the sexes. The eggs of both sexes will live even if unsupplemented by those of the opposite sex, though this supplementation is necessary for healthy growth. The female egg requires rich food and moves slowly, while the male egg requires light food and moves with great rapidity. This is the only difference between them. If it is possible to apply to man, as it is to plants and the lower animals, this principle of selection, the food that the mother of a male would have to take would be only as much in amount as would satisfy her hunger without giving very much sustenance, while to produce females, very rich and sustaining food would be required. I consider that the power of sex selection is a necessary one, and that it will certainly be made a practical thing sooner or later."

OBITUARY.

DOCTOR JOSEPH O'DWYER.

BY W. P. NORTHRUP, M.D.,
OF NEW YORK;
ATTENDING PHYSICIAN TO THE NEW YORK FOUNDLING HOSPITAL.

DR. JOSEPH O'DWYER, the inventor of intubation, was born at Cleveland, Ohio, October 12, 1841, and died at New York, January 7, 1898.

His boyhood was spent in Canada, near London, in which city he attended school. His first studies in medicine were with his preceptor, Dr. Anderson of London, Canada, about 1863. He came to New York and entered the College of Physicians and Surgeons in 1864, and was graduated in 1866. Immediately after graduation he became an interne in the Charity Hospital of New York City, under the then new arrangement by which this institution had its own interne staff, entirely separate from Bellevue. Among his associates forming the new staff were Drs. Leroy M. Yale, F. A. Castle, and P. A. Callan. The visiting staff comprised among its numbers Drs. J. Lewis Smith, Loomis, Flint, Van Buren, and Sayre.

During his service at the Charity Hospital there appeared in New York an epidemic of cholera, the hospital for which was located on Blackwell's Island. Dr. O'Dwyer was placed in charge of this institution—it is generally supposed he volunteered for this service, and it is accurately known that upon him, in his isolated quarantine, the commissioners most confidently relied. During his service typhus fever also appeared as an epidemic. This disease Dr. O'Dwyer contracted. His case was a rather severe one, but after a long illness he recovered without permanent injury to his constitution. He was fond of saying he knew the very hour of his infection. It occurred during an early morning visit, when he was called before breakfast to see a man in a small cell in the penitentiary who had been taken sick during the night. The room was close, and he spent some time examining the patient. Promptly on the day the incubation period expired Dr. O'Dwyer became ill with the disease.

During 1868-9 he became examining physician for the

hospitals under the commissioners of Charities and Corrections. His duties were the distribution of applicants to the various hospitals, to Bellevue and to Charity. During this service classes in physical diagnosis were permitted, and he often, in later life, referred with pleasure to this work. In this year (1868) Dr. O'Dwyer opened his office, on Second avenue near Fifty-fifth street, with Dr. Schoonover. During 1872 he moved to Lexington avenue near Sixty-fifth street, and began the part of his life which brought him into connection with the New York Foundling Asylum (1873) and to the study of intubation.

It was in 1880 that Dr. O'Dwyer "began to think" on the subject of intubation. Tracheotomy was in such bad repute at the Foundling Hospital, with a record of one hundred per cent. of deaths, that the physicians as well as Sisters of Charity saw no excuse for further torturing the children. The first fruit of his "intubation thinking" was a wire spring, which quickly gave way to a spring bivalve speculum. Then came the changes to a "tube of plain oval form," tubes with collar and constriction to receive the vocal cords, and tubes with retaining swell, a tilting back of the upper portion of the tube, thickening and blunting of the lower end, etc., recently detailed by the inventor in an article, entitled "The Evolution of Intubation."[1]

After five or possibly six years of work, thinking and trying, Dr. O'Dwyer reluctantly consented to operate upon patients in private practice. His fourth case was in a prominent family in the practice of the writer. This occurred during the first week of January, 1886. It will be remembered that he began "thinking" on intubation in 1880. Dr. O'Dwyer has occupied in recent years many positions of honor and responsibility, *viz.*, Consulting Physician to Willard Parker Hospital, Lecturer on Intubation at the Post-Graduate Medical School and Hospital, and later at Bellevue Hospital Medical College; Attending Physician to St. Vincent's Hospital and to the New York Foundling Hospital (during twenty-five years), President of the American Pediatric Society, Member of the Council of the Society for Relief of Widows and Orphans of Medical Men, and a member of the Physician's Mutual Aid Association; Consulting Physician to Seton Hospital, besides many medical societiest and the New York Academy of Medicine.

Dr. O'Dwyer was a devout Roman Catholic, the fond father of four boys, a devoted husband, and during the last ten years of his life a constant mourner of his dead wife. He was lonely, retiring, easily hurt by harsh criticism, a poor sleeper, growing year by year more feeble, and struggling harder and harder to get sleep. He was a martyr to intubation. Thinking on its development by day grew into thinking at night. The anxieties of intubation cases, before the use of "antitoxin," no one can know who has not tried to dismiss such a case from mind and to sleep—till the night-bell rings, and it is at once understood that either the tube must be reinserted or removed from a choking child.

[1] O'Dwyer, *Archives of Pediatrics*, June, 1896.

Intubation is O'Dwyer's monument. It is equally true that it killed him.

To the close friends of this good and great man intubation seems but an incident of his life. His general good judgment, his well-thought-out opinions, his candor, and his unbending honesty, the simplicity and purity of his life, these rise up in mind to form the memory of him. If to a close companion for fifteen years an unbridled expression may be allowed because it is true and spontaneous, it is this: O'Dwyer's was the sweetest soul God ever gave a man.

CORRESPONDENCE.

TAPEWORM IN THE ABDOMINAL CAVITY.

To the Editor of the MEDICAL NEWS.

DEAR SIR: In your issue of December 4th I find a letter from Dr. W. F. Saybolt of Wooster University in which he mentions having found a tapeworm in the peritoneal cavity of a live rabbit, and supposing the possibility of such an occurrence being the cause of intestinal perforation in the human being.

In November, 1892, I published the details of a celiotomy for supposed extra-uterine pregnancy, during which I found a tapeworm in the abdominal cavity that had escaped by means of a large ragged opening in the small intestine. The intestine was resected, 2½ inches being cut away. The patient made a satisfactory recovery, and is alive and well to-day. It is interesting to note that all the symptoms were singularly like those of ruptured extra-uterine pregnancy, and this experience adds further confirmation of the repeatedly made observation that the abdominal cavity never ceases to contribute its full share of surgical surprises. The tapeworm was twenty-eight feet in length, and the manner in which it caused destruction of the intestinal wall is the only noteworthy observation to be made in the case. It must have become entangled or rolled into a ball, and in its efforts to free itself caused pressure and gangrene.

FAY M. DUNLAP, M.D.

BLOOMINGTON, ILL., December 15, 1897.

OUR PHILADELPHIA LETTER.

[From our Special Correspondent.]

SECTION ON GENERAL MEDICINE OF THE COLLEGE OF PHYSICIANS OF PHILADELPHIA—PHILADELPHIA COUNTY MEDICAL SOCIETY—PATHOLOGICAL SOCIETY OF PHILADELPHIA—DR. KEEN'S ILLNESS—RESIGNATIONS FROM THE MEDICO-CHIRURGICAL COLLEGE FACULTY AND BOARD OF TRUSTEES—ALUMNI OF THE JEFFERSON MEDICAL COLLEGE—A TRAINING-SCHOOL FOR NURSES AT ST. CHRISTOPHER'S HOSPITAL—THE INCREASE IN ENTERIC FEVER.

PHILADELPHIA, January, 15, 1898.

AT the last stated meeting of the Section on General Medicine of the College of Physicians of Philadelphia held January 10, 1898, Dr. William G. Spiller showed *two cases of hysteric hemiplegia*, and *one of hysteric tremor*. The first case of hysteric hemiplegia occurred in a middle-aged man, the onset of whose disease w first manifested by weakness and numbness of the left leg occurring intermittently in attacks of short duration. Later well-developed zones of hyperesthesia and many other hysteric signs supervened, together with paralysis of the left leg and numbness of the left side. Under appropriate electrotherapeusis the patient greatly improved. The second case of this kind was a woman, thirty-six years of age, who some months after a fall, which occurred six years ago, began to complain of irregular pains, weakness of the left leg, which four years afterward spread to the left arm, tenderness in the left inguinal region, and unilateral hyperesthesia; there was a hysteric gait, the knee-jerks were normal, and there were neither contractures nor facial involvement. This patient also improved under treatment by electricity. The third case was that of a woman who, after having received a fright, began to have uncontrollable twitchings of the left arm and leg, the twitchings later becoming generalized and choreiform in character; on the left side of the entire body there were anesthesia, general weakness, tenderness in the inguinal and mammary regions, increase of the knee-jerk with diminution of many other reflexes, and contraction of the visual fields with preservation of the corneal reflexes.

Dr. Frederick A. Packard reported *a case of stricture of the esophagus* following typhoid fever. The patient was a man who, late in the course of the fever, found great difficulty in swallowing capsules containing sulphocarbolate of zinc. For two months the dysphagia was provoked by attempts to swallow any food other than liquids, and the patient became enfeebled and much reduced in weight. Following frequent passage of bougies, the stricture, which at first measured 2 mm. ($\frac{1}{12}$-inch) in diameter, was sufficiently dilated to relieve the difficulty in deglutition, and the patient rapidly gained in strength and weight. Dr. D. J. M. Miller reported an instance of *a large syphiloma of the liver*, which completely disappeared under the use of "mixed treatment." It was of interest to note that the tumor increased or decreased in size according to the discontinuance or continuance of the administration of the potassium iodid and mercury.

At the last stated meeting of the Philadelphia County Medical Society, held January 12, 1898, Dr. A. Ferree Witmer read an interesting paper on *the clinical aspect of the occupation neuroses*, in which he considered such conditions as writer's cramp, reader's cramp, and the condition somewhat similar to that which occurs in telegraphers as the result of long-continued overuse of the muscles of the forearm and hand. The speakers thought that writer's cramp was due to a cortical lesion rather than to local trouble, and mentioned as predisposing causes urate poisoning, lack of development of the nervous system, and hereditary influences. As a prophylactic the vertical system of handwriting was recommended, and for curative effects absolute rest of the hand and arm, massage, appropriate finger-exercises, and intramuscular injections of strychnin were advocated. Reader's cramp was described as a peculiar twitching of the eyelids, most often more marked on the right side, due to nerve-tire. Drs. Edward Martin and F. W. Patterson read a paper on the *sterilization of surgical instruments with paraform*, and demonstrated the method in detail with a number of different apparatus. Catheters were sterilized by placing them on trays in a closed tin or wooden box upon the bottom of which the powdered paraform was spread. After having been exposed to the paraform vapor for twenty-four hours it was found that the bougies were absolutely sterile, even if they had been purposely contaminated with septic material before the test. This paper was based upon one hundred experiments with the sterilization of instruments by various approved methods, of which paraform only had proved absolutely reliable. Dr. W. S. Forbes read a communication on the *technic and results of an original operation for the liberation of the ring-finger in musicians* by dividing the extensor communis digitorum muscle.

At the last meeting of the Pathological Society of Philadelphia, held January 13, 1898, a valuable paper on *chorio-epithelioma, or the so-called deciduoma malignum* was read by Dr. H. L. Williams. The condition, he said, is observed in women under thirty years of age, during pregnancy, or after abortion, and is characterized clinically by a sudden, gushing hemorrhage from the uterus, a widely dilated os, and an enlargement of the uterus, with a soft, friable condition of its walls. Metastases frequently occur; in the greater percentage of cases, involving the vagina; next frequently, the lungs. Of twenty operations in cases of chorio-epithelioma, collected by the speaker, three died as the immediate result of the operation, three died within six months after the operation, and the remaining fourteen were free from symptoms at the present time. Dr. Williams then went on to describe the gross pathology and the histology of the condition, and took occasion to point out that an absolute diagnosis may always be made by microscopically examining the fragments removed from the uterus during curettage. Dr. Alfred Stengel described a *rare case of cirrhosis of the liver with jaundice and staphylococcic infection of the blood*, occurring in an alcoholic dying from an acute toxemia; and also showed a specimen of gall-stone with enormous distention of the biliary ducts.

The condition of Dr. W. W. Keen, who for a week past has been seriously ill with septicema due to accidental infection while holding an autopsy on a patient who died of peritonitis, is so much improved that his attending physicians have pronounced him out of danger.

During the last two weeks two members of the faculty and a member of the board of trustees of the Medico-Chirurgical College have resigned, the latest resignation being that of Dr. W. Frank Haehlen, professor of obstetrics. It is rumored that these changes in the faculty and trustees of this institution are to be followed by others in the not distant future. The names of the successors to the chairs of Drs. Sajous and Haehlen have not as yet been made public.

The last scientific meeting of the Philadelphia Chapter of the Alumni Association of the Jefferson Medical College was held January 11, 1898, the speaker of the evening being Dr. J. Chalmers Da Costa, who read a paper on *tuberculosis of the kidney*. At the close of the meeting the members of the Association were tendered a luncheon by Dr. Addinell Hewson. At the annual business meeting of the general Alumni Association of this institution, January 15, 1898, the following officers were elected: President, Dr. William H. Warder; vice-presidents, Drs. John Strobel, I. P. Strittmatter, George McClellan, and George Morehouse; corresponding secretary, Dr. Thomas G. Ashton; recording secretary, Dr. Wilmer Krusen; treasurer, Dr. E. L. Vansant. After the meeting the members were entertained by Dr. W. J. Hearn.

The managers of St. Christopher's Hospital for Children have decided to establish a training-school for nurses in connection with this institution. Miss Edith Mayou has resigned her position as head-nurse of the Royal Victoria Hospital of Montreal to assume direction of the new school.

The largest number of new cases of enteric fever yet reported for any week since the present prevalence of the disease in this city are reported this week, the total number for the week ending January 15th, being 201, or 36 more than last week, with 17 deaths. There were 96 new cases of diphtheria, with 24 deaths; and 62 new cases of scarlet fever, with 6 deaths. The total number of deaths from all causes for the week was 489, an increase of 15 over the number reported last week, and a decrease of 21 from the record of the corresponding week of 1896.

OUR BERLIN LETTER.

[From our Special Correspondent.]

ORGANIC CARDIAC AND VASCULAR LESIONS FROM THE USE OF TOBACCO—A CASE OF NITROBENZOL POISONING—SOME NEW NAMES FOR OLD AILMENTS —THE NEW EDITOR OF THE "ARCHIVES FOR ANATOMY AND PHYSIOLOGY."

BERLIN, January 14, 1898.

MUCH more importance is attached here, one cannot help but think, to the organic cardiac and vascular lesions due to the use of tobacco than is usual in America. A "tobacco heart," with us, is regarded somewhat in the light of a functional cardiac neurosis whose improvement immediately follows abjuration of the habit. Professors Mendel and Leyden each happen to have introduced the subject at clinics during the past week. Professor Leyden says that tobacco indulged in to excess undoubtedly causes myocarditis with true fatty degeneration of cardiac muscular fibers. He admits that the harmfulness of the tobacco habit used to be much overestimated in Berlin, but thinks that generally the tendency of the profession is not to realize how permanent may be the cardiac injury its use may entail.

In Traube's time here it was considered an act of pupilary piety to refer a great many heart symptoms in smokers to the use of the weed. Traube himself had an organic heart lesion which was often the occasion of a good deal of annoyance to him. He insisted on attributing his cardiac symptoms to the use of tobacco, though he never quite gave up his pipe. His persistence in the self-illusion is all the more surprising as his heart trouble was complicated by a kidney affection which etiologically was intimately connected with it. Professor Frentzel afterward had something of the same opinion of his own case, and both are striking examples of how subjectivity of symptoms is apt to ruin accuracy of diagnosis even in great diagnosticians.

Professor Mendel has noted in a large number of cases of heavy smokers that the arteries become thickened, hardened, and tortuous long before the atrophic changes of old age begin to be manifested. He has especially noted this arteriosclerotic condition in persons between thirty and forty-five years of age, as he believes, from over-indulgence in tobacco. Professor Mendel himself is a smoker, so that there would seem to be no question of any unreasonable fanatic opposition to "the pipe that soothes" in his rather startling bit of clinical experience. Professor Leyden does not smoke, which may somewhat decrease the value of his opinion in the matter. He assured his students the other day, however, that he perfectly remembered the acute toxic effects of tobacco on one who was unused to it, though he considered that this was a chapter in the toxic effects which did not require elaboration before medical students.

Cases of nitrobenzol poisoning are growing more and more frequent as the economy of the use of this artificial coal-tar product, instead of the more expensive genuine oil of bitter almonds, in the manufacture of soaps, perfumes, etc., becomes clearer. A carefully observed case of poisoning by it has just been reported from Professor Furbringer's clinic at the Friedrichshain Hospital (*Deutsche medicinische Wochenschrift*). Curiously enough the case corresponds exactly in the manner of ingestion of the poison with another odd case described sometime ago. Both patients were draymen, who, while hauling the large flasks in which the nitrobenzol is shipped, took an unknown quantity of the liquid in order to find out what it was like.

In the last case death occurred within five days. A febrile temperature of between 39° and 46° C. (102.5° to 104° F.) persisted until the fatal termination. Though the blood was almost tar-like in consistency and black in color, no changes could be found in its cellular elements. There were no differences in size, shape, or color of the red corpuscles, no poikilocytes, or micro- or macrocytes. There was no leucocytic reaction to be observed and no noticeable change in the white cells, except, perhaps, a lessened tendency to ameboid movements.

Spectroscopic examination showed absolutely normal blood. There were at no time during the five days, though they were carefully looked for, the two dark absorption bands of meth-hemoglobin, which have been found in some other cases. On the other hand, the spectral bands of oxyhemoglobin were present. There was a reducing substance in the urine which gave a reaction with all the ordinary sugar tests, bismuth as well as copper. There was no blood in the urine, however, and no albumin. The autopsy produced absolutely negative results, except for the presence of the black, tar-like blood. There is evidently here some important discoveries awaiting some one whose opportunities and investigating spirit will enable him to solve the mystery of the fatality of the poison.

With the problem would seem to be involved certain

questions as to the physiologic functions of blood plasma which are important in their bearings on clinical medicine in a field that is as yet practically unworked. In the case in question intense trophic disturbances were evidently at work, though apparently none of the cellular elements of the blood were involved. Though in principle alcohol would seem to be contraindicated, the poison being an analogue of the alcohols, and therapeutists advise against its use, in this, as in other cases of like nature, alcohol seemed to be the drug which accomplished most in regulating the circulatory mechanism and in relieving the symptoms of intense depression which developed.

Sometimes one is surprised to find how much more important an old friend may seem in a new dress, and the same thing would seem to be true for some familiar ailments and the new terms applied to them. Careful analysis by the specialists of the disturbances of speech has separated various forms of what used to be plain stammering, and furnished new terms derived from the Greek. Inability to properly pronounce the letter "g" is called paragammatismus, the letter "r," pararhotismus, "l," paralambdismus. The difficulty of enunciating "s," which has been known to ordinary mortals for many a day, now becomes the scientific parasigmatismus. It will surely soothe the mother's anxious heart much better to know that her young hopeful is suffering from one of these "ismuses" than that he merely stammers or lisps.

Some defects which used to be considered somewhat more the result of intellectual hebetude or of pigritia indurata (the medical term for chronic laziness) are being arranged in the same category. The unconquerable defect which some people have of not arranging their words according to the usually accepted rules of syntax becomes in this way an intellectual ailment—agrammatismus. The corresponding defect of not always arranging the letters of words according to the usual rules of spelling, becomes an orpara-orthographismus. As this latter is in many cases undoubtedly a psychic ailment which no amount of hard work seems able to entirely eradicate, perhaps the new classification of these things as real mental defects is, after all, a rational one.

Upon the death of Professor Du Bois Reymond the Physiological Society of Berlin assumed the editorship of the Physiologic Department of the *Archives of Anatomy and Physiology* which he had held. Professor His is the editor of the Anatomic Department. With the beginning of 1898 Professor Engelman, who succeeded Du Bois Reymond in the chair of physiology at Berlin, assumes the editorship of the department which his predecessor had so ably managed for so long a time.

Recovery from Chloroform Poisoning by the Use of Large Doses of Strychnin.—REID (*Brit. Med. Jour.*, November 20, 1897) details a case of chloroform poisoning in which ½-grain of strychnin was injected subcutaneously in the course of three hours. By this means, as well as by artificial respiration and the use of an electric current of fifty volts (one pole of the battery being placed over the respiratory center and the other over the ensiform cartilage), the patient was kept breathing until the effect of the chloroform had passed away.

TRANSACTIONS OF FOREIGN SOCIETIES

London.

ATROPHY OF THE KIDNEY CAUSED BY OBSTRUCTION OF THE URETER—NEGATIVE ACTION OF SEWER-AIR IN RAISING THE TOXICITY OF DIPHTHERIA BACILLI—CAUSES OF THE VARIATIONS IN THE SIZES AND SHAPE OF THE COLI BACILLUS—OBSTRUCTION OF LABOR BY OVARIAN TUMORS IN THE PELVIS—SOME CASES OF PANCREATIC CYST—DEATH FROM INTESTINAL TOXEMIA—FIFTEEN CONSECUTIVE CASES OF INTUSSUSCEPTION.

AT a meeting of the Pathological Society, December 7th, BRADFORD spoke of *atrophy of the kidney caused by obstruction of the ureter*. With such a result in mind experiments were performed upon dogs. One ureter was ligatured in two places and divided. From ten to forty days later it was brought to the surface and sutured in the skin. When it was opened about two ounces of fluid was evacuated. The fluid was clear in nine cases and purulent in three. The animals were killed at periods varying from seven to fifty days after the second operation. In each case the kidney, the ureter of which had been tied, was found to have resumed its normal shape, but had shrunken to one-fourth its usual size. Microscopically, it could be seen that some tubules had disappeared, but the main cause of the atrophy was the crowding together of the tubules and the small size of their cells. The length of time during which drainage was allowed to go on before the animal was killed did not appear to have much influence on the degree of atrophy.

SHATTOCK read a paper on the *negative action of sewer-air in raising the toxicity of non-virulent diphtheria bacilli*. It has frequently been surmised that the inhalation of sewer-air determines the occurrence of diphtheria, although diphtheria bacilli cannot be conveyed in this medium since they are not disengaged by evaporation from the fluids in which they are grown. It is possible that a non-virulent diphtheria bacillus such as is present in the throats of many individuals may, in consequence of the inhalation of sewer-air, become virulent and give rise to diphtheria in the throat. In order to determine this point the author had grown non-virulent diphtheria bacilli in Duclaux flasks in broth, and over the surface of the medium sewer-air was continuously and slowly drawn by means of a water-pump. The only noticeable effect was a retardation of the growth of the bacilli. Their virulence was not increased, as was proven by subcutaneous injections in guinea-pigs. Shattock regards these results as interesting, although, as he stated, they do not exhaust the question

HASLAM discussed the *causes of the variations in the size and shape of the coli bacillus*. These variations, according to his experiments, are due to the different media upon which the bacillus is grown. For example, if in a glucose solution the nitrogenous matter is increased, he finds a corresponding increase of the longer forms of the bacillus. Growths on glucose with less proteid matter produce shorter forms, etc.

At a meeting of the Obstetrical Society, December 1st, MCKERRON read a paper on the *obstruction of labor by ovarian tumors in the pelvis.* One hundred and eighty-three cases had been collected in which ovarian tumors occupied the pelvis during labor. As shown by recent publications there is a wide difference of opinion as to the most satisfactory treatment of this complication. The reader drew the following practical conclusions: Reposition should in all cases be first attempted. When it fails a selection should be made, according to circumstances, from the following operative measures: Puncture, Cæsarian section, abdominal or vaginal oophorectomy.

At a meeting of the Medical Society, December 13th, DORAN described a *pancreatic cyst* occurring in a woman aged twenty-four years, which was *successfully treated by anterior incision and drainage.* The tumor was situated in the lesser peritoneal cavity, the lesser omentum and stomach formed the front of its capsule, and the transverse mesocolon was entirely below it. The fistula discharged for five months and then closed spontaneously. Stress was laid upon the surgical importance of defining peritoneal relations and the exact attachments of the cysts during operation. Such a cyst may lie in the lesser peritoneal cavity, in the fold of the transverse mesocolon, or in the general peritoneal cavity. When it occupies the lesser peritoneal cavity it has probably burst through the peritoneum in front of the pancreas. This would account for the complete freedom of the ascending layer of the transverse mesocolon, which is found entirely below the cyst in many of these cases. When a pedicle is formed, even if it includes the tail of the pancreas itself, total removal of the cyst is justifiable. Removal of a sessile cyst, on the other hand, involves risk of damage to the splenic and other large vessels and to small arteries and veins in the friable pancreatic tissue. The statistics of drainage in the treatment of sessile cysts seem very satisfactory.

ROLLESTON and TURNER contributed the notes of a *case of peripancreatic cyst.* The patient was a man aged thirty years, who complained of epigastric pain of six-months duration. During five months the feces had been clay-colored. Jaundice had existed three months. Examination showed a tense tumor containing thirty ounces of dark-brown fluid; no bile or pancreatic ferments were found therein. Although the cyst evidently arose in the neighborhood of the pancreas it was not immediately connected with it. Still it may have had its origin in a pancreatic hemorrhage. The cyst was tapped, drained, and the patient made a good recovery.

MALCOLM excised a *multilocular cyst of the tail of the pancreas* which simulated hydronephrosis. There was much difficulty in arresting the hemorrhage, but this being finally accomplished, the abdomen was closed without drainage.

At a meeting of the Clinical Society, December 10th, GOULD read a paper on a *case of acute intestinal obstruction relieved by operation, in which death from intestinal toxemia occurred on the ninth day.* The patient was a man aged forty-three years. The operation was performed on the fourth day, and a coil of small intestines twisted upon itself was found adherent in the pelvis. The intestine was liberated and gas and fluid intestinal matter at once passed into the cecum. On the following day the patient passed gas and a small amount of fecal matter by the rectum, and two days later he had a large evacuation of the bowels. In spite of this favorable symptoms, intestinal matter was regurgitated into the stomach, from which organ it was several times removed by means of a tube. Afterward the patient took fluid food well, and there were no signs of peritonitis; but gradually he passed into a condition of stupor, deepening into coma, accompanied by a slightly quickened pulse, quickened, deep, and noisy respiration, a subnormal temperature which was lower in the rectum than in the axilla, profuse diarrhea, the motions being of a peculiar odor, and of a grey-green color. The skin was covered was a dark erythematous rash. These symptoms reached their maximum on the sixth day after the operation. Four pints of a saline fluid were injected into a vein and immediately all the symptoms passed away. He relapsed next day, and saline fluid was again injected with marked benefit. Two days later he again become unconscious and died comatose in spite of a third injection of salt and water. The urine throughout the illness contained a great excess of indican, and another chromogen whose nature was not determined.

COLMAN mentioned a case in which *intestinal toxemia caused mental excitement, and not coma,* as in the preceding case. The patient was a woman forty years of age, who had a large fecal impaction in the ascending colon. Under treatment the mass became softer and she began to pass fecal matter in considerable quantity But on the third day she become delirious. She had no knowledge of her surroundings, and had hallucinations of hearing and vision which took the form of animals running about her bed, which, however, did not terrify but only amused her. There was no history of abuse of alcohol or of the administration of belladonna. Her temperature was low and her pulse even. By means of frequent enemata the bowel was completely emptied and the delirium entirely passed away.

BARKER read a paper on *fifteen consecutive cases of intussusception,* in eight of which injections were tried and failed, and subsequent events showed that in twelve of the fifteen reduction could not possibly have been effected by injection, even had it been employed when the patients were first seen. Unless, therefore, a case is seen a few hours after the onset of the symptoms, it is safer to at once proceed to open the abdomen. The danger of ventral hernia may be reduced by making a very small incision. An incision long enough to admit one finger is often sufficient.

Berlin.

A REMARKABLY PROLONGED CASE OF STAPHYLOCOCCIC INFECTION—RELATION BETWEEN OVER-FATNESS AND DIABETES—AN APPARATUS WHICH CURES MIGRAINE IN THREE MINUTES.

At a meeting of the Medical Society, December 1st, WOHLGEMUTH narrated a *remarkably prolonged case of staphylococcic infection.* The patient, a man aged fifty-six years, was operated upon for hemorrhoids. Catheterization was necessary, and cystitis and epididymitis followed. As he slowly recovered from these troubles suppurative inflammation developed in the left sternoclavicular articulation, requiring incision. Six months later an abscess developed in the right gluteal muscle, with spondylitis of the fourth and fifth dorsal vertebræ, for which a plaster jacket was applied. Fourteen months after the original infection there was purulent and bloody expectoration, in which no tubercle bacilli could be demonstrated. For the next three years there were occasional attacks of pain in various portions of the body, and stiffness of the muscles so that at times walking was almost impossible. Five years after the infection, without apparent cause, an abscess developed in the right thigh, from which there was evacuated a greenish pus containing the staphlococcus albus in pure culture. In similar cases which run a more acute course, staphylococcus aureus has been found.

HIRSCHFELD called attention to the *relation between overfatness and diabetes.* It often happens that very fat people will show glucose in their urine after a meal containing a fairly large quantity of sugar. Hirschfeld found that the glucose disappeared from the urine of those fleshly diabetic patients who were being treated for obesity, though not placed upon a strict diabetic diet. Instead of receiving 10 ounces of hydrocarbons per day, they were receiving only 3⅓ ounces, and an abundance of active exercise was prescribed. The speaker expressed the opinion that the glycosuria which so often follows traumatic neuroses is due to an excessive diet combined with a lack of active exercise. There would seem to be some relation between obesity and diabetes.

HANSEMANN said that in *seventy per cent. of diabetic patients he had found some alterations in the pancreas.* Of especial interest in this connection is a lipomatosis of the pancreas which, like that of the capsule of the kidney or of the heart, may exist either in connection with the general excess of fat, or, on the other hand, may be found in lean individuals. In such a condition little is to hoped for from treatment, for it is scarcely to be supposed that if the fat tissue has taken the place of the pancreatic tissue to any great extent, that a regeneration of this organ can occur.

At the session of December 8th, EWER showed an *apparatus which by slight, very rapid, and equal vibrations of the body is able to cure within two or three minutes all nervous pain, especially migraine.* The apparatus is operated by electricity, and consists of a small motor whose core revolves with great rapidity. This core at one end is bent a little from its center, so that with each revolution it strikes a rubber knob, giving to it a little thrust. If this knob is held against the surface of the body the rapid revolution of the motor transmits to it a quick trembling, with the relief of pain above mentioned. The form of the instrument may be altered according to the portion of the body upon which it is to be used.

***To Remove Callosities.*—**

℞ Liq. potass. } aa . . . . ʒ i
Tinct. iodini }
Glycerini . . . . . . ℥ ss
Aquæ . . . . . . ℥ i.

M. Sig. Paint the affected parts night and morning.

SOCIETY PROCEEDINGS.

THE NEW YORK ACADEMY OF MEDICINE.—SECTION ON GYNECOLOGY AND OBSTETRICS.

Stated Meeting, Held November 24, 1897.

DR. SIMON MARX, M. D., in the Chair.

ECTOPIC GESTATION, COMPLICATED BY TYPHOID FEVER.

DR. JOSEPH BRETTAUER showed specimens removed on the same day from two cases of ectopic gestation. The patient in the first case was twenty-nine years of age, the mother of two children. Operation was performed August 17, 1897, partial rupture having occurred. A large amount of fluid blood was removed from the abdominal cavity. The patient did well until the fourth day when the temperature ran up to 105° F., and the pulse to 160. The woman, however, did not present the appearance of a patient suffering from acute septic infection. On the following day the temperature fell to 100° F., and the pulse to 112, the general condition was improved, and the symptoms of the preceding day were ascribed to absorption of the serum which was left in the abdominal cavity. The patient continued to improve until September 2d, when the temperature suddenly rose to 105° F., and violent headache was complained of. The following morning there was a chill which lasted twenty minutes and was followed by a temperature of 106° F. Physical examination failed to reveal anything which would account for the high temperature. There was no exudate, no resistance whatever in the pelvis, the uterus was freely movable, the abdomen perfectly flat, and the wound had healed by first intention. As the spleen was found to be somewhat enlarged, malaria was suspected and a specimen of blood was examined for the plasmodium, with a negative result. A consultant was called in who found the spleen much enlarged and a number of typical rose-colored spots upon the chest and abdomen; there was also a dicrotic pulse. Widal's test was employed, but with a negative result. On September 5th the patient was removed to the city. The temperature at that time was 103° F. in the evening and 101.5° F. in the morning, and this rise and fall continued until the 12th, when it became normal and remained so. In view of the constant negative results of Widal's test the diagnosis of typhoid fever was not clearly established, but the speaker was, nevertheless, inclined to regard the condition as one of typhoid fever, possibly of an abortive type. The fact that the patient was taken sick at a summer-resort, where typhoid fever occurred at the time quite epidemically, was in a small measure responsible for this conclusion.

The second specimen showed a ruptured tubal pregnancy removed from a patient on the same day as that upon which the first was operated upon, and, although gestation had apparently continued over three months in this case, the fetus was only about three-fourths of an inch long, its growth having evidently been arrested by hemorrhage into the wall of the unruptured tube as was clearly shown in the specimen.

VAGINAL ENTEROCELE.

DR. PHILANDER A. HARRIS of Paterson, N. J., presented a case of vaginal enterocele. The patient was a married woman, twenty-four years of age, the mother of three children, and she has complained since the birth of her last child of a constant bearing-down sensation in the vagina, accompanied by a "dragging," which she refers to the umbilical region. These symptoms are especially distressing when she is on her feet, and in doing her work she is obliged to occasionally stop and lie down for a time. About a year ago an operation for repair of the perineum and of the cervex uteri was performed in Chicago. This, however, did not relieve the symptoms, and her condition has since become much worse. Physical examination shows a bulging of the posterior cul-de-sac which appears at the vulva. There is no rectocele or cystocele.

At the request of DR. HARRIS, the Chairman appointed DRS. GARRIGUES, BOLDT, and BRETTAUER a committee to examine the patient.

DR. HENRY J. GARRIGUES reported as follows: We found a protrusion of the posterior vaginal wall which extends down to the vulva and which at first sight resembles an exaggerated rectocele. Upon further examination we found that this protrusion leads into a transverse opening, large enough to admit three fingers, in the pelvic floor behind the cervex. There is no doubt as to the diagnosis of vaginal enterocele.

FIBROSARCOMA OF THE UTERUS.

DR. GEORGE H. BALLERAY of Paterson, N. J., exhibited a specimen of fibrosarcoma of the uterus which he had removed by vaginal hysterectomy from a patient sixty-two years of age. Menstruation had ceased fifteen years ago, and there were no symptoms referable to the uterus until last March, when a discharge of blood from the vagina was noticed which continued up to the time of the operation. The patient was in fairly good condition, but showed the effect of loss of blood. Vaginal examination revealed a small mass to the right of the uterus, the latter being small and still movable. The patient was a nullipara with an extremely narrow vagina, and much difficulty was experienced in performing the operation, it being necessary to divide the perineum and make an incision anteriorly before it was possible to bring down the uterus. A cyst containing bloody serum was found in the posterior part of the mass, and it was ruptured during removal. Clamps were exclusively employed, although the speaker said it was his usual custom to clamp only the lower segment of the broad ligament, retrovert the uterus, and tie the remaining portion of the ligament. The patient is at present in good condition and promises to make a speedy recovery.

DR. HIRAM N. VINEBERG: I would like to ask if a microscopic examination has been made in this case.

DR. BALLERAY: No examination with the microscope has been made as yet. The diagnosis was made entirely from the clinical history which pointed strongly to malignant disease. My experience with the microscope has not been reassuring, and my confidence in this method of making a diagnosis has been rudely shaken—so much so that I would rather trust to the clinical history than to a microscopist's report in a case of this kind. However, the specimen will be submitted to a pathologist.

DR. VINEBERG: I agree with Dr. Balleray that he did perfectly right in this case without a microscopic examination having been made. The diagnosis, however, can be verified by a pathologic examination. If this cannot be relied upon, we will have to go back on our pathology altogether.

KRAUT'S DRY-BED.

DR. FISCHER presented an apparatus, which consists of a wicker bassinet so arranged that a rubber bag within it receives the urine and feces of the child. The same principle has also been applied to invalid beds for cases in which there is incontinence of urine and feces. These beds are in use in many hospitals in Europe.

REPORT OF A CASE OF NEPHRECTOMY FOR STRICTURE OF THE RIGHT URETER AND EARLY TUBERCULOSIS OF THE KIDNEY.

DR. HIRAM H. VINEBERG reported such a case and exhibited the specimen. The patient was a woman, forty-eight years of age, married twelve years, the mother of five children, and she had passed the menopause four years previously. The symptoms began six months ago, and consisted of pain in the back and loins accompanied by nausea and vomiting. Three months later she came under the observation of Dr. Manges who administered methylene blue with apparently good effect at first. At this time a small quantity of pus was found in the urine. The patient also complained of pain in the hypogastric region extending to the right lumbar region. Micturition which had been frequent from the beginning, now becam still more so, and was very annoying. When seen by th speaker the right kidney could not be distinctly palpate and certainly was not enlarged, but a cord-like structur as large as a lead-pencil was made out in the anterio vaginal fornix, running upward and to the right. Thi apparently was the thickened right ureter. Cystoscopi examination with the patient in the knee-chest positio showed the left ureteral orifice seemingly normal excep that there was a small bleeding-point near it. The righ orifice was swollen and irregular in outline and presente the appearance of a nipple. A number of small, re spots were scattered over the lining membrane of th bladder. Upon introducing a catheter into the left urete clear urine was withdrawn, but even a small-sized ureter sound could not be made to enter the right ureter on ac count of a stricture about one inch from the outlet. diagnosis of stricture of the right ureter and localized cys titis was made, and the latter was treated by applications nitrate of silver with the result that the frequent mictur tion and hypogastric pain were relieved. At this tim repeated examination of the urine did not reveal tuberc bacilli, and the patient's condition improved so much th complete recovery was looked for. In August, howeve she was seized with a severe attack of pain in the rig iliac region which terminated with a discharge of blood urine. Urinalysis disclosed nothing to indicate the pre ence of stone, and another cystoscopic examination showe the right ureteral orifice in the same condition as before and the bladder surface perfectly normal. A tuberculous condition of the kidney was suspected and the patient advised to go to Baltimore to consult Dr. Howard A. Kelly. The latter made a diagnosis of stricture of the right ureter and advised operation and removal of the kidney if the symptoms could not be relieved in any other way. Operation was performed in October at St. Mark's Hospital, the right kidney being removed after it was ascertained that it did not contain a stone. The patient made a good recovery.

The specimen showed a kidney neither long nor narrow; length, 11 cm.; circumference at lower pole. 13 cm.; at upper pole, 10.5 cm. Upon making a longitudinal section two abscesses were disclosed, one, about the size of a small bean, situated immediately beneath the capsule in the cortical layer at the junction of the middle with the upper third; the other, about the size of a split pea, situated just internal to the first, but still in the cortex of the kidney; the wall of the smaller abscess was corrugated like that of a corpus luteum. The pus in these abscesses contained tubercle bacilli in abundance. A short distance above the site of the abscesses, in the cortex directly beneath the capsule, was a group of millary tubercles. The pelvis of the kidney, as well as the upper part of the ureter, was normal in appearance.

DR. H. J. BOLDT: This case has interested me very much. It is fortunate that the woman developed stricture of the ureter which gave rise to the symptoms which lead to the condition of the kidney being discovered. I recently observed a case of tuberculosis of the kidney, but there was no stricture of the ureter. The diagnosis was made by the enormous dilatation of the ureter which was ascertainable by palpation. The bladder was also affected, and was evidently the primary seat of the disease, as was probably the case in Dr. Vineberg's patient. In my case there was not enough thickening of the bladder end of the ureter to make it apparent on palpation. The prognosis is good when the patient is seen early and a radical operation performed.

DR. THOMAS H. MANLEY: I have taken considerable interest in this subject of tuberculosis of the kidney, and, in view of the fact that in the case under discussion pus-corpuscles were found in the urine, it seems to me that this should have led to a diagnosis of tuberculous kidney and a more conservative operation. If the disease was localized, the abscess could have been curetted and treated like any other abscess, and recovery would have followed.

DR. VINEBERG: In answer to Dr. Boldt I would say that at the first examination some thickening of the ureter was detected, and I was fairly confident that there was some trouble there. In regard to the frequent micturition, this was one of the first symptoms, but at the same time there was a cystitis present. This symptom disappeared when the latter condition was treated.

As to the criticism made by Dr. Manley, I can only say that the stricture of the ureter alone would have necessitated the removal of the kidney. Apart from that the kidney was extensively adherent to the perirenal fat, there were two abscess cavities, and a general tuberculous condition of the whole organ, and I do not think that justice would have been done to the patient if the kidney had not been removed.

DR. MANLEY then read the paper of the evening, entitled

SOME SPECIAL FEATURES IN HERNIA AND HERNIATED CONDITIONS IN THE FEMALE.

The author dealt with the subject in the most exhaustive manner, giving in detail the statistics of numerous authorities as to the relative frequency of the different forms of hernia in the male and female subject at the various periods of life, and he emphasized the necessity of carefully recording the sex and age of the patient and the symptoms when reporting cases in order to make such records of future value. According to his deductions, congenital hernia is more frequently found in male than in female infants, but the female is much more prone to develop hernia, especially the umbilical variety, in later life on account of increasing relaxation of the abdominal muscles incident to child-bearing. Hernia in the male is generally congenital. Strangulation is more apt to occur in femoral hernia, and the operative mortality is greater in this than in any other variety. In speaking of hernia following operation, the author quoted Bland Sutton's statement that abdominal section often leaves a condition far more serious than the one for which it was performed.

DR. GARRIGUES: As to the relation between sex and hernia, inguinal hernia is much more common in the male, and the reason for this is undoubtedly the fact that in man the inguinal canal is so much larger than it is in woman on account of the passage of the spermatic cord through this canal. On the other hand, femoral hernia is much more common in women because of the relaxation of the abdominal wall in all directions due to child-bearing, and also because of the difference in anatomic structure. The female pelvis is much flatter and more horizontal than that of the male, consequently Poupart's ligament is relatively longer and tends to make the femoral canal wider and consequently weaker. This anatomic difference acts as a predisposing factor in the development of femoral hernia. In regard to umbilical hernia, this condition is frequently found in new-born children of both sexes. In later life it is more common in women. Inasmuch as distention of the abdomen by pregnancy is such a fruitful cause of hernia in women, one would expect to find this condition in cases where unusual stretching of the abdominal walls has been caused by multiple pregnancy and hydramnion, and yet such is not the case. Femoral hernia in the male is often due to varicocele. The large swollen vein distends the crural canal, and thus favors the passage of the gut through it.

In regard to the relative value of abdominal and vaginal hysterectomy, it is often claimed by the adherents of the latter method that one of the advantages connected with it is that the danger of abdominal hernia is obviated. I personally know of a case in which vaginal enterocele followed hysterectomy *per vaginam*, and the fact that this does occur after vaginal incision should make those who favor this method exercise great caution. It is a safe plan to keep the patient in bed for three weeks subsequent to operation in order that the vaginal wound may be completely healed.

As to the ventral hernia, this is fortunately becoming constantly more unfrequent after abdominal operation because care is taken to unite separately the different structures of the abdominal walls, and also because the drainage-tube is used very much less now than formally. In regard to the prevention of hernia, I take it to be very desirable as a prophylactic measure that women should strengthen their abdominal muscles, and for this purpose I would call especial attention to the value of bicycling. In regard to treatment, in my opinion it is better to perform a radical operation than to apply a truss. The operation for radical cure is not dangerous. Dr. De Garmo has reported 250 operations of this nature without a single death.

DR. HERMANN L. COLLYER: In my experience umbilical hernia in women is most often due to pregnancy. I have also seen many cases of inguinal hernia in the female. Recently there came under my observation a case of vaginal hernia occurring after vaginal hysterectomy. In these cases, however, it will generally be found that the intestine is adherent and cannot prolapse very much. To my mind, all hernia should be operated upon, palliative treatment being employed only until such time as the patient makes up his or her mind to submit to operation.

DR. BRETTAUER: The author did not refer to that form of hernia which occurs after Alexander's operation. I have seen eleven cases of this kind. All came under observation at the clinic and in all healing of the wound was by granulation. I have here a photograph of one of the patients which shows such a condition in its extreme form.

NEW YORK NEUROLOGICAL SOCIETY.

Stated Meeting, Held December 7, 1897.

THE President, B. SACHS, M.D., in the Chair.

TOXIC TREMOR AND HYSTERIA IN A MALE.

DR. J. ARTHUR BOOTH presented a man whom he had first seen one week before at the French Hospital. The patient, sixty-one years of age, had been engaged up to 1885 as a mirror polisher, using mercury, and since then in the same occupation, but using silver instead of mercury. His family history is negative as regard nervous disease. At the age of twenty-two years he contracted syphilis, and was treated for this for some time. He then enjoyed good health up to thirteen years ago. At this time he fell on the street with both lower and upper extremities in a state of clonic spasm. He was taken to the Boston City Hospital, and subsequently was under the care of Professor Charcot for several months. He returned to this country during 1887, and resumed his work of mirror polishing, using silver. He has had three or four attacks of tremor. The present illness began November 17th after having worked very hard for some time previously. The tremors presented by the patient, the speaker said, certainly resembles those observed in cases of mercurial poisoning. A very slight tap on the body would set up a pitiable degree of reflex tremor. There is no nystagmus, but there is slight ataxia. It was found that the tremor is greatly increased when attention is drawn to him, and for this reason it seemed not improbable that there is a hysteric element in the case. There are no bladder or rectal symptoms.

DR. W. M. LESZYNSKY said that the disease seems to be a functional one added to the evident toxic tremor. The fact that he had had such attacks and had recovered from them would seem to confirm this view.

NEURITIS FOLLOWING AN INFECTED VACCINATION.

DR. W. B. NOYES presented an infant who had been vaccinated last spring, the wound becoming infected. When the bandages had been removed, it had been found that the child could not move the arm. Examination showed that the deltoid, biceps, and the muscles supplied by the ulnar nerve were involved. They did not react to faradism, but gave the reaction of degeneration. The case seemed to him, at the time, to be a neuritis resulting from an infected wound; but two other opinions had been offered, *viz.*, that it was the result of tight bandaging and that the child had had an attack of anterior poliomyelitis. The condition had developed within two weeks after the vaccination, and the power of motion in the arm had been largely recovered. There was no history of constitutional disturbance. His own opinion was, that the case is one of ascending neuritis involving the circumflex, ulnar, and musculocutaneous nerves.

PULMONARY TUBERCULOSIS AND TABES DORSALIS IN THE SAME PATIENT.

DR. FRAENKEL presented a man, thirty-nine years o[f] age, unmarried, whose family history was negative. Abou[t] ten years before he had contracted syphilis, but enjoye[d] fairly good health up to two years ago. At this time h[e] had repeated hemorrhages from the lungs, and rapidl[y] developed the signs and symptoms of pulmonary tubercu[-] losis. On admission to the Montefiore Home, May, 1896 there were present pronounced physical signs of pulmo[-] nary tuberculosis, and of a large cavity at one apex, an[d] death seemed imminent. The left pupil was but slightl[y] responsive to light. The temperature never rose abov[e] 98.5° F., or the pulse above 80. He steadily improve[d] up to May, 1897, at which time his sputum still containe[d] tubercle bacilli, but his condition was in every way better The signs of the cavity had disappeared. His pupils wer[e] unequal, and the left was myopic. The scapular, ab[-] dominal, gluteal, and plantar reflexes were exaggerate[d] on both sides. The left patellar knee-jerk was markedl[y] diminished. There was no evidence of ataxia or of inco[-] ordination. On November 18, 1897, physical examina[-] tion showed the thoracic organs to be in about the sam[e] condition. The patient then complained for the first tim[e] of occasional shooting pains in the left lower extremit[y]. The sexual appetite was markedly diminished. The le[ft] knee-jerk was greatly reduced. The three points of in[-] terest were: (1) The marked unilateral character of th[e] symptoms; (2) the combination of tuberculosis and tab[es] —a very rare condition, and (3) the apparent mildness [of] both diseases.

DR. NOYES said that the case appeared to be one of fibroid phthisis. Non-progressive tabes is due rather to a collection of connective tissue than to any actual degeneration of the posterior columns. These two conditions are occasionally associated, and the case presented is probably an example of this.

TIC CONVULSIF.

DR. WILLIAM HIRSCH presented a young man having tic convulsif. The doctor had first seen him about a year ago, and the symptoms had not changed materially since then. The object in presenting the patient was to demonstrate a certain relation between his symptoms and the psychic condition present. On tapping the cheek, the patient makes a number of grimaces. The fact that the symptoms had not changed was in marked contrast with what is observed in hysteria. This patient had had articular rheumatism, followed by endocarditis and the development of mitral insufficiency. Shortly afterward he had developed the neurosis in question.

WRY-NECK AND ASYMMETRY OF THE FACE.

DR. GRAEME M. HAMMOND presented for DR. MEIROWITZ a boy sixteen years of age, who had come under observation for the relief of what appeared to be a wry-neck. As far back as could be remembered the head had been deflected to the left, but he had never experienced any pain in the neck or elsewhere. There had been no twitching or jerking. Examination showed that the head deviated to the left; the left half of the face exhibited a perceptible slope from above downward to the left eyebrow; the side of the nose, the angle of the mouth, and the angle of the jaw were all higher than the corresponding points on the right side. The muscles of the neck were distinctly hypertrophied. The skull over the parietal region showed a perceptible flattening, not observed on the other side. The movements of the head were free in all directions. The hair curved to the left side. There was no disturbance of the cranial nerves, and no hemiatrophy, and the intelligence was normal. There was no family history of similar defects.

DR. FRAENKEL remarked that cases of congenital wry-neck had been explained as resulting from a lessened developmental resistance on one side.

DR. ONUF said that in most cases of congenital wry-neck there is this asymmetry of the face. He was not sure that pressure is alone responsible for the unequal development; it would hardly explain the asymmetric development of the ear. The atrophy seemed to him to be possibly the result of twisting of the carotid artery on one side, with a consequent interference with the nutrition on that side.

ENORMOUS HYDROCEPHALUS.

DR. F. PETERSON presented the brain from such a case, one of the largest observed during many years at the Randall's Island Hospital. The patient was a woman of twenty years, who, in the early stages, had had a left hemiplegia and imbecility. As the disease progressed she became diplegic and completely idiotic. The following are the measurements of the head: Circumference, 63.5 cm.; approximate volume, 1714 c.cm.; naso-occipital arc, 47 cm.; nasobregmatic arc, 16.5 cm.; bregmato-lambdoid arc, 19 cm.; binauricular arc, 50 cm.; antero-posterior diameter, 19.5 cm.; greatest transverse diameter, 18.5 cm.; length-breadth index, 94.8 per cent.; binauricular diameter, 12 cm.; auriculobregmatic radii, 20 cm.; facial length, 11.2 cm.; empiric greatest height, 17.7 cm.; height Beta-x, 19.2 cm. At the autopsy the sutures were found fully united and the fontanels perfectly closed. The skull-bones averaged 8 mm. in thickness. The dura in was not anywhere adherent. There was very little fluid the dura. Nearly all of the fluid was in the ventricles of the brain, there being more on the right side than on the left, for the right hemisphere had become in part membranous. Five pints of clear serum was removed from the ventricles. The third and fourth ventricles partook to some extent in the dilatation. It was unfortunate that through a mishap the brain was so injured that the patency of the foramen of Magendie could not be determined. Dr. Peterson said that, in his experience, it was difficult to examine this foramen, and apparently impossible to demonstrate the presence in any human being of the foramina of Mierzejewsky. It is very important in all cases of chronic hydrocephalus to examine, if possible, the foramen of Magendie, and not only that, but to determine the patency of of the aqueduct of Sylvius and of the foramen of Monroe. He had, with Dr. Blake, at the anatomic laboratory of the College of Physicians and Surgeons, examined the brain of a ten-year-old hydrocephalic of Randall's Island, and, in this instance at least, had determined definitely the permeability of the foramina mentioned, and also of the aqueduct.

ABSCESS OF THE BRAIN.

DR. PETERSON presented a specimen showing an abscess of the brain, operation having been attempted for its relief. The case had been first observed on September 3, 1897, in the service of Dr. Brown of the Mountainside Hospital, ar Montclair, N. J. The patient was a male, forty-one years of age, who, in an attempt at suicide, had struck his head upon a rusty spike and had sustained a compound depressed fracture in the right occipital region, very near the middle line. He was trephined, and the depressed bone removed. The dura was found uninjured, and was not touched. The wound became slightly infected, but aside from moderate fever no symptoms of importance appeared until two days before he had first seen the man, *i.e.*, about two weeks after operation. He then gradually developed within twenty-four hours a left hemiplegia, with left hemi-anesthesia. Examination showed complete paralysis of the left arm and leg, with considerable anesthesia over the paralyzed limbs; slight analgesia in some places, and hyperalgesia in others. The plantar and cremasteric reflexes were normal. The knee-jerks were subtypical, slightly greater on the left side. The mind was clear. There was no aphasia, no involvement of the face or tongue. There was no evidence, in pupils or pulse, of intracranial pressure, and no symptoms of cortical irritation. The temporal half of the field of vision of the left eye was lost. The right seemed normal. He heard a watch at only half the distance with the left ear as compared with the right. Taste was normal on both sides of the tongue. The fundus seemed slightly cloudy. A diagnosis was made of abscess deep in the brain in the region of the posterior limb of the internal capsule. The surgeon was advised to trephine in the parietal region, considerably back of the motor area, and insert an exploring-needle down into the supposed site of the abscess should the patient grow worse. Two days later this was done. The abscess was found at the site suggested, and was drained. The temperature became normal, the anesthesia disappeared, and the patient moved his left hand; but a few days later he suddenly became worse and died. The brain was sent to Dr. Peterson for examination. He found the dura very sclerotic over the site of the original injury close to the superior longitudinal sinus. The convolutions of the right hemisphere were considerably flattened. There was no meningitis. Deep in the interior of the right hemisphere was an abscess about the size of a hen's egg.

HEMIATROPHY OF THE BRAIN.

DR. PETERSON then presented a specimen showing apparent hemiatrophy of the brain. The brain was that of a Randall's Island patient, a man thirty years of age, who had been in the idiot asylum for several years. A history of the origin of his trouble could not be obtained. He was a large, heavy man, with a hemiplegia (the arm being much worse than the leg), and had frequent and severe attacks of general epileptic convulsions. While able to be about, he was dull and stupid, and in intelligence would be placed in the grade of moderate idiocy. He died in an epileptic fit. There was nothing abnormal in the other organs of his body, but the brain presented the condition of marked right hemiatrophy. There was very slight evidence of microgyria, the convolutions differing as regards normality from those of the opposite side in being somewhat smaller. The membranes over the right hemisphere were, perhaps, somewhat thicker than over the left. An examination of the vessels at the base of the brain showed that the blood-supply was apparently equal on the two sides. It was undoubtedly a lack of development through some obscure and early pathologic process.

A CASE OF AMIATROPHIC LATERAL SCLEROSIS—SUPPLEMENTARY REPORT.

DR. WILLIAM HIRSCH said that on October 1, 1895, he had presented to the Society a case of this kind. The patient was forty-three years of age, and had had poliomyelitis at the age of twenty. The clinical symptoms were such that at that time they had been traced to an old scar in the left anterior horn in the cervical region. The process must have approached the left pyramidal tract, and then, after affecting the right horn, spread over the right pyramidal tract, causing a spastic condition of the right leg. In the discussion which followed the presentation of the case, it was claimed that it was one of ordinary progressive muscular atrophy. But further clinical observation showed that such was not the case. The man died June 3, 1897, and Dr. Hirsch was now able to present microscopic specimens of the spinal cord in different regions, proving the correctness of his diagnosis. He said that in these specimens one could see the connective tissue spreading from the anterior horn to the left pyramidal tract, and the latter converted into connective tissue. The cells in the anterior horns had been destroyed; the connective tissue had formed all through the lateral tract. In the cervical region one bundle of connective tissue had spread backward into the posterior columns, as he had previously diagnosticated. Deep degeneration of the pyramidal tracts could be followed down to the lumbar region.

DR. HAMMOND asked how he would differentiate these specimens from progressive muscular atrophy.

DR. HIRSCH replied that the specimens showed that the case was not one of ordinary degeneration of the lateral tracts, but that the connective tissue grew horizontally from the anterior horn to the side. Furthermore, ordinary progressive muscular atrophy is a symmetric disease.

DR. HAMMOND said that in three unquestioned cases of progressive muscular atrophy which had been under his observation, there had been a typical degeneration of the pyramidal tracts. On looking up the subject, he had found that Gowers made the statement that he had not seen a case of progressive muscular atrophy in which the pyramidal tracts had not been extensively affected. It is true that in the specimen presented, one horn is affected more than the other, nevertheless, both horns are involved.

DR. C. L. DANA thought the sections looked very much like specimens from a case of progressive muscular atrophy. If the pathologic change were not one of degeneration of the horns and lateral columns, he would like to know what Dr. Hirsch thought it really was.

THERAPEUTIC HINTS.

An Ointment for Mumps.—

℞		
Ichthyol } Plumbi iodi }	aa	gr. xlviii
Ammon. chloridi		gr. xxx
Vaselini		℥ i.

M. Ft. ung. Sig. Apply with friction over swollen glands three times daily.

To Allay Pruritus in Eczema of the Scalp the following is recommended:

℞		
Ac. salicyl.		gr. vi
Menthol.		gr. xii
Ol. lini } Aq. calcis }	aa	℥ i.

M. Sig. For external use.—*Steinhardt.*

For Facial Erysipelas.—

℞		
Ac. carbolici } Tr. iodi } Alcohol. }	aa	ʒ i
Ol. terebinth.		ʒ ii
Glycerini		ʒ iii.

M. Sig. Paint over affected parts.

THE MEDICAL NEWS.

A WEEKLY JOURNAL OF MEDICAL SCIENCE.

VOL. LXXII. NEW YORK, SATURDAY, JANUARY 29, 1898. NO. 5.

ORIGINAL ARTICLES.

THE PRESENT STATUS OF VAGINAL OPERATIONS FOR DISEASES OF THE PELVIC ORGANS.[1]

BY EDWIN B. CRAGIN, M.D.,
OF NEW YORK;
ASSISTANT GYNECOLOGIST TO ROOSEVELT HOSPITAL.

THE time has come for a careful revision of our experience with vaginal operations and a calm judgment of their utility. The new operation, so attractive to a large number of the profession, has gradually lost its newness, and with a considerable mass of evidence, *pro and con*, presented from different sections of this country and from abroad, we are now in a position to ask and answer the question: Are we better able to treat patients suffering with diseases of the pelvic organs now than we were before the resurrection and extension, under the stimulating influence of the French surgeons, of the operation tried years ago and abandoned by Thomas, Gilmore, Battey, and others?

By the vaginal operation is meant the direction of attack and procedure in different operations upon the pelvic organs—draining abscesses or inflammatory exudates; removing tumors, the uterus, or the appendages.

It is only natural that after years had been spent in perfecting technic and developing dexterity in the abdominal operation a change so radical as that involved in the vaginal method should meet with opposition. Objections, the operation has, and now after several years of experience with it, we know something of the objections, something of what the limits of the operation should be.

It is said that the vaginal operation is a difficult one, and this must be admitted even by those who favor vaginal work and use this route in a large proportion of their cases. It certainly requires more practice to become familiar with it than the abdominal operation; but here as elsewhere experience removes the difficulties and practice gives dexterity.

Certain dangers have been emphasized as being more marked in vaginal than in abdominal work. Of these, hemorrhage and injury to the neighboring viscera, with resulting fistulæ, have been made especially prominent. It must be confessed that there has been ground for criticism in the early work of almost all who have tried and practised the vaginal method, and occasionally one has been obliged to open the abdomen to check bleeding, the control of which he did not feel sure of from below. As experience has increased, however, and we have better learned to judge the class of cases suitable for vaginal attack, the control of hemorrhage has been found to cause little, if any, more trouble than in abdominal operations.

Rectal fistulæ during one's early experience with vaginal work occurs perhaps with rather greater frequency than when operating through a large abdominal wound with the patient in the Trendelenberg position. The differential feel between rectum and distended Fallopian tube is not always appreciated with ease. Even the entrance into the peritoneum through the posterior vaginal fornix, in one's early work, sometimes gives trouble, especially when the pouch of Douglas is obliterated by adhesions, and in our efforts to separate these adhesions the rectum has been injured. Experience and the selection of cases suitable for the method have helped largely to overcome this complication, and it is generally conceded that even if a fistula does occur, as a rule, it closes spontaneously in a short time.

Thus far we have spoken chiefly of the disadvantages of the method and of its complications. Why should one wish to employ the vaginal operation if it is more difficult for the operator? Because we believe that in properly selected cases the operation is accompanied by less shock, the mortality is less, the convalescence is smoother, and even if the occurrence of hernia in a properly conducted abdominal operation is rare, it must be admitted that in the vaginal method it is still more rare; the writer has never met with one in his own experience. Although the avoidance of an abdominal cicatrix is not a matter of great importance, if the operation can be equally well performed without one, it is usually appreciated by the patient. The rapidity of convalescence and the shortness of time which the patient is required to be kept in bed are sometimes emphasized by enthusiastic advocates of the vaginal operation; but in the opinion of the writer, although the patients feel like getting out of bed sooner than in the abdominal operation, they should not be allowed to do so for at least two weeks. A firm cicatrix, absorption of exudate, and the future welfare of the patient

[1] Read at the Ninety-second Annual Meeting of the Medical Society of the State of New York, held at Albany, N. Y., January 25, 26, 27, 1898.

are certainly more promoted by rest and quiet than by any attempt to see how early the patient can leave the bed.

In certain cases the vaginal operation has marked advantages, and in our discussion of the subject the most important feature is the selection of cases for which the operation is suited. The writer, on looking over the record of his vaginal work, found included in the list, aside from operations for the removal of the uterus and appendages, such operations as removal of the vermiform appendix, removal of a displaced left kidney, myomectomy at the fundus of the uterus, etc. Certainly the possibilities of the vaginal method are great, but the question before us as conscientious surgeons is not what *can* be done through the vagina, but what, in the interest of the patient, *can best* be done in this way.

It is only natural that in testing the merits of a new operation we should extend its use into fields whose boundaries riper experience tells us had better not be crossed. In my early vaginal work a number of patients were operated upon by this route in which the uterus appeared to be so healthy that its removal did not seem indicated in spite of the removal of both appendages. Although the results were good, experience and observation lead me to think that, except in the case of small ovarian tumors, *if the uterus is not to be removed*, the abdominal operation is to be preferred for the removal of one or both appendages. Small ovarian cysts and prolapsed diseased ovaries, requiring removal, form a class of cases often well adapted to the vaginal operation. Except in these instances, however, I believe that unilateral disease of the appendages is best dealt with from above, where the organs may be more thoroughly inspected, and those which are not to be removed may be left in the best possible condition for the future welfare of the patient. These are general rules, and many exceptions may occur. A woman with a roomy vagina and a thick, fat abdominal wall, with the mass to be removed lying low in the pelvis, is a favorable subject for vaginal work.

The vaginal operation has been tried in different phases of ectopic gestation, but experience proves that except in cases in which rupture has taken place some time previously and the resulting hematocele is well encapsulated, the abdominal operation is the one to be preferred. Many operations have been tried through the vagina for the correction of posterior displacements of the uterus, but on account of frequent dystocia among those in whom pregnancy has followed the operation, vaginal fixation of the uterus has been largely abandoned. Vaginal shortening of the round ligaments at present has rather a brighter outlook, but experience with it has been s limited that judgment must be reserved.

Into the general question of whether it is ac visable after resection of a portion of a disease ovary or tube to leave the remainder, if apparentl healthy, I shall not enter, but will only say that this conservative work upon the appendages is to b done, most operators are agreed that it is bett done from above than from below.

A class of cases in which the vaginal operatio has proved of great service to the writer compris women who are pregnant and whose parturie canals are obstructed by tumors which cannot b raised out of the pelvis. I have three times ob served this condition, and by vaginal removal of th tumor have enabled the patient to be delivered of living child.

There are three groups of cases in which th vaginal operation has proven, in my experience, great boon to suffering women:

1. Pus cases in which removal of the uterus an appendages is indicated.
2. Cases in which exudate indicates drainage with out the removal of any organ.
3. Small fibromyomata.

The question of whether hysterectomy is indicate in every double salpingo-oophorectomy will not b discussed in this paper. Suffice it to say, that th profession are pretty generally in accord that the are many cases of double pyosalpinx in which th uterus, enlarged, the seat of a marked endometriti perhaps with cervix lacerated, had better be sacr ficed if both appendages are removed. Experien seems to justify this conclusion, and it is just in the cases in which the vaginal operation, with its lessen shock, lessened handling of the intestines, and mo complete drainage, finds its most perfect adaptatio

Puerperal septicemia does not often indicate hy terectomy, but there are a few cases, which, in t latter part of the puerperium, about the end of t first month, present pus foci in the uterine walls in the appendages, or in both together. Here aga vaginal hysterectomy has found a useful field. T writer has operated upon four such patients, saving t and losing two, a better result, I believe, than wou have been obtained by the abdominal operation.

It has long been a familiar fact that patients p foundly septic do not endure extensive operatio well; and it has long been the practice of ma men, in cases in which there are large collections pus, to drain the abscesses through the vagina a wait until the patient recovers from her sepsis bef subjecting her to the radical operation. This c tainly is a rational procedure, and its adoption I saved many lives by requiring, at a later date, a l extensive operation than would have been needed early, and sometimes by obviating the necessity of a subsequent operation.

Thanks to the work of Henrotin of Chicago, we have found that in the relatively acute cases, before the formation of much or any pus, a great deal may be accomplished by vaginal incision, breaking up the adhesions about the appendages, and draining freely through the vagina. In one case, in which was threatened an extensive peritonitis from infected, retained secundines, the writer, by curettage of the uterus, vaginal incision, separation of the adhesions about the appendages, and free vaginal drainage, secured a rapid convalescence with no permanent damage to the tubes and ovaries. Two patients with pelvic peritonitis and exudate in the pouch of Douglas and about the appendages, with physical signs as nearly alike as two cases could be, were placed by me in adjoining beds in a hospital ward. In one a vaginal incision was made in the posterior fornix, adhesions were broken up, and the pelvis was drained with gauze; the other was subjected to the usual routine treatment of vaginal douches, boroglycerid tampons, and counter-irritation. The former patient convalesced and left the hospital in just about half the time required by the latter. Of course it cannot be proven that the two cases were absolutely alike, but the symptoms and physical signs resembled one another closely, and the rapid symptomatic cure in one by means of drainage was in marked contrast to that of the other. The writer would not be understood as recommending vaginal incision in every case of pelvic peritonitis, but when there is present evidence of fluid exudate in the pelvis, vaginal incision and drainage will, I believe, shorten the convalescence and lessen the damage to the appendages.

Whether fibromyomata of the uterus should be attacked through the vagina depends upon their size and location in the uterus. If myomectomy is to be performed, unless the tumor is situated in the lower uterine segment, or in the cervix, the abdominal route should have the preference. If hysterectomy is to be done, and the uterus and tumors together do not form a mass larger than a pregnant uterus of three or four months, the vaginal operation, with or without morcellation, has advantages so marked that one has only to watch the convalescence in such cases to be impressed with the fact that patients thus operated upon present but little more reaction than from a plastic operation for the repair of cervix and perineum.

Into the technic of the operation I shall only go far enough to emphasize the value of (1) morcellation, (2) the Mikulicz drain, and (3) ligatures. Those who have not tried and practised morcellation in some form or other in the course of a vaginal hysterectomy with an enlarged uterus, have certainly not availed themselves of their opportunities. The facility which is thus given the operator in acquiring needed space for work, and in reaching parts hitherto beyond his reach can only be appreciated by those who have tried it. In the case of a fibroid uterus, with pus in tube or ovary, morcellation proves of especial value; as, after the removal of the cervix and middle third of the uterus, and the splitting of the fundus, the fingers, or even the hand if it is small, may be introduced into the pelvis and the appendages enucleated. It is probably familiar to nearly all that the secret of success in morcellation lies in the fact that steady traction upon the uterus, with a reliable volsella affixed above the part to be removed, controls hemorrhage.

In all cases requiring drainage after vaginal hysterectomy, the principle of the Mikulicz pouch carried out in the following manner has given me most excellent service: A square handkerchief-shaped piece of gauze is opened out by an assistant and held in front of the vulva; a blunt instrument, like a sponge-holder is placed by the operator against the center of this gauze and pushed on into the pelvis. The fingers of the operator are now substituted for this instrument and carried up on one side until he feels that he is above the highest pedicle of that side. The end of a long narrow strip of gauze is then passed along the finger, of course within the pouch, until it too is carefully placed above and against the highest pedicle; enough of the same long narrow strip is inserted to loosely fill that half of the pelvis. The fingers are then introduced above the pedicles on the other side and the same process repeated either with a part of the same long strip or with another. In this way the intestines are kept away from the field of operation, drainage is secured, and the strip of gauze may be gradually withdrawn from the pouch with scarcely any disturbance to the patient; the pouch collapses as its contents are removed and may be withdrawn as desired.

The profession is divided in the choice of clamps or ligatures as a means of controlling hemorrhage. It undoubtedly is often a great convenience to use clamps at various stages of the operation, but the impression seems to be gaining ground that the comfort of the patient is better provided for if the clamps, when used, are replaced by ligatures before the patient leaves the table. In my own practice it is a very rare exception if clamps are left on when the patient leaves the operating-room.

In conclusion we believe:

1. That there are many conditions in the pelvis not suited for the vaginal operation.

2. That care is required in the selection of cases for this work.

3. That small fibromyomata and small ovarian tumors are often well suited for vaginal attack.

4. That in pus cases indicating hysterectomy, and in cases requiring drainage, the vaginal operation has great advantages.

5. That in answering the question presented at the beginning of this paper we must admit that we are much better able to treat and cure patients suffering with disease of the pelvic organs now, than we were before the development of the vaginal operation.

OTITIS MEDIA PURULENTA; ITS COMPLICATIONS AND TREATMENT.[1]

BY GORHAM BACON, M.D.,
OF NEW YORK;
PROFESSOR OF OTOLOGY IN THE NEW YORK UNIVERSITY MEDICAL COLLEGE; AURAL SURGEON TO THE NEW YORK EYE AND EAR INFIRMARY.

I SHALL only endeavor, in the short time before me this evening, to refer in a general way to the more important symptoms of purulent otitis media, both acute and chronic, and to the complications of this disease. The subject is such an inexhaustible one that it will only be possible to touch on a few of the most important points. The causes of acute purulent otitis media are cold, influenza, the exanthematous diseases, diphtheria, typhus and typhoid fever, bronchitis, cerebrospinal meningitis, pneumonia, tuberculosis, the puerperal state, syphilis, sea-bathing, injuries to the auditory canal and drumhead from blows, falls, the improper use of instruments, and the application of caustic solutions. The use of the nasal douche, and sniffing up of salt and water for nasal catarrh, frequently cause otitis media. Dentition plays an important rôle, as children during this period very often have acute otitis media which subsides after the eruption of a tooth. Adenoid growths and enlarged tonsils should also be mentioned among the causes of this disease. As a rule, this form of inflammation begins in the nasopharynx and extends by means of the Eustachian tube to the middle ear.

Scarlet fever, measles, diphtheria, and influenza are responsible for most of the cases of acute as well as of chronic otitis media, so that it is of the greatest importance that the ears should be frequently examined during the course of one of these diseases. Prompt and early treatment will often effect a cure. Neglect of treatment, or "letting the ears take care of themselves," results, as a rule, in chronic purulent otitis media with caries of the ossicula and other complications. Besides pain and tinnitus there is present more or less febrile disturbance until rupture of the drumhead occurs. The temperature in children is apt to be very high, and the commencement of an attack is sometimes ushered in by a convulsion or severe vomiting, so that a diagnosis of meningitis has occasionally been made in such cases. In the tuberculous form, perforation of the drumhead occurs without pain, and in such, the drumhead and middle ear are, as a rule, quite pale in color.

The pain, after the discharge appears, is usually much less severe, and children who a short time before were screaming on account of its severity, suddenly fall asleep, while the temperature is apt to drop several degrees. When the pain persists after the ear has begun to discharge it is probable that the periosteum of the external meatus or the mastoid cells are involved. The most frequent seat of perforation is in the lower anterior or posterior quadrant, although in some instances it is observed in Shrapnell's membrane. The inflammation is apt to be of a much more severe type and run a more protracted course in patients who are scrofulous, or who have, or have recently had, scarlet fever, measles, diphtheria, or influenza. Acute purulent otitis media may terminate in recovery with or without permanent loss of hearing, or may become chronic.

It is most important in the acute inflammatory stage of purulent otitis media to at once apply the artificial leech close to the tragus, and thus endeavor to abort the disease by antiphlogistic measures. If, in spite of this treatment, the pain persists, or bulging of the drumhead occurs, we should at once make a free incision in the drumhead, but never a small opening with a paracentesis needle, as was formerly advised. A physician should never incise the drumhead unless he is able to see the membrana tympani by means of a good illumination with head mirror and speculum. During the course of scarlatina, measles, diphtheria, influenza, typhus, and typhoid fever, the ear should be constantly examined, and as soon as it is evident that there is fluid in the tympanic cavity it should be at once evacuated by means of a free incision in the drumhead. It should be the object in all cases in which micro-organisms are present in the discharge to use antiseptic solutions (preferably the bichlorid of mercury, 1–3000). The same treatment should be applied to the nasopharynx and nares by means of an atomizer. It should then be the endeavor to drain the middle ear as thoroughly as possible, and for this purpose, in addition to irrigating the canal, a strip of iodoform gauze should be pushed down to the drumhead and renewed as often as necessary.

If a free incision is not made and proper drainage from the middle ear established, there is then gre

[1] Read at a meeting of the New York Academy of Medicine, December 2, 1897.

danger that the acute purulent otitis media will become chronic. The pus not having a free exit forms caseous masses in the attic and antrum, and caries of the ossicles and inflammation of the mastoid cells is the result. In that form of inflammation limited mostly to the attic and Prussak's spaces, it is imperative, during the early stage, that several incisions should be at once made in Shrapnell's membrane, otherwise the pus cannot escape, and will be apt to cause caries of the ossicula, and the disease thus becomes chronic. When the latter condition results the surgeon should endeavor to thoroughly drain the cavity by enlarging the opening, if this be too small, and to wash out by means of the middle-ear syringe all secretion in this part of the tympanic cavity. Here bichlorid of mercury solutions are again indicated. Granulations should be destroyed by applications of chromic acid or by the use of curettes. If in spite of local treatment the discharge continues, a cure may undoubtedly be effected in a certain number of cases by excision of carious ossicles and remains of the drumhead, and by scraping and curetting the attic. There are, however, a large number of cases of long-standing suppuration in which removal of the ossicles will not effect a cure, and in such it becomes necessary to cut down on the antrum, from behind the auricle, and perforate the bone with chisels and mallet. Thus, the antrum may be reached and cheesy matter, which so often collects in this cavity, may be removed.

As a result of the acute and chronic forms of otitis media the following complications are liable to occur: Granulations and polypi; caries of the ossicula and temporal bone; cholesteatoma; mastoid disease; suppurative meningitis; epidural abscess; cerebral abscess (temporo-sphenoidal and cerebellar); pyemia; septicemia, and facial erysipelas. I have reported two cases in which facial erysipelas was secondary to acute otitis media. In both patients the general health was impaired. Disease of the mastoid cells may occur as a sequel of acute otitis media purulenta, or may develop in connection with the chronic form of the disease. There have been, according to my experience, many more cases of mastoid disease since influenza made its appearance in this city. It was formerly the exception for the mastoid cells to be simultaneously involved in a case of acute otitis media. Of late years this condition of affairs has been very frequent.

If, during the course of acute otitis media, the temperature remains high after the drumhead has been incised and the mastoid cells opened, the possibility of the existence of a latent pneumonia, or of some other complication, especially sinus thrombosis, should be considered. I have recently observed two cases in which pneumonia was the cause of the high temperature. I have also reported a case of acute otitis media and mastoid disease in which the temperature was very high and remained so until four molar teeth made their appearance. When mastoid disease exists, the temperature may vary from 99.5° to 104° or 105° F. As a rule, the temperature in simple uncomplicated cases is lower in adults than in children. A patient with extensive caries of the mastoid cells and with a carious opening into the cranial cavity may have a temperature but slightly above the normal, so that a comparatively low temperature does not necessarily signify that the case is not one of considerable gravity. Teething infants may present a temperature of 105° F., which is due to an otitis media. Puncture of the drumhead will cause a drop of several degrees in the temperature. When the perforation closes too suddenly the fever is apt to recur. In a case of measles in which both drumheads were bulging and tenderness on pressure existed behind the mastoid, with a temperature of 104° F., a free incision in both drumheads caused the temperature to suddenly fall to 100° F. An operation on the mastoid process should never be deferred until redness and edema of the tissues over the mastoid have appeared and the auricle stands out prominently from the head.

If a patient is observed who has had an acute purulent otitis media for at least a week or ten days, and an examination shows a bulging of the upper wall of the auditory canal and drumhead, and there is pain on pressure over the mastoid antrum or tip, and, further, if there is some elevation of temperature (frequently very slight), and especially if there is a profuse discharge, these symptoms, taken together, are very characteristic of mastoid inflammation. The condition of both mastoid processes should always be compared, because in some persons pressure made over the normal mastoid will cause pain. Edema and swelling of the tissues over this bone and pain on pressure also occur in cases of furuncle of the external meatus; an examination of the auditory canal will, of course, exclude this.

When acute inflammation of the mastoid cells occurs in connection with chronic purulent otitis media it is usually advisable to at once open the cells; otherwise some more serious complication may develop, such as lateral sinus thrombosis or cerebral abscess. In the first stage of secondary mastoid inflammation, after a free incision has been made in the upper and posterior portion of the membrana tympani, the artificial leech should be applied just over the antrum and tip. The Leiter coil should then be immediately adjusted, as cold is one of the best means of reducing the inflammation. The coil should not be left on longer than forty-eight hours, for, if at the end of that time the pain persists and other symptoms of mastoid disease are present an immediate operation is advisable. Just here I cannot too strongly protest against the frequent use of blisters for these conditions, a practice which only tends, I think, to aggravate the trouble. When an operation has been decided upon, a long incision should be made close to the auricle and extending from the mastoid tip to the upper border of the pinna, so that the entire mastoid process may be inspected. This incision may be enlarged in different directions if an intracranial complication exists. In acute cases it is not always necessary to remove the entire cortex, for the disease may be limited to one portion of the mastoid cells. It must not be forgotten, however, that when pus is not found in the antrum and upper part of the mastoid it may be contained in the tip. In such cases perforation of the tip frequently occurs, and if an operation is not immediately performed the pus will burrow down the neck beneath the deep fascia and possibly give rise to septicemia or pyemia. In all cases of mastoid disease occurring in connection with chronic purulent otitis media, the entire outer wall of the mastoid process should be removed and every pneumatic cell explored.

I sometimes inflate the ears by means of Politzer's method, when the perforation in the drumhead is large and the more acute symptoms have subsided, in order to remove the secretion from the middle ear. It is much better, however, to use a catheter if only one ear be affected, for fear of forcing pathogenic organisms into the normal ear. When caries of the tympanic roof has occurred, a collection of pus is frequently found between the bony wall and the dura, or this complication may be followed by an abscess in the temporo-sphenoidal lobe of the brain. In mastoid disease it is quite common to find erosion of the bony wall just over the lateral sinus, the sinus embedded in pus, and granulations or an abscess may be found in the cerebellum. Cases of extradural abscess are much more frequently observed than abscesses in the temporo-sphenoidal lobe or cerebellum. Cerebral abscess almost always occurs in connection with chronic purulent otitis media, although I have reported one case of temporo-sphenoidal abscess which followed acute otitis media.

The first stage of abscess is usually marked by irregular symptoms, such as irritability, pain, nausea or vomiting, and frequently the discharge from the ear becomes scanty or stops altogether. The occurrence of a change in a patient's disposition, *viz.*, a talkative person becoming morose, or *vice versa*, is another symptom of importance. The patient frequently complains of chilly sensations. As the disease progresses the cerebration becomes dull and the patient appears stupid and restless. When pus has formed in the brain the most important symptoms are a distinct lowering of the pulse-rate and a temperature either slightly above normal or subnormal. There are exceptions to this rule, for I have reported a case of temporo-sphenoidal abscess in which the pulse was rapid and the temperature very high, with marked fluctuations, so that thrombus of the lateral sinus was suspected.

When aphasia develops in a patient with a chronic purulent otitis media of the left side, it is fairly certain, if the patient be right-handed, that there is a collection of pus in the temporo-sphenoidal lobe. I believe this symptom to be of the greatest diagnostic value—optical aphasia, so-called and described by Freund, Pick, and Starr. Severe headache is also usually an important symptom. Inflammation of the optic nerve may or may not be present. It is more frequently observed in cases of cerebellar than of temporosphenoidal abscess. The mastoid cells are often found to be dense and ivory-like in cases of cerebral abscess. This seems to me an important point, for in such the pus is likely to perforate the tympanic roof, and thus cause an extradural abscess or an abscess in the temporo-sphenoidal lobe. Percussion of the skull on the affected side frequently causes pain, and Macewen has called attention to the fact that there is a difference in the percussion note on the side of the head in which the abscess is located. Other symptoms sometimes noticed are digestive disturbances, increase of reflexes in the limbs of the side opposite to the abscess, a difference in the size of the pupils, and facial paralysis.

In cerebellar abscess, the most characteristic symptoms besides slow pulse and low temperature are severe headache, nausea, vomiting, vertigo, a staggering gait, and facial paralysis. Facial paralysis may be due to pressure on the facial nerve in the pons. It must also be remembered that the nerve may be affected in its course through the middle ear. I have observed a case in which the pulse was slow and the patient had vertigo, vomiting, deafness, severe headache, etc., so that a diagnosis of cerebellar abscess was made. When the antrum was opened the semicircular canals were carious, which fact accounted for the symptoms. It is very important to thoroughly examine the external auditory canals in all cases of suspected cerebral abscess; for instance, in the case of a child who was brought to my clinic a short time ago, and who had characteristic symptoms of cerebellar abscess, including choked discs with retinitis, removal of granulations from the middle ears, with the establishment of proper drainage effected a cure. The choked discs and retinitis disappeared.

When thrombosis of the lateral sinus exists, the more prominent symptoms are severe headache, high temperature with decided fluctuations, nausea, vomiting, and rigors. Over-distension of the superficial veins in the mastoid region, with swelling of the tissues around the mastoid tip, are sometimes observed. When the internal jugular becomes involved there will be tenderness on pressure along the course of this vein, and it will also present a cord-like feel. Some of the deeper veins of the neck may also become thrombosed. At a late stage the cervical glands sometimes become enlarged. When an operation is postponed too long, pulmonary infarctions develop which in the early stage do not give rise to physical signs, and also general infection results; hence, the occurrence of septicemia and pyemia.

In all cases of brain complication, due to acute and chronic otitis media, the surgeon should first of all open the mastoid antrum and make this the starting-point of the operation; for it is in this cavity that the micro-organisms exist and where they rapidly fructify as long as the soil is fertile. Antiseptics injected into the middle ear do not reach them. The various cocci and bacilli found in the nasopharynx enter the tympanic cavity through the Eustachian tube. It is possible, however, for a purulent discharge in the ear to escape into the nasopharynx and cause a pneumonia, or if swallowed, the patient may have as a result a foul-smelling diarrhea.

The tympanic roof should be explored for a carious opening. If found, this should be enlarged and the bone just above the antrum cut away with forceps so that the dura in the middle cranial fossa may be thoroughly explored. From this point an exploring-needle may be introduced into the temporo-spenoidal lobe if brain abscess be suspected. If the symptoms point to thrombus of the lateral sinus, the latter may be quickly exposed by cutting away the bone with chisels and forceps. In some cases a thrombus will be found in the sinus even when a needle has been introduced and fluid blood withdrawn, and also when the sinus pulsates. In such cases, it is necessary to open it with a bistoury. This may be done if everything required to plug the sinus in case of hemorrhage be at hand. If the indications point to abscess in the cerebellum, the sinus should always be first uncovered, and then the opening may be enlarged posteriorly and the cerebellum explored for pus.

The question of ligating the internal jugular vein, whenever a thrombus is found in the latter, is a point still unsettled. My own opinion is that it is unnecessary to do this if it is possible to establish a free flow of blood in each end or the divided sinus. Pressure should be made on the neck from below upward along the course of the internal jugular vein in order to remove any thrombi in the lower end of the lateral sinus. A probe should be passed to the torcular and jugular bulb if necessary. If the flow of blood cannot be reestablished from the lower end of the sinus, it then becomes necessary to ligate the internal jugular vein, especially if there be tenderness or a cord-like induration along the vein. For fear of injuring some vessel in the brain it is better to use an instrument devised by Horsley rather than a sharp-pointed exploring-needle. I have never seen any bad results from exploring the different parts of the brain, if the operation is carefully performed and under strictly aseptic conditions.

All operations on the cranial cavity should be performed at an early stage of the disease if we wish to meet with success, and as rapidly as possible, for in many instances, I believe that patients are anesthetized for too long a time. I use the burrs recommended by Macewen in some cases, but, as a rule, I find that I can work more quickly with gouges, drills, and forceps. After evacuating the pus in a brain abscess great care should be exercised in syringing the cavity. A boracic-acid solution should be used, and afterward iodoform gauze loosely packed in the cavity. I prefer the gauze method of draining the abscess cavity to the use of drainage-tubes. In some cases in which the mastoid process is sclerosed, it will be necessary to remove a button of bone with the trephine in order to perform the operation as speedily as possible.

THE EARLY DIAGNOSIS AND TREATMENT OF EXTRA-UTERINE PREGNANCY.

By G. H. BALLERAY, M.D.,
OF NEWARK, N. J.;
GYNECOLOGIST TO THE PATERSON GENERAL HOSPITAL AND TO ST. JOSEPH'S HOSPITAL, PATERSON, N. J.; OBSTETRICIAN TO THE MATERNITY HOSPITAL, PATERSON, N. J.

UNTIL within the last fifteen years extra-uterine pregnancy was considered to be of such rare occurrence that most practitioners did not think it worth while to study the signs and symptoms which indicate the presence of this condition. Of late, however, a growing interest is being manifested in regard to its cause, diagnosis, and treatment. The cause of ectopic pregnancy is admitted to be some abnormal condition of the Fallopian tube, and it is generally conceded that almost all cases of extra-uterine gestation are primarily tubal—the almost endless variety described by the older writers being but accidental modifications of tubal pregnancy. We are indebted to Lawson Tait for the elucidation of this subject, and I think it may be truthfully said of him that he has accomplished more than any other man in placing the pathology of extra-uterine pregnancy upon a rational basis. Not only has he clearly pointed out the pathology of ectopic pregnancy, but by example he has taught us how to successfully treat this serious condition. My remarks will be limited to the diagnosis and treatment of extra-uterine pregnancy in the early months; its diagnosis and treatment at, or after, full term is so thoroughly considered in several classic works that it would be useless to repeat it here. Moreover, my personal experience in this class of cases is limited to a small number, and does not entitle me to treat the subject from a practical standpoint. The diagnosis of ectopic pregnancy in the early months, before the rupture of the sac, may present considerable difficulty, but that it is impossible, as some writers have claimed, is very far from true. I do not claim to possess any special diagnostic skill, and yet I have been able to diagnose extra-uterine gestation at this time on several occasions—the diagnosis in each case being verified by abdominal section. In this connection the two following cases may be interesting:

CASE I.—Mrs. W., aged twenty-seven years, the mother of one child, nine months old. I was called to see the patient by Dr. Vroom of Ridgewood, N. J., on March 7, 1896. The patient's previous pregnancy had terminated during June, 1895, the only thing abnormal being that she flowed considerably at the time, and continued to lose a good deal of blood during the two subsequent weeks. After the birth of her child she did not menstruate until December 8, 1895. The flow continued nearly ten days and was rather profuse. The next menstrual period occurred January 8, 1896, and continued about the same length of time. Her third period came on March 6, 1896, and continued until I saw her on the 17th. The flow was at times rather profuse, and was accompanied by colicky pains in the abdomen, which were occasionally so severe as to require the use of morphin in moderately large doses.

The patient was very pale and anemic, and her pulse was rather frequent and soft; but she looked bright and cheerful and seemed to think that both her medical attendant and her husband were unnecessarily anxious in regard to her condition. On vaginal examination, I found the cervix enlarged and soft and the os uteri patulous.

The uterus, by conjoined manipulation, was found to be crowded over to the right side of the pelvis by a resilient mass situated to the left, and posterior to the uterus. The mass seemed to be about the size of a duck's egg and was not movable. The conclusion reached was that the case was one of left tubal pregnancy—the tube being firmly bound down by pelvic adhesions. I stated my opinion to Dr. Vroom, and urged the necessity of the immediate removal of the patient to the hospital, in order that she might be operated upon without delay should rupture of the sac occur. The patient's husband, an exceptionally intelligent man, having been informed of the nature of the case, took measures to have her carefully removed the same afternoon to the Paterson General Hospital, the understanding being that I would operate upon her as soon as she had recovered from the fatigue of the journey—probably within forty-eight hours.

The following day Dr. Henry C. Coe of New York saw the case in consultation with me, and concurred in the diagnosis and the propriety of an early operation. Accordingly, assisted by my colleague, Dr. I. L. Leal, and in the presence of Drs. H. C. Coe, Wm. Blundell, E. J. Marsh, and others, I opened the abdominal cavity. The left Fallopian tube, the seat of an ectopic gestation, was found to be greatly enlarged and bound down by adhesions to the posterior face of the broad ligament, and also to the rectum and small intestines. The adhesions were carefully broken down, and the mass ligated and excised. On examination, the right tube was found dilated into a sac about two inches in diameter, but free from adhesions; it was also removed. On subsequent examination it was found to contain a fetus which had probably reached the tenth week of development. The pelvic cavity was carefully cleansed, a glass drainage-tube inserted, and the abdominal wound closed. The patient suffered severely from shock for about eighteen hours. She then began to rally and made an excellent recovery.

The points of interest in this case are as follows: (1) That it was a case of double extra-uterine pregnancy; (2) that the diagnosis was based upon the physical signs alone, the history being entirely negative, and (3) the evident advantage of the use of the drainage-tube. The presence of the drainage-tube enabled me to correctly interpret the symptoms which the patient presented a few hours after operation. These symptoms were extreme pallor, and coldness of the surface, including the face, very rapid and feeble pulse, widely dilated pupils, and sighing, almost gasping, respiration, with constant restlessness. The "air-hunger" was marked. A careful examination of the drainage-tube showed that there was no hemorrhage, only a moderate amount of bloody serum being discharged. The treatment consisted in keeping the foot of the bed elevated, application of warmth to the surface, administration, *per rectum* of hot saline solution containing a large proportion of brandy, and the hypodermic injection of strychnin and enough morphin to allay restlessness. Under this treatment the shock gradually passed away and the patient rapidly progressed toward recovery So strongly did the symptoms point to the occurrence of hemorrhage that had it not been for the presence of the drainage-tube I should have been sorely tempted to reopen the abdomen, and such course would in all probability have resulted fatally

CASE II.—I was called on the evening of March 31, 1896, by Dr. Homer Sylvester, then House Surgeon at St. Joseph's Hospital, Paterson, N. J., to see Mrs. R., a ward patient, admitted a few hours previously. Dr. Sylvester informed me that he thought the case one of ectopic pregnancy. The patient was a poorly nourished woman, thirty-two years of age, the mother of five children, the last child being two years old. She had last menstruated normally three months previously. She had then gone over two months without any menstrual flow. Three weeks before admission to the hospital she began to have a slight bloody discharge from the vagina, attended by colicky pains in the lower part of the abdomen. The pains and bloody discharge would occasionally cease for two or three days and then recur and continue three or four days. At no time was the pain sufficiently severe to confine her to bed, and the bloody discharge was never profuse. At times the blood which escaped from the vagina was clotted, and the patient thought she had noticed a shreddy substance in the clots expelled. Her pulse varied from 86 to 94 per minute, and was soft and compressible; the temperature was 99° F. Physical examination disclosed a mass to the left, and posterior to the uterus; it was not movable and displaced the uterus slightly upward and to the right. By means of conjoined manipulation the body of the uterus was found somewhat enlarged. The cervix was enlarged and presented that peculiar softness which is the rule in the early stages of pregnancy. A diagnosis of extra-uterine pregnancy was made.

From the immobility of the mass, I was satisfied that the Fallopian tube, the seat of the ectopic gestation, was firmly bound down in the pelvis by adhesions. As it was late in the evening, and as I had several important engagements for the following day, I fixed on the day after for operation, it being understood that Dr. Sylvester should at once notify me should symptoms of rupture occur in the meantime. At 9.30 A.M. on the the morning of April 2, 1896, I went to the hospital prepared to operate. I learned that about four hours previously there had been an unfavorable change in the patient's condition. She had been seized with pain in the lower part of the abdomen, and shortly after the pulse became much more frequent than it had been before. I found her with a pulse of 120, lips somewhat blanched, temperature 98° F., and complaining of some pain in the abdomen. I concluded that the fetal sac had ruptured, and that a moderate hemorrhage into the peritoneal cavity had occurred. Stimulants and anodynes having already been administered, and the field of operation having been prepared, the patient was anesthetized and taken to the operating-room. With the assistance of my colleague, Dr. Jas. W. Smith, and in the presence of the hospital staff, I opened the abdomen. About a quart of blood (fluid and clotted) was found in the peritoneal cavity. The fetal sac, except at the point of rupture, was adherent to the rectum, small intestine, and posterior surface of the broad ligament. The adhesions were carefully separated and the sac removed. As the right ovary and tube were diseased, they were removed. The peritoneal cavity was flushed with a hot saline solution and thoroughly cleansed. A glass drainage-tube was then inserted, and the abdominal wound closed. Under the influence of stimulating enemata, the patient reacted well. The drainage-tube was removed on the third day, and the patient left the hospital in good condition at the end of the fourth week.

The points of interest in this case are: the typical history; the diagnosis before rupture, and the emphasizing of the importance of prompt action as soon as the diagnosis is made.

Under less favorable conditions, the loss of time which occurred in this case between the diagnosis and the operation might have resulted disastrously. On subsequent examination the fetal sac was found to contain both fetus and placenta, together with a small amount of clotted blood.

It is highly important that the physician engaged in general practice should be fully alive to the comparative frequency of extra-uterine pregnancy. He will then be on the alert, and will not be liable to overlook the condition simply because it does not present the whole array of classic symptoms. It is he who generally sees the case first, and upon his early recognition of its true nature will often depend the issues of life or death.

Some idea of the comparative frequency of ectopic pregnancy may be gathered from the fact that according to the records of the Paterson General Hospital (which as its name implies is a general hospital, and not a special institution for women) seven women have been operated upon for ruptured tubal pregnancy during the past eight months. These were all cases of rupture into the peritoneal cavity. A case in which rupture occurred between the layers of the broad ligament was also admitted during this period. This patient was not operated upon, and she recovered. During the past year, within a single month, the writer operated successfully in three cases of tubal pregnancy, and within a few weeks thereafter saw, with two medical gentlemen of large experience, two other patients who were actually moribund when first seen, and were, therefore, not operated upon. In neither case had the physician in attendance suspected the true nature, although the symptoms in both, as described by the medical attendants, were almost pathognomonic.

Diagnosis.—The diagnosis of ectopic pregnancy in the early months, before rupture of the fetal sac, is based upon the history and the physical findings. In a certain proportion of cases the history is such as to create a strong presumption in favor of the presence of this condition; on the other hand, the history is often misleading, and in a large proportion of cases there is absolutely no history beyond the fact that the woman presented the usual symptoms of pregnancy and believed herself to be normally pregnant. In the latter case rupture of the sac is the first indication that anything abnormal exists. This terrible accident may then suddenly occur absolutely without premonition. It was formerly believed that extra-uterine pregnancy occurred almost invariably in women who had previously been sterile; *i. e.*, who either had never been pregnant or had not borne a child for a long period prior to the occurrence of the abnormal gestation. That sterile women are more likely to become subjects of extra-uterine pregnancy than those who have frequently borne children is probably true, but, at the bedside, neither previous sterility nor fecundity should be allowed to enter as a factor in the diagnosis. It should be remembered that all women during the child-bearing period are liable to the occurrence of extra-uterine pregnancy. If this is borne in mind fewer blunders in diagnosis will occur; and fewer lives will be sacrificed by that criminal procrastination which defers until too late the only rational means of saving the patient's life.

In a typical case the history of the patient is about as follows: There has been cessation of the menses for one, two, or three months, during which time the patient may or may not have experienced some of the symptoms which are supposed by her to be indicative of the occurrence of pregnancy, *viz.*, such as morning sickness, tingling sensations in the breasts, etc. After a time, varying in different cases, she begins to experience colicky pains in the lower part of the abdomen, accompanied by a discharge of more or less blood from the vagina. The blood is sometimes fluid, sometimes clotted, and occasionally shreddy substances are noticed in the discharge by the patient or by those in attendance. Mixed with the vaginal discharge a membranous mass, resembling a cast of the uterine cavity, is occasionally expelled. These symptoms (loss of blood and colicky pains) may disappear to again recur at intervals of a few days, or the flow of blood may be almost continuous and the colicky pains rarely absent for more than a few hours at a time, although they may not be sufficiently severe to confine the patient to bed, or require the administration of anodynes. The flow of blood is rarely profuse, almost never resembling the active bleeding accompanying an early abortion. The typical symptoms, then, are amenorrhea, followed by irregular discharge of blood from the vagina, recurrent colicky pains in the lower part of the abdomen, and occasionally the discharge of portions of deciduous membrane.

Upon physical examination, the uterus will generally be found enlarged if gestation has continued beyond the second month. The softness of the cervix, which is so marked, as a rule, in normal pregnancy, is not always present in ectopic gestation. I have observed it in three cases. In multiparæ the os is sometimes patulous. On one side of, and sometimes behind the uterus, a soft, resilient mass, varying in size according to the stage of the pregnancy, can usually be detected. On careful bimanual examination, it is found to be very close to the body of the uterus, and seems to crowd the organ somewhat to the opposite side of the pelvis. It is, as a rule, not difficult to make out that it is not continuous with the body of the uterus. Examination, *per rectum*, sometimes unables the practitioner to correctly appreciate the relations of the tumor.

The changes in the breasts, characteristic of pregnancy, may or may not be present. In a case presenting the history and physical signs detailed above, there should not be much hesitation on the part of the practitioner in coming to a conclusion in regard to the presence of ectopic pregnancy. If, however, he remains in doubt, an anesthetic should be administered and another careful examination made. Emptying of the bladder and rectum should precede this examination; as, indeed, it should all examinations of the female pelvic organs.

Differential Diagnosis.—The following hints may aid in the differential diagnosis between early ectopic pregnancy and the conditions for which it is likely to be mistaken. In retroflexion and lateroflexion of the gravid uterus, the tumor behind or to one side of the cervix is continuous with it. The cervix is enlarged and softened, and the fundus not in its normal position behind the pubes. There is no colicky pain, and no bloody vaginal discharge—unless an abortion is impending, or has recently occurred. In hydrosalpinx, pyosalpinx, ovarian abscess, small adherent ovarian cyst, and small cysts of the broad ligament, the uterus is not enlarged, and the usual signs and symptoms of pregnancy are absent unless a normal pregnancy coexists. Recurrent colicky pains and irregular bloody discharges from the vagina are not usual accompaniments of these conditions.

In acute pyosalpinx and ovarian abscess, more or less constant pain and tenderness on pressure are present, accompanied by elevation of temperature. In small myomata, the body of the uterus is enlarged, but the menstrual flow is not suppressed, and there is no semi-fluctuating or boggy mass on either side of the uterus.

Early pregnancy in the rudimentary horn of a malformed uterus, cannot be differentiated from ectopic pregnancy; nor is it essential that it should be, as the treatment is operative in both. Pregnancy in one horn of a well-formed bicornuate uterus may be distinguished from ectopic pregnancy only in cases in which a vaginal or cervical septum exists. In the absence of this distinguishing feature the diagnosis must remain doubtful. From pregnancy in one-half of a double uterus, the differential diagnosis may be easily made, if, in addition to a well-formed double uterus, there is a double vagina. In a case which I saw with my colleague, Dr. Harris, this condition obtained. The patient had symptoms which made the physician apprehensive of the existence of ectopic pregnancy, but after a careful examination it was concluded that the pregnancy had occurred in the right half of the uterus. Both cervices were well developed; and the os uteri of each was normal in appearance. Our determination to wait was rewarded in a few days by a verification of the diagnosis; for the patient aborted.

In a case in which, after careful bimanual examination, serious doubt exists as to whether the pregnancy is intra- or extra-uterine, the use of the sound has been recommended in order to ascertain whether or not the uterus is empty. While the use of the sound may be justifiable in certain cases, its indiscriminate employment cannot be too strongly deprecated.

There are two other conditions which, according to some authors, may be confounded with early ectopic pregnancy, *viz.*, hematoma of the broad ligament, and hematosalpinx. The writer has not referred to these conditions, for the reason that he believes that Bland Sutton is right when he says that nearly all cases of hematosalpinx are the result of a blighted tubal pregnancy, and as regards hematoma of the broad ligament, it is the writer's belief that in ninety per cent. of the cases this condition is the result of rupture of an early tubal pregnancy into the cellular tissue between the layers of the broad ligament.

The diagnosis after rupture of the gestation-sac is based upon the evidences of abdominal shock and concealed hemorrhage. Violent pain in the lower part of the abdomen, followed by symptoms of collapse, is the rule in all cases of intraperitoneal rupture attended by profuse hemorrhage. When the hemorrhage is less profuse the symptoms of collapse come on more slowly. Cases in which the Fallopian tube, the seat of the ectopic gestation, is perfectly free in the pelvic cavity previous to rupture, are, as a rule, attended by more profuse hemorrhage than those in which the tube is bound to surrounding structures by adhesions. The hemorrhage is generally out of proportion to the development of the gestation-sac; the earlier the rupture occurs the more rapidly fatal the hemorrhage.

The two following cases will illustrate these points:

CASE III.—I was called by Dr. Flitcroft, May 3, 1894, at 11 A.M., to see Mrs. V., a German, aged twenty-eight years. The patient had never been pregnant before, although she had been married eight years. Her last menstruation had occurred three months previously. When she was first seen by Dr. Flitcroft, a few hours before my visit, she complained of severe pain in the lower part of the abdomen, and there was a slight bloody discharge from the vagina. The doctor made a vaginal examination, and, finding no dilatation of the os uteri, concluded that the case was merely one of threatened abortion. After having given directions as regards the management of the patient, and requested the attendants to send for him should she become worse, he left the house. When he was called the second time he found the patient still complaining of pain in the abdomen, though it was not as severe as it had been at the beginning of the attack. Her countenance, however, had changed, and her pulse was more frequent and weaker than it had been at his first visit. The os uteri was not dilated. The doctor concluded that there was something seriously wrong with the patient, and requested me to see her with him. I found her with a pulse of 126, skin cool, face pale, but not anxious.

She was a short, fat woman; and, on inquiry, I learned that previous to the attack she had had a very florid complexion. The results of a vaginal examination were negative. No swelling of any kind could be detected on either side, or posterior to the uterus.

I expressed to Dr. Flitcroft the opinion that the case was one of ruptured tubal pregnancy, and that an operation should be performed without delay. He heartily concurred in this opinion, and expressed surprise that he should not have made the diagnosis himself in view of his previous experience.[1]

As the environments of the patient were such as to preclude the possibility of operating upon her in her own home, she was removed as quickly as possible to the Paterson General Hospital. As showing how very important it is not to waste any time in this class of cases, I will state that in the time which it took to remove the patient to the hospital the change for the worse in her condition was really alarming. Her pulse rose to 156, and the surface was cold and covered with perspiration. She appeared to be moribund, and yet the time occupied in her removal was less than two hours. Hot saline solution and brandy was injected into the rectum, the field of operation quickly prepared, and the patient anesthetized and taken to the operating-room. Assisted by Dr. Jas. W. Smith, I performed abdominal section.

As soon as the peritoneum was incised fluid blood

[1] Dr. Flitcroft had had within two years the unique experience of being present at the bedside of a patient at the moment of rupture of a tubal pregnancy. The patient was conversing cheerfully with the doctor when she was suddenly seized with an agonizing pain in the abdomen, and very soon afterward showed symptoms of collapse. Dr. Flitcroft called to his aid Dr. C. S. Van Riper, who promptly opened the abdomen and removed the ruptured gestation-sac. A large amount of blood was found in the peritoneal cavity. The patient recovered.

welled up from the abdominal cavity and ran down upon the floor of the operating-room. I quickly passed my fingers down through the mass of blood-clot into the pelvic cavity, and found that the ruptured gestation-sac was the left Fallopian tube. This was brought up into view through the incision, when it was observed that there was a rent in its walls through which the fetus had escaped, and from which bright-red blood poured in a constant stream. A figure-of-eight ligature was applied and the sac cut away. The abdominal and pelvic cavities were cleansed of blood, flushed with hot saline solution, and the abdominal wound closed. A three-months' fetus was found among the blood-clots; the placenta had been retained within the sac and was removed with it. It was estimated that more than a gallon of blood had been removed from the peritoneal cavity. Although the patient's condition was desperate at the time of operation, she rallied under the influence of active stimulation, and made an excellent recovery.

CASE IV.—Mrs. R., aged twenty-three years, married nine months, was admitted to the Paterson General Hospital, January 21, 1897. The history was that she had been seized with violent pain in the abdomen the evening previous to admission, and had gradually gone into the condition of collapse in which she reached the hospital. Shortly after she was taken ill she was seen by Dr. John T. Gillson, but when the doctor was informed by the patient that she had menstruated regularly—the last time only three weeks previously—he dismissed the idea of ectopic pregnancy from his mind, and attributed the pain to some form of intestinal disturbance. When he saw her the following morning he became convinced that intraperitoneal hemorrhage was going on, and sent her to the hospital. I was at the hospital when she was admitted, and the senior house-surgeon requested me to see her at once. She was almost pulseless, and death seemed imminent. The extreme pallor of the surface and waxy appearance of the lips, taken in connection with the sudden onset of the attack, in a person previously in robust health, left no doubt in my mind as to the existence of intra-abdominal hemorrhage. The result of a vaginal examination was entirely negative—nothing abnormal could be detected.

The rectum being found empty, a stimulating enema of hot saline solution and brandy was at once administered, and the field of operation having been prepared, abdominal section was performed. On opening the peritoneal cavity a large quantity of fluid blood escaped. The whole abdominal and pelvic cavities were filled with clotted blood. The right Fallopian tube was the source of the hemorrhage and was removed, together with the ovary, which was cystic. The ectopic sac was situated almost at the fimbriated end of the tube, and was lined by a rather thick membrane. Its size, when collapsed, would indicate that before rupture it was no larger than a hazelnut. In spite of active stimulation, the patient never rallied and died within twenty-four hours.

In this case the exsanguination was complete, an[d] no amount of saline solution could take the place o[f] the blood lost. Had this patient been operated upo[n] early there is every reason to believe that she woul[d] have recovered. Her history, however, was mis-leading, and her physician was at first deceived b[y] it. In this and the preceding case the fetal sac wa[s] entirely free from adhesions to surrounding parts.

When rupture occurs between the layers of th[e] broad ligament the evidences of shock and loss o[f] blood may be marked, but rarely to the same exten[t] as when it occurs into the peritoneal cavity. Th[e] differential diagnosis rests upon the result of a phys-ical examination. A large, soft, boggy mass i[s] found on one side, and posterior to the uterus. Th[e] uterus is crowded to the opposite side, and the cer-vix is pushed under the pubes, and, in a large pro-portion of cases, the os uteri seems to point directl[y] upward. I know of no other condition which give[s] rise to this particular form of uterine displacement[.] I regard it as a sign of the greatest diagnostic value[.] If a physician previously makes a vaginal examina-tion and detects a small mass on one side of th[e] uterus, its sudden increase in size, accompanied b[y] symptoms of shock and concealed bleeding, can b[e] due but to one cause, *viz.*, intraligamentous rupture with hemorrhage between the layers of the broa[d] ligament. When rupture of an early tubal preg-nancy into the peritoneal cavity occurs, any smal[l] mass, situated on one side of the uterus, which ma[y] have been previously detected, will generally b[e] found to have disappeared, unless the pregnant tub[e] is bound down by adhesions, and the effused bloo[d] to a certain extent, encapsulated. The treatment [of] extra-uterine pregnancy should be purely surgical, a[ll] other methods should be condemned as both inefficie[nt] and dangerous. If the diagnosis is made before ru[p]-ture has occurred, the abdomen should be opened an[d] the gestation sac removed. If rupture has alread[y] occurred, not a moment should be lost in resorting t[o] abdominal section, for a very brief delay may resu[lt] in the death of the patient from hemorrhage. Whe[n] the abdomen is opened there is generally an escap[e] of fluid blood and the pelvis is found filled wit[h] blood-clots, through which the surgeon passes h[is] fingers to the fundus of the uterus, and then alon[g] the broad ligament on each side until the site of t[he] gestation-sac is determined. The sac is immediatel[y] brought to the surface, securely ligated at its bas[e] and cut away. The abdominal and pelvic caviti[es] are then flushed with hot saline solution, and sponge[d] until free of blood. If the sac is found adherent t[o] surrounding structures the use of a drainage-tube wi[ll] add to the patient's changes of recovery. If t[he] hemorrhage has been great, and the patient is mu[ch] depressed, hot saline solution should be injected into the rectum. Brandy or good whisky may be given with the saline solution, and may also be given by the mouth in small doses frequently repeated, and in very hot water, as hot as the patient can bear. Morphin and strychnin administered hypodermically are generally indicated. When the patient has reacted her strength should be supported by nutritious liquid diet.

Intraligamentous Rupture.—When rupture of an early tubal pregnancy occurs and the fetus (fetal débris) and effused blood escape between the layers of the broad ligament, constituting what was formerly known as extraperitoneal hematocele, but now designated hematoma of the broad ligament, the interests of the patient will be best secured by letting her alone. These cases, as a rule, are fatal only through the officiousness of the medical attendant. If the patient be kept quiet, and trust put in *meditrix naturæ*, it will generally be found that at the end of a few weeks the effused blood and fetal remains have been absorbed, and that nothing is left but a slight thickening of the broad ligament on the affected side.

The only exception to this rule occurs in cases in which suppuration of the hematoma supervenes, or in those very exceptional instances in which, after primary intraligamentous rupture, secondary rupture through the roof of the broad ligament into the peritoneal cavity occurs. Cases of the latter class demand prompt and decisive action. The abdomen must be opened, the cavity of the broad ligament emptied of clots and packed with iodoform gauze, an end of which should be brought out through an opening in the vagina for drainage. The rent in the roof of the broad ligament may then be closed with a fine catgut suture. If the hemorrhage cannot be controlled in this manner, hysterectomy should be performed. In suppurating hematoma of the broad ligament, vaginal section, washing of the cavity with a disinfectant solution, and gauze drainage are indicated. It will be observed that in the treatment of ectopic pregnancy in the early months, abdominal section is the only method which I have advised. My reasons for so doing are, in the first place, my personal experience is limited entirely to this operation, and, in the second, I fail to appreciate the advantages of operation by the vaginal route which are claimed by the advocates of that method. The operation through the abdominal wall gives more room for work; the manipulations are performed under the guidance of the sense of sight, as well as touch, and in cases of intraperitoneal rupture, with the accumulation of large quantities of clotted blood in the abdominal and pelvic cavities, the cleansing of the peritoneal cavity can be more quickly and effectually performed.

Summary.—The points which I wish to emphasize are as follows:

1. Early ectopic pregnancy may be diagnosed before rupture has occurred, provided an opportunity to make a careful examination be afforded.

2. In the differentiation of early ectopic pregnancy from conditions which simulate it, a painstaking examination *per vaginam* and *per rectum*, under anesthesia, offers the best chance of making a correct diagnosis.

3. The use of the uterine sound as a means of diagnosis may be permissible in cases of grave doubt as to whether the pregnancy is intra- or extra-uterine; but its indiscriminate employment cannot be too strongly condemned.

4. In case of grave doubt as to whether or not early ectopic pregnancy be present, but when the presumption is strongly in favor of its existence, exploratory abdominal section is not only permissible, but imperative.

5. Abdominal possesses many advantages over vaginal section, and should, therefore, always be the operation of election in this class of cases.

6. All cases of early ectopic pregnancy, except those in which intraligamentous rupture has occurred, should be operated upon as soon as the diagnosis is made. Procrastination may mean death to the patient.

VIBRATORY THERAPEUTICS.

BY FREDERICK PETERSON, M.D.,
OF NEW YORK;
PROFESSOR OF INSANITY IN THE WOMAN'S MEDICAL COLLEGE; VISITING NEUROLOGIST TO THE CITY HOSPITAL.

IN view of the well-deserved attention during recent years to the various so-called natural methods of treating disease, such as massage exercises, hydrotherapy, dietetics, and the like, I have thought it well to add my experience to that of several others in regard to the rather novel method of treatment of nervous diseases by means of vibration. Vibration may properly be divided into two classes, *viz.*, mechanical and kinetic. The former is obtained by means of a variety of vibrating mechanical apparatus. The term kinetic seems to me applicable to the finer variety of vibration induced by some force such as electricity, an example of which is afforded by the sinusoidal current.

Mechanical vibration for therapeutic purposes was in use long before any mention of it found place in medical literature; for its value was recognized by the earliest of the originators of the Swedish system of gymnastics and massage. It was practised before Zander devised mechanical apparatus for the purpose. It seems to have been as late as 1878 before it attracted the attention of physicians and was made the object of investigation both as to therapeutic value and mode of action. Thus, in the same year appeared Horvath's[1] article on "The Influence of Rest and Movement upon Life," and the article by Vigouroux[2] upon "The Results of Vibratory Treatment of Nervous Diseases in the Service of Charcot at the Salpêtrière." The next reference to the subject was made two years later by Mortimer Granville, who applied vibration to the treatment of neuralgia, and he invented a vibrating hammer for application of vibration to affected nerve trunks. He published brief articles during 1880 and 1881 in the *Lancet*, and, during 1882 and 1883, in the *British Medical Journal*, but his brochure, entitled "Nerve Vibration and Excitation as Agents in the Treatment of Functional Disorders and Organic Disease," was not published until 1883. Baudet published an article on the treatment of pain by mechanical vibration in *Progrès Médical*, February 5, 1881. With the exception of an occasional biologic reference to the subject, such as Reinke's article in *Pflüger's Archiv*, 1880, on the influence of mechanical shaking on the development of certain fungi, and one or two others mentioned by Meltzer in his paper on "The Importance of Vibration to Cell-life" (*New York Medical Journal*, December 24, 1892), nothing appeared in medical literature in relation to vibration until Charcot (*Prog. Méd.*, p. 149, 1892) and Gilles de la Tourette (*N. iconog. de la Salpêt.*, p. 265, 1892) introduced the matter again to the profession with considerable acclaim. Outside of strictly medical circles, however, vibratory therapeutics had continued to develop, and before Charcot's paper was published the vibrating machine invented in Sweden by Liedbeck had been in use and even covered by an American patent as early as 1890.

W. B. Tomson published a brief note in the *Lancet*, i, p. 1299, 1890, entitled "General Appreciation of Vibration as a Sense Extraordinary," citing the cases of two deaf persons with remarkable sensitiveness to vibration; an interesting note from a speculative point of view, because the nervous system does seem to be often susceptible in an extraordinary degree to mechanical vibration. Morselli, during 1892 and 1893, wrote upon mechanical vibration as a means of cure of nervous and mental diseases, and his work is especially interesting and valuable (*Terap. Mod. Padova*, 1892, vi, 568, and also *Boll. d. r. Accad. med. di Genova*, 1893, 33).

With the exception of a paper by Dr. Patrick in the *Chicago Medical Recorder* during 1894, the above constitutes all I have been able to find in medical literature on vibratory therapeutics.

Regarding the apparatus used for the purpose, Larat and Gautier made for Charcot and Gilles de la Tourette the *casque vibrant* and the *fauteuil trepidant* employed by them. The *casque vibrant* is simply a metal helmet upon the top of which is fixed a small electric motor, its trembling motion being communicated by this means to the whole head. The *fauteuil trepidant* or shaking chair was constructed especially for cases of paralysis agitans, but is also used for other purposes, and is merely a chair mechanically adjusted to simulate the tremor of a train or omnibus.

In my own practice I have employed three varieties of apparatus. The first is a modification of the one in use at the Salpêtrière. It was made for me by Messrs. Waite & Bartlett of New York, and consists of a small motor with an eccentric adjustment to regulate the force and frequency of the tremor. This motor is fixed upon the head by means of clasps and a strap (Fig. 1).

FIG. 1.

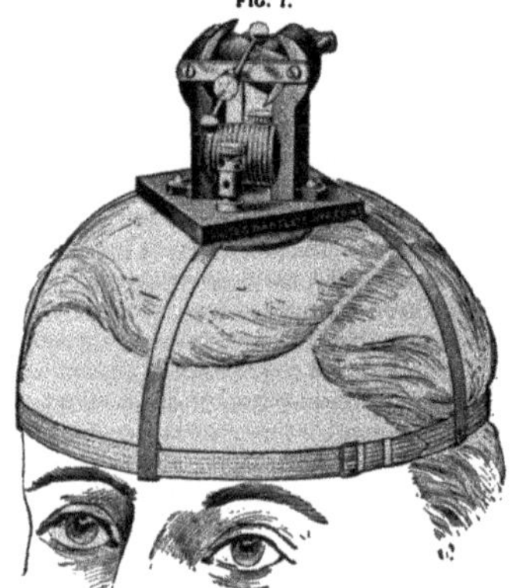

Electric vibrator for the head.

Another instrument made for me by the same firm is modeled upon the electric engraving-tool. It consists of a rod with an up and down movement affixed to the same motor used for vibrating the head. With this apparatus the trunks of nerves may be tapped and vibrated with any degree of frequency required (Fig. 2).

The third and best apparatus is one which may be used for administering vibration to any part of the body, to a nerve trunk, to the eye, the larynx, the head, a limb, the spinal column, and with any degree of force or frequency desired. It is an adaption

[1] *Pflüger's Arch.*, 1878, p. 125.
[2] *Prog. Méd.*, 1878, p. 746.

of the Swedish Liedbeck machine, but is operated by electricity (Fig. 3).

The effects of vibration will vary with the degree

FIG. 2.

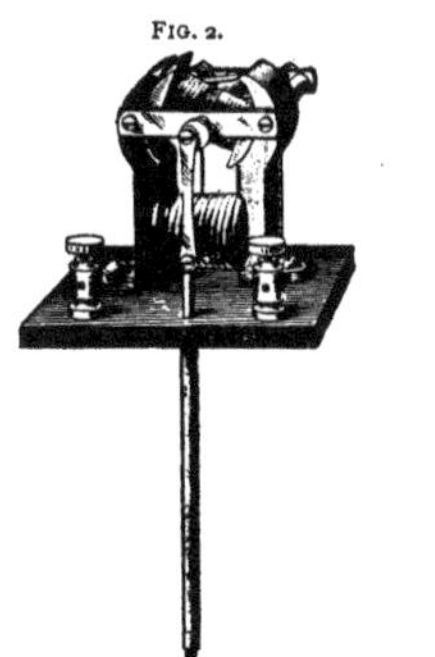

Electric vibrator for nerve trunks.

and duration of the application. A harmful effect may be induced by too prolonged vibration, while

FIG. 3.

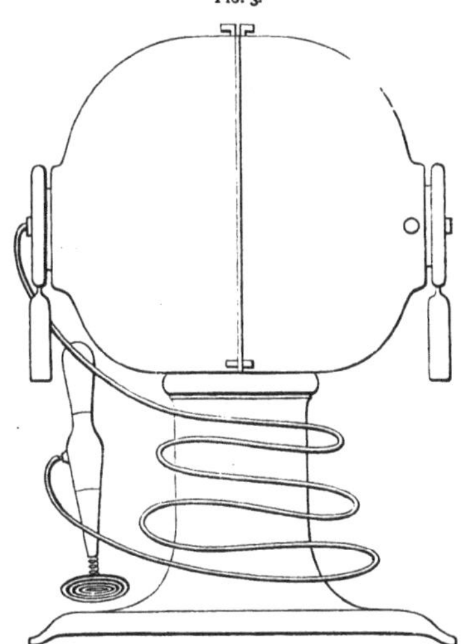

Leidbeck's electric vibrator for general use. It is provided with a number of terminals suitable for application to any part of the body.

moderate vibration has a favorable action, as shown by Meltzer in his experiments on the influence of shaking upon micro-organisms. Prolonged shaking destroyed the germs. Meltzer assumes, and rightly it appears to me, that shaking produces a vibration in the physiologic units of cells. It may be considered an established fact that one of the direct effects of vibration is to modify nutrition in the part treated. Growth is stimulated by mild vibration; strong vibration causes rapid katabolism. The chief virtue of this form of therapeusis lies in its influence upon the nervous system. Applied to the head, the whole skull-wall is shaken, together with the brain, and in a few minutes a pleasant torpor or lassitude is experienced with a tendency to sleep. A ten-minutes' séance will often induce a sound night's sleep in insomnia, and the Charcot school has claimed that eight to ten such séances completely cure insomnia when it is not due to organic brain disease. During the séance a dim monotonous murmur is heard in the ears. On cessation of the tremor sometimes a light vertigo is experienced. Applied to the spine or to large nerve trunks, a similar restful feeling is induced with an inclination to drowsiness. In fact, the effect upon the nervous system is that of a powerful sedative. This is borne out by its use in paralysis agitans, and I can corroborate the statements of the Charcot school that it causes the tremor to diminish, lessens the rigidity, and above all causes the disappearance of one of the nearly insupportable symptoms of Parkinson's disease, the general feeling ot restlessness, malaise, and fatigue. I have tried it in some of the neuralgias of peripheral nerves, in neurasthenic and hysteric conditions and in headaches, I have also made use of vibration in hysteric aphonia and in obstinate ringing in the ears. In all of these conditions its therapeutic effects were marked and valuable.

CLINICAL MEMORANDUM.

A PERSONAL EXPERIENCE IN RENAL SURGERY.

BY ROBERT F. WEIR, M.D.,
OF NEW YORK;
PROFESSOR OF SURGERY IN THE COLLEGE OF PHYSICIANS AND SURGEONS, AND SURGEON TO THE NEW YORK HOSPITAL;
WITH THE COLLABORATION OF
EDWARD M. FOOTE, M.D.,
OF NEW YORK;
SURGEON TO THE RANDALL'S ISLAND HOSPITALS.

(Continued from page 111.)

ABSCESS OF THE KIDNEY.

IN this group of cases are found two of traumatic origin, both of which were treated by means of nephrotomy. The result in one case, a recent one, was perfect. The other patient died within four days of suppression of the urine, and it was found that of the injured kidney only a fragment remained, and that the other one was affected by a diffuse suppurative inflammation. Following these instances, are two of idiopathic abscess, in one of which, originating in a gonorrhea, coli bacillus was extensively found in the minute multiple abscesses of the extirpated organ. Both patients did well after nephrectomy.

Surgical aid has not, I believe, until recently been extended to that form of renal sepsis which is mentioned under the title of "surgical kidney," or suppurative interstitial nephritis. By this is meant the acute infection which often occurs in this viscus from a rapidly ascending inflammation, and which shows itself at the autopsy, for it is always fatal in its results, as a swollen and congested kidney studded with numerous pus foci. The smallest of these are not visible to the eye, but microscopically groups of pus-cells are found between the tubules. Larger purulent streaks surrounded by zones of congestion are also often seen running parallel to the tubules. Great numbers of miliary abscesses may be seen or felt on palpation. In the living kidney it is sometimes difficult to recognize the small purulent collections because of the bleeding of the incised kidney, though their touch often aids the ineffectual vision. Therefore, from its great interest, I venture to report, in a condensed form, the following history of a case of this kind, previously published,[1] wherein the nephrectomy saved the patient's life. It marked an advance in renal surgery, and has since been followed in several instances by German colleagues.

CASE XIX. *Multiple Septic Abscesses of Kidney (Acute Surgical Kidney)—Nephrectomy—Recovery.*—Henry D., aged twenty-five years, entered New York Hospital, March 28, 1894, with a history of nephritis existing for four years, following scarlet fever. One year before admission he had had gonorrhea, and again three months before he had had a second attack of the same disease, the last invading his bladder. The cystitis improved, but twelve days before entrance to the hospital it grew worse, with the development of chills and fever, nausea and vomiting, and pain in the right lumbar region. On April 3d, when I saw him by request of his medical adviser, Dr. P. R. Bolton, he was in a serious condition, with an irregular temperature ranging from 101° to 105°F., and an acid urine containing pus and about twelve per cent. of albumin by volume. The right kidney was very tender and slightly enlarged.

April 4th, by means of König's curved incision, the kidney was exposed. No pus could be obtained by aspiration, but an incision was made into the organ, which was twice its normal size, deeply congested, and softened. It was then seen to be riddled with minute abscesses, and was removed after ligation of the pedicle and ureter with floss silk. The cavity was packed with gauze, and the wound partially closed. The patient left the operating-room in good condition, but collapsed within two hours. Under vigorous stimulation his condition improved, and he gradually became convalescent. The ligature separated within one month. Six weeks after the operation there was still a small amount of pus in the urine, and about eight or ten per cent. of albumin by volume, but there were no symptoms referable to the bladder. He was discharged in good condition with a superficial granulating wound in his loin. Cultures from the nephritic abscesses developed colonies of the bacillus coli communis, but none of the gonococcus. The kidney measured 14x6.5x4.5 inches. The patient made a complete recovery, and when heard from, three weeks later, was in good condition.

In this patient, the mass of symptoms being confined to one side, led me to believe that the infection was limited to this kidney alone. This determined the extirpation. As to the frequency one may expect to find an infection of this character similarly located, the investigation I made of the material of New York and St. Luke's hospitals showed that in forty-five cases of true surgical kidney (large single or multiple abscesses and those of chronic form being excluded), in six instances it presented itself as a one-sided lesion. Malherbe and Bazy also found twenty-six cases of this disease in which six were one-sided. In other words, in about seventeen per cent. of all the cases the affection is confined to one kidney. Even if both sides are affected a double incision might give the otherwise doomed patient a chance.

CASE XX. *Laceration of the Kidney—Pyelonephritis—Nephrotomy—Recovery.*—Mary O., aged twenty-six years, married, was admitted to New York Hospital, October 6, 1884. During the previous May she had had a miscarriage, with persistent uterine hemorrhages and attacks of abdominal inflammation. Her symptoms had disappeared by August 15th. One month later, just after a menstrual period, she again began to have pain in the abdomen, with nausea and fever. Urination was frequent and painful, and the urine contained pus, casts, and blood. The patient denied having received any injury. A needle thrust into a swelling in the right iliac region drew pus. The nature of the swelling, which extended from the liver almost to the ilium and was nearly five inches broad, was in doubt. A second and third punctures, made on different days, produced only blood.

Meanwhile her condition was comfortable and the urine nearly normal, though the temperature continued to reach 105° F. each day. On the fifth day after entrance pus was again obtained, and the patient was etherized for operation. Her physician, who was present to witness the operation, then furnished the important information that ten days before coming to the hospital Mrs. P. was kicked in the side by a person whom she was unwilling to implicate, and that for two days she passed bloody urine. In the hope that the abscess might be perinephritic an incision was made over the outer border of the tumor. This proved to be an unfavorable point of attack, and after the peritoneum had been opened and the inflamed kidney palpated the wound was closed and an incision made along the edge of the quadratus lumborum muscle. There was no perinephritic deposit of pus, but the kidney, when exposed, was found so softened by suppuration that the finger could easily be poked through it in one place into a gangrenous cavity, while a jagged rent ran from this downward along the border of the organ, evidently a laceration from the kick she had received. The cavity was drained, and within one month the wound was entirely healed. The tumor rapidly diminished from the time of operation, but two months afterward there was still some hardness at the region of its lower portion, due presumably to post-operative perinephritic inflammation.

CASE XXI. *Laceration of the Kidney—Perinephritic Abscess and Renal Fistula—Nephrotomy and Subsequent Nephrectomy—Death.*—Bernard M., aged twenty years, entered New York Hospital during the fall of 1886. Three years previously he had fallen six feet and struck his right side upon an iron bar. Hematuria, followed by local pain, swelling, and fever showed an in-

[1] Weir, *Trans. Am. Surg. Ass.*, vol. 12, p. 121, 1894.

jury to the kidney, resulting in an abscess. An incision was made into this by my colleague, Dr. Bull, and a large amount of pus evacuated. The resulting sinus healed, but subsequently opened several times. Since July, 1886, the pain in the flank and in the rectum prevented the patient from going about. Examination showed a large fistulous opening in the right loin midway between the ribs and ilium. From this, a probe passed nine inches downward into the iliac fossa along a tract which was both indurated and tender. Near this fistula was another leading toward the kidney to a depth of four inches. These openings discharged from four to six ounces of pus daily. Rectal examination was negative. The urine was slightly albuminous, and contained a few pus-cells. The daily excretion was from fifty to sixty ounces. The patient's condition was poor. He was steadily deteriorating in general health.

Under ether, a curved incision passing through both fistulæ was made through tissues matted together by old inflammation, and a cavity was opened through the thin wall of which the movements of the abdominal viscera were plainly felt. The sinus into the iliac fossa was then laid open, and another one extending into the pelvis was also drained. Examination of the cavity with an electric lamp showed a rent in its wall three inches long through which the liver and gall-bladder were visible. As no kidney had as yet been found, search was made for it through this opening into the peritoneal cavity, but no trace of it was discovered. The rent was closed with catgut sutures, and the wounds filled with gauze. Death occurred four days later. There was a marked rise of temperature forty-eight hours after the operation, followed by persistent vomiting and almost complete suppression of urine.

At the autopsy, the left kidney was found in a state of acute suppurative interstitial inflammation with pus under its capsule. There was no peritonitis. The lower two-thirds of the right kidney had entirely disappeared. The upper portion of the cavity referred to was formed by what was left of the kidney. In this cavity were two sponges, which had been crowded in to control hemorrhage, and had been left *in situ*. One of them was firmly adherent. They had not given any foul odor to the discharge. The sinus leading into the pelvis terminated behind in a pus-cavity, which led to the bladder and rectum and also extended through the right sacrosciatic notch, outside of which pus had collected to the amount of nearly two ounces.[1]

CASE XXII. *Pyonephrosis — Nephrotomy — Recovery.*—Emma T., aged forty years, suffered some months from indefinite dragging pains, followed by a sudden attack of severe lumbar pain in the right side. After this attack a tumor was for the first time observed, and the patient entered the hospital. In the right lower quadrant of the abdominal cavity could be detected a tumor the size of a child's head, not moving on respiration, and nearer than usual to the median line. The urine was of neutral reaction, had a mucus sediment, a specific gravity of 1014, and contained a trace of albumin. There were a few leucocytes and epithelial cells in the sediment. Owing to some doubt as to the origin of the tumor, on October 4, 1896, a small exploratory incision was made and showed it to be a greatly dilated kidney. The abdominal wound was closed, and the usual curved incision made in the loin. The sides of the wound were smeared with Whitehead's solution of tincture of benzoin and iodoform, and the kidney incised. About three pints of pus escaped. A probe was passed eighteen inches down the ureter, but it could not be detected in the bladder. There was no evidence of stone. The kidney was drained by means of iodoform gauze and two rubber tubes, and the wound partially sutured.

Recovery from the operation ensued. The wound discharged much pus and was dressed daily. Within fifteen days one tube was removed, and the other within about four weeks. Within eight weeks the lumbar wound had entirely healed, and the patient went home. For a time after the operation the urine was free from pus and albumin; but within a month, when the discharge from the loin had greatly diminished, there was a daily passage of forty-two to fifty-two ounces of urine containing a trace of albumin and having a mucopurulent sediment of from one to two ounces. In December, 1897, the patient was in excellent health, suffering no pain on the affected side, and urinating clear urine four or five times daily. There was no enlargement of the kidney to be felt, and no weakness of the cicatrix.

HYDRONEPHROSIS.

In the days of the Lister spray, now nearly forgotten, though less than twenty years have passed, a patient (Case XXIII.) came to me complaining of a lumbar swelling which proved, upon aspiration, to be a hydronephrosis. This puncture was followed by an incision and drainage, and after several superficial abscesses had been opened in the cicatrix the patient recovered. The case has been already reported,[1] but it is here again epitomized, not only for the sake of completing the record, but also for its historic interest, since, somewhat to my surprise, it has been recorded by Brodeur[2] as the first operation ever resorted to for a hydronephrosis. Two other cases, in each of which the tumor was of large size, are also in our list, one of which was before the date of Fenger's suggestion to save the kidney, if possible, by anastomosing the ureter below the stenosis to the renal pelvis above. The second one, however, in my judgment, promised so little, that extirpation was resorted to. Indeed, I do not think when such a thinned and interstitially changed renal substance is met with, as in a large hydronephrosis, any benefit can be obtained by conservative means. With hydronephrosis confined to the pelvis or only moderately involving the kidney tissue anastomotic procedures come properly into use.

CASE XXIII. *Hydronephrosis — Nephrotomy—Recovery.*—John W., aged twenty-one years. Soon after an attack of vague abdominal pain he noticed a slight swelling in the left iliac region, and when he entered New York Hospital, November 1, 1878, the tumefaction extended well up the side and downward to the ilium. Two ounces of limpid fluid, of a specific gravity of 1012, was withdrawn. No urea nor echinococcic hooklets were found in it. A second tapping, withdrawing twelve ounces of fluid, resulted in similar findings.

As the tumor increased to a considerable size, an

---

[1] There has been omitted from the above list of kidney lacerations one which occurred in a girl aged eleven years, who fell twenty feet, striking the left side on a bar. Laparotomy was resorted to twenty hours later, as her general condition warranted interference for the supposed displaced intestine. Much blood was found in the peritoneal cavity, and the kidney was found to be dislocated downward with its hilus and ureter torn across, the artery remaining intact, forming a huge hematoma. This organ was removed, but the bleeding still continued. A further search revealed that the blood came from a badly torn spleen. The damage necessitated the removal of this gland. Temporary improvement with death at the end of nine hours was the result.

[1] Weir, *Med. Record*, March 13, 1880.

[2] Brodeur, "De l'Intervention Chirurgicale Dans Les Affections Du Rein, 1886."

incision was made, December 20, 1878, in the loin, as for lumbar colotomy, and a dilated kidney exposed. This was punctured to the depth of one-quarter of an inch, and two pints of a semi-transparent fluid freely escaped. A drainage-tube was inserted, the outer end of which communicated with a rubber bag filled with carbolized sponges, covered with carbolized jute. The operation was made under carbolic spray. The following day the ureter was explored by my flexible metallic probe, used then for the first time, to a depth of nine inches from the surface wound, but no calculus was found. During April, 1879, the drainage-tube was removed, and the wound was allowed to close. Four times an abscess formed in the scar, and was lanced. After that recovery was complete. There were no symptoms referable to the urinary tract, and no tumor could be felt. All attempts to learn the subsequent history of this patient have failed.

CASE XXIV. *Hydronephrosis — Nephrectomy — Recovery.*—Joseph G., aged fifteen years, presented the following history: For a long time he had noticed that his abdomen was growing larger, particularly on the right side, but there was no pain, and no urinary symptoms. There had been increasing loss of flesh and strength, but no history of colic or ureteral obstruction. March 7, 1891, two months before his entrance to New York Hospital, the greatly dilated hydronephrotic sac had been incised in the lumbar region by my colleague, Dr. W. T. Bull, and several pints of a clear fluid evacuated. The urine before the nephrotomy had been pale, alkalin, of a specific gravity of 1013, and with a faint trace of albumin, but no sediment. The hydronephrotic fluid was of a specific gravity of 1009, and contained about one-half the amount of urea contained in normal urine.

The sinus persisted, discharging freely, and led to a cavity capable of holding 1½ pints of fluid, and on May 9, 1891, the sinus was enlarged above and below to a width of four-fifths of an inch, and its cavity exposed. It was found to consist of a thin-walled sac, with occasional traces of kidney tissue, reaching from the iliac fossa to the diaphragm. It was dissected out, its vessels and ureter, the last being an obliterated cord for more than two inches, separately tied, and the organ removed. The patient made a good recovery. At first, the quantity of urine voided from the bladder was below the normal, as it had been before this second operation, but soon it increased in amount from thirty-six to forty-five ounces daily. It contained a few casts for some days.

The patient gained flesh and strength, and left the hospital three weeks after the nephrectomy in good condition with the wound completely closed. He was seen during December, 1897, in good health. The scar was double, the straight one being along the quadratus lumborum muscle, and the oblique one parallel to the twelfth rib and about five inches long. Between the anterior end of this and the rib, on coughing and expulsive effort, a decided hernial bulging could be observed. However, no muscular weakness could be felt on that side.

CASE XXV. *Hydronephrosis — Nephrectomy — Recovery.*—Miss B., aged twenty-two years, a patient of Dr. A. Cushier, noticed, four years before operation, a swelling in the right lumbar region. This increased with, and was accompanied by, a dragging sensation in the back, and occasional attacks of sharp pain, but no urinary symptoms. Upon entrance to the hospital, the temperature was 99.8° F.; respiration, 22, and pulse, 80. The urine had a specific gravity of 1023. It was acid, without albumin or sugar, and its sediment presented nothing abnormal. The swelling in the lumbar region was the size of a cocoanut.

October 19, 1896, the tumor was exposed by a crescentic incision. It proved to be a large hydronephrotic cyst of the kidney. With a trocar and canula about twenty ounces of clear urinous fluid was withdrawn, and the cyst was opened. A long flexible probe inserted into the ureter, down to brim of the pelvis, detected no stricture, nor was the cause of the hydronephrosis discovered. Some difficulty was encountered in passing the probe, but much help was given by turning the dilated kidney inside out until the pelvis was recognized. As the kidney substance was generally reduced to an extreme thinness, and as it was much degenerated, it was determined to extirpate the organ. It was readily detached from its bed, and after the vessels and ureter were ligated, it was removed. As is my late custom after a nephrectomy, the cavity of the wound was lined with a Mikulicz "bag," or layer of iodoform gauze, six-tenths per cent., and inside of this was packed quite forcibly sundry handkerchiefs of sterile gauze, the ends of which emerged from the unsewed portion of the wound. This controls admirably any oozing, and the interior packing is removed at the end of one or two days, and the iodoform gauze a little later. The patient made a good recovery, except for a moderate sero-hemorrhagic discharge into the dressings, which occurred within the first twenty-four hours and persisted as a bloody grumous discharge for ten days. There was at first a very small amount of urine passed, but this reached thirty-eight ounces on the third day, and was nearly normal in character, having only a slight trace of albumin, which later disappeared.

The examination of the excised kidney showed it to be greatly distended and hydronephrotic, and to be made up of several cysts. The kidney tissue left was slight in amount and showed to a marked degree, on microscopic examination, chronic inflammatory changes. The ligature remained attached for seven weeks, and was only removed by means of my rubber-ball tractor,[1] which need not be described as it has been superseded by the better methods of Cleveland and Grad, to be referred to later. The patient was heard from fifteen months afterward, and she had gained in strength and was in good condition.

(To be continued.)

THERAPEUTIC NOTES.

Treatment of Metrorrhagia.—CONNERY (*Intercollegiate Med. Jour.*, December, 1897) speaks of the importance of an exact knowledge of the cause of metrorrhagia before treatment is attempted. He calls attention to the fact that cardiac, hepatic, or renal diseases have frequently produced metrorrhagia, although uterine disorder has been absent or slight. In such cases diaphoretic remedies should be given, according to the condition of the patient. Reliable remedies for checking hemorrhage are few. Hydrastis Canadensis is of value in many cases, and is too little known. Quinin and strychnin administered alone or in combination will often arrest hemorrhage in cases associated with debility. Absolute rest in a horizontal position and vaginal douches with the water at a temperature of 110° to 115° F., will often suffice to control hemorrhage. If in spite of treatment the bleeding continues without assignable cause, the cavity of the uterus should be explored; for a bleeding polyp or submucous fibroid has been known to produce death by loss of blood, although in itself it may be a comparatively trivial affair.

[1] Weir, MED. NEWS, April 3, 1897.

THE MEDICAL NEWS.

A WEEKLY JOURNAL

OF MEDICAL SCIENCE.

COMMUNICATIONS are invited from all parts of the world. Original articles contributed *exclusively* to THE MEDICAL NEWS will after publication be liberally paid for (accounts being rendered quarterly), or 250 reprints will be furnished in place of other remuneration. When necessary to elucidate the text, illustrations will be engraved from drawings or photographs furnished by the author. Manuscripts should be typewritten.

Address the Editor: J. RIDDLE GOFFE, M.D.,
No. 111 FIFTH AVENUE (corner of 18th St.), NEW YORK.

Subscription Price, including postage in U. S. and Canada.

PER ANNUM IN ADVANCE	$4.00
SINGLE COPIES	.10
WITH THE AMERICAN JOURNAL OF THE MEDICAL SCIENCES, PER ANNUM	7.50

Subscriptions may begin at any date. The safest mode of remittance is by bank check or postal money order, drawn to the order of the undersigned. When neither is accessible, remittances may be made, at the risk of the publishers, by forwarding in *registered* letters.

LEA BROTHERS & CO.,
No. 111 FIFTH AVENUE (corner of 18th St.), NEW YORK,
AND NOS. 706, 708 & 710 SANSOM ST., PHILADELPHIA.

SATURDAY, JANUARY 29, 1898.

PHILADELPHIA'S TYPHOID-FEVER EPIDEMIC; WHERE DOES THE RESPONSIBILITY LIE?

PHILADELPHIA, at the present moment, furnishes the unfortunate spectacle of a community of considerably more than one million souls needlessly plunged into a rapidly spreading and thus far unchecked epidemic of enteric fever, and absolutely helpless to rid herself of the pest because of the refusal of her city legislators to cooperate with the health authorities, and to provide a water-supply which may be used with safety. For months, yes, for years, Common and Select Councils, the governing bodies of that city, have been importuned to pass an ordinance for the establishment of a filtration-plant. The long-standing high mortality in Philadelphia from typhoid fever should have resulted years ago in the erection of filtering-stations and adequate storage-basins for the improvement of the water-supply, but the members of Councils, true to their traditions as professional politicians, have steadfastly declined to provide these safeguards to the health of citizens whose interests they are popularly supposed to represent—failed to provide the safeguard simply and solely because they were unable to effect among themselves, in taking such a step, a sufficiently remunerative plan for the division of the spoils attending the undertaking; for is not such remuneration, after all, the actual *raison d'être* of the vast majority of city law-makers of this brand? Thus it is that through the criminal neglect of this group of spoilsmen the present epidemic of enteric fever, for an epidemic it certainly is, has been needlessly inflicted upon our neighbors in Philadelphia, who must suffer physical ills and loss of life, unable to avert the danger by appeals to their representatives in Councils, and chafing under an injustice which carries with it a feeling of personal insult to every self-respecting citizen.

Since the beginning of the present outbreak, the first week of last December, 1134 new cases of enteric fever have been reported in the City of Philadelphia, and of this number 675 have occurred during the first four weeks of the new year, or an average of more than 168 new cases weekly up to the present time. As a striking comparison, we may state that during two weeks of the present month New York City—exclusive of Brooklyn, etc.—with a population twice that of Philadelphia, reported a total of 36 new cases of typhoid, while Philadelphia for the corresponding period, reported no less than 366 new cases! To further the comparison, two wards in the infected district of Philadelphia, having a combined total population of 100,000, in *one* week surpassed the total roll of enteric-fever cases reported among the 2,000,000 inhabitants of New York City for a period of *two* weeks. To make the contrast still plainer, in one recent week in New York City, only six new cases of typhoid were reported from the densely populated tenement districts below Fourteenth street, where the nature of the surroundings and mode of life offer every advantage to the development of filth-diseases. On the other hand, the section of Philadelphia in which typhoid is most prevalent is an area not of crowded tenements and of indifferent hygienic environment, but of separate, small dwellings, occupied, as a rule, each by a single family, and pronounced by the corps of health inspectors, which have just investigated the neighborhood, admirably drained and perfect as to all sanitary appliances.

As to the cause of the epidemic there is no uncertainty. The Schuylkill River, from which the greater part of Philadelphia's water-supply is derived, is polluted from end to end, and this foul, sewage-laden water is served, unpurified, to the patient tax-payer. Last November an accident occurred by which sewage was pumped directly into a reservoir, and thence into the city water-mains to the consumer; and this accident seems to have been a principal cause of the present outbreak. It is also known that further up the river typhoid is on the increase, and this adds another factor to the cause of the epidemic. But to enumerate these causes is of no avail. The Schuylkill is polluted, and every one has known the fact for years. Every one also knows that the practical remedy for the situation is either through filtration or an entirely new source of the water-supply. The majority of voters expressed in unmistakable terms their approval of filtration by the creation of a loan-bill last fall which empowered the city to borrow a large sum for general municipal improvements, including the sum of $3,700,000 for the immediate improvement and filtration of the water-supply; and yet, in spite of the fact that money is available for the project, that the people urgently favor it, and that the city health-officers heartily endorse the scheme, Councils persist in ignoring the situation, and criminally delay the appropriation of the money at their disposal to provide adequate filtration-plants for the city. Pleas, arguments, and merited censure on the part of the citizens at large, the daily press, and the medical profession, have failed to convince this body of its imperative duty, and the members continue to snap their thumbs at measures of public safety by suggesting that an appeal be made to the Government for aid in dealing with the epidemic, instead of acting without hesitancy in accord with the demands made upon them from every side. They richly deserve for their utter incompetency in all legislation save that pertaining to their individual enrichment, the desecration which is heaped upon them by the entire community.

THE BROOKLYN WATER-SUPPLY LABORATORY ABOLISHED.

WE regret to notice that the Rockville Center Research-Depot has been abolished by the Board of Health. It was established a little over a year ago, with infinite pains, by the then Commissioner of Health for Brooklyn, Dr. Emery, and was doing good work for the protection of the water-supply at a comparatively slight outlay of public money. It was the contention of Dr. Emery that the proper location for an institution of this nature is upon the watershed itself and that the chemic and bacteriologic researches should be accompanied by frequent inspections of all suspected feeders and ponds. The investigations have been conducted by Dr. H. Hill, formerly in the employ of the Louisville Water-Supply Commission, an expert in bacteriology, assisted by Dr. Ellms, chemist. Dr. Ezra H. Wilson, who recently resigned from the Health Department to give his sole attention to the work of the Hoagland Laboratory, was for a time in charge of the Rockville biologic work, but latterly was appointed to the honorary position of consulting bacteriologist. The names of these three officials are signed to an important report of two hundred pages setting forth the organization and results of the laboratory. This report is replete with tabular and other technical matters, and will be especially valuable to water-biologists and engineers; it may without exaggeration be characterized as a "State paper" of permanent value. As the new charter of New York City places the sanitary supervision of the water-supplies in the Board of Health, it is to be hoped, that this important function will not be slighted. It is beyond doubt a mistaken policy to neglect this line of sanitary work until the water becomes suspected or polluted, and popular panic and outcry, to say nothing of decimating epidemics, make its resumption necessary. It is true that there is a water laboratory belonging to the Water Bureau of the Borough of Brooklyn, but it is located remote from the water sources, being within the "city limits," near Prospect Park. That kind of a research-department, however, cannot be considered as competent to "fill the bill," and furthermore its position as an appendage to the Wate Bureau—where quantity rather than quality is eve the criterion—is unfortunate from the sanitary stand point. It is a relic of antiquated methods which doe not inspire confidence.

"HOW TO ELEVATE THE PROFESSION IN TH COUNTRY."

WHILE the city physician is disturbed by the dis pensary abuse, which threatens to take away hi livelihood, his country brother is menaced, accord ing to a writer in the *Charlotte Medical Journal*, by a still more dreadful fate—self-extermination. This writer speaks especially of North Georgia and East Tennessee, where the customary fee for obstetric cases is $5, and other charges in about the same proportion. It is justly maintained that the larger the territory in which a man practises, the more difficult it is for him to keep up with his profession, and the writer tells us that we ought to express neither surprise nor resentment when we learn that one of his colleagues (a "Doc," as he calls him) attempted to perform craniotomy with his pocket-knife and a pair of rusty scissors. By and by Nature delivered the woman and the baby lived for a week before yielding to the effects of craniotomy.

One cannot help sympathizing with a writer who says: "I don't see how a physician can wait on a case of obstetrics aseptically and antiseptically, and keep his eyes on the case till all danger of septicemia is past for $5, the case being anywhere from two to eight miles from his office."

But even this sad condition has its remedy, and when the doctor returns with (out?) his V., he writes: "I believe that if the Legislature would pass a law making it a penitentiary offence for a physician to wait on a case of obstetrics for less than $10, in the country, they would do more to benefit humanity and to evolute the world toward what God intends it shall be than was ever done before at a single stroke."

ECHOES AND NEWS.

Mothers' and Babies' Hospital of New York.—It is reported that this vigorous young infant has secured a lease of the building owned by Dr. T. Gaillard Thomas and recently occupied by him as a private sanitarium.

Smallpox in the United States.—The Marine Hospital Service reports the existence of an epidemic of smallpox at Birmingham, Ala. One hundred and thirty-one patients with this disease are now under treatment at that place.

Damages for a Druggist's Mistake.—The Supreme Court of Brooklyn, N. Y., recently awarded a verdict of $5000 to a widow for the accidental poisoning of her husband by a druggist who sold oxalic acid for Carlsbad salts.

Sudden Death of a Physician.—The death by shooting of Dr. Charles B. Day of Glencoe, Minn., is reported by telegram. He was an alumnus, of the class of 1889, of the College of Physicians and Surgeons of New York.

A Brooklyn Appointment.—Dr. John Griffin has been appointed to a commissionership in the Brooklyn Department of Public Instruction, a position formerly held by him for many years. Dr. Griffin was for a period of four years the health-officer of that city.

The Meeting of the State Society.—The recent meeting of the State Society at Albany was marked by a large attendance, and the members evinced great interest in proposed medical laws, the Dispensary Bill coming in for a large share of their attention.

The Obstetrical Society of Cincinnati.—At a recent meeting of this society the following officers were elected: President, Dr. E. S. McKee; vice-president, Dr. W. D. Porter; recording secretary, Dr. Wm. Gillespie; corresponding secretary, Dr. M. A. Tate; treasurer, Dr. George E. Jones; librarian, Dr. Bonnifield.

A Celestial Remedy.—A "hedge doctor," a kind of quack in Ireland, was being examined at an inquest on his treatment of a patient who had died. "I gave him ipecacuanha," he said. "You might just as well have given him the Aurora Borealis," said the coroner. "Indade, yer honor, and that's just what I should have given him next, if he hadn't died."

A Free Supply of Diphtheria Antitoxin for the Sick Poor of London.—The London Metropolitan Asylums Board has resolved that a supply of antitoxin shall be placed in the hands of the medical officer of health under its control for free distribution to any general practitioner who may be called upon to attend and treat patients unable to obtain admission into the board's hospitals. The board has made arrangements for a supply of antitoxic serum from the laboratories of the Royal College of Physicians and Surgeons.

Cure for Hog Cholera.—The Chief of the Bureau of Animal Industry, Dr. D. E. Salmon, has submitted his report upon the experiments made in the treatment of hog cholera with antitoxic serum. The report shows the most encouraging results. The cost of the serum is only 10 cents per head for animals treated, and inasmuch as the losses from hog cholera are enormous it is proposed to ask Congress to appropriate funds to enable the department to furnish 2,000,000 doses of the serum during the coming year.

Resolutions upon the Death of Dr. O'Dwyer.—Resolutions upon the death of Dr. O'Dwyer have been placed upon the minutes of all the various institutions with which he was connected. Copies of these tributes have been received for publication by the MEDICAL NEWS. They are so similar in their character that their publication hardly seems necessary. The glowing tribute published in the MEDICAL NEWS of last week, together with the announcement of the resolutions above referred to, afford becoming recognition of the loss sustained by the profession in the death of Dr. O'Dwyer.

Quinin in India.—Brigade Surgeon Lieutenant-Colonel George King, of the Indian Army, has gained his reputation as Superintendent of the Royal Botanic Gardens at Calcutta, particularly in connection with the practical cultivation of quinin. The British Government formerly imported yearly $250,000 worth of quinin until, after many experiments, Dr. King succeeded in the cultivation of the cinchona tree. There are now 4,000,000 trees in Bengal and every rural post-office in India sells a five-grain packet of the drug for half a cent, while the government makes about $3500 a year out of the profits.

Christian Science.—A "practitioner" of Christian Science of Kansas City, has recently been fined for not reporting a case of diphtheria to the Board of Health of that place. After a course of "Christian Science" the little patient having the disease died. The judge, before whom the case was tried, is reported to have said that "the methods of Christian Science in attempting to heal are frequently akin to murder." He might have gone a bit farther and said: "are murder," and then not have been very wide of the mark. The question is, how long will a civilized community tolerate this variety of baneful charlatanry?

Deaths after Christenings and Funerals in Winter.—At a recent London coroner's inquest the fact was brought out that in two cases children had died from pneumonia after having been taken to church to be christened. The coroner said he was in the habit of warning parents that all very young children should be most carefully wrapped up when they are taken out of the house, in winter weather, for any such purpose. Then, again, winter funerals are not without their dangers, as is pointed out by one of our contemporaries in the following paragraph: "Do not take off your hat at a funeral in winter when standing by the grave." At the funeral of Sir Frank Lockwood, M. P., a few weeks ago, another influential member of the Liberal Party, Mr. Charles Harrison, took cold and died within two days.

France Encourages Paternity.—The National Society for the Increase of the Population of France has just held an extraordinary meeting under the presidence of M. Jacques Bertillon. A resolution, adopted unanimously, was to the effect that as forty-seven of the General Councils of France had approved the program of the society, all electors at the coming general elections in the spring of 1898, and especially those who are the fathers of families, should be invited to demand of their candidates, to whatever political party they might belong, to inscribe in their program: (1) A reduction of taxation in proportion to the number of children; (2) the application of the same principle in all financial laws and in the succession duties; (3) the favoring by the State of large families from an administrative and military point of view.

Ambulance System in Jeopardy.—The ambulance system of the Borough of Brooklyn is in a position of uncertainty regarding its supply of the sinews of war. It is understood that the new charter of our greater city makes no provision for the appropriation that was for many years granted by the Board of Estimate. At seven of the hospitals ambulance stations are maintained at considerable cost, for the support of which the authorities have been in the habit of granting $1200 per annum. New legislation will probably be necessary to make it possible for this aid to be continued. The so-called city ambulances, three in number, were maintained by the health-officer at an annual cost of about $8000, inclusive of supplies. If the first interpretation of the new charter is correct there are no funds available for, or convertible to, the support of this branch of the public service.

Death-Rate of the Spanish Army in Cuba.—Inspector-General Losada, of the Spanish forces in Cuba, issued his official report about the middle of last month in which is indicated losses almost without precedent in modern times. His report shows that out of the 200,000 soldiers sent by Spain to put down the insurrection in the island from the beginning of February, 1895, to the beginning of December of the year just terminated, not more than 53,-000 (a little over one-fourth) are at this moment fit for active service. The 147,000 are either dead or sent back to the motherland ill or wounded. The causes of this unprecedented death-rate and sick-list are (besides casualties in action) mainly three: (1) the inappropriateness of the clothing furnished to the European troops; (2) fatigue; and (3) lack of food. "The report, which does not apparently err on the score of reticence, paints a lurid picture of military service in the chief Spanish colony. Under successive generals the three-years' campaign, in spite of numberless Royalist "victories," leaves Cuba as precarious a Spanish possession as ever; while a whole generation must intervene before island and motherland alike can recover from the loss of blood, property, and treasures.

Yellow Fever and the Philadelphia Local Quarantine.—I was recently and quite confidently reported in the lay press of Philadelphia that yellow fever had succeeded in passing the Government Quarantine-Station at Reedy Island (see "Our Philadelphia Letter" of this week), i consequence of which the competency of the Marine Hospital Service to properly guard the City of Philadelphia from imported infections has been seriously questioned That the report in question is fallacious we confidentl believe, and not without good ground, as the followin statement from Surgeon-General Wyman of the Marin Hospital Service will prove: "The Government Quarantine-Station at Reedy Island is located near the middle o the Delaware River. Occasionally the ice is so thic that it is impossible to board incoming vessels at thi point, and at such times a medical officer is sent to boar vessels in the harbor near Philadelphia from the revenu cutter. The local quarantine-station is situated at Marcus Hook some miles above the Reedy Island station. O January 19th the schooner 'Tingue' entered the harbo and was stopped at Marcus Hook, and it was stated b the Philadelphia papers that this vessel had cases of yel low fever on board. A medical officer of the Marin Hospital Service, an expert on yellow fever, was at onc sent to make an investigation, and reported that 'th cases are not yellow fever.' Furthermore, the 'Tingue would have been inspected by a national officer befor being allowed to enter the port." Signed, W. WYMAN Surgeon-General, Marine Hospital Service.

CORRESPONDENCE.

OUR PHILADELPHIA LETTER.

[From our Special Correspondent.]

A SENSATION IN QUARANTINE CIRCLES—ERADICATION OF BOVINE TUBERCULOSIS—CHARITY FOR WIDOWS AND CHILDREN OF DECEASED PHYSICIANS—PROFESSIONAL POLITICS AND THE HEALTH-OFFICER OF PHILADELPHIA—CONTROL OF THE EPIDEMIC OF ENTERIC FEVER—MENTAL CONDITION OF A YOUTHFUL MURDERER—DR. PEPPER'S ILLNESS—CÆSARIAN SECTION—CONGENITAL MALFORMATION OF GENITALIA—FIBROID TUMORS—TYPHOID FEVER ON THE INCREASE.

PHILADELPHIA, January 22, 1898.

QUITE *a sensation in local quarantine circles* was caused a few days ago by the arrival in the Delaware River of a vessel from a West Indian port with, it was said, yellow-fever cases aboard. Official reticence masks the true nature of the infection, but the general trend of public opinion stamps the infection yellow fever, particularly because of the fact that this disease is just at present epidemic at Jamaica, from which island the vessel hails. Yellow fever or not, the ease with which the ship managed to pass the lower river quarantine-stations to be finally held up by the State inspectors of vessels at a point just below the city has called down some caustic criticism upon the present régime at the Marine Hospital Quarantine Station in Delaware Bay, through whose fingers the fever ship slipped with so little effort. The incident illustrates, too, the fact that Philadelphia is none too well protected from the ravages of imported epidemics, and that our triple quarantine system is none too elaborate if the health of the city is to be maintained. [See "Echoes and News," page 150, for reply of the Marine Hospital Service.—ED.]

The report to the Department of Agriculture on the work carried on by Dr. Leonard Pearson, the State Veterinarian, and his associates, *in eradicating bovine tuberculosis and other contagious diseases of animals*, shows that during 1897, 16,000 animals were subjected to the tuberculin test, with the result that 2500 were condemned as tuberculous and killed. The same report also shows that equally important work has been done by these officials in dealing with the recent local outbreak of anthrax in the western part of the State, and that thorough investigations have been pursued for the purpose of eradicating rabies, hog cholera, and other animal infections.

At a meeting to be held on January 26th, at the College of Physicians, the members of the Mutual Aid Association of the Philadelphia County Medical Society hope to arouse a more general interest among both the medical profession and the laity in the efforts being made by the association *in extending the hand of charity to the indigent widows and families of deceased physicians*. At this meeting Dr. Charles A. Leale, President of the New York Society for the Relief of Widows and Orphans of Medical Men, will give an account of the work pursued by that body; Dr. A. F. Currier of New York will deliver an address on "The Fifty-five Years of the New York Society for the Relief of Widows and Orphans of Medical Men." Other prominent speakers of the evening will be the Rev. Dr. Charles Wood, the Rev. Dr. Joseph Krauskopf, and Drs. Edward Jackson, Charles Hermon Thomas, and John B. Roberts. At the close of the meeting a reception will be tendered the invited guests by the Association, at the University Club.

At a business meeting of the Philadelphia County Medical Society, held January 19th, the following important resolution, *apropos* of the *fight now being made to divorce from professional politics the position of Health-Officer of Philadelphia*, was adopted: "*Resolved*, That the Philadelphia County Medical Society believes that the best interests of the City of Philadelphia and of the State of Pennsylvania will be conserved by the appointment of an educated physician as Health-Officer. *Resolved*, That the secretary forward to the Governor of Pennsylvania a copy of this resolution, with the request that he give thoughtful consideration to the opinion of the society thus formally expressed." Regarding the necessity for taking *immediate steps to control the widespread epidemic of enteric fever* now prevailing in this city, the society "*Resolved*, That a committee be appointed to wait upon the mayor and councils and urge the necessity of immediate steps for the filtration of the water-supply of the city, in view of its responsibility for the prevalence of typhoid fever in the city." The society then took up the question of the publication in a medical periodical of its proceedings, and it was voted to enter into a contract for the present year with *The Philadelphia Polyclinic* by which this journal, on mutually advantageous terms, is to undertake the publication in its columns of the proceedings of the society, at regular intervals. The contract of a similar nature heretofore existing with *The Medical and Surgical Reporter* was abrogated. The following officers for the ensuing year were elected: President, Dr. Edward Jackson; first vice-president, Dr. S. Solis-Cohen; second vice-president, Dr. John H. Musser; secretary, Dr. John Lindsay; assistant secretary, Dr. Elwood R. Kirby; treasurer, Dr. Collier L. Bower; censor, Dr. William M. Welch. Six new members were elected, and the names of thirty-seven candidates for membership were reported favorably by the Censors.

Drs. Thomas J. Morton and John B. Chapin, the well-known alienists, have been appointed by the Court to *examine into the mental condition of Samuel Henderson, the fifteen-year-old murderer*, the revolting details of whose crime has already been given wide publicity by the daily press. The inquiry into the matter is to begin at once, and it is thought that the expert report rendered will largely influence the course to be taken by the authorities when the case comes to trial.

DR. WILLIAM PEPPER, *who has lately been confined to his house with an attack of la grippe*, has so far convalesced that he is able to undertake a journey to the South where he expects to fully recuperate. During his absence Dr. Alfred Stengel is filling the Chair of Practice of Medicine in the University of Pennsylvania.

The condition of Dr. Theophilus Parvin *is so serious that grave doubts of his recovery are expressed*. It is said that recent vesical complications and pulmonary edema have supervened to complicate the renal lesions from which he suffers. The lectures on obstetrics at the Jefferson Medical College are being delivered by Dr. Edward P. Davis, during Dr. Parvin's absence.

The appointment of Dr. W. E. Robertson *as demonstrator of bacteriology* in the Medico-Chirugical College is announced.

Commencing with the current number the *International Medical Magazine is to be published under a new management.* The editorship of this journal, formerly under the charge of Dr. Henry W. Cattell, has been assumed by Dr. Walter L. Pyle. It is understood that the general plan and scope of the *International* will remain unchanged.

At the last stated meeting of the Section on Gynecology of the College of Physicians of Philadelphia, held January 20th, Dr. G. M. Boyd read a paper on *Cæsarian section a second time, because of contracted pelvis—Cæsarian section, because of coxalgic pelvis.* Dr. J. M. Baldy presented a communication on *congenital malformation of genitalia*, and described a case in which absence of uterus and adnexa were associated with a rudimentary vagina, in a young woman, otherwise perfectly developed, and who had never menstrated; the speaker also made some *remarks on fibroid tumors*, and exhibited specimens of such growths. Dr. J. B. Shober reported a *double celiotomy for appendicitis and retroversion of the uterus*, in which he first did an operation for the excision of a diseased vermiform appendix, and then an abdominal section in the median line to correct a retroverted uterus by the method of ventral suspension; the patient made a good recovery, although for a time obstinate and serious intestinal paresis was present.

Despite the efforts of the Board of Health and despite the fact that the general sanitary condition of the city is reported good, *typhoid fever is on the increase in the infected districts*, and has begun to spread more generally through other parts of the city. It is conceded by all that the cause of the epidemic is the pollution of the water-supply. The new cases of typhoid for the week ending January 22d, numbered 212, as against 201 for the preceding week. The deaths from this cause reached a total of 23 cases, or 6 more than reported last week. There were 119 new cases of diphtheria reported, or 23 more than last week, with 20 deaths; and 62 new cases of scarlet fever, exactly the same number that occurred last week, with 2 deaths. Of the 461 deaths from all causes during the past week 147 were of children under five years of age.

OUR BERLIN LETTER.

[From our Special Correspondent.]

GERMAN MEDICAL OPINIONS ON ROTHELN—THE PRESENT STATE OF CLINICAL HEMOGLOBINOMETRY—PROFESSOR GERHARDT ON THE GRUBER-WIDAL-SERUM REACTION IN TYPHOID—PROFESSOR SALKOWSKI AND THE XANTHIN BODIES IN THE URINE.

BERLIN, January 20, 1898.

GERMAN measles, "*Rötheln*," occurs just often enough in America to make opinions as to its etiology and contagiousness interesting. Some recent opinions on the matter from Dr. Blaschko, whose opportunities for observations of the disease have been excellent, appeared in the last number of the *Therapeutische Monatshefte*, and his opinion seems to be more or less that of the profession here generally. Rötheln is not considered to be an independent disease with a specific etiology of its own, though this is not a universal opinion. The bacterial cause of measles is, of course, not as yet known, but it is considered that when it is discovered it will be found that rötheln is caused by a degenerate form of the bacterial cause of measles. As to contagiousness, Dr. Blaschko does not consider that the liability to contagion, even for the immediate members of the family, is sufficient to require isolation of the patient. He considers that other children of the family may be allowed to continue attendance at school without endangering their fellow pupils. Epidemics of rotheln spread in this way, it would seem, have not been observed in Germany.

As to treatment, all the indications are met by a bland diet, rest in bed during three to four days, and a weeks' confinement to the house. After two weeks the patients may resume attendance at school. Complications, Dr. Blaschko has never seen, and when they are reported to have occurred he believes that the cases were not really what should be called rotheln, but rather genuine measles, or at times scarlet fever.

The present position of the clinical pathology of the blood is strikingly unsettled, or at least would appear so from the rather varied and generally unsatisfactory positions taken by prominent clinicians. Grawitz is giving a course of lectures on blood pathology from the clinician's standpoint, which represent, I suppose, some of the best and most advanced scientific thought of the day on the subject. He never talks of the estimation of hemoglobin by any of the old methods. Notwithstanding all the ingenuity spent on supposed instruments of precision, and recent supposed important modifications of them, one never hears of either the instrument of Fleischl or Gowers, but always of the dried substance of the blood, *i.e.*, of the weight of the residue remaining after evaporation.

The use of this method shows at least one thing very clearly: that the blood plasma undergoes much greater change during the course of certain blood diseases than has usually been thought to be true. In chlorosis, for instance, the ratio of watery constituents in the cells and in the plasma of the blood does not always show coincident changes from the normal. Usually the amount of watery constituents of the cells is proportionately much greater in chlorotic conditions than that in the plasma. This holds true, as a rule too, for pernicious anemia, but there are cases of both affections in which the plasma shares in the hydremic change, and these cases are of especially bad prognosis. It seems probable that the near future will see certain changes in the ordinarily accepted division of blood diseases as at present taught, the modications being founded on the important changes in the plasma which are not yet systematized.

Professor Gerhardt, in talking of the *estimation of hemoglobin*, recently said that so much discredit had been thrown on ordinary methods of estimation that the practitioner scarcely knew what to adopt. He suggested that the simple test of Professor Martins is probably as good as any until the clinical-blood pathologists have settled among themselves whether instrumental color hemoglobinometry, the weighing of the dried substance of the blood, or the estimation of the specific gravity of the blood, is to be regarded as the best test of its hemoglobin contents.

Professor Martins places a drop of blood from the patient upon a handkerchief, and beside it, a drop of normal blood. A little experience enables one to judge with sufficient exactness for all clinical purposes how much the hemoglobin is reduced in the pathologic specimen. A series of specimens may be kept for some time for comparison, and the degree of improvement in the chlorotic condition fairly judged.

Professor Gerhardt's opinion, by the way, of what is called very generally here in Germany the *Gruber-Widal reaction in typhoid fever*, does not concede to it much practical value for the practitioner. The precise precautions necessary for its proper use, the fresh typhoid culture, the careful exact dilution, he thinks almost impracticable for general employment. Then, in many cases, the patient's history cannot be obtained with sufficient exactness to be absolutely sure about preceding attacks of typhoid, and besides the possibility of a second attack cannot be excluded in such cases. In certain cases even normal serum gives the reaction, while in certain others the reaction does not occur at a period sufficiently early in the disease to make it of diagnostic value.

On the whole, while its positive presence is not always conclusive, a negative reaction is not absolutely exclusive for typhoid. It is only in certain crucial cases that such a diagnostic aid is required, but in these cases surrounding circumstances are, as a rule, so dubiously significative that it is only an absolutely pathognomonic sign that is of practical value. As it is, the Gruber-Widal reaction gives no more assurance for the diagnosis than does the Diazo reaction, and that, after a period of enthusiastic popularity, has sunk into almost complete desuetude. What Professor Potain called some time ago the diagnostic problem of the end of the century—a means of diagnosing with certainty doubtful cases of typhoid fever still remains to be solved.

It has been known for some time that Professor Salkowski, in the chemical laboratory of the Pathological Institute, was at work on tests for the exact determination and *the significance of the xanthin bodies in the urine.* Since Horbaczewski's ground-breaking work with regard to the fate of the metabolic products of the cell-nuclei, especially of the nuclei of the leucocytes, the subject of the xanthin bodies has attracted a good deal of attention. The demonstration that uric acid and the xanthin bases are the end-products, not of systemic nutritional metabolism, but of tissue metabolism, especially of the leucocytes, was one of the most important steps of late years toward the solution of the mysterious processes of vital chemism.

According to Horbaczewski, there is a complete parallelism between the number of leucocytes and the amount of uric acid and xanthin bases excreted in the urine. Not long ago the whole field of physiologic and pathologic leucocytosis lay temptingly open, and soon a number of articles appeared on this subject. Most of them were not encouragingly scientific, and some were neither consistent with themselves nor with others along the same line. Something of the fault lay with the present tests for the xanthin bodies in the urine, and the inadequate means of separating them with certainty from uric acid and its derivatives, so that further work from a practical scientific chemist was eagerly anticipated.

Meanwhile, Neusser's description of the perinuclear basophilic granulations of leucocytes—the little bodies surrounding the nucleus which stained with triple stain are of a blackish blue—added to the interest of the question of nuclear metabolism, while diverting it to another phase of the process. These little bodies, evidently products of nuclear metabolism, some one of the steps perhaps of the oxidation processes which are known to connect nuclein with uric acid, might give important data for the solution of the questions at issue. Then Kolisch, working in Neusser's clinic in Vienna, claimed to have found a constant relation between these perinuclear basophilic granulations and the xanthin bodies in the urine. He even considered that the so-called uric-acid diatheses are not due to uric acid, or at least are not connected with variations of excretion of uric acid in the urine, but with the amount of the xanthin bodies. Gout, in other words, is not a manifestation of a uric-acid diathesis, but, so to speak, of a xanthin base diathesis. This part of his work has not only not been confirmed, but would seem to be thoroughly disproved. The interest in the xanthin bodies remained, however. Professor Salkowski's article in a recent number of *Pflügger's Archives for Physiology* will be eagerly welcomed. His silver method of precipitating the xanthin bodies and of separating them completely from uric acid would seem to fill the long felt want. While other tests have given extremely large amounts of xanthin as present, and besides, have shown extensive variations in supposedly healthy individuals where no reason could be found for it, this seems to give regular reliable results. The percentage of the xanthin bodies to uric acid present is much smaller than has been given by other workers. On the whole, Professor Salkowski does not think that these bodies deserve as much interest as has been devoted to them, and considers that important conclusions as to nuclear metabolism and the chemic vital processes of nuclear life do not lie hidden in our lack of knowledge of these bodies.

TRANSACTIONS OF FOREIGN SOCIETIES.

Paris.

ADVANTAGES AND DISADVANTAGES OF MASSAGE IN THE TREATMENT OF FRESH FRACTURES — EARLY DIAGNOSIS OF TUBERCULOUS AFFECTIONS OF THE CHEST BY THE AID OF SKIASCOPY—GASTRO-ENTEROSTOMY FOR ULCER OF THE STOMACH —THE HOSPITAL CONTAGION OF TYPHOID FEVER—PROTEOLYTIC POWER OF THE DUODENUM.

LUCAS-CHAMPIONNIERE showed before the Academy of Medicine, December 21, 1897, a young man who had sustained a comminuted fracture of the lower end of the humerus, the result of a fall. The first four days after the injury the arm was put in a splint; then it was kept in a sling only, and after eighteen days even this was discarded. From the very first day *there was a daily application of massage*, and as soon as the union was sufficiently firm there was also daily passive motion. Recovery was perfect. This surgeon holds to the idea that immobilization, far from favoring the repair of the tissues, as was formerly believed, in reality retards it. SEE stated that massage is useful in the treatment of fractures because it increases the activity of the absorption of the effusion, as union of the bone cannot take place until after this absorption is complete. The same end may be obtained more rapidly, and with less difficulty than by massage, by the application of a rubber bandage. PEAN said that massage ought not to be employed from the first except in those cases of fracture in which there is no displacement of the fragments. In most fractures some immobilizing apparatus is necessary for a time, in order to maintain perfect reduction. It is only after such preliminary treatment that massage is permissible in these cases.

KELSCH spoke of the *early diagnosis of tuberculous affections of the chest by the aid of radioscopy*. His observations were based upon the examination of 124 young patients with various thoracic diseases, thought clinically to be non-tuberculous. The result was negative in 73 instances. In 51 patients the apices of the lungs were found to be less permeable, and transmitted the rays less readily than in the normal, or the glands of the posterior mediastinum, or the pleura, were thickened, and there was partial ankylosis of the diaphragm. As these regions are those in which tuberculous processes begin it is reasonable to suppose that at least in some of these cases tuberculosis existed. This is in accord with the deductions reached through autopsies, *viz.*, that from 20 to 45 per cent. of young subjects present latent tuberculous lesions.

RENAUT illustrated by photographs, December 28th, the ease and certainty with which a differential diagnosis may be made between syringomyelia and rheumatism of the hand when the Röntgen-rays are employed.

WALTHER, RICARD, and KIRMISSON at the session of December 22d, described cases in which large cysts of the neck were removed, expressing the opinion that such cysts are of a venous rather than of a lymphatic origin as is usually supposed to be the case.

TUFFIER announced that he had three times performed *gastro-enterostomy for ulcer of the stomach*. Two of the patients so operated upon recovered. One died from septicemia starting from a gangrenous focus in the liver due to the gastric ulcer, inflammatory changes having glued these two organs together. The reason for operation in this case was uncontrollable hematemesis, as it was in one of the successful cases. In the third case there was thought to be a perforation, but at operation it was found that the symptoms were due to localized peritonitis caused by the ulcer, although the stomach wall had not given way. The good results which follow gastro-enterostomy in such cases are perhaps due to the complete rest given the stomach, and also to the fact that food is retained in this organ only a short time.

At the session of December 29th, HARTMANN stated that he had once performed gastro-enterostomy for hematemesis. Vomiting of blood ceased, but the patient died several days later. As far as known, this operation has been performed in 12 such cases, the result being 4 recoveries and 8 deaths. This is not very encouraging, and when one considers that immediate death from a large hemorrhage is rare, and that patients often recover when treated by means of decubitus, restricted diet, and ligatures to the limbs, it is doubtful if the operation is one to be recommended.

At the Medical Society of the Hospitals, December 17th, NETTER spoke of the *hospital contagion of typhoid fever*. From 1892 to 1895, 27 cases of typhoid fever developed in the Trousseau Hospital. Twelve of these cases were in nurses, and of these 10 were on the night force. In one case, which recently occurred, the proof was conclusive that the contagion was the result of contact with linen soiled by typhoid dejecta. These cases seem to conclusively prove the contagiousness of typhoid fever, but it does not seem necessary on this account to isolate patients having this disease.

LEMOINE mentioned an instance in which there was only a single typhoid-fever patient in the hospital ward; nevertheless, several patients convalescent from acute articular rheumatism all developed typhoid fever. As these patients made use of the same bed-pan, it seemed probable that the disease was transmitted in this manner. ŒTTINGER mentioned a similar instance in which transmission of contagion seemed to have occurred from th[e] infected tip of a fountain-syringe used for all the patients. The infection was not necessarily direct through the rec[-]tum, but more likely through the soiling of the hands o[f] the attendants with the fecal matter. Several member[s] of the society narrated similar instances.

At a session of the Biological Society, December 18th PACHON described experiments by which he had prove[d] that the *duodenum possesses a digestive power of its ow[n] with respect to albumin*. If thirty cubic centimeters [of] coagulated egg albumin be introduced into the duodenu[m] of a fasting dog and kept there by means of ligatures, it wi[ll] be almost completely digested within six hours. If, befor[e] it is introduced, the duodenum is roughly handled so th[at] submucous ecchymoses are produced it will not be d[i-]gested at all. This shows that the digestion cannot be a[t-]tributed to the pancreatic juice, but is the result of the pr[o-]teolytic action of the duodenum itself.

Vienna.

BACTERIOLOGIC ORIGIN OF TYMPANITES UTERI[—] RESULTS OF OPERATIVE TREATMENT OF LUPUS[—] MECHANICAL TREATMENT OF OBESITY—TEMP[O-]RARY UTERINE DISPLACEMENT POSSIBLY DUE [TO] MUSCULAR CONTRACTION.

At the Imperial Royal Society of Physicians, Decem[-]ber 10th, LINDENTHAL discussed *bacteriologic inv[es-]tigations in tampanites uteri*. This condition was f[or-]merly supposed to be due to putrefaction of the embry[o]. It has, however, been observed while the embryo s[…]

lives, and is at present regarded as of microbic origin. It has been sometimes ascribed to the action of the coli bacillus, although this microbe is not capable of producing gas except in the presence of sugar. In four cases of tympanites of the uterus, Lindenthal demonstrated the presence of different organisms. In every case, however, he found an anaerobic bacillus which was capable of producing gas in large quantities in a short time, and seemed to be related to the bacillus of malignant edema.

At the session of December 17th, LANG pointed out the *good results which may be obtained by the operative treatment of lupus.* Of thirty-five patients whose histories he followed for several years, twenty-seven were permanently cured. The various methods of covering defects by means of flaps give more permanent results than Thiersch grafts; for, although the immediate results of the latter method are most satisfactory, yet the subsequent shrinkage of the grafts may cause trouble.

At the College of Doctors of Medicine, December 6th, WINTERNITZ spoke of *mechanical cures for obesity.* Banting's cure consists in an almost exclusively albuminous diet. Ebstein allows a certain amount of fat. These and other similar methods are starvation cures, and it is questionable whether such can be carried out without injury. Thyroid extract reduces the fat by hastening the combustion of the intermediate products of metamorphosis. This would be the ideal treatment if it too were not accompanied by disturbances of the general system. There are, however, purely physical methods for increasing the combustion of fat; one of these is increase of muscular activity. If this is pushed to a degree, the temperature of the body is raised, anemia results, and there is a reduced capability of exertion. This may be avoided by artificially cooling the body before the muscles are called into play. If a patient is treated for several days with cold sponge baths, followed by steam baths, the skin is soon brought into such a condition that this increase of temperature is avoided. Profuse excretion of sweat also assists in reducing the fat. After the steam bath the patient takes a bath in a tub, and then the prescribed walk. Later massage is administered. This series of manipulations may be repeated twice, or in some cases, three times daily. After the steam bath some patients are at once put into a cold tub-bath. By this treatment Winternitz, within a few weeks, can bring about a loss in weight of forty-five pounds without weakening his patient and without altering the diet to any great extent.

At the session of the Medical Club of December 15th, SCHUTZ stated that in certain cases backward displacement of the uterus disappears spontaneously. This suggested the thought that the *uterus might be temporarily displaceed by spastic contraction of certain muscles.* While there is no clinical evidence to sustain this idea it appears that Douglas' pouch is sometimes of such form that muscular contraction would be able to draw the uterus backward.

Camphor as an Antigalactagogue.—HERRGOTT reports a remarkable diminution in the secretion of milk as a result of the employment of camphor internally in 3-grain doses, three times daily for three days.

SOCIETY PROCEEDINGS.

MEDICAL SOCIETY OF THE STATE OF NEW YORK.

Ninety-Second Annual Meeting, Held at Albany, N. Y., January 25, 26, and 27, 1898.

FIRST DAY—JANUARY 25TH.

MORNING SESSION.

THE meeting was called to order by the President, SENECA D. POWELL, M.D., of New York, after which prayer was offered by the Rev. Charles A. Richmond of Albany. The President then delivered his

INAUGURAL ADDRESS,

in which he said in part: In inaugurating your Ninety-second Annual Meeting, it becomes my pleasant duty to report that the affairs of the Society throughout the State are prosperous, and that the same excellent conditions reported by my predecessors continue at the present time. We are united in our brotherhood, contented with our affiliations, honored in our government, and enjoy the blessings of harmony. The only shadow which has fallen upon us is the shadow of death, twelve of our fellow members having died during the past year.

The Merrit A. Cash Prize, as at present applied, is of no advantage to the Society, and some steps should be taken to utilize it in a practical manner.

The work of the State Board of Examiners in controlling the practice of medicine shows that there has been no negligence on its part in endeavoring to maintain the standard of the profession. Of the 862 candidates for license to practise who have been examined, 627 were accepted and 235 rejected, an average of about twenty-two per cent. This would also show that the standard of our medical colleges has been raised. No worthy man is debarred from practice.

The law in regard to the sale of poisons is defective; for not a day passes but the daily papers contain reports of one or more deaths from carbolic-acid poisoning, the drug having been taken by mistake, and suicides by this agent are of frequent occurrence. The Medical Society of the State of New York should see that the people are protected not only from criminal intent, but from the impulse of self-destruction which comes to those so burdened that they know not which way to turn.

I hesitate to recommend any new legislation; for, as a rule, the less governed we are, the better. It is our duty to protect the sick and suffering, rich and poor, not only from the quack and charlatan but from the ill-educated doctor who cares nothing for science and practises medicine with none but pecuniary ends in view.

The annual report of the treasurer was then read. The receipts during the year amounted to $5558.63; disbursements, $2680.98; balance on hand, $2877.65.

The annual report of the Committee on Legislation was also read. The report detailed the work of that committee during the past year, it having chiefly consisted in successfully opposing bills which, becoming laws, would have been harmful to the profession. Among them was the Optician's Bill, and the attempt of the New York State Medical Association to obtain representation in the State Board of Medical Examiners. The bill exempting from examination practitioners from other States who desire to practise in the State of New York was defeated, as was also the bill providing for a State Veterinarian, thus retaining the examination and sanitary supervision of cattle in the hands of the State Board of Health. The bill abolishing the office of coroner and the Dispensary Bill, in regard to which the committee exerted itself to secure favorable action, failed to become laws. The Midwifery Bill and the bill for the regulation of expert testimony were not presented in time to be acted upon by the last legislature.

The annual report of the State Board of Medical Examiners was then read:

The report of the Regents' Office on this subject as annually presented to the public is a *résumé* of the work of the academic year ending July 31st of each year. The following figures, therefore, unless otherwise stated, bear upon the academic year ending July 31, 1897:

Total number of candidates, 862; accepted, 627; rejected, 27.2 per cent. State Board, 801; accepted, 580; rejected, 27.5 per cent. Homeopathic Board, 47; accepted, 37; rejected, 21.2 per cent. Eclectic Board, 14; accepted, 10; rejected, 28.5 per cent.

Five examinations were held during the academic year, *viz.*: in September, 1896; January, April, May, and June, 1897.

Since September 1, 1891, 37 examinations in all have been held, and from a list of 3290 candidates, 3102 were examined; of these latter 2399 were duly licensed, the total rejections being 703, or 22.68 per cent. The average rejections for the above period were as follows: State Board, 19.3 per cent.; Homeopathic Board, 16.5 per cent.; Eclectic Board, 26.7 per cent.

Most of the rejected candidates have subsequently been reexamined, in some cases repeatedly, as evidenced by the fact that of the 3103 examined only 181, or 7 per cent., have eventually failed to secure a license. Since September 1, 1891, 1192 physicians have applied for endorsement of their credentials under the several exemptions in the law providing for the correction of a legal registration, of which number all but 143, or 12 per cent., furnished satisfactory legal claim to such right. The figures as above given are an indication only as to the results obtained by those who *a priori* were fitted to enter the examinations. This entrance test in itself has been of sufficiently high standard to debar many persons from even being admitted to our examinations. Hence, it will be safe to assume that more than 30 per cent. of those who actually applied and of those who were actually examined were refused even admission to examination for licenses to practice.

The total number of candidates examined during the year who were graduates of New York institutions was 545, and it is a pleasure to again be able to make the statement that their examination papers were more satisfactory than those which were presented by graduates of medical schools outside the State, the ratio being as two to one.

A clause in the law permits New York State's Boards of Medical Examiners to endorse licenses obtained in other States whenever the requirements of New York State shall be equalled in all particulars. Up to the present time we have felt ourselves unable to recommend the endorsement of licenses obtained in other States because, although in many the New York standard is approximated, the preliminary requirements as well as the rigorous system of examinations here do not obtain. We do not care to lower our standard. The Medical Society of the State of New York has placed itself on record as opposed to any such step, and the lawmakers up to the present time have conformed to its wishes in this particular, considering it unfair to our own graduates to admit licentiates from other States on lower general standards than are required of our own candidates. A proposition has been made, however, to amend the law so that reciprocity may be carried on between States where, because of the non-existence of the excellent safeguard possessed by us in our Regents' body, similar tests cannot be applied by such States. The substance of the proposal is that each case be judged upon its individual merits, thus: A candidate from another State presented himself to the Regents for the endorsement of a license shall prove (1) that he has the preliminary academic requirements; (2) that he has attended four full courses of lectures at a school of medicine recognized by this State as of good standing; (3) that he was licensed by a State Board of Medical Examiners whose examination-tests are equal to ours; (4) that we have access to examination-records to prove that he was properly marked as proficient; (5) that the methods of examination conducted at the time he applied for a license in a foreign State were properly safeguarded. It is the belief that it would be only the part of justice to endorse the license of such an one. At the present time w[e] are charged with undue severity in this particular, and [a] willingness on the part of those interested to consider thi[s] question in all its bearings would show that at least w[e] are open to conviction. It is a cause for congratulatio[n] that all the medical colleges of the State have displaye[d] commendable zeal in elevating their standards, prolong[-]ing their courses of study, and adding to their professo[r]ships.

Fifteen invited guests were present, and upon resolu[-]tion were welcomed to all the privileges of the meeting.

DR. WEY, Chairman of the Committee on By-Law[s] reported adversely upon an amendment proposed at t[he] last meeting to change the place of meeting of the Socie[ty] to New York City, Buffalo, and Albany, alternately, an[d] the time of meeting to the first Tuesday in Februar[y]. This amendment was thoroughly discussed later in e[x]ecutive session, and was lost by a standing vote of 35 [to] 40. Albany will, therefore, continue to be the Mecca [of] the Society.

DR. WENDELL C. PHILLIPS of New York County re[ad] a paper, entitled

EAR MANIFESTATIONS IN GENERAL DISEASE.

The author said that although all diseases, especia[lly] the exanthemata, which lead to a debilitated conditi[on]

are apt to be accompanied or followed by ear manifestations. The subject has received but little attention. Cases were cited in which middle-ear disease accompanied malaria, syphilis, neurasthenia, scarlet fever, etc., and one was mentioned in which the ear trouble simulated the symptoms of typhoid fever. Adenoid growths in the pharynx was given as a frequent cause of middle-ear disease and consequent deafness, and statistics were quoted to show that many deaf mutes have such adenoid growths. Carious teeth was also mentioned as a cause of ear complications. The author showed a new ear speculum and electric light combined, which had been devised by Dr. Nichol of New York.

DISCUSSION.

DR. LUCIEN HOWE of Erie County: I cannot let this excellent paper pass without some word of comment to emphasize what has been said about the importance of ear manifestations in general diseases. The terrible results which follow neglect in cases of this kind should make us very careful not to overlook the condition. It is in the beginning that treatment will accomplish the best results.

DR. HOLT of Portland, Me.: In scarlet fever the ear should always be treated, and an ear affection arising at this time should never be allowed to continue until it becomes chronic. The time to treat the ear is when the discharge begins. The ear is sometimes involved in cases of Bright's disease, but, in such instances, little relief can be afforded. During the course of the acute diseases of childhood the general practitioner should always give attention to the ear.

DR. JOHN O. ROE of Monroe County then read a paper upon

CASES OF ACUTE NON-DIPHTHERITIC INFLAMMATION OF THE LARYNX REQUIRING THE PROLONGED RETENTION OF THE INTUBATION-TUBE.

The paper gave in detail the case of a child, thirteen months old, who was attacked by a slight croupy cough, apparently the result of a cold. There was some difficulty of respiration, which increased to such an extent that on the third day an intubation-tube was introduced. It was then thought that the child was suffering from laryngeal diphtheria, but repeated bacteriologic examination did not show the Klebs-Löffler bacillus, although numerous micro-organisms were found. The tube was worn during six weeks on account of the dyspnea, being repeatedly expelled and re-inserted.

A similar case, occurring in a little girl three years of age, was also cited. Complete recovery followed in both instances, but there was hoarseness and aphonia for a time after the removal of the tube. The author referred to two cases occurring in the practice of the late Dr. O'Dwyer, in which the tube was worn respectively ten and eleven months. Both of these were cases of diphtheria.

THE REPORT OF A CASE OF UNUSUAL CONTRACTION OF THE VISUAL FIELD AND DISORDER OF THE COLOR SENSE FOLLOWING AN INJURY,

was the title of a paper read by DR. T. F. C. VAN ALLEN of Albany County.

The patient was a man twenty-six years of age, a painter, who while at work was thrown from his scaffold by the breaking of a rope. He sustained a dislocation of the right shoulder, a fracture of the right humerus, and a cut on the head. There was no evidence of fracture of the skull. The eyelids became swollen and ecchymosed after the accident, but the vision seemed good. The patient made a slow recovery. Five weeks after the injury he found that in reading his eyes became tired within a few minutes, and that the text appeared blurred. Six months after the accident he was not able to distinguish colors, and, on this account, came under the speaker's observation. Examination showed that the intra-ocular tension was not increased; R. V. 20/40; L. V. 20/30; neither pupil responded to reflected light until the mirror was brought very close to the eye. There was considerable contraction of the visual field. His perception of red was good, but he could not distinguish blue from green. The man was of good habits, so alcoholic and tobacco amblyopia were excluded. Therefore, the author considered the condition due to the concussion and nervous shock resulting from the fall. Examination four years after the accident showed R. V. 20/30; L. V. 20/30; the visual field for white and yellow was increased; field for blue and green defective; field for red not very far from normal. He sees fairly well, but has difficulty in matching colors in a dim light.

DR. C. B. HERRICK of Rensselaer County, then read a paper, entitled

THE RAILWAY SURGEON AND HIS WORK.

The railway surgeon has become a specialist because of a demand for special services in this line. In the United States more than a million men are employed on railroads and of these 40,000 are injured annually. The injuries which the railway surgeon is called upon to treat differ from others in that they have been inflicted by enormous weights in motion, the crushing force of which is tremendous. The degree of severity of the injury depends largely upon the speed of the object which causes it, a train going at a slow rate of speed causing a crush, whereas one going faster will limit the injury to the wound itself. Owing to the elasticity of the skin it is possible for a train to pass over a man's leg without causing any external wound, and the general practitioner is often misled into to thinking that no serious injury has been inflicted, when in fact, it is so great as to frequently impair the tissues to such a degree that vitality is lost and repair impossible. The railway surgeon is conservative, especially when injuries of the upper extremities are concerned. When the lower extremities are involved it is possible to be too conservative. As the men employed on railroads usually have families dependent upon them, it is impracticable to subject them to prolonged treatment in the effort to save a crushed foot, and in such a case it is better to amputate at once. In amputating it should always be remembered that an artificial limb can usually be best fitted in proportion to the length of the stump. The conditions met with in the work of the railway surgeon are favorable to sepsis. The hand of the railroad man is covered with oil and cinders, and dirt of all kinds is often carried into a wound at the time of infliction. Accidents, too, are apt to occur in unfrequented places and often in inclement weather, all of which reduces the chances for recovery. Railway surgeons were first employed in the West where hospitals are widely separated, and now they are found all over the world. It has also been recognized that prompt attention to wounds is all important; therefore, emergency packets have been placed upon all trains to be used by a physician if there is one at hand, if not, by one of the train-hands, all of whom have been taught what to do in emergencies. They have also been instructed as to the best way to transport an injured man. On some roads a hospital-car is provided which at all times is kept in readiness to go where it is required.

The railway surgeon is constantly considering the proper sanitation of cars, recognizing as he does the great danger of infection being carried in this way. The examination of employees as to their fitness is also one of his duties. There are six thousand railway surgeons in the United States.

A paper, entitled

THE RIVALS OF THE PHYSICIAN IN PRACTICE,

was read by REYNOLD W. WILCOX, M.D., of New York County.

Considering the conditions under which medical men work, the author said, it is not surprising that they have so much to complain of. It is hardly realized how many hangers-on and camp-followers there are. This is probably due to what is said to be the American love of a title; there are many who want to be called "Doctor," and, if they cannot reach that height, some of them are willing to be dubbed "Doc." All medical men are familiar with the "Doc" of the corner drug-store—the prescribing apothecary who repeats prescriptions without the physician's permission, who gives to somebody else a prescription originally given to a different person, who substitutes preparations of his own manufacture for those ordered in a prescription. It seems as though such "physicians" will continue to increase in number to the end of time. There seems no way to confine the labors of these people to the legitimate business of compounding physicians' prescriptions. Then, again, there is the instrument-maker, but he has learned that a truss will not accomplish much for the patient when placed over a bubo or an undescended testicle. Of late years the physician has had to contend with the trained nurse, who prescribes for the members of the family of her patient, and the massage operators and bath attendants, who are always ready to give advice. Curiously enough, the veterinary surgeon is the only individual who will not prescribe for a human being, in spite of the fact that he is much better able to do so than many who do. The reason of all this is found in the fact that the physician works in an altruistic way, thinking only of the good of the people and not recognizing the commercial side of his affairs.

AFTERNOON SESSION.

DR. JOHN H. PRYOR of Erie County read a paper, entitled

WHAT SHALL THE STATE AND COUNTY DO FOR THE CONSUMPTIVE?

In the State of New York 13,000 persons die of consumption every year. In Buffalo alone the annual death-rate from this disease reaches nearly 500. These figures show the frightful loss of life due to tuberculosis and the necessity for measures which reduce the death-rate. Besides those who lose their lives, many are incapacitated by this disease. The popular belief that tuberculosis is an incurable affection is incorrect. Intelligent treatment, instituted early, and proper environment, will accomplish much in cases of incipient consumption. The well-to-do victims of tuberculosis seek change of climate, and thereby gain the best chance of recovery. The majority of the cases occur among the poor, and they are the real sufferers—struggling along until they can no longer work and then seeking relief. Special hospitals for these patients should be established in which they can have pure air, sunlight, and space for indoor exercise when advisable. Open-air life and nourishing food will be the means of cure in many cases of incipient consumption. Such a hospital should not be connected with an almshouse, as was recently attempted at Buffalo; it should be situated where the most beneficial climate can be obtained, and in this State there is none better than that of the Adirondacks. Ill-managed charity ignores the class of cases in question, while provision has been made for poor persons suffering from other diseases. It is the duty of the State to care for poor consumptives, many of whom, sooner or later, become public charges, and it would be better to make them dependent, say, for eighteen months during the curable stage of the disease, at a probable cost of $300, and then restoring them to a condition in which they can care for themselves, than to allow them to become incurable.

DR. WILLIAM WARREN POTTER of Erie County then read a paper, entitled

THE ADVANTAGES OF STATE CONTROL IN MEDICINE, WITH RESULTS OBSERVED.

The first attempt to place the practice of medicine under State control was made by the Medical Faculty of the University of Buffalo in 1864, and nothing came of it. In 1883 the project was again revived, also in Buffalo, by the Medical Society of the County of Erie. A bill was then framed and placed in the hands of a committee which debated the question for two years before presenting it the Legislature It was not until June 5, 1890, that such a bill was passed, and the examiner appointed by the Board of Regents were not named until March 11, 1891. Practically four-years' work was lost by the Exemption Bill (passed at the instance of 900 medical students in the State) which provided that those who began the study of medicine previous to June 5, 1890, should be exempt from examination. At present the original bill is still in force, although many assaults have been made upon it by those antagonistic to laws governing the practice of medicine.

DR. R. C. M. PAGE of New York County read a paper on

ANEMIA

(which will appear in a later issue of THE MEDICAL NEWS).

DR. J. B. RANSOM of Clinton County read a paper on

EXPERT MEDICAL TESTIMONY.

Reference was made to a decision recently given in an Illinois court to the effect that a medical man must testify when called upon to do so, just as if he were an ordinary witness. This point the writer has contested three times in this State, refusing in each instance to answer a hypothetic question, and he considers the subject of regulating expert medical testimony one of the most important of the day. He suggested that medical experts be appointed by the Court, not more than three in number; that they be permitted access to all the papers in the case and to the defendant in the presence of the other experts, and be allowed to examine medical witnesses as to their knowledge. They should then set forth their opinion in writing, signed by all three, provided they agree on essential points, or should render individual reports in case of important disagreement. If counsel demands it, these experts may be sworn as witnesses to give testimony in the manner deemed proper by the Court. Such experts should be especially qualified for the purpose and examined for fitness by the Board of Regents, and they should be remunerated for their services, in amounts to be decided by the judge. Examination by the Board of Regents should be necessary before a man is given a certificate of qualification, and he should have practised medicine in this State not less than five years and be trained in the speciality in regard to which he expects to testify. The function of the expert witness is entirely different from that of the ordinary witness, and for that reason he should form part of the Court; his testimony should be judicial and not partisan. This plan would result in (1) the protection of the people; (2) the protection of the accused, and (3) the protection of the profession. No change in the present method, however, can be hoped for without the cooperation of the legal profession.

DISCUSSION.

DR. EVARTS M. MORRELL of New York County: I doubt if there is any subject which has excited more interest than the regulation of expert medical testimony. One of the reasons why so much ridicule has been heaped upon medical experts by the newspapers is because it often happens that a man is called to the witness stand to testify in a line of work with which he is not familiar, and in this way casts a slur upon the whole profession. Let me give a word of advice: Charge a good fee for expert medical testimony. Do not consent to testify for a small fee. The services of a physician are worth as much, and often more than those of a lawyer, and yet most people expect us to testify for a pittance.

DR. A. WALTER SUITER of Herkimer County: It has been my lot to have had some connection with the Committee on Legislation for a number of years past, and, therefore, I have become interested in this question which engages the attention, not alone of the medical profession, but of the legal profession as well. Being chairman of the committee which framed the bill, I endeavored to make some impression favorable to it when it was presented to the Reference Committee of the Legislature. I was at once met by the remark that the bill was not constitutional, in that it provided an expert for the prosecution and none for the defendant; that, if the defendant accepted the expert provided by the Court, he would not be able to call for any other, for he would then be placed in the position of attacking his own witness, which, of course, was ridiculous and compelled us to withdraw the bill. Various other bills have been prepared in other States, notably Illinois and Minnesota, providing that expert witnesses be appointed by the judge. These bills have all failed. I confess that I am very much discouraged. I do not think it is possible for any judge to make such an appointment without bias. I certainly think that experts should be properly qualified by examination and certificates from, the Board of Regents.

DR. LANDON CARTER GRAY of New York County: We really do not need to regulate expert testimony. What we do require is education of the lawyers. It is within the province of the lawyer to ascertain the qualifications which an expert should possess. It is owing to the lack of education on the part of members of the legal profession that incompetent men are allowed to testify. Selection of experts by the judge is a bad plan, for they know very little about physicians. Moreover, because of the political consideration with which he is burdened the judge is perhaps the worst man in the world to select an expert. It would be better if such a bill provided that the judge select an expert from a list prepared by the Board of Regents, but even this plan has serious disadvantages. I am sorry to say, but it is nevertheless a fact, that in some of our large cities there are a number of our professional brethren who are nothing more or less than blackmailers. They foist themselves into every case, and, if they are not selected by the lawyers, immediately go to the other side and without pay, perhaps, testify for that side in order to show the lawyers who did not employ them that they are powerful men.

DR. JOHN T. WHEELER of Columbia County read a paper on

THE COLD-WATER TREATMENT OF TYPHOID FEVER IN PRIVATE PRACTICE

(which will appear in a future issue of the MEDICAL NEWS).

DR. HENRY L. ELSNER of Onondaga County read a paper, entitled

THE VAGARIES AND WANDERINGS OF GALL-STONES, WITH CLINICAL REPORTS

(which will also appear in a future issue of the MEDICAL NEWS).

DR. EDWARD D. FISHER of New York County read a paper, entitled

PARALYSIS, PROGNOSIS, AND TREATMENT.

The author treated the subject under four divisions, *viz.*: (1) cerebral, (2) spinal, (3) peripheral, and (4) muscular dystrophy. The first form is caused by meningeal or intracranial hemorrhage, thrombosis, tumors, injuries, etc. It is generally unilateral. The second form is due to disease of the anterior horns of the spinal cord, and is usually caused by inflammation, acute or chronic, hemorrhage, new growths, injuries, compression, spinal fracture, etc. Its principal characteristic is the wasting or atrophy of the muscles. The third variety is usually caused by constitutional dyscrasiæ, such as rheumatism or gout, lead poisoning, etc., and is associated with marked sensory symptoms. The fourth form, the cause of which is obscure, is apparently a developmental defect due to heredity. Prognosis is unfavorable in all varieties except the peripheral form. The treatment advised consisted of the application of electricity and massage.

EVENING SESSION.

The evening was devoted to a symposium illustrating the practical application of the X-ray in medicine and surgery. The exhibition was in charge of Dr. Arthur L. Fisk of New York County, and the program consisted of a display of X-ray apparatus, and an instructive and interesting illustration of its uses by Dr. Samuel Lloyd of New York County. Dr. Francis H. Williams of Boston followed with an interesting account of his application of the X-ray in medical cases. The author contended that in diseases of the heart, such as hypertrophy and dilatation, and in diseases of the lungs and pleura, more especially tuberculosis, emphysema, pleurisy, and empyema, more definite information can be obtained by the use of the X-ray than from percussion and auscultation. He recounted a case in which the progress of a tuberculous invasion of the lungs was accurately followed from its inception to the end. The use of the X-ray in surgery was entertainingly and attractively illustrated by stereopticon views of skiagrams of many complicated bone injuries by Dr. Fisk. Dr. William Hailes, Jr., of Albany County illustrated his clinical experiences with the X-ray and improved methods of microscopic projection.

SECOND DAY—JANUARY 26TH.

MORNING SESSION.

DR. E. F. BRUSH of Westchester County read a paper, entitled

THE IMPORTANCE OF THE HYGIENIC MANAGEMENT OF DAIRIES

(which will appear in a later issue of the MEDICAL NEWS,)

DR. N. H. HEATH of Erie County then read a paper on

THE MUNICIPAL CONTROL OF THE MILK-SUPPLY OF CITIES.

The officers for the ensuing year as reported by the nominating committee are as follows: President, Dr. John O. Roe of Rochester; vice-president, Dr. E. F. Brush of Mt. Vernon; secretary, Dr. F. C. Curtis of Albany; treasurer, Dr. C. H. Porter of Albany. The members of the various standing committees were generally retained, except those of the Committee on Prize Essays.

(To be continued.)

REVIEWS.

VITA MEDICA: Chapters of Medical Life and Work. By SIR BENJAMIN WARD RICHARDSON, M.D., LL.D., F.R.S. Longmans, Green & Co., 39 Paternoster Row, London, 1897.

THIS book will be welcomed by all who have followed the career or the teachings of its distinguished author, and they are many. The book does not profess to be an autobiography, but a reminiscence of the prominent events of the actor's life, in which not only are the serious affairs of life considered, but many interesting anecdotes are narrated. The book was evidently designed to be part of the Jubilee celebration of Queen Victoria's reign; indeed, it opens with a touching picture of the final leave-taking of the author's invalid mother on the day following the Queen's coronation, and was finished, as narrated in a note inserted by the author's son, "on November 18th, 1896, just before eight o'clock in the evening. At ten o'clock he was seized with the illness which ended fatally on Saturday morning, November 21st."

Sir Benjamin evidently took a serious view of life from his earliest cogitations, and a consciousness of the duties and responsibilities of a medical practitioner characterizes all that he writes. The volume makes very interesting and instructive reading.

THERAPEUTIC HINTS.

In Chronic Conjunctivitis, in addition to the correction of such possible causes as errors of refraction, a naso-pharyngitis, or an inflammation of the lachrymal sac, and attention to the condition of the general health, BERRY recommends for mild cases one of the following lotions:

℞		
	Ac. tannici	gr. ii–iv
	Sod. biboratis	ʒ i
	Glycerini	ʒ ii
	Aq. camphoræ	℥ iv.

M. Sig. External use;

℞		
	Ichthyol	♏ xx
	Aq. sambuci } aa	
	Aq. dest. }	℥ ii.

M. Sig. External use.

To Remove Comedones.—Moisten a towel with the following lotion and apply to the affected areas, with friction, several times daily:

℞		
	Kaolini	℥ ii
	Glycerini	℥ iss
	Ac. acetici	℥ i
	Ol. odorat.	q. s.

M. Sig. External use.

For Pharyngitis Sicca.—

℞		
	Ac. carbolici	ʒ i
	Tr. iodi	♏ v
	Tr. aloes	♏ vii
	Tr. opii	gtt. x
	Glycerini	℥ i.

M. Sig. By means of an atomizer apply to the pharynx several times daily.

THE MEDICAL NEWS.
A WEEKLY JOURNAL OF MEDICAL SCIENCE.

VOL. LXXII. NEW YORK, SATURDAY, FEBRUARY 5, 1898. NO. 6.

ORIGINAL ARTICLES.

ANEMIA.[1]

BY R. C. M. PAGE, M.D.,
OF NEW YORK;
PROFESSOR OF GENERAL MEDICINE AND DISEASES OF THE CHEST IN THE NEW YORK POLYCLINIC.

ANEMIA should be regarded as a condition secondary to some other affection rather than as a primary disease. The term itself is somewhat ambiguous, and is not infrequently used regardless of its real significance. For this reason we may assume at the outset that anemia signifies deficiency of red corpuscles or aglobulia. Then let us include under this head all such forms as hydremia, spanemia, and the like. When, however, there is increase of white corpuscles as well as deficiency of the red, then the condition is no longer one of simple anemia, but rather leukemia. The latter condition, as is well known, is always associated with hypertrophic enlargement of the spleen, in which there is an increase in the elements composing the normal splenic pulp. This disease is also called leucocythemia, and in all cases observed by me it has occurred in men from tropical or sub-tropical climates who had been subject to repeated attacks of intermittent fever.

In Hodgkin's disease, or lymphadenoma, the spleen is also enlarged, but this is due to two causes: First and most commonly, the increase in size of the spleen is caused by adventitious growths in its substance resembling mutton suet on section. In these cases there is simply anemia, but exceptionally the spleen is enlarged partly by hypertrophy of its normal elements and partly by the presence of adventitious growths. When this obtains we find not only anemia but also leukemia, as was observed in a case sent to me last year by Dr. W. N. Hubbard of the Out-Door Department of Bellevue Hospital. The disease is characterized not only by increase in the size of the spleen, but also by widespread enlargement of the lymphatic glands, usually beginning in the neck and extending into the axilla, groin, and elsewhere. I believe, also, clinically speaking, that this affection may be regarded as malignant.

The term chlorosis is indiscriminately used by most physicians and many authors to express the anemic condition, regardless of age or sex. I believe, however, with Dr. T. Gaillard Thomas, that it should be restricted to young girls, and only those who have not menstruated. It is true that such girls are usually anemic, but not necessarily so. Once establish the menstrual function and the chlorosis, or "green sickness," as it really signifies, disappears.

Pernicious anemia is a progressive disease first so-named by Biermer in 1871. Here we find simply diminution of red blood-corpuscles, many of which also become deformed without increase of the white, nor is there enlargement of the spleen. I have seen many more cases in the hospitals of Europe than in this country, and nearly always among women, especially women from twenty to forty years of age, and after repeated pregnancies. Chronic wasting diseases and certain uterine disorders may also cause the affection, but in some instances there appears to be no known cause. As in all cases of marked anemia there are the usual basic systolic heart murmurs and the venous hum heard over the neck. A valuable point in the diagnosis, as suggested by Dr. W. H. Thomson, is the presence of fever. The temperature varies from 100° to 101° F. The patient gradually declines, but death is generally due to some intercurrent disease, notably tuberculous nephritis, accompanied by marked dropsy. The pathology of pernicious anemia is not exactly known, but on account of capillary hemorrhages in the retina and other localities one is lead to suspect some disturbance of the sympathetic nervous system with consequent vasomotor irregularity. The disease is uniformly fatal, so that nothing more can be done than to attempt to prolong the patient's life by stimulants and highly nutritious food. Having very briefly alluded to leukemia, lymphadenomia, chlorosis, and pernicious anemia, I may now consider the chief subject of this paper, *viz.*, simple anemia.

As already said at the outset anemia may be regarded as a secondary condition rather than as a primary disease. It is, however, termed idiopathic anemia by some as well as simple or ordinary anemia. Perhaps insufficient food and overwork, especially when accompanied by bad hygienic surroundings, form the most frequent combination of circumstances which give rise to this affection. It is also due to excessive loss of blood from any cause, and frequently occurs during convalescence from severe sickness, as typhoid fever and the like—but there is one way in which

[1] Read at the Ninety-second Annual Meeting of the Medical Society of the State of New York, held at Albany, N. Y., January 25, 26, and 27, 1898.

anemia is brought about to which I wish especially to call attention, as first observed by Meinert of Dresden a few years ago. It is due to increased functional activity of the spleen from vasomotor disturbance of the nutrient vessels of that organ caused by prolapse of the stomach and bowels (gastroptosis, enteroptosis). We find the condition referred to chiefly among women with lax abdominal walls, such as those who have borne children, and those who, in following the prevailing fashion, wear clothing which presses down the stomach and bowels as well as the liver. We all know how common is what Strümpell calls the corset liver. In prolapse of the stomach the spleen is held firmly in position by the suspensory ligament. This allows traction on the splenic plexus formed by branches from the right semilunar ganglia of the sympathetic nervous system. These never accompany the splenic artery and its branches into the substance of the spleen. The traction on the splenic sympathetic nerve causes irritation, with consequent vasomotor disturbance of the nutrient vessels of the spleen, with increased activity of that organ. As an example of such irritation the increased heart-action in exophthalmic goiter may be given.

Accompanying the increased functional activity of the spleen there is generally some enlargement of this organ and also an increase in the number of white corpuscles of the blood without noticeable diminution of the red. Such a case could not, therefore, be called one of leukemia, but rather simple anemia. I have reason to believe that this condition of the spleen in simple anemia exists much more frequently than is generally supposed. After treating a patient for simple anemia for a length of time by ordinary methods I have been astonished at the lack of improvement. On examination, in such cases, I have invariably found slight enlargement of the spleen. These cases almost invariably occur among women. Instances of marked enlargement of the spleen are not referred to here, but I regard the spleen as sufficiently enlarged to require attention whenever it gives rise to marked dulness on percussion over the axillary line from the ninth to the eleventh ribs, with the patient in the erect position. In fact, it is a good rule when treating a patient for anemia to always begin by carefully examining the condition of the spleen.

Should improvement be slow and enlargement of the spleen suspected various remedies have been suggested with a view to lessening its size. To this end, while sufficient food of a highly nutritious order is indicated, excess is to be avoided, as well as a residence in a malarious locality. Ill-fitting dress should be remedied, and, as for drugs, I have found the internal administration of the iodid of potassium, with arsenic and an occasional positi dose of quinin, and, of course, the constant empl ment of some preparation of iron, to be most cient. Combined with this the surface over spleen should be rubbed every other night at b time with the iodid of mercury ointment (gr. ii ℥ i). Red-oxid-of-mercury ointment may be u instead.

While administering iron the bowels, if necessa should be regulated by some simple remedy, as t action of the iron will then be much more satisf tory. It is also well to remember that it is ofte good rule to stop all such medication during m struation.

THE COLD-WATER TREATMENT OF TYPHO FEVER IN PRIVATE PRACTICE.[1]

BY JOHN T. WHEELER, M.D.,
OF CHATHAM, N. Y.

THE experience of the profession with the Bra treatment of typhoid fever is a striking illustrati of the fact that something more than scientific me is needed in a therapeutic measure to secure its g eral adoption. The proof is ample that cold tubbi is the ideal treatment at the present state of kno edge, yet probably not one case in twenty in priv practice is treated by this means to-day. Hum nature, which has always to be reckoned with in art, has rendered against it a verdict of "too heroic and declares its preference for something perh more dangerous, but less distressing. Neverthel the Brand treatment is a magnificent achieveme and to it we owe, if not a rule of practice, the tablishment of certain therapeutic principles wh are the bed-rock of all sound antipyretic treatme

Typhoid fever is a disease which varies so muc severity in different localities and different epid ics and is, moreover, so complex in character th report by a single observer of a series of succes cases can never be conclusive as to the merits c particular line of treatment. It so happens tha have all my life employed cold sponge-bathing in treatment of typhoid fever, and, furthermore, I h never used any other treatment. My one hund and twenty odd cases cover my entire professi experience of twenty-three years. The one loca in which I have resided is not favored as to m ness of climate, and the series of years includes eral epidemics of decided severity, so that the eral average of my cases would represent a average of the severity of the disease in question

It may be a subject for wonderment that a man sh practise medicine during the past quarter of a cen

[1] Read at the Ninety-second Annual Meeting of the Me Society of the State of New York, held at Albany, N. Y., Ja 25, 26, and 27, 1898.

and not in all that time be tempted to use some of the many remedies commonly employed in the treatment of typhoid fever. I adopted cold-water sponging in 1875, at a time when it was still regarded in my section as a daring innovation. It was a revelation to me then to begin the treatment of a delirious typhoid patient, sliding down in his bed, reeking with sweat, and with teeth covered with sordes, and, after a few days of bathing, see his expressionless face begin to show a sense of consciousness and comfort. I was successful in those early cases, and my success continued afterward, so that I never cared, and perhaps never dared, to try drug treatment. I have had but one fatal case. If, then, my uniform success is not fortuitous, it is entitled to be taken as fairly direct evidence as to the merit of cold sponging. Perhaps I might better stop here with the mere statement of the results of the treatment in my hands, since I lay no claim to originality in the technic of bathing nor in the discovery of any new principle. But there seems to be no one method of applying the milder forms of bathing, so that I may venture to emphasize one or two points which I have learned to regard as of special value, and to discuss also a point in general management which, more than any other, I think important.

We may consider typhoid fever, for the present purpose, as the result of the action of a toxin upon the living organism, manifesting itself by high temperature and its consequences, and by depression of the nervous system. Cold-water bathing does not, of course, destroy the toxin, but combats its effects in two ways: (1) by the lowering of temperature through the abstraction of heat, and (2) by the stimulation of the nerve-centers, thus maintaining functional activity and nutritive integrity by means of thermic and mechanical shock.

Mechanical shock or friction operates in two ways: (1) It excites the vasodilator nerves and so determines a free flow of blood to the periphery, thereby counteracting the danger of internal congestion which the application of cold water alone would produce, and also by bringing more heated blood to the surface to be cooled by the water, and (2) it stimulates the cutaneous nerves over a wide area, thereby reflexly stimulating the entire nervous system.

In making a greater use of friction than is commonly done, both for the good it can do by itself in stimulating the nerves and also in counteracting the circulatory disturbances due to prolonged use of the cold water, lies the point in which my practice may differ from that of many who employ the cold sponge. To have secured the same sum-total of heat abstraction and nerve stimulation by decreasing the intensity of the cold applications, and at the same time increasing their frequency and duration, is where, in common with those who employ cold sponging, I seem to have secured the advantages of cold tubbing without its drawbacks. To have become convinced of the supreme importance of bringing every available weapon in our armamentarium, balneopathic and otherwise, into prompt and energetic action at the onset of the disease is, to my mind, after the bath, the most influential factor in my success in the treatment of typhoid fever. If to this be added the fact that I am sure I have killed no one with veratrum viride or antipyrin, I have included, perhaps, all the features which distinguish my individual practice.

Briefly stated, my plan of bathing is this: I order that a bath be given every two hours during the day as soon as the diagnosis is made. The bath is continued from fifteen to forty-five minutes, according to the severity of the case. In a certain proportion of atypical cases with severe onset I use the bath almost continuously, hour after hour, and also in any case in which the response to the treatment is not satisfactory. I meet obstinacy of symptoms by persistency of treatment. At an early stage, with a heart yet strong, and with the free use of friction, this vigorous plan of treatment is possible.

I do not regard elevation of temperature as a criterion of the urgency of bathing, or depend upon the fall in temperature as a measure of hydrotherapeutic effect. The stimulation of the nervous system is the main thing to be accomplished.

The temperature of the bath should be a compromise in which the feelings of the patient, his strength, severity of symptoms, duration of bath, and amount of rubbing are determining factors; but oftenest it will be found that after a little the coldest water consistent with comfort is sufficient to meet the requirements. Weakened subjects with feeble peripheral circulation receive a preliminary rubbing in place of whisky or a hot drink. Friction, which brings blood to the surface and makes a patient feel warmer and causes him to accept his bath gratefully, does not of itself raise the temperature. Friction alone often quiets restlessness and puts the patient to sleep. Cases which by the tenth day are of mild type, however turbulent and threatening previously, are left without other treatment than good nursing. With two exceptions, I have regarded my aborted cases as instances of a mistaken diagnosis.

Hemorrhage from the bowels is a contraindication to bathing, a complicating pneumonia, not necessarily, and a bronchitis not at all. Every case must be considered individually, and much may be learned from and trusted to the observations of a nurse. She soon acquires a proper conception of the theory of the use of the bath, from discovering that it is her work which keeps down the delirium, puts the patient to sleep, and cures the bronchitis; and, further, she learns to increase or relax her efforts with a definite and rational aim. Cases occur, however, which tax the vitality of subjects to the utmost and call for every kind of accessory support.

Next in importance to the bath itself is its early employment. The critical period of typhoid fever is not in the third or fourth week; it is in the first, and the battle is to be won or lost at this time.

Any one who plays whist knows that, although the interest centers toward the close on the fall of the last two or three tricks which win the hand, it is mainly the opening lead which determines the final issue, and in this fever it is equally true that that which culminates at the close is only a resultant of forces put in operation at the beginning. The daily damage from the typhoid toxin is no greater in any one day of the twenty-eight days of the fever than another, but the accumulated effect is more obvious toward the end. In fulminating cases the damage from the toxin is very great in the first week, yet I have come to regard such cases as ultimately mild, so certainly will persistent bathing break the power of the toxin to injure the organism.

The gastro-intestinal disorders of the first week are toxic. They are the first significant expression of lowered nerve tone. Calomel in small doses for a laxative effect, and strychnia and muriatic acid are helpful, but it is the sponging and rubbing which stop the vomiting, clear the tongue, and restore the appetite. To get the digestive apparatus in good order for the severe demands which are to be made upon it before it becomes functionally weakened is a matter of timely opportunity. I do not begin maximum feeding until assured on this point.

With bathing promptly begun during the first week I feel an almost positive assurance that the disease will be marked by a mild course. By this means the metabolic processes of the body are regulated so as to increase its resistance to the inroads of the disease; we have won Nature to our side in maintaining the strength and the general nutrition.

---

*THE VAGARIES AND WANDERINGS OF GALL-STONES, WITH CLINICAL REPORTS.**

BY HENRY L. ELSNER, M.D.,
OF SYRACUSE, N. Y.;
PROFESSOR OF THE SCIENCE AND ART OF MEDICINE, AND CLINICAL MEDICINE IN THE SYRACUSE MEDICAL COLLEGE.

THE vagaries and wanderings of gall-stones, as exemplified in the cases which I am about to report, have seemed of sufficient interest to merit attention.

The fact has been conclusively proven by clir and *post-mortem* experiences that in a large nun of cases in which gall-stones are ultimately fo their presence was originally unsuspected. The agnosis of cholelithiasis is often made with g difficulty, for there are so many conditions w simulate the presence of gall-stones that the d nostician is frequently puzzled. The various m festations of the symptom complex, associated paroxysmal pain in the upper abdominal regi many of the so-called gastralgias and enteral often prove to be a typical example of ch lithiasis. The prompt acceptance of the trutl this statement promises, if acted upon by the d nostician, to bring relief and cure to many; a clusion justified by the brilliant results recently tained in the field of hepatic and biliary surg This hope for the future is accentuated by the haustive studies and the growing literature on subject to which I will refer later.

CASE I.—On March 20, 1895, Mrs. F., a fifty-seven years, the mother of three children, sulted me on account of repeated acute pains w were referred to the upper abdominal regions. She a woman who had always been obliged to work h and had been actively engaged in her house duties since her marriage. Careful inquiry into history revealed the fact that she had suffered repeated attacks of gall-stone colic. These were lowed by great tenderness in the right hypochonc region, and a moderate amount of jaundice. diagnosis of cholelithiasis had never been m hence, gall-stones had not been looked for in stools. Between her attacks of gall-stone colic after her recovery from the acute symptoms suffered continuously from indigestion, both ga and intestinal. On March 25, 1895, after a se and characteristic attack, several small faceted culi were found in a stool. The usual symptom ready mentioned followed this attack, but the pa appeared more tired and weaker than ever be From March 25, 1895, until July 1st of the year, with progressive emaciation and anorexia had repeated attacks of severe biliary pain, none of which did careful search show the pres of gall-stones in the stools.

The tenderness over the right half of the ep trium and right hypochondrium was constantly ent. The patient became more emaciated, von a great deal, suffered from almost continuous pa the region of the stomach and liver, and on Jul 1895, a hard swelling about the size of a haz was palpable near the border of the epigastric right hypochondriac regions. This was tender seemed to be slightly movable. Examination o blood showed hemoglobin, fifty per cent.; red bl corpuscles reduced to 3,000,000 per c.mm.; n crease in the number of, or change in, the w blood-corpuscles. The symptoms now seeme most entirely referable to the stomach, and prom

---

*Read at the Ninety-second Annual Meeting of the Medical Society of the State of New York, held at Albany, N. Y., January 25, 26, and 27, 1898.

me to make an examination of the contents of this organ. After a test meal, on July 15, 1895, there was found complete absence of free hydrochloric acid, though pepsin and rennet were present, as was also a small quantity of lactic acid; there was a moderate amount of bile, and the total acidity was .025 per cent. Inflation of the stomach showed marked dilatation, with a tumor about the size of an ordinary egg occupying the normal position of the pylorus, and showing a considerable lateral movement during the inflation.

Taking the history into consideration, the increasing cachexia, the result of the chemic examination of the stomach contents, the dilated stomach found on inflation, the tumor occupying the normal position of the pylorus, its increase in size during the weeks preceding the final examination, the blood count, and low hemoglobin percentage, I was prompted to diagnose carcinoma of the pylorus associated with gall-stones. Repeated examination of the stomach contents failed to give results different from those first obtained. At no time did congo or tropeolin paper, or the Gunzburg test show the presence of free hydrochloric acid. The patient's suffering now became continuous, the tumor was at all times palpable, there was increasing splashing of the stomach contents, there was more or less peristaltic unrest, and the picture of carcinoma with constriction at the pylorus seemed complete. There was at no time more than a moderate amount of jaundice. The urine was of normal specific gravity, occasionally contained a trace of bile salts and pigment, but never albumin or sugar. An unfavorable prognosis was given, and, from day to day, the patient grew weaker and more wretched.

In this condition she continued until October 1, 1896, *a period of fifteen months after the recognition of the tumor, during which time the latter was always palpable*. At this time she was seized with violent pain which radiated throughout the upper half of the abdomen, and during my temporary absence from the city another physician was called to see her who partially relieved her by means of hypodermic injections of morphin. During the first week of October, 1896, symptoms of partial intestinal obstruction were manifested. There was considerable hiccough, increasing weakness of the pulse —which until the present time had been of good quality—while the tumor was no longer palpable. During my visit on October 8, 1896, I noticed a characteristic coiling of a portion of the intestine into a sausage-shaped mass in the upper part of the abdomen, stretching from the right to the left side, across the lower border of the epigastrium. This coiling continued for about sixty seconds, when it disappeared after an audible gurgling, with the relief of the acute pain. On the following day the symptoms were in no measure relieved, though the patient had passed some flatus *per rectum*, the tumor was not palpable, the upper abdominal regions were tympanitic, there was more or less vomiting of a dirty, green, and at times brown-colored, sour-smelling fluid, the coiling of the intestine had increased, and about four feet of intestine could be seen through the abdominal walls, sausage-shaped, tense before it collapsed after a characteristic gurgling in the upper part of the abdomen.

Deep palpation now showed the presence of a hard mass in front of the tense intestine, the size and shape of which corresponded exactly with that of the tumor originally found in the region of the pylorus. The nature of this tumor was no longer a matter of doubt, for I had concluded that we had an enormous gall-stone impacted in the gall-bladder simulating the symptoms of pyloric cancer. That this had been dislodged was no longer doubtful. The movable mass in its progress downward was giving rise to partial intestinal obstruction and increased coiling of the small intestine. On October 13, 1896, we were enabled to empty the colon by means of high rectal injections without making any impression upon the symptoms referable to the small intestine. The strength of the patient continued about the same, the temperature ranging between 97.9° F. and normal; the tongue throughout was moist and stained by the vomited matter. On October 14, 1896, the coiling seemed to involve the entire length of the small intestine which could be seen, as before, through the abdominal walls distinctly sausage-shaped, and the different coils could be moved upon each other. The increase of coiling seemed to justify a delay in instituting surgical interference, I concluded that obstruction was not complete, and that the obstructing mass was movable, as shown by the increased length of the intestine involved from day to day. I felt that if the strength of the patient would permit we might wait until the offender was safely passed into the large intestine by Nature's effort.

On the morning of October 16, 1896, with Dr. Coe of Syracuse, the patient was visited for the purpose of determining a method of hastening the passage of the mass. On entering the room our patient received us cheerfully. She informed us of the fact that after a night of considerable suffering from rectal tenesmus, without coiling of the small intestine, she had passed an enormous stony mass, which she had left in the vessel, where Dr. Coe and I found it. It proved to be a gall-stone, composed mainly of cholesterin. Its circumference was 13 cm. (5½ inches), its length 7.5 cm. (3 inches), and its weight was 368 grains. There were no further symptoms referable to the abdominal organs, the patient gained strength and flesh, and after a few weeks she resumed her household duties. The stomach, while still somewhat dilated, performed its functions satisfactorily, and to all appearances the patient was fully restored to health.

About eleven months after the passage of this enormous gall-stone and during my absence from the city, my assistant, Dr. Kieffer, attended the patient for what was considered an acute indigestion. There were no pains characteristic of gall-stone colic. Four days after this visit the patient sent a gall-stone to my office which she had passed after considerable rectal spasm. It weighed 240 grains, was 5 cm. (2 inches) long, and 7.5 cm. (3 inches) in circumference. Since the passage of this last gall-stone the patient has remained well.

From a diagnostic, as well as from a pathologic standpoint, this case is full of interest. The complete clinical picture of cancer of the pylorus, coupled with cholelithiasis was presented. No other diagnosis seemed justified when we considered the previous history, the repeated attacks of gall-stone colic, the final tumor persisting for months, with gastrectasia, the characteristic displacement of the mass to the right and its upward movement on inflation of the stomach, and finally, the results of the analysis of the stomach-contents, with the emaciation and cachexia. With these conditions present, the gall-stone disease was readily considered to be of secondary importance. The irregular forms of gall-stones, as Naunyn has forcibly demonstrated, by prolonged incarceration may give rise to a variety of pathologic complications, the most serious of which are attribntable to added infection or ulcerative changes. In the case reported the enormous gall-stone which finally gave rise to partial intestinal obstruction, had filled the gall-bladder, which organ, as the result of protective and adhesive inflammation, became adherent to the duodenum. The pylorus was sufficiently distorted by traction and thickening to suffer ultimate constriction with consecutive gastrectasia. After fifteen months of retention in its capsules, the offender escaped by an ulcerative process through a fistulous opening into the duodenum, the free peritoneum being well protected. In its descent downward the stone was arrested at various points, causing obstruction with increasing intestinal coiling, and all of the other symptoms mentioned. The final unique feature of the case was the passage of the stone eleven months after the disappearance of the tumor, without the usual painful symptoms. Undoubtedly this stone originally formed a part of the misleading tumor, but it had found during its detention—and after the escape of the first large stone—a suitable resting-place in a diverticulum of the adherent gall-bladder, a condition pictured by Riedel.[1] Finally the stone escaped through the patent fistula into the duodenum. The fact that the last stone did not give rise to symptoms is by no means surprising, for incarcerated stones have frequently been found without having been suspected in spite of the fact that great local mischief had been done. Many of these unsuspected cases are associated with malignant disease. The writer has several times found innumerable concretions in the smallest branches of the hepatic ducts without a single symptom referable to the liver.

It will be profitable in connection with this case to consider three points: (1) The simulation of pyloric carcinoma. (2) The ulcerative process causing the gall-bladder-duodenal-fistula. (3) The final intestinal obstruction (incomplete).

1. The simulation of pyloric carcinoma which continued in this case during fifteen months is not entirely without parallel. Simulation was made easy by the presence of the tumor, the ultimate production of stenosis of the pylorus, and dilatation of the stomach. Eminent clinicians have been mislead in similar instances.

Pepper[3] reports a case in which there was a gall-stone of unusual dimensions which simulated scirrhus of the pylorus with all of the symptoms of cancer of the stomach, including persistent vomiting and great irritability of the stomach. The patient died three weeks after coming to the notice of the physician, some six months after the commencement of the illness. "The tumor felt during life, in the pyloric region, proved to be a large gall-stone completely filling the bladder and molded to its shape. The gall-bladder itself, however, was perfectly healthy, as was also the liver and its ducts. The surface of the stone was unusually smooth, of a light yellowish color; it weighed a little more than half an ounce, and measured two inches in its greatest circumference, and in length it was two and one-half inches. Portions of the small intestine were agglutinated together; their walls were adherent in several places, and they connected with each other through ulcerative openings. The stomach was perfectly healthy." Other parallel cases are reported by Miles,[3] Fiedler,[4] Ross,[5] Hale White,[6] and Ogle.[7]

In all of these cases, as in the case reported by the writer, there was gastrectasia and a palpable tumor. In the case reported by Miles, there were evidences of fermentation of the stomach contents. In the cases of Fiedler and Ross there was vomiting of blood. In all of these cases the authors mentioned made during life a positive diagnosis of cancer of the pylorus. Naunyn[8] reports a case which he observed in Königsberg, in which a tumor persisted during seven months in the region of the pylorus. At first it grew rapidly, then suddenly disappeared. While it was palpable there was persistent vomiting. After one year there was recurrence of the tumor, recurrence of vomiting, persistent pain in the right hypochondrium, gastrectasia, fermentation, increasing cachexia, and finally coma and death. At the *post-mortem* an enormous gall-stone was found, and it entirely filled the gall-bladder; there was ulceration of the adherent duodenum, the gall-bladder itself was ulcerated in spots; besides the communication with the duodenum there was a fistula leading from the gall-bladder into the colon.

Fiedler's case was that of a woman sixty-six years

complete or partial intestinal obstruction deserves more than passing notice. With the disappearance of the original tumor, and the appearance of intestinal distention and the gurgling followed by immediate collapse of the tube, came the suspicion that the offender was a gall-stone of considerable size. The literature relating to intestinal obstruction due to gall-stones is by no means meager, and the possibility of its occurrence must not be forgotten. In fact, we must conclude that the occurrence of intestinal obstruction, after the passage of gall-stones from the gall-bladder into the intestine, is surprisingly frequent, owing to the large size of these stones. Thus, Courvoisier[16] reports ileus in twenty-eight of seventy-three cases, or 38.3 per cent.

We are frequently misled in our diagnosis because of the fact that gall-stones find their way into the intestinal tract through fistulous openings without producing symptoms until the sudden occurrence of obstruction. The differential diagnosis of the cause of the obstruction in this class of cases cannot possibly be made. Mayo Robson[17] reports cases of acute intestinal obstruction from gall-stones, in some of which recovery followed operation, in others the stones, after a number of days, were passed *per rectum*. In one case reported by Gray[18] obstruction continued twelve days before the stone was dislodged. Craigie[19] reports a case in which intestinal obstruction continued nine days, at the end of which time the stone was passed and the patient recovered.

The prognosis is much more serious when ileus follows gall-bladder-duodenal-fistulæ then when the opening is into the colon. Of thirty fatal cases, twenty-eight were due to gall-bladder-duodenal-fistula, and only two to gall-bladder-colon-perforation (Naunyn[20]). If a gall-stone finds its way directly into the duodenum through the common duct there is but little danger of intestinal obstruction. The rarity of ulceration of stones large enough to cause intestinal obstruction through the choledochus walls is emphasized by Courvoisier[21]. He found in thirty-six cases in which large stones entered the intestine and in which *post-mortems* had been made, that in three the stones had escaped through the common duct.

The expectant treatment, in the writer's case, seemed justified because it was reasonably certain that a gall-stone was present, and that it was slowly moving along. Robson[22] says, "If it were possible to be certain that a gall-stone is the cause of the block, the expectant form of treatment would be fully justified, since the probability, arguing from published cases, is that the gall-stone will eventually pass." The same author suggests that in those cases offering "diagnostic difficulties" the surgeon is accepting "great responsibility in waiting for Nature's cure." Naunyn[23] makes the statement, after considering the results of thirteen operations for ileus due to gall-stones—of which number only one resulted in recovery—that laparotomy is not to be recommended, and in over fifty per cent. of the cases recovery results without operation; that frequently the condition yields after from seven to nine days of obstruction, and as operators will always be encouraged by these facts, they will rarely operate early, hence they will find, with late operations, necrosis of the intestinal wall and circumscribed peritonitis. Langenbuch[24] takes a more extreme view of this question. He makes the unqualified statement that "gall-stone obstruction is a surgical disease, the treatment of which is to be entrusted to the physician only during a very short period."

CASE II.—On September 12, 1897, I saw Miss W., aged twenty years, a student, in consultation with Drs. Easton and Kellogg of Syracuse. Her family history was negative. Prior to January, 1897, she had been in good health. While in Chicago shortly after January 1, 1897, she was taken with fever and evidences of tonsillitis, and finally more or less pain in the upper abdominal regions, marked gastroduodenal disturbance, rapid pulse, and, after a few days, repeated chills, which observed a periodicity, recurring at intervals of from twelve to twenty-four hours, without (at this time) noticeable jaundice. The physician in attendance during her stay in Chicago considered her trouble to be of malarial origin, and treated her accordingly. She remained in bed five weeks, had not then convalesced completely, but continued to complain of vague symptoms, malaise, and a generally reduced condition, when, in March, 1897, she was suddenly seized with severe lancinating pains in the right hypochondrium, which continued acute during two hours. Her symptoms of gastrohepatic disturbance now became continuous, and she had had at intervals of a few weeks, when Drs. Easton and Kellogg saw her, what to them seemed characteristic attacks of gall-stone colic.

On August 9, 1897, she became jaundiced. Dr. Easton attended the patient in Syracuse. She had with each attack of colic more or less elevation of temperature, usually between 100° and 101° F. A sharp rise of temperature, averaging 103° F., followed the more acute exacerbations of what had now become a chronic condition. Jaundice persisted, and became more intense with each paroxysm of pain. Her temperature was at no time normal, being usually slightly elevated. Between the attacks her pulse was at all times alarmingly rapid, without encouraging arterial tone. The urine had been examined and found bile-tinged, without albumin, and negative in other respects.

I found the patient in a typhoid condition. The tongue was characteristic; pulse varied in frequency from 110 to 120; at one time during the consultation it fell to 100 per minute. Temperature, 100° F. There was intense jaundice, with all evidences (subjective and objective) of profound infection associated with disease of the gall-bladder and bile-ducts. The intestines were distended with gas. The most acute suffering on pressure was located in the region of the gall-bladder.

Physical Examination.—There was nothing noteworthy in the thorax. The abdomen was tympanitic and tender to pressure. Careful examination revealed a mass corresponding in size to a goose-egg, which gave fluctuation on deep pressure. This tumor moved up and down with respiration. The liver dulness was slightly increased. The spleen was somewhat enlarged.

A diagnosis of infectious cholecystitis, cholangitis, empyema of the gall-bladder, and associated gall-stone was made. We concluded that in all probability there was occlusion of the common duct. Immediate operation was recommended. Dr. Easton took the patient to New York, where on September 20, 1897, Dr. Lange operated, opening the gall-bladder, which was found filled with pus. A gall-stone the size of a beach-nut was found in the gall-bladder. The cystic duct was occluded. The common duct was palpated, found hard, thickened, but no stone could be felt in it. It was not disturbed. Following this operation there was slight improvement. Whatever discharge finally escaped through the wound proved to be the secretion of the gall-bladder only. The temperature was lowered, there was less jaundice, though this was not materially changed.

About October 1, 1897, the patient had a chill, after severe biliary colic requiring morphia for its relief. The pulse again became rapid, fever high, and the icterus decidedly deepened. The stools continued putty-colored. The patient's condition warranted the conclusion that the common duct was still obstructed, and that there was either hardened mucus and pus, or gall-stones which had been forced to the obstruction, giving rise to the characteristic pain of biliary colic. The deep jaundice and other increasing positive evidences of obstruction of the common duct prompted Dr. Lange to undertake a second operation on October 6, 1897. On opening the common duct no stone was found in spite of careful search, but a cicatricial contraction was felt at the point of entrance into the duodenum. A new opening was made into the duodenum, and an anastomosis was then established between the common duct and the intestine. Dr. Lange reported everything progressing favorably for five days, when, after the removal of the tampon, the suture line leaked, and for about one week bile and duodenal contents escaped through the wound. The general condition of the patient suffered materially. Finally, the skilful surgeon by means of persistent posture on the left side, and an improvised tamponade succeeded in healing the wound. There were no further symptoms of obstruction. The discharge once checked, the jaundice disappeared, and recovery was uninterrupted. A fistula opening into the gall-bladder has remained, but the discharge from this is but slight, nothing more than a trace of mucus daily, and causing no inconvenience. This can be overcome later if indications demand it.

In the hands of a less experienced surgeon, this young life would in all probability have been lost. The case is as interesting in its pathologic as in its surgical aspect. The history strengthens the more recent views which attribute to infection an important rôle in the causation of pathologic changes within the bile passages, and in the production of gall-stones. The primary illness associated with tonsillitis in January, 1897, was a far-reaching infection; this spread from the intestine, where there may have been a duodenal ulcer in the region of the papilla, to the bile passages and gall-bladder, causing cholangitis, cholecystitis, and gall-stone formation, with empyema of the gall-bladder and consecutive occlusion of the cystic and common ducts, the latter due to deep ulcerative or inflammatory changes. The enlargement of the spleen found at the consultation on September 12, 1897, strengthens these conclusions.

Dr. Lange wrote: "I was also under the impression that the pancreatic duct was dilated, and formed, with the end of the common duct, a rather large cavity, into which I was able to pass my finger behind the posterior wall of the duodenum."

The great interest in this case is centered in the unique obstruction of both the common and cystic ducts, as the result of violent infectious cholecystitis and cholangitis. Such cases are exceedingly rare. I have thoroughly searched the authorities on this subject at my command, and find no cases which seem to correspond exactly with the one here reported. In the large proportion of choledochus strictures reported the duct was much dilated, resembling at times the gall-bladder. Langenbuch[25] reports four cases of common-duct stricture in which choledochostomy was performed. In each of these there was enormous cystic dilatation of the common duct, which in each case had been opened and drained; the respective operators supposed that they were dealing with a distended gall-bladder, never suspecting the distension of the common duct. In two of these cases the autopsies proved the fallacy of the operators' conclusions (Helferich and Ahlfeld[26]).

In the case of Levy[27] the duct was bent upon itself, distended, and mistaken for the gall-bladder. In the fourth case (Quenu[28]) a large abscess was opened which was not connected with the gall-bladder, but was, according to Terrier, in all probability connected with the common duct. Yörsen[29], during a laparotomy, found a swelling the size of an apple, which, owing to its position, he supposed to be the gall-bladder. He opened the mass, after stitching it to the abdominal walls, and gave exit to foul-smelling pus and gall-stones. The patient died the following day. It was demonstrated that the common duct had been fastened to the parietal peritoneum—the gall-bladder was not involved. Kocher[30] was the first to avail himself of the original suggestion of Langenbuch. The latter had called attention to the possibility of establishing an anastomosis between the common duct and the duodenum, the operation which Lange performed in the case reported.

Kocher's case was one in which a gall-stone was impacted in the common duct. He was fearful that lithotrity might fail; he therefore introduced his sutures into the duodenum and common duct with the idea of ultimately uniting these if necessary. The stone yielded and the anastomosis was not made. Besides this case, in which choledocho-duodenostomy had been performed, I find one reported by Riedel.[31] In this case the operation was performed for impacted stone, which the operator could not reach in the common duct. He made an anastomosis between the common duct and the duodenum. The stitches gave way, owing to the thin choledochus wall. The patient died of peritonitis. Sprengel[32] reports recovery in a case in which he first did a laparotomy and attempted to push a stone impacted in the common duct into the duodenum. In this he failed, and closed the abdomen. Three weeks after this operation he made a second attempt, and completed the operation with a choledocho-duodenostomy.

Terrier[33] and Kocher[34] each report a case in which the anastomosis became necessary in complicated constriction from gall-stone, and in which the patients made a happy recovery. Czerny[35] reports a case in which he united an enormously dilated and constricted common duct, by means of the Murphy button, with the duodenum. The case is supposed to have terminated favorably.

Cases in which there has been obstruction to the outflow of bile, from the choledochus into the duodenum, and in which the simpler operation of chollecysto-enterostomy has been successfully accomplished, do not concern us in considering the case reported. Anastomosis between the gall-bladder and duodenum is to be preferred, provided the former will serve as a canal to return the bile from the common duct above the constriction to the intestine. It has occasionally been found impossible to establish the communication with the duodenum, hence the colon has been made the receptacle of the diverted bile. The suspicion of ulcer of the duodenum, expressed in considering the pathology of the case reported, is justified by a statement made by Langenbuch,[36] in which he mentions the possibility of cicatricial contraction of the common duct following duodenal ulcer; but he fails to mention a case. Courvoisier[37] has collected sixty-two cases of obliteration of the choledochus. Of this number seventeen were congenital. The majority of these were due to fetal inflammation; in all probability most of these were of specific origin. Cholelithiasis was found to be the more frequent cause of constriction of the common duct after birth, and was found in twenty-three cases. In one case reported by Archambault,[38] there was obliteration of the common duct due to a typhoid process propagated from the intestine. A case of Richard's[39] is reported in which there was a benign stricture of the pylorus which involved the common duct in the cicatricial contraction. Musser and Keen[40] report a case of common-duct obliteration due to chronic enteritis, and make mention of the "closure of the ducts" by the "healing of an ulcer in the duct or at the duodenal orifice." Courvoisier's list contains three cases[41], [42], [43], in which traumatism was supposed to have caused obliteration of the choledochus. In the remaining cases reported by Courvoisier, the histories do not justify positive conclusions as to the origin of the obliteration of the duct, but the compiler adds, "the thought which one must always entertain in connection with these cases is that irritation from gall-stone descent is the more probable cause, though this cannot be proven."

CASE III.—In this case a man, aged about fifty-five years, was seen in consultation with Dr. George R. Kinne, and the patient presented all of the symptoms of grave abdominal disease. There were no evidences of stenosis or intestinal obstruction, but all of the usual symptoms of malignant disease of the mesenteric glands, with more or less pancreatic indigestion. There were no symptoms referable to the gall-bladder; the patient had never had gall-stone colic. Emaciation was progressive and after the lapse of six months he died of asthenia. There was a suspicious dulness in the upper part of the epigastrium.

The *post-mortem* revealed the fact that a gall-stone had quietly burrowed its way from the cystic duct into the retroperitoneal space, and had found a resting place in a dense connective tissue capsule back of the pancreas. There were evidences (in uneven dilatations of the fistulous tract) of incarceration at several points during the progress of the stone to its final resting place.*

CASE IV.—The patient was a man, aged sixty years, who came to Syracuse from the lumber regions of Michigan. He had had repeated attacks of vague abdominal pains, and had often suffered from intermittent malarial fever. On one occasion, about two years before he came to Syracuse, he had a severe attack of what, in the light of subsequent developments, must be considered gall-stone colic. He seemed to recover from the acute attack, but was never free from pain in the right lumbar region. After a few months he developed a train of symptoms referable to the genito-urinary organs, particularly the right kidney. At one time he claims to have had free hematuria. Subsequently, the color of his urine became dirty brown and flaky. Emaciation was progressive. He finally became cachectic, and when I saw him was almost moribund. About two weeks after my first visit he passed a small calculus, *per urethram*, which fell into the vessel and was not saved. The urine contained bile, blood, pus, and albumin. He died four weeks after his arrival in Syracuse.

The *post-mortem* disclosed a fistulous tract leading from the gall-bladder into an abscess the size of an orange, and from this to the pelvis of the right kidney, in which we found an enormous cholesterin gall-stone. The gall-bladder wall was thickened and contained three good sized gall-stones. The abscess was surrounded by a dense mass of connective tissue. The kidney tissue was infiltrated and presented a characteristic yellowish-brown appearance.

Courvoisier[44] reports seven cases of urinary fistulæ associated with gall-stones; six of these were found in women. In one of these cases, reported by Pelletan and Barraud,[45] 200 stones passed the urethra within eight days. In this case the last stone became caught in the urethra, but was easily pushed on from the vagina. The patient recovered. An abstract of the histories of these cases makes very interesting reading and can be found in Langenbuch's[46] recently published work.

Experience has convinced me that in many cases cholelithiasis, with or without colic, is early associated with localized peritonitis. This may, in some instances, be a fortunate occurrence for the patient where ulceration finally takes place, but in a number of cases consecutive adhesions with distortion and displacement of the gall-bladder and adherent intestine have caused insuperable obstacles to the performance of life-saving surgical operations, and have given rise to annoying symptoms.

CASE V.—Patient, female, aged thirty years, seen in consultation on June 21, 1895, with the late Dr. Magee. She had all of the symptoms of impaction of a gall-stone in the common duct, with associated localized peritonitis and infection. In spite of the fact that both Dr. Magee and I insisted upon immediate operation, other consultants doubting our diagnosis the operation was delayed until the woman was practically moribund. Dr. Magee opened the abdomen, found dense adhesion of the gall-bladder to the duodenum. The parts were drawn backward and downward. The common duct could be distinctly felt filled with enormous gall-stones, but surgical relief was made impossible by the depth of

* Only three cases of retroperitoneal perforation were found in the collection reported by Courvoisier.

the parts and their changed anatomic relations. The patient died. The *post-mortem* showed three stones closely packed in the common duct, the surface of which was ulcerated and the duct itself enormously distended, besides the conditions mentioned.

In many cases pain in the region of the gall-bladder, after the passage of gall-stones, becomes persistent. This symptom is due to adhesions of the gall-bladder to the surrounding parts and to traction. Mayo Robson[47] reports cases of this kind in which he operated, overcoming adhesions, to the great relief of his patient. These operations were undertaken for the removal of suspected gall-stones. My list of cases includes a considerable number in which gall-stones found exit through the abdominal wall. The point of perforation was usually in the neighborhood of the umbilicus. These cases present no unique features, and I will not dilate upon them. One of these, however, is interesting from the fact that the patient is now seventy-seven years of age, and that during the past twenty years she has passed innumerable biliary calculi through an opening in the abdominal wall, which closes, as a rule, within a few weeks after the passage of a stone. Her general health does not seem to suffer in consequence of these occurrences.

CASE VI.—Patient, Mrs. H., aged fifty-six years, was first seen in consultation with Dr. Doust. In this case there was a history of gall-stone disease, with repeated attacks of colic, dating back twenty-five years. When I saw her on October 19, 1897, she was deeply jaundiced and had all of the symptoms of gall-stone impaction in the common duct. There were also evidences of an enlarged gall-bladder and liver.

During the course of a few weeks the patient passed a large number of small gall-stones, without relief of her symptoms. On December 9, 1897, I again saw her in consultation with Drs. Doust and Breese, when a fistulous tract was found at a point about two inches below the free border of the ribs on a line drawn from the right sternoclavicular articulation. Within a few days after this visit Dr. Breese examined the patient under ether. He opened the sinus, through which yellowish pus had escaped, but failed to find an opening from this into the gall-bladder.

On January 14, 1898, Dr. Breese again opened the abdomen. He found the gall-bladder everywhere adherent and hard. Pressure on the surface of the gall-bladder gave a peculiar grating. The anterior wall was converted into dense cicatricial tissue and was continuous with the liver, from which it could not be separated. The cystic duct was obliterated and converted into a dense mass of infiltrated tissue. The pancreas was hard. The adhesions were so dense and the changes so far reaching that the surgeon could see no way of overcoming the obstruction; hence, the abdomen was closed. At the *post-mortem* the gall-bladder was found to contain 601 small pyramidal hard white stones. The induration of the common and cystic ducts had an appearance suspicious of carcinoma. There were a few enlarged glands to be seen back of the gall-bladder. The mural abscess was probably due to the escape of one of the small stones, after which the gall-bladder closed and detached itself from the parietal peritoneum. The hepatic duct was obliterated at its junction with the cystic. The ducts above the obliteration were enormously dilated and were filled with bile.

My clinical experiences have demonstrated the fact that gall-stone colic is not entirely without danger from sudden heart failure. In elderly people the association of gall-stone disease with myocardial degeneration is not at all uncommon. In some of these cases I have also observed associated diabetes. In a case seen a number of years ago the patient, who had had repeated attacks of gall-stone colic, was suddenly seized during one of these with violent precordial pain, and immediately expired. The *post-mortem* examination showed well-marked myocardial degeneration, dilatation of the heart, with partial rupture in the anterior wall of the left ventricle. A gall-stone the size of an ordinary marble was found impacted in the cystic duct. In a number of my cases of persistent jaundice due to long-continued gall-stone impaction, alarming brain symptoms developed. In one of these an old man became violently insane. The insanity yielded with the relief of the obstruction and the disappearance of the jaundice. A similar case was recently seen in consultation with Dr. Jacobson, in which prolonged cholemia due to obstruction of the common duct caused confusional insanity.

Gall-bladder infection from the presence of the bacillus typhosus, also the involvement of the bile ducts in a similar process, or suppurative cholangitis, with and without gall-stone formation, have been observed by the writer, but these cases cannot be considered at this time. An attack of gall-stone colic masked the early diagnosis of a case of typhoid fever seen with Dr. Joy at Casenovia a few months ago. A coachman, who had previously suffered from gall-stones, while driving was suddenly seized with high fever and the usual pains of an ordinary bilious colic. He had been feeling badly for several days before the attack. Great tenderness over the region of the gall-bladder persisted, with slight jaundice and evidences of localized peritonitis. The high fever was entirely out of proportion to the extent of the local peritonitis. We found, as the disease progressed and time was given for diagnosis, that he had typhoid complicated with cholelithiasis. The patient recovered.

Only once have I found *post-mortem* the ball-valve gall-stone in the common duct in the diverticulum of Vater, a condition which has been so thoroughly described by Osler[48]. I have seen several recoveries after recurring symptoms of partial obstruction of the common duct, with occasional marked exacerbation and deepening of jaundice. These cases were usually accompanied with the intermittent hepatic fever described by Charcot, which led me to believe that I was dealing with a ball-valve gall-stone in the common duct.

Since the appearance of Courvoisier's, Naunyn's, and Mayo Robson's elaborate monographs, Riedel's work in 1892, in which his statistics showed a successful issue in ninety per cent. of gall-stone operations, the monumental work of Langenbuch, recently published in the *Deutsche Chirurgie*, and the convincing paper read by Lange[49] of New York at Johns Hopkins', the duty of the diagnostician has been made plain. The symptoms of all cases of cholelithiasis demand correct interpretation at the earliest possible moment. I have attempted to demonstrate, both by clinical and pathologic data, that processes which are protective may at the same time seriously interfere with the surgeon's results. I feel justified in concluding that the persistence of gall-stone symptoms demand the same concerted action of physician and surgeon that has so promptly succeeded in reducing the mortality from appendicitis. The surgeon will always require the physician's knowledge of pathology in these cases and possibly some of his conservatism to guide him, but together, they will ultimately find themselves breaking loose from extreme views to meet on vantage ground where deliberate judgment and sound reasoning will prevail.

BIBLIOGRAPHY.

[1] Riedel, Figure 2, "Erfahraungen uber die Gallensteine Krankheit, etc.," p. 5, Berlin, 1892.
[2] Pepper, *Amer. Jour. Med. Sciences*, vol. xxxiii, p. 13, 1857.
[3] Miles, *London Lancet*, vol. i, 1861.
[4] Fiedler, "Ueber Gallensteine," *Wiener Medic. Blatter*, 1880; No. 49. u. *Jahresberichte d. Gesellsch. für Natur Heilkunde in Dresden*, p. 121–136, 1879.
[5] Ross, *British Med. Jour.*, vol. i, p. 251, 1885.
[6] White, Hale, *Trans. Path. Soc. Lond.*, vol. xxxvii, p. 280, 1886; *British Med. Jour.*, vol. ii, p. 903, 1886.
[7] Ogle, *St. George's Hosp. Reports*, 1868.
[8] Naunyn, "Klink der Cholelithiasis," p. 142, Leipzig, 1892.
[9] Naunyn, *loc. cit.*, p. 143.
[10] Bartholin, "Obstetrics," 54, p. 243.
[11] Beaussier, *Jour. de Med. Chir. Pharm*. tome 32, Fevr., p. 163, 1770.
[12] Walter, J. G., *Mus. Anat.*, *loc. cit.*, I., p. 125, No. 250.
[13] Blumenbach, *Med. Bibl.*, Bd. I, p. 121, 1783.
[14] Courvoisier, "Casuistisch-Statistische Beitrage zur Pathologie und Chirurgie der Gallenwege," p. 84, Leipzig.
[15] Courvoisier, *loc. cit.*, p. 83.
[16] Courvoisier, *loc. cit.*, p. 101–110.
[17] Robson, Mayo, "On Gall-stones and Their Treatment," Cassell and Company, p. 92, 1892; *Medical and Chirurgical Soc.*, pp. 52–53, 1895.
[18] Gray, *Trans. Lond. Clin. Soc.*, vol. iv, p. 194.
[19] Craigie, *Edinburgh Medical and Surg. Jour.*, vol. xxii, 1824.
[20] Naunyn, *loc. cit.*, p. 144.
[21] Courvoisier, *loc. cit.*, p. 104.
[22] Robson, *loc. cit.*, p. 107.
[23] Naunyn, *loc. cit.*, p. 173.
[24] Langenbuch, "Chirurgie der Leber und Gallenblase," ii, p. 233. Theill, Stuttgart, 1897.
[25] Langenbuch, *loc. cit.*, pp. 341–342.
[26] Helferich and Ahlfeld, quoted by Langenbuch, *loc. cit.*, p. 342.
[27] Levy, quoted by Langenbuch, *loc. cit.*, p. 342.
[28] Quenu, quoted by Langenbuch, *loc. cit.*, p. 341.
[29] Yörsen, quoted by Langenbuch, *loc. cit.*, p. 342.
[30] Kocher, quoted by Langenbuch, *loc. cit.*, p. 342.
[31] Riedel, *loc. cit.*, p. 119.
[32] Sprengel, quoted by Langenbuch, *loc. cit.*, p. 342.
[33] Terrier, quoted by Langenbuch, *loc. cit.*, p. 342.
[34] Kocher, quoted by Langenbuch, *loc. cit.*, p. 342.
[35] Czerny, quoted by Langenbuch, *loc. cit.*, p. 342.
[36] Langenbuch, *loc. cit.*, p. 180.
[37] Courvoisier, *loc. cit.*, pp. 52–53.
[38] Archambault, *Bull. Soc. Anat.*, p. 90, 1852.
[39] Richards, *Bull. Soc. Anat.*, p. 82, 1846.
[40] Musser and Keen, *Am. Jour. Med. Sciences*, pp. 339–342, October, 1884.
[41] Andral, *Clin Med.*, p. 534, obs. 49 L, p. 526, obs. 50.
[42] Maurer, *Acta phys. med. Acad.*, Bd. viii, p. 363; Cals. Nat., Norimbg., 1748.
[43] Hufeland, *Jour d. prakt. Arzneikundl*, Bd. ix, 3 stuck, p. 105, Berlin, 1813.
[44] Courvoisier, *loc. cit.*, p. 106, etc.
[45] Pelletan and Barraud, Pelletan (Barraud, Batillat.), *Jour. de Chimie med., de Pharm. et de Toxicol.*, ii ser., t. 2, pp. 593–600, 653–669, 1836.
[46] Langenbuch, *loc. cit.*, p. 234.
[47] Robson, Mayo, *loc. cit.*, pp. 216–217.
[48] Osler, *Lond. Lancet*, vol. i, p. 1319, 1897.
[49] Lange, *Johns Hopkins Hosp. Bulletin*, p. 29, February, 1897.

CLINICAL MEMORANDUM.

A PERSONAL EXPERIENCE IN RENAL SURGERY.

BY ROBERT F. WEIR, M.D.,
OF NEW YORK;
PROFESSOR OF SURGERY IN THE COLLEGE OF PHYSICIANS AND SURGEONS, AND SURGEON TO THE NEW YORK HOSPITAL;
WITH THE COLLABORATION OF
EDWARD M. FOOTE, M.D.,
OF NEW YORK;
SURGEON TO THE RANDALL'S ISLAND HOSPITALS.

(Continued from page 146.)

TUBERCULOSIS.

THE possibility of an early diagnosis of this form of renal infection has been much increased during the past few years, and especially by the use of the cystoscope. This instrument will some day perhaps settle the much-disputed question as to whether the kidney affection is primary or secondary to tuberculosis of the bladder, prostate, etc. It was formerly the almost universal opinion, from clinical data alone, that the infection traveled upward through the ureter. Donnadieu,[1] in a comprehensive article, showed some time ago the difficulty of deciding the question at an autopsy, when the lesions found in both kidney and bladder are usually caseous, so that it is impracticable to speak of their relative age. He quotes Guyon as saying he had observed but one case of uncomplicated renal tuberculosis. Since that time, however,

[1] *Arch. clin. de Bordeaux*, November, 1892.

numerous instances of undoubted primary renal tuberculosis have been reported, among them being an interesting one of Thorel's.[1]

More commonly, however, the kidney is secondarily infected from a previously existing pulmonary tuberculosis. This occurs in from thirty-four per cent. (Brown) to fifty per cent. (Morris, Steinthal) of the cases. The miliary form of infection presents in about one-third of the instances, and then usually invades, according to many writers, both kidneys. This, however, I am inclined to doubt. In the other two-thirds the involvement was found more advanced; that is to say, it is presented in the form of caseous deposits, and, what is of surgical importance, about one-half of these lesions were confined to one kidney. In cases of all kinds of a somewhat chronic form which admit and demand surgical attention, and which have arisen in distant tuberculous foci or in other parts of the genito-urinary tract, *e.g.*, the testis, prostate, and bladder, it has been demonstrated that the renal lesions are one-sided in about one-half of the cases (Steinthal, twelve out of twenty-four cases).

The localization of lesions in both kidneys is more apt, according to Dickinson, to be found in children under twelve years of age, for in twenty-eight cases reported by him it occurred nineteen times in both kidneys and nine times in a single kidney. In persons over twelve years of age, however, the tuberculous invasion was found to be confined to one kidney in thirty-eight instances out of sixty-seven cases. With the aid of the expert cystoscopist not only will the diagnosis be earlier and oftentimes more certainly determined, but its one-sided character can positively be arrived at, and also important information may be obtained as to the condition of the bladder[2]—often a doubtful point because the irritation of the renal discharge often simulates a calculus, a tumor, or a tuberculous cystitis. From the aid derived from this mode of examination, with its ureteral interrogation, earlier operation becomes, not only possible, but greatly advantageous in sparing the bladder and the opposite kidney from probable secondary infection. This is self-evident, and to it, it is hardly necessary to allude. Of far more weight is the following question: Having accomplished the extirpation of a tuberculous kidney, or having performed nephrotomy for the relief of an abscess or abscesses, what final result may be expected? Experience has accumulated much clinical data in answer to this question, though a large amount is not of as positive a character as one might wish. Albarran, for instance, reports eight nephrectomies for tuberculosis with one death from the operation. Of the remainder, five patients were living and in good condition from fifteen to thirty months afterward. He also performed nephrotomy eleven times for tuberculous abscess, eight of these patients dying three to seven months thereafter. This, with him, is an argument against the procedure and in favor of primary nephrectomy. Guyon recently reported twenty primary nephrectomies for tuberculosis, resulting in eleven deaths and seven absolute cures. Israel reported at the Moscow Congress twenty nephrectomies for tuberculosis with eight deaths. Of the twelve in which operation was successful, six patients were alive and well two years and over, and six were living one year thereafter. One does not find much collected information on this point, and on the finer one, of any proper appreciation of the value of extirpations in the beginning of a tuberculous renal lesion, we can find little or nothing of service. In most of the cases so far published there have been advanced lesions, and to a certain extent associated damage to the ureter, and even to the bladder, which organs have been either left untouched surgically to be cured by Nature's subsequent efforts (which are, I believe, as potent an influence for good in the genito-urinary tract as in the lungs), or have been dealt with by a later surgical attack (Kelly, Israel, and others). Suffice it to say, that if a patient complains of lumbar pain, with a sense of weight and dragging, extending to the inguinal region, with some nausea and anorexia and slight emaciation, though without the characteristic symptoms of renal colic, renal sand, renal catarrh, or malignant disease, pyelitis, pyonephrosis or hydronephrosis, the urinary sediment should be frequently and carefully examined for tubercle bacilli by a competent bacteriologist, and an early cystoscopic examination and catheterization of the ureters should be methodically carried out. On the microscopic demonstration of tubercle bacilli alone, however, too much dependence should not be placed; for Leyden[1] has recently stated, and in this opinion several authorities concur, that the tubercle bacillus so closely resembles in appearance and staining properties the smegma bacillus, which is often found in urine, and almost always in cystitic urine, that the microscopic evidence should always be confirmed by inoculation experiments. Pousson[2] gives a beautiful description of a case in which he was able to follow the history for months, through what he called the hemorrhagic stage, and into the purulent stage, for he believes that many cases of "renal phthisis," like many of "pulmonary phthisis," pass through an era of congestion and hemorrhage before one of suppuration develops. Such instances might be multiplied. Even though no bacilli are found in the urinary sediment the cystoscope may show congestion of one ureteral opening, or circumscribed patches of inflammation or superficial ulceration, between this and the urethra. Moreover, by the analysis of the urine from each kidney, which may thus be obtained, positive evidence will often be furnished of the state of both kidneys, and early nephrotomy may be performed if necessary. The success which may be expected to follow such treatment is illustrated in a case recently reported by Meyer.[3] On the other hand the difficulties frequently associated with such examinations were brought out in a case of my own in which the same acknowledged expert kindly officiated and only obtained knowledge of the condition of each kidney after six protracted trials (Case XV.). Un-

[1] *Deut. Arch. klin. Med.*, vol. lv, p. 449, 1895.

[2] Kelly (*Annals of Surgery*, January, 1898) has shown that an endoscopic tube may be introduced in the male bladder, and with the patient in the knee-chest position the viscus becomes distended with air, as in women, and its interior may then be fairly well explored. This is a cheaper, easier, and readier method than that in which the cystoscope is used.

[1] *Berl. klin. Wochenschr.*, No. 17, 1896.

[2] *Gaz. Hebdom. de Méd. et de Chir.*, vol. xxxii, p. 278, 1895.

[3] MED. NEWS, vol. lxx, p. 545, 1897.

fortunately, in only two of the nine cases of renal tuberculosis in which I have been called upon to operate was the patient observed at so early a stage as has just been indicated. In one of them (Case XXIX.) the illness was said to be of only three-months' duration, but in this case as well as in others presenting a history of illness lasting from one to several years, the kidney was thoroughly diseased and its condition was diagnosed by ordinary means. In six of these cases an attempt was made to relieve the symptoms by means of nephrotomy, either as an end in itself when the tuberculous nature of the trouble was not absolutely established, or to enable the patient to get into a better condition for a subsequent nephrectomy, a procedure which, though frowned upon by Albarran, is, I still believe, of decided benefit in certain cases. Twice with me, nephrotomy has been followed by a permanent cure. These cases (Nos. XXVI. and XXVII.), from the associated symptoms of tuberculous arthritis, cough, etc., were considered to be tuberculous and they are so classified. The patients were seen in robust health eight and nine years after operation. In both the sinus in the operative area remained open two years and then healed permanently. In another patient, upon whom nephrotomy was performed, the sinus healed only to reopen, and in this instance, as well as in three others, the continued fever, purulent urine, and general emaciation rendered necessary the more radical nephrectomy. Of the six patients from whom I removed the kidney for tuberculosis, one (Case XXIX.) survived this operation only a short time. One died suddenly within a month from complete suppression of urine, and four are in good health to-day, twenty-eight, sixteen, fourteen, and eight months respectively, after the date of the operation.

Although success may rarely follow the lesser operation of nephrotomy, it is not unknown, and only last year Vanderveer[1] described a case in which he drained and irrigated a tuberculous abscess of one kidney, and obtained an apparently perfect cure, the wound healing and the urine becoming normal. Israel[2] has also recently reported a case in which he successfully removed a portion of one kidney for tuberculosis, stopping the hemorrhage by digital compression.[3] However, in most cases there are multiple tuberculous foci, solid or in abscess form, and the necessity for removal of the entire organ exists. Thus, in Case XXXII., wherein half the bladder was at first removed for tuberculous infection, with a nephrotomy for renal abscess, though there was a complete closure of the lumbar wound this apparent cure was of brief duration. The sinus reopened, and it was necessary to remove the disorganized kidney. In a few months thereafter the patient made rapid gain in weight, and when seen one year afterward, he weighed seventy pounds more than at the time of his last operation, and at this time both renal and bladder incisions were closed, and further, tubercle bacilli were not to be found in the urine, which was clear and passed every two or three hours, thus marking the capacity of his diminished bladder.

[1] *Trans. Am. Surg. Ass'n*, vol. xiv, p. 113, 1896.
[2] *Deut. med. Wochenschr.*, vol. xxii, p. 22, 1896.
[3] *Jour. Cut. and Genito-Ur. Dis.*, vol. xiii, p. 33, 1895.

The removal of a tuberculous ureter has been proposed and carried out, first by Reynier[1] in 1893, and in 1896 by Kelly,[2] either through an abdominal incision or by a lumbar nephrectomy, the upper part of the ureter being removed with the kidney and the lower part by a prerectal or vaginal incision; or—the operation which Kelly now prefers—by an oblique incision parallel to, but somewhat above, Poupart's ligament. Through this opening the peritoneum may be peeled off and pushed up until the kidney and the entire ureter are dissected out extraperitoneally. A similar procedure was commended by Reynier. This ureterectomy may be performed at the time of the nephrectomy or left to a later time. Occasionally a thickened ureter, under such circumstances presumably tuberculous, will not cause further trouble. This was the condition in Case XXXIV. The depressed condition of the patient at the termination of the operation, a nephrectomy, compelled me to leave *in situ* a much thickened and obviously involved ureter; but her great improvement in health leads to the belief that Nature's powers have been able to neutralize the remaining infection. A similar condition of ureteral involvement was left untouched in Case XXXI., and has apparently been safely cared for by the *vis medicatrix naturæ*.

CASE XXVI. *Tuberculosis (?)—Pyonephrosis—Nephrotomy—Recovery.*—Mary F., aged twenty-three years, noticed during the nine months previous to coming under observation a decreased quantity of urine, some vesical irritation, and later, pain; and more recently, a smooth swelling in the right loin. Micturition increased up to fifteen times daily. Once a small amount of blood followed urination. Cough and night-sweats had existed for two months. The urine was acid, of a specific gravity of 1028, and contained no albumin. Its sediment consisted of pus-cells, epithelium, and calcic oxalate crystals. No tubercle bacilli were found.

May 24, 1888, a three-inch oblique incision exposed the distended right kidney. A needle drew pus, and by an incision made into its pelvis, ten ounces of pus was evacuated. No calculus was found. A drainage-tube was left in position. The patient made an excellent recovery. The flow of urine through the wound quickly ceased, and on her discharge from the hospital, three weeks after the operation, the sinus was not apparently more than an inch deep. It, however, remained open for nearly two years and then healed under the persistent use of injections of diluted tincture of iodin. Eighteen months after the nephrotomy the patient developed a tuberculous abscess of the lower end of the tibia, which continued two years, but which terminated in recovery. She was last seen during December, 1897, and was in good health. The kidney was still slightly enlarged. The scar was firm, and there was no weakness of the lumbar region or yielding on expulsive effort. This case was doubtless one of tuberculous abscess, though this could not be proven by the demonstration of the bacillus.

CASE XXVII. *Tuberculous Abscesses of Kidney—Nephrotomy—Recovery.*—Florence S., aged twenty-five years, entered New York Hospital, July 17, 1888, and presented a tuberculous family history and a personal history of an illness of sixteen months, marked by persistent cough and expectoration, by painful and frequent

[1] Reynier, *Rev. de Chirurgie*, p. 272, 1893.
[2] *Bulletin Johns Hopkins Hosp.*, February and March, 1896. See also Hartmann, *Rev. de Chir.*, Nov., 1897; and Gerster and McCosh, *Annals of Surg.*, Sept., 1897.

micturition, and pain in the right loin. These symptoms were increasing, and were associated with decided loss of strength. Examination showed two rounded masses in the right lumbar region, connected, and rather tender, and projecting below the liver. The general condition of the patient was bad.

July 18th the right kidney was exposed by a slightly oblique incision and aspirated. Pus was withdrawn, and an incision into its pelvis showed the kidney to contain numerous abscesses. The intervening septa were broken down, and about a pint of pus evacuated. The kidney was irrigated, and a drainage-tube inserted. The general condition of the patient was somewhat improved by the operation, though suppuration and fever continued. The amount of pus in the urine became less and the tumor gradually shrank in size. When the patient was discharged from the hospital, about eight weeks after operation, the urine still contained pus, and occasionally blood, and the sinus in the loin had not closed. This remained open nearly two years, the discharge of pus growing less. Improvement was hastened by injections into the sinus of tincture of iodin and water (one part to three). Since the wound healed the patient has enjoyed good health. She was last seen during December, 1897, having gained greatly in weight. In this case there was also, most probably, a tuberculous infection, though such was not satisfactorily proven.

CASE XXVIII. *Tuberculous Abscesses of the Kidney—Nephrotomy—Subsequent Nephrectomy—Death.*—Mary D., aged twenty-five years, entered New York Hospital during May, 1892, with a history of cystitis of one-year's duration. Eight months after the beginning of her illness she married, and from that time grew much worse, having involuntary micturition and loss of strength. Ten days before entering the hospital her physician discovered a round, smooth, and slightly fluctuating tumor in the right side of the abdomen, and in its lowest portion it was covered by the distended colon. The urine was full of pus.

May 25, 1892, a four-inch transverse incision was made in the right lumbar region and the greatly distended kidney was exposed. It was incised, and three distinct abscess cavities were washed out and drained. The amount of kidney substance remaining seemed very small. Plenty of gauze was used for drainage. The pus from the kidney contained staphylococci, but no tubercle bacilli. The patient did not rally well after the operation, and it was noticed that the kidney remained much enlarged. There was a daily fever of about 102° F. June 13th, Dr. Bull, who was in charge of the service in my absence, explored the sinus, broke into more abscess cavities, and inserted two large rubber drains. Still the condition of the patient did not improve, and six weeks later Dr. Stimson removed the purulent kidney. The patient could not, however, stand the shock of the operation, and died the following day.

The extirpated kidney measured 18x6x4 cm. Its surface was smooth, but bulging in many places. The lining of its pelvis was everywhere in a state of cheesy degeneration, and numerous similar areas were scattered through the kidney substance, many of which were in communication with the pelvis of the organ. The microscopic appearances were those of tuberculosis.

CASE XXIX. *Tuberculosis of the Kidney—Abdominal Nephrectomy—Recovery.*—Frances G., aged nineteen years, was seized in December, 1893, with a sharp pain in the right lumbar region, without known cause. This was followed by fever. The pain and fever continued, though there was but slight tenderness over the affected region. There was increased frequency of micturition. Three months after the initial symptoms a movable tender tumor the size of a cocoanut was discovered in the right side of the abdomen, reaching below the umbilicus, and leaving a space between it and the ribs above. The urine was of a specific gravity of 1008, and contained a trace of albumin and some pus and blood-cells. On account of the rather unusual position and from the size of the tumor, an exploratory laparotomy was performed March 17, 1894. A two-inch incision over the tumor disclosed a displaced kidney, which was nodular and greatly enlarged. The peritoneum was incised, external to the ascending colon, and peeled off the kidney, which organ was freed and lifted out of its bed. The pedicle was ligated with catgut, the ureter and vessels being separated for that purpose. A counter-opening for drainage was then made in the lumbar region, and both openings in the peritoneum were closed by sutures, as was the laparotomy wound. There was a quick recovery from the operation. The abdominal wound healed by first intention, and within eighteen days the patient was up and passing daily about forty ounces of urine. Examination of the urine showed that it still contained a large amount of albumin, some blood, casts, and many tubercle bacilli.

Three weeks after the operation occasional vomiting occurred and persisted. The quantity of urine decreased steadily, and the patient died in the middle of the fourth week in uremic convulsions. No autopsy was permitted. The extirpated kidney showed several caseous abscesses and ulceration of its pelvis.

CASE XXX. *Tuberculous Pyonephrosis—Nephrotomy—Subsequent Nephrectomy—Recovery.*—Lilly C., aged twenty years, began to have pain in the left side of the abdomen during the summer of 1893. The following spring she had a severe attack of cystitis with pus and blood in the urine, and suffered on several occasions from intense pain in the left lumbar region. These symptoms grew worse, and there was also pain in the right side and in the back. For two weeks before her entrance to the hospital, December 20, 1894, she had noticed a swelling in the right side of the abdomen. Physical examination showed her to be pale, thin, and weak, with a temperature varying from 99° to 104° F. Nearly the whole of the right upper quadrant of the abdomen was occupied by a soft, fluctuating, tender swelling, apparently due to a distended kidney. The urine was light colored and cloudy, though acid, and was of a specific gravity of 1018, and contained eighteen per cent. of albumin by volume. It also contained much pus.

December 23, 1894, a slightly oblique incision was made in the right loin, and the kidney was exposed and incised. A great quantity of pus escaped, especially after the septa between the walls of the numerous abscesses were broken through. On account of free hemorrhage the cavity was firmly packed with gauze. After the operation the patient became somewhat more comfortable, but the urine still contained about ten per cent. of albumin, and the temperature elevations continued, though not so high as before. Nephrectomy was, therefore, performed January 5, 1895. From the lower end of the former wound a transverse incision was made forward, and the kidney exposed, dissected free, and removed, the pedicle being ligated with silk. The fresh wound was sutured and a gauze drain placed in the old opening. On the fifth day the gauze was removed and the cavity irrigated. Three weeks after the operation the patient still had an afternoon temperature of 102.5° F., but her general condition seemed much improved, and the urine contained only occasionally a slight trace of albumin. February 17th tubercle bacilli were demonstrated in the urine. There was also vesical tenesmus, an afternoon fever, and the general condition was not good. By her own request the patient was removed to her home. The ligature of the pedicle had not come away. Death followed six weeks later, about three months after the operation. The excised kidney was found to present the lesions of the various stages of tuberculosis. It was evident that the other kidney was likewise involved in the infection.

CASE XXXI. *Lumbar Sinus—Tuberculosis of Kidney—Nephrectomy—Recovery.*—Eugene L., aged twenty-two years, entered New York Hospital, October 29, 1895. He had received a kick in the left lumbar region when seventeen years of age, and thereafter there was always more or less pain in that situation. Two weeks after the accident a tender and hard swelling formed, which grew softer in time, and after two years was opened and a quantity of pus evacuated. For a year the sinus persisted and then closed in part, with increase in pain. During April, 1895, it was scraped, and it then gradually closed so that for the five months preceding the operation shortly to be described there was no discharge at all. Pain during this time was growing constantly worse, so that the patient had now been disabled for some months. Otherwise the health had been good; there were no disorders of digestion, no symptoms referable to the bladder, and no chills. There had been a loss of ten pounds in weight in the year preceding admission to the hospital. Examination of the urine showed it to be absolutely normal, except that the sediment contained the crystals of triple phosphates and ammonium urates.

October 30, 1895, a transverse incision was made midway between the crest of the ilium and the last rib, and to gain more space another incision was made directly upward from the middle of the first. In dissecting free the adherent kidney both the pleural and the peritoneal cavities were accidentally opened, and were immediately closed by stitches of fine catgut and silk. No immediate or secondary bad effects followed the accident, which may be considered, from the experience of others, as well as my own, to be usually without unfavorable sequelæ. The kidney was entirely separated and finally brought out through the wound, and it was found to be riddled with abscesses. Its pedicle was ligated *en masse* with strong silk, and the kidney was removed. The transverse incision was sutured, and the other left open for the abundant gauze drains.

Recovery from the operation was prompt. The urine contained a little albumin for a few days, but this entirely disappeared later. The dressing was changed on the second day and the drains were removed on the fifth day. No symptoms developed referable to either the pleural or peritoneal cavity. Six weeks after operation the patient left the hospital much improved in health. There was still a small sinus in the loin. The kidney was not much enlarged, but was almost entirely composed of cheesy and calcareous material separated by fibrous septa. No renal tissue was apparent on gross inspection. Microscopically a few shrunken tubercles were found in the fibrous tissue, but the diagnosis of tuberculosis was not absolutely verified by the pathologic examination.

CASE XXXII. *Extensive Tuberculosis of the Bladder and Kidney—Resection of One-half of the Bladder—Nephrotomy—Nephrectomy—Recovery.*—Frederick T., aged forty-four years. For two and one-half years this patient suffered from attacks of renal colic on the right side, the pain extending from the lumbar region into the pelvis. The attacks increased in severity, and were accompanied by nausea and frequency of micturition. The urine contained much mucus and blood; it was acid, of a specific gravity of 1024, with ten per cent. of albumin (by volume), and its sediment contained blood and pus. By palpation, the bladder seemed somewhat thickened and very tender.

June 12, 1896, a cystoscopic examination was made, and a tumor was seen to occupy the posterior wall of the bladder. Suprapubic cystotomy was performed. The tumor was soft and sessile and bled readily. It occupied the posterior wall of the bladder, covering an area about 1½ inches in diameter, and reaching to within ½ an inch of the ureteral openings. The peritoneum was dissected off from the bladder to the prostate, and on each side to the vas deferens; then a triangular portion of the whole thickness of the bladder, including the new growth, was resected, the incisions being everywhere in the healthy portions of the bladder-wall. Thus, the bladder between the ureters and the whole top, making about one-half of the viscus, was removed. In peeling off the peritoneum two openings were torn in it. These were promptly closed with silk. The hemorrhage from the divided bladder-wall was quite free, but it was quickly controlled by the catgut sutures, which, passing through the entire thickness of the bladder, closed its posterior portion to the summit, which was left unsutured. Gauze packing was then placed between the sutured bladder and the stripped-off peritoneum, and a Mikulicz drain was inserted in the bladder itself. By a lumbar incision the right kidney, which two days before had been recognized as enlarged, was then opened, and three ounces of pus evacuated from its pelvis. Drainage was here secured by gauze and a rubber tube. The wounds were dressed daily. The gauze in the bladder was soaked daily with Thiersch's solution. It was removed on the fifth day. Within ten weeks both wounds had completely healed. The bladder held two ounces of injected fluid. Eleven weeks after the operation the patient passed a black silk suture covered with phosphates. All the others used were of catgut. This one had accidentally been applied. August 29th he left the hospital and went home, returning two months later somewhat emaciated, and with lumbar and suprapubic sinuses now open and discharging pus and urine. On several occasions the urine was examined for tubercle bacilli; once with a positive result. The vesical sinus was also found to be tuberculous. There was an afternoon rise of temperature of 100° to 104° F. The kidney-tumor was still marked and tender.

Nephrectomy was determined upon as affording him a chance of relief, and November 25, 1896, the old lumbar scar was incised, and as the adhesions were extensive, the kidney was peeled out of its capsule. The vessels and ureter were tied together with strong silk. The wound was partially sutured and drained with gauze packing. The division of the ureter showed suspicious thickening, and as far down as it could be palpated it was found to be much enlarged. The patient's condition, however, did not permit extirpation of the affected ureter. Examination of the kidney showed it to contain numerous tuberculous abscesses. To overcome the tardy separation of the ligature on the pedicle of the kidney it was tied around a small flattened rubber ball, and the tension thus secured by the elasticity of the rubber brought it away in about five days.[1]

Six months later the patient had vastly improved. He had gained forty pounds in weight. The suprapubic fistula was still open, but contracted to the size of a needle. The urine was retained for two hours and discharged in the day time entirely through the urethra. By night there was often leakage. The urine was still cloudy, but less so.

[1] Weir, "The Extraction of Too Long Retained Silk and Silk-worm-gut Ligatures and Sutures," the MEDICAL NEWS, April 3, 1897.

It was acid and contained two per cent. of albumin (by volume), and was of a specific gravity of 1020. No enlarged ureter could be felt on palpation.

December 8, 1897, the patient again reported for inspection. He had gained ninety pounds, and weighed more than he ever had before. He said that he could hold his urine from two to three hours, and when discharged it was clear. Two examinations of the urine failed to detect any bacilli. Both the lumbar and suprapubic wounds had solidly healed.

CASE XXXIII. *Tuberculous Pyonephrosis—Nephrotomy—Subsequent Nephrectomy—Recovery.*—Mamie D., aged twenty-seven years, gave birth to her only child when she was twenty years old, and was afterward troubled with attacks of pain in the right side, with occasional chills and fever. During March, 1896, six months later, she entered New York Hospital, where a diagnosis of probable pyosalpinx was made by my predecessor, and on September 24, 1896, an exploratory laparotomy was performed. Nothing warranting the removal of a tube was found, and the wound was closed. On my return to duty on October 1st, I found that the pain had continued, and was then referred to the region of the right kidney, which could be palpated bimanually and was tender on pressure. The urine was cloudy, acid, and of a specific gravity of 1015, and contained five per cent. of albumin (by volume). The sediment contained abundant pus and blood-cells. October 10th an enlargement of the right kidney could be clearly defined, and a curved lumbar incision was made, the organ in question being exposed and incised. Three or four ounces of pus escaped, the cultures from which contained the bacillus coli commune, and staphylococcus aureus. The wound was drained with gauze and not sutured. On the fourth day after operation there was a sharp rise of temperature, which then recurred daily, and was at first considered to be due to the drainage, which was not entirely satisfactory. This was corrected, and four weeks later the gauze packing was discontinued. There then remained but a small sinus. Meanwhile every afternoon there was a daily temperature of 101°-103° F., and the urine contained from one to four ounces of pus. The patient's condition was rapidly deteriorating. Nephrectomy was, therefore, decided upon, and performed December 31, 1896.

At the operation the finger was thrust into the old sinus and much pus escaped. The incision was then prolonged above the crest of the ilium and the kidney dissected out by means of the fingers. The pedicle was clamped and tied, the ligature including the loop of a galvanocautery in order to subsequently divide and release the silk ligature (Cleveland's method). There was left on the stump about three-fourths of an inch of kidney substance. A rent in the diaphragm, near the tip of the twelfth rib, was sutured with catgut. A Mikulicz drain of iodoform and sterilized gauze was tightly packed into the wound. The patient was a good deal depressed by the operation, but rallied under stimulating treatment.

January 1, 1897, the patient passed 25 ounces of urine of a specific gravity of 1028, and containing only a trace of albumin. On the succeeding days the amounts were 47, 54, 66, 67, 48, 43, 30, 21 ounces, and from then on the quantity varied from 25 to 45 ounces daily. On the third day the packing was all removed, except the outer layer of gauze. On the fifth day, the wire loop was burned through the ligature, which was then removed. Recovery was slow, and there continued to be a daily afternoon temperature of 100° to 102° F. The patient left the hospital February 15, 1897. The last urinary examination showed the urine to be turbid, acid, of a specific gravity of 1012, and free from albumin. There were a few pus-cells and several tubercle bacilli in the sediment. There was a line of unhealthy granulations in the loin about three inches long into which a probe sank a couple of inches in several places, though no distinct sinus seemed to exist. Pressure over the pedicle and ureter was painful. The extirpated kidney measured 10x5x3 cm., and contained several abscesses and hemorrhagic areas. Microscopic sections showed typical tuberculous lesions throughout nearly the whole organ. The patient was reported January 1, 1898, as improving steadily, but until then the fear existed that the remaining kidney was similarly affected.

CASE XXXIV. *Tuberculous Pyonephrosis—Nephrectomy—Recovery.*—Alice B., aged twenty years, kindly referred to me by Dr. Messoner, presented a history of gradually progressive loss of flesh and strength during the previous two years, and without assignable cause. There was more or less constant pain in the right lumbar region, and an increased frequency of micturition, with very great tenesmus. Lately there had been noticed a plainly palpable tumor occupying the seat of the right kidney. There was an afternoon fever, sometimes reaching 104° F. The patient had hip disease at the age of ten years, with multiple bone abscesses, and somewhat later a tuberculous ulceration of the sternum. The urine, of which from 50 to 60 ounces were passed in the twenty-four hours, was pale, and contained a stringy sediment, albumin, and pus.

June 15, 1897, lumbar nephrectomy was performed by the usual curved König's incision. The kidney was exposed and freed without difficulty; its pedicle was ligated and the organ removed. The ureter was separately ligated with catgut. In order to facilitate the removal of the silk ligature from the pedicle at will, Grad's[1] procedure was adopted. On the sixth day, the ligature was untied by means of the tractor threads and removed with ease.

The temperature fell after the removal of the badly diseased kidney, and except for a most annoying irritability of the bladder which various remedies failed to benefit the patient made a good though slow convalescence. Five days after the operation, when it was possible to measure the urine, it being then passed in amounts of an ounce or less, the daily quantity was 41 ounces. From this time on this amount varied from 35 to 55 ounces. Vesical pain and tenesmus continued to annoy the patient long after she was up, and after the wound in the loin had healed. November 5, 1897, five months after the nephrectomy, she had gained in weight and in the ability to retain the urine, and the scar in the loin, which once opened after closing, was solid and not tender.

The kidney in this case was filled with large caseous nodules of tuberculosis, with almost total destruction of the renal substance. Tubercle bacilli were found in large quantities.

(To be continued.)

MEDICAL PROGRESS.

A Case of Rabies with a Prolonged Incubation.—FELTZ and ARCHAMBAUD (*Gaz. Heb. de Med. et de Chir.*, September 30, 1897) give the notes of a case of rabies occurring in a young man, aged twenty years, who died in wild delirium within thirty-six hours after the initial symptoms of the disease appeared. No history of a dog bite was obtained, and the correct diagnosis, although suspected, was not fully established until after death. Then, in questioning the parents, it transpired that the young man had been

[1] *Amer. Gynec. and Obstet. Jour.*, February, 1897.

bitten in the mouth six months previously. The animal by which the bite was inflicted was found to have rabies, and a child bitten by it was treated at the Pasteur Institute and recovered. The case of the young man is remarkable on account of the long period which elapsed between the slight bite of the dog, and the fatal disease of the man. There was no possibility that fear caused the illness, as neither the patient nor the parents suspected its nature until after death had occurred.

In this connection it is interesting to note that POTTEVIN (*Centralb. für Bakter., etc.*, October, 1897) says that during 1896, 1308 persons were treated at the Pasteur Institute of whom 4 died, giving a mortality of 0.3 per cent., and making the total mortality since 1886 a fraction under 1 per cent. Bites in the face gave a larger mortality than wounds of other parts of the body. Since the establishment of the Institute 3096 foreigners and 15,549 natives have been treated in the Paris institution. It will thus be seen that the number of persons treated last year is considerably below the average for the ten years in which the Institute has been open. This is due, no doubt, to the establishment of similar institutions in other cities rather than to the fact that treatment for rabies is becoming unpopular.

An Official Employment of Formaldehyd Disinfection.—DR. MACKENZIE of Leith, Scotland, was one of the first medical officers of health to employ the formalin spray system for room-disinfection. He reports that he has found that the general results of the spray disinfection with formalin are entirely satisfactory. "Of some 400 houses, or rooms, disinfected, I can say that not in any instance has infection been contracted after spraying. In one or two instances the fever was caught before spraying, and developed symptoms on the same day as the house was disinfected. But in this case the original patient had remained at home. But where the patient is removed and the house disinfected, a second case is practically unknown. Further, a hospital pavilion was used from September, 1896, to May, 1897, for scarlet fever—say about 120 cases. I had the pavilion sprayed with two-per-cent. formalin solution, and a week afterward, or less, placed patients with measles there. During three months of measles, about thirty cases, not a single suspicious sore throat, rash, or indication of scarlet fever occurred. Similar experiments have been repeated with a smallpox ward, several times in diphtheria wards, erysipelas wards, etc. In no case have I found any suspicion of infection. The precise facts will be published later in the annual report for 1897."

Removal of Foreign Body from the Trachea by Means of a Tube:—SEVESTRE and BONNUS (*Rev. de Therapeut.*, December 1, 1897) were called upon to treat an infant who had sucked into its trachea a small glass bead. A tube was passed through the larynx and the foreign body was expelled through it. If this maneuver had not been successful tracheotomy would of necessity have been performed.

Cure of Prolapse of the Female Urethra.—WOHLGEMUTH (*Deut. med. Wochenschr.*, November 4, 1897) has been most successful in his treatment of obstinate cases of prolapse of the female urethra by means of the thermo-cautery. The cauterizations should extend radially, that is, they should be made in the longitudinal axis of the urethra, and should extend throughout the whole of its thickness. By the cicatricial contraction which follows, the prolapse is completely obliterated, though in some instances repeated applications are necessary. The advantages of this simple procedure are: the fact that it requires no especial antiseptic precautions; that it obviates the necessity of leaving a catheter in the bladder, and that there is no danger from hemorrhage during the operation.

THERAPEUTIC NOTES.

Treatment of Chronic Ulcers of the Legs.—LANGSEORFF (*Centralbl. f. Chirurg.*, November 20, 1897) has treated over 200 ulcers of the leg, without a single failure, by means of the following method. The leg is rubbed with green soap, washed and dried. The ulcers are then dusted thickly with calomel, which is stirred to a paste with a wet cotton swab. Fine salt is then dusted upon the paste, and is in turn mixed with it. By this means corrosive sublimate is formed which in its nascent state acts very energetically, and for three or four hours causes a strong burning sensation, which in a nervous patient may require a morphin injection. On the following day the granulations are completely burned off, and there is presented a clean wound, with possibly a small slough in its center, which soon separates. Pain has entirely disappeared. Under a stimulating salve containing turpentine, and with as complete rest in bed as is possible, the ulcer is quickly covered with epithelium. Only occasionally is it necessary to touch excessive granulations with a crystal of cupric sulphate. It sometimes happens that the ulcer partially closes and then the healing process comes to a standstill. In these cases a solid salve is spread upon a visiting-card and bound firmly upon the ulcer. From the effect of the moisture the callosities quickly dissolve and the growth of epithelium is resumed. In only two cases of the series were Thiersch grafts found necessary. After healing is complete the leg and foot are covered with zinc salve as high as the knee. This dressing is left in position two weeks. A good effect is also produced by this treatment in eczema of the lower extremities associated with numberless minute granulating ulcers. In these cases the calomel and salt are mixed to a paste, and spread upon the leg which has previously been scrubbed with green soap and water to remove all fat from the ulcers.

For Alopecia Areata.—PANICHI (*Centralbl. f. die gesammte Ther.*, December, 1897) treats alopecia areata with a mixture of three or four parts of a solution of carbolic acid, and six or seven parts of tincture of cantharides. This mixture is not only rubbed daily on the bald areas, but is injected by means of a syringe into the skin every four to six days, so as to exert an influence directly upon the hair-follicles.

THE MEDICAL NEWS.

A WEEKLY JOURNAL

OF MEDICAL SCIENCE.

COMMUNICATIONS are invited from all parts of the world. Original articles contributed *exclusively* to THE MEDICAL NEWS will after publication be liberally paid for (accounts being rendered quarterly), or 250 reprints will be furnished in place of other remuneration. When necessary to elucidate the text, illustrations will be engraved from drawings or photographs furnished by the author. Manuscripts should be typewritten.

Address the Editor: J. RIDDLE GOFFE, M.D.,

No. 111 FIFTH AVENUE (corner of 18th St.), NEW YORK.

Subscription Price, including postage in U. S. and Canada.

PER ANNUM IN ADVANCE $4.00
SINGLE COPIES 10
WITH THE AMERICAN JOURNAL OF THE MEDICAL SCIENCES, PER ANNUM 7.50

Subscriptions may begin at any date. The safest mode of remittance is by bank check or postal money order, drawn to the order of the undersigned. When neither is accessible, remittances may be made, at the risk of the publishers, by forwarding in *registered* letters.

LEA BROTHERS & CO.,

No. 111 FIFTH AVENUE (corner of 18th St.), NEW YORK, AND NOS. 706, 708 & 710 SANSOM ST., PHILADELPHIA.

SATURDAY, FEBRUARY 5, 1898.

A NEW TERROR FOR MEDICAL STUDENTS.

UNDER this heading the *Medical Press* depicts the discomfort the medical student is destined to experience when called upon to discuss, in his final examination, the diagnosis which he has formed of an injured joint by the aid of his trembling fingers, when confronted by a shadow on the screen of a fluoroscope, which in all probability will display appearances very much at variance with his previously expressed opinion. It is trying enough, remarks this writer, to be asked, with one's brain still in a muddle from the final "crams" to identify the various organs and tissues which are exposed to view in an artfully dissected subject, but it will be vastly more disconcerting to be required to outline and describe the organs by the aid of an X-ray screen. A further extension of the present curriculum may become necessary to enable the student to familiarize himself with the various innovations in matters diagnostic, and the time is probably not far distant when X-ray diagnosis will become a special item of medical education. A stage later, the candidate may be shown a pulsating something dimly visible through the thoracic cage, and asked to say whether it is the heart, the aorta, or an aneurism.

On first thought, this all impresses one as being something only possible in the very remote future, but to those attendants at the recent meeting of the Medical Society of the State of New York who had the good fortune to witness the demonstration of the X-ray and its use in surgery and in medicine, it was evident that the experience described by the writer in the *Medical Press* awaits the medical student at no distant day. The practical use of the X-ray in surgery is now quite familiar to all advanced surgeons, but its usefulness in medicine as an aid in securing greater exactness in discovering the extent and nature of pathologic lesions in the organs and soft tissues, as demonstrated by Dr. Francis H. Williams of Boston, awakened no little surprise. Indeed, his skiagrams, showing the presence of tuberculous deposits, pleuritic exudates, and the delicate differential diagnosis between a dilated and a hypertrophied heart, were marvels of expert skiagraphy and a convincing demonstration of his contention that more definite information can be obtained in regard to these and similar conditions by the use of the X-ray than by percussion and auscultation.

THE SCOPE OF THE MARINE HOSPITAL SERVICE.

IT is often stated by those who are opposed to the Marine Hospital Service, and it is uttered with all the solemnity of a final pronunciamento, that the Service was originally established to care for sick and disabled seamen, and is, therefore, incapable of performing other or allied functions. When this had been uttered, the final blow was thought to have been dealt to the Service by those who are interested in opposing its development.

That it was originally established for the purpose named is true, but to assign that as a reason why it is incapable of performing other functions is both unimportant and superficial. The care of sick and disabled seamen brings the officers of the Service into intimate relations with the hygiene and sanitation of ships, and the history of the Service abounds with records of investigations made into these subjects, which are so closely allied to quarantine. Long before the Marine Hospital Service was entrusted with the duties of enforcing National quarantine laws, its officers had made both official and unofficial investigations into the cleanliness of ships, the hygiene of the forecastle, sanitation of crews, examination of the food-supply of deep-sea vessels, all of which may be found in the annual reports, which have been issued for the past quarter of a century. So far from disqualifying officers for the work of a public-health service, particularly in its relation to maritime quarantine, the intimate and almost indispensable connection with the functions of a public-health service peculiarly fits the officers for the performance of such duty, and the active participation by them in such work during the period named makes them what unbiased persons regard them to be—the only corps of medical men in this country specially skilled in the class of work in question. The very foundation of a system of safeguards for the National health is a protection of the interior of the country from the introduction of contagious disease from without. The Service which, since its foundation, has dealt with "men that go down to the sea in ships," and with the condition of ships themselves, is the one best fitted by long and practical experience to deal with the question of maritime quarantine.

This is not all. Along the line of natural development The Marine Hospital Service has progressed, by direct authority of Congress, in other fields of investigation and execution in respect to public-health functions, and besides its original work of caring for sick and disabled seamen (of which over fifty thousand are treated annually), keeping officers in touch with active professional work, it has performed its functions as the Federal agency in the management of quarantine; undertaken investigation of smallpox by direction of Congress, the results of which study are ready for publication; has collected and published data respecting health and mortality statistics throughout the United States and the world, the last by the reports of the Consular service. It has also been engaged for the past year or more in experiments in car sanitation with respect to communicable diseases; has conducted investigations concerning the pollution of water-supplies; peformed pioneer work in this country in respect to diphtheritic antitoxin and formaldehyd disinfection; and two of the officers are now in Havana, Cuba, by detail of the President, conducting an investigation into the causation of yellow fever. These varied duties which it has performed and is now performing, certainly indicate the variety of its work in connection with public health service. Its hygienic laboratory is one of the best equipped in the country, and here every year, in turn, several officers receive instruction bearing upon the advances in hygiene, bacteriology, and allied sciences. These facts should certainly satisfy any reasonable professional man that the scope of the Service is sufficiently varied, and that it is entitled to the sympathy and support of the medical profession throughout the country in its development and progress.

Any movement which has for its cardinal text the relegation of the Marine Hospital Service, which has done so much pioneer work in the interests of public health, to a secondary or even more obscure position in the ambitious plans of its enemies will not meet with a responsive chord in the minds of the majority.

The Service is developing in the exact direction which the promoters of the proposed Department of Public Health expect to attain by one act of legislation.

The Senate, upon the recommendation of its Committee on Public Health and Quarantine, has already indefinitely postponed two bills for the establishment of a Department of Public Health, and favorably reported the Caffery bill, which imposes additional powers and duties upon the Marine Hospital Service. In view of the state of the National finances and the improbability of Congress assenting to the large and indefinite expenditure necessary for the establishment of a Department of Public Health, it seems to us that the profession should turn its attention to developing and supporting the Marine Hospital Service as the public health service *de jure* as well as *de facto*, and that those who are now, as we think, mistakenly, if honestly, expending their efforts in the attempt to create a Department of Public Health should join with their fellows in strengthening the hands of their professional brothers in the Marine Hospital Service who have been so long and faithfully serving the public.

ECHOES AND NEWS.

Death of Dr. Pean.—The death of Dr. Jules Emile Pean, the eminent surgeon and gynecologist, is announced as occurring in Paris on the 30th ult.

Typhoid Fever in Jersey City.—During the past month more than seventy-three cases of typhoid fever have been reported in Jersey City. Dr. Thomas H. Atkinson is one of the latest victims, and his condition is very critical.

Concentration in the New York City Board of Health.—The Board of Health has abolished the local boards of Newtown, Jamaica, Hempstead, and Flushing, and removed all their employees with the exception of Dr. P. J. Maynard, health-officer of Flushing.

Smallpox in the South.—At Atlanta, Ga., the health authorities seem to have checked the spread of smallpox, only twelve new cases being reported there during the week ending January 29th. In Alabama the disease is on the increase, and 175 cases were reported to the Board of Health during that period of time.

Officers of the New York Medical League.—At the recent annual meeting of the New York Medical League, the following officers were elected: President, Joseph E. Janvrin; vice-president, F. R. Sturgis; recording-secretary, J. C. Schminke; corresponding-secretary, Douglas H. Stewart; treasurer, E. Eliot Harris.

Memorial Services to Mr. Ernest Hart.—A memorial service was held on Tuesday, January 11th, at Mary-le-Bone Parish Church, London, and the address was delivered by Canon Barnett, who tenderly reviewed Mr. Hart's career and admiringly depicted the manysidedness of his activity. A large number of scientific and medical men were in attendance, and thus paid this last mark of respect. At the conclusion of the service the body was removed to Woking for cremation.

The New York Physicians' Mutual Aid Association.—At the annual meeting of this association, held January 26, 1898, the following officers were chosen for the ensuing year: President, Daniel Lewis; first vice-president, J. W. Hyde; second vice-president, W. F. Mittendorf; recording secretary, J. V. D. Young; treasurer, Robert Campbell. The report of the treasurer showed a permanent fund of $31,000, being an increase of $2100 during the year. The membership at present numbers 1451, showing an increase of 100 despite the numerous deaths during the past twelve months.

Houses of Ill-fame under the Guise of Massage Establishments.—This form of deception and vice has been carried on in London for a number of years. It is one of the most subtle, insinuating evils with which the detectives and police of that city have had to deal. The first suspicion that it had invaded our country and endeavored to establish itself here was aroused by the recent account of the case of a young girl from Buffalo, N. Y., who was lured from her home by an advertisement purporting to come from a massage establishment in New York City. On account of what she saw and the insults offered her in the house, she fled in terror, and later became insane.

The Dispensary Bill before the New York Legislature.—The bill of the Medical Society of the County of New York, recently introduced into the Legislature, has been advanced to its second reading. There is every prospect that it will pass the Legislature without serious opposition. The bill was not presented in the New York State Medical Society for endorsement, and no action upon this bill, was, therefore, taken by that society. It is reported, however, that the chairman of the new Legislative Committee of the State Society is strongly opposed to the measure. In consequence of which it would be wise for the friends of the bill to interview this gentleman promptly.

The New York State Board of Charities and the Dispensary Abuse.—The annual report of this organization recently presented to the Legislature urges that immediate steps be taken to stop the abuses of medical aid at the dispensaries, especially in New York City. The report estimates that 1,208,173 cases have been treated, and 1,938,637 prescriptions filled at the dispensaries of the Borough of Manhattan during the past year. The Board advances the idea that if one-half the thought and energy that are wasted in making the poor of our great cities dependent were used to encourage habits of industry and a spirit of independence, the condition of the destitute poor would be materially improved. New and larger buildings for Gouverneur, Harlem, and Fordham Hospitals are recommended.

The Medical Society of the County of New York and the Board of Health.—Representatives of the County Society appeared before the Board of Health, January 26th to present arguments in favor of restricting the powers of the latter organization. They contended that consumption should be removed from the list of contagious diseases, and the Board's power to sell vaccine and antitoxin should be taken away. Dr. Satterthwaite's antiquated argument that an effort which had been made in Naples over one hundred years ago to control and restrict the spread of consumption accomplished nothing, had little convincing effect. In regard to the manufacture and sale of antitoxin, President Straus of the Board of Health maintained that the only way to keep a good supply of antitoxin always on hand was to keep the laboratories in operation all the time. Consequently there must be a surplus, and it would be wasteful to throw this surplus away. The sale of it was a legitimate effort to reduce the expenses in the protection of the city against diphtheria and smallpox.

Discovery of an Agglutination Test in the Diagnosis of Yellow Fever.—The news comes from New Orleans that Drs. P. E. Archinard and R. S. Woodson of the United States Army have discovered an agglutination test to be used in the diagnosis of yellow fever. The test is made in the following manner: A drop of blood is taken from the lobe of the ear of the patient and dissolved in twenty times its volume of sterilized water. This is then placed in a culture-tube containing yellow-fever germs which have been active and increasing for twenty-four hours. In from five to thirty minutes after the drop of suspected blood dissolved in twenty times its volume is put into the culture-tube, the germs in the blood become agglutinated and motility ceases entirely, which shows that the blood is that of a yellow-fever patient. If, however, agglutination does not take place, yellow fever is not present. The yellow-fever germ has been found in between eighty-seven and ninety per cent. of the cases in which this test has been employed, therefore it must be superior to that of Sanarelli by means of which the germ was found in only forty-seven per cent. of the cases.

Special Meeting of the New York County Medical Society.—At a special meeting of this Society, held Monday evening, January 31st, the question whether it was advisable to prohibit or to license midwives was discussed in a general debate which continued for two hours. The general sentiment seemed to be in favor of abolishing such a guild as the midwives, but even those who most strongly favored this idea were quite positive in their opinions that such a measure could not be passed through the Legislature. Other speakers, and these formed no insignificant minority, were in favor of educating and improving midwives, and after submitting them to a course of study and examination to license them. This contention was based upon the statement that parturition is a physiologic process in the vast majority of cases, that only the services of a nurse or midwife are required, and that the class of people who employ midwives cannot afford the services of a physician. The second order of business was the resolution calling upon Dr. D. B. St. John Roosa to explain his recent public statements in the New York *Tribune* regarding the action of the Society and of its committee appointed to appear before the Board of Estimate and Apportionment in reference to granting public funds to private institutions. After various obstructive parliamentary proceedings, Dr. Roosa explained that his characterization of the action of the Society as a "snap vote" was in accordance with Webster's definition of the term, "as something done sharply, quickly, abruptly"; that in using the word, he had not intended to reflect disparagingly upon the action of the Society. In regard to his statement that the Committee knowingly disobeyed the instructions of the Society, this he believed to be true, assurance of which he had from two or three members of the Committee. As the meeting was a special one called for the purpose of discussing the bill concerning midwives and to listen to Dr. Roosa's explanation, no action could be taken. Dr. Roosa's explanation was received with attention and courtesy, and the meeting adjourned.

SPECIAL RESOLUTIONS.

RESOLUTIONS UNANIMOUSLY ADOPTED BY THE MEDICAL BOARD OF BELLEVUE HOSPITAL AT A REGULAR MEETING, FEBRUARY 1, 1898.

WHEREAS, in the opinion of this Board, the Health Department of New York has rendered great public service by the measures which it has taken to check the spread of infectious diseases, including tuberculosis, and by the zeal with which it has promoted scientific research, and

WHEREAS, there has been introduced in the State Senate a bill known as Senate Bill No. 5, which, if it becomes a law, will greatly restrict the field of work of the Health Department and hamper it in its efforts to secure improved sanitation for the citizens of New York, therefore, be it

Resolved, That this Board do humbly protest against Senate Bill No. 5, believing that its passage would work great injury to the interests of this community;

Resolved, That these resolutions be spread upon the minutes of this Board, and that copies be transmitted to the Senate Committee on Cities, to the New York City Health Department, and to the medical journals of this city.

OBITUARY.

THEOPHILUS PARVIN, A.M., M.D.

DR. THEOPHILUS PARVIN died at Philadelphia on the morning of January 29, 1898. He had been seriously ill for a month from cardiac asthma. Pulmonary edema, associated with renal complications, was the direct cause of his death. Dr. Parvin, whose life was devoted to the teaching of obstetrics and allied branches, at different periods of his career occupied chairs in the Ohio State Medical College at Cincinnati, in the University of Lowell, in the Indianapolis Medical College, and in the Jefferson Medical College, in which latter institution he was Professor of Obstetrics and Diseases of Women and Children at the time of his death. He was an honorary member of a number of Continental and British obstetrical societies, and has always been a prominent contributor to obstetric literature.

Dr. Parvin was born of American parentage at Buenos Ayres, Argentine Republic, in 1829, but from his earliest childhood the greater part of his life was spent in Philadelphia. He graduated from the Medical Department of the University of Pennsylvania in 1852, after having taken his arts' degree five years previously at the University of Indiana. As a mark of respect to Dr. Parvin, the lectures at the Jefferson Medical College were suspended on the day of his death, and resolutions of regret were passed by the trustees and faculty of the college, by the student body, and by the Theophilus Parvin Obstetrical Society.

CORRESPONDENCE.

OUR PHILADELPHIA LETTER.

[From our Special Correspondent.]

COMMON COUNCILS AND THE FILTRATION ORDINANCE—MORE RESIGNATIONS AT THE MEDICO-CHIRURGICAL COLLEGE—TO PROSECUTE INCOMPETENT DRUGGISTS—DELEGATION TO THE BOSTON CITY HOSPITAL—DR. WILLIAM PEPPER FOR MAYOR—GERMAN HOSPITAL—PHILADELPHIA NEUROLOGICAL SOCIETY.

PHILADELPHIA, January 29, 1898.

ANOTHER instance of the depraved personnel of the Common Councils of the City of Philadelphia is found in the action of that body of politicians in refusing a few days ago, in the face of the present disgraceful typhoid outbreak, to pass the popular loan-bill authorizing *water-filtration*—refusing, by fifty-three votes, to redeem themselves in the eyes of the public and to make what atonement lay in their power for the already large and wanton waste of human life which their past obstructionary tactics have caused. The fifty-three councilmen who succeeded in defeating the passage of the proposed filtration ordinance were the individuals who are now known to favor the passage of another bill, now pending, forcing the city to purchase at a tremendous sum the rights of a private water-company; but the responsibility of more deaths from typhoid, due to their criminal delay, rests like a feather upon their shoulders in view of the individual enrichment to be derived from their support of this speculative syndicate's interests. The *Public Ledger*, a newspaper whose conservatism and reliability make its opinions authoritative, says editorially of this incident, that "nothing more infamous has occurred in the municipal history of Philadelphia," and directly charges the politicians referred to with a gross betrayal of trust, with an endeavor to squander public funds on useless purchases of water-rights, and with every moral responsibility for the delay in providing relief from the present epidemic. Charges of this kind from a newspaper like the *Ledger* are convincing, especially when the full names of the accused are printed along with the charge, as this paper has done. The scorn of the *Ledger* is echoed by every decent paper in the city, but they seem powerless, every one, to effect the slightest reform. Dr. A. C. Abbott, Director of the Bacteriological Laboratory of the Board of Health, after a thorough investigation of the epidemic, attributes the cause to infected drinking-water. The new cases of typhoid for the present week (January 29th) reach a total of 212. The deaths during the week numbered 10, or 13 less than last week. This makes a total of 1346 cases since the beginning of the epidemic last December, and of 887 cases during the first five weeks of this year. Meanwhile, the Board of Health remarks, in official notices, "Boil the drinking-water."

The *numerous resignations* which have been received of late from members of the faculty and board of trustees of the Medico-Chirurgical College were augmented a few days ago by the resignation of Mr. Charles W. Bergner, president of the board of trustees of this institution. Anent the latest change many spicy comments, *pro and con*, have been heard from those interested. Mr. Bergner states that his resignation was prompted by a change in the financial policy of the school, whereby it was proposed to guarantee to the professor of surgery, Dr. W. L. Rodman, a large yearly salary for a term of years. This change of policy he deemed unwise, inasmuch as to none of the other "practical" chairs are salaries attached, and he, therefore, sent in his resignation. The faculty have issued a public statement declaring that the situation was wholly misrepresented by the late president of the board of trustees, and further, a member of the faculty goes so far as to state without reserve that Mr. Bergner's resignation was requested in the interests of the school. Whatever the cause of the disagreement, the fact is apparent to the public, who have been acquainted for a week past with details galore of the fuss, that the ferment which they have scented points to a decided undercurrent of antagonism among a number of the authorities, lay and medical, of the college. To recapitulate, the "Medico-Chi." has within four weeks been deprived by resignation of the services of a professor of laryngology and dean, of a professor of obstetrics, of two trustees, and of a hospital superintendent. Truly, these are troublous times for this young institution, though it boasts of an appallingly costly operating arena, and of enormous State appropriations for its hospitals!

The State Pharmaceutical Board has determined to employ an agent to ferret out evidence leading to the *prosecution of violators of the pharmacy law* in this State, and it is said that especial attention will be directed to the incompetent compounding of physician's prescriptions by unqualified assistants. At the recent examinations held by the Board in this city, 134 candidates for licenses to practise pharmacy in Pennsylvania were examined, of whom but 39 passed. Of the 98 applicants for certificates as qualified assistants 42 were successful.

With the object of embodying in the additions to be made to the Municipal Hospital every modern facility of proven value, a delegation consisting of Dr. A. C. Abbott, director of the City Bacteriological Laboratory, Dr. Woodward of the Board of Health, Dr. W. M. Welch, physician in charge of the Municipal Hospital, and other city officials have gone to Boston, to make an *inspection of the Boston City Hospital*. The new building of this institution, which is considered one of the best equipped in America, will be studied by the delegation with a view of adopting its best features in the construction of the new wings to be added to the Philadelphia institution.

It is rumored that Dr. William Pepper will be presented as the next *candidate for the mayoralty of this city*. Dr. Pepper's public spirit and his wide interests in matters for the welfare of the community, together with his well-known executive ability, unite to qualify him for a public trust of this kind.

At a recent meeting of the board of trustees of the *German Hospital*, it was decided to divide the work of the institution into five departments, and the following were elected to assume charge: Chief of the medical department, Dr. James C. Wilson, with Drs. Harvey Shoemaker and Henry F. Page as assistants; chief of the surgical department, Dr. John B. Deaver, with Drs. George G. Ross and A. D. Whiting as assistants; chief of the ophthalmologic department, Dr. Charles Turnbull, with Drs. Edward K. Perrine and William T. Shoemaker as assistants; chief of the marine department, Dr. Fairfax Irwin, United States Marine Hospital Service; chief of the laryngological and aural department, Dr. Arthur A. Bliss. Dr. Adam Trau was elected consulting physician, and Dr. Carl Frese was re-elected medical superintendent.

At the last meeting of the Philadelphia Neurological Society, held January 24th, Dr. F. X. Dercum exhibited a case of *hemialgia* in a patient who for two years had had pain in increasing severity, first beginning in the right knee and at present involving the right lateral half of the body. The patient had been an iron worker, and said that for a number of years he was obliged to expose his right side to intense heat. There was also present tremor of both quadriceps extensors and the right gastrocnemius, and weakness of the right leg, together with some haziness of the optic discs, more marked on the right side. The disease was considered some anomalous lesion, probably of the basal ganglia. Dr. William Pepper, Jr., presented two specimens for Dr. Charles K. Mills, the first, a brain showing *bilateral symmetric softening of the internal capsule*, from a patient of advanced years who presented symptoms of syncope and hemiplegia of the left, and later of the right side; the second specimen was a *cerebellar tumor* from a patient whose most prominent symptoms had been occipital headache, mental hebetude, and a staggering gait. Dr. Pepper presented for Dr. F. X. Dercum a specimen of *large cerebral abscess* of the superior parietal lobule, from a patient who had during life stupor, convulsions, right-sided hemiplegia, and intermittent high temperature ranges, but without ocular manifestations. Dr. J. W. McConnell reported a case of *neuritis of the fifth nerve*, which was followed by the development of herpes in this situation, and later by an eczematous eruption over the course of the nerve. The affection, which was of three-weeks' duration, was considered due to influenza. Dr. J. H. W. Rhein reported a case of *unilateral flushing and sweating of the face* in a young woman of hysteric tendency, in whom these phenomena were accompanied by swelling of the right arm, and by pain in the right hand and arm, probably induced by exertion. The following officers to serve for the present year were then elected: President, Dr. F. X. Dercum; vice-presidents, Drs. Wharton Sinkler and H. A. Hare; secretary, Dr. William G. Spiller; treasurer, Dr. Guy Hinsdale.

The total number of deaths reported in this city for the week ending January 29th was 458, a decrease of 3 from those of last week, and a decrease of 98 from the corresponding period of last year. Of the total, 143 were of children under five years of age. There were 121 new cases of diphtheria, with 28 deaths; 52 new cases of scarlet fever, with no deaths; and, as has been before noted, 212 new cases of enteric fever, with 10 deaths.

OUR BERLIN LETTER.

[From our Special Correspondent.]

REGULATION OF PRIVAT-DOCENTS, AND SCIENTIFIC FREEDOM AT THE GERMAN UNIVERSITIES—TREATMENT OF MIGRAINE BY THE VIBRATORY CHAIR—PROFESSOR STOHR AND THE MICROTOME DISEASE—THE VIRCHOW JUBILEE BANQUET.

BERLIN, January 27, 1898.

THE recent introduction of a bill in the German Reichstag *making the privat-docents responsible to the Ministry for their teachings*, instead of to the university faculties, as heretofore, is evidently going to cause a renewal of the storm of opposition which greeted a similar measure some time ago. Professors at the German universities owe their positions to government appointment, and receive their salaries practically as employees of the Educational Department of the Empire. They are responsible to the government, therefore, for their teachings, and may be readily "rounded up" if they, perchance, show a tendency to kick over the traces of what the Minister may consider conservative opinion in science and politics. Usually, however, by the time a man has become an ordinary professor at a German university he has either become so staid and conservative that disciplinary regulation is unnecessary or his work has made his position so assured that a certain liberty of thought is allowed.

It is quite different with the young privat-docents. They owe their positions to the faculty of the University, being qualified as private teachers by special examination. For their private opinions they are responsible to no one; for what they teach, only to the University faculty. In matters of theoretic opinion faculties are apt to be notably lenient in their judgment of teachers, especially in these later times, and so the privat-docents have become thorns in more than one minister's side. Some of them have dared to hold and publicly express social-democratic views—the term over here for certain very reprehensible opinions as to liberty and equality which are contained in our Declaration of Independence.

They have not taught such views because they are not teaching in departments in which it would be possible. Their example, however, cannot but be contagious, because some of their views have the unfortunate pervasiveness of truth. There are said to be especially two or three of the younger men in Berlin at whose heads the proposed regulations are aimed. One is teaching integral and differential calculus and units of measurement in electricity, and another histology—not very promising subjects when handled scientifically (and that the men in question are not scientific no one has even hinted), for the propaganda of social democracy. The serious thing is that these young men hold views which a paternal government considers subversive in tendency, and it wishes the right to dictate the opinions which shall obtain at the University, even outside of the class-room.

The protests against a previous measure of the same nature came from some of Germany's greatest teachers. Virchow pointed out that Germany owed her superiority in intellectual matters to the enthusiastic devotion of her young men to scientific pursuits. The privat-docents, entirely independent of authority in a way, but with a career to work out, have devoted themselves to purely scientific investigation and theoretic speculation in a manner which has brought out what was best in them. As a consequence the government has always had ready at hand plenteous elaborated material from which to select the members of university faculties. France and Italy have begun to realize that it is the lack of this body of free lances in science and philosophy which has kept the originality of their rising men in the background, and recent modifications of their existing educational institutions are along the lines of imitation of German university customs in the matter.

On the whole Virchow's plea for the present status—the freedom of privat-docents from government influence and from the thought of currying favor with ministers, is worthy of the man who in his own privat-docent days (they celebrated his jubilee last week) thought it advisable to accept a position away from Berlin at Würzburg because of the opposition aroused in government circles by some of his liberal views during the revolution of 1848. Notwithstanding government efforts and exaggerated tendencies toward paternalism, it seems probable that such views will prevail. After all, as has been pointed out, their constitution provides for "freedom of scientific thought and teaching."

The situation of the matter here in Germany is not without its lesson for other countries, even for those in which there is no question of government interference. Too often the weight of influence of university trustees is thrown into the scale of a so-called conservatism that is sometimes a meddlesome opportunism. Recent events in university life in America point out that the precious heritage of free teaching in political science at least may be sadly encroached upon. Such an example is contagious, and one is apt to wonder if an overweening respect for tradition is to be the watchword in other sciences and what the results of such a policy would be. The protest on the part of universities here against the threatened encroachment on the liberty of teaching cannot but be re-echoed sympathetically by teachers all over the world and, as here, by none more cordially than by medical men who realize how much groundless authority and tradition may stand for.

At a recent meeting of the Berlin Medical Society, Dr. Ewer exhibited a model of a new apparatus, which its inventor calls a "Tremulor," *for the vibratory treatment of migraine*. It consists of a chair in which the patient sits while vibratory motions, rhythmic in character, are communicated to the body, especially to the head. It has been used with excellent results in a number of cases here in Berlin, and the apparatus has been found of use, too, in certain peripheral neuralgias in which the vibrations may be communicated to the affected nerve.

The theory of the curative effect of vibration would seem to be twofold: a tonic stimulation of nerve-endings and trunks by direct and reflex irritation, and a variation in the circulatory conditions which prevail in the part, with consequent changes in the nutritional metabolic processes. The invention would seem to be the application to separate parts of the body of Charcot's vibratory chair, which is still in use at the Salpêtrière in the treatment of certain neuroses. Charcot took the hint for his invention from the number of neuralgic patients, who claimed that a ride on the railroad did them good. For many cases of paralysis agitans this is said to prove an excellent remedy for the feeling of intense constraint which accompanies the muscular rigidity that has of late years came to be pointed out as almost the most characteristic symptom of the disease.

Professor Stöhr has an article in the last number of the *Archives for Microscopical Anatomy*, which is interesting from several points of view. It is his first article since the acceptance of Kölliker's chair at Würzburg, and will, therefore, be followed with unusual interest by the many who have always looked for the contributions from the Anatomical Laboratory of the University of Würzburg as representing the forefront of progress in anatomic science. The article is in itself very striking, because it would seem to be a *demonstration of the falsity of the position still held by some histologists that it is from cells of epithelial origin that the lymphoid elements in the intestine come*. There would seem to be as little scientific probability of the cells of one special form of tissue ever changing into another as of finding one species of animal changing into another. Professor Stöhr's article would also seem to be a distinct contribution to the question of the origin of leucocytes—that interesting subject which underlies so much that is yet to be known of the physiologic properties of the blood, and a question which has become only more interesting as the battle of serum immunity and phagocytosis continues to attract so much attention.

At the end of the article are some striking remarks on the disease which causes so much dry rot among the pretty systems of the histologist and the pathologic anatomist—*the microtome disease*. The microtome has undoubtedly been the greatest discovery, next to the microscope itself, for microscopic science, but it has, in Professor Stöhr's words, "been the occasion of some of the most egregious errors, and has furnished seeming support to the most erroneous theories." It is extremely difficult in hardened and imbedded specimens to know exactly the positions which sections occupied *in vivo*. "Too often," to quote Professor Stöhr, "when it is fondly hoped that sections are perpendicular to a given plane, they are oblique or tangential." As sections are now cut extremely thin, countless false pictures are found, and selected ones from among them will furnish ample grounds for the support of almost any favorite theory which the investigator has started out to prove. The plea for greater openness to conviction on the part of scientific observers is evident, but men are only men, and error will creep in. The much more important reflection for the practical medical man would seem to be that pretty theories, even when founded on supposedly scientific data, require ample confirmation before they can be accepted as truth.

On Wednesday evening, December 29th, representatives from all the German universities greeted Professor Virchow at *the banquet held in honor of his jubilee as a teacher*. The grand old man of medicine received the ovation tendered him with a modesty all his own. For him there would seem to be but two things in his career which he looks back upon with personal gratification: One is that he has been able to accomplish something, though he insists himself, more by the direction he has given other's studies than by what he has done himself, in placing modern medicine on the secure foundation of a scientific pathology, and the other is that this work in pathology turned the attention of the medical world toward German medicine. Two talismans there were for him in his younger days—his country, his university. The felicitations extended so plentifully to him he insists on sharing with his German colleagues, and his toast is: "*Alma mater*, just about to enter upon the most glorious part of her history, in a new century, with the new clinics, museums, and laboratories which are already in course of erection for her."

Donation to the London Hospital.—The London Hospital has received an offer of $125,000 to defray the expense of a new out-patient department. The offer is accompanied by two conditions, *viz.*, (1) that the patients shall contribute a small sum toward the cost of medicines, and (2) that letters of admission shall be abolished.

SOCIETY PROCEEDINGS.

MEDICAL SOCIETY OF THE STATE OF NEW YORK.

Ninety-Second Annual Meeting, Held at Albany, N. Y., January 25, 26, and 27, 1898.

SECOND DAY—JANUARY 26TH.

MORNING SESSION.

(Continued from page 160.)

DR. E. F. BRUSH of Westchester County read a paper, entitled

THE IMPORTANCE OF THE HYGIENIC MANAGEMENT OF DAIRIES

(which will appear in a future issue of the MEDICAL NEWS).

DR. W. H. HEATH of Erie County then read a paper on

THE MUNICIPAL CONTROL OF THE MILK-SUPPLY IN CITIES AND VILLAGES.

The author brought out the fact that although milkmen in cities are obliged to obtain a license to sell milk nothing of the kind is required of dairymen. The State Board of Health is wofully negligent in this respect. A high standard should be adopted, and sustained by stringent rules enforced by the State. Infected milk from diseased animals should be guarded against by veterinary examination of the herds at regular intervals. Contamination after milking should be prevented by absolute cleanliness of the dairy. Dairy inspection should be enforced, particularly with regard to the following points: (1) Character of the herds, as to breed, health, and whether or not subjected to veterinary examination; (2) method of cleansing utensils, and the length of time devoted to cooling of the milk—an important point; (3) water-supply; (4) character of the employees.

A milk-house should be sufficiently large and constructed of such material that it can be flushed and cleansed. There should be no communication with stable, living-room, or water-closet. The storage and cooling-room should be scrupulously clean, should open to the outer air, and should not have any sewer or drain connection. Rules containing explicit directions as to the cleansing of cans, utensils, etc., should be adopted, and conspicuously posted in the milk-room. Cans should bear tags on which is marked the date and hour of milking, and no milk should be sold which is more than twenty-four hours old. No disinfectants should be used in a dairy. Any dairyman who does not conduct his dairy on these lines should be deprived of his license.

DR. HERMAN E. HAYD of Erie County read a paper, entitled

SOME POINTS IN THE TECHNIC OF THE ALEXANDER OPERATION.

The author advocates the operation in which the ligament is picked up at the external ring, and lays particular stress upon the necessity of saving the knuckle of fat which appears at the external opening, as he considers this an important landmark. He then cuts off the ends of the ligament and transfixes the cord through a thick portion of the muscle, taking care not to draw the suture too tightly in approximating the pillars, believing that too much stricture upon the poorly nourished cord is apt to favor suppuration. He deprecates all operations which open the canal, as he is convinced that such a course is unnecessary, complicates the procedure, and favors the production of hernia.

DR. EDWIN B. CRAGIN of New York County read a paper on

THE PRESENT STATUS OF VAGINAL OPERATIONS FOR DISEASES OF THE PELVIC ORGANS. (See MEDICAL NEWS, January 29, 1898.)

DR. W. E. FORD of Oneida County read a paper, entitled

THE REMOTE CONSEQUENCES OF EXCESSIVE UTERINE HEMORRHAGE.

Sudden losses of blood of considerable amount are not especially dangerous. In these cases the blood-count shows great diminution of red cells, two million or even less to the cubic millimeter, but restoration to the normal five million speedily occurs. Shock seems to be in proportion to the diminution in the number of red cells. After childbirth the blood-count does not show much change from the normal, but when a laceration occurs which extends above the internal os the loss of blood is likely to be large during the labor and to continue afterward. The degeneration of the endometrium in these cases often protracts the hemorrhage. As a result of the constant leaking of blood, the local degeneration gives rise to a neurosis which results in a painful and sensitive uterus. This state is followed by neurasthenia in many instances, even though there has been little inflammatory trouble. These are the cases in which ordinary trachelorrhaphy fails to cure the nervous symptoms. Amputation of the cervix is a better operation in these cases. Small lacerations not extending above the interal os often require no treatment whatever, but if inflammation be present cicatrization surely follows, then curetting combined with ordinary trachelorrhaphy is necessary to cure the patient. In these last-mentioned types nervous symptoms are not usually presented, which is due, as the author believes, to the fact that there has been less loss of blood. A study of a large number of cases in which nervous symptoms were prominent leads to the belief that persistent hemorrhage only precedes menorrhagia. Nervous symptoms should not be attributed to reflex conditions. The blood-count in most of these cases, even when the patient is pale, thin, and nervous, shows that there is no true anemia; a record of blood-counts in several cases showed that only rarely does the number of red cells fall below 4,500,000 and the amount of hemoglobin below eighty-five per cent. Women with bleeding fibroids and cancer of the uterus present true secondary anemia, and nervous symptoms in such cases are not nearly as frequent or severe as in cases in which there has been continuous hemorrhage from high tears. The reason why so many women apply for treatment of lacerations several years after childbirth is that true neuralgia is an ultimate result of continuous degeneration, thus differing from the processes of inflammation which manifest their results much sooner. Hence, hemorrhage ought to receive more consideration and pure inflammations less in estimating the causes which produce neurasthenia uteri. All tears which open the internal os should be repaired before the neuralgic condition results. Too much should not be promised in long-standing cases from simple trachelorrhaphy. Microscopic studies of the blood show why iron tonics do not relieve the nervous symptoms of women having high cervical tears. The author then contrasted the blood-counts in these cases with those of an entirely different class of patients—young women with delayed or suppressed menstruation. In these latter iron is of little value, and in such a blood-count shows that real anemia does not exist.

DR. J. RIDDLE GOFFE of New York County then read a paper, entitled

THE ANATOMY AND FUNCTION OF THE PELVIC FLOOR IN WOMEN, AND THE OPERATION FOR REPAIR OF INJURIES DUE TO PARTURITION

(which will appear in a later issue of the MEDICAL NEWS).

DISCUSSION.

DR. GEORGE M. EDEBOHLS of New York County: It is a matter of congratulation to me to hear those who are familiar with Alexander's operation commend it so highly. It has always seemed to me irrational to open a woman's abdomen and create adhesions in cases of movable retroversion, and I am glad that the still small voice of conscience is making itself heard, and that operators have begun to consider it almost criminal to open the pelvic cavity, either from above or below, for this purpose. Alexander's operation will accomplish all that is necessary in these cases. I know of no one who performs the operation better than Dr. Kellogg of Battle Creek, Mich., who fastens the ligaments to the fascia. The only objection to his method is that the ligaments are placed in an unnatural position. The operation as performed by Dr. Hayd is the old operation of picking up the ligament at the external ring where it is weak and apt to tear as it is pulled out. Within the canal it is well developed. There is no danger of the ligament parting if the canal is opened before the ligament is picked up. This may be objected to as tending to weaken the inguinal canal, but such is not the case if the wound is closed by the Bassini method.

DR. W. GILL WYLIE of New York County: I agree with the last speaker that in simple cases Alexander's operation is an ideal one and much to be preferred to that in which the uterus is attached to the abdominal wall—a method that is somewhat obselete. I think, however, that Alexander's operation should only be performed by men skilful enough to be able to do it without opening the inguinal canal.

In regard to Dr. Cragin's paper, I think the status of the vaginal operation is now fixed. Nowadays, everyone does vaginal work, and only time will tell whether the vaginal is to be preferred to the abdominal route. Both methods are equally good in the hands of the expert, and the death-rate is not greater in one than in the other. In regard to the comparative value of ligatures and clamps, good results may be obtained by the use of either. Personally, I prefer the clamps. I now use them altogether, employing five or six pairs, because I think they leave the vagina in a better condition than when ligatures are employed. There is not that shortening of the vagina which sometimes follows the use of ligatures.

I was much interested in the paper of Dr. Goffe on the perineum, although I cannot agree with him in regard to the function of the transversus perinei muscle. My idea is that it is a very active muscle, and that it retracts and everts the mouth of the vagina when the perineum is lacerated. It is because the general surgeon does not understand the action of this muscle that he sews up a perineum improperly. As described by Dr. Goffe, I should think that a good deal of this everted tissue would be included in the stitches, and a bad result follow.

DR. ALBERT VANDER VEER of Albany County: I believe it is the consensus of opinion that Alexander's operation is indicated in cases of retroversion in which the uterus is movable. The suggestions of Dr. Hayd are worthy of careful consideration. I think, however, that the operation is performed in many cases in which it is not required. It may be avoided by palliative treatment, and by having the patient systematically assume the knee-chest position.

In regard to Dr. Cragin's paper, I think that the operator who is not familiar with vaginal work had better turn his attention to something besides surgery. I was one of the first to do the vaginal operation; eighteen years ago I removed a fibroid tumor through the vagina. The cases should, however, be carefully selected, and the position of the appendages ascertained before making the vaginal incision.

Dr. Ford's paper is one which goes home to the average practitioner. Many of the patients to whom he referred may be relieved by a proper line of treatment, and let me say right here that a great deal of benefit may be derived by these patients from the use of the bicycle. When trachelorrhaphy is indicated, all the hard cicatricial tissue in the angles of the tear should be removed as pointed out by Dr. Emmet.

Dr. Goffe's paper deals with the old muscle over which we have struggled many years. He has brought it out very clearly by his illustrations on the blackboard, and in a manner which must impress the obstetrician with its importance.

DR. FORD: In regard to Dr. Goffe's operation, I have been employing a method in which the silver wire sutures are passed, *not* through the mucous membrane, but about a quarter of an inch within the denuded surface, a deep bite being taken by the needle before it is brought out on the opposite side, and making a figure-of-eight as it is crossed there, pulling up the perineum to its normal position.

DR. GEORGE M. EDEBOHLS of New York County then read a paper, entitled

INVESTIGATION AND EXPLORATION OF THE OTHER KIDNEY IN CONTEMPLATED NEPHRECTOMY.

A knowledge of the presence and condition of the other kidney is of the first importance when nephrectomy is contemplated; inasmuch as there are cases on record in which autopsy proved that the kidney removed was the only one present. Palpation will usually determine the existence of the kidneys, although an enlarged gall-bladder has been known to be mistaken for the right kidney. It is difficult, however, to ascertain the condition of the kidney by palpation alone. Cystoscopy and catheterization of the ureters are of great value in this respect, although not always entirely satisfactory, nor should the danger of carrying infection to a healthy kidney be forgotten. Collecting separately the urine of each kidney will often throw light upon the condition. As a final resort, incision down upon, and exploration of, the opposite kidney may be performed before completing a nephrectomy. This procedure was first practised by the author in 1894, and he has employed it in two additional cases since that time.

DISCUSSION.

DR. WILLY MEYER of New York County: I think Dr. Edebohls' paper is of immense importance. A surgeon cannot feel easy when he removes a kidney unless he knows that the remaining organ is healthy, and every method must be employed to determine this point. In these cases cystoscopy and ureteral catherization should be employed. If the mouth of one of the ureters is found to be ulcerated, its kidney is probably diseased and the other healthy; for I am convinced that as a rule inflammatory conditions and tuberculous disease are ascending and not descending. Should these means fail, I recommend suprapubic cystotomy and direct ocular inspection of the bladder with the patient in the Trendelenburg posture. The ureters may also be catheterized at this time, the catheters being left *in situ* twenty-four hours, if necessary, to determine if both kidneys secrete healthy urine.

DR. P. M. WISE, of Albany County read a paper, entitled

THE PAST, PRESENT, AND PROSPECTIVE METHODS OF TREATMENT OF INSANITY IN THE STATE OF NEW YORK.

After briefly reviewing the treatment of insanity in the past, the author criticized the lack of instruction in the medical schools on the subject, and stated: "At the present time, when one of every two hundred of the population is insane, and the insane diathesis so permeates society that we dare not estimate its extent numerically, the schools dismiss the subject in almost a flippant manner." He referred to the small interest taken by physicians throughout the State in the hospitals maintained by the latter. State care means a uniform standard of care and treatment for those requiring segregation, and 19,000 of the 21,000 insane are at present properly domiciled. In two years, if the present policy be supported by the Legislature, all insane persons will be provided for. The foremost object of this great State charity is the restoration of the insane to health, and during the past year 1800 insane patients under State charge have been discharged in a condition to be useful. If the incurable forms of insanity were deducted from original admissions, sixty per cent. of the remainder would be shown to have recovered.

The author maintained that the present practice in the standard hospitals was abreast of medical progress, and that the changed condition for the better in asylums was due to rational methods of treatment, and not to suppression, as formerly. He called the attention of physicians to the dangers of narcotism in the early treatment of the insane, and said that the preservation of household quiet had resulted in disaster. The removal of mind-poisons was dwelt upon as well as the toxic effect of sense-irritation upon the excited brain. The present principles of treatment in hospitals are founded upon the removal of active causes—toxins, irritation of the nervous mechanism from all sources, and the improvement of the general health. The governmental policy is based upon the truism that every patient cured relieves the State from maintaining one person for a period of twelve years, which is the average duration of insane life. He referred to the unfavorable character of the cases now admitted, and also to the fact that the expectancy of curability is decreasing. The over-worked, over-stimulated, over-fed, immoral, and misguided are in greater excess than formerly. Resistance is weakened through heredity, and the weapons of attack are increasing. The cooperative plan has been adopted in the State Hospital for the Insane, and an experience gained at one State institution is available to all. This is shown in the pathologic work which is united for all the hospitals, and this plan has met such general favor that it is being followed by other States and foreign countries. He predicted marked advances in pathology as a result of recent technical methods which permit examination nearer the border-line of health and disease. Toward the consummation of this result the hospital system for the insane is working. He referred to the advantage enjoyed by the general physician in observing cases in the earliest stages, and to the relation of the physician to the prevention of insanity. Upon him must depend almost wholly whatever checks are exercised by society in the present almost universal destruction of nervous energy and resistance.

DISCUSSION.

DR. LANDON CARTER GRAY of New York County: I have been very much interested in this paper, and think we may all agree with the author in believing that the treatment of the insane in the State hospitals has undergone a very great improvement, and that an intelligent effort is being made to do what is best; still (in a spirit of meditation and not of criticism), I would like to have Dr. Wise's opinion of certain inherent defects in the present system. In the first place, it is a significant fact that in spite of the millions which have been annually spent upon these State institutions in the State of New York, not a single text-book, not a single new discovery in pathology, not a single new demarcation of symptoms, and nothing new in therapeutics has come from any man connected with them. This must be due to an inherent defect in the State care of the insane. If you or I want to study something in medicine or surgery we visit a medical center, go to hospitals, begin at the bottom of the ladder, wash sponges for six months, and at the end of that time we have charge of fifty or sixty patients, although still not in charge of them, for there is a visiting physician who comes in every day and directs the treatment; but we live in an atmosphere of medical teaching, therefore we learn. Precisely the reverse of this state of affairs is found in the case of the study of insanity. The men who receive appointments to insane asylums did not formerly have to pass a competitive examination, although I am happy to say that such is now necessary. They do not live in a medical center. They are isolated, and live in what is practically a large insane boarding-house, away from the clash of intellect which makes the mind keen and the man ambitious. Therefore, it seems to me that the system is defective. I am no reformer, and I do not know how the difficulty can be remedied. A gentleman who is in a position such as that held by Dr. Wise should use his efforts to change all this. What is done with the great wealth of clinical material? It should be the duty of the State to supply every clinic within its territory with the material required. It is the duty of the State to encourage and make easy the visiting of competent men who wish to study neurology and psychology. So far, knowledge of these subjects has been largely anatomic and pathologic. It is just beginning to be understood clinically, and it is very important that this knowledge should be extended.

DR. WISE: I will admit that some of the criticisms made by the last speaker have a substantial basis. It cannot be denied that the hospitals of this State are defective in many respects. I very much deprecate the fact that nothing new in therapeutics has emanated from these institutions, and yet whatever additions we have had to psychiatrics has resulted from the work of persons connected with such institutions. The tendencies are certainly in the right direction, and steady progress would be secured by the hearty cooperation of the workers outside the institutions. The insane hospitals are isolated, it is true, but this is from necessity; and yet I believe that the material which is in these hospitals should be used in teaching. Insane asylums have only just emerged from municipal control, and I think that sooner or later the efforts of the Lunacy Commission will result in permitting this material to be used in medical schools.

AFTERNOON SESSION.

DR. HERMAN MYNTER of Erie County read a paper, entitled

A YEAR'S WORK IN APPENDICITIS.

The author said he considered all classifications of appendicitis artificial, but, for clinical purposes, he divides the affection into simple catarrhal appendicitis, ulcerative appendicitis, with or without perforation, and septic appendicitis, with or without abscess. More deaths occur as a result of appendicitis than from any other abdominal disease. The prognosis is unfavorable when medical treatment is employed, the death-rate being between 16 and 20 per cent. Of those patients treated medically who recover, 50 per cent. suffer relapses. The mortality in those cases in which treatment is surgical depends upon whether or not the operation is performed at an early stage.

DR. A. M. PHELPS, of New York County then read a paper on

CONGENITAL DISLOCATION OF THE SHOULDER BACKWARD, WITH A REPORT OF SEVEN CASES AND AN OPERATION FOR ITS RELIEF.

The first case of this kind which was seen by the author was brought to him in April, 1895, at which time only six similar cases had been recorded. Such cases are generally supposed to be instances of unrecognized dislocation existing from birth. The author discovered not only dislocation but fracture of the glenoid in five of his cases, and believes the injury is directly due to traumatism inflicted by the accoucheur at the time of birth. In but one other case had operative treatment been employed before the author's first operation was reported. Operation was performed in all of his cases save two; in one, that of a child nine weeks old, he was able to reduce the dislocation without opening the joint, and a second refused operation. In the remaining five cases the joint was opened by incision, the dislocation reduced, and the head of the bone excised in order to make allowance for the shortening of the muscles due to the long-standing dislocation. The retaining capsule was then cut away, a drainage-tube inserted, and the wound closed. A slight paralysis will remain on account of injury received by the nerve from the same violence which preduced the dislocation. When the joint alone is injured, the results are fairly good, although motion is always slightly limited. The arm should be put up in a rotated position.

DISCUSSION.

DR. LEWIS A. WEIGEL of Monroe County: This subject is very important to the general practitioner and obstetrician, for there is no doubt that the condition in question is very often unrecognized. Within the past two weeks I have seen three cases of so-called "obstetric paralysis," and in two of them I am sure there is a dislocation: for the palm of the hand points backward—a diagnostic sign of this condition. I am prepared to endorse the author's statement that in nearly every case the injury is due to violence inflicted at birth. It is also my opinion that in some cases the paralysis is due to injury to the central nervous system at this time. In these cases there is always presented a history of difficult labor, long compression of the head followed by difficult delivery of the shoulders. In one of the cases which I recently saw there was asymmetry of the face, which would indicate central injury.

The author has referred to shortening of the arm as a result of the dislocation proper. It seems to me that it is possible that in a certain number of cases this shortening is due to arrested growth and atrophic change. I believe also that the paralysis is due to injury to the nerve. Before subjecting patients having this condition to operation, an accurate knowledge of the condition should be obtained by means of fluoroscopic examination and X-ray photographs.

DR. PHELPS: Regardless of whether paralysis exists

in a given case I would invariably reduce the dislocation, for this is the only means of placing the muscles in their normal position. In regard to the etiology, I think there can be no doubt that the condition is due to violence on the part of the accoucheur. In the cases I have operated upon I have found evidence of fracture, fragments being detected in three of them.

DR. REGINALD H. SAYRE of New York County then read a paper, entitled

THE TREATMENT OF RACHITIC DEFORMITIES.

The author advocated the early treatment of the rachitic condition in order to prevent deformities. The etiology of the disease is not well understood. It generally develops shortly after birth, and is supposed to be due to dietetic and hygienic factors. There is also some hereditary tendency which causes the disease to develop in some children and not in others. There are decided changes in the long bones, which become soft and flexible. Later, they become extremely hard. "Pigeon-toeing" is a conservative effort on the part of a child who is rachitic, because it finds that it can best support the weight of its body by turning in the toes. This should not be corrected, for it will take care of itself when the general condition is improved by proper diet, hygienic surroundings, and constitutional treatment. Cod-liver oil is excellent. Phosphorus has also been recommended, but the author has not seen good results follow its administration. If patients are seen early and treated in this way, but slight deformity will result. When the bones are markedly soft, the child should not be allowed to stand on its feet. In the case of an infant it should be placed in a wire basket or upon a padded board. The legs of older children should be put up in plaster of Paris, which is better than any apparatus. When seen in a late stage, after the bones have become hard, the deformity must be corrected by breaking or cutting the bone and putting the limb in a plaster-cast.

DISCUSSION ON THE MANAGEMENT OF HYPERTROPHY OF THE PROSTATE GLAND AND ITS COMPLICATIONS.

DR. L. BOLTON BANGS of New York County, opened the discussion with a paper, entitled

GENERAL CONSIDERATIONS AND CATHETER LIFE

(which will appear in a later issue of the MEDICAL NEWS).

DR. SAMUEL ALEXANDER of New York then read a paper, entitled

PROSTATECTOMY AND PROSTATOTOMY, SUPRAPUBIC AND PERINEAL,

in which he gave the results obtained in 205 operations. The author stated that in the majority of cases of hypertrophy of the prostate, operation is not required, palliative treatment being all that is necessary. The value of regular catheterization cannot be over-estimated, and too little attention is given to instructing the patient how the catheter should be used. In those cases in which the catheter fails to give relief, owing to the shape or size of the enlarged prostate, operation should be performed; but catheterization should be employed in every instance until it fails. Operation is indicated (1) when spontaneous urination is impossible, (2) when there is marked and constant vesical irritation, (3) when the amount of residual urine is steadily and surely increasing, (4) when catheterization is becoming more and more difficult, (5) when catheterization is followed by severe cystitis, (6) in cases of cystitis which resist all treatment, and (7) when the patient refuses to use the catheter. The author prefers the suprapubic operation as giving better results in regard to reestablishing voluntary urination. The death-rate is also less than that which follows the perineal operation. When drainage is required, the latter operation is the better. The condition of the kidneys at the time of operation should always be ascertained, as this is a most important factor in determining the result. The entire obstruction should be removed or failure will be sure to follow. Cystitis is not a contraindication to the operation.

DR. WILLY MEYER of New York County continued the discussion with a paper, entitled

BOTTINI'S GALVANOCAUSTIC RADICAL TREATMENT, AND THE PALLIATIVE TREATMENT OF HYPERTROPHY OF THE PROSTATE.

The author advocated the use of this method in the conservative treatment of the condition in question before operation is resorted to. He exhibited the instrument, which consists of a hollow metal catheter in which is hidden a small platinum knife which is made to emerge by the turning of a screw placed at the lower end of the instrument. A scale on the handle also shows the extent of the cutting surface exposed. The amount of current employed to heat the knife is regulated by a rheostat. The technic is simple. The bladder is first completely emptied. If irritation be present, the urethra is cocainized. The current is turned on before the instrument is inserted. Two or three grooves are made at the site of the enlargement of the prostate. The author has employed the method three times with good results. The cases, however, must be carefully selected.

DR. L. S. PILCHER of Kings County read a paper, entitled

CASTRATION FOR THE RELIEF OF HYPERTROPHIED PROSTATE,

in which he recommended the employment of this procedure in place of prostatectomy or prostatotomy. It requires no special skill and gives most satisfactory results.

DR. E. L. KEYES of New York County read a paper on

STONE ASSOCIATED WITH HYPERTROPHY OF THE PROSTATE.

The author alluded to the fact that in a discussion before the Society six years ago he advocated litholapaxy whenever practicable, whether or not the prostate be enlarged. He had then stated his belief that even in the case of a very small stone, when the prostatic condition is a main factor in the general morbid state, that it might be wise to insist on suprapubic lithotomy in order that partial prostatectomy might be performed—the patient's necessity being converted into the surgeon's opportunity—

and this opinion, which he still holds as a result of growing experience, is based upon the following facts: (1) lithotrity is a maneuver of the specialist. A general surgeon will perform lithotomy, cystotomy, or prostatectomy as well as, and often better, than a genito-urinary specialist. This is not so in the case of litholapaxy, which, therefore, can never become a general operation; (2) even the expert lithotritist cannot, for mechanical reasons, remove every fragment or grasp a final flat piece of stone from the deep *bas fond* in some cases of enlarged prostate. Even if he could, such removal would not and does not relieve the subjective symptoms, but rather aggravates them in some instances; (3) even suprapubic lithotomy, in which the entire stone is removed, does not *necessarily* relieve the symptoms, although it usually does so in great part. Suprapubic lithotomy *plus* partial prostatectomy does not *necessarily* relieve unless the vesicle orifice of the urethra be lowered and all bar-like obstructions removed.

The author stated that in France the Guyon school is returning to an advocacy of catheter-life, and is not advising prostatectomy. The operation is too severe to be generally advocated. Vasectomy is not at all reliable. Castration has been much overdone, and is not so devoid of risk to the patient's body and danger to his mind as might at first appear. Bottini's operation has not yet been tested and cannot be pronounced upon.

The following conclusions were reached: (1) When stone complicates enlarged prostate, if the condition of the latter be such that were the stone absent no operation would be called for, the question is to be solved by deciding whether the obstructive quality of the prostatic enlargement, the size of the bar, the depth of the *bas fond*, the irritability of the prostatic urethra and its resentment of instrumental interference, are sufficient to make litholapaxy impossible or to make it possible only at the expense of leaving the patient worse off than before. If such conditions obtain the stone should be removed by the knife. (2) In short, the question is one of diagnosis by the searcher, the cystoscope, rectal touch, and the tentative testing of the prostatic urethra with instruments. (3) The mere size of the prostate is not a factor in the problem. (4) The size or position of the stone is not a factor, except in the case of encysted stone, or one too large to be grasped by the lithotrite, or in the case of a foreign body. The size of the stone alone is relatively an argument against litholapaxy, since the symptoms in such a condition must be ascribed rather to the prostate than to the foreign body. (5) If lithotomy be performed, the suprapubic route is to be preferred, since this opens the door for more perfect work, and allows the surgeon to remove obstructions such as the third lobe, interstitial growths, outstanding horse-collar enlargements, bar, and to *lower the vesicle end* of the urethral floor, thus accomplishing all that could be done by a more extensive prostatectomy without very seriously increasing the operative risk. (6) Finally, here as elsewhere in surgery, the only safe, practical guide is surgical judgment based upon diagnosis guided by experience.

DISCUSSION.

DR. PILCHER: The presentation of the subject and the conclusions arrived at have been given in a masterly manner by Dr. Keyes which must commend them to our judgment. I have traveled over the same road and have come to the same conclusions—we must resort in some cases to suprapubic cystotomy for the removal of the obstruction to urination. It is the extreme danger which follows this bloody interference with the prostate when the bladder is opened which has caused me to advocate removal of the testicles, although I appreciate the enormous objection which may be raised against this procedure. I think, however, that this objection is exaggerated, and can be obviated altogether. I am not a partisan of any one method, and have merely contributed my own personal experience.

EVENING SESSION.

ANNIVERSARY ADDRESS BY THE PRESIDENT.

THE OBLIGATIONS OF THE PHYSICIAN AND THE LAYMAN TO EACH OTHER.

"There is a general tendency affecting all grades of people toward that which will create a sensation, and the advancement of science having disturbed very materially our old creeds, we have been disposed to accept those which seem newer and which seem akin to the marvelous. This is evidenced by the success of the traveling doctor who goes from place to place, heralded by posters and trumpets, and who cries his wares and his miraculous cures from the house-tops. The old-time doctor is passing away, and in his place we have the up-to-date medical man who, having imbibed his share of the spirit of the times, is losing in many respects more than he gains. It is his work which has reduced the death-rate in our largest cities to the lowest point in the history of the land, and which has built up the magnificent fortunes of life-insurance institutions.

"There is an unidentified something in the make-up of the medical man which you do not find in any other citizen. I speak of that jealousy which exists between himself and his brother practitioner, which makes him give free medical attendance to a patient who is not able to pay the fee demanded by him, but who is able to pay a smaller fee to his less successful brother. I doubt very much if any legal act could be devised to meet such emergencies, but if the members of the medical profession would respect the rights and privileges of each and every individual of their august body, and would see to it that no act of theirs would tend to jeopardize the interest of another, then would come the solution of this entire difficulty without the intervention of law.

"I am not a believer in reducing the practice of medicine to the status of a trade. I do not believe that the profession should organize itself into a trade's union for the furtherance of the interests of its members professionally, politically, and financially; but I do believe that there should be that honesty and respect for others' rights which should make men realize the justice or injustice which has been dispensed to their predecessors before serving in the capacity of successors. My special point is, that if we do not sustain honorable members in their expectation of just and courteous treatment we injure and degrade the profession itself."

THIRD DAY—JANUARY 27TH.

MORNING SESSION.

The Committee on Nominations announced the following committees:

Committee on Arrangements: Samuel B. Ward of Albany, Reynold W. Wilcox of New York, W. J. Nellis of Albany.

Committee on By-laws: H. D. Wey of Elmira, Nathan Jacobson of Syracuse, F. C. Curtis of Albany.

Committee on Prize Essay: Joshua M. Van Cott of Brooklyn, Andrew McFarlane of Albany, George McNaughton of Brooklyn, W. S. Cheesman of Auburn.

Committee on Publication: F. G. Curtis of Albany, Daniel Lewis of New York, C. H. Porter of Albany, W. W. Potter of Syracuse.

Committee on Hygiene: Henry R. Hopkins of Buffalo, A. H. Bartley of Brooklyn, C. E. Bruce of New York, J. M. Mosher of Oneonta, H. F. Hart of Shrub Oak, George Seymour of Utica.

Committee on Legislation: Frank Van Fleet of New York, Arthur G. Root of Albany, Eugene Wende of Buffalo.

Committee on Ethics: Evarts M. Morrell of Yonkers, George McNaughton of Brooklyn, Lewis A. Weigel of Rochester.

State Board of Examiners: Eugene Beach of Gloversville, H. D. Wey of Elmira, J. P. Creveling of Auburn, Daniel Lewis of New York.

DR. T. D. CROTHERS of Hartford, Conn., read a paper on the

TREATMENT OF DELIRIUM TREMENS,

in which he stated that the condition is due to alcoholic injury to the brain-centers, in some cases to the action of bacteria, and to auto-intoxication from various constitutional diseases. The principal indication in treatment is the induction of sleep. The use of strong opiates and hypnotics, especially chloral, are to be deprecated on account of the depressant after effects. The use of alcohol should be at once stopped, in spite of the widespread belief that its immediate withdrawal will cause death in some instances. Many of the cardiac stimulants are dangerous, and it is best to avoid their use. Elimination is of first importance. To favor this the hot bath is most essential. In private practice a blanket sweat will answer the purpose, and free diaphoresis should be kept up for two or three days. The employment of diaphoretic drugs should never be substituted for external applications. Calomel, followed by salines, should be administered. If restraint is necessary, it should be mild and alternated with liberty in order that the muscular excitement may be worked off. But little food should be given until the period of sleep comes on. The classic delirium tremens of the text-books is rarely seen. The old writers do not mention the dementia and melancholia which often follow the continued use of alcohol. A new chapter should be written on the pathology and treatment of this form of delirium. The large number of deaths which annually occur in police stations among persons who are found comatose on the street, is due to ignorance in caring for them.

DR. H. S. DRAYTON of New York County then read a paper, entitled

INTRATRACHEAL INJECTIONS IN DISEASES OF THE BRONCHIAL TUBES AND LUNGS.

This mode of treatment was first suggested in 1840 by Dr. Horace Green of New York, and elicited much adverse criticism at that time, the method being denounced as cruel. Later experiments have shown that the pulmonary mucous membrane is capable of absorbing liquids without irritation and without interference with respiration. The difficulty of manipulating the instruments is overcome by good illumination, a knowledge of the laryngeal region, a steady hand, and practice. A syringe holding half an ounce, devised by Dr. Joseph Muer of New York, is employed, to which is attached a curved metal tube about six inches long. If there is irritability of the throat, a spray of cocain may be first used, but this is rarely necessary. The syringe having been charged, the patient is instructed to sit upright and grasp the tongue with the right hand, drawing it well forward, at the same time opening the mouth wide and throwing back the head. The tube is then introduced and the injection made. This is more easily done with the aid of the mirror. Three injections of one dram each are given at a sitting, such material being used as will act adversely on the bacteria and produce a soothing effect as well as a mild stimulation; for instance, olive oil, glycerin, methol, eucalyptol, camphor, etc.

In the absence of the retiring President, the Vice-president introduced the newly elected President, Dr. John O. Roe.

Upon taking the Chair, DR. ROE said: "Ever since I was first sent as a delegate to a meeting of this Society, nearly twenty years ago, it has been my privilege to attend its annual meetings, and the profit which I have acquired in so doing I hope I may be able to return to the general stock of its medical knowledge. I will endeavor to show my appreciation of the preferment shown me by my zeal in the future, and, with your assistance, I will hope to make the next meeting as successful as those of the past. I thank you cordially for the honor conferred upon me, and wish you all a year of health, happiness, and prosperity."

The meeting was then declared adjourned.

THERAPEUTIC HINTS.

For Blepharitis Marginalis.—

℞ Ichthyol . . . . . ♏. xiv
Ung. zinci oxidi . . . . ℥ ss.

M. Ft. ung. Sig. Apply to corners of closed eyelids.

For Pulmonary Edema in Children it is recommended to give one to three drops of the tincture of strophanthus every three hours. Diuresis is produced and the edema is quickly diminished.

THE MEDICAL NEWS.

A WEEKLY JOURNAL OF MEDICAL SCIENCE.

VOL. LXXII. NEW YORK, SATURDAY, FEBRUARY 12, 1898. No. 7.

ORIGINAL ARTICLES.

CATHETER LIFE, AND SOME REMARKS ON THE ETIOLOGY OF HYPERTROPHY OF THE PROSTATE GLAND.[1]

BY L. BOLTON BANGS, M.D.,
OF NEW YORK;
CONSULTING SURGEON TO ST. LUKE'S HOSPITAL, ETC.

SIR HENRY THOMPSON states that an enlargement of the prostate gland of moderate degree occurs in one out of every three males who reach middle age; (2) that twenty per cent. of all men have fibrous tumors of the prostate previous to the fiftieth year of life; (3) that after the age of fifty years one man in every eight has marked enlargement of this gland, and finally (4), that the disease rarely begins later than the seventy-fifth year of life. Reginald Harrison states that one-third of the male population of the world who have passed the age of fifty-five years are the subjects of prostatic hypertrophy. The question naturally arises, why should the health of such a large proportion of men begin to be undermined by a harassing, and sometimes alarming, series of symptoms, at a period of life when they ought to be the most comfortable, and capable of their greatest and best work? There must be some cause, very general in its application, and it has been attempted to discover this in the analogy between these pathologic conditions of the prostate and fibroid degenerations of the uterus. I think a sufficient objection to this proposition is found in the very fact that while so many men begin to suffer from the affection in question when on the "down hill" side of life, the great majority of females, on the contrary, after forty-five years of age, enjoy a condition of comfort, and go on to an equable, satisfactory old age. Moreover, the function of the two organs is entirely dissimilar, and, as might be expected, the pathologic conditions, with the exception of the cases in which fibroid tumors have developed, are also entirely dissimilar.

In the great majority of cases of hypertrophied prostate the disease begins and remains in the glandular tissue, the other structures becoming secondarily involved. This view explains the absorption of the prostate which occurs in some cases after its function has been abrogated by the operation of castration. From these considerations, and from careful observation extending over several years, I am warranted in the statement that the first steps in enlargement of the prostate take place in youth. Admitting that general systemic conditions such as gout, rheumatism, and general atherosis may account for some cases, I claim that the chronic irritation and hyperemia, due to excessive function of the gland, often commencing in early life, and maintained during the vigorous period of existence, is sufficient to account for the largest proportion of those who suffer from this malady. It is interesting to find what a history may be developed by careful cross-questioning, even when it would be least expected, of some excessive or unphysiologic use of the prostate, which, starting in youth from ignorance, extends all the way through life to the time when symptoms, more or less severe, call attention to the existence of a urinary affection, and compel such a one to seek the aid of a physician. The subject is so immense and so complicated that in the limited time allotted me it can only be lightly touched, leaving to some subsequent occasion its consideration in detail.

Some, and occasionally all of the following elements enter into the etiology of hypertrophied prostate: (1) the habit of masturbation during childhood, caused either by some local irritation or by the teachings of bad companions; (2) possible and probable associations in the developmental years (that is, from twelve to twenty) with lewd women; or, the ignorant and foolish associations of young persons of the opposite sexes in which the male, though wrong is not intended, is kept in a state of constant or frequently recurring sexual excitement; (3) then, according to the moral status of the individual, follows (or accompanies) adultery or fornication, usually under the conditions of alcoholic stimulation and licentiousness; (4) if marriage occurs, these habits being already established, there is invariably excess. Subsequently there is apt to be objection to the birth of children, and then some unnatural or unphysiologic expedient to prevent conception is resorted to, generally on the part of the male, and this is persisted in oftentimes during years, until symptoms arise which call the attention of the subject to his sexual apparatus. At this period the symptoms may be of a minor grade, and, an intermission in the habits taking place, graver

[1] Read at the Ninety-second Annual Meeting of the Medical Society of the State of New York, held at Albany, N. Y., January 25, 26, and 27, 1898.

symptoms are not presented until later in life, although in the meantime the hyperemia, which has existed from youth, has caused the gradual development of the tissues composing the prostate. Even at this point in the individual's life, if the advice of the physician is sought, a greater or lesser degree of prostatic enlargement will be found to be present. Therefore, I believe that I am correct in the observation that a certain degree of hypertrophy of the prostate is present in many men long before it is suspected. Although surgeons have not considered it generally necessary to explore the bladder of young men (say about forty years of age) for residual urine, they have often been surprised to find many men retaining a small but varying proportion of the contents of the bladder. In some of these cases it cannot be said that at this period of life a self-perpetuating enlargement is presented, because, in many, treatment is successful, and it is even possible by proper remedial applications to effect a reduction in the size of the already enlarged gland, but if the presence of residual urine is to be regarded as one of the symptoms of hypertrophy of the prostate, this condition will be found present oftener than is suspected.

Usually the first evidence of the existence of prostatic hypertrophy is a sense of irritation at or about the neck of the bladder and some variation from the normal sexual condition. Such a patient may at times experience a sense of fulness in the perineum, but unless there has been an acute inflammation of the prostatic urethra there is usually no pain incident to the early stages of this affection. As time goes on a slight increase in frequency of urination may be noticed, and also a little tardiness in starting the urine. The stream of urine is not usually changed in volume, although at times it may be somewhat smaller than usual, and this fact should be borne in mind in differentiating this affection from stricture of the urethra. Gradually, with occasional intercurrent exacerbations, the calls to urinate become more frequent, but following micturition there is a sense of relief, and the individual is not aware that he does not completely empty the bladder and that the latter is gradually becoming fuller and fuller. At this time he may complain of a dull pain over the sacrum or in the lumbar region, which is generally treated as "rheumatism" by means of domestic remedies. Still later the bladder becomes distended, the hydrostatic pressure gradually thins its muscular layers, and there is now more or less atony of this viscus, as manifested by a slow, feeble, dribbling stream of urine. There may also be a relaxation of the cut-off muscles surrounding the neck of the bladder and prostatic urethra. This permits a small quantity of urine to enter the urethra, and then there may be a constant and tormenting desire to urinate, with perhaps involuntary evacuations of a few drops, or even a decided "overflow." The latter is apt to take place at night, during the relaxation of sleep, and the individual has the added misfortune and mortification of wetting his bed. At this juncture, if not before, medical advice is usually sought, and the question arises in the mind of the attending physician,—what is the cause of this frequency and perhaps involuntary urination? It will not do to say that such a patient has "incontinence of urine," and prescribe alkalies and diuretics, for these would only make matters worse by increasing the volume of fluid in the already over-distended bladder.

If an adult presents the series of symptoms which have been narrated, and especially if he has the nocturnal involuntary urination, a careful and discriminating diagnosis must be made; for these symptoms point to some obstruction which the bladder has long been endeavoring to overcome. Stricture of the urethra must be excluded by eliciting the patient's history, and by a careful and aseptic exploration of the urethra with the *bougie à boule* and sound. The latter may take the place of a searcher at this point in the examination and furnish evidence of an obstruction at the neck of the bladder, either by failure to enter the viscus, or by the amount of rotation or depression of the handle required before feeling its point free in the bladder. In general, a searcher after the Sir Henry Thompson pattern is the best exploring instrument, and will often enable the physician to outline the prostate with great accuracy. The passage of a catheter into the bladder, and the discovery of a varying amount of urine remaining after the patient has been requested to urinate and expel all that he can spontaneously, will usually make the diagnosis clear, especially if added to the evidence furnished by the searcher. The simple passage of a catheter into a supposedly empty bladder may often suffice to establish the diagnosis, but cannot be relied upon in a doubtful case; for enlarged prostate is not the only cause of residual urine. Digital examination of the prostate by the rectum should supplement the examination, and may reveal a large, full-lobed, or swollen and sensitive prostate gland, but the diagnosis of retention due to hypertrophy of the latter should not be based upon this method alone. Here it should be remarked, that at this period a new series of symptoms is liable to be manifested from the possible advent of urethral fever, or cystitis, or both.

It should be remembered that it is not the presence of residual urine alone that is dangerous, although when large in quantity such may cause a serious condition of vesical atony, with perhaps a secondary dilatation of the ureters and congestion of the kidneys from back pressure. The presence of residual urine always renders the bladder liable to infections. Normal urine does not necessarily cause inflammation of the bladder, but residual urine, and the consequent congestion due to the efforts of the bladder to expel its contents, prepares the way for the development of infection of the bladder. From the foregoing it follows that the first introduction of a catheter into the bladder of a patient presenting these symptoms should be regarded as a surgical operation, and must be conducted with the most scrupulous attention to surgical details. The meatus and penis should be carefully scrubbed with soap and water. Clean towels if obtainable, if not, sterilized gauze, should be so placed as to surround the penis. The hands of the operator should be carefully prepared with soap and water, and finally scrubbed in pure alcohol. Then the penis and the urethra should be irrigated with an antiseptic solution, and for convenience and ready adaptability, a solution of salicylic acid (gr. viii to Oi) may be used. Then the catheter, which has been previously sterilized with formaldehyd gas or formalin solution, should be removed from its wrappings of gauze, smeared quickly with a sterile lubricant, and, maintaining a current through it of the antiseptic solution, should be carefully and gently introduced. The lubricant which I prefer is made for me by Van Horn & Ellison of New York, and is composed of Irish moss, with the addition of eucalyptol (1–1000) and formalin (1–2000). The first introduction of the catheter into a bladder in which there is presumably residual urine is so important and may mean so much to the patient that, in my opinion, he (or some member of his family) should be previously informed that although every precaution will be taken, there is a possibility of infection of the bladder and consequent cystitis.

In regard to catheters, one should be chosen which will be easily admitted by the meatus. It should be a soft rubber instrument with a solid tip, and its introduction should be made with the utmost slowness and gentleness. The urethra is the habitat of micro-organisms, many, but not all, non-pathogenic, and the urethra and bladder will be made more vulnerable and liable to infection in proportion to the damage to the epithelium which is caused by the introduction of the instrument in question. Moreover, if there be any reason to suspect that the individual has any catarrhal condition of the colon or rectum, or if he has been liable to chronic constipation, the first use of the catheter should be postponed, if possible, even for diagnostic purposes, until the bowels have been thoroughly emptied by free catharsis or by a high enema, and perhaps irrigated with a weak solution of chlorinated soda. This is for the purpose of preventing infection of the bladder by the development of the bacillus coli communis.

The foregoing diagnostic suggestions are made with a case in mind in which there is yet spontaneous urination. If, however, the case presented is one in which complete retention has suddenly occurred, the patient, not being able to pass any urine except perhaps in drops, and whose agonizing attempts to evacuate the contents of his bladder are producing an aggravation of all his symptoms, no delay, excepting the reasonable time which should be allotted to the preparation of instruments, can be permitted. Relief must be speedily attained or the condition may become serious. Absolute cleanliness is, of course, essential. Though one form of catheter may not suffice, the first one to be tried is the soft and flexible instrument such as previously described. Its passage may be facilitated by the previous introduction of 20 to 30 minims of a four- to eight-per-cent. solution of eucain after the urethra has been irrigated. Eucain is somewhat slower in its action than cocain, and six or eight minutes should be allowed for its absorption before local anesthesia will be obtained.

If the soft catheter fails—on gentle manipulation—to enter the sensitive and swollen prostatic urethra, then resort may be had to one, either with an angle at the end (*coudé*), or one with two angles (*bi-coudé*), or to one with a curve and also a tapering, bulb-pointed end, known as the "natural-curve catheter," and which has been of the greatest use to me. Even these may fail, and then resort may be had to other forms, or to a carefully sterilized silver instrument with a large long curve—known as the prostatic curve. But if these successive steps cause traumatism of the urethra, as evidenced by a few drops of blood oozing from the meatus, and it is manifest that the manipulations are to be prolonged, I advise, in view of the safety of the patient, that all instrumental attempts by the way of the urethra should be discontinued, and the over-loaded bladder relieved by suprapubic aspiration. Of course, it is needless to say that this procedure should be undertaken with the same careful sterilization of the hands and of the area of puncture, and equal care in the preparation of the aspirating-needle, as in any other surgical operation. Aspiration may be repeated as often as once in four or six hours when carefully conducted, without damage, and with great relief to the patient. A high enema should be given, and in the intervals between the aspirations hot antiseptic irrigations of the urethra should be instituted, together with hot irrigations of the prostate through the rectum by means of Kemp's tube. These will aid materially in reducing the congestion of the prostate, which added to the chronic state of hypertrophy, has resulted in the sudden attack of retention. In this way a certain amount of spontaneous urination may be restored, but in many cases this will be deferred indefinitely. At this time the conditions are so acute that no attempt should be made to massage the prostate, but subsequently digital massage of the prostate through the rectum will help to relieve the over-loaded blood-vessels of the gland and facilitate the introduction to the "catheter life," which in all probability must now begin.

The question of prolonged drainage of the bladder is, in my opinion, to be considered at this stage only in case the bladder becomes infected, and when the latter cannot be made clean or obtain rest by means of irrigation. This operation can only be considered in relation to a given case, and must be determined upon by the judgment of a competent surgeon.

In order to consider the details of "catheter life" a broad or general grouping of the cases may be made into those in which there is more or less spontaneous urination, and those in which the individual is absolutely dependent upon the catheter. As the latter class is the more important, let us follow the case of a patient to whom we have been called in the emergency of complete retention. Generally, within two or three days, and aided by the measures which have been instituted, the congestion will have subsided sufficiently to enable the introduction of a catheter. Unless great care is exercised in the first few introductions of the instrument minute traumatisms of the prostatic urethra may occur, and the patient suffer so keenly that he dreads the time when the instrument must be passed. This suffering may be modified, of course, by the use each time of the eucain solution, but in the intervals between catheterization something must be done to relieve the sensitiveness. There are several suggestions which may be followed, such, for example, as the continuation of the hot irrigations which were being used during the acute stage, and this same hot antiseptic solution should be allowed to flow through the urethra each time the catheter is used. Massage of the prostate may be instituted with great comfort to the patient, but must not be performed violently or continued too long at each time. Subsequently a weak solution of nitrate of silver, not over 1–5000, to begin with, and gradually increased in strength, may be applied to the whole of the deep urethra, and especially at the bulbomembranous junction, by means of an instrument which will gently distend the urethra at the same time the application is made; or, else by injecting the solution through a catheter of a size which has been found to enter with the least pain; also, the careful and gentle introduction of a sterilized steel sound, smeared with iodoform emulsion, will be found to relieve this extreme sensitiveness. If, in spite of care, gentleness, and patient effort, the hyperesthesia remains, and especially in those cases in which not even a measure of spontaneous urination is restored, or in which infection of the bladder has occurred, and a persistent and painful cystitis persists, some operative procedure must be considered. The first of these, in my opinion, is drainage of the bladder, and though this part of the subject will be presented by my colleague, Dr. Willy Meyer, I may be permitted to say at this time, that whether my opinion in regard to "drainage" being the first operation to consider will be changed by the re-awakened galvanocautery treatment remains to be seen. I shall make some observations in regard to the latter, and trust that my experience combined with that of others, will enable us to ascertain its merits.

To proceed with the consideration of those cases in which "catheter life" is to be led, we will now assume that the irritability of the urethra has subsided and that the catheter can be painlessly introduced. The patient may now be taught to introduce the instrument himself, and also the care of the catheter, etc.; but, first and foremost, the principles upon which depend the maintenance of a sterile bladder and urethra must be forcibly impressed upon him. If at all intelligent, he can understand (since the knowledge in regard to micro-organisms has become so widespread) that he may easily poison *himself*, and that if he does there will follow a long train of complications, the result of an infected bladder. In general it may be said that if the urine remains sterile the catheter may be passed at the patient's convenience, but this should be done once in six hours at least, leaving a longer interval at night, but depending somewhat on how long the individual sleeps.

Many a prostatic patient with sterile urine, and yet dependent upon the catheter for emptying his bladder, will sleep eight or even ten hours without being awakened by a desire to urinate. So long as the urine remains clear and sterile no necessity for washing the bladder exists. Even after the patient has become established in the habit of using the catheter and has acquired the skill and facility which many of these patients do, he should visit his physician at regular stated intervals, in order that the first evidence, even though slight, of infection may be ascertained and, if possible, immediately remedied.

Unfortunately, many of these individuals become so self-confident and so satisfied with their condition that infection occurs insidiously, increases gradually, and suddenly there is an explosion of cystitis, which may or may not be accompanied by an intercurrent prostatitis. I am in the habit of humorously informing such patients that they should periodically submit themselves to the inspection of their medical advisers on the same principle as that with which they cheerfully pay the fire-insurance premiums upon their property.

In case cystitis has supervened, what shall be done? During the acute stage the patient should be put to bed, placed upon a milk or light diet, and an antiseptic administered by the mouth which will be eliminated with the urine. I am now well pleased with the use of benzosol for the purpose. It may be given in 2- or 3-grain doses as often as every two hours, but I have given it in 5-grain doses without resulting harm. It is usually well-borne, does not set free carbolic acid like salol, and in the intestines (chiefly) is transformed into guaiacol and benzoic acid. The use of Kemp's tube is also indicated in this stage. Now resort may be had to irrigation of the bladder, and if the patient is seen early enough the effect of the infection may be aborted by careful washing of the bladder with a stronger solution of nitrate of silver than I have mentioned.

It is surprising sometimes to see how a threatened severe attack may be modified by the introduction into the bladder of a solution of nitrate of silver of even a strength of 1–1000. Here let me say that this must be gently accomplished. The bladder-walls are congested and are contracting more frequently and vigorously than normal, sometimes with a marked degree of tenesmus, and if a large quantity of fluid is injected or allowed to run in with force, the affection will be aggravated. It is best to be content to inject only an ounce or two ounces of the solution, allow it to run out, and then repeat the injection. The first effect is an irritation. The patients experience what some of them jocosely call a "red-pepper" feeling, but they receive so much relief that they often ask for a repetition of the "red pepper." If this does not give the expected relief, then frequent ablution of the bladder—that is to say, three, four, or even more times a day if the urethra will bear the introduction of the catheter, with a mild antiseptic solution, must be resorted to. The first effect of the solution upon the mucous membrane must be studied, and sometimes it may be necessary to employ such a mild irrigating fluid as normal salt solution, which may be made extemporaneously by dissolving one dram of chemically pure chlorid of sodium in a pint of hot, sterile water. As the case becomes more chronic and the bladder less sensitive, irrigations may be less frequently employed and the fluids used may be varied according to the amount of pus and mucus present. Once in three or four days the physician may use the solutions of nitrate of silver as suggested.

In the consideration of those cases in which a certain degree of spontaneous urination remains, the first question which presents is, what rule shall govern the employment of the catheter? This depends largely upon the amount of residual urine, that is to say, the average amount of urine which remains in the bladder after each active urination, and upon the sensibity of the latter organ. In many cases there is no accumulation of urine beyond this average amount which remains at or about two ounces, excepting during some intercurrent affection of the prostate which may cause an increase in the degree of obstruction. If the residual urine is normal in quality, that is to say, is not infected, is normally acid, contains no crystalline elements — in other words, if of a bland, non-irritating character, the bladder does not resent its presence, remains quiescent, and the patient is not conscious of any irritability of the viscus. In such subjects, and under such conditions, it is not necessary to use the catheter at all, but if the urine changes in quality, and especially if there are obscure pains over the sacrum or in the pelvis, then it may become necessary to withdraw even this small amount of urine—particularly at night, in order that refreshing and undisturbed sleep may be obtained. In some individuals, even one ounce or less of residual urine, if the latter, though sterile, be abnormal in other respects, will irritate the bladder, and therefore should be withdrawn.

As has already been remarked, in these cases of sterile urine it is not necessary to resort to washing the bladder; but after the bladder has become infected the question arises how often shall it be irrigated. Only general directions can be given in answer to this question. The repetition of washing will depend largely upon the amount of pus and mucus present in the urine, upon the frequency with which the patient is called upon to urinate, and also upon the general irritability of the nervous system of the individual. Some persons require daily ablution; others, once in two or three days, and others again, not oftener than one irrigation a week. The interval should be that which suffices to keep the patient comfortable—thus, many men continue for years to urinate but once in four or five hours, and are not disturbed at all during the night. After the patient has learned to introduce the catheter the most important instructions which can be given him are as to the care of this instrument. The form and kind of catheter having been adapted to the individual, directions which will keep it aseptic must be strenuously enforced by the physician, and rigidly followed by the patient. In my experience, these directions in order to be adhered to by the patient under all conditions, must be simple. Even in the case of medical men who are the subjects of prostatic hypertrophy, and who from their calling are supposed to know the value of thorough asepsis, I have found it necessary to make the directions as simple as possible, in order that they might be followed. Heretofore, thorough washing of the catheter with soap and water after each use, and then immediately before its use, steeping the instrument in boiling water and then in the solution which is used for washing the bladder, has proved satisfactory in some respects, but of course not entirely so. Here I may say that the general intelligence of the patient and the resistance of his tissues have much to do with the prevention of infection.

Unquestionably, a simple but efficient and non-destructible method of rendering and maintaining catheters thoroughly aseptic has long been required, as well as a means which can be readily employed by our patients. It seems to me that the question of catheter antisepsis has been solved by the application of formaldehyd. To this purpose many experiments have been made with this gas, but its employment is not, as yet, within the reach of everybody. I employ in my office a Lilly's apparatus which generates the gas directly from wood alcohol, and catheters and other instruments may be exposed to its influence for hours. Lately my attention has been called to a fallacy in the use of the gas, and I may be allowed to quote from a recent paper by Dr. Park of the Health Board of New York City, who made some observations upon the diffusibility of the gas in long-closed tubes, such as we may consider a catheter to be. For example, he filled a glass tube with colonies of bacteria and noted that those at the extreme end of the tube were not touched by the gas. He drew the inference that although the gas entered each end of the catheter there might be a zone in its center untouched by it. Hence, it appears that a current is necessary for the transmission of the gas through the catheter or to the end opposite to that at which the generation of the gas occurs. Therefore, since the polymer of the gas, known as paraform, which is in the form of powder or tablets, and which volatilizes, has been used for the purpose of maintaining catheters sterile while suspended in glass tubes or in boxes, this source of failure should be remembered.

In order to ascertain whether the solution of formaldehyd called formalin (a forty-per-cent. solution of the gas) would answer the purpose, and to ascertain the strength of the solution necessary to render catheters sterile, I took three catheters which had been used by patients; one which had been used for the purpose of withdrawing sterile urine, and only used three or four times; another which had been used by a patient for some mouths, but whose bladder was infected; and a third which had been in use nearly two years in a moderately infected bladder. These catheters had all been treated in the same way by the persons who used them; that is to say, they had been carefully washed in soap and water immediately after use, then steeped in boiling water, and also steeped in boiling water immediately before being passed into the urethra. In the first instrument referred to staphylococci were found—a non-pathogenic and a large pathogenic bacillus; in the second, a large coccus and a diplococcus, the latter differing morphologically from the gonococcus of Neisser; in the third, staphylococci and streptococci, and a large spore-bearing non-pathogenic bacillus were found. A one-per-cent. solution of formalin was used. This killed all pathogenic germs after fifteen-minutes' immersion, but it should be observed that in sterilizing catheters in the liquid formalin care should be taken to see that the air confined inside is displaced (by the liquid) by a process of stripping or milking. This I regard as highly important, and desire to call especial attention to it.

From the foregoing may be deduced the following general directions, which must be rigidly followed by the patient:

The soft catheter with solid tip is the best to use if possible. If a rigid one is required, one made of elastic webbing, with a curve or bend at the point which will be the most comfortable for the patient, is preferable. A new catheter must be treated with the same care as to cleanliness and asepsis as one which has been in use. If possible it should be exposed to the vapor of formaldehyd; if not, it should be immersed in a solution of formalin (one- to two-per-cent.) during at least fifteen minutes. Then it should be rolled in a strip of bichlorid gauze or placed between the folds of a perfectly clean towel. Each catheter should be kept in a separate receptacle or closed drawer where dust cannot find access to it, and where it cannot be handled except by the person who is to use it. If the patient's necessities require that the instrument must be carried about with him, it should be kept wrapped in several layers of bichlorid gauze, and outside of this should be placed a wrapping of "waxed" (parafin) or parchment paper held firmly by rubber elastic bands. At the time of use the patient must thoroughly clean his hands and rinse his fingers in pure alcohol, of which he should always have a quantity on hand. In the meantime the catheter should be lying in the formalin solution. Then, after shaking it and wiping off any drops which may remain upon it with a piece of clean gauze (to avoid irritation of the urethra with the solution), and smearing it with the lubricant already referred to, it may be gently introduced. Immediately after use the catheter should be thoroughly washed with soap and water, steeped in the solution of formalin and then carefully put away in gauze or clean towels in readiness for the next use. If the individual is dependent upon his catheter, and in consequence must have one at his place of business, it is well to provide one sterile instrument for home and another for office use—to be cleaned as well as possible immediately after using and then put away for thorough sterilization on return to the base of supplies.

I have a patient who has a rule never to use one catheter more than a week. He buys them by the dozen, is very particular in their care, and at the week's end throws the catheter away and starts in with a new one. He maintains his bladder in an admirable condition, and I may say that I rarely see him, though he comes in for an occasional inspection, and feels well repaid for the care which he exercises.

SOME OF THE DANGERS SURROUNDING THE DAIRY.[1]

BY E. F. BRUSH, M.D.,
OF MT. VERNON, N. Y.

IF the dairy is suggested to the every-day urban citizen, his imagination immediately conjures up the fair and buxom milkmaid, the foaming pail, the breath of the sweet-smelling kine, luscious cream for his oatmeal and strawberries, golden pats of butter, and bountiful, innocent sweetness, milk and honey. It may be owing to this sentimental idea of the dairy that so many take kindly to raw milk, while having at the same time an abhorrence at even the thought of eating raw meat from the same animal; when, actually, the danger of contagion, disease, and the ingestion of impurities are far greater from the milk than the meat. Few people, I believe, realize the menace which lies in the milk-supply of cities. Milk which is dangerous, and perhaps deadly poisonous, appears just as innocent, innocuous, and deliciously nourishing as the fluid that is so in truth.

In many of the dairies supplying milk for food nearly everything is either totally wrong or not quite right enough to produce a wholesome product. It is well known that the dairy cow is subject to numerous grave diseases, and many of her maladies are, we know, the same as those which afflict the human race, and it is also an established fact that any disease in the cow affects her milk perniciously. Every one who observes current literature on the subject knows that there are several articles of absolutely refuse material which are used as food for the dairy cow, while she is expected to give in return one of the highest types of food for human use. The cow is necessarily a delicate creature. What condition may be imagined, except actual disease, that is more opposed to robustness, vigor, and hardihood to withstand the shock of cruelty, bad food, and dirty surroundings than maternity and lactation? The cow, while giving us milk almost constantly, at the same time sustains a fetus; and so it is only reasonable to affirm that the dairy cow must receive solicitous attention, gentle treatment, and absolute cleanliness in her surroundings and feeding if it is expected that she will supply milk fit for human food. It was long ago discovered that what affects the mother affects the nursling, sometimes even so far as to cause the death of the latter.

Unfortunately, it is the exception to find a dairy in which the cows are treated kindly and fed or housed in a cleanly manner. At the present time health authorities appear to recognize nothing but tuberculosis as the sum total of all the disease and danger contained in the improperly managed dairy. The sources of possible contamination which surround the milk after it is drawn from the cow are many and serious on the majority of dairy-farms as they are conducted at the present time, and it is this part of the hygiene of the dairy to which I particularly wish to call attention now, because this branch of the subject receives everywhere less attention than it deserves, and I believe that when we are able to exclude the diseases which arise from milk-contamination in the dairy, outside the cow, we will be better able to trace some of the epidemics which find origin in the animal herself. Until all the dangers of the dairy are recognized many of the more grave and menacing ills cannot be remedied.

It must be remembered, in considering milk, that there is no other article of food just like it. There is no food, fluid or solid, which presents so many favorable conditions for the absorption of the tangible material of disease and for its preservation and multiplication, and in no other instance is a medium found for the conveyance of infection by which so much harm can be accomplished in such a very short time. Of course, a certain degree of heat will disinfect milk, but even a high temperature will not eliminate the toxins already contained therein.

[1] Read at the Ninety-second Annual Meeting of the Medical Society of the State of New York, held at Albany, N. Y., January 25, 26, and 27, 1898.

We are constantly searching for a specific remedy for scarlet fever and other often fatal diseases of childhood, while frequently permitting the bacterial cause of these diseases to be fed to our children in their milk. Many of the diseases of infancy may be rendered much less frequent or even altogether eradicated by proper attention to the hygiene of the dairy, and I believe that the achievement of success in this line is being delayed by the futile efforts of well-meaning physicians, who imagine that they are correcting the evils of a bad milk-supply by modifying, Pasteurizing, sterilizing, adding animal and chemical compounds, and by otherwise changing the character of the milk.

Around every dairy is a multitude of dangers—dangers, unfortunately, which are not always appreciated or avoided, and hence culminate in disaster. There are many other animals about the dairy besides the cow which menace the dairy product, often as seriously as a diseased cow herself. Horses, dogs, cats, rats, mice, and fowls undoubtedly are often the direct means of infecting milk, and of thus passing contagion along to the human race.

Cats loll and purr around many dairies all day, and it is a very common thing to see a wheezy old cat lapping warm milk from a pail or other milk container. These animals are known to succumb to a throat trouble which appears identical with human diphtheria, and it is also known that they die from many tuberculous forms of disease. So it is not unreasonable to ascribe contagion to these animals when they are allowed the freedom of the diary. Dogs prowl about the farm day and night, and very often depend upon the carcasses of dead animals for their living. Cows, horses, and pigs often die of septic and contagious diseases; the carcasses are hauled into the woods or fields, away from the house, and there left exposed as meat for the farmer's dogs. These dogs come back and lap the milk from the pail, lick the empty milk vessels which are never properly cleaned; and can there be doubt that the milk is thus infected? Where this danger exists in a dairy it is practically unlimited. Rats and mice infest the ordinary dairy; they get into the milk and the milk-vessels. These animals also have their diseases, and, therefore, the element of danger and disease from these pests must be acknowledged. The poultry around the farm are sometimes very numerous, and not always healthy. The diseases to which they are subject are many, and, owing to their high, normal body temperature (108° F.) there is no other animal which so readily becomes tuberculous or which dies so quickly from this disease. On some dairy farms the hens are everywhere, in the cow stable, in the milk-house, in the dwelling-house, and even in the milk-pails. The dairyman, as a rule, has a family of children who are often attacked with the grave diseases of childhood. The milking vessels are frequently washed in the house, and not unusually there is a close connection between the house and the dairy, and sometimes the living-house is, itself, used as a dairy-house. It requires no argument to point out the dangers here; in fact, numerous epidemics have been traced to such a source.

Those who milk the cows are not always free from disease; often we see the milker with hands that are cracked or sore. One of the dirtiest habits which exist in many dairies is that of wetting a cow's teats to lubricate them, to make the milking process easier to the milker. This custom, not rare, unfortunately, is the most common nasty habit permitted in many dairies. If it were not for the good that is sure to follow the agitation of these matters I should hesitate to record that I have myself seen milkers spit upon their hands to wet the teats before they began milking, and then, when there was a certain quantity of milk in the pail, dip their dirty hands into it, and keep the teats dripping wet during the whole process of milking. Cow's teats should not be wetted in any manner, especially in winter, even to wash off dirt if it is already there. This should be removed with a brush or a dry towel. Wetting of the teats very often leads to chapping, and chapping to cracks, and these cracks often become running sores from the constant irritation of the milking process.

In these days of bottled milk the danger of spreading contagion is vastly increased. Bottles which go into rooms where children are suffering from any of the contagious diseases must be a source of danger if they are not subsequently sterilized. Quite recently I had occasion to visit a man who did a large bottled-milk business in New York City. The milk came in wagons from the upper part of Westchester County, and he had a horse-stable half way between his source of supply and New York. Here his horses were changed. All the milk came to this stable in cans, and the empty bottles came back here from New York to be washed. He had two wooden troughs in this stable, and a stove with a large kettle to heat water, and the bottles were washed here in lukewarm water with sal soda, rinsed with cold water, and then filled from the cans.

I think, if some of us followed these bottles around and had seen where some had been, we would want them pretty well steamed and sterilized before we drank milk from them. It is often a source of wonderment to me why we do not have more direct and palpable evidence of trouble arising from just this state of affairs. Of course, there are unfortunate results from this sort of carelessness; but how much or how little we are not always able to say. We ought to be able to prevent it by insisting that all milk containers be sterilized with steam under pressure after each usage.

When the dangerous elements are recognized and eliminated from the dairy, then it only requires that the cows be healthy, properly fed and cared for, in order that we may have milk fit to drink and to feed to the baby, without the intervention of the chemist or any of the prevailing laboratory methods, which at the best are only questionable makeshifts.

A GROUP OF AGED PATIENTS.

BY J. H. EMERSON, M.D.,
OF NEW YORK.

ONE morning last winter I had occasion to call upon four patients whose united ages amounted to 346 years, and in thinking over others, whom I had recently seen, I realized that there were enough who were over eighty years of age to form a rather interesting group. I have, therefore, written down such facts as constitute sketches, rather than detailed or complete histories, of a few of them, in an effort to trace such features referable to advanced age as they present in common, and to give some account of their management. I hope in this way to furnish a topic for discussion, and, it may be, reach some generalizations of clinical utility as to phases of disease, and some of the demands of treatment, in the aged.

CASE I.—Female, aged ninety years. The patient lived the ordinary life of a well-to-do woman in society, spending the winter in New York and the summer at Newport until the autumn of 1884, when she returned to town on the last day of October, exhausted, feeble, and breathless, so that she was barely able to mount the single flight of stairs to her bedroom. I found a feeble and dilated heart, albuminous and phosphatic urine, and subsequently casts. The patient was short in stature, and at this time very stout. Under the influence of rest in bed, with the administration of mercurials and digitalis, attention to the bowels and diet, and good nursing, she gradually recovered from the most urgent and distressing symptoms, and attained a great measure of comfort. During this period she lost, it is true, the greater part of her flesh, and also her muscular strength, so that although in the following summer she went out of town to a place but a few miles off, it was necessary to bring her back the whole distance in a carriage, and since then she has remained on one floor of her house, occupying a north room during the hot weather, and a south room the rest of the year, but for many years now never leaving her bed except when lifted out to have it made.

The physical ailments which I had to encounter in this case were, in addition to the feeble heart and degenerated kidneys, an umbilical hernia, which would occasionally escape in spite of a bandage constantly worn, a lateral as well as angular curvature of the spine in the dorsal region, an obstinate constipation of the bowels, and of late years a pyelitis, with probably the development of a sac in relation either with the pelvis of the kidney or with the ureter. Thus, the urine will sometimes remain clear and free for months; then will come a period of pain, nausea, vomiting, and perhaps some febrile movement with very scanty elimination, and sometimes the presence of a large mass in the left side of the abdomen.

Relief comes only with free urination, sometimes about one-third part of the excretion for days together consisting of tenacious, phosphatic, purulent matter. These complications, especially those arising from bowels and kidneys, very often lead to acute disturbances of the stomach, with sometimes an irritating salivation, but more frequently nausea, constant gaseous eructations, vomiting, and syncope, so that when these attacks are threatening the nurse keeps mustard and ammonia ready for instant use, hot water at hand, and the hypodermic syringe ready charged with brandy or tincture of digitalis. The prompt use of these measures has again and again rescued the patient from profound syncope before the nearest physician could reach her. Then she enjoys long periods of placid comfort, lying from morning till night propped up on her left elbow with many a little cushion, holding her paper or book, reading everything that is new and entertaining, and keeping up the most lively interest in all the affairs of the city and the great world. The left pectoralis major muscle, meantime, has acquired a surprising strength and firmness in her otherwise emaciated frame.

Of course the treatment has long contemplated nothing but such regulation of the bowels as will keep the stomach available for sufficient supplies of food and the meeting of emergencies as they arise; for the heart is quite equal to the minimum demands which are made upon it by one who rests absolutely in bed all the time, whose passions are all in abeyance, and whose stomach is never overloaded with food. The question of feeding has often been quite puzzling, but the solution of it has always been aided by finding how very small the actual demands of her system are. The proportion of alcohol has been gradually increased. Many changes have been made from time to time, but for months past the following has been the almost unvaried dietary: During twenty-four hours she takes two cups of black tea, being about half milk, one piece of zwieback, one lady finger, one soft-boiled egg, two cups of bouillon, and sometimes the soft part of a baked apple. She also disposes of one gallon of brandy in six weeks and one bottle of sherry a week, making about three ounces of the former, and three and one-half ounces of the latter *per diem*.

CASE II.—Female, who died about January 1, 1897, in her ninety-first year, and whose case I have already mentioned before this society. Her death was directly due to the development of malignant disease of the stomach, and, probably, of the large intestine, which had followed upon the cancerous degeneration of what Dr. Abbe referred to as an explosion cyst, originally a cystic tumor, over the left scapula, and which had remained an unhealed ulcer during four or five years. When she came under my charge, about three and a half years ago, I learned that she had been using during many years suppositories of opium and extract of belladonna, the dose not having been increased, however, since it was originally prescribed, nor did she increase it till about two years ago, when she doubled it, and after that took daily a dose of 2¼ grains of opium, and ¼ grain of extract of belladonna. She had also, many years ago, been treated with nitrate of silver to an extent which had left a permanent stain upon her lips and cheeks. Her arteries were rigid, she had both mitral and aortic heart murmurs, and the urine showed a slight but constant quantity of albumin.

Having always been in the habit of indulging her taste for rich food she suffered much from indigestion and lack of appetite, troubles which were naturally increased by the constipation due to her opium habit. She would often pass a number of days without an evacuation of the bowels, and then relieve herself by a process of excavation aided by enemata. These methods had resulted in an atonic state of the large intestine, so that no ordinary dose of cathartics produced anything but discomfort. Finally, I succeeded in producing evacuation of the bowels by means of capsules of blue mass, extract of colocynth, and ipecac., to which, at Dr. A. A. Smith's suggestion, I added extract of cascara.

About the end of last October, however, epigastric pain and tenderness, with occasional vomiting, which shortly showed a coffee-ground character, and the detection of a small mass in the epigastrium to the right of the median line warranted the diagnosis of malignant disease of the stomach. From this time treatment had to be limited to the administration of such concentrated food as she could be persuaded to swallow, including liberal quantities of brandy. She was also given cathartics and narcotics. The adjustment of the latter proved to be a most difficult problem, both on account of her long addiction to opium and of the profound depression produced by doses sufficient to cause sleep. She could not sleep without opiates, and the pain also demanded their use, yet she absolutely refused to go to bed. She would at the utmost spend but a few hours lying on the sofa, but most of the entire day and night sitting up in her chair and resisting in every way she could all efforts to make her sleep, to the despair of her nurses. I had actually twice to hold and etherize her, which secured several hours' sleep.

If a sufficient dose of morphin was given to procure a few hours' sleep, the succeeding period was marked by hopeless depression of spirits, with constant restlessness and fear of impending death. Coffee, lavender, bromids, codein, Squibb's liquor opii compositus, and chlorodyn, proved useless either to stimulate her, or to prolong in moderate degree the narcotic effect of the morphin. So that ultimately, for some weeks, she received at about 9 P.M. one of the suppositories, followed, about midnight, by a hypodermic injection of ¼-grain of morphin, and about 3 or 4 A.M. either a second suppository or ⅛-grain more morphin, with, for a while, trional instead of a second dose of morphin. Such medication had to be suspended now and then to allow of the administration of cathartics, although toward the end there was a diarrhea, which was regarded as evidence that some portion of the intestinal canal below the stomach had become involved in the disease.

CASE III.—Male, aged eighty-two years, has a feeble heart, slightly enlarged, but no valvular lesions. His urine contains a small smount of albumin, but casts have not been found. The earliest symptoms of failing health began to be noticeable some nine years ago, and were, a gradually increasing slowness of gait, leading to shortness of breath and a tendency to puff, or a prolonged expiration, accompanied by a whistling noise. He frequently had to stop and lean against a railing until he gained breath or force enough to go on. A very slight acclivity materially increased the trouble, and one reason why he can walk more comfortably at his home in the country is because the town in which it is situated is almost absolutely level. By degrees, however, this dyspnea became noticeable even when he was sitting in his own library, more particularly if he tried to talk, of if his visitors were many, or if they bored him. Close attention was paid to his diet, for he had been accustomed to hearty and rather rich food. Regular action of the bowels was readily secured, and from time to time I gave small doses of calomel.

The lungs have presented symptoms of emphysema, but of the senile or so-called atrophic type, without asthma, or more than occasional and moderate bronchial catarrh, though there are often fine râles on inspiration in the lower lobes of the lungs posteriorly. He has never suffered from orthopnea, always finding comfort in the recumbent posture. The most serious intercurrent attack he has had occurred two years ago, when he suffered for some weeks with atony of the large intestine, accompanied by some pain and irregular action of the bowels, and leading to great debility. As a result of this he gave up his house where his library and dining-room were two stories away from his bedroom, and took a large apartment fronting on Central Park, where he has an abundance of air and light, and all rooms on one floor. Here, under the care of a competent woman attendant, he lives with all the comforts his physical disabilities will allow.

So far I have said little of his medical treatment. I have found it impracticable to give him iodids, and although Dr. Loomis, who saw him in consultation, urged them, a further trial proved them to be so disagreeable to him that I gave them up.

Various other preparations, burning of niter paper, etc., have but moderate effect in relieving the dyspnea, and the best results have been obtained from a pretty steady administration of small doses of digitalis, strophanthus, and belladonna, in varying proportions. One of the most interesting features of this case has been the gradual change in disposition. From having been as a practising lawyer a man of positive convictions, ready to say a sharp thing even at the expense of another's feelings, showing often his rough side to those about him, and liking to do his own work in his own way he has gradually grown more genial and gracious in speech and manner, craves sympathy, is absolutely submissive to medical authority or the suggestions of his nurse, and seems to find nothing more distasteful than making up his mind to do a new thing or to exert himself physically or mentally. Often he will smile, but shake his head at the proposition that he should go even into the next room. Meanwhile he gives freely to charity, and takes pleasure in seeing his friends who call upon him.

CASE IV.—Female, aged eighty-nine years, presents another instance of varied pathological conditions and much suffering, which still have not prevented the attainment of great age. She has suffered over twenty years from convulsive tic, for five years from chronic inflammation of the subcutaneous connective tissue of the legs below the knee, with occasional eczema and obstinate ulcers, making her a prisoner in her room, and three years ago she had an attack of pneumonia which was interesting in three particulars, *viz.*: she recovered from it; the confinement to bed cured the ulcers on her leg, and third, she learned the use of whisky, from which she has since been unwilling to part. It may be thought, naturally enough, that this is not a record particularly creditable to the physician in charge, but I had called in, for surgical consultation, two members of the Clinical Society; had exhausted my own resources on the *ulcera cruris*, and yet they healed only during the confinement to bed made necessary by the pneumonia, to reappear when she was again able to be upon her feet.

In spite of the demonstration afforded by this experience, no persuasion or exercise of professional authority have sufficed to make her consent to another period of repose in bed. The case furnishes an unhappy instance of a narrow and undisciplined mind, a prey to many an old-time superstition and prejudice, of personal vanity which has grown ridiculous and pitiful with advancing years, and of the evil resulting from the want of personal cleanliness, when the dim eye of age will not recognize its deficiencies, and the attentions of hired attendants and of affectionate relatives are alike wanting or rejected.

As further illustrations of conditions which call for our attention among octogenarians, let me mention very briefly the following cases:

CASE V.—Female, aged eighty-three years, now drawing to the end of a life of many trials, which culminated for her personally five years ago in an apoplexy and right hemiplegia. The conditions which persisted were an emotional state with frequent tears, and that form of aphasia in which simple phrases come easily but in which the special word to tell the incident which made an impression upon the mind will not come, on which follow disappointment and hopeless attempts until the faint hold on the idea is entirely lost. There were also some contraction of the forearm and a dragging foot. A placid temperament, a good digestion, sound heart and kidneys, supplemented by good nursing, have prolonged the scene until now increasing drowsiness and debility point to an early fatal termination.

CASE VI.—Male, aged eighty-two years. This patient last fall presented a large ischiorectal abscess, the third development of the kind within twenty years, but it healed so promptly following simple incision and drainage that no more radical treatment seemed warranted. He has long had a bronchial catarrh, with some dilatation of the tubes, and twice has had acute exacerbations which required confinement to bed. From early life he has had an irritable bladder, which has made him somewhat of a recluse, and prevented him from doing many things that would otherwise have been attractive. But he does not seek treatment for it, having apparently made up his mind that it is a thing to be endured rather than cured. In spite of his age he still occasionally visits the Produce Exchange, of which he was until recently an active member.

CASE VII.—Female, over ninety years of age, has been under my observation but a short time. About eighteen months ago she fell and injured the right thigh, so that she now has to walk with a cane, but fortunately escaped a fracture. About six weeks ago she had what must have been an embolism of some artery of the brain, for she suddenly found herself unable to rise from her chair on account of weakness of the left leg. This was only temporary, although the left arm was of but little use for several days. These symptoms had passed off when I saw her, but I found the most rigid arteries I ever felt. The heart sounds gave evidence of both mitral and aortic disease, while the urine contained a small amount of albumin, but no other evidence of renal degeneration. Both eyes are cataractous, so that she can with difficulty recognize a person who enters the room. Her mind is still alert and intelligent, and it is surprising to see how briskly she can walk in the street, supported on her son's arm, or go about her own apartment unaided. The simplest directions as to diet and the regulation of the bowels, together with the administration of small doses of nitroglycerin, have contributed materially to her comfort.

CASE VIII.—A Quaker maiden, ninety-one years of age, two years ago came comfortably through an attack of erysipelas involving the head and most of the trunk. It began at the left nipple in an excoriated area, connecting with a small sinus from which a scanty purulent discharge constantly flowed. The excoriation healed under applications of oxid-of-zinc ointment, and the discharge ceased. Since then it has been useful to her to take about an ounce of whisky daily in divided doses. Another indulgence, from which she will not be parted, even while ill, is candy, of which she secures a supply for daily use. She dozes away much of her day but is bright and sociable at meal times. A year ago she went to the photographers to have her likeness taken, and spent last summer at Nantucket.

CASE IX.—Female. I desire to mention this case because of the long endurance of malignant disease, the patient dying about a year ago at the age of eighty-one years, after having suffered twenty-four years from an epithelioma, which she first showed me during 1872. It began in the skin of the forehead, a little to the right of the median line, extended down to the root of the nose, to the right eyelid, and ultimately to the orbit. Dr. Prudden found it a typical epithelioma in 1883. At that time I did a plastic operation upon it. I subsequently used various caustic applications, curettings, etc. Dr. Sands operated upon her once, and Dr. Weir twice. After the last operation, which was four or five years before her death, it was surprising to see the comfort she derived and the degree to which the ulcerated surface diminished under the persistent use of a bichlorid lotion, followed by free powdering with iodoform. This patient also had a large fatty tumor in the right axilla.

In reviewing the points of interest presented by these cases, I think there are several which are noticeable and characteristic of the one feature they have in common,—I mean the advanced age of the patients. Thus, all of them are the subjects of more than one marked pathological condition. Persons who reach eighty, much more those who reach ninety years, must be endowed with more than ordinary capacity for enduring the minor ills of life, and the same vitality doubtless stands them in good stead when more serious diseases develop; so that on examining such patients it need not surprise us to find a tolerance of disease in important organs to which the more vulnerable would long before have succumbed. As akin to this, and largely accountable for it, I would place that absence or blunting of acute sensibility, which is a trait of the aged. In earlier life, the functions of all the organs are vigorously and actively performed, the impressions upon all the senses are sharply felt, and meet with a quick response in either mental or muscular activity, giving the keen zest to healthy existence. But the man who has lived through three score years and ten begins to realize that his affairs will go on pretty well even if he does not hurry and drive to accomplish them. So many little stimuli have affected him that a degree of tolerance has been established. There comes a time when even Ulysses or Gladstone no longer cares,

> "To drink delight of battle with his peers."

He is satisfied with a placid and uneventful course of life, and finds his recompense in diminished anxiety, less wear and tear, fewer demands on failing powers. He gets a glimpse of the twilight of the gods. If the restlessness of earlier years is maintained, if the old man insists on keeping up the activities and sharing the responsibilities and even the pleasures of middle life, it soon appears that he is not availing himself of the prerogatives to which his years entitle him, and fretfulness and impatience add largely to the physician's difficulties in treating the patient. The gentle amelioration of the temperament and the restful calm that comes from it, are well illustrated in Cases I. and III., and the opposite in Cases II. and IV.

When finally we come to consider what lessons of treatment may be learned from the observation of these aged patients I would first emphasize the value of repose, a striking instance of which is furnished by Case I., in which an overtaxed heart, even in the presence of many and serious complications, has been able to perform its functions with comfort for many years. Next, and as a most important agent in securing the restful life, comes a good nurse, able to take up and bear the many personal cares our patient has long been feeling as a burden. And among the first duties of the nurse, the faithful performance of which may be more manifest, perhaps, to friends and physician than to the patient, will be keeping him or her clean. I have known wondrous changes, appreciable by more than one sense, wrought by such simple care given to those whose own senses were dulled by advanced age. Then, too, the physician must be willing to hold his hand. It is seldom that what is called active treatment is required. He must be satisfied to let many matters take their course, must be content to alleviate rather than cure, to advise against a resort to surgical measures which might be clearly indicated in similar conditions in younger persons.

The nutritive demands of these patients are apt to be small, and it must be recognized that alcoholics in some shape are almost always needed. The small amount of food, the fact that much of it is taken in a concentrated form, the want of active exercise, all contribute to sluggish action of the bowels, and the simpler laxatives are matters of almost daily necessity.

An Extraordinary Case of Extra-Genital Chancre.—At a meeting of the Ophthalmologic Section of the College of Physicians of Philadelphia, held January 18, 1898, Dr. G. E. de Schweinitz described and exhibited a water-color sketch of a case of chancre of the conjunctiva in a physician who became infected during the delivery of a pregnant woman. The physician's face was spattered by some of the discharge, and was hastily wiped off with her apron by an officious bystander. The diagnosis was not made till the lymphatic glands of the face and neck became swollen and the specific eruption appeared on chest and limbs. Under antisyphilitic treatment the ulcer which had appeared on the conjunctiva rapidly healed and all symptoms disappeared.

CLINICAL MEMORANDUM.

A PERSONAL EXPERIENCE IN RENAL SURGERY.

BY ROBERT F. WEIR, M.D.,
OF NEW YORK;
PROFESSOR OF SURGERY IN THE COLLEGE OF PHYSICIANS AND SURGEONS, AND SURGEON TO THE NEW YORK HOSPITAL;
WITH THE COLLABORATION OF
EDWARD M. FOOTE, M.D.,
OF NEW YORK;
SURGEON TO THE RANDALL'S ISLAND HOSPITALS.

(Concluded from page 177.)

CYSTS.

WHILE renal cysts, sometimes containing large amounts of fluid and generally single, are found, and presumably are acquired, yet it is believed that the multiple cysts or the veritable general cystic degenerations of the kidney are of congenital origin or begin in early life, and that both kidneys are usually simultaneously involved, though not always to the same extent. Occasionally this transformation with its innumerable cysts is encountered in but a single kidney, but this is so rare that surgical action should not be based on this fact alone. The ordinary cysts—that is to say, those which are few in number and comparatively small, and in which decided renal tissue may be seen to intervene between them—do not call for surgical interference, though they occasionally attain such size as to necessitate operative relief. The hemorrhagic tendencies, with the increased tension which often supervenes and produces renal pain, are usually not to be diagnosed until a surgical puncture or an incision has been made—sometimes not until after a nephrectomy has been performed, as in Case III.

Concerning the true multiple cystic degeneration, an example is given in Case XXXV., in which a surgical error was made. From a too imperfect examination of the other kidney, its rounded inferior end having only been palpated, the deduction of one sound kidney was made and the nephrectomy accomplished. It proved afterward that the remaining kidney, though effective in a previous easy condition of life for carrying on the necessary urinary secretion, yet, with the additional load of elimination, it failed almost entirely, and the patient, though recovering from the operation, died uremic not long thereafter.

While in this instance no difficulty in diagnosis arose as soon as the kidney was exposed, yet I have since seen in consultation with a colleague an example in which, after the kidney had been exposed by a lumbar incision, great difficulty was experienced in determining whether the irregular knobbed masses yielding bloody fluid on puncture were due to multiple cysts or to a neoplasm. Under the impression that the latter existed, nephrectomy was resorted to with a fatal result. The accepted rule of surgery in these cases is that extirpation is not justifiable.

CASE XXXV. *Multilocular Cyst of the Kidney—Nephrectomy—Recovery.*—Caroline B., aged thirty-four years, entered New York Hospital January 7, 1890, with a history of constant and increasing pain during the four previous months, associated with the discovery of a round, smooth swelling in the left loin. Examination showed the left side of the abdomen to be occupied by a solid nodular mass of variable consistency, which reached nearly to the pelvis, and was quite immovable. On consultation, it was supposed to be an enlarged spleen or a retroperitoneal growth. The urine was pale, acid, of a specific gravity of 1010, and contained a trace of albumin. There were no casts, but an abundance of renal cells.

January 10, 1890, a vertical incision was made at the outer edge of the rectus muscle. Upon opening the abdomen the tumor projected itself through the wound and was recognized as a multicystic kidney. It was so badly diseased that it was removed, especially as palpation showed the right kidney to be comparatively free from disease. Gauze was used for drainage.

Although the patient had received only ¼ grain of morphia (by hypodermic injection before the operation), her respirations fell to 4 per minute afterward, and her condition was critical for a time. She also vomited a good deal for several days, but finally recovered, and left the hospital in five weeks after the operation, the wound being not quite healed at the time.

The extirpated kidney was made up of a mass of cysts. It weighed 1038 grams and measured 25x12x10 cm. The vessels and ureter were normal. The individual cysts varied in size from a minute speck to 5 cm. in diameter. Their contents were clear, grayish, and even opaque and black (Fig. 3). The patient, it was afterward learned, made but indifferent progress after leaving the hospital, and some three months later developed edema and died from uremic convulsions. The autopsy showed that the right kidney was moderately enlarged, but that it had also undergone marked cystic degeneration.

FIG. 3.

Multiple cystoma of the kidney.

CASE XXXVI. *Supposed Appendicitis—Cyst of the Kidney—Multiple Abscesses—Transperitoneal Nephrectomy—Death.*—Alice H., aged thirty-three years, concluded a pregnancy by a normal labor two months before entrance to the hospital. No symptoms were noticed until two days before operation, when there was a pain in the right side, increasing in severity, and followed by a chill and vomiting. Slight vesical tenesmus was noticed.

There was an ill-defined mass reaching from just below the ribs, downward, beyond the anterior superior spine of the ilium, and toward the median line. It was most tender at its lower margin, and dull on percussion, and did not present a clear outline. The abdominal walls were very thick. The patient had a temperature of 102.6° F., and a pulse of 116. The urine was acid, of a specific gravity of 1020, and contained ten per cent. of albumin by volume, and a moderate amount of pus. The diagnosis was doubtful. It lay between appendicitis, with a high-lying abscess, or a ruptured gall-bladder, or renal suppuration.

December 19, 1895, a vertical incision was made over the lower part of the tumor—to meet the probability of its being an appendical abscess. The appendix was found to be normal. The tumor was then ascertained to originate in the kidney, and the abdominal incision was therefore enlarged upward and the peritoneum over the kidney incised, peeled back, and sewed to the divided peritoneum of the wound. Aspiration revealed a large cyst containing urine; and as the kidney was evidently further diseased, the ureter was tied with one strong silk ligature and the vessels with another, and the kidney removed. During the manipulation the ligature on the vessels slipped, and considerable blood was lost before it was replaced. A lumbar incision was made for drainage, and the posterior peritoneum stitched together over the bed of the kidney, and the abdominal wound closed. Despite stimulation, hot enemata, and an intravenous injection of saline solution (14 ounces), the patient died within twelve hours.

The extirpated kidney contained numerous small abscesses, especially in its lower two-thirds (of acute origin), and above this there was a large thin-walled interstitial cyst lined with a dense membrane. The renal tissue was the seat of parenchymatous and interstitial inflammation. No autopsy was permitted.[1]

NEW GROWTHS.

The outlook for a patient with a malignant growth of the kidney is grave indeed. As far as is known Kocher was the first surgeon who was able to save such a patient by removal of the diseased organ. That was over twenty years ago. Since then some hundreds of attempts have been made in the same direction, but usually without encouraging results. Up to 1890 a large proportion of the patients operated upon (fifty-two to sixty-six per cent., according to different authors) died from the effects of the operation itself. Since then the results have been better, and according to Wagner the mortality from operation is now not more than twenty to twenty-five per cent. in the hands of the most expert surgeons. Individuals have recorded still better results; for instance, Israel had a mortality from operation of only 12.5 per cent. in twenty-four cases. In the malignant growths in children, which are principally sarcoma, Walker[2] reported a mortality from the operation of thirty-seven per cent. None of these results take into account the deaths from recurrence, but granting that almost all of the patients operated upon succumb either to the operation or to the disease, an operation, in adults, is still advisable, and is indicated in those cases in which the patient's condition is favorable; for thereby a period of comparative comfort of from two to four or even more years is gained, as well as the possibility of a radical cure. In children, however, out of 60 nephrectomies only 4 patients survived a period of 3 years, a result that almost prohibits operation. When one turns to the published histories of these cases to ascertain which were *absolutely unfitted for operation*, it appears that the decision must rest, aside from the patient's general condition, not on the size of the tumor, nor on its duration, but on the amount of existing adhesions. A neoplastic kidney with adhesions is hard to remove, and its dissection is often long and dangerous; so that these patients frequently die from shock and loss of blood. If the operation is successful the patient is also certain to die, either from a continuation of the growth in the vicinity, or from metastatic deposits formed before the removal of the primary focus of the disease.

[1] I now believe that the forward extension of König's incision would have sufficed in this case.

[2] Walker, *Annals of Surgery*, November, 1897.

An early diagnosis is here, as in all malignant growths, most important, and in the case of the kidney it is especially difficult to make. The presence of a tumor may be the first sign observed. Thus, in a case reported by Rovsing,[1] a woman, aged forty-five years, had noticed a swelling in the side, where she had had some pain during four months. The urine was absolutely normal, and the tumor movable. Under these circumstances an easy operation was expected, but the adhesions about the upper part of the kidney were so firm that it was torn in two in the attempt to remove it, and the patient died from shock and loss of blood within six hours.

If the growth originates in the lower part of the kidney, both diagnosis and operation are rendered easier.[2] Unfortunately this is not apt to be the case, for the majority of tumors begin either in the suprarenal capsule and grow into the kidney, or else in the upper part of the kidney itself. Even when a tumor is palpable a diagnosis is by no means certain. One of the most difficult of diagnoses lies between a malignant growth and multilocular cystoma. Even when the latter is bilateral, as it usually is, it may still be palpable only on one side. Here an exploratory incision is the readiest method of deciding the question. When a cystoma or an adherent carcinoma is found, the wound should be at once closed. In some cases a quantitative estimation of the amount of urea excreted in the twenty-four hours may be significant. If cystic or neoplastic degeneration has reached any marked degree, the urea elimination will be so decreased that it will be useless to think of any radical operation.

Other cases of malignant tumors are associated with hematuria. This symptom, again, may be very deceptive; for instead of the painless, constant hemorrhage which we might expect, the blood often comes intermittently, with colic, and with the association of urates and uric-acid crystals or even small bits of gravel, so that the diagnosis of nephrolithiasis is often erroneously made. The loss of weight, the presence in the urine of abnormal varieties of cells, or bits of tumor tissue, frequently will suffice to clear up a case; but these distinctive signs are often wanting in the early stages, and an exploratory operation may be required to establish an absolute diagnosis. Therefore, in every unexplained hematuria, one ought to think of the possibility of a malignant tumor of the kidney.

CASE XXXVII.—*Adenocarcinoma of the Kidney—Abdominal Nephrectomy — Death.* — Charles H., aged thirty-three years, a burly butcher, was suddenly seized with cutting pain in the left lumbar region, and passed a quantity of bloody urine. Similar attacks occurred at not very long intervals, and he frequently passed gravel. In the second year from the first attack the symptoms became much aggravated, pain in the loin was almost constant, and the patient became worn out from loss of blood and suffering. A tumor was noticed in the left flank extending from a point three inches external to the umbilicus, upward and backward under the ribs. It was slightly movable bimanually, and seemed to be abou

[1] *Arch. f. klin. Chir.*, xlix, p. 412.

[2] Israel, *Ber. klin. Wochenschr.*, vol. 26, p. 125.

seven inches thick. The urine contained no abnormal elements except blood.

December 2, 1886, an exploratory incision was made in the left loin and the kidney exposed. No calculus could be felt either by thorough palpation or by thrusting a hat-pin into the kidney at several points. The diagnosis of sarcoma was made, and it was evident that the kidney was too much enlarged to be removed by a lumbar incision. It was, therefore, decided to resort later to abdominal section for its extirpation. Estimation of the urea showed a diminished excretion, the daily amounts ranging from 219 to 240 grains. This decreased excretion is said by Thiriar to be characteristic of malignant tumors.

January 20, 1887, an incision five inches long was made along the outer margin of the left rectus, the abdomen opened, the intestines pushed aside, and the peritoneum covering the kidney to the outer side of the descending colon incised. The diseased kidney was readily dissected free with the fingers, and its pedicle was tied *en masse* with floss silk. A heavy clamp was placed on the vessels between the ligature and the kidney, and the latter was removed. By the slipping of the clamp a vein which was not included in the ligature bled freely, but it was easily seized and tied (an advantage of the abdominal method of nephrectomy). Considerable bleeding took place for a time from the fibrous envelop of the kidney, but the total amount of hemorrhage was in no way alarming. The lumbar scar was reopened for drainage, and a rubber tube was led through it to the site of the kidney. The rents in the posterior and anterior layers of the peritoneum were then closed, and the wound in the abdominal wall approximated by silver wire and catgut sutures. On account of gastric irritation no fluid was introduced into the stomach during the following week, during which time nourishment was administered *per rectum*.

The amount of urine passed was as follows: First day, 8 ounces; second day, 20 ounces, and somewhat bloody; urea, 1.01 per cent.; specific gravity, 1020; third day, 49 ounces; fourth day, 88 ounces. After that it gradually subsided until the daily amount was 50 ounces, the urea being still below normal; though of greater amount than before operation. The patient recovered without incident. The extirpated kidney measured 9x5½ inches, and weighed 21 ounces. It was invaded by a tumor about as large as the fist, which was everywhere marked off by a distinct capsule. Microscopically it was found to be an adenoma. The patient remained well for a year when a recurrence took place from which he succumbed eighteen months after the nephrectomy.

CASE XXXVIII. *Sarcoma of the Kidney—Nephrotomy—Death.*—James L., aged seven years, was seen by me with Dr. J. B. Hunter, January, 1886. There was a history of failing health, some irritability of the bladder, but no hemorrhage or pus in the urine, though diminished urea was observed in a late examination. Three weeks before, his physician had recognized a swelling in the left upper half of the abdomen, which, when seen by me, was the size of a cocoanut, projecting downward to the umbilicus, very slightly movable, painless, and not at all tender. It could also be felt in the loin. A few days previously, an aspirator-needle had been introduced, and through it about one-half ounce of a slightly turbid deep yellow fluid and a little fresh blood had been withdrawn. It was hoped that a cyst or hydronephrosis existed, though his pallor and weakness were greater than should accompany such affections. Early in March a lumbar exploratory excision was made, but the repetition of aspiration on the exposed posterior surface of the enlarged kidney did not show any cyst. An incision was made into the soft mass, which appeared sarcomatous. The hemorrhage from the incision proved very troublesome, and by the time it was arrested no thoughts of anterior nephrotomy could be entertained. So much was the little patient weakened by the operative effort added to that of the disease, that he succumbed twenty-six hours thereafter. No autopsy was granted.

CASE XXXIX. *Carcinoma of the Kidney—Abdominal Nephrectomy—Death.*—Alexander P., aged fifty years, sent me by Dr. Ross of Montreal, entered St. Luke's Hospital February 27, 1891. The family history was unimportant, except that one sister died suddenly of cerebral tumor, and an aunt of cancer. Since 1888 the patient had suffered from indigestion with vomiting and slight jaundice, growing gradually worse with slight loss of flesh and strength. The year previous to admission, he had noticed a fulness on the right side of the abdomen accompanied by some pain, and the presence of a tumor was determined by several physicians. There were no urinary symptoms. The urine was acid, of a specific gravity of 1024, and contained a trace of albumin, but no sugar. In the sediment were a few leucocytes. The swelling in the right side was found to lie partly behind the distended colon, and a diagnosis of retroperitoneal cyst, probably connected with the kidney, was made.

March 2, 1891, the abdomen was opened by an incision along the outer margin of the right rectus muscle and a heart-shaped tumor exposed, which was adherent to the omentum and intestines.

The adhesions were separated, and the posterior peritoneum which covered it was divided. In the attempt to peel off the peritoneum to attach it to the anterior abdominal wall, and thus close off the peritoneal cavity, the tumor was ruptured, and about one quart of greenish inodorous fluid escaped in among the intestines from a cyst of the kidney. The cyst and kidney were removed after ligation of ureter and blood-vessels. A lumbar incision was made for a drainage-tube, and the abdomen closed, after cleansing and uniting its posterior divided layers.

The patient stood the operation well, but died within eight days of suppurative peritonitis. The kidney was found upon examination to contain a large cyst about five inches in diameter, from the wall of which projected masses which microscopic examination showed to be cancerous. The substance of the kidney itself was nearly normal.

METHOD OF OPERATION.

The lumbar incision as described in the cases cited, that is to say, a cut extending from the twelfth rib downward parallel to the edge of the quadratus lumborum muscle, and then, when near the ilium, curving forward as far as the anterior superior spine, or further if necessary, is, on the whole, the most satisfactory of the various incisions I have employed. Its length forward enables the operator to meet promptly accidents and complications. This incision is called König's, but is also claimed by Ancona. The muscular layers of the anterior portion of the incision are divided rather than separated, as has been suggested by Abbe, until the peritoneum is reached, and then the surgeon will have free access, not only to the kidney and its vessels, but also to the ureter, etc. The value of such an incision was well illustrated in Case XVIII., in which a torn vena cava was promptly recognized and sutured without difficulty.

The success previously alluded to (obtained in my last ten nephrectomies, performed during the past two years with but a single fatal result, and the last six of which were consecutively successful) I largely attribute to the complete view of the operative field which follows even a freer extension of this incision anteriorly than in my earlier cases. The mortality, however, in the total of my twenty-five cases of nephrectomy herewith presented, is twenty-eight per cent.; which is only slightly better than the percentage in 180 cases recently presented by Tuffier, Israel, Newman, and Hamill, their mortality being thirty per cent. In their cases the lumbar incision was generally employed. Emphasis is again laid on the preference for division of the muscular layers of the abdomen: for though it is theoretically true that this separation of the muscles and their subsequent replacement affords a more solid wall, yet the usual method of carefully suturing in layers the divided abdominal fascia and muscles up to the vertical leg of the incision, and even a part of this if judgment so inclines, restores very happily the *status quo ante*. Moreover, in the comparatively few instances in which a certain amount of weakness and yielding of the cicatrix has resulted in a lumbar hernial bulging, it has usually shown itself in the vertical scar, that is to say where the drainage gauze had been left; and in none of these instances has the patient expressed any discomfort or inability from the weakness of the abdominal wall. Inquiry has been particularly made upon this point, as reference to the cases will show.[1]

For the removal of large tumors the anterior abdominal incision along the outer edge of the rectus abdominis muscle has been occasionally chosen. This is usually carried out as in ordinary abdominal work; but sometimes, when it has been revealed, as in Case XXXVIII., that a cyst is associated with the neoplasm, and once when an abscess was included in a tumor, the divided posterior edges of the peritoneum were attached at numerous points to that of the abdominal wound, thus shutting off the peritoneal cavity, and the extirpation of the diseased kidney accomplished by the so-called transperitoneal method. Anterior or abdominal nephrectomy is known to be more dangerous than lumbar, but it allows, of all operations, the best access to the vessels, etc., though since the increased prolongation forward of the lumbar incision, the anterior route with me has ceased to be employed. The difference in mortality of the two methods, lumbar and abdominal, has been given by Tuffier as twenty-eight per cent. in the former, and thirty-six per cent. in the latter.

For exploring the kidney or ureter for a suspected calculus, a few details may properly be discussed. The liberation and separation of such kidneys, particularly if not enlarged by abscess, may be accomplished, especially on the right side, so freely that the affected organ can as a rule be brought into and even out of the wound to allow careful palpation, and if exploration with the finger be decided upon, as it should be rather than relying upon untrustworthy prodding with needles, the pedicle of the kidney may be slipped between the second and third fingers of the left hand which will at the same time not only support and hold steady the kidney but facilitates compression of its vessels, so that when the exploratory incision is made into its substance to reach the pelvis with the introduced finger and sound, but little bleeding will occur. Usually the hemorrhage is not severe, even when compression is not employed; but I have once, under such circumstances, been compelled to plug the wound and postpone further examination for three or four days. At the close of such an exploration, with or without the extraction of a calculus as the case may be, it is my custom to pack the renal pelvis with a wick or string of iodoform or sterile gauze, and to suture the kidney wound with deep catgut stitches except at the point of exit of the gauze.

This same lifting-out of the kidney renders possible the better use of the X-rays for the detection of small calculi, as has been lately suggested by Fenwick, and already alluded to under "renal calculus."

The examination of the ureter for a moderate distance is easy by the operative incision described above. This will permit its palpation for two or three inches below the crest of the ilium. Internally the ureter may be examined through the incised kidney. When the lower end of the latter is strongly tilted or pulled up, by a ligature passed through it a flexible steel probe may be introduced and pushed through the whole length of the ureter. This requires a probe much longer than is anticipated. I have lengthened my own probe (after a number of trials) to twenty-three inches. It requires from nineteen to twenty three inches of the probe to reach the bladder from the loi[n] incision. Only once have I been able to feel the prob[e] end in the bladder by means of a sound introduced throug[h] the urethra, though in a number of instances it has bee[n] passed to its full length. The advantage of a metallic instrument in the detection of a calculus is evident, as wel[l] as is its greater ease of introduction. It is, however, no[t] easy to pass such an instrument into the ureter in all cases. One cannot always find the ureteral orifice in the renal pelvis. For help in this endeavor, I employ open-ended catheters of various curves (Fig. 1), through which, when introduced into the kidney pelvis, the flexible probe is carrie[d] and swept about in search of the desired outlet. When th[e] probe is engaged in the canal, the catheter is slipped over i[ts] distal end and removed, and the probe is gently pushe[d] onward. The length of the ureters, from the pelvis [of] the kidney to the bladder, varies from 26 to 34 cm. (1[0] to 14 inches) according to Huntington and to Funkel,[1] bu[t] the ureters are easily stretched. On exploration, when th[e] ureters were normal, I have often found the length abo[ve] given to be exceeded by reason of this extensibility, whic[h] is brought about by the resistance offered to the passag[e] of a probe, even though flexible, through these doubl[y] curved tubes.

When a cyst or cavity is a large one, turning the dilate[d] and thinned kidney inside out as was done in Case XXV[.] will aid in finding the ureteral opening. The difficulty [is] sometimes great in appreciating an obstacle in the urete[r] and one should, before condemning a kidney to extirp[ation,]

[1] Since the above was written Dr. A. McCosh exhibited, at a meeting of the Surgical Society, a patient with lumbar hernia following nephrectomy, which, emerging from the vertical portion of the incision through an opening one-half inch in diameter, gave great discomfort and demanded surgical interference.

tion, either open the pelvis for exploration, either digital or otherwise, or pass a catheter from the bladder to the kidney (Albarran); or, as I propose doing in my next case, incise the ureter fairly low down in the lumbar wound, and from this point of entrance explore the kidney.

In ligating the renal pedicle the ureter is separately secured with fine catgut, and commonly the vessels are tied *en masse*. Strong silk is used in preference to thick catgut, the sterilization of which is often doubtful. Lately, care has been taken to employ a method which will permit the withdrawal of the ligatures from the third to the seventh day after the operation, as may be determined upon. To this end is followed either the plan of Cleveland[1] of enclosing in the ligature the wire loop of a galvano-cautery, or that of Grad[2] of placing in each turn of the knot a releasing pull-thread. I have employed each of these contrivances with the happiest results, preferring, however, the latter for its simplicity.

I also venture to call attention again to the temporary packing of the large cavity left after a nephrectomy. (See Case XXV.) This not only controls the hemorrhage very well but drains most efficiently. The central packing is removed within from twenty-four to forty-eight hours,

FIG. 4. FIG. 5.

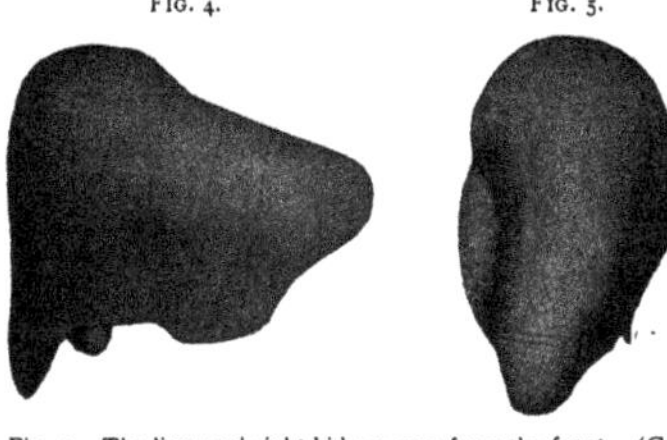

Fig. 4.—The liver and right kidney seen from the front. (Cunningham.)
Fig. 5.—A profile view of the liver and kidney. (Cunningham.)

and the exterior layer, constituting the Mikulicz bag, comes away on traction before the ligature is removed. In all renal operations anesthesia by ether is preferred to that by chloroform, as the latter has been fully shown by my own observations, as well as by those of others, to affect the kidney more seriously than does ether.[3]

A final word on the subject of the detection of renal enlargement. A long experience has convinced me that when, on the right side particularly, the kidney can be palpated on bimanual examination, it is either an enlarged kidney or a movable one. If the latter, beside the usual means of displacing and replacing it, it is always advisable to put the patient in an erect posture, resting the hips against the edge of a table, and then leaning forward with the hands or head against a support. This relaxes the abdominal walls and permits an easy repetition of the bimanual test. In all varieties of renal and gall-bladder enlargements, etc., I have frequently had much success in placing the patient in a sitting posture, in bed, leaning forward, with the hands clasping the legs above the ankles, which similarly relaxes the abdominal walls, and allows the surgeon's hands to pass well backward beyond the edges of the ribs, and well over the under surface of the liver.

In confirmation that a normal kidney is not to be felt anteriorly below the liver, I ask attention to the accompanying diagrams (Figs. 4 and 5) of results obtained by Professor Cunningham of Dublin.[1] Here it will be seen that such a small portion of the kidney projects below the liver as to be only rarely palpable. The recent investigations of Brewer also confirm this statement. Myles, in the article just quoted, also shows clearly the risk of probing a kidney of normal size or only one moderately enlarged through the skin; for there is risk, not only that the needle may perforate the peritoneum, but that a vessel or intestine may be punctured.

[1] Weir, MEDICAL NEWS, April 3, 1897.
[2] *Amer. Gyne. and Obstet. Jour.*, February, 1897.
[3] Weir, *N. Y. Med. Jour.*, November 16, 1895.

[1] Myles, *op. cit.*

MEDICAL PROGRESS.

Two Cases of Sarcoma Cured without Operation.—OWENS (*New Orleans Med. and Surg. Jour.*, July, 1897) reports two cases of sarcoma of the leg below the knee in which complete cure followed injections of the mixed toxins of erysipelas and the bacillus prodigiosus. Sixty-three injections were employed in each case, the smallest dose being one-half a minim and the largest 10 minims. In one case, the diagnosis was confirmed by a microscopic examination, the tumor being a giant-celled sarcoma of the tibia following a contusion.

The Disappearance of Warts.—ROUSSEL (*The Med. Press and Circular*, November 3, 1897) takes up the question of the disappearance of warts and mentions a great number of instances, undoubtedly accurate, in which warts have disappeared within a few days after the application of the most ridiculous remedies, such as the liver of the male goat, the skin of a serpent, the soles of old shoes steeped in wine, rancid bacon, salt water, etc., etc. According to this writer, the theory of suggestion is the only one which will explain the disappearance of warts immediately after such varied treatment. Bonjour employs suggestion with intention, making a few cabalistic passes and telling the patient that the warts will disappear. Thus far, his prediction has never failed. The word suggestion does not reveal to us the intimate mechanism of the nervous centers, but it is sufficiently clear to be understood by all medical men. That an impression of a psychic order can bring about a durable anatomic modification of the papillary bodies is of extreme interest to all reflective minds.

THERAPEUTIC NOTES.

Vulvovaginitis in Children.—COMBY (*Jour. de Méd. de Paris*, October 3, 1897) says that the vulvovaginitis of little girls is almost always of a specific character, but almost never of venereal origin, being acquired in an innocent manner from towels, sponges, etc. External application of small douches are not sufficient to meet the indications. It is necessary to employ prolonged irrigations through a small flexible catheter or tube; for instance, a quart or more of a strong antiseptic solution, such as corrosive sublimate, 1–10,000 or 5000, permanganate of potash, 1–4000 or 2000, or even 1–1000. With a weak antiseptic solution it requires from two to six months to cure a vulvovaginitis. With a strong solution this may be accomplished in fifteen days. If the affection is very intense, the irrigations should be made three times daily, and as improvement is manifested the number may be reduced to two each day, one a day, one every two days, twice a week, etc. In simple vulvitis strong injections will do no good. The only treatment required is to bathe the vulva with plain boiled water, or a weak solution of boric acid, two or three times daily, and to powder the parts, or to smear them with some hydrophilic ointment.

In all cases the toilet of the diseased parts should be most carefully directed, and the possibility of the conveyance of the contagion to other children should be kept in mind. The general health of the patient will also require attention.

Treatment of Enuresis.—MARTIN (*The Med. Press and Circular*, December 15, 1897) gave a boy, aged seven years, who for some months had been in the habit of wetting his bed three or four times each night, the following mixture:

℞		
	Potass bromid.	ʒ ij
	Tinct. belladonnæ	ʒ ij
	Tinct. chloroformi co.	ʒ j
	Aq. ad.	℥ vj.

M. ʒ ss. at 4 P.M., and a second dose at bedtime.

From the time when this was first administered there was no recurrence of the enuresis. The patient, in this case, was an active-brained boy, of athletic disposition, who was keenly alive to the desirability of overcoming his habit, but who had been unable to do so in spite of all endeavors. There was no phimosis, no adhesions, and no collection of matter beneath the foreskin to explain the constant recurrence of the affection. There were no symptoms referable to the bladder, no history of worms nor intestinal irritation, and the patient was not accustomed to lie on his back. The source of the mischief seemed to be in the direction of some form of cerebral excitement. The cure was perfect up to the time of report, about one month after the medicine was first given.

Treatment of Tuberculous Cystitis.—BANZET (*Centralb. für die Gesammte. Ther.*, November, 1897) recommends irrigation of the bladder with corrosive sublimate solution in cases of tuberculous cystitis. In his experience remarkable results have followed the use of this treatment, although he does not pretend to explain exactly how they are produced. Other antiseptics employed for a similar purpose, such as iodoform, lactic acid, sulphate of copper, formaldehyd, carbon dioxid, creosote, etc., have not given, in his hands, equally good results. The sublimate is used at first in a solution of 1 to 5000, and only after a considerable time is the strength increased to 1 to 4000, or even to 1 to 3000. A rapid increase in concentration may produce pain and hemorrhage. Thirty-nine patients were treated in this manner, and of these he considered six as entirely cured. Injections of guaiacol also gave good results. They have an anesthetic influence upon the mucous membrane of the bladder which is very grateful to the patient. If the pain cannot be relieved by medical measures, operations are necessary, of which suprapubic cystotomy, peritoneal drainage, and curetting may be mentioned. Curetting the neck of the bladder in a male may be performed through a minute perineal opening, and in the female through the urethra. This slight operation associated with subsequent drainage often produces remarkable relief. This method of treatment is preferable to suprapubic cystotomy in these cases.

There are, from a bacteriologic standpoint, two classes of cases of tuberculous cystitis. Those in which a great many bacilli are found in the urine, and those in which very few are found, or, possibly, no micro-organisms at all. Therapeutically, cases of the latter form are much more easily influenced by injections of corrosive sublimate. These may be cured in a short time. However, in the more severe forms the disease may be brought to a standstill, or even cured under favorable conditions. Naturally, general should be combined with local treatment.

Difficulties of the First Dentition.—In troubles due to teething, CHOMPRET (*Rev. de Therapeut.*, December 1, 1897) recommends that the mouth be frequently washed from early infancy up, with a solution of chloral hydrate, one per cent., an analgesic and antiseptic preparation with only feeble toxic power. Pruritus may be allayed by frequent rubbing of the gums with the following mixture:

℞		
	Cocain hydrochlor.	gr. ij
	Chloroformi	gr. xv
	Glycerini	ʒ v
	Aq. rosæ	gtt. vj.

For coryza, the nose should be irrigated with a lukewarm solution of boric acid or chloral hydrate. If the gums are distended they should be lanced. If necessary, tonic treatment should be employed.

Preventive Treatment of Alopecia.—DEICHLER (*La Méd. Moderne*, November 6, 1897) points out the need of the organism of gelatinous and colloid substances if the hair and nails are to be kept in a healthy and active condition. He prescribes, for those of his patients who are troubled with premature loss of hair, soups made of the bones of young animals, or of commercial gelatin which contains gelatinous matter from the fibrous as well as the osseous tissues. When the patients have taken these articles regularly for a few days there is a noticeable change in the condition of the hair and nails. The nails become clearer and smoother, and the hair becomes stronger and shows less tendency to drop out. With this general treatment should be combined local treatment of the scalp, and, in the opinion of this author, frequent washing of the head with soap is one of the most useful procedures.

THE MEDICAL NEWS.

A WEEKLY JOURNAL

OF MEDICAL SCIENCE.

COMMUNICATIONS are invited from all parts of the world. Original articles contributed *exclusively* to THE MEDICAL NEWS will after publication be liberally paid for (accounts being rendered quarterly), or 250 reprints will be furnished in place of other remuneration. When necessary to elucidate the text, illustrations will be engraved from drawings or photographs furnished by the author. Manuscripts should be typewritten.

Address the Editor: J. RIDDLE GOFFE, M.D.,
No. 111 FIFTH AVENUE (corner of 18th St.), NEW YORK.

Subscription Price, including postage in U. S. and Canada.

PER ANNUM IN ADVANCE	$4.00
SINGLE COPIES	.10
WITH THE AMERICAN JOURNAL OF THE MEDICAL SCIENCES, PER ANNUM	7.50

Subscriptions may begin at any date. The safest mode of remittance is by bank check or postal money order, drawn to the order of the undersigned. When neither is accessible, remittances may be made, at the risk of the publishers, by forwarding in *registered* letters.

LEA BROTHERS & CO.,
NO. 111 FIFTH AVENUE (corner of 18th St.), NEW YORK,
AND NOS. 706, 708 & 710 SANSOM ST., PHILADELPHIA.

SATURDAY, FEBRUARY 12, 1898.

THE NEW YORK CITY BOARD OF HEALTH AND THE MEDICAL PROFESSION.

AT a recent meeting of the Medical Society of the County of New York the question whether midwives should be educated and licensed or abolished was presented for discussion. Finally a resolution was offered demanding that a bill be introduced in the Legislature which would "wipe out" the guild of midwives, whereupon one man had the insight and the courage to rise and insist that by the endorsement of such a resolution the Society would simply make itself ridiculous not only in the eyes of the community but of the entire State of New York. This warning appealed to the good sense of the Society, and the resolution was voted down.

At the present time there is a bill before the Legislature restricting the powers and acts of the New York City Board of Health. It is to be regretted that some one has not the foresight and the courage to declare with convincing force that the provisions of this bill are designed to make the profession of New York City ridiculous, not only in the eyes of the local profession, but also of the entire country. He who stands in the way of progress in these latter days, sooner or later is overthrown, and the wise course for the medical profession is to regulate and direct progressive forces when possible rather than endeavor to obstruct and suppress.

It has long been recognized and deplored that there does not exist in this country a scientific, disinterested, authoritative, governmental department of medicine whose duty it should be to declare officially the remedial efficiency of new drugs, to test the quality of all pharmaceutic and bacteriologic preparations, and so guarantee to the physician the efficiency of the agents constituting his armamentarium. Quietly, unostentatiously, almost unconsciously, there has grown up in our midst just such an authority, controlled and animated by a true scientific spirit, free from bias and personal aggrandizement. Clearly reference is here made to the New York Board of Health. The quality of the work done in its laboratory is recognized by all scientific men as of the first order. It has not only enabled the profession of New York to have at its disposal the best facilities for ensuring the bacteriologic diagnosis of diphtheria, but has also placed in its hands the best antidiphtheritic serum to be had anywhere in the world. It has not only kept abreast of the most advanced scientific ideas but in many instances has been the leader. As a matter of fact the first diphtheritic serum which was manufactured in this country was produced at the laboratory of the New York City Board of Health. With a most commendable conception of its duty to humanity it opened the doors of its laboratory to representatives from other boards of health throughout the country and to employes of firms which have now become producers of bacteriologic products. It thus appears that the New York Board of Health has been a school of instruction from which knowledge of modern bacteriologic methods has been disseminated all over the country. It has also steadily kept before it the fact that serum-therapeusis is still in the experimental stage and offers unlimited opportunities for improvement. By means of carefully conducted experiments the quality of antitoxic serum was steadily improved in its laboratory until it actually surpassed that made in any other laboratory in the world.

It can be said, without danger of contradiction, that diphtheria antitoxin, which is now accepted the world over as a specific in diphtheria, would certainly not have been used in this city or State to anything like the extent it is now employed had it not been for the pioneer work of the New York City Health Department. All the producers of reliable antitoxin in this country are directly indebted to the laboratories of this Department for assistance in the production of this remedy, if, indeed, they are not wholly dependent upon it for the instruction and encouragement they received there. The virulent cultures which were obtained by this Department were sought by all biologic laboratories, not only in this country, but even by those of England, France, and Germany. Not only has this laboratory thus surpassed the laboratories of the world in procuring the best grade of diphtheria antitoxin, but it has improved by its investigations the quality of vaccine lymph and the methods of its preservation. With the glycerinated vaccine pulp now employed by the Board of Health such results are obtained in primary vaccination as surpass all previous experience. In more than 20,000 primary vaccinations made by the employes of this department during the past year, and which were subsequently inspected, nearly ninety-nine per cent. of successful results were obtained. As to the propriety of the Department undertaking this work, it may be said that vaccine virus is produced by or directly under the immediate supervision of the government in Great Britain and every other country on the European continent. There is no other producer of vaccine virus in New York State.

All antitoxins other than diphtheria antitoxin are as yet largely experimental. No commercial house can afford financially to undertake and carry on such experimental investigations as are necessary to determine the methods of production and the value of the efficiency of such unstable products. They will produce and offer for sale only such preparations as are profitable to them directly or indirectly, and as there are only three producers of diphtheria antitoxin in this country, the probabilities are that if the New York City Board of Health is restrained from manufacturing this product the price will soon be placed at such a figure as to be beyond the reach of all except the very rich.

More might be said in justification of the high estimate we have placed upon the work of the New York City Board of Health: of its production of streptococcic and tetanus antitoxins; of its thoroughly systematic and scientific methods of controlling the spread of pulmonary tuberculosis; of its high position as an authority in pronouncing upon the quality of biologic products manufactured in other laboratories, and, finally, of its superb results secured in reducing the death-rate in the city of New York to a percentage unparalleled in its history. Is it not the duty rather of the medical profession of this city, of the State, and, indeed, of the entire country, to encourage and maintain the permanent establishment of this magnificently organized institution?

The feature of the bill now before the Legislature which appeals universally to the medical profession is the clause removing a political disability from members of the medical profession, *viz.*: the inability under the old law for a member of the medical profession to hold the position of president of the Board of Health. This political disability was an indignity offered to the medical profession which all with justice resented, and, therefore, gave cordial approval to a measure which restored medical men to a political equality with their fellows. But attached to this bill there have crept in numerous modifying clauses as riders, which, if enacted into law, will so cripple the Board of Health as to incapacitate it for a continuance of the work which, as we have said, has called forth not only the admiration of this community, but of the world.

Is it not, therefore, the duty of the medical profession to cast its powerful influence against this bill and so witness to the community that they are ready, as ever, for the benefit of humanity, to carry preventive medicine to the very fullest limit justified by modern science.

SOME CONSIDERATIONS OF THE BILL RESTRICTING THE POWERS OF THE BOARD OF HEALTH.

THE framers of this bill, by one of its provisions, assume to determine for all time what diseases shall be regarded by the sanitary authorities as infectious, contagious, or pestilential, and in so doing have excluded such diseases as the plague, relapsing fever, puerperal fever, tuberculosis, leprosy, contagious influenza (*la grippe*), epidemic dysentery, and all the contagious diseases of the eye and skin.

Under the provisions of this bill the Department of Health of New York would be powerless to act (until special legislation was obtained) in the presence of an epidemic of relapsing fever, or the introduction into the city of the bubonic plague from the East, which is possible at any time.

The chief purpose of the provision specifying what diseases should be regarded as contagious or infectious is to exclude tuberculosis or consumption from the list of the diseases over which the Health Department has power to exercise supervision; yet the contention that tuberculosis is not infectious is limited to a few, and the statistics of the world show that it destroys more lives than all the other infectious diseases combined. Nearly one-seventh of all deaths throughout the civilized world are due to tuberculosis, and nearly one-fourth of all deaths among the adult population are due to this disease, and yet the framers of this bill would exclude this scourge from the possibility of supervision by the sanitary authorities.

The provisions of the present law as now enforced can in no wise work a serious hardship to the unfortunate sufferer from the disease, and the enforcement of its provisions, it is believed, will be followed by a marked diminution in the number of cases of this affection in New York.

The sanitary authorities under the present law require that all cases of pulmonary tuberculosis shall be reported to the Health Department, and that to prevent infection measures shall be taken to render the sputum of such patients harmless. No inspection is made in cases under the care of physicians. Those who are too poor to employ a physician are visited by inspectors of the Health Department and printed instructions as to the methods of preventing infection are left with the patient and his family. The Health Department is also empowered to provide hospital accommodations for such patients as are too poor to obtain medical aid, and whose condition and environment require that that they should receive such assistance. There are turned away from the general hospitals in this city each week from fifty to seventy cases of pulmonary tuberculosis chiefly because of lack of accommodation in these institutions. It is to provide for such as they that the Health Department has received during the last year $60,000 from the municipality. This is to be expended for the care of patients admitted to various institutions at the request of the Health Department and who cannot be provided for in the various public hospitals. This bill would probibit the Department of Health from assisting in any way in the care of these persons.

The assertion has been frequently made that it is the intention of the sanitary authorities to isolate and segregate from the community cases of pulmonary tuberculosis, and to provide special hospitals for the accommodation of patients suffering from this disease, these hospitals to be under the care of the Health Department, and the treatment to be directed by its officers. The sanitary authorities have frequently denied that such is the purpose of the Health Department, and have repeatedly stated that they do not propose to carry out any such plan. It is their purpose to educate the public whose interest is the greatest to prevent the spread of pulmonary consumption, so that they may be enabled to carry out the simple measures necessary to accomplish this, and they do not propose to establish special hospitals under the management of the Department. That the present law and the methods used to enforce it have the sympathy and approval of the public and of scientific medical men, cannot be doubted. No sufficient argument has yet been advanced to show the necessity of the proposed changes in the law. The bill now under consideration, if enacted into a law, would remove the safeguards aimed to prevent the spread of consumption in New York, and this the people will justly resent.

THE BRITISH MEDICAL COUNCIL.

VICTOR HORSLEY has been recently elected one of the Representatives on the General Medical Council of Great Britain.

The General Medical Council is a sort of board of examiners and licensing, and is composed of eight members chosen by the medical colleges of England, eight by the colleges of Scotland, five by the colleges of Ireland, five nominated by Her Majesty, and five elected by the medical fraternity at large; the latter are known as direct representatives, and are, as a rule, chosen from among the general practitioners of the smaller towns. The members who represent the colleges are nicknamed "academic respectabilities," while those named by the Queen are called "their officials."

Horsley's election was a close one. his strongest

opponent being Michael Foster, the eminent physiologist.

The election is conducted by letter vote. In the present instance about 22,000 voting papers were sent out to the registered physicians of Great Britain and Ireland and a return requested within a certain time. Only 14,000 availed themselves of the opportunity. Several hundred ballots were ruled out because of improper marking, lateness, etc. Horsley received 7000 votes and Foster 6100; a few hundred were divided among the remaining candidates. While the General Council has very limited powers, the general practitioner looks to it for all sorts of things. According to one prominent medical journal the physicians regard it "as a kind of fairy god-mother whose business it is to provide silver spoons for her professional children, and to shield them generally from the slings and arrows of outrageous Fortune."

The Council provides for the entrance examination of students in medicine and examines them again before registering them as practitioners. Its real title is "General Council of Medical Education and Registration of the United Kingdom." Sir Richard Quain is its presiding officer.

It has only been a few years that the general profession has had direct representation in this council, and those who uphold the system are afraid that if in future elections so large a proportion of the profession abstain from voting as obtained in the present instance, the privilege will be taken away from them. Of the 22,000 voting papers distributed, 8000 (or considerably more than one-third) were not returned. The election occurs once in seven years; the present election was made to fill the unexpired term of a member who had resigned.

ECHOES AND NEWS.

Exsection of the Stomach.—Unsuccessful attempts have been made by surgeons in St. Louis and Milwaukee to repeat the operation of total excision of the stomach, which was successfully carried out by Dr. Schatter of Zurich.—*Science.*

The Dispensary Bill.—The Senate Committee on Public Health has reported favorably on the Dispensary Bill introduced by Senator Sullivan in the New York Legislature. One amendment to it was made, providing that the action of the State Board of Charities may be reviewed by the Supreme Court of the State.

New Editor of the British Medical Journal.—At a recent meeting of the Council of the British Medical Association, the assistant editor, Dr. Dawson Williams, who for seventeen years has been connected editorially with the journal, was unanimously appointed editor. Mr. C. Louis Taylor, who has been sub-editor for the last eleven years, was appointed assistant editor.

Epidemics at Barre, Vt.—The news comes from Rutland that 170 cases of diphtheria and 130 cases of typhoid fever have been reported in Barre, Washington County, which has a population of only 4000. A large number of deaths have occurred. The State Board of Health is making an investigation as to the cause of the double epidemic.

"Faith Cure" in Indiana.—Advices have been received from Indianapolis that warrants have been issued for the arrest of "Dr." J. L. Stevenson and Samuel Fuller, leaders of the "Christian Scientists" in Jackson township, on the charge of manslaughter. They are held responsible for the deaths of a child of the former and the wife of the latter, both of whom died without receiving medical attention.

The Voluntary Determination of Sex a Proprietary Idea.—It is reported from Vienna that Professor Schenk has prepared a paper in which he describes his system for determining the question of sex. The rights to publish this pamphlet have been sold in Germany for $10,000. There is a stipulation, however, that it shall not be published until the American and English rights have been disposed of.

Hospital Sued for Damages.—According to a decision recently rendered by Justice Goldfogle in the Fifth New York District Court, charitable institutions are not responsible for damages which may be inflicted by their agents and servants. A suit in which this decision was rendered was brought against Roosevelt Hospital, New York, by a man whose bicycle was demolished by an ambulance belonging to that institution.

Plague Measures in Bombay.—Recent despatches from India say that quarantine barriers are being established in all the towns against the Bombay exodus. The Governor, fearing that the plague will increase rapidly within a few weeks, and that the penning up of the large population will result in a panic, has issued an order inviting those affected to remove themselves and their families to a camp on the islands across the harbor. Regiments have been ordered to Bombay for plague duty.

Register of Licensed Physicians Practising in Illinois.—The twentieth annual report of the Illinois State Board of Health to be published soon will contain an official register of all licensed physicians practising in Illinois. The secretary of the Board, Dr. J. A. Egan, in order to ensure accuracy, requests that every physician entitled to the privilege who desires his name and address correctly reported to send the information to him on a postal-card at once, mentioning number and date of certificate.

Radical Treatment of Smallpox at the Immigration Bureau.—A case of smallpox was recently discovered in the detention quarters of the Immigration Bureau at New York.

The patient was a Russian, who arrived on January 22nd from Rotterdam. He was at once sent to the Riverside Hospital, and the detention-room, articles of clothing and bedding were fumigated, and the ninety other detained immigrants and those of the employes who had come in contact with the patient were vaccinated.

Indian Plague Riots.—Recent news from Bombay indicates the steadily advancing increase of the bubonic plague. The superstition and opposition of the native population are serious bars to the application of sanitary measures. In the neighborhood of Bombay fatal riots have been occasioned by the efforts of the health authorities to prevent the spread of the disease. The rioters have killed a hospital assistant, burned the segregation camp, wrecked the post-office, and cut the telegraph wires.

Professional Opinion Regarding the Board of Health Bill.—It is gradually becoming known that a strong, intelligent branch of the profession of New York is opposed to the Brush Bill now before the Legislature. Evidences of this are rapidly becoming apparent. Dr. Jacobi has placed himself upon record as opposed to the bill by resigning from the Special Committee of the County Medical Society appointed to consider the bill. Resolutions in opposition to the measure have been unanimously passed by the visiting-staffs of Bellevue, New York, Presbyterian, Roosevelt, and St. Luke's Hospitals, and the Hospital for Contagious Diseases.

The New Philadelphia Health-Officer.—Dr. Benjamin Lee secretary of the State Board of Health and of the State Quarantine Board, was recently appointed by the Governor Health-Officer of Philadelphia, to fill the vacancy caused by the resignation of Theodore Stulb. Dr. Lee was graduated from the Medical Department of the University of New York in 1856, and formerly resided in this city, but removed to Philadelphia in 1866. He is widely known as a specialist in orthopedic surgery, nervous affections, and mechanical therapeutics. He introduced the method of self-suspension in the treatment of spinal affections, and has contributed many valuable papers on the special departments to which he has given time and study as well as to the science of public health.

The Society of the Alumni of Charity (New York City) Hospital.—The eighth annual reunion and banquet of this Society was held at the Savoy Hotel, New York City, on the evening of February 2, 1898. From a social as well as a gastronomic standpoint, the gathering was a most delightful affair. About 150 covers were laid, and some of the members journeyed many miles in order to be present. In addition to the usual postprandial speeches and good stories, the Society indulged in the unusual experience of listening to a serious discussion of the dispensary question by the Reverend Dr. Greer. In response to the circular letters which were sent out asking for personal information, 150 answers were received, from which it is learned that 25 of the alumni are now either professors or instructors in medical schools, 6 are authors of standard books, and the writers of articles for medical journals are as numerous as the members themselves. Some of the members were found located as far north as the Klondike and others as far south as South America. They are scattered through twenty-two States of the Union; one alumnus is located in Japan and one in China. The following officers were announced for the ensuing year: President, Walter B. Johnson; vice-president, W. L. Stowell; secretary, Charles J. Proben; treasurer, Henry M. Schroeder; editor, A. T. Muzzy.

The Status of the Marine Hospital Service as a National Quarantine Board.—The Senate Committee on Public Health and National Quarantine, in its report on the Senate bills concerning a national quarantine submitted to it, says "It has not been satisfactorily shown that the yellow fever which entered the United States last summer at a point on the Gulf coast near Ship Island occurred by reason of the carelessness or negligence of the officers on duty at the Ship Island Quarantine Station. The fever first appeared at Ocean Springs, a few miles from the Station, but it is unjust to conclude on the ground of propinquity alone that it came through Ship Island. In our opinion it is wise and necessary to retain the present system of quarantine under the management of the Marine Hospital Service, with its hospitals, quarantine stations, improved apparatus for the investigation of disease germs, and corps of officers, twenty-five per cent. of whom have experience in the prevention and treatment of infectious diseases, and especially of yellow fever. It may be found expedient hereafter to expand the service into that of a department, but to do so now would mean the useless expenditure of money and the destruction of the only systematic antagonism to the invasion of contagious disease. While we believe that the quarantine jurisdiction of the Marine Hospital Service should be retained, we are clearly of the opinion that its powers should be enlarged and made more distinct and uniform. No timidity nor adherence to technicalities should prevent the adoption of any measures which are necessary to exclude contagious diseases from our shores. The experience of past years, and especially of last summer, demonstrate the absolute and immediate necessity of so amending existing laws as to enlarge and concentrate the powers of the Marine Hospital Service, so that the present sporadic and conflicting condition, in which there is constant friction and collision between Federal and State officials, shall be changed, and the exclusive, ultimate control be given to one authority."

The Source of the Yellow-Fever Epidemic Definitely Determined.—The committee of the Mississippi Legislature appointed to investigate the yellow fever of last summer has made its report, after having visited Ocean Springs, Biloxi, and other coast towns where the fever prevailed. It finds, beyond all question, that the yellow fever originated at Ocean Springs, Miss., but not from the United States Marine Hospital Quarantine Station at Ship Island, as was supposed, and it also declares that that quarantine station is not a menace or a danger to the health of the people of the Gulf Coast or of the South. Those who did not think that the fever originated at Ship Island, and was communicated by the quarantine officials to the mainland, held that it was introduced by Cuban refugees who met at Ocean Springs in June to arrange for a filibustering expedition to Cuba, and one of whose members died of a mysterious disease and was buried at Ocean Springs. This very generally accepted theory is disproved by the Mississippi legislative committee, which finds that yellow fever was introduced into this country much earlier than it was supposed—as early, indeed, as April—and that it came, not from Cuba, but from Guatemala. The existence of yellow fever was not discovered at Ocean Springs until September 6th, and hitherto the utmost researches have not traced it back beyond the end of July. The committee finds that yellow fever prevailed during four months at Ocean Springs, and that it was introduced into this country by a Mississippi family, who had been temporarily in Guatemala and who came to the United States on the Central-American steamer "Breakwater." Their baggage was neither fumigated nor disinfected, and they went direct to Ocean Springs, where one of them was taken sick with fever. Within a few days other cases of fever appeared in their immediate neighborhood, and from that time a disease of the same character prevailed at Ocean Springs until the end of the summer, although it was not diagnosticated as yellow fever until September. The committee attributes the introduction of the yellow fever to the fact that the quarantines of the Gulf States against the West Indies and Central America go into effect on May 1st, whereas the "Breakwater" brought the disease into the country in April—before the quarantine was put in operation. This shows the necessity for early quarantine in order to assure protection. The epidemic of 1878 was brought into this country long before the quarantine was put in force, the steamer "Emily B. Souder," which brought it, arriving in March. The committee also investigated the amount of damage done by the yellow-fever scare, and found it to be greater than estimated. The loss to business in the State during the prevalence of the scare was from twenty-five to forty per cent., and property on Mississippi Sound has shrunk 30 per cent. in value because of the fever. The expense of the various quarantines in vogue was found to run as high as $5000 in many of the counties.

CORRESPONDENCE.

PRIVATE DISPENSARIES.

To the Editor of the MEDICAL NEWS.

DEAR SIR: Before writing a word on the subject of this letter an apology is tendered to your readers. I write for information in regard to the small *flat dispensaries* springing up all over the East Side of this city. It appears that these places (one can hardly call them dispensaries) are run entirely as private affairs; in the sense that the physician in charge tries to turn each case officeward. He may be anxious for patients because he is connected with some large clinical institution and wishes to hand material to his professor for students to examine. Go through East Seventy-third street between Second and Third avenues and you will find the words "Dispensary, Walk In," in a window, but on the door it reads, "*Office, East Seventy-eighth street.* Again, try Eightieth street between First and Second avenues, or Eighty-third street between First avenue and Avenue A, or Ninety-fourth street, and many other streets, and see what games our very professional brethren are playing. District physicians find daily, bottles of medicine in the poor man's home without any doctor's name attached thereto, for which the patient has paid from 10 to 25 cents each. The composition of these mixtures is, as a rule, R. and S. Co., or aquæ crotonis, with, perhaps, some bitter added for flavor. Is there no law, legislation, or remedy which can save the ignorant classes from this species of medical fraud?

E. C. CHAMBERLIN, M.D.

NEW YORK, January 11, 1897.

OUR PHILADELPHIA LETTER.

[From our Special Correspondent.]

DISPENSARY ABUSE—THE TYPHOID SITUATION—THE COLLEGE OF PHYSICIANS' ATTITUDE TOWARDS FILTRATION OF THE WATER-SUPPLY, AND THE PLACARDING OF HOUSES BY THE BOARD OF HEALTH—LEGALITY OF THE COMPULSORY VACCINATION LAW CONTESTED—A SETBACK TO THE BAKE-SHOP REGULATIONS—REPORT OF CONTAGIOUS DISEASES FOR 1897—DR. W. W. KEEN—DR. FRANK HAEHNLEN—THAT $100,000 APPROPRIATION FOR THE JEFFERSON HOSPITAL—A BEQUEST TO THE PENNSYLVANIA HOSPITAL—DR. EVANS' WILL AGAIN.

PHILADELPHIA, February 5, 1898.

A SIGNIFICANT step in the movement to suppress "hospitalism" in this city was taken at a special meeting at the Charity Hospital on February 5th, to protest against the indiscriminate gratuitous treatment of patients by hospitals and dispensaries. Resolutions were adopted requesting the Philadelphia County Medical Society to confer with the Board of Charities and Correction and with the boards of managers of Philadelphia hospitals, with a view to adopting measures for the restriction of the evil. Dr. Frederick Holme Wiggin of New York City, read a paper on "The Abuse of Medical Charity in New York," and suggested that charitable institutions be placed under the strict control of a State board of charities. Addresses were also made by Drs. Horace Y. Evans, A. B. Hirsh, and others. The statements made by the several speakers at this meeting may be considered to voice the general sentiment of Philadelphia medical men on the dispensary question, which, with the multiplication of hospitals, has grown to be a matter of serious import. The present step is but an indication of what is soon to follow, for your correspondent is informed by reliable persons that the abuse is to be thoroughly ventilated, and that, as soon as the requisite data and statistics have been collected, a determined fight against the evil is to be made both by local discussion of the subject and by State legislation.

A comparative reading of this week's mortality report of the Board of Health shows that enteric fever is still prevalent in this city to an unusual extent, although it is gratifying to be able to state that the returns for the week reach a slightly smaller total than last week. There were 199 new cases of typhoid fever reported for the week just ended (February 5th), with 16 deaths from this cause, as compared with 212 new cases and 10 deaths from the preceding seven days. In the nine weeks which have elapsed since the present outbreak, over fifteen hundred new cases, more than one hundred of which proved fatal, have occurred; and during the first six weeks of the present year almost eleven hundred new cases were reported. The chain of evidence presented by the report of Dr. A. C. Abbott, Director of the Bacteriologic Laboratory of the Board of Health, leaves no doubt concerning the pollution of the water-supply; although, as was expected, he was unable to demonstrate the presence of the specific cause of typhoid fever in the samples of water examined. The detection of the colon bacillus in some of the suspected water is direct proof that the Schuylkill water is polluted with excreta from the human intestinal tract.

At the last meeting of the College of Physicians of Philadelphia, February 2d, two topics of importance to the community at large, the immediate improvement of the city water-supply, and the obnoxious custom of placarding houses in which contagious diseases are present, were acted upon. Relating to the first, the following resolutions were unanimously adopted: "WHEREAS, The College of Physicians of Philadelphia believes that improvement in the water-supply is essential to the city's health, and even if a pure and ample source were at hand it can never be possible while the water is drawn from populous districts, to avoid all chances of contamination, nor to secure it without years of waiting; therefore, be it *Resolved*, That this college declares itself most strongly in favor of filtration of the city's water; that it believes that this should be done at the earliest possible moment, and to so much of the water-supply as money can be made available for. And further be it *Resolved*, That this college considers it unwise, undesirable, and dangerous to the conservation of the public health to permit such important municipal functions as the supply or filtering of the water of the city to be in the control of any body of men other than the government of the City of Philadelphia."

It is interesting to observe that the college has, in this latter paragraph, unmistakably recognized the fact that the control of Philadelphia's water-supply lies entirely in the power of a large clicque of politicians hostile to any reform, for reasons best understood by themselves, unmindful of the loss of life which daily adds to the monument of shame against them, and prostituting their pledges as representatives of the constituents electing them to office. A committee consisting of Drs. J. K. Mitchell, A. C. Abbott, and D. D. Stewart was appointed to present the above resolutions to the city Councils. The second topic, that of placarding with yellow signs houses in which contagious diseases are present, aroused much discussion on both sides, and gave rise to a good deal of caustic criticism of the methods of the Board of Health at present in vogue, while the board itself, came in for a full share of the college's disapproval. Dr. Arthur V. Meigs opened the subject with a paper, entitled "Reasons Why the Placarding of Houses in Which There Are Persons Suffering with Scarlet Fever and Some Other Contagious Diseases Should Not Be Continued." He declared that the custom of placarding houses is not only a source of great inconvenience, but even an inquisitorial interference with the private rights of families. He referred to the fact that in reality in many cases the non-enforcement of the law had made it a dead-letter, and he characterized the members of the Board of Health, with two exceptions, as being ignorant of the requirements of their office, mentioning, in passing, that their dereliction of duty was a matter of general admission. Dr. Meigs' statements were endorsed by many other Fellows of the college, and views concurring largely with his own were expressed by Drs. James Tyson, Henry R. Wharton, Morris J. Lewis, and others. Among those who deprecated the expression of extreme views in this matter were Drs. H. A. Hare, A. C. Abbott, and H. B. Pease, all of whom favored a more moderate view of the subject. The outcome of the discussion, during the course of which the methods pursued by the Board of Health were analyzed and criticised with no gloved hand, was the passing of a resolution appointing a committee, composed of Drs. S. Solis-Cohen, Wharton H. Sinkler, and F. A. Packard, to wait upon the Board of Health to represent to this body the opinion of the college on the subject under discussion, and to ask that the board discontinue the present custom of placarding all houses in which are cases of contagious disease.

The constitutionality of the Pennsylvania compulsory vaccination law is being contested in the Blair County courts of this State, where the local courts have issued a mandamus against the School Directors of the City of Altoona, requiring them to show cause why the children of the contesting party should not be admitted to the public schools of that city without a certificate of successful vaccination. The importance of the decision to be rendered in this case cannot be overestimated, for an endorsement of the present law in this test-case should effectually silence the protests of the antivaccinationists, and should show to their fellows in absurdity, the antivivisectionists and the faith-curists, that laws are laws, notwithstanding their many loud and hysteric clamorings for a revision of the statutes to suit their delusions.

Another law which has recently been contested on the grounds of its unconstitutionality is the "bake-shop law," which Judge Willson this week characterized as "meaningless and absurd," at the same time handing down an opinion quashing the indictments against three bake-shop owners charged with its violation. The "bake-shop law," which went into effect last summer, has already proved a valuable means for the control of the sanitary arrangements of bakeries and for protecting the health of the consumer and of the bake-shop employe, and it is hoped that Judge Willson's opinion will be speedily reversed by the Supreme Court, to which the Commonwealth will at once appeal. Pending this final decision, the State Factory Inspector, Mr. Campbell, has announced that he intends to continue to prosecute all violators of the law.

The report of Medical Inspector J. H. Taylor shows that during the year 1897 there occurred in this city 5031 cases of diphtheria, 3553 cases of scarlet fever, and

2994 cases of enteric fever, this being, as compared to the year 1896, an increase of 1840 cases of diphtheria, of 2511 cases of scarlet fever, and of 505 cases of enteric fever. Last year there was an increase of 369 in the number of deaths from diphtheria, an increase of 221 in deaths from scarlet fever, and a decrease of a single case in deaths from enteric fever. During the years there were 2388 deaths from pulmonary tuberculosis reported, or a decrease of 136 from the preceding year.

Dr. W. W. Keen, who has been convalescing at Cape May from his recent illness, has returned to the city, and expects to be able in the near future to resume his professional duties. Another medical man who has been on the sick-list is Dr. Frank Haehnlen, late of the Medico-Chirurgical College, who is again quite restored to health.

The doubt existing in the minds of the trustees of the Jefferson Medical College and Hospital as to whether a change in the building plans of the hospital of that institution would disbar them from the use of the State appropriation of $100,000 granted them last year, has been dispelled by the announcement of the State Attorney-General that the change may be made without invalidating the appropriation. The new site for the hospital, which the institution intends to erect during the coming spring, has not yet been definitely decided upon.

The Pennsylvania Hospital has been left the sum of $50,000 by the will of Josephine M. Ayer of Lowell, Massachusetts. If we mistake not, this Mrs. Ayer is the widow of the Ayer of sarsaparilla notoriety, concerning whom, however, comment is unnecessary, in view of the munificence of his relict.

The uncertainty regarding the bequest made by the late Dr. Evans to found a dental institute and museum in this city has been cleared up by the receipt of copies of the document by the mayor. The city authorities immediately took legal steps for the incorporation of a trust to execute the will, and an appropriation has been asked, under the terms of the will, to protect the city's interests by retaining counsel in Paris. Just how large the bequest is, has not yet been announced, but it is said on good authority that the sum is not far from $2,500,000.

The total number of deaths occurring in this city for the week ending February 5th, was 451, a decrease of 7 from last week, and a decrease of 54 compared to the corresponding week of 1897. New cases of diphtheria numbered 93, with 23 deaths; and of scarlet fever, 56, with 6 deaths. Of the total number of deaths reported 142 were of children under five years of age.

OUR PRAGUE LETTER.

[From our Special Correspondent.]

THE POLITICAL SITUATION AND THE GERMAN UNIVERSITY OF PRAGUE—PROFESSOR VON JAKSCH'S NEW CLINIC—MEDICAL OPPORTUNITIES AT PRAGUE.

PRAGUE, February 3, 1898.

DURING December the eyes of Europe were turned Prague-ward to observe the result of the race disturbances in the Bohemian capital. For awhile it looked as though vacillating Austrian policy would allow serious injury of life and property to be inflicted upon the Germans in Prague before stern military regulations would put an end to the rioting and wanton destruction. In the early days of December hostile Czechic mobs surged around the German University buildings. The handsome laboratories of the Medical Department especially attracted the attention of the thoroughly aroused populace. The buildings bore the hated name "German," and the mob, thoughtless of the good work which had been accomplished in them, set about their wanton destruction.

There was no question of opposition, the police for the time being were too few to be able to protect the endangered property, and the work of destruction went on almost unhindered. The chemic, anatomic, and pathologic institutes suffered most. Windows were smashed with stones which went crashing through show cases in museums ruining valuable specimens and preparations. The pathologic-Anatomic Museum of Professor Chiari especially suffered in this way. Not content with the damage already done the mob broke into the lower floors of some of the buildings and proceeded with their destructive work—the anatomic room of the professor of legal medicine was almost ruined.

For several days there were repetitions of the outrages It was deemed advisable to dismiss the students of the German University Medical Department for the Christmas holidays early in December. A declaration of what was practically martial law and the hasty importation of Austrian troops from other parts of the Empire, brought the rioters to their senses. Collisions between the troops and the populace did not occur to any serious extent, and gradually the old town again became quiet. Every occasion was taken to make impressive demonstrations of the presence of additional troops, and with the desired quieting effect.

It is still considered advisable to place special guards around the German University medical buildings on holidays when the presence of large numbers of the working classes on the street might prove an occasion for further violence and destruction. In the early days some demonstrations were made by the mob before the houses of German professors, and in one or two instances these were such as to endanger the lives of the occupants, Professors Germak and Goldschmidt of the Medico-Legal and Chemic Departments being especially singled out, but on the whole the rising was distinctly racial in character and very little of personal animosity entered into it.

At Prague it is a tradition that the prominent men of party suffer for the ideas of the party. The old town possesses the unenviable distinction of having two council-rooms, from the windows of which councillors have been, on two separate occasions, flung to destruction. On the whole the mixture of elements which compose the Prague populace are just such as are not prone to take counsel, but act first and think about it, perhaps repentantly, afterward. Everything now seems thoroughly quiet. The presence of the additional soldiers on t streets is the only sign of the previous trouble. The German University reopened on January 10th, as usual.

The same day the diet of the Bohemian representatives for the province convened, and the last remnants of the martial law which had been allowed to remain in force up to that time was declared inactive.

The Czechs are fearful of losing, in the unsettled state of Austrian politics, the language rights so recently acquired by Austrian law, and are intent on making their feelings in the matter clear. The Czechish journals here in Prague have been fomenting racial discord, and a number of their issues have been suppressed.

For a while it seemed as though the German University might leave Prague for good. There are examples in history for such a course of action. The University of Leipzig owes its foundation to the withdrawal of German professors and students from the University of Prague nearly five hundred years ago, because the reigning king of Bohemia proposed to limit the privileges of foreign students attending the University. At a meeting of the representatives of German feeling in educational matters, held on the 28th of December last, it was proposed to transfer the present German University of Prague to Eger. Here, not far from the Bavarian boundary line, in the midst of a thoroughly German population, it was thought that it would regain its old prestige. It has gradually lost ground beside its vigorous young rival, the Bohemian University here, and under present circumstances many of the young Germans of Bohemia go either to Vienna or to one of the universities of Germany.

The expense of such a removal was an almost insurmountable obstacle. Generous offers were made, but universities are no longer, as in the olden days, merely a corps of professors and a body of students. Lecture-rooms, laboratories, hospitals, and libraries are now absolutely essential for teaching-purposes, and all these cannot be called up in a day, even when there are unlimited financial resources, which there are not—for educational purposes—in any place in Austria. Then too, to abandon Prague just now would look too much like abandoning their standards in the face of the enemy. So it is settled; the German University will remain here, and with the memory of the work which has been done within her walls, the medical world can only wish her the meed of success she so richly deserves.

Meantime, medical matters are not at a standstill. Professor von Jaksch's new clinic is being rapidly pushed to completion, and will probably be ready for partial occupancy by the time of the opening of the summer semester and entirely completed for the next winter semester. It contains some features, as might be expected since Professor von Jaksch himself has had a hand in the drawing of the plans, which seem worthy of special mention. Here in Prague, where the various contagious diseases may be expected to turn up at almost any time, owing to the unsanitary conditions prevalent, it is very necessary to guard against their introduction into the hospital wards. For all patients with fever who are admitted there is a reception ward in which they are observed for twenty-four hours, or until such time as it is absolutely sure what the condition really is. Everywhere one finds the glazed walls, the rounded corners, and the oiled floors, which admit of thorough antiseptic cleaning.

All the wards are so arranged that no beds are placed against the walls, and no patient faces the glaring light from windows directly in front of him, but has the light fal from behind. The large, high, airy, thoroughly lighted, and ventilated wards are much more suggestive of our American hospitals than one usually sees over here. There is, besides, a recreation and a retiring-room for nurses—a feature which is almost unique in German medical institutions, and a pregnant sign that they are beginning to realize that if they would have a better class of women as nurses they must take pattern after English and American ideas, and afford them better treatment than they are accustomed to receive.

It is typical of Professor von Jaksch, and of some of the methods he has been the means of introducing into practical medicine, that the laboratories in connection with the wards should be large, commodious, inviting rooms. For all the instruments of precision a special room, centrally located as regards the laboratories, has been erected. It has special walls arising directly from the foundations, with sliding-doors which will not slam, and with special arrangements in windows and doors to prevent the entrance of dust. It is hoped, thus by lessening vibration and preventing jarring, and to as great an extent as possible the presence of dust, that even hospital scales, polariscopes, spectroscopes, etc., will really be what is expected of them, instruments of scientific precision.

Prague as it is, with its large and varied clinical material, with a teaching staff that contains some of the great names in German medicine, and with its magnificent opportunities in obstetrics, is likely to remain for many years the Mecca of a good many foreign medical students. One cannot but think that many an American who comes abroad for medical studies misses the golden opportunities to be had in many a smaller university town because he comes with the idea that his studies must be most effective if made in one of the great capitals, where the harvest indeed is great, but the laborers are legion.

TRANSACTIONS OF FOREIGN SOCIETIES.

Berlin.

TREATMENT BY MOVEMENTS IN DISEASES OF THE NERVOUS SYSTEM—NEURALGIA CURED BY INJECTIONS OF OSMIC ACID—PROPHYLACTIC VALUE OF PERIODIC SWEATS.

GOLDSCHEIDER addressed the Union for Internal Medicine, December 13th, on the subject of *treatment by movements in nervous diseases.* He has applied the theories of Frankel and Leyden in the treatment of numerous tabetic patients, who are able to learn, by using what is left of their sensibility, and particularly with the help of their eyes and muscular sense, to perform many coordinated movements which has become impossible for them without this practice. Those patients who are already bedridden must begin with simple movements, and must be protected from overdoing, as they have no means of knowing when their muscles are exhausted. The general nutrition must also be kept up as well as possible. When patients are still able to go about, the treatment should consist not so much in complicated motions like walking, but in very simple ones, such as touching with the toes a given point. No especial apparatus is necessary. The pauses between the periods of exercise should be long to avoid overdoing; and it is well to tone up the muscles at the same time with massage and electricity, and to bandage the joints with flannel, to prevent over-extension. The speaker said that he had observed good results from this treatment in many diseases besides tabes. In the intention tremor of multiple sclerosis, which is really an ataxic symptom and is closely related to tabes, the effect of exercise is prompt. Here attempts are made to touch a certain point with the finger. The disease itself is of course not affected. In chorea, in writer's camp, and in different paralyses, improvement also follows these regular daily exercises.

KANN had tried the treatment in some thirty cases of tabes, and in three of muliple sclerosis, with excellent results. The requisites for success are patient and persistance on the part of both doctor and patient. Exercises should be carried out for an hour or two at a time, with long pauses for rest, and treatment continued for three or four months. In hemiplegias treatment should not be delayed more than four weeks after the beginning of the attack.

FRANCK presented two women who had suffered from *trigeminal neuralgia*, and whom he had *cured by injections of a watery solution of osmic acid*, 1 to 1.5 per cent. Sometimes a single injection suffices; but if the nerve is not found by the first injection, it is necessary to repeat the attempt. The injection itself is painful, but it is followed by anesthesia in the region of distribution of the nerve. EULENBERG endorsed this treatment, cautioning the members to always have a freshly prepared solution, as solutions of osmic acid decompose easily.

At the session of this Society December 20th, JARISLOWSKI said that the *prophylactic value of periodic sweats*, which is claimed by Ziegelroth, is not yet proved. They have a great value in stimulating and cleansing the skin. For some persons the steam baths are more to be recommended, and for other Russian baths. He cautioned against too long continuance of a steam bath.

BELOW spoke of the use which is made of sweats in the tropics to cure syphilis, by allowing patients to lie in heated river or sea sand. This treatment increases the pigmentation of the skin, as sun baths do. This effect of heat, without sunlight, upon the pigment of the skin ought to be further studied.

Medical Anachronism in Fiction.—Harry Thurston Peck, Professor of Latin at Columbia University, in a review of "Quo Vadis" says: "There is an anachronism involved in the introduction at the end of the ninth chapter of a freedman 'with his face marked with smallpox;' for no mention of smallpox in Europe is found till four hundred years after the period described in 'Quo Vadis,' and no Roman author speaks of such a disease."

SOCIETY PROCEEDINGS.

NEW YORK NEUROLOGICAL SOCIETY.

Stated Meeting, Held January 4, 1898.

THE President, B. SACHS, M.D., in the Chair.

RACHITIS; PETIT MAL; ARRHYTHMIA OF THE HEART.

DR. WILLIAM HIRSH presented two boys, brothers, one being six, and the other, three years of age. When each one was a year old a severe epileptic attack occurred, and this was succeeded by frequent attacks of *petit mal*. Almost immediately after the first attack the father noticed something wrong with the eyes. Examination now shows an internal strabismus, apparently due to a paralysis of the right external rectus muscle. Both boys are very markedly rachitic, and in both the heart's action is of that type which the Germans call "gallop rhythm." Both boys present in like degree that scaly condition of the skin, termed ichthyosis. In the eyes of both children there is a condition identical with that described in the adult as "choked disc." Both children exhibit choreiform movements, and both are idiotic. The speaker said that there does not seem to be a single lesion which will explain all these symptoms. There is no history or other evidence of syphilis. A little girl of the family, born between these two children, is well developed, both physically and mentally. The father and mother are cousins.

DR. LANDON CARTER GRAY remarked that attacks of *petit mal* in rachitic and choreic children are by no means uncommon. These cases usually recover under a treatment which improves the general nutrition.

DR. W. H. THOMSON remarked that the rhythm of the heart appeared to be due to hypertrophy of the right ventricle.

DR. HIRSCH replied that these cases are peculiar, because of the existence of choked disc, absence of patellar reflexes, and the peculiar rhythm of the heart.

A CASE OF PROGRESSIVE MUSCULAR ATROPHY.

DR. FREDERICK PETERSON presented a case of this kind. It was that of a girl of eighteen years who, at the age of seven years, had an attack of measles, six months after which she began to drag the right foot, and shortly afterward the left. There is no hereditary taint of any kind in the family, and except the measles she has never had any disease peculiar to childhood. Her drop-foot led to the application of orthopedic treatment for several years, though the weakness and wasting in the legs below the knees grew gradually worse in spite of such treatment. Two years ago she noticed beginning wasting and weakness in the hands. She had never had any pains in the hands, arms, legs, or feet. Examination shows the condition at the present time to be as follows: Pupils and eye muscles are normal. There is slight scoliosis; shoulder and arm muscles well developed and normal; thigh and hip muscles well developed and normal. She presents double *main en griffe* and double talipes varus with drop-foot. There is reaction of degeneration in all the intrinsic muscles of both hands, and in the muscles of the legs below the knees. There are no sensory changes whatever. The plantar reflexes are present. The knee-jerks are absent. She sways on standing. There is no incoordination of the muscles. Her general health is excellent. She presents, therefore, all the typical features of the peroneal form of progressive muscular atrophy; *viz.:* perfect preservation of the general health, remarkable contrast between the tapering wasted extremities and the well-developed muscles about the extremities where they are attached to the body, protrusion of the internal femoral condyles, garter-like atrophy of the legs below the kneecaps, talipes varus, *main en griffe*, fibrillary tremor, equine gait, and a tramping movement on standing in one one place (like a horse in a stall). There are fewer than sixty cases of this form of progressive muscular atrophy on record, and some of these, at least, are not genuine, but probably poliomyelitis. The seven autopsies recorded show that the lesion is a multiple neuritis, so that this—the Charcot-Marie-Tooth form—is a connecting link between the Duchenne-Aran or spinal type of progressive muscular atropies and the primary muscular dystrophies.

DR. SACHS said he believed he had been first in America to describe this disease. He had first seen it in two brothers, and the cases had been published in *Brain* in 1890. He had proposed at that time to regard the disease as the "leg" type in contradistinction to the "hand" type of progressive muscular atrophy. Only two months ago another case came under his observation. In almost all of the reported cases the extensor muscle of the great-toe was the first part affected. The last autopsy reported, one made by Oppenheim, showed that there is positively no change in any part of the central nervous system, and that it is after all a disease of the muscles—in other words, that it may be as closely allied to the dystrophies as to the spinal diseases.

A CASE OF PROGRESSIVE MUSCULAR DYSTROPHY.

DR. W. H. CASWELL presented a man, twenty-seven years of age, a silk weaver by occupation. His family history is negative. For some years he had had weakness of the arms. There is no history of serious illness or of syphilitic infection. Examination shows a decided hollowing of the thorax in the infraclavicular region, and the shoulders are carried more forward and inward than usual. Some of the muscles about the arm and shoulder are atrophied and others hypertrophied. He can only extend the arms laterally to the horizontal, but another person easily raises them above his head. The right half of the face presents a flatness and weakness. Electric examination shows faradic contraction in all the muscles, though diminished in those which are atrophied. There is no reaction of degeneration anywhere. The case, therefore, is one of progressive muscular dystrophy of the facio-scapulo-humeral type.

DR. L. STIEGLITZ said that he had had this case under observation for some months. He wished to direct attention to the changes around the orbit. The palpebral fissure on the left side is larger than on the right. At times, if the patient looks down, the lid of the left eye will not immediately follow the movement of the eyeball—Gräfe's symptom. In these cases he thought the face was involved very much oftener than Erb originally believed. When the face is involved, it is not usually affected symmetrically—an important point in differentiation.

BLINDNESS FOLLOWING CRYING.

DR. W. B. NOYES presented a little girl of eight years, having a negative family history. Four years ago, after a good deal of crying, the sight began to fail, and in four months she was blind. The child had had headache, right internal strabismus for a few weeks, and occasional vomiting, but no fever. Examination showed double optic atrophy. With the symptoms just narrated a clinical picture is formed which might have been taken for that of a brain tumor. The vision is reduced to the mere perception of light. The child is in good general health. His own idea is that the child originally had a subacute meningitis, which gradually involved the optic nerves.

DR. W. M. LESZYNSKY said that primary optic atrophy is very rare in children, and he is, therefore, inclined to believe that a localized basilar meningitis had been the primary condition. Some years ago he had presented to the Society a case showing this form of meningitis, although it did not involve the eyes. The cases are not very uncommon, and are liable to follow the exanthemata. At the time of reporting his case, he had referred to the one reported by Hobb of Zürich, in which the diagnosis had been confirmed by autopsy.

DR. MARY PUTNAM JACOBI asked if the presence of tubercle could be entirely excluded.

DR. NOYES replied that he could not bring himself to believe that this child had tuberculosis, but that she had been infected with syphilis is barely possible.

TORTICOLLIS SUCCESSFULLY TREATED WITH CONIUM.

DR. GRAEME H. HAMMOND presented a young man who had developed torticollis during last March, and in whom the spastic condition was still present when he first came under observation during September of last year. The patient was now taking 90 drops of the tincture of conium three times daily, and exhibited none of the toxic symptoms of the drug. No improvement had been observed until the dose had been increased to about 40 minims three times daily.

DR. H. ALLEN STARR said that he had had a case which was very much improved by the same treatment after the dose had been increased to 30 minims three times daily.

DR. W. H. THOMSON said that a very prominent oculist had caused the death of a patient suffering from blepharospasm by giving him 25 drops of the tincture of conium.

DR. GRAY said that more than one fatal case from the use of this drug had been reported; the trouble seemed to be that it was impossible to obtain a stable and reliable product. If, therefore, he happened to secure a good preparation for a given case, he endeavored to continue the use of the particular specimen until the patient recovered.

DR. HAMMOND said that most of the fluid extracts of conium found in drug-stores are almost inert. He always specified "Squibb's, and always began with a dose of 4 drops, and increased the dose by one drop daily. The system soon becomes tolerant of the drug.

AN UNUSUAL CASE OF RECURRENT MULTIPLE NEURITIS OF UNCERTAIN CAUSATION, WITH PARALYSIS OF THE PHRENIC NERVE.

DR. M. ALLEN STARR said that in cases of paralysis from multiple neuritis developing subsequently to the acute infectious diseases, there is rarely any tenderness along the nerves. It is only in the more severe cases that any cranial involvement is observed. Disturbance of respiration, from involvement of the diaphragm, is the rarest of all, and naturally is of the gravest significance.

The patient who forms the subject of the present report first noticed during 1892 a clumsiness of his hands, and shortly afterward he was unable to stand. There had been no preceding sore throat. Within three weeks he was unable to use his hands, walk, or stand alone. Control of the bladder and rectum was normal. During October, 1892, he was seen by Dr. Starr at St. Luke's Hospital, and then had total paralysis of all the muscles below the knees and elbows, with considerable atrophy of these muscles, and loss of faradic excitability. The trunk muscles had not escaped. There was partial wrist- and foot-drop, but no sensory disturbances. After a month he was able to go home, though he could not stand alone. 'In July he was reported as having fully recovered. In August, 1894, he was readmitted in about the same condition as at first. The second attack began during July of that year, with an almost total parralysis, as before. In September he developed a multiple neuritis. The next month he was able to leave the hospital, and the following April reported that he had regained complete power of all his muscles. On September 20, 1897, he came to Dr. Starr's office complaining of some numbness in the fingers and toes. There was slight anesthesia in the fingers up to the second joints. His appearance was that of a young athlete. In the course of a month there was absolute total paalysis of all the muscles of all the extremities, with rapid atrophy and loss of faradic reaction; he could not sit up, and his speech was noticeably thick. Early in October, while in the hospital, deglutition became affected; then the respiration suddenly became unnatural, and it was found that there was no spontaneous action of the diaphragm. This lasted two weeks, and he could sleep but little during this time because of the necessarily conscious effort at respiration. The diaphragm gradually resumed its functions during the following month and improvement advanced rapidly in all of the muscles. At the present time he is able to walk with the aid of crutches.

This case, Dr. Starr said, presented many of the features of diphtheritic multiple neuritis, yet he had not been able to find any recorded cases of this form of neuritis in which there had been a recurrence. Gowers states that involvement of the pneumogastric a second time in alcoholic neuritis is almost uniformly fatal. The causation of the multiple neuritis in this case could not be easily determined. It is easy to rule out alcoholism. Diphtheria was suspected, but careful questioning failed to elicit any history bearing on this point. Cultures were made from the throat on several occasions, and bacilli were found, similar to the Löffler bacillus, but injections of these cultures into guinea-pigs gave entirely negative results.

DR. SACHS reported a case of recurrent multiple neuritis of syphilitic origin that he had had under observation for a number of years. The patient was a man, thirty-five years of age, temperate in all his habits, who had been married two years. There was a history of a syphilitic infection three years previously, in 1892. During October, 1895, he first noticed difficulty in going up and down stairs, and this was quickly followed by marked paresis of both lower extremities, considerable atrophy of the anterior thigh and also of the tibial muscles. The knee-jerks were entirely absent; there was no evidence of spasticity, and there was good control of bladder and rectum. Under a course of mercurial inunction improvement was immediate, and early in 1896 he was able to go about as well as before the illness began. The patient again consulted him in May, 1897, because of a slight left ptosis. This disappeared after a course of inunctions. In November, 1897, he complained of numbness in the left hand and fingers. Examination showed the power of the hand to be almost nil. There was gradual involvement of the musculo-spiral, median, and ulnar nerves, with loss of faradic response. All these symptoms pointed to the neuritic character of the affection. He had seen only one other case which at all resembled this one.

DR. HIRSCH asked if the spleen had been enlarged in Dr. Starr's case, and whether the blood had been examined for the malarial plasmodium. He recalled one case of multiple neuritis occurring from paludal infection, as demonstrated by the presence of the plasmodium in the blood. He had seen a case at Professor A. Fränkel's clinic, in which there were two attacks of multiple neuritis, finally ending in tabes. He thought a number of cases were on record in which tabes had been preceded by a history of multiple neuritis. This seemed to confirm the theory of Leyden, that tabes originates, not in the posterior columns, but in the ganglia.

DR. STARR replied that malaria had been excluded in his case by examination of the blood, and that the spleen had been of normal size.

DR. HAMMOND said that he now had under treatment a patient whose case is similar to the one reported by Dr. Starr. After having been in the hospital for a few days the patient's symptoms had all been aggravated, following two distinct paroxysms of intermittent fever, except that there was no return of the paralysis of respiration. This man had had chills and fever at intervals for fifteen years previously, and his original attack had occurred shortly after a paroxysm of this disease.

DR. MARY PUTNAM-JACOBI remarked that in the last number of *Brain* Fleming had reported a case of multiple alcoholic neuritis, occurring in an alcoholic subject, in which at the end of three months there had been involvement of the phrenic nerve, and death had ensued after six hours of most intense dyspnea. The autopsy showed a degeneration of the phrenic nerve, and also hemorrhages into the anterior horns of the spinal cord.

DR. FRAENKEL said that he had under observation two cases similar to the one reported by Dr. Starr. One entered the Montefiore Home about three years ago—a case of poisoning by snuff. He returned twice with a new and more severe attack. The second case was that of a man, forty-four years of age, who had had three attacks of multiple neuritis. Each time the relapse had followed his return to a house the walls of which were covered with green wall-paper, thus establishing a possible source of arsenic poisoning.

DR. SACHS said that he could recall one case of multiple neuritis, exactly like Dr. Starr's, in which intense dyspnea had been a prominent symptom, death occurring with unusual suddenness. In the case that he had just reported, the ptosis was mentioned simply to prove that the entire nervous system was affected by the syphilis; the ptosis might be due to peripheral disease.

BRAIN TUMOR—PRESENTATION OF A PATIENT AND OF A SPECIMEN.

DR. FRAENKEL presented a little boy, seven and one-half years old, in whom there was facial asymmetry—most noticeable when he smiled. The skull was also asymmetric, and there was enlargement of the cervical and inguinal lymph-nodes. There were no knee- or elbow-jerks, and the muscles of the right half of the body were more flabby than those of the other side. During July, 1896, he began to have attacks of vomiting and severe headache, and became dull and drowsy, and a right facial palsy developed. On examination, the right angle of the mouth was found to have dropped, and he had an ataxic-hemiplegic gait. He showed mental hebetude, and his speech was slow and stammering. There was distinct tumefaction of the right optic disc; the right facial nerve appeared paralyzed in all its branches, and the motor power of the right upper extremity was diminished. A diagnosis was made of subcortical brain tumor, probably in or near the optic thalamus. Mercurial inunctions and the internal administration of iodid of potassium soon caused improvement in all the symptoms. After three weeks the subjective and most of the objective symptoms had disappeared.

Dr. Fränkel then presented a brain, removed from a man twenty-nine years of age, who had been admitted to the Montefiore Home on August 20, 1895, suffering from pulmonary tuberculosis. There was a moderate lesion at the apex of each lung. Examination showed edema of the lower extremities, anemia, lesions of both lungs and enlargement of the liver. The skull was asymmetric. The most prominent feature was the facial expression; the left eyelid drooped and the eyeball was injected. The right facial nerve was found to be normal. The patient performed all the motor functions with the left facial nerve, and with unnecessary force. The tongue was dry and furred, and not tremulous. The knee-jerks were very much diminished. There was no ataxia. He was given mercurial inunctions, and iodid of potassium was administered internally. After two weeks he complained of vertigo, and developed a typical cerebellar gait. Treatment was continued three weeks longer, at which time most of the symptoms had disappeared. The diagnosis seemed to lie between meningitis and a tumor at the base of the brain—in the posterior fossa. The patient finally died in uremic coma. The autopsy was made by Dr. William Vissman. No abnormalities of the spinal cord or of the dura mater of the brain were found. At the base of the brain were a number of grayish-white nodules, the exact nature of which had not yet been determined. The anatomic diagnosis was tuberculous meningitis of the base of the brain, pulmonary tuberculosis, and the nervous affection was thought to be entirely functional. Tubercle bacilli were never found in the sputum.

Dr. Fränkel was of the opinion that the first case was specific, and that in the second the lesion was undoubtedly tuberculous. The specimen showed that it had, for the most part, disappeared.

REVIEWS.

LECTURES ON THE MALARIAL FEVERS. By WILLIAM SYDNEY THAYER, M.D., Associate Professor of Medicine in the Johns Hopkins University. New York: D. Appleton & Co., 1897.

So widely known is Dr. Thayer's original work in the study of the malarial fevers that a new contribution on the subject from his pen is quite likely to invite attention and interest. The reader of his lectures will not be disappointed. The subject is presented here with a facility born of actual knowledge, with a scientific instinct that is developed on the first page, and with a literary grace so charming that one is inclined to believe that the author's previous work will be eclipsed by the present.

Beginning with a thorough historic review of the literature of the disease, Dr. Thayer points out the poor choice of name for the malarial parasite, the "plasmodium malariæ," and utters the hope that it may soon be permanently replaced by a title more appropriate. He emphasizes the necessity of knowing well the histology of the normal blood before attempting to study that of disease. He leads us next into the detailed methods of staining and studying malarial blood, and discusses the distribution and transmission of the parasite. It is interesting to note that the author doubts the transmission of the disease from mother to child, and he cites an instructive case in defense of his view. The clinical appearances of malaria, its sequelæ and complications, are next considered, and are followed by a thorough discussion on treatment, a chapter which was, unfortunately, all too short in the monograph of Thayer and Hewetson, but whose excellence in the present work wholly atones for that omission. A chapter on general pathology and one on diagnosis complete the book.

The work of the Johns Hopkins school in setting aside "malaria" as a diagnosis of self-satisfaction will, in the course of time, be appreciated by the profession, and the present work can only tend to enhance this scientific effort.

ing. The tenth and succeeding editions will find an abundance of readers.

THE AMERICAN TEXT-BOOK OF OPERATIVE DENTISTRY. Edited by EDWARD C. KIRK, D.D.S., Dean of the Dentistry Department, University of Pennsylvania. Philadelphia and New York: Lea Brothers & Co., 1897.

THIS is a system by fifteen authorities on subjects relating to dentistry. Appended is a list of the contributors, with the subjects treated:

R. R. Andrews writes on the embryology and histology of the dental tissues; Henry H. Burchard, on plastic fillings, their properties, uses, and manipulations; including a history of amalgam, its physical properties, giving diagrams and tables of its shrinkage, expansion, etc.; the treatment and filling of root canals; the pathologic conditions which obtain, and the therapeutic agents and materials used in their treatment. Dento-alveolar abcesses, their causes, pathology and morbid anatomy, with diagrams by Dr. Black, together with the latest methods of treatment, are next considered. Local anesthetics and tooth extraction are the succeeding topics discussed.

Calvin S. Case discusses the development of esthetic facial contours, and William E. Christensen writes of inlays, the setting of porcelain cavity stoppers, the process of forming and fusing porcelain inlays by the use of the Downir crown furnace, and the Custer electric furnace. Dwight M. Clapp considers combination fillings. M. H. Cryer writes on the extraction of teeth and surgical anatomy of the maxillæ; the treatment of abnormalities, with instruments and accessories employed.

Edwin T. Darby is the author of the operation of filling cavities with metallic foils and their modifications. Clark L. Goddard discusses care of the deciduous teeth, and the character of the filling materials for the same. S. H. Guilford writes on the preparation of cavities, with descriptions of instruments used.

THERAPEUTIC HINTS.

For Chloasma.—

℞ Hydrarg. bichlor. . . . . gr. viii
Ammon. chlorid. . . . . gr. xlviii
Spts. rect. . . . . . ʒ vi
Inf. hamamelidis . . . ℥ iii.

M. Sig. Apply small compresses wet with this solution to pigmented spots.

For the Arrest of Acute Coryza at its onset, the following powder is recommended:

℞ Salol . . . . gr. xv
Ac. salicyl. . . . . . . gr. iii
Ac. tannici . . . . . . gr. i
Ac. borici . . . . . . ʒ i.

M. Sig. Use hourly as a snuff for half a day.

For Gonorrheal Epididymitis.—Apply locally the following ointment:

℞ Guaiacol . . . . ʒ ii
Lanolini }
Resorbin } aa . . . . . . ʒ iii.

M. Ft. ung. Sig. For external use.

A fifty-per-cent. solution of guaiacol in glycerin may be used instead of the above. After the inflammation is subdued it is advised to substitute ichthyol ointment as a resorbent.

For Acne Indurata.—

℞ Plumbi nitrat. . . . . . gr. xv
Ung. petrolati . . . . . ℥ i.

M. Sig. Apply twice daily.

Administration of Cod-liver Oil.—The following formula is recommended by BRICEMORET:

℞ Ol. morrhuæ . . . . . ℥ vii
Syr. tolutani . . . . . ℥ iiiss
Tinct. tolutanæ . . . . . gtt. vi
Ol. caryophylli . . . . . gtt. i.

M. Sig. One tablespoonful two or three times daily. To be well shaken before using.

THE MEDICAL NEWS.

A WEEKLY JOURNAL OF MEDICAL SCIENCE.

VOL. LXXII. NEW YORK, SATURDAY, FEBRUARY 19, 1898. No. 8.

ORIGINAL ARTICLES.

CHOLELITHIASIS, WITH REPORT OF CASES.

BY A. MORGAN CARTLEDGE, M.D.,
OF LOUISVILLE, KY.;
PROFESSOR OF GYNECOLOGY AND ABDOMINAL SURGERY IN THE LOUISVILLE MEDICAL COLLEGE, ETC.

THE importance of this subject seems to be just dawning upon the profession, and it is certain that its history, as written at the close of the next decade, will record one of the most brilliant epochs in surgery. When it is considered that on an average probably one out of every ten persons is at some period of life afflicted with gall-stones, the great frequency of pathologic processes of the biliary ducts, including the gall-bladder, will be appreciated. The old are most prone to have gall-stones, also persons the subject of preexisting disease in this region, such as cancer of the liver and adjacent structures. Women are more frequently affected than men—in the proportion of five to two. Tight-lacing has been considered a cause of cholelithiasis, but sedentary occupation with its attending torpor of secretion and excretion is probably largely responsible for this difference in the frequency of the affection in men and women.

The essential pathology of gall-stone formation consists in an altered condition of the mucous membrane of the bile passages. Once there is destruction of the epithelium, as from extension of inflammatory processes of the duodenum, or from invasion of the ducts by the bacillus coli communis, or from circulatory disturbances resulting from the mechanical pressure of growths, the conditions are at once created for a deposit of cholesterin, carbonate of lime, and bile pigment. The nucleus of such deposits, as well as much of the component mass, often consists of dead epithelial cells and inspissated mucus from the preexisting catarrhal inflammation. The well-known tendency of Americans to so-called gastric and duodenal catarrh, induced by peculiarities of living, such as rapid eating and exertion at a time when large quantities of food are still in the process of digestion, would seem to render them especially liable to this affection.

In detecting the presence of gall-stones too much stress must not be laid upon the presence or absence of jaundice. As a matter of fact most of the patients with gall-stones who apply to physicians for relief have never had jaundice; hence, in the past, they received treatment for something else, the true nature of the disease never being recognized. Severe pain in the right hypochondrium and epigastrium followed by jaundice, which usually passes away in a few days, marks the passage of a gall-stone so plainly that no diagnostic skill is required to surmise the nature of the condition. Or, again, severe sudden pain followed by continuous jaundice usually indicates an impacted calculus in the common bile duct. These are matters of common observation, and need not be dwelt upon in dealing with the symptomatology of the disease. The point in recognizing gall-stones which most deserves consideration is, that such symptoms as have already been enumerated probably do not exist in more than one-tenth the number of cases which come under the observation of the physician. Many patients suffer years with gall-stones in the gall-bladder which are too large to pass the cystic duct; such calculi, of course, never become engaged in the common duct, and so jaundice is not produced. Such cases are most often characterized by attacks of pain, usually requiring several hours or days to attain the greatest severity, with a variable period of persistence, followed by complete relief, the pain subsiding rather suddenly. The explanation of such attacks is to be found in the occlusion of the cystic, or gall-bladder duct, by the stone or stones and the distension of the gall-bladder with mucus. As soon as the passage is cleared by shifting of the stones, the result of the paroxysmal efforts of the muscular gall-bladder, the mucus escapes into the common duct and quiet ensues until the occurrence of another attack.

The pathology of this condition is confined to the gall-bladder and its duct, and from the ease with which the affection may be dealt with, it is especially important to recognize it before the graver complications of common-duct obstruction ensue. During the attacks of cystic-duct obstruction a careful search will usually reveal the enlarged and distended gall-bladder. If we would carefully examine these patients, instead of following the routine practice of calling the disease an attack of colic or indigestion and giving a dose of morphin, we would often establish a diagnosis of gall-stones in the gall-bladder at a time when operation would give the most brilliant results, and at a time when such treatment may be truthfully said to be preventive of the dangers of gall-stones.

Another and very frequent form of this disease is that in which the stones are very small and very numerous. I have removed more than fourteen hundred distinct but small calculi from a gall-bladder. In such cases one or more stones are passed every day or every few days, and the cystic duct being much smaller than the common duct the little stones usually pass very easily without producing jaundice. However, they give rise to a slight pain and feeling of discomfort, especially in the epigastric region, which lasts from a few minutes to an hour or more. I believe that patients having this form of the affection have been given a large proportion of all the pepsin and other lauded digestive agents which have ever been manufactured.

To recapitulate this part of the subject: (1) We recognize the presence of gall-stones attended with sudden severe pain and jaundice, or by obstruction either temporary or permanant of the common duct; (2) calculi confined to the gall-bladder and cystic duct attended with periodic pain without jaundice and characterized by a tumor composed of the distended gall-bladder in its usual situation (such cystic accumulations vary in size from that of a hen's egg to that of the human head). Occasionally the cystic-duct obstruction fails to be relieved, and the greatly distended gall-bladder may rupture, or, what is most common, become inflamed and adherent to adjacent organs, or to the anterior parieties; (3) cases characterized by slight pain in the epigastrium of varying intensity and duration, but without tumor or jaundice.

In competent hands the surgery of the gall-bladder is to-day the most satisfactory in its results of all abdominal work, and when we reflect how often it could be made preventive of the dread consequences of calculus disease, it should urge us to a due appreciation of the great advantages to be derived from a recognition of gall-stones, if possible before jaundice has become a symptom.

A brief history of fourteen cases subjected to operation is appended. Of these the calculi occupied the gall-bladder, or cystic duct, or both, in thirteen patients. In one case the common duct was alone the seat of obstruction. This was the only fatal case in the series, and in it jaundice had existed during eight months.

CASE I.—Mrs. B., aged thirty-six years, the wife of a physician, presented a history of periodic pain of a very severe character in the hypogastric region. Examinations by many physicians failed to determine the cause of her sufferings. There was no jaundice. In the absence of anything more conclusive her trouble was finally diagnosed and treated as gastric neuralgia.

September 19, 1892, I was requested to see her in consultation with her physician and Dr. Scott. The latter, having seen her the previous day, made a diagnosis of over-distended gall-bladder from impaction of stones in the cystic duct. During this last attack, which was most severe, requiring partial chloroform anesthesia for three days, there was a slight degree of jaundice. On examination of the patient I could detect a small tumor, about three inches in length by two inches in width, in the region usually occupied by a distended gall-bladder.

Operation was performed the following day, September 20th. A vertical incision was made at the outer border of the right rectus muscle, extending from the costal arch down to the lowest point of the tumor. The gall-bladder was found very tense and free from adhesions. By aspiration two ounces of clear mucus was withdrawn. The gall-bladder was incised, and several large stones removed, mostly from the cystic duct. The last of these stones was so deeply placed as to impinge upon the common duct, thus causing the slight jaundice from which she suffered. The gall-bladder was stitched to the parietal peritoneum, drained with a rubber tube, and the abdomen closed. Her recovery was afebrile, rapid, and uneventful. Bile flowed freely through the fistula for ten days, after which time its discharge ceased. Her health has been perfect ever since.

CASE II.—Mrs. K., aged twenty-five years. Four weeks previously she had been seized with severe pain in the region of the stomach and gall-bladder, which lasted the greater portion of the night, and necessitated morphia, hypodermically, for its relief.

An incision was made as in Case I. The gall-bladder was found to be at least five inches in length and very tense; it was about the shape of a large sausage. The fundus was drawn up into the abdominal wound, a flat sponge placed behind it, and an incision made through which was evacuated about six ounces of clear mucus. Twenty-four calculi, varying in size from that of a small chestnut to a half pea, were removed from the gall-bladder and cystic duct. A drainage-tube was inserted after stitching the gall-bladder to the parietal wound. Bile flowed for about twelve days afterward from the fistula, when the latter closed spontaneously. The patient did not require any opiate, and made a rapid and complete recovery. She has since remained in excellent health.

CASE III.—Mrs. S., aged twenty-six years, the wife of a physician, had suffered three years with recurring paroxysms of pain. A small tumor was noticed two years before in the region of the gall-bladder, and it was attended with circumscribed peritonitis. The trouble at this time was thought to be mesenteric tuberculosis. The history was somewhat obscure. There had been marked impairment of the general health, with gradual enlargement of the tumor mentioned. Vomiting was a common symptom. There was no jaundice. The shape of the enlargement was not that of an over-distended gall-bladder, and, moreover, its situation was not typical, being too far to the right and a little too high up. This enlargement was broadest at the base and not at the fundus. Cystic degeneration of the kidney had been diagnosed. After careful and repeated examination of the patient I believed the trouble to be calculus impaction in the cystic duct. Operation revealed an enlarged gall-bladder with numerous adhesions. The border of the liver was drawn down, very much thinned, and adherent over most of the tumor. The gall-bladder was found to contain three or four ounces of normal secretion. This was drawn off, and five very large calculi found impacted in the duct, causing complete occlusion. These calculi were quite as large as the largest chestnuts. The gall-bladder was stitched in the usual way to the abdominal parietes and drained. The patient made an uninterrupted recovery, and has since experienced the greatest improvement in general health.

CASE IV.[1]—The patient, a physician, aged thirty-two years, had always been very fat, his usual weight being 217 pounds. He presented a history of never having been ill until two years previously. While making a visit to a patient he was seized with severe pain in the region of the gall-bladder, which he at once thought was an attack of biliary colic. This lasted for some time, finally passing off. The subsequent history was that he had numerous attacks of the same kind but of varying severity. During the spring of 1894 he had an attack which was much more severe than usual, since which time he had almost constant pain and was incapacitated for performance of professional duties. Later in the spring he thought he detected an enlargement in the region of the gall-bladder. This became very tender. June 1st he took to his bed. He was under the treatment of his partner in practice. One day he felt, as he described it, something "give way," and he began vomiting large quantities of pus and bile, and actually vomited gall-stones. This was followed by several large bowel evacuations of the same fluid during the course of ten or twelve hours, and in the dejecta were numerous particles of gall-stone débris, together with about one and one-half ounces of sand-like material. His own diagnosis was proven by the operation to have been entirely corrrect, *viz.;* that he had an over-distended gall-bladder, which had become inflamed and adherent to the duodenum into which it had finally broken. After this "giving way," as he called it, he suffered the most intense pain; there was loss of appetite amounting almost to complete anorexia; there was constant pain which confined him to his bed; he became emaciated, falling off in weight to about 160 pounds. In the meantime, he contracted the morphin habit, and, during the late summer months, daily took six or seven grains of this drug when the pain was most severe.

[1] The history of this case is of great importance as showing the probable outcome in the majority, if left to themselves. It also proves that calculus impaction or other impermeable occlusion of the cystic duct must eventually lead to one of two things: Either rupture of the attenuated, over-distended gall-bladder into the peritoneal cavity occurs, followed by inflammation, suppuration, and adhesion to some part of the alimentary canal, or adhesion to the abdominal walls takes place, through which the contents of the gall-bladder are ultimately evacuated.

As I have said, his own diagnosis was absolutely correct, as was demonstrated by the operation, *viz.:* an obstructed gall-bladder containing calculi, adherent and fixed very high up toward the duodenum with which it had a fistulous communication—a natural cholecystenterostomy, but which, on account of the pathologic material still remaining, failed to give relief. Jaundice was present in varying degree from time to time throughout the course of the disease, and evidently corresponded to the passage of some of the calculous débris by way of the common duct. On opening the abdomen the first thing which came into view at the notch of the liver was a thick mass of adherent omentum. I incised this, and gently pushing it out of the way, came down to the under surface of the edge of the liver, but could not locate the gall-bladder. A hard mass was finally detected high up beneath the diaphragm, and after a great deal of trouble I finally isolated the gall-bladder, which was little larger than my thumb and enclosed by numerous adhesions. A further separation of the adhesions brought into view the attachment to the duodenum, it being very high up, probably above the point of entrance of the common duct. The adhesions to the duodenum were very firm. The question was, as I was working high up under the ribs, at least four inches from the point where I would have to make an attachment of the gall-bladder to the parietal peritoneum, whether or not I should carry out my original purpose and establish a fistula through which the débris could be discharged, and allow the communication between the gall-bladder and the duodenum to heal. After great difficulty I succeeded in getting the fundus of the gall-bladder down, and stitched it to the highest part of the wound, which was nearly in the middle line over about what would normally correspond to the situation of the pylorus. I scooped out a large number of small calculi and débris, and placed a drainage-tube in the wound, packing gauze around it, fearing, as there was much tension, that the sutures might give way. The patient rallied nicely from the operation, and on the second day great quantities of this sand-like material were discharged through the drainage-tube. On the third day the whole dressing was for the first time saturated with bile. While the pain continued during the first few days after the operation, yet it was much less marked, and by the sixth day the patient was quite comfortable. The wound healed; his general health is almost perfectly restored, and everything promises a complete recovery.

CASE V.—A woman, aged thirty years, was first seen in consultation. The history was that the patient had suffered more or less continuously with abdominal pain, with paroxysms of greater severity, for about one year. Jaundice was not present. There was some emaciation, and a tumor the size of a fetal head, occupying the gall-bladder region, was detected. A diagnosis of over-distended gall-bladder from obstruction of the cystic duct was reached.

The usual incision being made at the outer border of the right rectus muscle, there was disclosed the largest distended gall-bladder that I have ever seen, it being quite as large as a child's head. The contents consisted simply of normal mucus. Its enormous weight had drawn it down on a line with the umbilicus. I incised the sac after drawing off part of the fluid, and, passing my finger down into it could at first feel nothing. Passing a finger down to the junction of the cystic and common ducts in the peritoneal cavity, I could feel a large calculus impacted at about the junction of the cystic with the common duct. On again putting my finger into the gall-bladder I could feel the stone, the folds of the duct intervening, but could not bring my finger in contact with it. After drawing up the gall-bladder and putting its walls on the stretch, I was barely able, with the tip of my little finger, to touch a small part of the surface of the stone, but could not move it. With the fingers of the left hand underneath and outside, I could not impart any motion to it. I felt sure there was a constriction on either side of the calculus, and it seemed positive that it was thoroughly impacted or encysted, as I was absolutely unable to move it by my first manipulations. Fully fifteen minutes were consumed in extracting the stone; several times it seemed necessary to incise the duct from the outside and in this way remove the calculus. Finally, however, the distal side of the duct was sufficiently dilated to allow the passage of the stone. The specimen looked much more like a urinary than a biliary calculus. It was very large and of a color that I have never seen before in a gall-stone, being almost white and extremely hard. The gall-bladder was stitched in the usual way, and bile flowed freely through the fistulous opening within eight hours after the operation. This continued for six or eight hours, when it ceased, and has never returned up to the present time, although a small fistula, discharging mucus, has remained. Adhesion of the stricture has probably occurred at the site of the stone, thus cutting off communication between the common duct and the gall-bladder. If the little mucus fistula persists, I shall enlarge the wound and excise the gall-bladder, which in this case can be of no use to the patient.

CASE VI.—A man, aged forty years, five years ago was seized with severe abdominal pain, which was diagnosed by the attending physician as being due to the passage of a gall-stone. Since that time he has had repeated attacks of a similar character, attended with slight jaundice. Within the past year he has not had jaundice, but the paroxysms of pain have been much more frequent than formerly. I saw him November 7, 1894, when he was confined to bed with severe and almost continuous pain in the region of the gall-bladder; temperature, 101° F.; pulse, 100, vomiting and loss of appetite being present. Examination revealed a large tumor below the margin of the ribs on the right side, very broad at its base, and extending as low as the umbilicus. This tumor was quite tender. A diagnosis of over-distended gall-bladder with inflammation was reached.

The usual incision was made. The omentum was found adherent to the fundus of the gall-bladder. The gall-bladder was intensely congested, and presented the evidence of an acute, engrafted upon a chronic, inflammation. Aspiration revealed the presence of pus. After protection with sponges, and having the patient turned upon his side, the gall-bladder was incised and three ounces of pus and twenty-five medium-sized calculi were extracted. There seemed to be complete occlusion of the cystic duct, all stones occupying the cavity of the gall-bladder. After irrigation and drainage of the latter it was sutured in the usual way.

The patient made an easy recovery, bile appearing in the wound on the fifth day. The fistula closed within a few weeks.

CASE VII.—Mrs. W., aged forty-four, married, had suffered a year with periodic pain in the epigastric region, usually lasting less than an hour and recurring almost daily, but with no definite regularity, and independent of any dietary restrictions. In fact, she had been treated during four months by the rest and milk treatment for indigestion. She was very nervous and tired of taking medicine for dyspepsia and gastralgia. February 13, 1896, an exploratory incision was made in the median line above the umbilicus. No abnormality of the stomach was found. The gall-bladder was filled with small calculi. Cholecystostomy was performed. The patient made a prompt recovery, with cure of the gastralgia. The fistula closed within three weeks.

CASE VIII.—Mr. H., policeman, aged thirty-seven years, suffered two years with periodic attacks of biliary colic, slight icterus, great itching of the skin accompanying each attack. Operation was performed April 2, 1896. The gall-bladder was found distended with small calculi (1407). Cholecystostomy; uncomplicated recovery; fistula closed within four weeks.

CASE IX.—Mrs. B., aged thirty-two years, married, enjoyed good health until three years ago. She had had repeated attacks of colic attended with jaundice, and had been treated for congestion of the liver. Eight months prior to the time I saw her she had been seized with a very severe attack of colic, with rapid and profound jaundice, which latter, with emaciation, has continued. Operation was performed, August 22, 1895. The gall-bladder was small, and did not contain calculi, nor were there any in the cystic duct. A single large stone was found embedded in the common duct near the duodenum, around which adhesions were numerous. After freeing the duct it was incised and the calculus removed. The incision was sutured first by fine catgut, and over this a continuous Lembert suture of silk was inserted. It seemed secure. A drain of gauze was carried from the suture-point to the lower angle of the wound. The time occupied in performing the operation was fifty minutes; reaction was very good. On the second day, the patient, a very self-willed woman, arose during the momentary absence of the nurse and crossed the room to where a pitcher of water had been left; she helped herself to this and returned to bed. The following night the dressing showed a bloody discharge of almost tarry consistency. The lower stitches were cut, and a large quantity of dark clotted blood removed from beneath the parietal peritoneum, but no definite point of bleeding ascertained. Liberal drainage was provided. The bloody oozing continued until death ensued from exhaustion at the end of the fourth day. No autopsy.[1]

CASE X.—Mrs. K., age thirty years, married, presented a history of many attacks of biliary colic during the previous four years. Last attack had been very severe in character. Operation was performed February 7, 1896. Cholecystotomy; removal of twenty-six calculi of various sizes. Easy convalescence; fistula did not close until the end of six months.

CASE XI.—Mrs. H., aged fifty-eight years, presented a history of much pain and soreness in the right hypochondrium during the previous five years. She recently had had some fever, but never jaundice; a large tumor in the region of the gall-bladder was easily detected. At the operation, February 14, 1896, the gall-bladder was found to contain a pint of pus and between sixty and seventy gall-stones. Cholecystotomy; bile discharged through the fistula on the second day; easy recovery; fistula closed five weeks after the operation.

CASE XII.—Mrs. S., aged thirty-three years, married, presented a tumor in region of the gall-bladder as large as a fetal head; little pain; never had had jaundice. Operation was performed May 25, 1896, and the gall-bladder was emptied of a quart of clear mucus and probably four hundred calculi, most of which were impacted in the cystic duct. Bile appeared through the fistula on evening of the first day after the operation; quick recovery; fistula closed within eighteen days.

The following case is, I believe, unique in the history of gall-stone operations:

CASE XIII.—Mrs. R., aged thirty-nine years, presented herself for treatment during April, 1896. She was much emaciated and was confined to her bed most of the time. She suffered great pain and tenderness in the region of the liver. She gave a history of having had pains in this region during several years, but the present illness dated back four months, at which time she had a chill, followed by fever, the latter being more or less continuous ever since. Examination revealed the presence of a large mass continuous with the liver and reaching as low down as the umbilicus. Careful palpation led me to believe that the enlargement was the liver.

Exploration, April 6, 1896. On opening the peritoneum the liver was found to be as low as the umbilicus, the abnormal position being the result of displacement rather than any increase in size. Attached to the inferior border of the right lobe of this organ, across its entire length, was the transverse colon. Beneath the liver was one inextricable mass bound down by omental, colonic, and duodenal adhesions. The mass was undoubtedly inflammatory, and, from the history of the case, I was satisfied that it contained pus. So great were the adhesions to the transverse colon that the liver was drawn down almost from beneath the ribs. The condition impressed me as probably being an abscess of the under surface of the liver. I did not think it wise to attempt a separation of the visceral adhesions which would contaminate the abdominal cavity with pus in a situation which it is impossible to drain satisfactorily. The superior (now anterior) surface of the liver was free and in no way adherent to the parietal peritoneum. I thrust an aspirator-needle through the lower border of the liver to a depth of three inches, and was rewarded by finding pus. The peritoneum was carefully packed with gauze around a space of liver surface two inches in diameter, the center corresponding to the aspiration-point. An incision one inch long was made into the liver, and deepened until the abscess was opened by means of forceps. Six or eight ounces of pus was evacuated, and the cavity of the abscess thoroughly washed through the opening in the liver. The soiled gauze was now removed and replaced by a coronet of fresh gauze, and a large rubber drain carried to the bottom of the abscess cavity. The upper part of the wound was closed by sutures. The patient made an uninterrupted recovery, the temperature falling almost immediately to the normal. The gauze dam was removed on the third day, and the abscess-cavity, which secreted surprisingly little, was irrigated daily.

The seventh day after the operation, after removing the sutures, I concluded to replace the rubber tube with a small strip of gauze, as there seemed so little discharge. In carrying the gauze through the liver into the abscess-cavity my probe came in contact with a hard substance, the click of which was unmistakably that of a calculus. Believing the liver adhesion to the anterior abdominal wall to be firm, I had the patient etherized, enlarged the tract with my finger, and delivered by means of urinary stone-forceps an enormous calculus nearly two inches in its longest diameter. The drainage-tube was replaced; bile appeared through the fistula four days later, the fistula closing on the twenty-third day after the primary operation. The patient made a rapid and complete recovery.[1]

CASE XIV.—Woman, aged forty-seven years, presented a history of many attacks of biliary colic, accompanied with jaundice. There was some tumefaction over the region of the gall-bladder. Operation was performed November 6, 1896. The right kidney was found displaced and adherent to the under-surface of the gall-bladder. Thirty-six stones were removed. Recovery ensued.

[1] I have assisted at two operations upon patients with common-duct obstruction, but without the marked cholemia of long standing which characterized this case, and the same method of suture and gauze drainage had been employed with perfect success. The operations were performed by my associate, Dr. James S. Chenoweth. It is significant that this unfortunate woman should have passed many stones, and lose her life from arrest, and common-duct impaction of the last one in her collection.

[1] This is the only case that I am aware of in which a gall-stone has been removed through the liver. Had I known the true condition at the primary operation it might not have terminated so favorably for my patient. Had this woman lived without operation, I have every reason to believe that the stone would have been discharged into the colon.

COLLES' FRACTURE AND THE ROENTGEN-RAYS[1]

BY CARL BECK, M.D.,
OF NEW YORK:
PROFESSOR OF SURGERY IN THE NEW YORK SCHOOL OF CLINICAL MEDICINE; SURGEON TO ST. MARK'S HOSPITAL, ETC.

COLLES' fracture is the commonest of all fractures, yet in regard to no other is there more difference of opinion as to treatment. Since the Röntgen-rays began their triumphant march from the modest town on the Main throughout the world, our knowledge of fractures and dislocations has been greatly enlarged, and our methods of treatment revolutionized. It may be safely said that treatises on this subject which were written before the Röntgen era have ceased to be regarded as authoritative. Following the new discovery great interest was at once concentrated on the much disputed classic fracture of the lower end of the radius, and it soon became evident that a much greater variety of the different types of this fracture (which represents ten per cent. of all fractures) exists than was ever anticipated before. As far as my own experience is concerned, I must admit that I never saw a case in which the diagnosis made

FIG. 1.

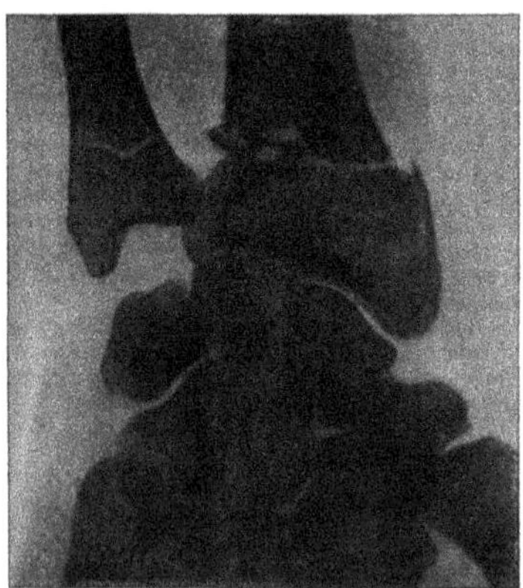

Colles' fracture with slight sideward displacement.

before a skiagram was taken was not more or less modified thereafter, especially when considerable effusion and swelling were present.

Since March, 1896, I have observed forty-four cases of Colles' fracture, all of which were skiagraphed. Most of the skiagrams revealed conditions not thoroughly anticipated when examined by the usual methods. One most surprising feature was that in nineteen of these cases *a distinct transverse fissure above the capitulum ulnæ* existed, without causing any apparent symptoms. In seven cases the styloid process of the ulna was entirely broken off. In some instances besides the typical transverse fracture there was also a vertical fracture of the radius,

FIG. 2.

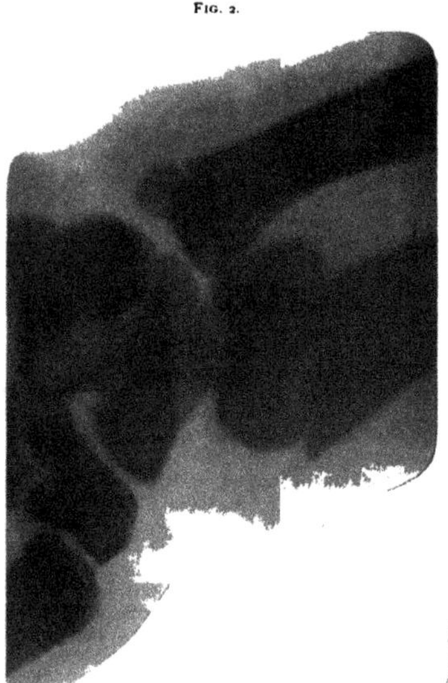

Fracture of left radius.

which reached into the radiocarpal joint. In fourteen cases there was no displacement in spite of the great extent of the lesion, the periosteum of the dorsal surface apparently having kept the fragments together.

The clearer our knowledge of a pathologic condition is the simpler and easier will be the indications of treatment. Surely there is a different plan to be pursued if there be a total separation of the lower end of the radius or only a fissure with little or no diastasis. It is of great importance to know the direction of the line of fracture and whether it extends into the joint. Another point which must be considered is whether or not there is any impaction. Sometimes there is a decided turning of the fractured end, its upper margin being forced toward the ulna

[1] Read at a meeting of the physicians of the German Poliklinik, October 29, 1897.

while the lateral margin protrudes and the joint-surface is directed upward to the dorsum. It is apparent that in all such cases unless thorough reduction is at once made the function of the wrist will never be restored; and *vice versa*, if the fracture-line extends upward from the volar side and downward to the dorsum, the displacement must occur in

FIG. 3.

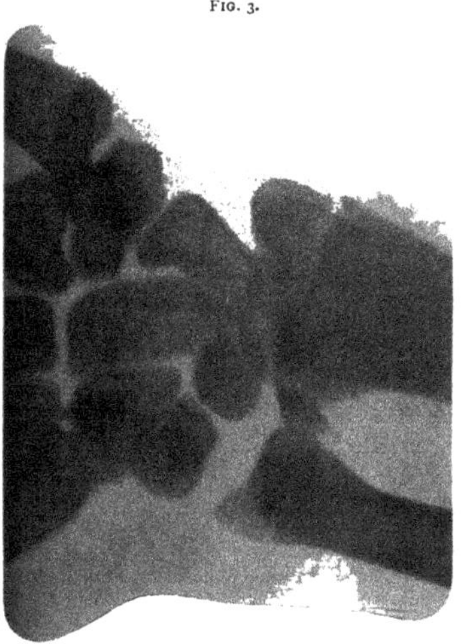

Fracture of right radius.

the opposite manner, the principle of reduction, however, remaining the same. If the direction of the fracture-line is oblique it generally extends into the joint—a point which has to be especially considered in the after-treatment. The method of reduction as well as of applying the dressing will also be modified when there is a fracture of the ulna or of its styloid process, or when a bone particle has been chipped off, as shown in Fig. 2. These lesions are often diagnosed with difficulty by ordinary methods, even when the manipulations are skilled, and are seldom recognized by any other means than by the Röntgen rays; but if the nature of the injury can be clearly studied on the photographic plate, the proper line of treatment is easily determined and may always be followed without subjecting the patient to unnecessary or tentative manipulations.

In the treatment of all fractures there are two very simple rules to be observed: (1) Replace a displaced fragment to its normal position, and (2) keep it there. If the skiagram does not show displacement there is, of course, no need of reduction. This explains why the results in certain cases of Colles' fracture are always good, no matter what sort of treatment is employed. In fact, if treated by a quack, whose ignorance leads him to treat the injury as a sprain with an ointment, poultice, or with "faith," often a better result is obtained in such ordinary cases than by the learned medical neophyte, who, after having made a most erudite diagnosis, immobilizes the joint for too long a period in his zeal to keep the fragments together; there will be no deformity, but adhesions will be formed, and the wrist will remain stiff or immobile. In such a case a patient, the motion of whose hand was not prevented by immobilization, would escape serious consequences. In all cases in which displacement is present of course a great amount of care and deliberation is necessary.

The first requirement, accurate reduction, may be carried out with little difficulty. If forced extension and downward pressure by the surgeon's thumb,

FIG. 4.

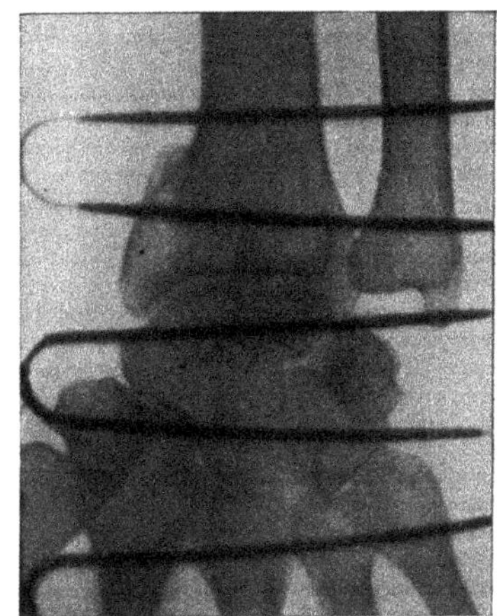

Colles' fracture with copious callous formation.

while counter-extension is used on the forearm, flexed rectangularly, should fail, anesthesia must be employed. But the more difficult thing is to keep the fragments well adjusted in a proper position. This I have always been able to secure by applying a long adaptable wire splint (Fig. 4) reaching at the flexor side of the arm from the tip of the fingers to the elbow, the splint being applied while forced traction is made. If the direction of the displacement is upward—*displacement à la fourchette*, a pad of adhesive plaster is attached to the dorsal integument above the fragment. Then a short narrow splint of wood is placed on the dorsal aspect of the arm, reaching from the metacarpo-phalangeal joint to four inches above the wrist, and is kept pressing down by the application of a gauze bandage. If the tendency of the displacement is downward the same procedure is carried out in the opposite manner, the wire splint being applied on the dorsal and the wooden splint and pad on the palmar side of the arm.

If the displacement be sideways, which is generally the case when there is a simultaneous injury of the ulna, the immobilization must be carried out on entirely different lines. The adhesive-plaster pad must then be applied laterally to the fragment, two long, narrow, wooden splints being used at the same time. One of these splints, being a little broader than the diameter of the bone, begins at the metacarpo-phalangeal joint of the thumb and the other at the same joint of the little finger. Both extend up to the elbow, the same as the long wire splint. If there should be any displacement to the opposite direction, the pad must be applied on the ulnar side. No dorsal splint is used in this variety. After the dressing is finished, the skiagram verifies the proper position of the fragments. If there be much swelling, wet applications may be advantageously used by pouring a solution of acetate of lead, for instance, upon the gauze bandage, the wire splint permitting penetration of the fluid.

It is of the greatest importance in such cases that the fragments, after being properly reduced, be kept *in situ*. The extremely strong ligamentum carpi volare never breaks, as Nélaton well demonstrated, and, therefore, it is in the first instance the *bone* which has to be taken care of.

If after the lapse of a week agglutination of the fragments is obtained and no deformity is evident, then the soft tissues must receive consideration. It is only then that short splints are in order. They consist of well-padded pieces of wood, extending from the metacarpo-phalangeal joint up to the middle of the forearm. After another week they extend only to the wrist, thus permitting free motion of the hand. The patient is told to move his fingers, as in playing the piano. After the third week massage treatment is indicated, active as well as passive motion of the joint being employed at the same time.

If all these points are observed, and if their proper execution is certified by the skiagram, surgical clinics will no longer furnish so much testimony of deformities and functional impairment following Colles' fracture. To illustrate some of the points alluded to, the following cases may be of interest:

CASE I.—In this case is shown (Fig. 1) a Colles' fracture with slight sideward displacement in a man, twenty years of age, three hours after the injury was sustained. The small splinters of bone, penetrating the soft tissues, are clearly evident. There is also a distinct fracture-line in the ulna.

CASE II.—In this instance is shown a fracture of both radii (Figs. 2 and 3) in a lad of seventeen years, five days after the injury had occurred. On the right (Fig. 3) there is considerable sideward displacement toward the ulna, thus representing a counterpart to Case I., in which the sideward displacement was in the opposite direction. In this case there is also a complete fracture of the ulna. On the left side (Fig. 2) may be seen two radial fragments. The larger one is not displaced, its fracture-line running into the joint. The small fragment is entirely severed and touches the inner surface of the ulna, which is broken transversely at its lower end. Four very small bone-splinters, piercing the soft tissues, can also be clearly recognized. Five days after the injury the patient was presented to an audience of about one hundred physicians, none of them being able to recognize an ulnar fracture, which, indeed, was hardly to be suspected, as the patient could not only walk about without a splint, but also did light work at the time, and was able to lift heavy objects from the floor. There was hardly any swelling and no visible deformity.

CASE III.—In this is shown (Fig. 4) a Colles' fracture, after two weeks, in a woman forty years of age. There is but slight deformity. On the day of the injury there was considerable displacement, which was corrected by an able surgeon. There is some copious callous formation, which induced the patient to believe that the "fracture was not set properly." The skiagram convinced her that she had been correctly treated.

Nothing may inculpate or exculpate a surgeon more than a good skiagram. In the May issue of the *International Medical Magazine* I published an illustration which showed an enormous amount of callous; it prevented pronation as well as supination so much that the case was pronounced to be one of vicious union. It was only the skiagram that exonerated the attending surgeon.

MIDWIVES.[1]

BY HENRY J. GARRIGUES, M.D.,
OF NEW YORK;
CONSULTING OBSTETRIC SURGEON TO THE MATERNITY HOSPITAL;
VISITING GYNECOLOGIST TO ST. MARK'S HOSPITAL, ETC.

DURING 1884 a bill was introduced in the State Legislature the aim of which was to grant a charter to a certain college of midwives in this city. After a heated discussion in the County Medical Society a resolution was passed in opposition to the enactment

[1] Read before the Section on Obstetrics and Gynecology of the New York Academy of Medicine, January 27, 1898.

of the bill referred to. Dr. Albert W. Warden and I were sent to Albany as delegates to confer with persons of influence in the matter, and the bill was eventually killed.

So far as I know, nothing has been done since that time to regulate the practice of midwifery in this city, but of late the question has been brought up in the Society of Medical Jurisprudence, and the hope was expressed that adequate legislation might be secured "to regulate the practice of midwifery by midwives in our Empire State."

In this State there are no general laws concerning midwives, and but two that are special, one for Erie County, and the other for the City of Rochester. The one for Erie County, in which is situated the City of Buffalo, was passed on May 22, 1885, and forms Chapter 320 of the laws of the State of New York for that year.

It prescribes that the county judge shall appoint a board of examiners in midwifery, to consist of five members who shall have been licensed to practice physic and surgery in this State. They shall on the first Tuesday of October and April of each year, and on such other days as said board may appoint, examine candidates of the age of twenty-one years or upward, possessed of good moral character, who shall present themselves to be examined for license to practise midwifery in the County of Erie; and shall, on receipt of $10, issue a certificate to any person so examined who shall be found by them to be properly qualified. The money received shall be applied to defray the expenses of the board.

The successful candidates are entitled, within the County of Erie, to practice midwifery in normal labors, and in no others; but such persons shall not in any case of labor use instruments of any kind, nor assist in labor by any artificial, forcible, or mechanical means, nor perform any version, nor attempt to remove adherent placenta, nor administer, prescribe, advise, or employ any poisonous or dangerous drug, herb, or medicine, nor attempt the treatment of disease, except when the attendance of a physician cannot be speedily procured, and in such cases such person shall at once and in the most speedy way procure the attendance of a physician. The board shall have power to recommend to the Judge of Erie County the revocation of a license, and said judge shall have power to revoke the same.

Any person who shall practise midwifery, or without the attendance of a physician when one can be procured, attend a case of labor within the County of Erie, without being duly authorized so to do under existing laws of this State, or without having received and recorded the certificate named above, and any person who shall violate any of the provisions of this act, shall be fined not less than $50 or more than $100, and shall forfeit any certificate theretofore granted under the provisions of this act.

The act regulating the practice of midwifery by others than legally authorized physicians in the City of Rochester forms Chapter 842 of the laws of the State of New York for 1895, and is, with slight modifications, a verbatim copy of the Erie County act. In Syracuse some time ago the local Board of Health passed a resolution compelling all midwives to register with the Clerk of Vital Statistics, but the County Clerk writes me that he does not think the city ordinance has been lived up to.

In regard to our own city, there is no law whatever regulating the practice of midwifery. The only restriction of any sort is contained in Section 5 of the Sanitary Code of the Board of Health, which requires midwives, as well as physicians, to register in the office of the Register. No qualifications whatever are or can be demanded of any person registering in that office as a midwife. Under the law, or absence of law, any person may practise midwifery.

There are at least five schools of midwifery in this city in which instruction is given and diplomas are issued.

This condition of things is certainly astounding in a civilized country at the end of the Nineteenth Century. Still, if the remedy is to be any kind of official recognition of midwives, and the establishment of one or more legally chartered colleges for midwives, or the appointment of examining boards with the right to grant certificates entitling the candidates to practise midwifery, then I prefer the present chaos, for the simple reason that it cannot last forever, and that it must lead to the enactment of a law by which midwifery, as all other branches of medical practice, is exclusively placed in the hands of the medical profession, where it belongs.

The conduct of labor used to be, and among uncivilized people still is, the exclusive domain of women. Originally any woman who had herself borne children assisted her friends during this ordeal, but in the course of time special authorized guilds of midwives were formed who alone possessed the right to practise the art, and who only called in a physician when they found themselves incapable of completing the delivery.

It was in the beginning of the Seventeenth Century that in Paris doctors first began to assume the direction of normal labor cases. As early as the year 1600 Charles Guillemeau and Honoré began to be in great request by most ladies of quality. Louyse Bourgeois deplores, of course, the immodesty and wantonness of the women of her day, which led them to prefer male physicians, even in ordinary labor.[1]

In England physicians were not employed in normal labors before the end of the last century, and

[1] Wm. Goodell: "A Sketch of the Life of Louyse Bourgeois," pp. 40-41. Philadelphia, 1876.

at first the so-called men-midwives met with great opposition. In Germany the old system obtained much longer, and to a great extent still exists, but it has become quite usual for well-to-do women to employ physicians instead of midwives. In Denmark, also, some years ago physicians began to be employed as accoucheurs.

The reason of this gradual domination of the field of midwifery by physicians is that the superiority of the new over the old system at once becomes manifest wherever it is tried.

I do not share the view of Louyse Bourgeois, who, with jealous eyes saw the advent of those dangerous competitors, and pretended it was only the wantonness of the coquettes that made them prefer the assistance of a physician to that of a midwife. Quite the contrary, many modest women have to conquer their natural aversion to the exposure of their person to the sight and touch of a male practitioner of midwifery, but they do so because experience has proved beyond contradiction the superiority of the physician over the midwife.

Of the thousands of midwives who have practised their art only four have given expression to their experience in printed books, three in France and one in Germany:

The oldest work is that of the above-mentioned Louyse Bourgeois (1609), but that of Charles Guillemean bears the same date. Justine Siegemundin published her "Königliche und Churbrandenburgsche Wehemutter" in 1690. Mme. Boivin dedicated her work in 1811 to Mme. Lachapelle, whose pupil she styles herself. In 1821 the latter published the first volume of her treatise on "The Art of Accouchement," the last two volumes of which were edited by her nephew, Antoine Dugès, Professor of Obstetrics at Montpellier.

Great as the experience and dexterity of these women may have been, the science and art of obstetrics is not a structure of their rearing, but of physiciaus, from Hippocrates down to the present time.

Obstetric work presents certain peculiarities which make it preeminently objectionable to tolerate its performance by half-taught or entirely ignorant persons. While in other branches of the healing art every case concerns the well-being or restoration to health of one human being, in obstetrics every case involves the fate of at least two individuals. Beside the specific services rendered by the obstetrician, at least three other specialties—internal medicine, surgery, and pediatrics — are more or less constantly involved. In no other department does prevention of evil play a similar rôle. For instance, a cross-presentation recognized before rupture of the membranes may be easily corrected by external version, and thus the necessity for difficult and dangerous operations at a later stage be averted. Very often the demand for immediate action is imperative, so that no time is left for examining books or consulting men of larger experience.

In no branch of the medical art has the inauguration of antiseptic measures wrought greater reduction in mortality. The records of the New York Maternity Hospital, from 1875 to 1883, show an average maternal mortality of 4.17 per cent., in some years running up to between six and seven per cent. During the last six months of this period it was eight per cent., and during the last month of the era referred to, even twenty per cent. After I had introduced strict autisepsis in that institution, the total mortality from 1884 to 1896 sank to 0.83 per cent., or less than one-fifth of what it formerly was.

So essential is antiseptic practice in obstetrics that, without much exaggeration, we may say that the term aseptic midwifery is synonymous with good midwifery, and likewise, septic midwifery with bad midwifery, no amount of personal skill being able in this department to counterbalance the risks connected with neglect of antiseptic precautions. In an apparently simple case the gravest operation may become necessary, and the choice of methods and results depend, first of all, on the aseptic condition of the genital tract.

In private practice the mortality is twice as large as in maternity hospitals, and, although we unfortunately cannot entirely exempt physicians from blame, this sad result is largely due to the employment of midwives. Even in European countries, with their strong governmental supervision, constant complaints are being uttered in regard to the inefficiency and short-comings of midwives. The average midwife is entirely incapable of foreseeing complications; and preach to her as much as you like, she will never grasp, still less carry out, the principles of antisepsis.

To take, as an example, one of the most common occurrences, a laceration of the perineum; if it is not of unusual dimensions the midwife may not be able to see it at all; or, if she observes the injury, she does not realize its importance, and it is to her advantage to conceal it. Thus, the patient is exposed to an infection which may cost her her life, or she may leave her bed possessing the germ of tedious gynecologic disease, while the honest physician will take proper measures to repair the injury, so that the woman regains her health and strength.

Children suffer still more from bad midwifery than their mothers. While still-births in Berlin occur in three per cent. of confinements, they reach nearly eight per cent. in New York. In New Jersey blindness due to ophthalmia neonatorum has increased five times more rapidly than the population.

Midwives not only do harm through their lack of obstetric knowledge, but they are most inveterate quacks. They treat, first of all, disturbances during the puerpery, later gynecologic diseases, then diseases of children, and are finally consulted in regard to almost everything. They never acknowledge their ignorance, and are always willing to give some advice. They administer potent drugs, such as ergot and opium. Their scarcely veiled advertisements in the newspapers show them to be willing abortionists; and since they have the right to give certificates of still-birth, who knows whether or not an infant's death is a natural one?

Although an evil, midwives are, however, in most countries a necessity, in view of the fact that physicians would be unable to find time to do the work. Not so here, where there is a superabundance of medical men. According to the last census the population of the United States on June 1, 1890, was 62,979,766; or, leaving out Alaska and the Indian Territory, 62,622,250. Of these 30,554,370 were females, only 15,742,636 of whom were of a child-bearing age (between fifteen and forty-nine years of age). At the same time there were 104,805 physicians and surgeons, which gives one physician for every 150 women of a child-bearing age; but women do not bear children every year; quite the contrary. We may estimate, even by a liberal calculation, that in America they, on an average, only give birth to four children in all; consequently, the number of women in the child-bearing period (thirty years) must be divided by about eight in order to find the average number of births *per annum*, which gives about nineteen confinements every year for each physician in the United States.

In the State of New York the total population was 5,997,853, of which 3,020,960 were females. Taking the proportion for the United States, this leaves 1,555,190 women of child-bearing age. Now, there were 11,139 physicians and surgeons, or 1 physician for every 139 women of child-bearing age, or an average of 17 births per annum in the State of New York.

In this city, that is the old New York as it existed when the last census was taken, the number of births becomes proportionally smaller. The total population was 1,515,301. Of these 767,722 were females, and by computation it is found that of these 395,556 were of a child-bearing age. As to physicians, the number of male physicians was 3206; that of the females is not specified, but the "Medical Directory" for 1897 shows that in that year there were 145, which gives a total of 3351 physicians and surgeons. Consequently there was one physician for every 118 women in the child-bearing age, or an average of but fifteen confinements yearly for each physician practising in the City of New York. Nobody will contend that physicians cannot easily attend to this number of confinements.[1]

Analogies cannot be drawn from European countries. New York has proportionally to the population nearly twice as many physicians as London, and the United States nearly three times as many as Great Britain. On the continent of Europe there are still fewer doctors, varying from about 1 in 2000 to 1 in 6,000 of the population.

Even the prejudice of those who object to the male accoucheur, can to a great extent be conciliated, as nowhere is there such a number of female physicians and nowhere better trained nurses than in this country. According to the above statistics there were in the United States 4557, in the State of New York, 693, and in the City of New York, 145 female physicians.

Another objection to the exclusive employment of physicians in confinements has been raised on financial grounds. Midwives, as a rule, charge a small fee, and some physicians a very large one for obstetric work, but with the great number of idle physicians, a woman can obtain the services of many a reputable practitioner during her confinement for the same price she pays to the midwife. And if she is too poor to pay even that modest sum, she can, at least in this city, with the greatest facility obtain gratuitous aid, either in a hospital or in her own home, as she may prefer. Of all medical charities none is so overdone as this. I am myself at the head of a department in a dispensary which sends an experienced accoucheur to the patient's home, and furnishes gratuitously all necessary materials, drugs, and medicines, and still only an insignificant number of women avail themselves of this privilege—freely advertised by means of a placard conspicuously placed in the dispensary referred to. What better proof can be offered that this form of charity is already much overdone?

Even in the country the physicians are able to attend to *all* labor cases, and, even if a woman cannot secure medical aid during her confinement, she is much better off when left alone or assisted by a friend than when provided with the services of a midwife.

Under these circumstances there might occasionally occur a tear of the perineum or a post-partum hemorrhage which might have been avoided by timely obstetric aid, but this danger is so small com-

[1] The State of Nebraska has set a good example by restricting all obstetric practice to those who have the degree, Doctor of Medicine.

pared with that of infection that it may be left out of consideration.

The institution of midwives is a remnant of barbaric times, a blot on our civilization, which ought to be wiped out as soon as possible. Since they have never been recognized by the State, except in a few minor instances, the attainment of such an object ought not to be difficult; but since they have been tolerated it would be necessary for the Legislature to enact a law declaring that only licensed physicians shall have the right to practise obstetrics.

The Legislature would not be justified in an endeavor to prevent one woman from assisting another in childbirth, any more than it would be in an effort to prevent one from advising the other to take a foot-bath, or to put a mustard plaster on her chest; but it certainly has the right to prevent a person from exposing a sign as a midwife and practising midwifery for a consideration. It would probably be necessary to respect the so called "vested rights" of those who at the time of the passage of the new law had been, by legal authority, engaged in the practice of midwifery.

It would be eminently proper for the Section of Gynecology and Obstetrics of this Academy to declare itself in favor of a bill restricting obstetric practice, after a certain date, to legally authorized practitioners of medicine; and it would be desirable to have such a bill indorsed by the Academy of Medicine, and by other societies.

If such a law cannot at present be obtained, it is better to leave the question of midwives as it is. Any law embodying a recognition of midwives and the establishment of colleges for their instruction would not only be injurious to the lawful and rational rights of the medical profession, but would result in great danger to the community at large. It would lead to a considerable increase in the number of midwives, while there would be unsurmountable difficulties in the way of legal supervision of them. If a demand for a law, such as the one I propose, be not acceded to by the legislators, the time is not far, when, nevertheless, it will surely be enacted, and any recognition or organization of midwives will only retard this happy hour, when our hopes in this matter will be realized.

As America has led the world in establishing colleges for the education of women physicians, let it also form the vanguard in a war of extermination against the pestiferous remnant of pre-antiseptic days, midwives, and schools of midwifery.

In accordance with the principle herein laid down I offer the following resolution, which I hope may receive favorable consideration from the Academy:

RESOLUTION.[1]

WHEREAS, midwifery, or obstetrics, is an important branch of medical science and art;

WHEREAS, midwives are not recognized by the State;

WHEREAS, Section 153 of the Laws of New York, 1893, Chapter 661, amended in 1895, prescribes penalties for any person who, without being then lawfully authorized to practise medicine within this State and so registered according to law . . . shall assume or advertise any title which shall show, or tend to show, that the person assuming or advertising the same is a practitioner of any of the branches of medicine;

WHEREAS, midwives by their ignorance and lack of cleanliness do great harm to parturient and lying-in women, and assume to administer potent drugs to them without the advice of a physician, and often treat sick women and children, and frequently are guilty of causing abortions.

Resolved, That the Section on Obstetrics and Gynecology strongly recommends the taking of immediate steps to secure the passage of a law providing for the supervision of all persons, not legally qualified physicians, now engaged in practising midwifery, and debarring from such practice all persons not proven to be competent and qualified; and also containing such provisions as, without conflicting with existing rights, shall tend to confine the practice of midwifery to qualified medical practitioners.

CLINICAL MEMORANDA.

A CASE OF FEVER WITH INTERCURREN PLEUROPNEUMONIA.[2]

BY PALMER C. COLE, M.D.,
OF NEW YORK.

DURING June of last year I was called to see H. G. male, aged thirty-two years. I reached his bedside a 12.30 A.M., and found him delirious and in a high fever temperature, 104.5 F.; pulse, 120. There was constan vomiting, and his conjunctiva was a deep yellow. Up t a few hours before he had been in apparent good health coming home in the evening at 9 P.M. after a hard day' work, eating a hearty supper, and about 10 P.M. he com menced to feel ill. At 11 P.M. he had a chill, and too 10 grains of quinin, a hypodermic injection of about 1½ grains of morphin, and went to bed. Vomiting and de lirium followed, in which condition I found him.

Subsequent investigation disclosed the fact that he wa addicted to the use of morphin, taking about a grain hy podermically every twenty-four hours, as he afterwar stated. Judging from symptoms, I concluded that th case was one of acute bilious fever complicated wit malaria. I prescribed calomel, soda, and sugar of mil (10 grains of each), to be followed by a seidlitz powde within a few hours if the bowels did not move. The cal

[1] Passed by the Section on Obstetrics and Gynecology of th New York Academy of Medicine, January 27, 1898.

[2] Read at a meeting of the Northwestern Medical and Surgic Society of New York, December 15, 1897.

omel and soda checked the vomiting, and the seidlitz powder was followed by five copious bilious evacuations. I now gave full doses of quinin, but observing no benefit from the administration of this drug, the dose was reduced the next day to 2 grains three times daily. I also slightly reduced his allowance of morphin, and, as the heart was weak, ordered strychnia sulph. gr. 1/60, and tr. digitalis, 1 minim, three times daily, to be taken alternately every four hours.

There was no improvement, and as I considered his condition critical Dr. Janeway was asked to see him in consultation. He was out of town, and the family called another physician who saw the patient without my knowledge, and who left me written advice to administer 10 grains of phenacetin every four hours, and also wrote that he would meet me the next day. The phenacetin was tried, with injurious results, causing emesis and loss of appetite. It was discontinued after the third dose and previous treatment resumed. The physician referred to was two hours and a half late in keeping his appointment, and in consequence I never met him.

On the morning of the fifth day incipient pneumonia of the left lung was detected. With this complication in a case in which the illness was already critical and the condition steadily growing more grave (pulse, 140; temperature, 104.6° F., respiration rapid, and a weak heart in spite of tonics and stimulants), I made up my mind there was but one hope, which lay in the application of the cold pack.

Having come to this conclusion, I sent for Dr. Simon Baruch.[1] Dr. Baruch was unable to meet me before 10 P.M., when examination showed that there was slight pleuritic effusion on the left side. Dr. Baruch advised the administration of 10 grains of calomel, which was at once given, and then the application of cold compresses was commenced under Dr. Baruch's personal supervision. The temperature of the water used was 65° F., and the compresses were renewed every hour. The cold pack in this case consisted of two heavy linen towels (without fringe, which is important) loosely stitched together and covered with white flannel. On removal the linen was thrown into a large tub of water kept at a temperature of 65° F., and the flannel was dried. The compresses extended from the neck to just below the base of the lungs.

In renewing compresses it is important that the patient *be not* raised in bed, but gently rolled over, a fresh compress taking the place of the one removed, and the patient gently rolled back. In addition to the application of the pack, the patient was sponged with cold water once or twice a day. Dr. Baruch met me the next morning, and, finding no improvement in the symptoms and no diminution of temperature, suggested the advisability of changing the packs every forty-five minutes. Though this was done, there was no improvement, but by evening the right lung was also invaded—without any increase of the affected area in the left, in which the condition seemed to remain stationary. The next morning, as the temperature and pulse were slowly climbing up, I ordered the cold compresses to be applied every half hour, but after about eight hours concluded such frequent changes were not beneficial, and returned to applications every forty-five minutes. This was continued for about eight days, by which time the temperature had fallen to 101° F.; respiration and heart-action decidedly improved, and then the cold compresses were stopped. Convalesence from this time on was slow but uneventful.

Morphin had been entirely withdrawn by the end of the second week, strychnin and digitalis taking its place, and when the patient finally resumed his work he was a well man. He had no recollection of what had occurred during a period of four weeks. He subsequently thanked me more for having cured him of his opium habit than for saving his life. I have not the slightest doubt that the patient owed his life to the persistent external use of cold water, and that under any other treatment he would have died.

[1] Twenty-five years ago I used cold sheets in typhoid fever, but had it not been for Dr. Baruch's invaluable papers and discussions on hydrotherapy, I should not have thought of applying this treatment in pneumonia.

RETROPHARYNGEAL ABSCESS ULCERATING INTO THE LEFT INTERNAL CAROTID ARTERY (?) FOLLOWED BY RIGHT-SIDED HEMIPLEGIA WITH APHASIA AND RECOVERY.

BY MELVIN M. FRANKLIN, M.D.,
OF NEW YORK;
SURGEON TO CHARITY HOSPITAL, AND TO THE OUT-PATIENT DEPARTMENT OF ST. JOSEPH'S HOSPITAL.

THIS case is reported because of its rather unique complications, the happy subsidence of ominous symptoms, and because of the extreme rarity with which such an affection is followed by restoration of health.

A. S., aged seven years, was first seen May 11, 1896. Upon examination it was found that the patient was suffering from a simple angina with very little tendency to any of the subjective symptoms of the affection; there was, however, a slight edema of the posterior wall of the pharynx. A gargle was prescribed, and it was ordered that the child be kept quiet. The next day I was hurriedly summoned, and found the patient in a state of collapse, with blood flowing from the nose and mouth. The child was stimulated with strychnia and atropin and the fluid extract of ergot was injected subcutaneously. Closer examination revealed a pulsating swelling on the left side of the neck. Ice and pressure were applied, and, as a coagulum had formed in the nose and the hemorrhage from the mouth had largely ceased (which might probably be explained by syncope), instead of looking immediately for the cause of the hemorrhage a pint of saline infusion was administered subcutaneously. After this the child's head was gently raised and the mouth opened, when blood was seen gushing from a point posterior to the left tonsillar pillar. With the view of applying pressure internally a soft catheter was introduced through the anterior, and brought out of the posterior nares, and a large piece of sponge was pulled tightly into the vault of the pharynx. The stimulants previously given now began to have some effect, and were continued at proper intervals, so that in the course of a couple of hours the child was in a fairly good condition. At four o'clock the same afternoon the patient was again visited, and the general condition found about the same, but aphasia, together with paralysis of the right side of the face and the right arm, was becoming marked. The paralysis rapidly developed until by six o'clock there was complete loss of sensibility and paralysis of the entire right side of the body, and also complete aphasia. The following morning the condition was much the same, with the exception of an increase in the pulse and a temperature of 101° F. For three days the general condition remained stationary, though the tumor in the side of the neck gradually disappeared. At the end of this time the nasal plugs were removed, after which there was some slight hemorrhage, but this was readily controlled by the use of local hemostatics. In the course of a month the child was able to be about, but could not walk unaided. Several months elapsed, however, before articulation was properly performed. At the present time (a year later) the patient has completely recovered the power of speech and suffers only from a slight disability in the use of the right arm and a talipes equinovarus, the latter being relieved by the use of proper apparatus.

As to the question from which artery the hemorrhage occurred, it is only necessary to glance at the subsequent symptoms to confirm the diagnosis of ulceration into the left internal carotid artery; for, explained in any other way, the case becomes a most remarkable pathologic coincidence. There is already in literature the report of a similar case which, unfortunately, terminated fatally. That the hemorrhage, in my case, should cease spotaneously seems highly improbable, although the nervous phenomena which followed point directly toward the establishment of the diagnosis named. It may be said that other causes than the one already suggested could have produced the hemiplegia, but why should two such unique morbid changes occur practically simultaneously, each bearing directly on the other, and yet so widely different in character? The condition might, again, have been caused by the marked ischemia resulting from the hemorrhage. Whether or not the paralysis was embolic in nature or due to cortical hemorrhage or thrombus, the chief causes of cerebral paralysis, it is difficult to determine, but without a previous constitutional diathesis it is most likely, in a child, to have been caused by an embolus of the middle cerebral artery—a terminal branch of the internal carotid.

SPECIAL ARTICLE.

THE LAPORTE CASE DUPLICATED IN WEST VIRGINIA.

BY T. A. HARRIS, M.D.,
OF PARKERSBURG, W. VA.

ON the 16th day of January, 1895, Dr. A. S. Keever of Belleville, accompanied by Dr. W. S. Keever of Parkersburg, called upon me at my house. Dr. A. S. Keever asked me to go down to the lower end of the County to operate upon a Mrs. Tice for ovarian tumor. The plan was to go to Belleville the next morning, from which point we were to go to Mr. Tice's house, eight miles from Belleville. Mrs. Tice was a patient of a Dr. Deem (of Tyner, Wood County, W. Va.). Dr. A. S. Keever stated to me at this time that he had seen Mrs. Tice the previous day (the 15th) in consultation with Dr. Deem, and that she had an ovarian tumor which Dr. Deem had previously tapped twice, but failed to empty the sac, as the fluid was too thick to run through the cannula. The little fluid that came away was of a dark, grumous character, and the small quantity removed did not make any impression upon the size of the woman's abdomen. He stated that there was no probability that pregnancy could be a complication, for, while he had made but little examination to determine this point, Dr. Deem had said that he had made a thorough examination and had repeatedly passed a sound into the uterus. They had agreed that she was suffering from blood poisoning and could live but a short time unless an operation was performed for the removal of the tumor.

I objected to going to the woman's house to operate, and stated that I thought the operation would be much more likely to succeed if the woman were first removed to Parkersburg, or even to Belleville. He said it was impossible to move her in her present condition, and he thought I would realize this when I saw her. He stated that it was a condition of emergency, and that if something was not at once done for her she would die, and that soon. I objected to doing the operation in this way, as I had but little expectation of its success, but as a matter of humanity I agreed that Dr. William Keever and I would go down the next morning and do the best we could for her. On the 17th, Dr. Keever and myself went down to Belleville, where we were joined by Dr. A. S. Keever: we rode eight miles up hill and down, over frozen roads and snow, to Mr. Tice's house. We found a small house with one fair-sized living-room, and one or two small rooms adjoining. In the living-room we found Mrs. Tice sitting in a chair; in the room was a bed and a stove. We expected to have met Dr. Deem there, but he had not yet arrived. I sat down by Mrs. Tice (the family were all strangers to me), made some superficial examination, and talked to her about her condition. She told me that the dropsy had been coming on during five or six months; that she had had a lump in her left side. She said that she was not able to lie down to sleep, but had sat in her chair during the last six weeks. The pulse was weak and frequent; temperature about 103° F. She had had chills; the skin was cool and moist; she presented the appearance and symptoms of one suffering not only from the presence of an abdominal tumor, which interfered with respiration, heart's action, and the functions of stomach and bowels, but also of a person suffering from toxemia, the source of which I took to be the tumor which had been tapped, but not emptied, and which was then, and had been for some time, leaking into the abdominal cavity from the hole made in it by the trocar. I told her that I thought we could relieve her of her trouble, but at the same time I explained to her the dangers and uncertainty of the operation which she would have to undergo. She said she wanted to be relieved of her present distressing condition, for she said she could not live as she was. She was willing and desirous that the operation be performed.

Dr. Deem not having arrived, we concluded to make all the necessary arrangements for the operation. By the time they could be completed we expected he would be on hand, as a messenger had been sent to his house, only a short distance away. We procured a table, and arranged it; the necessary vessels were provided, containing the antiseptics for the instruments and for the cleansing of the hands, etc.; also, towels soaked in antiseptic solutions. Mrs. Tice was placed upon the table for the purpose of a careful examination, and this without any anesthetic; the fact that an ovarian cyst filled the entire abdominal cavity was easily established; there was the mark of the trocar between the pubis and the umbilicus. The breasts were rather large and flabby, the areolæ being darkened in color and having numerous papillæ. Upon passing a finger into the vagina the os uteri was found sufficiently open to admit two fingers, and it projected between the labia so as to be plainly seen without the aid of either speculum or tenaculum. Presenting from within the uterus, just within the dilated os was the head of a dead fetus. At this time Dr. Deem arrived, and he was told of the condition of affairs, and was asked to make an examination, which he did. Then assisted by Dr. Wm. Keever, I proceeded to extract the dead fetus. The mouth of the womb was just within the external genitals, forced down by the pressure of the tumor above, and the efforts of Nature to expel the dead fetus.

In removing the fetus I introduced my fingers into the uterus, after making digital dilation, and with a small pair of forceps caught one foot and brought it down and out. In doing this the body was rotated within the uterus. Making some traction on this leg it came away at the hip-joint. The second leg came off in the same way. An arm, when drawn upon, parted at the elbow. It was plainly evident that the fetus was in a state of decomposition. Securing the pelvis of the fetus with a tenaculum, it was extracted, and the head retained within the uterus. I felt sure that with very slight traction the neck would part, and the head be left loose within the womb. I tried first the tenaculum, but this tore through the skull as it would through a piece of wet paper. I then asked for a blunt hook. Dr. A. S. Keever handed me a piece of ordinary wire slightly hooked at one end, which had been polished with a file and washed in an antiseptic solution. Guiding this wire with my finger, I thrust it into the skull which was just within the mouth of the womb, and extracted the head, the brain oozing out of the opening made by the tenaculum. The entire decomposing fetus had been extracted piecemeal. The cord was limp and flaccid, resembling a piece of tape; it easily parted from the fetus. The placenta was still adherent to the uterus, and was retained. No special effort was made to remove it for fear of hemorrhage from the flaccid uterus. I felt sure that coincident with the occurrence of uterine contractions the placenta would be expelled in the natural way, and also that I could not remove it at this time without the employment of more force than I felt was justifiable under the circumstances. During these procedures the woman laid upon the table without any anesthetic. She made little or no complaint of pain, and then only when I was dilating the mouth of the womb with my fingers.

Having cleansed everything connected with this part of the operation, we made a careful examination and found the woman in as good condition for the removal of the tumor as she was before the extraction of the dead fetus. As said before, up to this time, anesthesia had not been induced, as very little pain was complained of during the previous manipulations; the patient had not lost two ounces of blood, and was in full possession of all her faculties. It was decided to proceed with the operation for the removal of the ovarian tumor. Dr. A. S. Keever administered the anesthetic, while Dr. Wm. Keever prepared the surface of the body for operation, which he did with all antiseptic precautions, scrubbing the surface thoroughly with soap and water, shaving it with a razor, and then scrubbing it again with a solution of bichlorid of mercury, and finally applying towels wrung out in a solution of bichlorid. Everything now being ready, Dr. Wm. Keever and myself prepared ourselves by most thoroughly disinfecting our hands and arms. I took my place on one side of the table, Dr. Wm. Keever, as assistant, being on the other side, with Dr. Deem behind him to act in the capacity of general utility. Before the operation was begun Dr. Deem passed the catheter and drew off the urine.

Upon inspection of the abdomen it presented the appearance of a woman at about the eighth month of pregnancy. At a point about midway between the pubis and the umbilicus was seen the site of the puncture where tapping had been performed by Dr. Deem; the skin puncture had entirely healed. Making, then, an incision about five inches long between the navel and the pubis, the tense skin retracted and the tumor was disclosed, bearing upon its anterior surface the open pnucture of the trocar from which the cyst contents were slowly oozing. As there was already an opening in the tumor I did not think it necessary to try to empty it with a trocar at this stage; the opening in the abdominal wall was not long enough to allow so large a tumor to pass through it. The patient was brought near the edge of the table, and I seized the tumor with a pair of forceps at the point of puncture so as to close the opening. She was turned over on her side, nearly on her face, on the edge of the table. The tumor was then punctured with a bistoury, and its contents poured out into a bucket held by her father, assisted by Dr. Deem.

The cyst was multiocular and contained several smaller cysts within the large outer sac; these were successively punctured and emptied. When the tumor had been sufficiently emptied to allow it to be drawn out through the abdominal incision it was found to have no adhesion except a small pedicle connecting it with the left ovary. This pedicle was securely tied with a heavy silk ligature, and dropped back into the abdominal cavity. There being no adhesions, there was no weeping into the cavity. In the pelvis there was a small amount of what appeared to be leakage from the tumor, not more than a spoonful or two, which was carefully sponged out. The abdominal wound was sutured, dressed, and secured by a bandage, no drainage being provided. The woman was placed in bed, hot applications made to her body, and she gradually recovered from the influence of the anesthetic.

We remained in the house in all two or three hours. Before leaving I had quite a talk with the patient. She had entirely regained consciousness, and was not nauseated. She wanted to know if the tumor had been removed, how large it was, and asked various questions relating to herself. Her pulse and general condition were fairly good under the circumstances; temperature elevated, and skin warm. She expressed herself as being comfortable, and said it was a great relief to be able to lie down, and also that she "had some place to breathe now," respiration being much embarrassed previous to the operation. I parted with her expressing my hope and expectation that she would soon be well. She was left in charge of Drs. A. S. Keever and Deem. She was seen by them the next day, at which time, the placenta having become detached, it was removed and the uterus washed out with a disinfecting solution. She was at that time much in the same condition as before the operation; slightly weaker, and at times slightly delirious. Their prognosis was grave. She died before they met to see her the following day.

The case presents several points of unusual interest, the principal one being the unfavorable condition of the patient previous to operation; she was suffering from the well-marked symptoms of sepsis of such degree as would indicate an early fatal termination. She had been tapped for an ovarian cyst, which had not been emptied of its thick, dark, grumous contents, but was leaking into the abdominal cavity; whence, after undergoing decomposition, this material was absorbed into the general system, producing the blood-poisoning. She was at the same time carrying in her womb a dead and decomposing fetus of about four months. All the complications made a very unfavorable prognosis in an operation performed in a remote country house with few of the necessary comforts, and where she must be left to the nursing of well-meaning but ignorant relatives. It emphasizes the oft repeated advice, "Never tap an ovarian cyst unless you are prepared to operate for its removal." The presence of a dead fetus or a decomposing fetus is not often a complication of this operation. A notable thing, also, is the fact that the continual oozing of the fluid from a puncture of an unemptied cyst will prevent the adhesion of the cyst to the abdominal wall at the point of puncture.

But there is a point connected with this case of far greater interest to the medical profession in the State of West Virginia than anything furnished by its medical aspect. This case has been made the basis of a suit for malpractice against Drs. T. A. Harris, W. S. Keever, and A. S. Keever, and the damages laid at $10,000. The charge stripped of its verbiage is as follows: (1) That the fetus removed was alive; (2) that the mouth of the womb was cut open with a knife; (3) that the fetus was pulled out piecemeal and killed with a piece of rusty, unclean wire, which had been a piece of fencing wire; (4) that the placenta should have been removed at once; (5) that the operation for the removal of the ovarian tumor should not have been done at once, but some (an indefinite) time should have been allowed to elapse between the two (alleged capital) operations; (6) that in emptying the ovarian tumor of its contents a trocar should have been used, and it should not have been punctured with a knife; (7) that in puncturing it with a knife its contents were allowed to flow into the abdominal cavity; (8) that the abdominal cavity was not washed out with any chemic antiseptic.

These several charges were solemnly sworn to either by Dr. Deem or by Mr. Scott (the father of the woman) or by a Mrs. Canary (a relation of Mr. Scott's). When it was proposed to put on the witness stand the doctors concerned in the operation it was objected to by the prosecution, and an article was found in the Code of West Virginia which says, "that when one party to a suit is dead the other party shall not testify as to any communications or transactions had with the dead party." The learned judge in this case ruled that the term "transactions" applied to this case; that a surgical operation is a transaction; that the defense could not testify in their own behalf; could not give in detail the conversation which took place in Parkersburg, and which led to the operation; that Dr. A. S. Keever could not testify as to the conversation at his consultation with Dr. Deem two days before the operation, nor as to his examination of the patient at that time, nor as to his diagnosis made at that time; that neither Dr. Harris nor Dr. W. S. Keever could testify to what they said, saw, did, or thought within the room at the time of the operation upon Mrs. Tice, nor was Dr. A. S. Keever allowed to testify as to Mrs. Tice's condition the day after the operation, when he saw her for the last time, nor to testify to any conversation with Dr. Deem at that time. And it was further ruled among other things by the learned judge above referred to that no question should be put to any expert witness that was not based on the assumption that the evidence sworn to by the prosecution was true. The only persons present at the operation besides the doctors were the father of the woman, the grandmother, the husband, and a relative. Dr. Deem swore to certain of these charges as given above, Mr. Scott and Mrs. Canary swore to certain others; the grandmother was not produced as she was said to be out of the State. The husband did not testify as he is administrator of the estate of the deceased, and brought the suit. It was said that if he had testified the defendants might have been heard.

After the trial had continued ten days the jury disagreed, two being for the defense and ten for the prosecution. The case will, of course, be tried over again.

The comments I wish to make are as follows: No physician is safe in practising in West Virginia, if he loses a patient; it matters not whether the case be medical, surgical, or obstetric; if he is sued on the civil side of the court he will not be allowed to testify in his own behalf. If he is fortunate enough to be sued for a criminal act he may testify; no evidence of skill, ability, or experience will avail him, for the court holds that "The greater the ability and the more the experience the greater the responsibility." No legal process can be drawn that will relieve doctors from responsibility. The only help is to take disinterested witnesses to all surgical operations and cases of labor, or cases of serious illness, or to trust to the next Legislature to amend the law, or to give a different construction of the word "transactions" in the law referred to.

NOTE.—This case was again called for trial at the ensuing November term of the court. At that time the judge who had presided at the original trial was dead, and not one of the original attorneys in the case appeared for the plaintiff. He was represented by the stenographer of the original trial, and he pleaded that "he was unprepared for the trial and had not a witness present." The case was thrown out of court. During the session of the Legislature of 1897 the law was so amended as to allow physicians to testify in their own behalf. This same law, just as it was in West Virginia before being amended, is in the codes of a number of other States—notably in New York—a menace to all practitioners of medicine and surgery.

MEDICAL PROGRESS.

Rupture of the Callus in Fracture of the Patella.—BEGOUIN and AUDERODIAS (*Gaz. méd. de Paris*, October 23, 1897) have collected some of the published reports of fractured patellæ treated by the method advocated by Tilanus, *viz.*, by massage and early movements. They find that of thirty patients so treated, no less than seven suffered the accident of refracture through the callous. This percentage is so high that it must be taken into account in deciding on the best method of treatment of this condition. The two procedures which are to-day attracting the attention of surgeons are the methods of Tilanus, and the osseous suture. In point of view of rapidity of cure the former must give place to the latter; and when to this disadvantage is added the refracture of the callous in almost every fourth case treated by massage and early motion, the suture must be regarded as the method of choice.

A New Radical Operation for Inguinal Hernia.—BERNHARD (*Correspondenz-Bl. f. Schweiz. Aertzte*, November 1, 1897) advocates a new operation for the radical cure of inguinal hernia. The departure from previous operations consists in the separation of the testicle with its cord, the ablation of the tunica vaginalis, and the return of the organs in question to within the abdominal cavity, outside of the peritoneum. When this is accomplished, the accurate closure of the inguinal canal is comparatively a simple task. Bernhard has performed this operation upon two patients, each time with success. He has, of course, no means of knowing what the fate of the transplanted testicle may be. As a disadvantage of this method is mentioned the difficulty of diagnosis in case of a subsequent development in the transplanted testicle of such diseases as attack this organ, for instance, syphilis, tuberculosis, carcinoma, sarcoma, cysts, etc. A warning is given to those who perform this and other hernia operations to avoid, if possible, dividing the skin of the scrotum, as the probability of primary union is thereby much diminished.

Formula for Home Modification of Milk. — WESCOTT (*Archiv. of Pediat.*, January, 1898) is of the opinion that mixtures of cream and whole milk are more reliable and accurate than mixtures of cream and under-milk. He suggests the following simple and practicable formula:

Cream (12 per cent.) -	7 ounces, 2 drams
Whole milk - -	8 ounces, 1 dram
Lime water - -	2 ounces
Sugar of milk (dry) -	1¼ ounces
Water - - -	22 ounces, 5 drams.

This formula will give forty ounces of a mixture containing three per cent. of fat, six per cent. of sugar, and 1.5 per cent. of proteid. The advantage of a formula of this sort is that the fat and proteid may be gradually increased or diminished without frequent changing of the whole formula. To do this it is simply necessary to alter the amount of milk and cream in the mixture. Thus, in normal cases, a half ounce of milk may be added, that is, a teaspoonful more each day for four days in the week, this quantity to be maintained for the balance of the week. Then, if digestion is not disturbed the same increase may be directed for the next succeeding week, or possibly it may be necessary to omit the increase for a week—according to the condition of the child.

Disinfection of Houses with Formaldehyd. —JOHNSON (*Brit. Med. Jour.*, December 25, 1897) has obtained good results in disinfection of rooms by formaldehyd, liberating the gas under pressure from a mixture of equal parts of formalin, and twenty per cent. calcium chlorid solution. He has found formaldehyd lamps unsatisfactory. He also found it necessary to use larger quantities of formaldehyd than are generally advised, the best results being obtained upon using one pound of formaldehyd per 1000 cubic feet to be disinfected. At a cost of from twenty-five to thirty cents per pound the expense of disinfecting in this manner is not great for private houses. He made a number of experiments to determine the penetration of the gas in absolutely tight chambers, and in those having ordinary cracks. As a result, he has found it more serviceable to generate an excess of the vapor rather than to paste up cracks, though no large crevices or drafts should be permitted. For smaller articles the use of a portable chamber made of "enameled duck" having a projecting flap around the open end so as to be rolled up, with a corresponding flap of the cover, gave him good results.

On the Duration of Life of Epithelial Grafts.—WENTSCHER (*Centralbl. für Chir.*, January 8, 1898) has conducted experiments to determine the length of life of epithelial grafts outside the body. He preserved the grafts either in normal salt solutions, or dry, in sterilized gauze.

Later, these grafts were transplanted upon suitable surfaces (usually prepared by excision), such as granulating ulcers of the leg. The oldest graft which grew was twenty-two days old. Grafts which had been preserved dry for four weeks showed no evidences of growth after transplantation. Cold had very little effect upon them. It was found that grafts which had been kept frozen for fourteen hours, when thawed and placed upon a suitable surface grew without difficulty. Heat was more disastrous, a temperature of 50° C. (122° F.) in one case prevented the subsequent growth of a graft. Grafts are very easily affected by chemic influences. Even weak antiseptic solutions prevented their subsequent growth in every case, with one exception.

Soap as a Disinfectant.—TALBOT (*Diatet. and Hygien. Gaz.*, January, 1898) reviews the work of various experimentors and shows that soft soap in one-per-cent. solution is a valuable disinfectant for bacillus anthracis, cholera germs, for the bacteria of typhoid fever, and also for bacterium coli. Care, however, should be taken in the choice of potash soaps. The ordinary soft soap of commerce is often extremely unclean and possesses very little value. It is necessary to use a strong solution, and to wash the hands thoroughly with plenty of soap and water. Unfortunately, soap has no effect upon pus cocci. Almond soap was found to be more powerful than other varieties experimented with. It was also shown that soap containing antiseptics, *viz.:* benzol, carbolic acid, has less antiseptic power than the same amount of these substances without the soap. Therefore, the practice of manufacturing soaps with the addition of disinfectants is not founded on rational principles. The proper method of disinfecting the hands must still continue to be, first, washing them with soap, and afterward with the selected disinfectant.

Purulent Inflammation of the Fat Capsule of the Kidney.—MAASS (*Centrabl. f. d. Grenzgebiete d. Med. und Chir.*, December, 1897) draws some interesting conclusions from twenty-two cases of purulent inflammation of the fat capsule of the kidney. In all of these the perinephritic abscess was secondary to suppuration elsewhere. The source was usually in the kidney itself, although sometimes it was in an inflammation of the connective tissue of the pelvis. Such abscesses may also be secondary to inflammation in the thorax. The clinical symptoms are those of abscesses in general: fever, localized pain, pressure upon the colon, etc. The diagnosis is, in most instances, easy to make, especially if a tumor has formed in the lumbar region, or if edema of the skin presages the approach of pus; but in the very beginning of the trouble the diagnosis may be most difficult, even impossible. Treatment consists in evacuation of the pus by means of the most convenient incision. This is usually found to be an oblique one, beginning in the angle between the twelfth rib and the quadratus lumborum muscle and extending downward and forward a distance of seven or eight inches. The prognosis after operation is good. Sixteen of twenty-one patients treated by this method recovered.

Chronic Proctitis.—TALLEY (*Mathews' Quar. Jour. of Rect. and Gastro-Intes. Dis*, January, 1898) regrets that chronic proctitis has not yet received the study and attention which its importance demands. He insists that the only proper method of making a diagnosis of a rectal affection is by means of direct inspection. The use of Kelly's proctoscope, with a strong reflected light, will clear up many obscure cases. This instrument is better than a speculum and is less painful. In examination with a proctoscope the mucous membrane closes uniformly over the open end of the instrument as it is withdrawn. The patient may be placed in the lithotomy or knee-chest position, the latter being preferred when high examinations are to be made. Gonorrheal proctitis is common in prostitutes, the discharge from the vagina easily infecting the rectum, but is not found in men unless they practise pederasty. Non-specific chronic proctitis may occur as an acute inflammation, as a superficial ulceration, as a papillomatous vegetation, or it may involve the submucous tissue, causing proliferative stenosing proctitis. The main symptom of this former variety is slight tenesmus, with frequent mucopurulent stools, at times streaked with blood. The patient should be put to bed, and placed upon a bland diet. The sphincter muscle should be divulsed, and the ulcerated mucous membrane touched with a strong solution of nitrate of silver. The rectum should be irrigated daily with warm boric-acid solution. Injections of sweet oil and iodoform, and the introduction of suppositories of iodoform and boric acid are also grateful to the patient.

Proliferative stenosing proctitis never heals of itself. It may be treated palliatively by means of dilatation with rubber bougies, passed at intervals, though not oftener than every five days. If the stricture is very resistent an internal proctotomy should be performed to facilitate dilatation. This is an operation practically without danger when the stricture is not more than two inches above the external sphincter muscle. After division of the stricture divulsion of the rectum should be performed, and elastic bougies should be passed from time to time to avoid recurrence of the stenosis.

Recent Observations upon Cocain Poisoning.—GRIFFIN (*Phil. Med. Jour.*, January 8, 1898) calls attention to the variety of susceptibility and idiosyncrasy to cocain which different individuals present. Some patients who are acutely poisoned exhibit maniac excitement, while others are stupid. It is well known that poisoning has followed the use of a dose far short of the maximum therapeutic allowance, even .077 of a grain having caused serious symptoms. There are also instances in which a solution of a certain strength has been used without unpleasant effects, while a repetition of the same dose on a subsequent occasion has caused toxic symptoms. The injection of camphor dissolved in ether and the employment of artificial respiration have recently been extolled as the best treatment for the acute poisoning.

In chronic poisoning by cocain there is one symptom known as Magnan's sign, which is of considerable importance in establishing a diagnosis when the use of the drug is denied, and is also of importance in other cases as indicating to the physician the necessity for immediate discontinuance of the remedy. This sign is a hallucination of sensation, the patient complaining of feeling some foreign body beneath the skin. This is generally described as being small in size, and is usually ascribed to the presence of "sand," "worms," or "microbes."

THE MEDICAL NEWS.

A *WEEKLY JOURNAL*

OF MEDICAL SCIENCE.

COMMUNICATIONS are invited from all parts of the world. Original articles contributed *exclusively* to THE MEDICAL NEWS will after publication be liberally paid for (accounts being rendered quarterly), or 250 reprints will be furnished in place of other remuneration. When necessary to elucidate the text, illustrations will be engraved from drawings or photographs furnished by the author. Manuscripts should be typewritten.

Address the Editor: J. RIDDLE GOFFE, M.D.,
No. 111 FIFTH AVENUE (corner of 18th St.), NEW YORK.

Subscription Price, including postage in U. S. and Canada.

PER ANNUM IN ADVANCE	$4.00
SINGLE COPIES	.10
WITH THE AMERICAN JOURNAL OF THE MEDICAL SCIENCES, PER ANNUM	7.50

Subscriptions may begin at any date. The safest mode of remittance is by bank check or postal money order, drawn to the order of the undersigned. When neither is accessible, remittances may be made, at the risk of the publishers, by forwarding in *registered* etters.

LEA BROTHERS & CO.,
No. 111 FIFTH AVENUE (corner of 18th St.), NEW YORK,
AND NOS. 706, 708 & 710 SANSOM ST., PHILADELPHIA.

SATURDAY, FEBRUARY 19, 1898.

THE NEW YORK CITY BOARD OF HEALTH AND THE BRUSH BILL.

IN last week's issue we had occasion, in connection with the bill before the Legislature restricting the powers and acts of the Board of Health of New York City, to comment in general upon the excellence of the work of this board and the credit it had reflected upon the community and the country. One feature of the bill, that bearing upon the management of pulmonary tuberculosis, was treated in detail. Judging from the notices in the secular press and in some contemporary medical journals, there apparently exists such a shadowy notion in regard to the provisions of the Brush Bill that it seems wise to present more in detail the main features of this measure.

1. The clause in the former bill restricting the presidency of the Board of Health to a layman is stricken out, thus opening the possibility of that office being occupied by a member of the medical profession, although the health-officer of the port is debarred from holding the position. This provision seems eminently wise. There is no reason why the president of the board should not at times be a physician.

2. The board is reduced to five members, consisting of the health-officer of the port and four commissioners appointed by the mayor, two of whom shall be physicians. The president of the police board, who was formerly a member, is thus excluded. This provision is of little moment, and is as unnecessary of discussion as it was of insertion in the hill.

3. The term of service is changed from six to four years. This brings the tenure of office in correspondence with that of the mayor, and so savors more of politics than of statesmanship.

4. The clause empowering the board to produce diphtheria antitoxin or other antitoxins is stricken out, and all authority to relieve, by antitoxin treatment, persons suffering from diphtheria or other infectious disease is omitted, as well as the power of disinfection in these diseases. The cunning hand of some ardent opponent of antitoxin seems to be apparent here. As we read the revised bill, no authority to produce, to use, or to distribute antitoxin is given the board. Indeed, all detailed reference to diphtheria is stricken from the law, the disease simply being mentioned as one of the infectious, contagious, or pestilential diseases. What more startling announcement could come thundering in the ears of an intelligent community, to say nothing of those interested in and conversant with sanitary measures, than that there has been taken away from the sanitary authorities and the medical profession in conjunction therewith, the power and the privilege of reducing the death-rate of diphtheria in New York City from 35.2 per cent. during the four years preceding 1895 (when antitoxin was first employed) to 16.3 per cent. for the three years following that period, and to 14.6 per cent. during the year 1897? The medical profession of the city has come to rely so implicitly upon the diphtheria antitoxin of the Board of Health that during the past year 1100 cases of diphtheria were treated without charge by the Board of Health at the request of the attending physicians. These patients were reported by the physician in charge as being too poor to pay for his visits.

5. The power to afford gratuitous vaccination to and among the poor is retained, and the board is empowered "to procure and preserve pure vaccine lymph or virus." No authority is given to produce vaccine lymph, and yet, as shown in our editorial of last week, the Board of Health, by experimentation in its laboratories during the year 1896, brought

vaccine lymph to a higher standard of perfection than was previously known.

With all due consideration of the economic principle that subsidized institutions should not be allowed to compete with private enterprise, and with all respect to the private commercial drug-houses who supply the profession and the community with other high-grade pharmaceutic preparations, we would submit the proposition that in an enterprise involving so much scientific experimental work and in which so much is at stake, involving an almost complete revolution in the principle of therapeusis, an exception can justly be made. We trust, however, that the time is not far distant when the art of producing biologic products will have reached such a definite, settled basis as will permit commercial competition to be a sufficient motive, not only to maintain but to advance the excellence of these preparations. It is to be hoped also that when that time arrives sufficient public funds will be placed at the disposal of the Board of Health to enable it to carry on its laboratories without the necessity of selling any of its products. By private letters received from the H. K. Mulford Company and from Parke, Davis & Company assuring us that they are now producing the most highly concentrated product that has ever been offered to the medical profession, the realization of hopes in the direction referred to seems already at hand.

6. Every physician is obliged to report every birth occurring in this city at which he may be present under the penalty of a fine of $100. This is an apparent injustice. Physicians are frequently called to poor women for the purpose of correcting some malposition in obstetrics, for which they receive no remuneration whatever, and yet they are obliged to be at the expense and trouble of reporting such births or be fined $100. In England a fee of $1 is allowed for every birth reported.

7. On the same penalty for omission, physicians are required to report all cases of infectious, contagious, or pestilential disease within twenty-four hours after the nature of the disease is ascertained or suspected. The following diseases are named as being embraced in this classification: Measles, diphtheria, scarlet fever, smallpox, chickenpox, typhoid fever, typhus, cerebrospinal meningitis, Asiatic cholera, and yellow fever. Evidently the intent of this clause was to exclude pulmonary tuberculosis, but, in doing so, as was pointed out in these columns last week, a number of well-recognized infectious and contagious diseases have been omitted.

Several other minor changes have been made in the wording of the bill, but the provisions already mentioned are the principal ones requiring attention. With the exception of the clause first named, they all show ill-considered preparation and in their entirety so restrict the sphere of action of the health authorities as to menace the welfare and health of the community. The bill should be withdrawn.

WHAT'S IN A NAME?

It is a phrase often quoted that the rose by any other name would smell as sweet, and this saying not only has the advantage of being ancient but likewise truthful. Many persons interested in the development of a health service in this country have expressed a well-meaning and undoubtedly honest objection to the name of the Marine Hospital Service as indicative of a service caring for the public health.

It is true that the name Marine Hospital Service does not indicate specifically all the functions which this department performs. It was baptized 100 years ago by our respected forefathers, and that they did not have the gift of foresight and prophecy is not extraordinary. It is not always that christening produces results which entirely suits later conditions of life. A child may be baptized Napoleon Bonaparte Smith, and turn out to be a character more befitting the name of Peter Cooper Smith. The fact that he was christened Napoleon Bonaparte does not necessarily mean that he is expected to pass through the world performing the same sort of volcanic upheavals as his namesake, but it none the less cripples him in the performance of duties to which he is by training and instinct better fitted. The growth and development of the Marine Hospital Service in the line of its work as a public health service has been gradual and satisfactory. Were it specifically named The Public Health Service a closer designation of one of its important functions would probably be attained, but that it is not so designated is not an insuperable objection to its continuing in the performance of work which it has satisfactorily accomplished in the past, and is performing with equally good results in the present.

The health interests of Great Britian are under the supervision of the Local Government Board, a title which no one will claim indicates just what its duties are, but there seems to be no demand in England for a change of this title so long as the work is properly performed. The Department of the Interior scarcely describes the variety of work which is continually and satisfactorily being performed under this name. No one seriously undertakes to suggest changing the name of this department of the Government, because the title does not accurately express all its duties. In fact a common instance of misapplication of names is the term "quarantine service" or "quarantine station." This term originally meant a forty-days' detention of ships or persons coming from infected places, a regulation which does not exist at the present day, and has been entirely superseded by modern and intelligent methods of disinfection and control. It would be better to substitute another word for this wherever it occurs, but it has become so fixed in our vocabulary that its eradication would be impracticable.

The Marine Hospital Service is an old organization, and has made its reputation under its present name. The public are so used to it that if it were sailing under another name they would have to become educated to the fact that it was not a new organization that was doing its work. It is known from Maine to California and from the Lakes to the Gulf, as our political orators would say. There is no demand for a change of name, and but for the fact that it has been suggested by interested and well-meaning gentlemen who think it is a serious obstacle to the Service becoming the representative health organization of the country, it seems to us that the objection is unimportant, and has no bearing upon the real question. The Service performs its duties satisfactorily considering the limited powers at present entrusted to it, and so long as it does this there need be no discussion as to the colors under which it sails.

ECHOES AND NEWS.

A Medical Senator.—Dr. Samuel Pozzi, the eminent French gynecologist, has been elected Senator for Dordogne.

The Registration of Midwives.—Meetings in support of a bill providing for the registration of midwives are being held in various parts of England.

Fees in Insanity Cases.—In Kansas, jurors who serve in cases in which the sanity of an individual is to be determined, do not receive a fee unless they find a verdict of insanity.

Motor-Cradles.—The latest scientific addition to the nursery is the motor-cradle. It is a question, however, whether babies should be rocked either by machinery or by hand.

Typewriters' Cramp.—According to the *Phonetic Journal* one of its correspondents is suffering from this new form of occupation neurosis as a result of a too assiduous use of the typewriter.

Appointments at Mt. Sinai.—At a meeting of the Board of Directors of Mt. Sinai Hospital, New York, held February 13th, Drs. Morris Manges and Nathan E. Brill were appointed Visiting Physicians to the hospital.

Department of Hydrophobia.—A department of hydrophobia, similar to the Pasteur Institute in Paris, is to be added to the Institute for Infectious Diseases in Berlin, of which Robert Koch is director.

Deportations from State Hospitals.—During the past year the New York State Commission in Lunacy has sent to other States and countries 110 alien and non-resident inmates of the New York State hospitals.

Individual Drinking-cups.—The Columbus (Indiana) Health Board has issued an order requiring the pupils of the public schools to provide themselves with individual drinking-cups. The board is also in favor of individual communion services.

The American Medical Association and Dr. Busey.—Dr. Samuel C. Busey of Washington, who was appointed to deliver the address on State Medicine before the American Medical Association in Denver, has resigned the appointment on account of ill-health.

Medical Popes.—According to the *British Medical Journal*, several of the Roman Pontiffs were students of medicine in their youth, and one, John XXII., who reigned at Avignon from 1316 to 1334, was a qualified doctor according to modern ideas, and wrote medical works.

Louisiana's New Board of Health.—Governor Foster recently announced the appointment of the following gentlemen as members of the new State Board of Health: Drs. Edmond Souchon, John J. Castellanos, L. F. Reynaud, Luther Sexton, H. S. Lewis, Messrs. S. O. Thomas, J. W. Castles, J. D. Hill, and J. C. Denis.

Second Quinquennial Prize.—The second quinquennial prize of $1000 dollars will be awarded on January 1, 1900. This prize, under the will of the late Samuel D. Gross, M.D., is to be awarded every five years to the writer of the best original essay upon some subject in surgical pathology or surgical practice founded upon original investigations. The candidates must be American citizens.

Another Verdict for a Hospital. —Justice Stover, in the Supreme Court, New York City, recently dismissed a suit brought against the Montefiore Home by Alexander Burshell for $100,000 damages for the death of his son who was killed by falling through the elevator shaft while a patient at the Home. Justice Stover held that charitable institutions are not responsible for the acts of their employes.

Tennessee State Board of Health.—The death of Dr. J. Berrien Lindsley, as formerly announced, left vacant the responsible position of secretary of the State Board of Health, with which organization he had been connected many years. Dr. J. A. Albright, at that time president of the board, we learn, has resigned his office and has been elected to succeed Dr. Lindsley. Dr. Albright has our congratulations and best wishes.

Unmerited Criticism.—The *New York Medical Journal* calls attention to the fact that the *Journal de Médecine de Paris* for January 16th states that Mr. Cornelius Vanderbilt has employed Dr. Jean Charcot as his physician for a cruise upon his steam yacht, and remarks that it thinks Dr. Charcot does not do great honor to his father's name by accepting a place as physician and nurse which would be more suitable for an indigent student.

Opposition to the Dispensary Bill.—At a conference of representatives of dispensaries of Greater New York recently held, the bill to regulate dispensaries, now in the hands of the Committee on Cities, was opposed as being harmful and unwarranted. A resolution in opposition to the bill was carried by a vote of 41 to 2, the representatives of the Northeastern Dispensary and of the East Side Dispensary, respectively, alone voting in the negative.

The Brush Bill Condemned by Central Labor Union.—At a recent meeting of the Central Labor Union of New York, one of the delegates attacked the bill which cripples the work of the New York Board of Health by prohibiting the manufacture and sale of vaccine virus and antitoxin. He characterized the bill as vicious and a direct blow at the praiseworthy and successful efforts of the Board of Health in keeping down the death-rate. A resolution condemning the bill was passed, and it was ordered that a copy of the resolution be sent to each member of the Legislature.

Dr. Weir Mitchell's Novel.—According to the *Bookman* Dr. Mitchell's book "Hugh Wynne" is about the second in popularity at the present time. A review has appeared in the *Friend's Intelligencer* of Philadelphia, and also in pamphlet form, the avowed object of which is to correct some of the descriptions given in Dr. Mitchell's book of the manners and customs of the Friends at the time of the Revolution. The resultant of this is a sketch of the old-time Quakerdom of the City of Brotherly Love which might never have been brought out had it not been for the "mistakes" of Dr. Mitchell.

Obituary.—Dr. John Cronyn, one of Buffalo's prominent physicians, died there February 11th. Dr. Cronyn was born in Ireland, obtained his degree of M.D. at the University of Toronto, and settled in Buffalo in 185[illegible] He was an ex-President of the Medical Society of th State of New York.—Dr. George C. Briggs, a prominer Vermont physician, died in his carriage of heart disease at Burlington, Vt., February 11th. Dr. Briggs was sixty eight years old, was graduated from the University of Michigan School of Medicine, and for ten years was Pro fessor of Materia Medica in the University of Vermont

Kipling's Estimate of American and Other Practitioners.— Rudyard Kipling, the poet novelist, in an after-dinne speech at a banquet given in London to Sir Williar Gowers not long since, paid a graceful tribute to th heroism of the medical fraternity. He had mixed wit doctors, he said, the world over, and had seen them go ing to certain death with no hope of reward. He ha seen them handling cholera and smallpox, and, when dy ing therefrom, telegraphing for a substitute. He had see them, in America, manage a practice twenty miles in eac direction, driving horses through eight feet of snow t attend an operation ten miles away, digging their horse out of the snow and then proceeding on their way. Mr Kipling declared that it was one of the proudest things of his life to have been associated with "real fighting me of this class."

Charity Abuses in Michigan.—Recent information froi Detroit leads to a belief that an earnest effort will be mad there to combat the growing dispensary evil. In this re spect, as in many others, New York has set a good ex ample, which we are glad to know is being followed b our brethren throughout the country; though it is to b hoped that they will not injure the prospects of reform atory measures by an internecine strife such as at preser characterizes the position of New York physicians on th question of a bill to abolish medical charity abuses— measure of such vast importance, not only to physician but, on a general economic basis, to the people at larg In Michigan the abuse referred to seems especially rife the free dispensary of the University Hospital at An Arbor, and it is against this institution that criticism particularly leveled.

The Marine Hospital Service and National Quarantine.— It is somewhat gratifying, after several months spent l the MEDICAL NEWS in presenting the various aspects this subject, to note that the *New York Medical Journ* and the *Medical Record* have rallied to the support the Marine Hospital Service and united with the MED ICAL NEWS in indorsing the Caffery Bill establishing National Quarantine in charge of that department of go ernment. The quarantine convention recently held at M bile, Ala., discussed the various phases of quarantine in d tail, but failed to pass a resolution indorsing any of the bi now before Congress. Doubtless the discussion in the co vention was a source of enlightenment to the various i terests represented regarding the necessity of uniform in law and practice.

Smallpox in North Carolina.—This disease has be hovering along the southerly borders of the "Old No State" for several months. It has been said that as ma as thirty Georgian counties have been infected; the disease has also made its appearance at Rock Hill, S. C., but it was not known until quite recently that a case had entered the North State. That case was at last brought into Wilmington, in the person of a colored train-hand, whose "run" took him frequently into South Carolina. The editor of the *Bulletin* of the State Board of Health, Dr. Lewis, sounds a note of warning to the local health authorities that the time has come for each and all of them to proffer free vaccination in their respective precincts. He further remarks that the number of persons in that State who have never been vaccinated at all is so great that he and other sanitarians view the situation with alarm.

Dr. Kelsey and the Post-Graduate.—Dr. Charles B. Kelsey of New York recently applied to the Supreme Court of the city for a writ of mandamus directing the Board of Directors of the New York Post-Graduate Medical School and Hospital to reinstate him as professor of surgery in that institution, a position which he held from March, 1890, until January 27, 1898, when he was removed without a hearing by the Board of Directors of the institution. Charges of disloyalty toward the hospital had previously been preferred against him. Dr. Kelsey was removed by a vote of 6 to 1. The by-laws provide that a vote of three-fourths of the board, which numbers eleven, is necessary for a removal, so the question of the legality of the removal rests upon whether this means three-fourths of the whole Board, or three-fourths of those present and voting. Decision was reserved.

CORRESPONDENCE.

THE DISPENSARY BILL.

To the Editor of the MEDICAL NEWS.

DEAR SIR: Your allusion in a recent issue of the MEDICAL NEWS to my opposition to the Dispensary Bill seems to call for a reply on my part; indeed, I am glad to have this opportunity to place this bill before the medical profession in its true light.

In the first place, you are mistaken if you think the Chairman of the Legislative Committee of the Medical Society of the State of New York is the only person opposed to the measure under consideration, for my action is endorsed by the whole committee, by the officers of the State Society, and by the majority of the medical men of the State. It is safe to say that not one-fourth of the profession of the city of New York would endorse this bill if its true character were known; I doubt very much if you would. Let me place before you some of our objections to it:

This bill provides that after its passage all dispensaries must make application in writing, accompanied by such statements, verified by oath, as may be necessary, to the State Board of Charities for a license. If this board believes that the operations of said dispensary will be for the public good a license shall be issued; "but that no dispensary shall enter upon the execution, *or continue the prosecution* of its purpose unless licensed in this way."

The bill gives the State Board of Charities absolute power to make such rules governing dispensaries as it may deem proper, to alter or amend the same at will, and to revoke licenses at pleasure. In other words, it takes away from the medical profession and the Boards of Managers of all dispensaries in the State of New York any voice in the management of these institutions, and vests this power in a State Board, political in its character and subject to change at any time. Now we ask you and we ask the medical profession if this is just? Is this what we have been striving for for several years?

What would be the effect of a law of this kind? Under Chapter 771, Laws of 1895, the State Board of Charities has the right to maintain a general supervision over all institutions of a charitable or eleemosynary character, incorporated or unincorporated, whether State, county, or municipal, and to call upon the Attorney-General of the State, or the district attorney in any county, to enforce its rules; further than this no institution can receive money from the county or State if the State Board of Charities objects. Is this not power enough? With all this power, the State Board of Charities has done little or nothing! If the present dispensary bill should become a law is there any reason to suppose they would do any more? The law would in all probabilities become a dead letter, and the medical profession, instead of being benefited, would be prevented from doing anything further in its effort to remedy dispensary abuses. On the other hand, the State Board of Charities could, on October 1st, close every dispensary in the State of New York. When it comes to dispensaries in drug-stores and tenement-houses, we have little to say. If it is in the interest of the public to close them, we would be willing to assist any effort in that direction, but we will oppose to the end any effort the consequences of which would be to place a weapon so terrible in the hands of any State board. The dispensaries in the State would be in a constant condition of uncertainty, which would seriously cripple their usefulness; trust moneys, instead of being used to benefit the poor, would be diverted to purposes for which they were never intended; *i.e.*, defraying the expenses of endless litigations, and in the end the medical profession would receive the contumely it would deserve if it allowed so pernicious a measure to go unchallenged. The question is naturally asked if there is no way in which this matter can be adjusted, and in answer I beg to refer the members of the Medical Society of the County of New York to the minutes of the meeting of May 24, 1897. It is recorded that over seventy-seven per cent. of institutions of this city expressed their willingness to correct any abuses that might exist in the dispensaries. Let the medical profession of the State, through representatives of the State and county societies, get together and confer with the boards of managers of the various institutions, and with the State Board of Charities if necessary, and there is no doubt a satisfactory solution of this vexed question could be found which would be just to all concerned.

I believe I have said enough to show my position in this matter, but I voice the sentiment of the Legislative

Committee, if referred to, when I say that we feel that we would be false to the trust imposed in us if we did not protest against a bill so manifestly unjust to the medical profession and to the community at large as the present Dispensary Bill.

Very truly yours,
FRANK VAN FLEET,
Chairman of the Committee on Legislation of the Medical Society of the State of New York.

116 EAST EIGHTY-SECOND STREET,
NEW YORK, February 7, 1898.

VIBRATORY THERAPEUTICS.

To the Editor of the MEDICAL NEWS.

DEAR SIR: My attention has been called to a historic article on vibratory therapeutics from the pen of Dr. Frederick Peterson which appeared in a recent issue of the MEDICAL NEWS. Doubtless in the preparation of his article the writer was ignorant of the fact that in the second edition of my work upon nervous diseases (H. C. Lea's Sons, 1881) I described and depicted a vibrator of my invention which I had used since 1879. This, so far as I know, was the first *perculeur* in which electricity has been employed, and is, I believe, to-day the best, because of the fineness of its vibrations. Some years ago I purchased a motor instrument from Gaiffe of Paris, which is more compact than those the Doctor describes, and this, too, he appears not to have seen. After many years use of vibratory therapy I am now convinced that its value its greatly exaggerated, and depends more upon the creation of suggestion than anything else, in which conclusion I think I am supported by Dr. Dana, who has gone fully over the ground. This form of treatment has been so popular with hypochondriacs that a few years ago a company with a large capital was formed here to exploit a "household" vibrator, of which nothing is now heard.

ALLAN MCLANE HAMILTON, M.D.,
44 EAST TWENTY-NINTH STREET,
NEW YORK, December 29, 1898.

OUR PHILADELPHIA LETTER.

[From our Special Correspondent.]

THE INVESTIGATION OF HOSPITALISM—CONTAGIOUS DISEASES DURING 1897—THE STATE QUARANTINE —PHILADELPHIA HOSPITAL'S NEW BUILDING— THE DELIVERY OF MILK IN SEALED JARS—LUCIEN MOSS HOME FOR INCURABLES—MASS-MEETING IN FAVOR OF THE FILTRATION BILL.

PHILADELPHIA, February 12, 1898.

IT is difficult to conceive a more complex undertaking than the effort, now in its inception in this city, to eliminate "hospitalism." If undertaken in a spirit of fanaticism directed toward hospital physicians as a class, as seems the inclination of some agitators, the movement must surely stir up such hostility among this class of the medical profession that cooperation will be impossible, and the outcome will be profitless. On the other hand, if undertaken with conservatism and with the help of representative local medical societies, the evil may be remedied to the satisfaction of all. The movers in this pending attempt at reform must necessarily represent all classes of respectable regular physicians—the general practitioner, faculties of the medical schools, and the physicians connected with the various city hospitals. The officers of the Charity Hospital, who are the prime movers in this inquiry into the question of indiscriminate free treatment by hospitals, are inclined to adopt a rational and sensible method of procedure, by inviting the attention of the County Medical Society to their plans, and by asking this body to act with them in the matter. This is to be done at the next meeting of the Society, on February 23d, until which time the precise method of beginning the investigation must remain a matter of conjecture. Meanwhile, the daily press is taking up the matter, and throws open its columns to every one who may choose to express his views, with the result that fictitiously signed letters from holders of medical degrees (?) have begun a tirade against hospital physicians which cannot but reflect unjustly upon the objects of their disapproval; for how is the newspaper-reading public to discriminate in a matter of this sort? Undoubtedly hospital abuses exist, but they should be remedied by the profession itself, and an editorial throttle should be applied to the rantings of the many disgruntled correspondents whose anonymous expressions only retard real progress toward a solution of the difficulty, and help to breed in the minds of an impressionable public a preconceived biased view of the actual situation. Apropos of this topic, it may be remarked that Director Riter, of the Department of Public Safety of this city, has written to Dr. Frederick Holme Wiggin of New York demanding an explanation of a charge that "in some instances policemen are paid $1 or $2 for each patient they bring to the hospital," made by Dr. Wiggin in his address on the hospital question at last week's meeting at the Charity Hospital. The outcome of this will be watched with interest, for the charge has caused a sensation in local medical circles and in the police department.

The annual report of Dr. William M. Welch, physician in charge of the Municipal Hospital for Contagious Diseases, shows that during the year 1897 more patients were admitted to the hospital than during any previous year in its history, the number exceeding even the totals of 1871 and 1872, when smallpox was very prevalent here. Dr. Welch attributes this increase not to an extraordinary prevalence of contagious diseases last year, but to the strict enforcement by the health authorities of the law requiring the placarding of infected houses, with the alternative of removal of the infected inmates to the city's hospital, and to the growing popularity of this institution. The incease in the number of admissions to the Municipal Hospital during the last eight years is shown by the following summary: 1890, 52; 1891, 127; 1892, 480; 1893, 524; 1894, 810; 1895, 1191; 1896, 1252; 1897, 2179.

The quarantine officers of this State are protesting against the passage of a bill now before Congress which, should it become a law, would seriously interfere with the power of State quarantines, by allowing a vessel to enter port with a clean bill of health from the government quarantine officials, regardless of the certificates of the State and local authorities. Inasmuch as the Pennsylvania State Quarantine Service has proved its usefulness in numerous instances in which the government officers have passed vessels requiring a later detention, it does not seem that the passage of this pending bill is quite justified. Philadelphia, at any rate, does not feel that the power of her State and city authorities should be curtailed in such a summary manner.

The Board of Charities are endeavoring to secure for immediate use an appropriation of $60,000 from Councils to complete the new additions to the insane department of the Philadelphia Hospital. This sum, which, like the filtration bill is delayed by councilmanic inactivity, is urgently needed to provide heating apparatus for the new building, which cannot be occupied until this provision is made. The new building will afford accommodations for 1400 patients, while the present quarters of the insane department, which are intended for but 1050 inmates, actually contain 1340.

Arguments for and against the practice of delivering milk to customers in sealed glass jars, now largely adopted here, took place this week before the Board of Health. The question arose from a petition recently presented to the board by a local dairymen's association, asking for the passage of an ordinance prohibiting the distribution of milk in glass jars, on the ground that this custom tends toward the dissemination of disease. Thus far, the evidence produced by the complainants has not been of a very convincing nature, when opposed to arguments in favor of the glass-jar system by such authorities as Mr. William Gordon of the Walker-Gordon dairies; Dr. J. Cheston Morris, whose dairy-farm in Chester County is considered a model of its kind; Dr. Meade Bolton, of the New Jersey State Laboratory of Hygiene; and Dr. Ravenal, Bacteriologist of the Pennsylvania State Live Stock Sanitary Board. Another hearing will be given the oppositionists at a later date, and the Board of Health promises to make a thorough investigation of the whole matter before delivering an opinion.

The erection of the buildings of the Lucian Moss Home for Incurables of the Jewish Hospital will be commenced within a short time, the present delay being due to the auditing of the accounts of the donor, whose will is still under legal consideration. The Jewish Hospital received last week a gift of $10,000 to the endowment fund of the institution, in memory of the late Ida M. Fleisher.

That the people of Philadelphia have awakened to the fact that something must be immediately done to provide a pure water-supply was amply and emphatically demonstrated at a mass meeting held at Horticultural Hall, on February 12th, under the auspices of the City Organizations' Committee, for the purpose of forcing Councils, through public opinion, to remedy the trouble by at once passing a bill creating a loan for the establishment of a filtration-plant. Representatives from all classes of citizens were present at this meeting, and definite demands were made that immediate steps be taken to eradicate the present typhoid epidemic by providing a new water-supply for the city. Members representing the following bodies were present at this popular demonstration: the College of Physicians of Philadelphia, the Philadelphia County Medical Society, the Health Protective Association, the Board of Trade of Philadelphia, the Trades' League, the Civic Club, the New Century Club, the Union Labor League, and many other societies, building associations, and hospitals. Addresses were made by Frank J. Firth, chairman of the committee, by Judge Ashman, by Rabbi Krauskopf, by Dr. S. Solis Cohen, by William Waterall, and by Dr. John K. Mitchell. Resolutions were unanimously adopted for presentation to Councils, urging immediate action for the creation of a loan "for the purification and filtration of the city water-supply, under direct municipal control, ownership, and management, and in no other way." This is the second indication of the popular mind presented to the notice of the city legislators this week. On February 10th, Councils' Committee on Water gave a hearing to the views of representatives of local medical societies and municipal organizations, who joined forces for the occasion, to urge upon Councils the necessity for the installation of a filtration-plant at the earliest possible moment. At this hearing the following organizations were represented: the College of Physicians of Philadelphia, by Drs. John K. Mitchell, A. C. Abbott, and D. D. Stewart; the Philadelphia County Medical Society, by Drs. S. Solis-Cohen, Edward Jackson, and William M. Welch: the Municipal League, by George Burnham, Charles Richardson, Clinton Rogers Woodruff, and Hector McIntosh, and the City Organizations' Filtration Committee, by Frank J. Firth and J. Vaughan Merrick. Views similar to those expressed at the mass meeting at Horticultural Hall were laid before Councils' Committee on this occasion.

OUR PRAGUE LETTER.

[From our Special Correspondent.]

THE GERMAN UNIVERSITY OPENS ITS DOORS ONCE MORE — THE BOHEMIAN UNIVERSITY AND THE CZECHISH MOVEMENT—INFECTIOUS DISEASES IN PRAGUE—THE STATISTICS OF THE PRAGUE MATERNITY IN THE MIDST OF THE PREVAILING UNSANITARY CONDITIONS.

PRAGUE, February 11, 1898.

THE German University opened its doors once more after a six-weeks' interregnum on January 10th. Peace, at least for the time being, seems to have settled down over Prague, and the two universities, the German and the Bohemian, will continue their sessions side by side as before. It is officially announced that a new Czechish or Bohemian university is to be opened in Mähren (Moravia) before the end of the year. Though founded only in 1881 and the medical department only in 1884, the Bohemian University of Prague has now over 2300 students, of whom about 750 are engaged in the study of medicine. It has this large number not because it has attracted students from the German University, for the number of students at the latter institution has only decreased by about three hundred, but rather because the spirit of advance among the awakening Czechish people has attracted numbers of students to their university. The intellectual enthusiasm so notable among the other Slav peoples of northeastern Europe has touched the Czechs too, and with surprising results. From the medical faculty of the Bohemian University has come during recent years a series of scientific advances which have attracted worldwide attention.

Professor Hlawa's name is well known in pathologic anatomy, and from Professor Horbaczewski has come some of the most striking work of late years in physiologic chemistry. A series of text-books in Bohemian by the medical professors has served to fix the status of the language and give it a place in the scientific world which it did not have before.

The Bohemians insist that their language shall, equally with German, be the language of their courts of law, of government business, and of the officials who caused the late unpleasantness. The means employed—the riotous demonstration, the injury of the property of German citizens, and of the German University, cannot but be universally decried; the movement itself—a demand of their language rights for the sake of their nationality can scarcely fail to elicit sympathy from all sides. The rioting was the work of the ignorant, the mobile vulgus so hard to control, whom a demagogic press had worked to a frenzy because it seemed as though recent laws enacted in their favor might be declared legally inactive. The Czechish movement itself depends for its vitality upon a widely different class—a thoroughly determined, highly intellectual body of men who will not cease their endeavors until they have acquired for their country the autonomy which Hungary enjoys in the Austrian Empire.

Of this body of educated men and zealous patriots many are physicians who have been the apostles of the movement to the country people. Bohemia possesses a very large number of doctors, many of them young. About five years ago, between the Bohemian University with 1200 medical students and the German University with 800 there were altogether 2000 embryo doctors coming into existence each year. All of them were practically from Bohemia, all intending to practice within her borders, and yet Bohemia is but a small country. It can readily be understood then what a large and influential body of patriots they make. An interesting study in supply and demand is the gradual reduction of the number of medical students at both universities, until now scarcely 1000 are here. The number of law students has almost proportionately increased at both universities.

There is a lesson for the antivaccination agitators in the faces one sees so often on the streets of Prague. Much oftener than elsewhere in central or eastern Europe, at least, one comes across faces deeply pitted with pockmarks. Fifteen to twenty-five and more years ago, in the country districts of Bohemia there was great opposition to the enforcement of the vaccination regulations. This was shared in many cases by the natural leaders of the people, the schoolmasters, the local clergy, and the officeholders. The result was as might have been expected, a series of smallpox epidemics, some of them of very severe types.

Gradually the state of things altered. The spirit of advancement among the Czechs led to the general recognition of the foolhardiness of further refusal to accept what the world has long recognized—the immense benefits of vaccination. Curiously enough, the same reformation of feeling has not occurred among certain of the German rural populations, especially near the Bohemian boundaries, and I am credibly informed that now it is among this class of the population that smallpox continues to be more or less endemic; so it is likely enough that the striking lesson of the pockmarked faces in the streets of Prague will continue for some years to be a warning to those who, for reasons which it is not easy to understand, persist in their senseless opposition to vaccination in countries in which it is to be supposed that civilization is far enough advanced for the public to accept sanitary precautions at the bidding of science, and not oppose them for factitious, imaginary, and sentimental considerations.

Here, in Prague the lesson of the benefit of sanitary and hygienic precautions, from their absence, is extremely striking. All the infectious fevers find a place here at almost any season of the year. Typhoid rages because the water-supply is contaminated, and there are always a large number of patients with this disease under treatment in the hospital. Diphtheria and scarlet fever seem especially common, though the former, thanks to the serum treatment (in most cases they administer absolutely no other remedy), now claims less than one-third the number of victims it formerly did.

Owing to the unsanitary, overcrowded, uncleanly condition of the poorer classes, skin diseases seem to take on a special character. Impetigo is very common, and modifies other skin affections to a considerable extent. Rheumatism seems much more than ordinarily frequent. It takes on a great deal more than usual of the character of an infectious disease, and seems to be at times even directly contagious. Slight epidemics of it seem to have come under observation, and the cases are prone to occur in groups with definite relations to one another as regards time and place. Its analogy with pneumonia in these respects would seem to be much more outspoken here than elsewhere in Europe, though most of these peculiarities have been noticed by other clinicians, for instance, Eichhorst and Senator.

Influenza would seem to be endemic here, and cases are observed in the hospital wards every fall and winter, especially in which the diagnosis is made, not from the clinical symptoms and course of the disease alone, though these are extremely characteristic, but from the demonstration of the bacilli in the sputum. On the whole, the hygienic conditions here are just such as prevailed generally in Europe fifty years ago. Determined, well directed efforts which deserve the highest commendation are being made to change this state of affairs. Medical men head the movement, and the most advanced scientific principles are guiding the endeavor. Within a few years the whole aspect of things will have undergone a radical change for which Prague will be indebted to the medical profession. Meanwhile, Prague remains an *argumentum crucis* for the doubters of the benefits of modern hygienic and sanitary principles and their practical application.

Notwithstanding this utterly unsanitary condition of the poorer classes, Prague has a maternity hospital which can claim favorable comparison with any like institution in the world. With a mortality of considerably less than one per cent. for all cases received, and a morbidity that is wonderfully small, more than 3000 cases of confinement are conducted a year. The material is freely used for teaching purposes, but with such thoroughly antiseptic and aseptic precautions that in whole services of 300 to 500 cases treatment is carried out with total absence of fever, or, perhaps, fever is present only in such cases as have been treated and examined before being admitted to the hospital. The result is all the more marvelous when compared with the extremely high mortality which prevailed before the advent of modern obstetric methods. Prague, with all her disadvantages, continues to be the teacher of the world in obstetrics, and gives besides the striking lesson of how much may be accomplished, even under the most unfavorable circumstances, in ridding labor of its dangers.

TRANSACTIONS OF FOREIGN SOCIETIES.

London.

CYSTIC DISEASE OF THE LIVER AND KIDNEY—SEROTHERAPY OF TYPHOID FEVER—LARGE INTRAHEPATIC CALCULI IN SITU IN A CASE OF DIABETES—CONDITIONS OF THE OCCURRENCE OF LEPROSY IN CHINA AND THE EAST INDIES—PREVENTION OF ENTERIC FEVER.

AT a meeting of the Pathological Society, held December 21st, STILL read a paper on a *case of cystic disease of the liver and kidney in an infant* eight weeks old. He discussed the various theories which have been adduced to account for this condition, and particularly combatted that which ascribes the affection to inflammation. Inflammation of the liver would certainly produce jaundice, and further, the resulting fibrosis would be progressive. The case mentioned was without kidney signs of inflammation. The speaker regarded the condition as due to irregular development, there being overgrowth of the mesoblastic elements of the organ which leads to cystic dilation of the tubules and ducts of the kidneys and liver. ROLLESTON said that no theory would be satisfactory which did not also explain the occurrence of cysts in the brain, pancreas, liver, and kidneys, and he still thinks the inflammatory hypothesis the most satisfactory theory which has yet been advanced. PAYNE pointed out that whichever theory is adopted it is clear that the disease must begin at an early period of fetal life. If the ducts were obstructed just before birth there would be definite symptoms just as in the case of biliary cirrhosis. The process must begin before the secreting and excreting parts are connected.

At the meeting of January 4th, JOHNSON related the history of a case of *cystic disease of the kidneys and liver occurring in a woman aged fifty-three years.* Both kidneys were converted into masses of cysts, varying in size and containing clear or opalescent fluid. The liver was studded throughout with cysts, the largest being the size of a hazelnut. In other respects the liver was normal. The kidneys, however, gave evidence of inflammatory changes, considered by him to be of a secondary character. Johnson thinks that the appearances supported the view expressed by Still at the previous meeting, that the cystic change is to be regarded rather as a developmental error than as a result of inflammation.

AT this meeting BOKENHAM gave an account of researches bearing on the *serotherapy of typhoid fever.* While the serotherapy of diphtheria and tetanus depends upon the existence of a true antitoxic function of the remedial serum, no such function has yet been demonstrated as possessed by any known "antityphoid" or "antistreptococcic" serum, their good effects appearing to be due to bactericidal rather than to antitoxic power. Several methods of immunization have been employed; one consists of the use of virulent cultures; another the use of cultures which have been killed either by chloroform or some other antiseptic substance; a third, and the most satisfactory in some respects, consist of the use of filtrates of cultures grown in albuminous broth, and sterilized by heat.

As a result of his experiments upon horses, Bokenham summarizes as follows: (1) Non-toxic filtrates of fresh cultures have distinct immunizing powers; (2) the immunizing action is displayed toward both living and dead cultures; (3) the serum of an animal treated with filtrates of fresh cultures acquires agglutinative and bactericidal properties; (4) mixed with living cultures in sufficient proportion the serum renders them harmless, and (5) to a certain extent the serum has also protective and curative powers.

ROLLESTON showed large *intrahepatic calculi in situ* from a man, aged thirty-eight years, who died of diabetes and pulmonary tuberculosis, and had been jaundiced. It appeared possible that the extension of duodenal catarrh to the pancreatic duct had produced chronic pancreatitis, and that this in turn had caused diabetes. There were no calculi in the gall-bladder, and the cystic duct was not dilated, so that the intrahepatic calculi must have been formed *in situ.* Intrahepatic calculi existing alone and of large size are rare, as is the existence of cholelithiasis in diabetes.

At a meeting of the Epidemiological Society, December 17th, CANTLIE read a paper on the *physical and ethnologic conditions under which leprosy occurs in China, the East-Indian Archipelago, and Oceanica.* In this part of the world leprosy is essentially a Chinese disease, extending from its focus in the south-eastern provinces to every region visited by the lower class of Chinamen, and to no others. The Japanese, Malays, and some Mongolian races suffer in a less degree, but the aborigines, black and brown, have never known the disease, and, indeed, have in their languages no words for it. A rapid encroachment of the sand from the desert on the cultivated northern provinces of Asia drove the sturdy Manchus southwards, crowding out the weaker Chinamen of the south, and compelling them to seek employment beyond the seas. The coolies belonging to the poorest classes include many actual or incipient lepers who spread the disease in districts in which it was previously unknown, while the Chinese settlers are solely merchants, planters, or tradesmen. In China itself there are distinct leprous districts, not all of the country being affected. Among the eighteen provinces of the "Middle Kingdom," only six contain such leprous areas. The women of China are themselves active disseminators of the infection, "selling the disease," as they call it, in the belief that they can free themselves from it by coitus with a healthy man.

The Royal Medical and Chirurgical Society, on January 11th continued the discussion of the *prevention of enteric fever.* (See the MEDICAL NEWS, vol. 72, p. 59.) CORFIELD called attention to the fact that mortality from typhoid fever had been enormously reduced throughout the country since the passing of the Public Health Act of 1875, which led to the wide adoption of water methods in the disposal of feces, including the water-closet. London is probably the one city in all England in which water-closets and water-carriage of sewage are most universal, and the death-rate is less for London than for the whole of England and Wales. On the other hand, mortality is highest in the countries in which the water-system least prevails.

Some curious differences between the spread of typhoid fever and cholera are worth noting. Thus Lyons, France, is a town of cesspools, and typhoid fever is always prevalent there; yet, although cholera has been repeatedly introduced, the disease never spreads, and so well recognized is this fact, that the inhabitants of Paris and Marseilles flee to Lyons in time of danger. In his opinion, the air of the houses becomes contaminated from the underlying cesspools, and so favors the occurrence of typhoid fever. SEATON spoke of the reduction of sixty per cent. which has been effected in the mortality of typhoid fever. He thinks that the fundamental point in the prevention of epidemics is the strengthening of the sanitary authorities. Compulsory notification has proved one of the greatest safeguards in spite of the opposition to its enforcement.

LITTLE recommended for the prevention of typhoid epidemics: (1) universal notification, with compensation to any breadwinner prevented from following his or her occupation; (2) performance of clinical tests, such as Widals, by the local authorities, free of expense to the medical practitioner; (3) supervision of all public buildings, such as barracks, docks, railway-stations, hospitals, etc., by the local medical health-officer; (4) the water test should be insisted upon before any drains are even permitted; (5) municipal control of the water-supply with right of inspection back to the source; (6) inspection of the sources of the milk-supply; (7) all raw shell-fish should be regarded as "suspected"; (8) all cases should be treated in hospitals, under the charge of their own physicians; and last (9), typhoid excreta should not be applied to the soil.

WILLIAMS remarked that the distinct family proclivity to have the disease must not be lost sight of. In his opinion there is also a distinct race vulnerability, the Anglo-Saxon people being more prone to contract typhoid fever than the Southern races. He mentioned one town on the Mediterranean in which there are no drains, and the custom of the place is for each inhabitant to deposit his own feces outside the city wall, to be disintegrated by the elements, with the assistance of dogs, birds, and flies, and as yet typhoid fever is there almost unknown. SMITH said that the bacilli are present in the urine and feces for a considerable time after defervescence—at least two to four weeks—and that, therefore, the disinfection of these excrementitious matters ought to be continued throughout the convalescence. Burning is preferable to disinfection with strong antiseptic solutions.

In conclusion POORE said that he did not advocate the abolition of the water-closet in London, but that typhoid stools should be burnt to prevent contamination of the water; and that in the country it is best to put the excreta near the top of tilled humus. Merely digging a trench, filling it with excrement which is then covered with soil, is quite a different matter, and tends to preserve rather than to disintegrate the feces. The method advocated is by no means a new one, as it was commanded by Moses (Deut. xxiii, 13) that every one should go outside the camp to defecate, bearing with him a paddle with which lightly to cover the excrement.

SOCIETY PROCEEDINGS.

NORTHWESTERN MEDICAL AND SURGICAL SOCIETY OF NEW YORK.

Stated Meeting, Held Wednesday, December 15, 1897.

THE President, CHARLES L. DANA, M.D., in the Chair.

DR. P. C. COLE read the paper of the evening, entitled

A CASE OF FEVER WITH INTERCURRENT PLEURO-PNEUMONIA. (See page 236.)

DISCUSSION.

DR. SIMON BARUCH: I have so often spoken on this subject that I can add but little to what I have already said. I would, however, like to say that the author lays too much stress upon the fact that the temperature was not reduced until several days after the compresses were first employed. The object of the compress treatment is not the reduction of temperature, which is a secondary consideration in the treatment of infectious diseases. The principal thing is to counteract the toxemia which is overpowering the patient and doing damage to the organs which maintain life. This is accomplished by the action of the compresses on the peripheral cutaneous vessels. Dr. Hutchinson of Buffalo recently read a paper in which he refers to the "skin heart"—a very important discovery, I think. He is an expert in comparative anatomy and physiology, and has traced the skin heart from its rudimentary development and goes on to show that the cutaneous vessels possess the power of contracting and dilating, and that they are supplied with ganglionic centers which control this capacity. This was clinically demonstrated by Romberg some years ago, and by others since then. In my book it has been shown that the enfeeblement of the heart in infectious diseases is not so much due to failure of this organ—fatty degeneration—but rather to a failure of the cutaneous vessels to aid the circulation of the blood as they normally do. In the normal condition the circulation is maintained by the heart driving the blood into the vessels and capillaries, and the tone or resistance of these vessels furnishes what is known as arterial tension. This arterial tension is interfered with by the spastic contraction of the cutaneous vessels in typhoid fever and other infectious diseases. To overcome this failure of the peripheral vessels is the principal object of the cold compress. I do not use the cold bath in pneumonia because the disturbance which it involves would damage the inflamed lung and pleura. Quite a considerable reduction of temperature in pneumonia will follow even rather high temperature baths, *i.e.*, 85° F.; indeed, they often produce a greater fall than do baths at 65° F. The compress at 60° F., however, is an agent which I have found of value in stimulating the peripheral circulation, and thus enabling the heart to overcome the toxemia, although by this means the temperature is seldom reduced more than a degree or two. The compress treatment, like the Brand treatment of typhoid fever, is for the purpose of carrying the patient through the toxic period of the disease. The history of the case which Dr. Cole has narrated shows very clearly that this was accomplished. The patient did not begin to improve until the fifth or sixth day, when the natural life of the diplococcus ceased. The cold compresses maintained the patient's life until this period arrived—until the poison was eliminated. I like to dwell upon this fact because it is very generally misunderstood by the profession. Cold baths and compresses are not employed as antithermic agents. We have been taught so much about the danger of high temperature that we imagine that all that is necessary is to reduce this. If this were the case, we could accomplish the desired end by the use of antipyrin, and the result would be that the patient would be permitted to die with a normal temperature.

DR. J. H. FRUITNIGHT: I disclaim any criticism of Dr. Cole's diagnosis in the case under discussion, but it seems to me that it was from the commencement one of pneumonia and of a typhoid type. It is quite possible that the physical signs of pneumonia were not present on the first or second day. We observe such cases every day, especially in those in which the pathologic process begins in the center of the lung. I myself had an attack of typhoid-pneumonia which ran a somewhat similar course.

DR. A. R. ROBINSON: I agree with Dr. Fruitnight and believe the case was one of central pneumonia. In regard to the application of cold compresses, I read a paper before this Society fifteen years ago in which I advocated the use of the cold pack, in the manner employed in this case, in the bronchial pneumonia of children. I do not, however, entirely agree with Dr. Baruch in regard to the object gained by cold applications. I am of the opinion that benefit is to be derived from keeping the temperature down below what is clinically regarded as dangerous; nor do I think that all the indications in this affection are met by cold compresses alone. Treatment in such an infectious disease should be directed also toward elimination, so far as possible, of the toxin which caused the dangerous conditions. Elimination is demanded and this can best be accomplished by way of the kidneys rather than through the intestinal canal. Of course, if we can cause the skin to act also in this direction, so much the better.

DR. ROBERT A. MURRAY: The case is unusually interesting on account of the patient being an opium habitué. I have observed many of these cases, and have noticed that when they are attacked with pneumonia the disease does not frankly declare itself. I have tried to explain this by the fact that the pneumonia was a central one, but I have not always been able to believe that this was the case. The question, in these cases, also arises as to when the use of opium should be stopped. If we discontinue its use the patient is apt to die. Opium with them is a powerful support to the heart, and this is the reason why it is so hard to make them give it up. In treating these patients it is essential that the kidneys be made to act well. These patients should be given quantities of fluid so that the waste products may be washed away. It is also well to give calomel to clear out the intestines. It is a curious fact that many patients with opium-poisoning who are brought to the city hospitals develop a fatal pneumonia. This may be due to the cold effusions which are applied or to the exposure which the patients undergo. but it does seem that there is some relation between opium-poisoning and inflammation of the lungs.

In regard to cold-water applications in the treatment of pneumonia, they stimulate the patient and relieve the contraction of the capillaries, besides reducing the temperature. It is not well, however, to bring down the temperature too quickly. I have noticed that the patient makes a bad convalescence if this is done. I am a firm believer in the stimulating effect of carbonate of ammonia in these cases.

DR. CHARLES L. DANA: The pneumonia of the alcoholic or opium habitué is usually a mixed infection or else one due to the streptococcus; it is rarely croupous pneumonia. The lowered vitality of the patient as well as the intensity and mixture of the infection accounts for the mortality. Infection comes sometimes through the foulness of the mouth and the stuporous condition of the patient, which allows infected matter to penetrate into the lungs and stomach. I have watched and directed many kinds of special treatment for pneumonia in the wards of Bellevue Hospital, and I have found no one method which is superior to any other. The best results have been obtained when the patient had a watchful physician and nurse who met the symptoms as they arose. Oxygen seems to have a symptomatic value. In regard to the case under discussion, I agree with Dr. Fruitnight that it was one of pneumonia in the beginning. The treatment was certainly very successful, but I would not like to say positively that the cold packs saved the man's life, for I have seen recovery in many bad cases of pneumonia without the use of these packs.

DR. JOSEPH COLLINS: I would like to hear a general

expression of opinion of the members of this Society in regard to the use of oxygen in pneumonia. Doubtless there is an opinion abroad that the use of this gas is serviceable, but statistics are more valueless in this respect than in any other. The only way of getting at the facts is by means of personal experience. We have all employed oxygen. I have not only used it but have entirely discarded its employment in pneumonia, neurasthenia, and other diseases; for I regret to say that I have found it utterly worthless. I would like to ask Dr. Cole what his experience with this agent has been.

DR. DANA: There is no question but that oxygen produces good results symptomatically. The patient improves as he inhales it, and this is enough to justify its use. I know of only three remedies which will relieve the patient with pneumonia. One is oxygen; the second is the free use of cups, 80 or 100 being applied to the back; and the third is external applications—such as hot poultices of mustard and flour—which stimulate the circulation. In milder cases the use of stimulants like ammonia will have a good effect, and at times copious bleeding of an almost moribund patient will produce a marked improvement.

DR. L. DUNCAN BULKLEY: Twenty-five years ago, when I was a hospital interne, I had some experience with oxygen. We had an elaborate apparatus and employed it a great deal, but within six months we concluded that we had had enough of it, and its use was discontinued. The immediate results seemed to be good, but there was a disagreeable reaction afterward. In many cases we believed that this reaction was the cause of death. Since then my experience has confirmed this opinion.

DR. FRUITNIGHT: I do not think that oxygen should be discarded because it does not always save life. It gives immediate relief to a patient suffering from severe dyspnea. I have recently used it in two cases with marked benefit in each. At the Children's Hospital of St. John's Guild we have many cases of croupous pneumonia, and it always does good in those in which there is dyspnea and cyanosis. We use it there in combination with digitalis and strychnia.

DR. BARUCH: I used oxygen to a marked extent for eight or ten years, and ceased using it about six years ago. I always employ hydrotherapy in cases of pneumonia. I have the record of a case of pneumonia occurring in a girl eleven years of age, which was seen by Dr. Jacobi. The temperature was 106° F., and the pulse 160. The most powerful stimulants had been employed without effect. I stopped the use of poultices and gave her a full bath with the water at a temperature of 95° F. The temperature fell to 102° F.; she rallied, and the cyanosis, which was due to an enfeebled heart action, disappeared. She made a good recovery, though but two baths were given.

I would like to have the privilege of saying something about the remark made by Dr. Robinson to the effect that elimination is necessary in these cases and that cold compresses alone are not sufficient to meet the indications. The point in regard to elimination is a good one, but he has lost sight of the fact that baths and the wet pack aid largely in eliminating the poison. A quantity of fluid should also be given. I give my patients plenty of water to drink. I insist upon the administration of six or eight ounces of water every hour, and the same quantity of milk every other hour. It has been clinically demonstrated that the cold bath in typhoid fever increases the amount of urine. I have seen it increase to 120 ounces in the twenty-four hours in a boy of eighteen years suffering from typhoid fever, and it is often increased to sixty or eighty ounces in pneumonia. All these cases are due to infection, and, therefore, elimination should be the chief therapeutic aim. Both theory and practice show that this is accomplished by the treatment I have mentioned, *i. e.*, cold compresses, copious draughts of water, and the administration of strychnia and calomel.

DR. MURRAY: I do not think I could do without digitalis in the treatment of pneumonia. The edema of the lungs is often relieved by hypodermics of this drug. It is an exceedingly powerful agent, and is of great value when the heart is rapidly weakening. Nitroglycerin is of benefit in cases in which there is a cold, clammy perspiration; for it relieves the contraction of the capillaries and stimulates the respiratory circulation. I have been criticised for advocating blood-letting in pneumonia, but in Bellevue Hospital I have seen many lives saved by this procedure. This was accomplished by means of cups, as advised by Dr. Alonzo Clark. My experience has taught me that in pneumonia the symptoms and not the disease must be treated. In some cases I have used the cold bath with good results, and when I could not get the desired effect with this I have employed hot baths at a temperature of 108° to 110° F. Hot flannels applied to the chest are often of benefit in bringing a patient out of a condition of collapse.

DR. ROBERT H. GREENE: I agree with what has been said in condemnation of oxygen. I have employed it in a large number of cases of pneumonia, and have never seen good results follow its use, although it temporarily stimulates the circulation. The circulation afterward becomes more feeble, the month is made dry, and the patient becomes more exhausted. I have used all the heart stimulants, and the one which has given me the best results is musk. The great disadvantage of this drug is that it is very expensive. Personal experience has led me to believe that there is no medicine which has a curative effect in pneumonia. I have not employed cold baths or compresses in treating this disease, but I have used cold water with good results in cases of erysipelas in which the patient was in a condition of systemic toxemia. I am inclined to think that in selected cases, if properly applied, it would be of benefit in pneumonia.

DR. COLE in closing: Dr. Baruch thinks I have laid too much stress upon the reduction of temperature in the case reported. The pack was applied on the evening of the fifth day, and the temperature did not begin to go down until the morning of the eighth day, and did not reach 101° F. until the morning of the thirteenth day.

Dr. Taylor has asked how the pack is changed with

out disturbing the patient. This is a very simple matter. The patient is rolled over on the side, the pack is removed and a new one applied; the patient is then rolled over on the back and the compress is brought up from each side and fastened over the chest.

In regard to the diagnosis Dr. Fruitnight may be right. The case may have been one of typhoid-pneumonia in the beginning, but there was not the slightest symptom of it until the morning of the fifth day, although the patient had been seen four or five times during each previous twenty-four hours.

I employed oxygen some years ago, but cannot recall ever having obtained any benefit from its use. The after-effects are injurious. When there is cyanosis blood-letting, in my experience, is much more valuable. For years my greatest stand-by in the treatment of pneumonia has been the carbonate of ammonia. During the entire illness the bowels and kidneys should be kept open. In the case reported, in addition to the cold pack, the patient was sponged daily with cold water and then wiped dry, and was given quantities of water and milk. I agree with Dr. Robinson that this constant application of cold reduces the temperature.

More than forty years ago my sister and her husband (in command of his own vessel) were in China. My sister was attacked with pneumonia, and a surgeon from a British man-of-war was called in to attend her. After two- or three-days' attendance he was obliged to leave with his vessel, which had received orders to sail. The next day my sister's extremities, hands and feet, were cold, blue, and she was pulseless. Respiration was hurried and irregular. In desperation my brother-in-law called in a Chinese physician, none other being obtainable. This physician immediately bathed the thorax with hot water and then covered it with leeches, which were allowed to gorge themselves and drop off. My brother-in-law said he counted more than fifty. My sister recovered, and lived more than twenty-five years afterward. The Chinese physician recognized the need of blood-letting in the cyanotic stage of pneumonia, and by its prompt application undoubtedly saved my sister's life. How many of our physicians would have done the same, that is, drawn blood freely from a patient with pneumonia?

THE NEW YORK ACADEMY OF MEDICINE.—SECTION ON OBSTETRICS AND GYNECOLOGY.

Stated Meeting, Held January 27, 1898.

SIMON MARX, M.D., Chairman.

THE paper of the evening, entitled

MIDWIVES,

was read by HENRY J. GARRIGUES, M.D. (See page 232.)

DISCUSSION.

DR. POLK: In dealing with this question we must regard it from a high standpoint and a high plane. All the rights in the case must be taken into consideration. The people wish an educated service, and this they can obtain only through physicians, male and female. It seems to me that the duty of this Section is plain; the question is simply, Shall or shall we not have midwives? This is answered by the general feeling which exists throughout the community, in other words, there cannot be too much education; and this being the case, there is no reason why midwives should not be licensed to practise as doctors of medicine; they should be qualified in the usual way, that is, by obtaining a regular medical education.

DR. TUTTLE: I have been asked by the president of the County Society to come here to-night, though I do not understand why, as that body has not taken any action on this subject; therefore, I do not know how to represent it.

If I present my own opinion, I would say that midwives are a menace to public health and life. The women of our households should not, through ignorance, be entrusted in their hour of greatest trial to the hands of incompetent persons. It is no longer believed by any one that it is technically correct to speak of labor as a physiologic process. It is rarely so in the tenement districts of this city. I do not wish to characterize all midwives as immoral. The majority are honest, whole-souled women; but aside from all this the institution of midwives furnishes an opportunity to women of immoral character to enter the occupation of abortionist.

We, as physicians, have some rights; for instance, the right of self-preservation. This question should also be considered from our standpoint—the point of view of the physician. We should insist that the person who delivers our wives and sisters should be educated and competent.

DR. GRANDIN: My individual opinion in this matter is that the profession and the community should realize that the institution of midwives has no right to exist. I question the legality of its existence for the reason that the members of this guild are engaged in the practice of medicine. I take the ground that obstetrics is as much a part of medicine as pediatrics, and that any one wishing to practise midwifery should not be allowed to do so without passing the Regents' examination. The only thing to do in attempting to reform present conditions is to amend existing laws, thus giving midwives the right to practise or else to undertake their education—not in obstetrics alone, but in general medicine and surgery. In my opinion labor cannot be regarded as a physiologic process. Civilization has so altered woman that she is not now what she once was. During labor emergencies and complications may arise which require the judgment of an educated physician. Furthermore, the actual labor is not the only thing to be attended to; long before the advent of the expected confinement the condition of the heart, kidneys, and other organs should be under constant supervision, and such duties no midwife is competent to perform without having a regular medical education.

DR. BOLDT: I am personally in favor of abolishing the institution of midwives, but I am afraid, gentlemen, that unless an unusually strong amount of backing is brought to bear upon the Legislature, we will never be able to carry the point; and I feel we must devise some means to accomplish it gradually, if we wish to succeed at all. My views are entirely in accord with those of the reader of the paper. I certainly favor entire abolishment.

DR. VINEBERG: I hold a different view from what has been expressed by the majority of the speakers who have preceded me. I was sent here to confer. I should like to ask what opportunity is given to teach doctors to attend midwifery cases. If some of the terrible experiences which occur in the practice of midwives are depicted, why not describe some which occur in the practice of qualified physicians. I believe in thorough education, but not in a three-years' course. Now, for example, let us take a woman in the tenement district; a midwife will talk and wait with her; a qualified physician, under the same circumstances, will apply forceps. I do not think that midwives are a curse as they now exist. It behooves us to educate and to limit them. They cannot apply forceps or sew up a perineum, and they are obliged to send for a physician if they have a difficult case.

DR. GARRIGUES: In closing, I have only a few remarks to make. Most of the gentlemen who have spoken declare themselves in favor of abolishing the institution of midwives. It should be distinctly understood that the only way to obtain what we wish is by means of a law by which we can have supervision over those who are now practising midwifery. I have not said that female physicians would be able to do all the work of the midwives. What I said was that the profession, male and female, could attend to all cases of labor. It is only in cities of large population that midwives flourish. They are not recognized by any general law. I wish to emphasize one more point in regard to the economic side of the question. I have been informed that it is not only the poor who employ midwives, but others as well. Many midwives are paid as high as $20. The general run of poor people pay the midwife $5 for her services, and I am sure that there is a number of regular practitioners who would be willing to attend labor cases for that price.

REVIEWS.

SURGICAL PATHOLOGY AND PRINCIPLES. By J. JACKSON CLARKE, M.B., F.R.C.S., Assistant Surgeon at the N. W. London and City Orthopedic Hospitals. With 194 illustrations. London: Longmans Green & Co., 1897.

THE preface informs us that this work is based upon a course of demonstrations given to students. The book is divided into two parts. The first, a general consideration of the surgical principles, and the second, a description of the pathologic processes of the special tissues and organs. The plan adopted is an admirable one. The chapter on diseases of the bone is one of the best.

Whereas the part played by bacteria is not any too strongly emphasized, the clinical features are never lost sight of, and are always harmonized with what is pathologic. Therapeutic measures receive a casual reference. The illustrations throughout are rather conventional.

As a compend of this subject, elaborately treated in other works, this book ought to appeal to the medical student.

THERAPEUTIC HINTS.

For Erysipelas.—The intense burning pain is said to be relieved and the progress of the disease favorably influenced by the use of the following application:

℞ Aristol . . . . gr. xx
Collodii . . . . ℥ i.

M. Sig. Apply freely with a camel's-hair brush over and slightly beyond the inflamed area. This should be renewed as it scales off.

For Threadworms.—

℞ Santonin . . . . . . gr. ¼
Calomel . . . . . . gr. iss.

M. Ft. chart. No. I. Sig. Take one powder before breakfast every day for three days.

In addition a small quantity of the following ointment should be introduced into the rectum each night:

℞ Amyli glycerit. . . . . . ʒ ii
Ung. hydrarg. . . . . . ʒ i—*m.*

An Ointment for Enlarged Glands.—

℞ Ichthyol
Ung. hydrarg. } aa . . . . ʒ i
Ung. belladonnæ
Ung. petrolati . . . . . . ℥ ss.

M. Ft. ung. Sig. Apply night and morning over affected glands using friction till absorbed.

For Pertussis.—

℞ Tr. Belladonnæ . . . . . ʒ ss
Phenacetin . . . . . . ʒ i gr. xv
Spts. frumenti . . . . . ʒ iv
Ext. castaneæ fl. . . . . . ℥ ii.

M. Sig. To a child over one year of age administer ten drops every two to six hours; for a child of ten years the dose is one teaspoonful.

For Renal Colic.—

℞ Lycetol . . . . . . ʒ iss
Sod. bicarb. . . . . . gr. xlv.

M. Ft. chart. No. VI. Sig. Take one powder night and morning in a glass of mineral water.

For Acute Laryngitis.—After a calomel purge give the following:

℞ Tr. aconiti . . . . . . gtt. xii
Sod. brom. . . . . . ʒ ii
Syr. lactucarii . . . . . ℥ i
Aq. . . . . . q. s. ad. ℥ iii.

M. Sig. One teaspoonful every four hours.

For the Insomnia of Senile Dementia it is recommended to give from eight to sixteen grains of trional in a glass of hot milk at bedtime. A calm sleep of six to nine hours may be expected to follow the use of the drug.

For Favus.—

℞ Sulph. sublimat. . . . . . ℥ ss
Potass. carb. . . . . . . ʒ i
Ol. picis liq. } aa . . . . ℥ iss
Tinct. iodi
Adipis . . . . ℥ iii.

M. Sig. External use.

THE MEDICAL NEWS.

A WEEKLY JOURNAL OF MEDICAL SCIENCE.

VOL. LXXII. NEW YORK, SATURDAY, FEBRUARY 26, 1898. No. 9.

ORIGINAL ARTICLES.

THE TREATMENT OF DELIRIUM.[1]

BY JOSEPH COLLINS, M.D.,

OF NEW YORK;

PROFESSOR OF DISEASES OF THE MIND AND NERVOUS SYSTEM IN THE POST-GRADUATE MEDICAL SCHOOL; VISITING PHYSICIAN TO THE CITY HOSPITAL.

THE subject to which I ask attention is very comprehensive, and some of you may question the advisability of giving it consideration as an entity. I believe, however, that there is as much justification for discussing the treatment of delirium as there is for discussing fever, pain, headache, or constipation, which are usually considered individually, although all of them are symptoms. Moreover, although delirium is a symptom, occasionally it is the only one, or I might say the entire condition, demanding treatment.

Preliminary to a discussion of the treatment of delirium it is necessary to refer briefly to its nature and varieties.

Delirium is a general disturbance or perversion of consciousness characterized by an apparent exaltation of mental processes, which close examination, however, shows to be in reality a diminution or restriction in apperception, although association may be accelerated and in consequence seemingly enriched. It manifests itself in detail by some degree of mental irritation and confusion, by more or less transitory delusions and fleeting hallucinations, by disordered, senseless speech, and by motor unrest. It varies in intensity from the slightest so-called "flightiness," up to a most intense maniacal condition. I do not use the term delirium synonymously with insanity, although naturally admitting that the former presupposes an unsound mind during the time of its occurrence. I wish to speak principally of the temporary mental disturbance occurring with bodily diseases, and not at all of the more or less highly organized, fixed, or changeable deliria of paranoia, of chronic mania, melancholia, general paresis, and the like. In other words, in my own mind the term delirium is not given the wide application which the modern French writer accords it.

For the purpose of discussion, and in no way to be considered absolutely comprehensive, delirium may be classified into: Primary and secondary delirium.

Primary delirium, delirium acutum, delirium grave, is not a disease *sui generis*. In other words, it is not an individual affection, but a condition of varying mental disturbance, which occasionally attends different states of bodily disorder, such as collapse, intoxication, katatonia, etc., although it is often, if not always, dependent upon, or at least associated with, demonstrable changes in the cortex of the brain.

Secondary delirium is by far the more common and the less understood. It may be subdivided into the delirium of (1) infection, (2) intoxication, (3) exhaustion, (4) irritation (peripheral and central), and (5) senility.

The deliria of infection are more common in the young and in the able-bodied. They occur particularly with the diseases that are dependent upon specific organisms, such as typhoid fever, pneumonia, scarlet fever, yellow fever, puerperal fever, pyemia, etc., although delirium occurs with analogous diseases which have not yet been proven to be dependent upon specific organisms.

Deliria of intoxication may be subdivided into endogenous and exogenous. The endogenous comprise those dependent upon septic intoxicants, and are included under the head of sapremia, uremia, cholemia, diabetes, auto-intoxication, insolation, etc., while the exogenous include those due to alcohol, the drugs constituting the group of midriatics, morphin, cocain, mineral poisons, iodoform, and the like.

The deliria of exhaustion may be subdivided into those due to inanition, to acute anemia, such as results from hemorrhage, or from the presence in the blood of some powerful hemic dissociation substance, such as exalgine, the plasmodium of malignant forms of malaria, wasting diseases, excessive lactation, and the like.

The deliria of central or peripheral irritation may be subdivided into those due to local injury of the brain, such as blood clot from accidental trauma or surgical operation, to meningitis, acute encephalitis, or to other central diseases. The peripheral irritation or excitation which may be associated with delirium, is pain, a condition that could not be manifested without central interpretation. Delirium may also be due to, or associated with, states of central depression, such as those of epilepsy, hysteria, etc.

[1] Read at the meeting of the Northwestern Medical and Surgical Society of New York, January 19, 1898.

The delirium of senility requires no subdivision, for although it occurs under the apparent auspices of different exciting factors, it in reality is conditioned by the pathologic state of the vascular system incident to old age.

This classification will be found sufficiently comprehensive for practical purposes, and may afford a working basis for intelligent discussion of the subject. It may be remarked that no particular mention has been made of the delirium following surgical operations. This has been done advisedly because although such delirium is not of very infrequent occurrence, it is due to one of three things, *viz.:* to infection, intoxication, or exhaustion, and thus falls under one of the captions mentioned above.

The diagnosis of delirium is very easy, and the determination of its intensity or degree of severity depends only upon observation. But neither its diagnosis nor the determination of its severity is of any considerable service in suggesting appropriate therapy. This can only be decided upon when the causation and the pathologic associations of the delirium have been discovered. I shall very briefly take up in turn the varieties of delirium classified according to their causes as mentioned above. In discussing these varieties of delirium one has naturally an inclination to say something concerning their symptomatic individualities, and to speak of the morbid conditions which they accompany and are dependent upon. So far as possible I shall limit my remarks to their treatment, however.

The delirium of the disease which is now universally known as acute delirium, or delirium grave, resembles very much that which is associated with febrile diseases. It is ordinarily accompanied by considerable rise of temperature which has no definite course. great prostration, and by rapid development of an asthenic or typhoid state. The treatment ordinarily resolves itself into the fulfilment of two indications, *viz.:* the obtention of sleep and the maintenance of the patient's vitality. All accessory treatment should be contributory to these two ends. Without entering into a discussion concerning the virtues of the various sleep-producing measures, I trust that I shall be permitted to say that the first end in view may be more readily accomplished by the cold pack and the administration of sulphonal or trional in small doses, 10 to 20 grains, repeated every three hours, than by any other measure. When sulphonal and trional combined with the measures just enumerated fail to give the desired sleep, chloral hydrate may be given in full doses, but I never use it as the initial hypnotic in this condition unless there are some special indications. In those cases early attended by great restlessness and excitement, the cold pack is of signal service, both in conserving the patient's strength and in soothing him to a condition anticipatory of slumber. Personally, I am very adverse to the administration of drugs which produce hypnosis and coincident or subsequent depression, such as the bromids, opium, chloralamid, and hyoscyamin, although the latter is not usually rated as a hypnotic, but as a general motor sedative. Quite as important in the early stages, and much more so in the later, is the careful, judicious administration of partially or readily digested food in small quantities and of a temperature equal to that of the body. Specific enumeration of such nutriment does not seem necessary; but sufficient emphasis cannot be laid upon the fact that in reality the chances of recovery from an attack of acute delirium stand in definite relationship to the patient's capacity to retain and absorb food. Oftentimes it is necessary to indulge in forced feeding, and no time should be lost in resorting to the stomach tube. If the stomach will retain small quantities of nutriment, this method has great advantages over that of rectal feeding, no matter how carefully the latter is done. As in all acute asthenic conditions, stimulants must be given early, and this is one of the diseases in which alcohol supersedes in efficaciousness all other forms of stimulation. There should be no hesitancy in resorting to its early employment, and comparatively small experience soon teaches that more alcohol can be given with benefit in this disease than in any other form of intracranial lesion. In this, it is the exception to the rule which applies to the administration of alcoholic stimulants in diseases of the brain. Naturally, the details of treatment vary with the causative factors of the acute delirium.

Those cases of delirium which are complications or sequences of other diseases require a more varied therapy directed toward the latter. Formerly it was considered of prime importance to employ what may be called revulsive treatment, such as the administration of salines, the application of leeches to the scalp, and blisters behind the ears, but at the present day such measures are considered barbarous. The treatment may be summarized in a few words: Induce sleep, maintain nutrition, fight the progressive asthenia with stimulants, counteract the motorial unrest and fever with the cold pack, and carefully guard the period of convalescence. A good nurse is far more useful than an indifferent physician. The most important warning is: Never give motor depressants, even though apparently they are momentarily indicated. They are in reality therapeutic boomerangs. If it be borne in mind that in every case of delirium acutum, or delirium grave, we are dealing with acute parenchymatous encephalitis, we will rarely make the mistake of administering motor depressants to overcome motorial unrest.

The treatment of the deliria which I have called secondary is a very much more important subject to the general practitioner, for they are common concomitants of the diseases which he encounters. As has already been said, delirium frequently occurs with the infectious diseases, in many of the minor forms of which it is so slight and transitory that it requires no treatment. Such are the deliria occurring in young children with measles, infection of the gastro-intestinal tract, and bronchopneumonia. In other diseases, and particularly in typhoid fever, pneumonia, and scarlet fever, its early occurrence is a danger signal which should prompt immediate action. Initial delirum is not very common in typhoid fever, nor in pneumonia. When it occurs in the former, it manifests itself either in a mild form, preceded or accompanied by a degree of anxiety which is soon followed by depression, and what is colloquilly termed "flightiness." Such a mental state has absolutely no relationship to the temperature, and may even precede the occurrence of the latter. In other cases, the delirium is so severe as to constitute actual mania. These cases are likewise infrequently attended with high temperatures. They differ very materially both in their clinical manifestations and in their indications for treatment from the delirium which occurs during the third and fourth weeks of the disease. The former variety stands in direct relationship to the amount and intensity of infection, while the latter is frequently, but not always, an exhaustion delirium. The treatment of initial delirium of typhoid fever should be directed particularly to counteracting the effects of the infection on the nervous system, and, personally, I am convinced that no form of therapy meets the requirements so efficaciously as the administration of one or two large doses of calomel, followed by the injection of a large amount of saline solution into the intestines, or subcutaneously beneath the mammary gland. In two cases of typhoid fever with initial delirium, both of the acute maniacal form, the adoption of high rectal injections of warm saline solution was followed by most gratifying results, and had not such been the case I should not have had the lightest hesitation in using it subcutaneously. Its presence in the blood seems to have a beneficial influence in neutralizing or counteracting the pernicious action of the poisonous matters on the vital centers. The treatment of delirium occurring in the later stages of typhoid fever does not differ materially from the treatment of delirium due to other exhausting conditions.

In this connection I desire to say a few words concerning the relationship of fever to the occurrence of delirium, not alone in typhoid fever, but in other febrile diseases. There is a well-defined conviction in the minds of many physicians that the occurrence of delirium stands in definite relationship to the degree of febrility. Personally, I do not share this opinion, and am inclined to the view that fever *per se* plays absolutely no part in the genesis of delirium, and consequently that treatment directed immediately to the fever is of no avail in counteracting the delirium, except in so far as such treatment is operative against the factors upon which the delirum is dependent. I anticipate that this attitude may not receive the endorsement of those who advocate the most rational and most efficacious plan of treating infectious disease to-day, the plan which we may for brevity's sake call the hydric method.

If hyperthermia is in itself sufficient to cause delirium, this symptom should be a concomitant of hyperthermia artificially produced, and a common symptom of disease attended by high temperature. A few minutes' retrospection on the part of any one of us will, I believe, show that this is not a fact. For instance, witness the colossal rise of temperature which sometimes occurs in malarial infection, in rheumatism, and occasionally even in insolation, while the mental facilities remain unimpaired. On the contrary, the antithesis of delirium is quite as frequently the mental state in such cases. It cannot be legitimately said that because the application of cold water, according to the most approved plan, in the acute febrile diseases has a salutary action in preventing delirium and in controlling it when it does occur, that the hydric procedure prevents or overcomes the delirium by lowering the temperature. On the contrary, the cold water acts by facilitating the elimination of the poisons in the blood which are acting deleteriously upon the anterior poles of the cerebral hemisphere; it assists the blood to oxidize and consume these injurious products, and it stimulates the vital centers to renewed effort in their combat with the overwhelming agencies which are manifesting their peccant activities by enshrouding the sensorium. True it is that the hydric measures simultaneously reduce the temperature, and their beneficial effects on these two symptoms may be coincident, but this in no way should foster the belief that the two are interdependent. On the contrary, it seems to me that fever is conditioned by a mechanism quite apart from that which conditions delirium, and that to speak of febrile delirium to cover the deliria of infectious diseases is an unwarrantable assumption of the interdependency of these two symptoms.

Initial delirium in the pneumonia of the adult always means one of two things: the occurrence of the disease in an alcoholic subject, or an extremely severe infection. Occurring in the infant it suggests that we have to do not only with a severe infection but with an apical involvement as well. If alcoholism, or, better said, the alcoholic habit, can be excluded, the chances are that the patient has a streptococcus pneumonia, and not a diplococcus or tuberculous pneumonia, as initial delirium is of much more common occurrence in the former variety. As an indication for the election of therapy, it matters not very much upon what the delirium is dependent, as the treatment in every instance may be summarized in one word: stimulation, unless, indeed, the administration of a specific antitoxin be considered. The election of the stimulant, or combination of stimulants, may vary. If the patient be alcoholic, it will be necessary to continue administering to him the prop that served him so ill in times when he could make his own selection, and to combine it with strychnin; while in non-alcoholic cases the more diffusible stimulants and digitalis may be indicated. Here again it is necessary to say a word regarding the selection of a hypnotic. In children, and in non-alcoholic adults, chloral in small doses is the best hypnotic, especially in the beginning of the disease. At least, this has been my individual experience. For the insomnia and delirium occurring later in the course of the affection, and in alcoholics, sulphonal has served me more satisfactorily, possibly because it is always given in hot milk, which of itself is not inconsequential as a stimulant and sedative.

The deliria attending scarlet fever, and, in fact, I may say all of the eruptive diseases, are best counteracted in the early stages by the application of the ice cap and the cold pack. On account of the frequency of renal complications, and the widespread belief on the part of the laity that cold water makes the eruption "strike in," there is often great objection by parents when the cold pack is suggested, but I am sure that no other measure or combination of measures compares in efficaciousness with it in the treatment of this symptom, even though it is not associated with hyperthermia.

The delirium attending the severer infections, such as puerperal fever and pyemia, requires practically the same treatment as that accompanying septic pneumonia. In all of these, as in delirium acutum, sleep must be obtained at all hazards, and the prop of the patient's vitality, *viz.:* his nutrition, must be constantly bolstered. Here the mistake of giving motor-depressants, such as the bromids, chloral, and hyoscyamin, should, I believe, never be made. It should also be said that it matters not how maniacal the patient may become, mechanical restraint should not be employed except as a last resort. All mechanical restraint, with the exception of that which makes captive the legs alone impedes respiratory freedom, and thus becomes a very powerful influence in contributing to asthenic consolidation of the lungs. The restraining influence of one or more nurses, combined with the sleep-producing potency of 20 grains of sulphonal or trional, administered in hot milk or in some form of alcohol, is far more efficacious.

Passing now to a consideration of the deliria of intoxication, I shall say very little concerning the endogenous varieties, as the treatment here consists of efforts to overcome the source of the *materies morbi*, to counteract its effect upon the central nervous system, and to secure its elimination from the system. I have no faith in my ability to say anything that would interest or be worthy of attention concerning the treatment of sapremia, uremia, cholemia, diabetes, etc., and shall content myself in allowing these to pass without more direct attention than is contained in the general treatment of delirium. I may say parenthetically, however, that if two important facts be kept in mind concerning the toxic and autotoxic deliria the treatment will be very much simplified. These are: Nature should be assisted to get rid of at least some of the poison in the system, then strike at the source of the intoxication. If the latter be a wound that is filled with iodoform the removal of the latter is a very evident duty, but if the absorbent surface be the entire gastro-intestinal tract, and the *materies morbi*, the as yet unknown toxin which produces the clinical phenomena of insolation, the task is much more difficult. But, as will be said later, after all, the important matter first of all is to determine the pathologic association of the delirium.

In the treatment of deliria of exogenous origin I have had a considerable experience, and consequently some facts have been impressed upon me. Of the deliria having their origin in toxic substances coming from without, delirium tremens is the most important, because it is so frequently encountered and because it is so uniformly fatal after the first or second attack. All toxic deliria are associated with more or less profound asthenia, and the first aim of treatment should be the counteraction of this asthenia while simultaneously fulfilling a more pointed indication. In alcoholic subjects there has almost invariably been a prolonged and outrageous indulgence in substances which destroy the metabolic functions of the economy, and before measures can be taken to counteract the influence of the poison itself upon the nervous system the *primæ via*, and the avenues leading up to it, must be carefully attended to. Therefore, of paramount importance and antedating all other therapeutic indulgence is the introduction of small quantities of partially digested or predigested nourishment into the patient's alimentary tract. There should be no hesitation in resorting to uncommon avenues of introducing nourishment if the patient, because of anorexia, or under the dominancy of a delusion or hallucination, refuses food. I am so convinced that at least one-half of the patients in the early stages of delirium tremens would weather as satisfactorily the danger incident to their vice by this plan of treatment alone that I not infrequently employ it to the exclusion of all other treatment save that of some of the rapidly acting hypnotics which are not depressants. To cite one illustration: The last case of delirium tremens which I observed was in a man who is as yet under observation, and who came to me with a record of having consumed upward of a quart of whisky every day for seven previous months, in addition to from four to six grains of morphin, taken hypodermically. His mental and physical conditions mirrored the typical description of *mania a potu*, with a well-pronounced typhoid state. He received no other treatment than attention to his nutrition, such as suggested above, careful nursing, the use of the warm pack twice daily, and repeated doses of trional in small quantities, taken in hot milk. He made a good recovery, and at the end of a fortnight, being well advanced in the convalescent stage, the administration of strychnin in $\frac{1}{30}$-grain doses three times daily was begun.

I know how extremely common it is for physicians, when they find themselves face to face for the first time with a patient suffering from delirium tremens, to write a prescription containing about 15 grains of chloral, 30 of bromid, and from 3 to 6 drops of tincture of digitalis, and instruct that this be administered every four hours, and at the same time give more or less perfunctory instructions regarding the diet. At a subsequent visit, if the patient is very delirious and difficult to restrain, they give a hypodermic injection of morphin, and possibly leave orders that it be repeated, if necessary. Candor compels me to state that I have never been able to convince myself that such a combination does not very frequently, by adding to the patients asthenia and to the depravity of the blood, do more harm than good, and I confess that I should have to be pushed very hard before indulging in the administration of a mixture recommended in one of the most recent treatises on therapeutics. The writer of the article to which I allude says that it is his custom to give dram doses of the bromid of ammonium, 15 grains of chloral, and ¼ grain of morphin, in order to induce sleep. Such a mixture, it seems to me, has entirely too high a potentiality of dangerousness to give to any person, but particularly to one whose vitality is at a low ebb. As a matter of fact, I never use the bromid and chloral mixture, nor hyoscyamus, until four other hypnotics have failed me, the four being sulphonal, trional, paraldehyd, and chloralamid. If the stimulants, strychnin and digitalis, are properly used, and if the indications for maintaining the patient's strength as mentioned above are fulfilled, the depressant drugs will rarely be found necessary.

I am not inclined to the use of alcoholic stimulants in the treatment of delirium tremens, unless this condition is associated with pneumonia, as, unfortunately, it not infrequently is. When indications of this complication show themselves, whisky and brandy freely given will sometimes save the patient's life.

The delirium of exhaustion is the one which is the least frequently interpreted of all the deliria. It seems difficult for some to admit the reality of its occurrence, but although it is one of the rare forms, there can be no doubt of its existence. Its association suggests the indications for treatment, and there would be no difficulty in following out the proper therapeutic plan were it not that its recognition must grow out of a process of exclusion. The treatment is symptomatic, and should be directed particularly to overcoming exhaustion.

Senile delirium is in reality a delirium of exhaustion, remotely conditioned by pathologic changes of the blood-vessels, and immediately by disordered intracranial blood-supply. Its chief clinical characteristics are that it is of the so-called "busy," active kind, and it almost invariably occurs at night. During the day the patient may have customary mental lucidity. In addition to the ordinary measures to maintain the patient's nutrition, special precautions should be taken to prevent deleterious lowering of vitality in the early morning hours. If such a patient is taking one of the iodin salts and nitroglycerin, it is very advisable to give him a full dose on retiring, and also a liberal amount of warm peptonized milk and to repeat this once or twice during the night, even though it be necessary to awaken the patient. Alcoholic stimulants are likewise of signal service in preventing delirium of this nature. Their efficaciousness seems to be increased if administered in hot water or in hot milk. The value of dry heat to the extremities should not be overlooked.

The deliria of central or peripheral irritation is a very large subject. and one that I cannot attempt to handle in a brief consideration of this kind. From the slight experience which I have had with cerebral injuries, either accidental or surgical, I am inclined to the opinion that surgeons are more apt to seek the cause of the delirium in infection than they are in local irritation. There may be ample reasons for this, but nevertheless delirium is so frequently a symptom of meningeal and cerebral irritation, unattended with any considerable infection or intoxication, that its occurrence should cause no astonishment. When the irritation is of a post-traumatic origin, and the delirium is continuous, this should be sufficient justification to warrant operative interference.

The delirium associated with states of central depression, such as epilepsy and hysteria, demand the greatest circumspection in their diagnosis and interpretation. Psychic epilepsy, that is epilepsy in which the customary motor explosion, let us say, is replaced by psychic phenomena of an uncontrollable nature, is, proportionately to the ordinary epilepsy, rather uncommon; and this, perhaps, accounts for its lack of recognition when it does occur. The psychic equivalent may assume the form of delirium, even from the very beginning, or an epilepsy starting in as an ordinary motor-epilepsy may alternate in its explosions, one attack being externalized by a convulsion, another by a delirious state. The same is true of hysteria, although hysteric delirium is relatively more common than epileptic delirium. In this connection it may be well to say a word of the delirium which occasionally accompanies chorea, constituting chorea insaniens. Occasionally there is superadded to the typical symptoms of a severe Sydenham's chorea, a profound state of unsystematized delirium. It has been suggested by some writers that the delirium is the expression of an extensive encephalitis, it being known that in some cases of chorea which have proved fatal, vascular changes pointing to a mild degree of parenchymatous inflammation have been found. Personally, I am not inclined to this view. I believe that the delirium from which chorea insaniens takes its descriptive adjective is analogous and comparable to the delirium which is occasionally an accompaniment of rheumatism, and that its causation is to be sought for in the profound dissociation of the component parts of the blood occurring in both of these diseases.

The treatment of chorea insaniens would be very simple were it not for the profound vascular depravity behind the chorea, for this militates against the administration of a drug, exalgin, which if given in 3- to 5-grain doses and repeated every two or three hours, would soon stop the delirium, at least temporarily; but as exalgin tends to liberate the hemoglobin and thus act as a severe hemolytic, it should never be used. The general treatment of asthenic delirium, enforced rest in bed and the administration of small doses of bromid, suffices to control the attacks in most cases. This is one of the forms of deliria in which hyoscyamus should never be given.

The treatment of epileptic delirium is practically the treatment of status epilepticus, save that the necessity for giving stimulants, which is so patent in the latter condition, is not so urgent. In reality, the treatment is small doses of one of the bromid salts; let us say, 10 grains every hour or two, which with mechanical restraint, usually suffices to terminate an attack. The treatment of hysteric delirium oftentimes baffles every resource of the physician, and then after resisting them all, disappears spontaneously. The most potent element in its treatment is complete isolation and the application of cold packs, although in many of these cases the salts of hyoscyamin given in doses up to their full physiologic limit are of the greatest benefit.

General Remarks on the Treatment of Delirium.—After thus wandering over a very large subject, and touching here and there some of the more important points, I should like to ask indulgence for a few general remarks on the treatment of delirium, fully cognizant that therapeusis must vary in every case, and that the indications in one kind of delirium may not suffice or be sufficient in another. Nevertheless, there are a few underlying principles in the treatment of all deliria, and it is these which I shall here endeavor to lay down, prefacing my remarks by saying that, in the opinion of the writer, sedatives are used too frequently and too indiscriminatingly. Bromids, especially, are frequently given offhand, in large doses, and over quite an extended period, apparently forgetful of the fact that they may, by adding to the vascular depravity which is so often at the bottom of the delirium accompanying asthenic states, intensify and prolong the duration of the symptoms for which they are given.

The general indications in the treatment of delirium are first to secure sleep; second, to overcome motor unrest; third, to prop up and maintain the patient's vitality by contributing to his nutrition, and fourth, to discover and remove the cause upon which the delirium is dependent.

To meet the first indication hypnotics are almost always required, although it should never for a moment be forgotten that an hour's sleep induced by measures taken to fulfil the third condition is far more salutary than three-hours' sleep obtained by the use of a hypnotic. Moreover, that in many forms of asthenic delirium, whether the asthenia be induced by infection, intoxication, exhaustion, senility, or what not, sleep is more readily induced and maintained by measures directed immediately against the asthenia than against the insomnia. In the selection of a hypnotic the one least depressant to the patient's vitality and least apt to be followed by depression should always be given preference. The motor depressants should never be used in the delirium accompanying the asthenic state, except as the very last resort. In certain forms of sthenic delirium, and especially those in which a sedative effect cannot be produced by the external application of water, drugs which are motor depressants and at the same time hypnotics may be used with the greatest benefit. Of these, the alkaloids of hyoscyamus are the most available.

The second principle is that great care should be exercised in the application of mechanical restrain in all forms of asthenic delirium, lest the encroachment on respiratory capacity lead to pulmonary complications which jeopardize the life of the patient. Whenever possible, physical restraint is very much less dangerous.

Concerning the third principle, that of maintaining the patient's vitality, I have perhaps already said sufficient.

The meeting of the fourth indication, *viz.*: the discovery and removal of the cause of the delirium, is after all the most essential procedure in the treatment of this symptom. To do this the pathologic association must be determined, and then our ammunition leveled directly against it, while simultaneously the three first enumerated principles are guiding us in symptomatic therapy.

PNEUMOTOMY.

BY DUDLEY TAIT, M.D.,
AND
ALBERT ABRAMS, M.D.,
OF SAN FRANCISCO.

AFTER the invasion and conquest of the abdomen and head, surgeons have in recent years turned their attention to the numerous diseases of the chest which have baffled medical treatment. Although pneumotomy is mentioned as early as 1710 by Baglivus and advised by Börhave, Pouteau, and others, it is quite evident that the operation was undertaken unknowingly, in the rare cases in which the lesions resembled empyema or abscess of the chest-wall. Hence, as Terrier justly remarks in his masterly "Lessons on the Surgery of the Pleura and Lung," the caption pulmonary surgery should be reserved for those cases in which the chest-wall and pleura are deliberately traversed with the intention of attacking an intrapulmonary lesion." Truc's valuable monograph (1885) was the first important contribution to this subject. In 1894, Fabricans of Cracow tabulated all the cases in the literature of the previous twenty years, amounting to thirty-one cases of pneumotomy for abscess, and twenty-six for gangrene. The following year, with Reclus' admirable address before the French Surgical Congress, and the extensive discussions which followed it, the question assumed both a scientific and practical aspect. Of late, French surgeons have done much, by careful clinical, physiologic, and experimental investigation, to widen the heretofore very narrow limits of pulmonary surgery; and already many surgeons of prominence believe this branch of the art is near its greatest height, if only the indications promising complete success be counted (Paget, Kochler). When, however, we consider Delagéniere's audacious exploratory pleurotomy, which he places on the same footing as laparotomy and trepanation for exploratory purposes, we cannot refrain from suggesting that the limitations of pulmonary surgery are as yet undefined.

The great obstacle to progress in this direction is the absence of precision in pulmonary localization, and regarding this, it is to be hoped that surgeons will utilize the results obtained by Bouchard by means of the X-rays, which may justly be considered as valuable in the examination of the chest as in the diagnosis of bone lesions. We regard the illumination of the chest as of great diagnostic value in the detection of patches of consolidation which, in consequence of their diminished area or depth from the chest-wall, elude the results of percussion and auscultation.

The following case of pneumotomy is reported on account of several interesting clinical features, and also as partly illustrative of some of Delagéniere's suggestions in regard to the exploration and drainage of pulmonary lesions:

J. M., aged seven years, weight forty-four pounds. There was no history of tuberculosis in the family. Three weeks before, according to the statement of the attending physicians, the patient contracted croupous pneumonia, primarily involving the lower lobe of the right lung, and, subsequently, the lower and part of the upper lobe of the left lung. The pneumonia in the right lung underwent resolution, but the areas of consolidation in the upper portion of the lower lobe of the left lung persisted. The symptoms presented—night-sweats, fever, rapid and progressive emaciation, and occasional slight chills—were suggestive of an acute suppurative process involving the lung; temperature, 104° F.; pulse, 140; respiration, 24.

The first exploratory puncture, at the lowest portion of the area of dulness in the mid-axillary line, proved unsatisfactory; the second, at a higher and deeper point, revealed the presence of thick pus. The needle did not oscillate with the movements of respiration; which fact led us to affirm the presence of pleural adhesions directly over the affected portion of the lung. Pneumotomy was performed two hours later through a U-shaped incision of the skin and muscles. Nine cm. (3½ inches) of the seventh and eighth ribs, between the anterior axillary and scapular lines, were resected. The pleura was opened after a fruitless attempt at extrapleural palpation by Tuffier's method. With the use of retractors the entire region could be explored with the greatest ease and satisfaction. The only adhesions present were about 7 cm. (2¾ inches) above the opening. Inspection and *manual* exploration showed the lung to be free below the adhesions and markedly hepatized. There was no effusion in the costodiaphragmatic cul-de-sac. After shutting off the pleural cavity with gauze, the lung was incised to the depth of 3 cm. (1¼ inches), with the Paquelin cautery, heated to a dark-red color. About 75 c. c. (2½ oz.) of thick, non-fetid pus immediately escaped. The pulmonary opening was then increased, and the cavity found to extend upward toward the surface of the pleura. Its walls were covered with sphacelated tissue, but did not seem thickened. After breaking up a number of trabeculæ, and searching in vain for secondary purulent collections, the cavity was thoroughly swabbed and gently packed with gauze. The gauze in the pleural cavity was then removed, and the skin and muscle flap sutured. At no time during the operation was there any trouble from hemorrhage. Cultures were made from the pus, but, owing to an accident in the laboratory, the result remained doubtful.

After the operation there was an immediate improvement in the temperature, which fell 3° F.; the pulse and respiration were only slightly modified. Patient ceased to lose weight. Excepting the slow elimination of the sphacelated walls and the consequent tardy appearance of healthy granulations, the wound offered nothing of interest. Four weeks after the operation friction sounds could still be heard at the point already mentioned. One month later the wound had entirely closed, and nothing in or over either lung could be elicited by physical examination. Skiagraphy then revealed opacity at the base of the left lung, probably due to cicatrical tissue. The mobility of the lung border at this point was absent. The lower border of the lung on this side was 2 cm. (¾ of an inch) higher than the corresponding border of the right lung.

Although the exploring needle revealed the seat and nature of the pulmonary lesion, it was, nevertheless, misleading in regard to the pleural adhesions. The absence of oscillations may not, therefore, always indicate the existence of adhesions, a fact already mentioned by Quincke, Rochard, and Terrier. In the diagnosis of abscess of the lung, the results furnished by the exploring needle are frequently as unreliable as in other regions; the pus may be present and not escape through the needle, or the cavity may be nearly or entirely empty after an attack of coughing. On the other hand, the use of the needle is not devoid of danger; death from pneumothorax in a case of emphysema has been reported by Fränkel, and purulent pleurisy is mentioned as a complication by Israel, Pochat, and Winge. Exploratory puncture should, therefore, constitute the first step of the operation, serving as a guide to the seat of the intrapulmonary lesion.

It will be noticed that after finding the adhesions above the pleural opening it was, nevertheless, not considered proper to make a new incision and thus transfer the field of operation to a higher level immediately over the adhesions, as in a successful case reported by Bazy. If a similar plan had been adopted in the present case the object of the operation would not have been attained. The reasons for preferring the direct low pulmonary incision were: (1) the results of the exploratory puncture; (2) the desire to secure the best possible drainage, an indispensable element, as Delagéniere has so clearly demonstrated. Moreover, it was inferred that if the abscess extended to a point in the vicinity of the pleural adhesions it could be easily laid open by extending the pulmonary incision directly upward by means of the cautery.

Too much stress cannot be laid upon the facility afforded by a liberal resection of the ribs in all cases of exploration of the lungs. De Cerenville, Truc, Lauenstein, and many others have insisted upon this and have shown that the gravity of the operation is thereby diminished, and, in purulent intrapulmonary lesions, the retraction of the cavity and apposition of its walls greatly favored. This is especially true in abscesses of long standing, for in such cases the process of repair is notably influenced by an extensive sclerotic zone, chronic bronchitis, and dilatation. Simple resection of one or two ribs may then prove inadequate, and thoracoplasty by Schede's method becomes necessary. Cases of respiratory trouble attributed to extensive resection of ribs have been reported by various surgeons; but it is quite improbable that the accidents were caused by the procedure, for very much more extensive operations on the chest-wall have since been made without being followed by similar accidents (Terrier). Spinal deviation (Ollier) has likewise been mentioned as a sequel.

The stripping of the parietal pleura off from the ribs in Tuffier's method of extrapleural explorations is not as easily accomplished as may be imagined; it requires considerable practice on the cadaver. Terrier states that he saw Tuffier himself tear the pleura, but that no symptoms suggesting pneumothorax ensued. Lejars and Brun each report a failure with this method. Surgeons differ greatly regarding the extent of the pleural incision in pleural and pulmonary explorations. Bazy prefers a small opening sufficient to permit digital exploration; Delangéniere, in three successful cases, made a liberal opening through which the entire hand could be introduced. Terrier inclines toward the latter method. Truc holds that absence of adhesions over the pulmonary abscess constitutes an absolute indication against operation. This rule, although supported by some eminent surgeons (Quincke, Volkmann), is questionable, and happily passing into oblivion. Terrier justly remarks: "In either case one should unhesitatingly continue the operation and not be influenced by a condition of such meager interest." In the majority of cases the preliminary use of caustics (Quincke), iodoform gauze (Neuber), or needles (De Cerenville), in view of creating adhesions, may be condemned for very much the same reasons as all stomach and gall-bladder operations performed in two stages. Many surgeons advise suturing the two layers of pleura around the seat of operation before incising the lung (Godlee, Roun), but such a procedure must necessarily be restricted to a group of well localized, circumscribed lesions (gangrene and apical cavities especially). In the present case, it was thought wiser to first shut off the pleural cavity with gauze and explore the lung before suturing.

The avoidance of pneumothorax has greatly occupied all those interested in pulmonary surgery, and, although many expedients have been proposed, the question still awaits a practical solution. Quénu advises tracheotomy in cases of large opening of the pleural cavity; Delorme considers this procedure unjustifiable, and resorts to cocain anesthesia or incomplete choloform narcosis. Tuffier and Hallion, in a series of interesting and precise experiments, have demonstrated that a slight increase in the intrabronchial pressure does not interfere with the pulmonary or general circulation. Tuffier, therefore, rejects tracheotomy, which, in his opinion, is as dangerous as pneumotomy, and seeks to neutralize the retractility of the lung with laryngo-tracheal insufflations by means of a special laryngeal tube. Experience alone will determine the value of this ingenious method. More audacious than others, Delangéniere, the clever surgeon of Mans, does not anticipate much danger from pneumothorax, and in his exploratory pleurotomy, after resecting the eighth, ninth, and tenth ribs, he opens the pleura sufficiently to admit the entire hand; the lung is seized with forceps and secured to the parietal pleura. In considering this bold but nevertheless successful procedure, it becomes quite evident that operative pneumothorax is not as dangerous as heretofore believed. In the course of nephrectomy, the pleura has been accidentally incised, and a similar accident occurred while removing a hydatid cyst involving the convex surface of the liver. No alarming symptoms developed in either instance. In the present case the cautery, heated to a dark-red color, was used for incising the lung on account of the marked hyperemic condition. According to Terrier, the knife should be reserved for those cases of dense sclerosed tissue in which hemorrhage is not feared.

Whilst the possibility of recovery without operation is admitted in certain cases of abscess of the lung, either by absorption or by discharge into the air-passages, the fact, nevertheless, remains that basic cavities are frequently ill-drained through the bronchial passages; septic absorption is a common occurrence, and sudden suffocation due to rupture into a bronchus is not rare. Furthermore, in large cavities of the apical region, in spite of bronchial evacuation, the process of repair is greatly hindered and somestimes rendered impossible by the rigidity of the thoracic walls. In the present case, the septic condition constituted the primary indication for operation, and, judging from the absence of cough, the extensive sphacelated walls, and surrounding congested area, it may be safely said that nothing short of surgical interference would have been of the slightest value. As Reclus remarks, "Wherever there is an abscess there ought to be an operation; no need to wait for fever, septic absorption, and the resulting alarming condition. Delay is unjustifiable, save perhaps in very small abscesses draining easily and rapidly into the air-passages or in multiple abscesses requiring for their evacuation unwarrantable mangling of the chest. Fortunately, these latter cases are exceptional." Even if the intrapulmonary exploration proves negative in certain purulent lesions, the operation may, nevertheless, do good, for in numerous cases it has been noticed that the cavity subsequently ulcerated and broke through its wall at this point of least resistance. (Quincke, Reclus, and Groube.) As illustrative of this point, and also of the difficulties experienced in localizing lesions of the middle and lower part of the lungs, in spite of direct exploration, and, furthermore, as an example of the tolerance of the lung to traumatism, we recall a case under the care of a surgeon of this city, at the French Hospital, in 1893.

A man, aged forty years, contracted severe bronchitis a year previously, and at the time of admittance to the hospital expectorated large quantities of very fetid pus every morning. No tubercle bacilli were present. Physical examination pointed to a cavity in the lower portion of the right lung, with corresponding dry pleurisy. Ten cm. (4 inches) of the eighth and ninth ribs were resected in the axillary line, the pleura incised and found adherent. The Paquelin cautery was then sunk into the sclerosed lung to a depth of 2 to 3 cm. (about one inch) at two distinct points. Only a little air and mucus escaped. The wound was packed with gauze. The patient showed immediate signs of improvement, and within two months entirely recovered from the pulmonary trouble.

In the drainage of pulmonary lesions tubes should be used with circumspection; if allowed to remain long hemorrhage from ulceration of the blood-vessels may result, as illustrated in the cases reported by Walsham, Grainger Stewart, and Sutherland. Gauze, with or without a tube, is certainly to be preferred. Cases proving the great dangers resulting from irrigation in pulmonary surgery are quite numerous, and we firmly believe the same verdict holds equally good in surgery of the pleura.

SOME MANIFESTATIONS OF SYPHILIS IN THE UPPER RESPIRATORY TRACT, WITH REPORT OF A CASE OF CHANCRE OF THE NASAL SEPTUM.[1]

BY JOSEPH A. KENEFICK, M.D.,
OF NEW YORK;
ASSISTANT SURGEON IN THE THROAT DEPARTMENT OF THE MANHATTAN EYE, EAR, AND THROAT HOSPITAL; AURAL ASSISTANT SURGEON NEW YORK EYE AND EAR INFIRMARY.

IT is a most important fact to be borne in mind by every physician and surgeon that in the nose and throat are constantly found all the different lesions of syphilis, and at all periods of life, from the snuffling infant, with hereditary taint, to the external and internal deformities of the advanced disease. As eminent a physician as Professor Osler of Baltimore only recently made the significant statement before the New York Academy of Medicine that he had said to his students: "the only disease one must know thoroughly is syphilis; if one knew syphilis, one knew internal medicine."

While the usual genital lesion may attract but passing attention, and the characteristic cutaneous manifestations entirely escape detection, the comparatively insignificant nose or throat affection for which the patient seeks relief may be the first intimation of the true condition. This outlines an occurrence which is by no means infrequent; indeed, it is so common that my own experence in dispensary work has led me to determine the presence or absence of specific disease as almost the first step in diagnosis.

The diagnosis of syphilis in the nose is comparatively easy. The "snuffles" of the infant with inherited disease is quite characteristic, but by no means pathognomonic. Not all infants presenting this symptom are syphilitic, especially after the earlier months. Careful examination in this class of cases may disclose the presence of a foreign body or a diphtheritic membrane in the nasal chambers.

During last summer I observed a child at the Manhattan Eye and Ear Infirmary (Dr. Knight's clinic) who had snuffles. There was a brown sanious discharge from both nostrils, and a significant excoriation of the upper lip beneath the right meatus. Relief for this condition, which the mother called "chronic catarrh," had been sought in vain at various hospitals and dispensaries. A foreign body was found in the right nostril, which on removal proved to be a long piece of stout linen cord that had been introduced into the nose six months before. Complete relief promptly followed removal of the foreign body. It was evident from the history that the antisyphilitic treatment by inunction had been experimentally tried. On the following day another child was observed, who, to all outward appearances, presented the same condition and symptoms; and yet examination showed the presence of a diphtheritic membrane on the septum and inferior turbinate bone of the side most affected, and the Health Department reported that the case was one of true diphtheria.

Primary syphilis of the nose is not a very rare condition. Up to 1894 thirty-seven cases had been recorded, constituting between three and four per cent. of all cases of extragenital infection. In such cases the virus is undoubtedly introduced by means of the finger, and the chancre is nearly always situated on the septum, occasionally on the turbinate, and just within the nasal orifice. Characteristic mucous plaques are also found in the nose, though they rarely appear on the septum. When a secondary syphilis is observed, without evidence of initial lesion, but with a history of persistent obstructive rhinitis, one ought always to think of the nose as a possible seat of primary infection. Through the courtesy of Dr. C. H. Knight I am able to give the history of the following case, which was observed in his clinic at the New York Post-Graduate Hospital.

Marie W., German, aged thirty years, the mother of two healthy children, and whose husband, as far as she knew, was also healthy, had always been well up to three months before presenting herself for treatment. At this time she began to suffer from persistent stenosis of the left nostril, with pain and occasional slight bleeding. The affection had continued in spite of all sorts of local treatment.

Examination revealed a shelving ecchondrosis of the septum, a characteristic punched-out ulceration, with well-defined border—rounded and elevated, and a dirty, yellowish base. Marked hypertrophy of the inferior turbinate occluded the nostril. On lips, gums, soft palate, and right faucial pillar, were characteristic mucous patches. The usual adenitis was present, the submaxillary gland on the affected side being especially prominent and painful.

[1] Read at a meeting of the Harvard Medical Society of New York, December 18, 1897.

The patient had noticed great loss of hair during the previous two weeks. The case was diagnosed by Dr. Knight as one of chancre of the septum. Under specific treatment continued ten days the ulceration promptly healed, with marked improvement in the general and local conditions.

Between secondary and tertiary manifestations in the nose Dr. Hajek of Vienna recognizes certain difficulties of classification. He claims that an early periosteitis and chrondritis resulting in quick destruction of bone may sometimes occur, and that infiltrative gummatous syphilis may be observed as early as the sixth month of the disease. Erythema of the mucous membrane is the usual nasal accompaniment of secondary syphilis.

Tertiary syphilis of the nose, according to the usual classification, is observed only too often. The early treatment in these cases is always an interesting question, and one in which it is difficult to determine facts. My own impression is that with an early diagnosis and proper treatment, continued over a sufficient length of time, there should be practically no tertiary manifestations. When such occur they appear in the form of gummatous tumors or as a necrotic process most frequently involving the bony and cartilaginous septum, at first continuing quietly beneath the intact mucous membrane and later breaking down with great proliferation of granulation tissue. Finally, the process becomes purulent and the sequestri find their way out or remain until removed by a surgical procedure. Ultimately there is left a general nasal atrophy, accompanied by various external and internal deformities.

The diagnosis of nasal syphilis should be made from the history of the patient, the microscopic character of the new tissue, and from the result of specific treatment.

I have now under observation a woman who presented herself for treatment on account of nasal stenosis. A granular tumor growing from the septum had completely occluded both nostrils. There was no history or evidence of infection or dyscrasia of any sort. The pathologist reported that the specimen presented all the features of syphilitic granuloma. The growth is at present disappearing under the administration of syrup of hydriodic acid.

The history, gross and microscopic appearances of new growths in this region may be so misleading that general surgical measures should be resorted to only after great care and deliberation. A pathologist's "small, round-cell sarcoma" recurring after complete extirpation through the superior maxilla at the hands of the general surgeon, and melting away again under generous doses of potassium iodid is by no means an impossible occurrence.

The nasopharynx of young subjects not infrequently furnishes evidence of hereditary syphilis, taking on the form of obstruction and stenosis due to contraction of the soft parts from the presence of cicatricial tissue. Of primary syphilis in this region —the nasopharynx, the less said the better. Doubtless all have heard of that famous Eustachian catheter in Paris, which some years ago was discovered by Fournier, but not before it had contributed forty such cases to the literature.

Primary lesions of the lips and tongue are no longer rare. "Cold sores" and "canker sores" which resist the usual remedies should be regarded with suspicion. In the oropharynx is presented a field of great importance in the general physical examination of all patients. Careful inspection here will often show the presence of certain small stellate cicatrices in the mucous membrane which prove veritable X-rays in revealing an all important truth through the dense opacity of conflicting history and symptoms. Primary lesions in this region are not rare, and the danger of infection here is shown by a case reported by Julian, in which a girl of seventeen years had both tonsils infected from the nipples of a recently delivered woman who had received the disease from her husband. Arlau of Padua has reported a very interesting case of persistent angina of the left tonsil in a woman, thirty years of age, the mother of two healthy children, and of exceptionally good history. He finally excised the tonsil, which had broken down, and the operation disclosed the presence of a chancre in the depths of the tonsil. In such cases the tonsil becomes much indurated, and the neighboring glands, especially those on the affected side, become unusually large, dense, and tender.

The occurrence of secondary pharyngitis, usually means that the general disease has continued from six weeks to three or four months. I have often been surprised, however, to observe, a pharyngitis, presenting the usual secondary characteristics, yield to specific treatment when the history extended over a period of years. Here, also, no hard and fast lines can be drawn clinically between the different stages, and this should always be borne in mind in the determination of a proper method of treatment. As a rule, when there is found in the pharynx an excessive hyperemia, with an evenly distributed edematous swelling over the palate and fauces, and presenting a sharp line of demarcation, the presence of syphilis should be suspected. These appearances may, however, occur in other diseases, and the order of the secondary manifestations may also change. In a case in which syphilitic infection was doubtful, and in which I very carefully observed the symptoms, rapid disappearance of both tonsils by ulceration and without pain was the earliest secondary sign observed.

Tertiary manifestations occur in this location as gummata of the hard and soft parts, most frequently observed in a process of ulceration. They usually respond promptly to local and general treatment.

In the larynx the various manifestations of syphilis, simple catarrh, diffuse infiltrations, gumma, ulceration, cicatrices, with fibrous adhesions, parichrondritis, and paralysis all present certain characteristics which, together with the history, general examination, and results of treatment, make the diagnosis reasonably certain; under certain conditions, however, differentiation may be a problem presenting serious difficulty. In this connection a case reported by Dr. C. H. Knight[1] shows an interesting complication:

The patient, a young student, presented typical signs of tuberculous laryngitis, and the diagnosis was confirmed by the presence of tubercle bacilli in the sputum. The patient went to California where he at first improved but soon become worse. A suspicious ulceration developed in the pharynx, and under mixed treatment there was prompt and permanent improvement in the local as well as in the general condition.

With regard to treatment it would seem that all authorities are agreed upon mercury and iodin as the two great remedies, though they are doubtful as to the advisibility of using these drugs as reactionary agents, fearing the existence or non-existence of syphilis. The relation between early treatment and tertiary manifestations is another subject receiving serious attention and study by the great syphilographers of the day. In this connection, the difficulty of obtaining reliable data is obvious, and it will only be by means of the collective experience of many observers, covering a long period of time that such data will be obtainable.

Finally, in the physical examination of a patient about to receive mercurial treatment, an exact knowledge of the condition of the kidneys may be of vital importance; for next to the intestines these organs are chiefly concerned in the elimination of mercury. Brouardel of Paris reports an interesting case in this connection, in which a woman, after taking the first mercurial pill was seized with stomatitis and alarming uremic symptoms. On examination the kidneys were found to be diseased, in consequence of which the drug was not properly eliminated.

It seems possible that an examination of the urine at the beginning of treatment, and at frequent intervals during the course of the disease, might reduce the number of cases reported as "syphilitic nephritis."

[1] MEDICAL NEWS, June 5, 1897.

CLINICAL MEMORANDA.

REPORT OF THREE CASES OF ADIPOSIS DOLOROSA.

BY WILLIAM G. SPILLER, M.D.,
OF PHILADELPHIA;
PROFESSOR OF DISEASES OF THE NERVOUS SYSTEM IN THE PHILADELPHIA POLYCLINIC.

BUT a few cases of this disease, described and named by Dercum, have been reported, and it may be well to record three which the author has had the privilege of studying, even though nothing definite can be said concerning the pathology of the affection. Two of these cases have been studied with Dr. Dercum, and their histories have been obtained from him; the third was a patient of Dr. Mills. The writer is indebted to these gentlemen for the reports of the cases. Repeated opportunity for observation of Dercum's first case of adiposis dolorosa has also been given. All three patients, whose clinical histories are herewith published, are women, and at present, at least, the disease seems to be more common in the female sex.

FIG. 1.

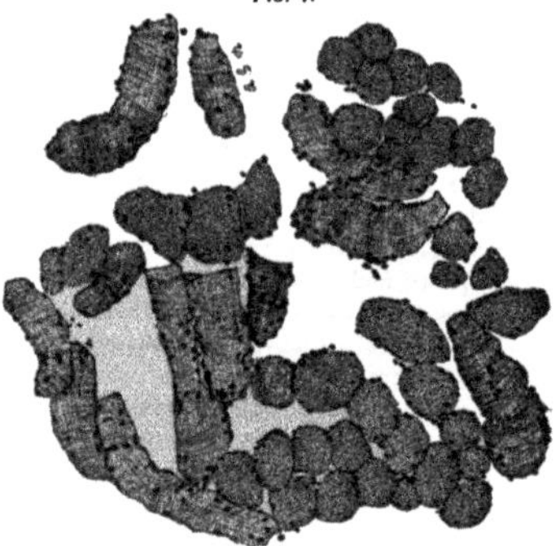

ross section of muscle from a case of adiposis dolorosa showing no appreciable change from the normal, except, perhaps, a slight enlargement of the nuclei.

CASE I.—Miss A. B., aged twenty-nine years, was referred by Dr. Rudolph Matas of New Orleans to Dr. Dercum. The family history was negative. Her father and three brothers were living and well. Her mother died in confinement. She had the various diseases of childhood, but never any nervous affection, and was well in early youth. The history of the present trouble was obtained from the patient herself, and is as follows:

About seven years ago, while walking along the street, she felt a sharp, sudden pain in the arch of the right foot. It was of a neuralgic nature and prevented her, for a few moments, from walking to a car. It continued for an hour or so and then disappeared for some days; but from that time on she was subject to more or less severe attacks of pain in the right foot. After a year or two, she consulted a physician who pronounced the disease rheumatism, and prescribed salicylic acid. Four years ago she noticed that her right lower limb was swollen at the ankle and also just above the knee. Finally, as she was not getting better, and observing that the entire extremity was growing noticeably larger, she went to another physician who also pronounced it "rheumatism of a neuralgic order" and prescribed salicylic acid. He directed her to bind her entire limb in a surgical bandage from the hip to the toes, to reduce the swelling. This she wore for about four weeks, but without satisfactory result.

At this time the pains in the leg were quite as severe as that in the foot, and they began to materially interfere with walking. Standing or walking markedly increased the pain. While in Canada last September she took a severe cold, and for two weeks could neither walk nor raise her right arm, as the pain also affected the right shoulder. Electricity, baths, massage, and a visit to Hot Springs all failed to make an impression upon the disease. Tingling sensations, at one time present in the toes of the right foot, disappeared, but in other respects the affection became more pronounced, the swellings increasing in size and number until the right limb was much larger than the left. In a letter from Dr. Matas the statement is made that at his first examination the pain was distinctly marked along the paths of the external cutaneous, anterior crural, and musculocutaneous nerves.

The clothing having been removed and the patient placed upon her back the right thigh was at once observed to be decidedly larger than the left. The left thigh and leg were full and well formed. The trunk, shoulders, and arms were also well rounded, but did not give the impression of obesity. In other words, the left leg, trunk, both shoulders, and arms were well formed and well proportioned. On palpating the right foot a small spot, exquisitely sensitive to pressure, was discovered immediately over the distal third of the instep, extending slightly over the first metatarsal bone and first interosseous space. It was not accompanied by any swelling. Behind the external malleolus another small area of tenderness was discovered, and here, in addition, a soft fatty swelling was observed. The circumference of the ankles, the tape lying over both malleoli, was a quarter of an inch greater in the right than in the left foot. By measurement the right leg was also found to be somewhat enlarged. Thus, at the junction of the upper and middle thirds, the right leg measured 13⅜ and the left 12¾ inches. The enlargement appeared to be diffuse and uniform; no nodules, defined masses, or painful areas were detected. The enlargement of the thigh was very striking and readily confirmed by measurement. At the junction of the lower and middle third the right thigh measured 19⅜ and the left 17⅞ inches. At the junction of the middle and upper thirds, the right thigh measured 22¾ and the left 22¼ inches. The middle third of the right thigh measured 21½ and the left 19¾ inches. The enlargement of the thigh was found on palpation to be unevenly distributed. Immediately over and above the internal condyle, for example, an area was found at which the enlargement was more pronounced, and which felt nodular or lumpy. At this situation great pain was elicited by pressure. Upon the outer aspect of the lower third, several small, nodular, painful masses were also detected. In addition several painful areas were found in the course of the external, middle, and internal cutaneous nerves.

Some enlargement was present above the thigh, that is, over the lumbar and also to some extent over the right gluteal region. The enlargement had taken place, as far as could be judged, only in the fatty tissue. Over the right iliac crest, and to some extent posteriorly, a striking enlargement about the size and shape of a large orange was noted. This mass presented the same nodular (worm-like) feel noted in other situations. It was exquisitely painful, and not sharply circumscribed, but shaded off into the adjacent fatty tissue. The soreness was so great as to prevent the patient from lying upon her back or upon the right side. The entire lateral aspect of the right buttock was very sensitive to pressure, the pain interfering with the patient's sitting in a chair. A soft, more or less circumscribed mass was found in the right popliteal space. No nodules were discovered in any other portion of the body save on the inner aspect of the left arm, where a small mass, the size of a large nut, was detected.

The patient was a well-nourished young woman with a rather good color. There was no history of hemorrhage from mucous surfaces, or of cough or dyspnea. There was no headache. Backache, however, has been present at various times. Menstruation was normal.

The patient stated that the pain was never absent in the fatty masses, and that they were always more or less tender. At times, however, great exacerbation of the pain occur. In other words, the pain was subject to paroxysmal exacerbation, and she had repeatedly observed during these periods that the various nodular swellings above described had a firmer and somewhat indurated feel and were distinctly increased in size. After the paroxysm of pain subsided the intensity of the swelling somewhat diminished, but it never entirely disappeared. She further stated that each attack of pain seemed to add permanently, though slightly, to the size of the swellings. It was evident, from the examination, that the swellings were in the fatty tissue. There was no involvement of the muscles or bones.

CASE II.—M. A., an unmarried woman, aged sixty-five years, born in Ireland, was admitted to the service of Dr. Dercum at the Philadelphia Hospital, November 25, 1896. She was a very stout woman, and complained of pain in her feet. Her mother died of dropsy at the age of fifty years; her father was drowned. Three brothers and three sisters died in infancy. One sister grew very stout after the menopause, and finally died of asthma.

The patient had always been very healthy. She denied alcoholism. Menstruation ceased at forty. She had formerly been thin, but began to grow gradually stout at about the age of forty. She worked in a laundry during twelve years, and at the end of this period began to have pain. The pain was first felt beneath the heels, especially on walking. This pain extended to the legs, and seemed to be in both flesh and joints, later involving the hips and right shoulder. Two years ago (1894) she noticed pain in the fatty tissue of the limbs and trunk. She had never vomited blood nor had hemorrhages; she had not had headache or vertigo. The pain in the fatty tissue was subject to paroxysmal exacerbations. She stated that she had grown much stouter since the pains began.

Tenderness and pain were elicited by pressure, and upon handling the fatty tissue of the arms, thighs, legs, buttocks, lumbar region, and back. Slight soreness was also detected over the abdomen, the right shoulder, and the right arm, both inner and outer aspects, and local weakness was also observed. The pain did not follow any nerve distribution, and there was no anesthesia. The response to tests for heat and cold was prompt and correct. The patellar reflexes were normal. The tongue was protruded in a straight line. The pupils were equal and normal. The patient complained of headache and pain during motion of the left hip-joint, the latter having continued three years. She had also a marked flush over the forehead. The obesity was very marked over the thighs, calves, abdomen, nates, and back. It was also very great in the arms, less marked in the forearms, and absent in the feet and hands. In the face there was no special deposit of fat and no pain. The same condition was present in the neck. The isthmus of the thyroid was exceedingly small. The presence of lumps was not noted in this case, as in Case I.

CASE III.—Mrs. A., aged forty-five, referred to Dr. Mills by Dr. Thomas Hay of Milwaukee. The patient stated that there was no history of a trouble similar to hers in her parents or in their families. Her mother had had rheumatism which caused a very different kind of pain. A daughter of the patient's was in delicate health, but did not have a similar disease, and her three children were healthy.

The patient had been corpulent twelve or fourteen years, and first began to gain fat when she was about thirty-five years old, after the birth of her last child. She weighed 116 pounds at the time of her marriage, and during the four years previous to coming under observation weighed about 192 pounds. After an attack of pain she was always more fleshy and could not wear her clothes. The pains began about four years ago, at a time when she was rapidly gaining fat. The history of the commencement of these pains is as follows:

The legs from the knees to the feet began to ache, especially at night, and she could not sleep. After three or four weeks she had a sensation as of worms creeping in the flesh below the knee, and this made her exceedingly nervous. She also had a sensation of a tight band wound about the right lower limb from the lower part of the thigh to the foot. The calves of the legs felt as if they would burst open.

These symptoms continued for several months until she had an attack of very severe pain with a sensation of burning in both lower limbs, attended by a difference in the degree of temperature on the outside and inside of the thighs, as tested by her own hand. About three months later the pains were felt in the right arm, and some months later in the left.

During the first attack she noticed small pea-like swellings beneath the skin of the thighs, legs, and feet, but not in the arms. She had had severe attacks of pain, attended by painful swellings, at irregular intervals, but had been free from them as long as two years at a time. About four years ago nodular swellings were noticed on both sides of each knee, but were more marked on the right limb. These gradually grew smaller. At one time she had a large lump in the left inguinal region, which increased in size and was more painful at her monthly periods. This subsequently disappeared. She had also, at one time, a painful swelling over the back of the left hand.

Massage benefited her greatly, and under treatment with thyroid extract she improved so much that she became much thinner, and last summer could walk a block and a half. Her headache, from which she suffered greatly four years ago, is at present much less severe.

This patient had never had pain in the face. Often during her attacks of pain the palms of the hands and the soles and sides of the feet were covered with blisters, and after the attacks were over the skin peeled "as in scarlet fever."

On examination the patient was found to be corpulent, but not nearly as heavy as the patient first described by Dercum. A small lump was found on the outer side of the right knee. She complained of much pain in the lower limbs and to a less extent in the upper. This pain was spontaneous and was increased by pressure, and did not follow the course of any nerve. The hands and feet were somewhat puffy, but did not pit on pressure. The face was not affected and was not tender to pressure, except above the eyes. The patellar reflex was obtained in the left leg, but not in the right, even by reinforcement. There was no ankle clonus. Sensation for pain and touch was everywhere normal. There was no limitation of the visual fields, as tested with the hands. Except over the coccyx there were no painful points along the spine. There was no inguinal tenderness (ovarian), but there was slight inflammatory tenderness on the right side, and still more tenderness on the left. The limbs were everywhere tender to touch, and the back and front of the trunk were also tender, but not to such a degree as the limbs.

A CASE OF INGUINAL HERNIA OF LARGE SIZE; CURE FOLLOWING AN UNUSUAL METHOD OF OPERATION.

BY A. ERNEST GALLANT, M.D.,
OF NEW YORK;
ASSISTANT, DEPARTMENT OF SURGERY, IN THE NEW YORK POLYCLINIC.

DURING April, 1895, Mrs. M. N., aged sixty-two years, was referred by Professor Van Arsdale from the Good Samaritan Dispensary to the Lebanon Hospital. Her history was as follows:

Twenty-six years ago, while at work, she felt a [illegible] and something seemed to give way in the left groin, following which a small mass made its appearance in the region referred to. With the birth of each of her [illegible] children the mass increased in size. During recent years she has had three attacks of so-called "strangulation," the last two occurring two months before admission to the hospital. Bandages and supports of various kinds had been tried, and failed to afford any relief. She finally became practically bedridden, and, fearing another period of complete obstipation, was willing to submit to any precedure offering a chance of relief.

The operation was performed May 22, 1895, an incision six inches long being made over the anterior part of the tumor. Later, the opening was enlarged upward and outward toward the anterior spine of the ileum in order to facilitate reduction and suturing. The thin-walled sac contained the greater portion of the transverse and descending colon and nearly all of the small intestine. A portion of the small intestine fifteen inches long was ad-

FIG. 1.

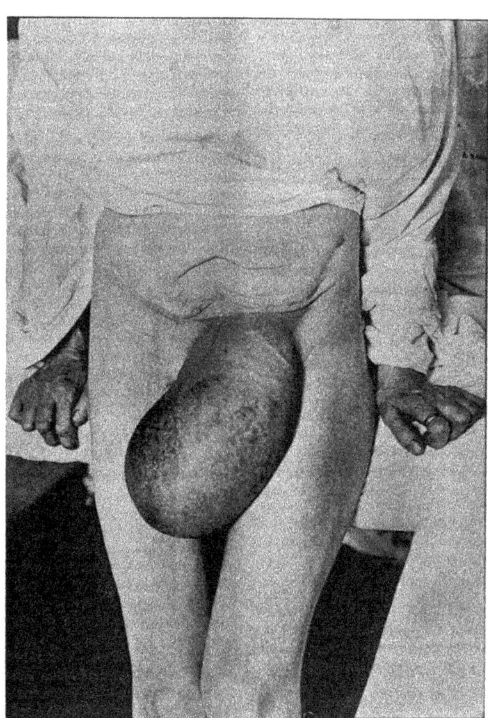

Inguinal hernia in a woman.

The condition previous to operation is well shown by the accompanying illustration (Fig. 1). Through the thickened inguinal ring the patient could reduce the mass to about one-half its usual size. She was examined by the members of the visiting staff of Lebanon Hospital, and all agreed that, in view of the liability to obstruction or strangulation, operative interference was justified, as likely to afford relief for a time at least, though cure could hardly be expected.

herent to the most pendulous portion of the sac, and was released with difficulty. The abdominal cavity, being relieved for so long a period of such a large portion of its contents, had contracted to such an extent that reduction was very difficult, and, when finally accomplished, made the abdominal walls as tense as a drum. While the intestines were being replaced, Dr. Parker Syms cut off the sac close to the groin, leaving only sufficient tissue to cover the wound.

Owing to the weakness of the patient's pulse, no attempt was made to cover the raw surface which remained after the separation of the adhesions. Anticipating very great abdominal tension it occurred to me that the following method of introducing the sutures could be more quickly applied, and perhaps more likely to hold than the usual method of uniting corresponding structures. Kangaroo tendon was employed for the buried sutures. The sutures were passed through the upper border of the wound, including the peritoneum, transversalis and external oblique muscles, and then, *inside the abdominal cavity*, through the peritoneum just above Poupart's ligament. The external oblique muscle and fascia were stitched edge to edge, *en masse*, to all the structures which compose Poupart's ligament. By this means the second tier of sutures overlapped the first by about one inch. The skin wound, twelve inches long, was sutured with silkworm gut.

On the afternoon of the second day after the operation the patient presented a marked degree of tympanites. Twelve doses of epsom salt, 1 dram each, were given. This was followed during the night by enemata of soapsuds, and later by a high injection of turpentine and sweet oil, but without affording any relief. At this time Dr. Syms telephoned that the patient was suffering from intestinal obstruction, and instructed me to operate for the relief of that condition. The abdomen was extremely distended, and the patient in great pain and fearing death.

After the removal of the dressing light friction was applied to the abdomen with the palm of the hand, beginning at the right iliac fossa, passing along the course of the colon to the opposite side, down to the region of the segmoid over the pubes. This maneuver was slowly and constantly repeated, and, after a few moments, the abdomen became less tense and the pain subsided. With the closed fist greater pressure was now exerted, and within fifteen minutes considerable gas was passed from the rectum. The patient expressed her appreciation of the relief afforded by kissing the hand of the masseur, shortly after which she went to sleep. During the day the bowels moved four times. No further difficulty was experienced. Healing of the wound took place by primary intention. The highest temperature reached at any time was 99.6° F.; pulse, 88. During the period of abdominal distention the respirations reached 52 per minute. Since leaving the hospital the patient has been able to attend to all her domestic duties, washing, ironing, scrubbing, etc.

During March, 1897, the patient changed her residence, and since then I have been unable to locate her, but at that time, twenty-one months after operation, she was in excellent condition.

This patient may be regarded as cured, and the writer feels that the good result was due to (1) the method of introducing the sutures, and (2) to the prompt relief of the intestinal distention by means of friction, a procedure which has proven useful in many cases.

A Victim to the Plague.—Madame Florence Morgan, the superintendent of the Plague Hospital at Bombay, recently died at that place of bubonic plague.

MEDICAL PROGRESS.

Tuberculous Ulcer of the Inner Surface of the Cheek.—CARRIERE (*Monats. f. Pract. Dermat.*, vol. XXVI., No. 1) describes the beginning of tuberculosis in a patient, aged thirty-seven years, who came to him for treatment of a slight abrasion on the inner surface of the left angle of the mouth. In the course of a few days this healed, leaving a somewhat elevated scar. Soon after, in this scar, an ulceration appeared and extended gradually backward 2.5 inches parallel to the margin of the teeth, where it presented the appearance of a raised lesion with sharp whitish edges. It was not painful, but was exquisitely tender if disturbed. The surrounding mucous membrane was normal in appearance. Tubercle bacilli were found to exist in the margin of the ulcer.

Amputation of the Leg below the Line of Demarcation.—ALLEN (*Med. Record*, December 25, 1897) describes a case of typhoid fever followed by gangrene of the left leg, apparently due to thrombosis. Owing to the very weak condition of the patient, amputation under an anesthetic was rejected as likely to prove fatal, and poultices were applied. As soon as demarcation was established, the patient was given a small dose of chloral, and without her knowledge the leg was amputated through the gangrenous tissue. Six months later, the flaps were split up, the bones divided at a higher plane and their ends covered. Union was this time primary, and the patient entirely recovered. This rather tedious method of procedure, in Allen's opinion, saved a patient who under any other plan of treatment would have succumbed.

THERAPEUTIC NOTES.

Antiseptic Treatment of Acute Otitis Media. — CHEATLE (*Pediatrics*, January, 1898) urges the importance of antiseptic treatment of the external meatus in cases of middle-ear trouble. The cartilaginous portion of the meatus teems with micro-organisms. The writer has observed that in acute otitis media puncture of the drum membrane is frequently followed by the escape of serosanguinous fluid without pus. Even if pus is present, if possible further infection should be prevented. The first thing to be done when consulted by such a patient is to purify the auricle and meatus. This is best performed by means of a 1–20 carbolic-acid solution. Small swabs of cotton are dipped in this, and with them the meatus is thoroughly scrubbed. The ear is also douched with a 1–40 carbolic-acid solution. When the meatus has been thus purified, a light plug is introduced into it, and a dressing and bandage applied. If it subsequently becomes necessary to puncture the membrane this may readily be accomplished without infection, and even if this does not become necessary, the dressing gives the ear functional rest, a point the value of which is not sufficiently appreciated. Carbolic acid is a particularly good disinfectant in these cases on account of its anesthetic property, and its power of penetration into fats. Patients with middle-ear disease, if treated in accordance with these principles, do very well indeed

THE MEDICAL NEWS.

A WEEKLY JOURNAL

OF MEDICAL SCIENCE.

COMMUNICATIONS are invited from all parts of the world. Original articles contributed *exclusively* to THE MEDICAL NEWS will after publication be liberally paid for (accounts being rendered quarterly), or 250 reprints will be furnished in place of other remuneration. When necessary to elucidate the text, illustrations will be engraved from drawings or photographs furnished by the author. Manuscripts should be typewritten.

Address the Editor: J. RIDDLE GOFFE, M.D.,
No. 111 FIFTH AVENUE (corner of 18th St.), NEW YORK.

Subscription Price, including postage in U. S. and Canada.

PER ANNUM IN ADVANCE	$4.00
SINGLE COPIES	.10
WITH THE AMERICAN JOURNAL OF THE MEDICAL SCIENCES, PER ANNUM	7.50

Subscriptions may begin at any date. The safest mode of remittance is by bank check or postal money order, drawn to the order of the undersigned. When neither is accessible, remittances may be made, at the risk of the publishers, by forwarding in *registered* letters.

LEA BROTHERS & CO.,
No. 111 FIFTH AVENUE (corner of 18th St.), NEW YORK,
AND NOS. 706, 708 & 710 SANSOM ST., PHILADELPHIA.

SATURDAY, FEBRUARY 26, 1898.

DOES PUBLICITY INCREASE CRIME?

WHEN the medical student reaches cardiac diseases in the course of his studies he frequently discovers that he has a systolic murmur or some other alarming symptom of heart disease. This fact is so well known that it has passed into that most ancient of all storehouses from which the college professor draws his jokes. Is this harmless form of "suggestion" a true index of the effect on the public of a constant presentation to their minds of the details of crime? Do the sensational reports of murders, of rape, of arson, incite other men and women to like deeds? Is crime infectious and contagious?

Warren, in discussing this subject in the January number of the *University Medical Magazine*, asserts that newspapers propagate crime in three ways: (1) by suggestion, (2) by creating an insane desire for newspaper notoriety, and (3) by placing a premium on crime. The newspaper stands in about the same relation to the public, according to this writer, as a hypnotist does to his subject; and while there is some doubt whether a hypnotist can by suggestion induce a person to commit crime unless he already has a leaning in that direction, still there are too many individuals who are willing to be persuaded into wrong-doing, especially if they hope to profit by it, to make that excuse of much avail.

As for the effect on the would-be criminal of seeing his name and photograph in the "Extra" of a penny print, there is much direct testimony that boys and others, who have committed some horrible crime such as train-wrecking, were impelled to it by the love of notoriety. Imagine yourself a criminal, considering the chances of being caught if you carry out a certain daring burglary. What would be the relative deterrent effect upon you of the methods of trial and publicity in this country, and, for instance, in Germany? The conditions here do not require description. On the other hand, in Germany, the prisoner drops out of existence, one may almost say, until the result of a secret trial has either released him or separated him still further from all contact with his fellows. It cannot be denied too, that in Germany the scarcity of mercy would have a still further deterrent effect upon intending criminals; but the difference in this respect in our own country is, in no small degree, the result of the habit we have grown into of looking upon a criminal trial as a contest, and if the criminal makes a plucky fight, or if the odds are heavily against him, the love of bravery and fair play, makes both jury and public unwilling to decide against him, irrespective of the crime which has brought him into the lists. The remedy for this state of affairs proposed by Warren, is to ask the representatives in Congress and in the Legislatures to pass laws prohibiting the publication of this class of news.

In the *Public Health Journal* for December, Humphrey of Oregon, takes up the increase of crime from a little different point of view. He too, admits the increase of crime (there were 48,834 murders and homicides in the United States in the ten years ending 1895), and laments the ineffectual means of prevention which are now employed. Impressed as he is with the fact that criminals to a great extent breed criminals, he advocates the asexualization of old offenders, as the most logical measure to protect the State from an ever-increasing number of individuals having a well-marked criminal tendency.

As to the practical outcome of such a law, he says: "Criminals would regard such a law with terror, and would rather take their chances against anything than having their procreative organs removed. I am aware that a great many will not agree with me, but I have the courage of my convictions and can afford to be criticized. Of all the criminals that should be so dealt with for the first offense are those who rape innocent women and girls. All other classes might be subjected to the operation of such a law on a second conviction."

The study of anthropology has proved the existence of a criminal type, with marked characteristics in anatomy and physiology. How fruitless to allow these parasites upon society to multiply, and then to spend millions in the attempt to alter these characteristics in the individuals of ever-recurring generations! And every year while the Government is performing this task of Sisyphus, thousands of good members of society are robbed and butchered by the degenerated who ought never to have been generated.

EXPERT MEDICAL WITNESSES.

A BILL has been introduced in the New York Legislature which aims to provide for the examination and appointment of medical expert witnesses in certain cases, and for the regulation of their compensation. The act is fostered, it is understood, by the Homeopathic State Medical Society.

The essential features of the bill are: That upon the trial of all indictments for felonies in a court of criminal jurisdiction, whenever it is made to appear to the Court that the trial will probably require the introduction of medical testimony, the Court may, upon application of either party, appoint such a number of experts—not less than three or more than five—as the Court shall deem proper. The presiding judge shall provisionally prepare a list of names of such persons as it may have reason to believe properly qualified, and shall cause any of these persons to be subpœnaed to appear at such time and place as the judge may order. They shall then be examined by the latter, touching their qualifications to serve as experts, and if they pass a satisfactory examination they may be employed; if they do not, they are at liberty to return to the duties of their profession, with which they believe themselves competent to cope and which the licensing faculty has deemed them fitted to perform.

If the individual who has been preemptorily summoned from his chosen labor satisfies the presiding judge that he has sufficient "expertness," he is to be paid from $10 to $100 a day for his servi depending upon the value which the all-wise S who then happens to wear the ermine puts upon services. He is also allowed mileage, the sam other witnesses. As the bill provides that exp may be summoned from without the State, it be well for experts living or sojourning in the O dent to enlarge their strong boxes and make p now for the repletion of their exchequers. only other feature of the bill which calls for remar that nothing in the act shall be construed to l or effect the right of either party to summon o expert witnesses—as many as they may be abl induce to give testimony on a contingency, or a basis.

No one will deny the opportunities of the ti nor the necessity of reform in the present met or want of method, of employing medical ex testimony. There has already been much us discussion on this topic, and it is not improbable in time a plan will be evolved which will be a g advance on that in vogue at the present day. regret, however, to say that the bill in question not contain a germ of laudable or legitimate ormation, and we hope sincerely that every ph cian who is interested in this matter and every ciety to whose Committee on Codes it will referred, will do all in their power to prevent enactment.

The first, if not the most serious, objection ra to the act is, that it leaves the power of appoint of experts in the hands of the presiding ju This individual may be deeply learned in the he may be profoundly versed in the humanities may be an honest, upright, judicial personage; wherefore should he know of the weary delving the realms of science, and of the years of stud labor on the part of physicians, whom he does know either by word or reputation, which give the right to be called "expert" by their pr sional brethren? As a matter of truth, he does know, nor in all human probability has he any bition to extend his knowledge in this direct One of the speakers discussing this subject at meeting of the State Society a few weeks ag Albany, said that it was notorious that judges lected their physicians from the ranks of the ho paths or the quacks, and it was the exception judge to have in his service a reputable, distinguished physician. If they cannot be relied upon to show greater wisdom in the selection of their family physicians why should they be expected to be more perspicacious and discriminative in behalf of the public?

A second objection to the bill, and one that more closely concerns the physician, is that no law that compels him to relinquish whatsoever he may be engrossed in, even though it be of the gravest import, and dance attendance upon a court which shall examine him as to his fitness to testify on a matter which may not be of the slightest interest to him, can be enforced. The "expert" may be called upon to give testimony that spares a human life, or to testify to facts that will keep in the hands of legitimate legatees millions of dollars, and for this service he is given $15, or $40, or even, if Magnanimity is sitting on the bench, $100. For this paltry sum he has burned the fires of his soul and pigmented his cortical cells, that a judge may rise up and call him expert. No wonder that the legal faculty look upon the doctor as an easy prey, when there are those amongst us who assume the rôle of reformers and put the value of a journeyman plumber's wages upon their services. Imagine employing Daniel Webster, Henry Clay, and Rufus Choate, in their day, or in ours, for from $10 to $100 a day. Shades and spirits of these immortals gather around and protect us! Yet this bill proposes to call, at any time or place, the leaders of the medical profession, the authorities of the day, and, after using them to their advantage, requite their services with a contemptible sum which not even the most inconsequential lawyer would deign to accept as a retainer.

And lastly, when the whole matter is simmered down, of what earthly benefit would the enactment of such a law be? It states specifically that either party may call as many experts as he sees fit. Modern Crœsus, accused of crime, may summon the flower and fruit of the medical faculty, and so bewilder his twelve peers sitting in judgment upon him that the trial would be an exact counterpart of those of to-day. On the other hand, an impecunious, miserable wretch, on trial for murder, might with her nescient wail, touch the sympathetic cord of a hysteric sisterhood, who, under the guidance of crafty counsel, would erect a psychic superstructure of fantastic epilepsy that, through the mediumship of outside experts, would sweep her from the electric chair.

If we are to have reform in the matter of expert medical testimony, let us have reform based upon sound reasoning and legitimate principles of equity and honesty.

MEDICAL POLITICS AT MOBILE.

WE had not given any credence to charges made in certain papers that the quarantine convention intended to be composed of delegates from the South Atlantic and Gulf States, which met in Mobile on February 9th, 10th, and 11th, was, as specifically charged by them, a "packed" convention conceived by persons inimical to a national quarantine, and incidentally opposed to the development of the Marine Hospital Service. The fair appearance of the call, the equable division of representation among the Southern States, and the high character of some of the gentlemen named as its leading spirits, seemed to forbid such a conclusion; but the reports which we have at hand from this meeting indicate that the elaborate program laid out by its astute managers to discuss the varied features of maritime and interstate quarantine and sanitation in general was nothing more or less than a Barmecide feast.

The ingenuous gentleman who went to the convention under the impression that he would hear scientific papers and discussions on the diagnosis of yellow fever, the sanitation of cars, baggage, and freight in times of epidemic, the disinfection of houses and other similar topics of vital interest, soon found that while the politics of the managers of the convention necessitated this masquerade to attract attendance, the real interest of its promoters was to secure an endorsement of the so-called American Medical Association bill to establish a Department of Public Health, and to denounce the Caffery bill which has been drawn in the interest of Federal quarantine. We learn that the Executive Committee, a self-appointed body, selected a permanent Chairman for the convention without giving the members the privilege of voting on the presiding officer, and that this same Chairman thereupon named a Committee on Resolutions, who were to formulate the sentiments of the convention upon the all-important point of national or State supremacy in quarantine matters.

Although this convention was to be composed of delegates from the South Atlantic and Gulf States, it was soon discovered that Illinois was represented by the editor of the *Journal of the American Medical Association*, and Wisconsin by the Chairman of the Committee of the American Medical Association, by which was formulated the bill designed to obliterate the Marine Hospital Service in national health matters. Delegates were also present from New York, Maryland, and Kentucky, and these gentlemen and the delegates from these three States were accorded equal privileges on the floor, and were appointed members of the Committee on Resolutions, a body of thirteen members, of which these constituted almost one-half. The rest was easy, and although the managers did not secure an endorsement of their bill, neither did it secure a denunciation of the Caffery bill, as there was a large minority, who, in their disappointment at the outcome of the convention, did not propose to be led further into a game which had become manifest at the close of the third day. One day of scientific discussion and two days of wire-pulling had opened their eyes to the meaning of the convention. What the convention resolved,—a sort of endorsement of national quarantine, with a reference to the reserved rights of States,—is highly unimportant even if it was unanimously passed. In fact, the New Orleans *Times-Democrat*, in its issue of February 12th, says editorially "unless Congress can do better for the South Atlantic and Gulf States than the convention proposes that it shall do," referring to these resolutions, "their liability to invasions of foreign disease will not be materially lessened."

ECHOES AND NEWS.

Monument to Tarnier.—The former pupils of the late Professor Tarnier have formed a committee to secure funds for the erection of a monument to his memory.

An Enormous Heart.—At an autopsy recently held in London (Eng.) to determine the cause of death in the case of a man, forty-six years of age, who had suddenly expired in an omnibus, it was discovered that his heart weighed forty-three ounces.

Another Achievement in Abdominal Surgery.—Mr. Frederick Treves, the English surgeon, recently removed the whole of that part of the bowel below the transverse colon, together with the anus, in a case of idiopathic dilatation of the colon in a child. The patient made a good recovery.

Hospital Service for Alaska.—A company known as the Alaska Sanitary Company has been organized under the laws of Illinois for the purpose of establishing a series of hospitals at all the important points in Alaska. The chief promoter of the enterprise is Dr. F. H. Booth. A two-story log structure has been erected at Dawson City as a hospital. The institution is under the charge of Father William Judge of Baltimore. It has twenty-six patients. At present the nursing is done by the miners, but six sisters of St. Anne are on their way from Montreal to act as nurses and teachers.

A New Location for Mt. Sinai Hospital.—A site consisting of twenty-five lots on Fifth avenue between One Hundred and One Hundred and First streets has recently been purchased by Mt. Sinai Hospital of New York, upon which a new building is to be erected in the near future.

Sterilization by Frying.—Olive oil at a temperature of 256° F., is recommended for sterilizing syringes and instruments. Immersion for an instant in the hot oil will completely sterilize an instrument, while to render a syringe germ free, it is only necessary to twice fill the barrel with oil at the temperature mentioned.

Funds for the Craig Epileptic Colony.—Among the bills recently passed by the New York Assembly is one appropriating $161,000 for the Craig Colony of Epileptics. This experiment in the management of epileptics may now be considered an established system, and the recognition of this fact by the State legislators is thus assuring it substantial aid.

The Middleton Goldsmith Lecture.—The Middleton Goldsmith lecture of the New York Pathological Society was delivered at the New York Academy of Medicine on Friday evening, February 25, 1898, by Professor William T. Sedgwick of Boston. The subject was: "The Establishment and Conservation of Purity in Public Water-supplies, Especially Those of Great Cities."

Expectoration Tracts.—The Women's Health Protective Associations in different parts of the country have extended their warfare against expectoration in public buildings and street-cars by the distribution of neat little cards which invite the attention of the offender against public health and cleanliness to the fact that expectoration is forbidden. These cards are already in use in Boston.

To Abolish Coroners.—The first county to seek to take advantage of the omission of any mention of the office of coroner in the new constitution is Ulster, and Assemblyman Tremper has introduced a bill abolishing the office in that county. The measure is now awaiting its final reading in the Assembly. If the bill passes, it is expected that a number of other counties will follow suit.

An Instrument with a History.—The museum of the Royal College of Surgeons of England has been enriched by a case of instruments which has a distinct historic value. The case contains a saw which bears this inscription: "The first subcutaneous osteotomy saw made by Mr. Blaise, and used by Mr. William Adams on December 1, 1869, in his first case of division of the neck of the femur."

"Undesirable Invalid's Bill."—According to the *Lancet*, this is the title of a bill which it is proposed to bring up for the second time before the House of Representatives of New Zealand, The bill is directed against the landing on the islands of patients afflicted with communicable diseases, and stringent measures are to be adopted with regard to those people already in the colony who are similarly afflicted. Foremost among such diseases is tuberculosis, and more particularly pulmonary tuberculosis.

Scarlet Fever from Milk.—Some cases of scarlatina at the Oranges, New Jersey, are reported to have been traced to a dairy conducted by a family, all the members of which have been, or are now, suffering from that disease. The dairy is at Northfield and has been taken in hand by the State Board of Health. The cows have been given a clean bill of health and are now at another farm. The nature of the attack was not understood by the family until the first patient, a person over sixty years of age, had passed into the desquamative stage.

Female Candidates for Fellowship.—Among the list of candidates for fellowship of the Royal College of Surgeons, Ireland, appear the names of three women who present all the qualifications prescribed by the College and recognized by the General Medical Council. In conformity with collegiate rules the applications will receive attention with a view to inquiry as to the eligibility of the applicants in other respects, and it is assumed that if no objection is then offered, they will be admitted to the examination. Whether they will achieve the fellowship is another question.

Improved Methods of House Disinfection.—The question of what to do with people who live in two or three rooms when a case of infectious disease necessitates closing these up for disinfecting purposes, has been solved in England. Upon the suggestion of the medical officer of health, Dr. Waldo, the vestry of St. George's, Southwark, have opened a receiving house for the reception of the temporarily homeless families. They are taken care of at the receiving house for eight hours, during which time they are given baths and their clothing is taken from them and disinfected.

Examinations in Hygiene.—Rutgers College is the first educational institution in this country to definitely recognize the specific qualifications of sanitarians. The college will conduct examinations and grant certificates in municipal hygiene to officers of local boards of health, sanitary inspectors, factory inspectors, plumbing inspectors, and to those who may seek appointments to these positions. The examinations, which will be held on the first Wednesday of the months of March, June, and October at the college buildings in New Brunswick, New Jersey, will be designed to test the fitness of persons who may by called upon to engage in the execution of the health laws.

Obituary.—Dr. John G. Truax died at his home in New York on February 16th of Bright's disease and heart failure. Dr. Truax was born in Oneida County, New York, in 1848. From the University of Michigan he went to Rush Medical College, Chicago, and was graduated from that institution in 1871. He came to New York in 1876. He was a brother of Judge Truax of the Supreme Court.—Dr. Robert A. Wheaton recently died of apoplexy at his home in St. Paul, Minn., at the age of thirty-five. He was a graduate of Harvard, and was professor of minor surgery in the University of Minnesota, and captain and assistant surgeon in the Minnesota National Guard.—Charles Todd Quintard, D.D., LL.D., Bishop of the Protestant Episcopal Diocese of Tennessee, died last week at Meridian, Ga., of heart failure. He was born in Stamford in 1824. After leaving Trinity School he studied medicine with Dr. James R. Wood and Dr. Valentine Mott, and was graduated from the University of the City of New York in 1847. He then removed to Athens, Ga., where he began the practice of medicine. In 1851 he was appointed professor of physiology and pathologic anatomy in the medical college at Memphis, Tenn., and was co-editor with Dr. Ayres P. Merrill of the *Memphis Medical Recorder*. In 1855 he was appointed a deacon in the Protestant Episcopal Church, and in January, 1857, became rector of the Calvary Church, Memphis. After the death of Bishop Otey in 1865, he was elected Bishop of Tennessee. He received the degree of doctor of divinity from Columbia in 1866, and that of doctor of laws from Cambridge (Eng.) in 1867.

Statement by Surgeon-General Wyman Regarding Ship Island Quarantine.—In a letter to the *Washington Post*, in reply to one asking for information in regard to the quarantine station on Ship Island, Miss., Surgeon-General Wyman says: "There is absolutely no place for the location of a quarantine off the coast of Mississippi to which greater objections cannot be made than are made to Ship Island. If a distance of twelve miles from the coast is an insuperable objection, then the quarantine stations at San Francisco and San Diego, Cal., Galveston and Sabine Pass, Tex., Mobile, Ala., Key West and Fernandia, Fla., Brunswick and South Atlantic Quarantine, Ga., Cape Fear Quarantine, N. C., and New York Quarantine all would have to be moved, for they are all nearer to the coast or to populated districts than is Ship Island. . . . Captain Laym of the Revenue Cutter Service and Surgeon Murray of the Marine Hospital Service were directed to visit the other islands in the Gulf, and reported under date, December, 19, 1883, that Ship Island was the best located and the only island which possessed the necessary advantages for a quarantine station. Nevertheless, in 1898 various influences brought about the act of Congress authorizing the removal of the station to some other island. This act of Congress gave authority, but was not mandatory in its language. A board was appointed March 10, 1888, to select a site for a new quarantine station, and though their orders required them to recommend some other site than Ship Island, the board went out of its way, in the fourth paragraph of its report, inserted at the suggestion of Dr. Wilkinson of Louisiana, to state as follows: 'There is no evidence to warrant the belief that the presence of the National Quarantine Station on Ship Island is a real source of danger to the inhabitants of the Gulf Coast, but all testimony points absolutely to the fact that the absence of an efficient quarantine service at that place will afford a probable inlet to contagious diseases into that vicinity.' This report was signed by Surgeon W. H. H. Hutton of the Marine Hospital Service; Captain J. H. Parker of the United States Revenue Cutter Service; Dr. J. W. Mabin of Biloxi, who represented Mississippi, and Dr. C. P. Wilkinson of the Louisiana State Board of Health. The Board reported that Chandeleur Island afforded the 'next best' location, and accordingly the station was removed there in 1889, and, all told, about $85,000 was expended in its establishment. Immediately thereafter, the State of Mississippi established a quarantine at the abandoned site, performed active work there inspecting and disinfecting vessels, charging the customary fees therefor, and continued to do so with some intermission until 1894, when the United States establishment was replaced on Ship Island."

CORRESPONDENCE.

OUR PHILADELPHIA LETTER.

[From our Special Correspondent.]

PUBLIC OPINION AND THE TYPHOID EPIDEMIC—A LOW DEATH-RATE FOR 1897—METHYLENE BLUE IN THE TREATMENT OF GONORRHEA—PAPILLARY NEOPLASMS OF THE ILEUM—THE OXYTOXIC INFLUENCE OF QUININ—A LARGE BEQUEST TO THE PENNSYLVANIA HOSPITAL—THE ALIENISTS' REPORT ON A BOY MURDERER.

PHILADELPHIA, February 19, 1898.

PUBLIC interest in the typhoid situation has to some extent abated, in the face of other topics of the hour, and in realization of the fact that all agitation for the abatement of the pest by help of the city legislators is exertion uselessly expended. The people have expressed convincingly their opinions in the press, in mass meetings, and before Councils themselves, but to absolutely no avail in so far as securing an appropriation for an improved water-supply is concerned. So the question begins to become uninteresting to some, apathetic to others, and a wholly useless topic for discussion to all—the public, by a long apprenticeship, have grown accustomed to the prevalence of enteric fever, and they are inclined to look on it just as they look on the other preventable infections diseases which we, in our much-heralded republican freedom, accept as necessary evils attending the present *fin-de-siècle* civilization. Public interest, it should be remarked, and not the interest of medical men, is on the wane. Physicians throughout the city continue to urge filtration, continue to demonstrate the wanton sacrifice in human lives which typhoid costs the city of Philadelphia, and continue to exert their every effort for the improvement of the situation, without, it must be confessed, very tangible hopes of success. It has narrowed down to this point: that Councils refuse absolutely to comply with the popular demand for filtration of the water-supply, and that the arguments of the people and of the medical profession may, like Tennyson's brook, run on forever, and never so much as wear the faintest indication of a groove of humanity or common sense in the cerebra of these "city fathers" of ours. The whole affair is disgusting to every fair-minded Philadelphian. The fever-pest still continues, with, however, a decrease during the last two weeks in the number of new cases, which improvement is offset by a much higher death-rate. During the week ending February 19th there were 156 new cases, with 17 deaths reported, as compared to 185 new cases, with 21 deaths, for the week of February 12th. Since the epidemic began 1839 new cases of typhoid, and 196 deaths from this cause have been reported to the Board of Health. Further comment is unnecessary to the intelligent; it is unconvincing to the opponents of the filtration bill.

In spite of the general increase in infectious diseases and of the increased death-rate from diphtheria and scarlet fever, the death-rate in Philadelphia for the year 1897 was but 18.72 per thousand inhabitants—the lowest rate for thirteen years. The total number of deaths from all causes and at all periods of life was 22,735, or a decrease of 1247 from the previous year. It is also gratifying to note that the death-rate last year in children under five years of age was the lowest ever attained here, the deaths at this period of life numbering 33.45 per cent. of the total number of deaths, in both adults and children, from all causes. This is attributed, in a large extent, to a better personal acquaintance on the part of parents with laws of sanitation and with hygienic measures, and to the extensive municipal improvements which have been made in the poorer districts of the city, where formerly improper drainage and careless house-inspection kept the infant mortality at a high figure. In this connection, also, the highest credit must be rendered to the various "fresh-air" organizations, such as the Red Bank Sanitarium and the Country Week Association, for their humane and indispensable labors in caring for thousands of the little ones of the alleys and slums during the heated months; the value of their work cannot be estimated too highly.

Horwitz, at the last meeting of the Philadelphia County Medical Society, related his experience with the treatment of gonorrhea with methylene blue combined with the oils of sandalwood and cinnamon and the oleo-resin of copaiba, together with urethral irrigations with permanganate of potassium solutions of a strength of from 1-2000 to 1-1000. Methylene blue was given usually in 2-grain doses three times daily, but as this quantity was found to produce strangury and slight diarrhea in about twenty-five per cent. of the patients to whom it was given, the dose, in such instances, was diminished one-half. The combination of powdered nutmeg seemed to prevent, in a measure, these untoward symptoms. It was invariably the rule that the urine of patients receiving methylene blue was colored by the drug. Bacteriologic studies of cases treated by this method showed that the addition of the analin to the other drugs greatly adds to their germicidal power on the gonococcus; this fact was also demonstrated with solutions of methylene blue alone. Of 105 cases of specific urethritis thus treated by Horwitz, 77 were cured within three-weeks' time, 16 required four weeks to complete the cure, and the remaining number recovered within seven weeks. In cases of non-specific urethritis, on the other hand, it was maintained that the employment of methylene blue was of no value.

F. A. Packard, at the last meeting of the Pathological Society of Philadelphia, exhibited several curious specimens of a papillary new growth of the serous surface of the ileum, from a child dead of tuberculous peritonitis. The neoplasms consisted of numerous slender, whitish processes, $\frac{1}{30}$-inch in width and about $\frac{1}{3}$-inch in length, and were distributed over the serous surface of the ileum at the middle of its course; they consisted, microscopically, of collections of loosely formed areolar tissue enveloped with a serous covering, and having a central arterial canal. Inasmuch as the growths conformed to no known histologic type, their exact character could not be determined.

L. J. Hammond, in a paper read before the Obstetrical Society of Philadelphia, at the last meeting of this body, expressed the belief that quinin exercises a decidedly tonic effect upon the propulsive powers of the uterus during labor, particularly in women whose general muscular development is deficient or atonic. He administered the drug to 100 cases of parturient women, giving half-hourly doses of 10 grains until 30 grains had been taken. Of the thirty-eight primiparæ to whom quinin was given, there was an increase in the frequency and force of the uterine contractions in thirty-five cases; of the sixty-two multiparæ, an increase in the propulsive power was noted in thirty-one instances.

By the will of the late George Plumer Smith, who recently died in this city, a large sum of money is left to the Pennsylvania Hospital, and smaller amounts to other city and State charitable institutions. The entire amount left by the late Mr. Smith is nearly three-quarters of a million dollars, of which sum the entire residuary estate, amounting to about $400,000, is bequeathed to the contributors of the Presbyterian Hospital. The sum of $10,000 is also left to the Presbyterian Hospital of this city.

The inquiry into the mental condition of Samuel Henderson, the boy murderer, has been completed by the alienists appointed by the District Attorney, Drs. Chapin and Morton. Contrary to general expectations, the precise nature of their report will, it is announced by the authorities, be withheld from the public until the case comes up for trial, the time for which has not yet been decided upon.

During the week ending February 19th, the number of deaths reported from all causes in this city was 491, or 15 less than reported last week, and 39 less than those of the corresponding week of last year. Of this number, 148 were of children under five years of age. There were 82 new cases of diphtheria reported, with 25 deaths—the same number of cases and of deaths as reported last week; scarlet-fever cases number 57, with 7 deaths from this cause.

OUR BERLIN LETTER.

[From our Special Correspondent.]

THE NEW CHARITÉ AS IT WILL BE WITHIN FIVE YEARS—A PASTEUR INSTITUTE FOR BERLIN AND WHAT IT MEANS AS TO THE TREATMENT OF RABIES—NEW MEDICAL JOURNALS—THE MEDICO-LEGAL DIFFERENTIATION OF DEATH BY FREEZING.

BERLIN, February 17, 1898.

THE last number of the *Charité Annalen* (the report of the principal hospital here in Berlin) contains an interesting account of the early days of the Charité. So much of Berlin medical history is contained in the wards of this old hospital that it will always have a place in medical lore. Virchow, Frerichs, Traube, to say nothing of many others, did their great work here. The most interesting part of this account, however, is the future of the Charité; for at the beginning of the Twentieth Century the University of Berlin will have in the new Charité, just about to be built, one of the largest, most modern, best-appointed, and best-equipped hospitals for teaching purposes in the world. This is the confessed aim of the present administration and the question of money is not to stand in the way.

Those acquainted with the present Charité know how much this is needed. Those who know other hospitals about Berlin, Moabit, Friedrichshain, or the Kaiser and Kaiserin Friedrich Kinderspital in Reinickerdorf, know what a model hospital the modern German institution may be. Special pride is taken in making the new Charité in every way worthy of the medical center of the world, as, of course, every good German (need I say most every one else) considers Berlin to be.

Some 10,000,000 marks ($2,500,000) are to be spent on improvement of the Charité within the next five years. Practically all of the old buildings are to disappear to make room for modern structures. Some of these are already under way. The new Pathological Institute, to cost 1,500,000 marks ($375,000), is nearly completed. It has been a pet project of Professor Virchow's for many years to have the erection of the new institute under his direction before his death. The arrangements of the building will be such that it will surpass any thing in this line so far erected. It is to be hoped that the veteran professor will not say his *nunc dimittis*, until, working for some years in the new laboratories, he has proved how great are the opportunities still left in pathology. The Laboratory of Pharmacology and Toxicology is also well under way. The Department for Mental and Nervous Diseases is soon to be begun. It is a sign of the times and of the amount of attention that is being devoted on all sides to diseases of the nervous system, that, after the Pathological Institute, this department comes next in the amount to be appropriated for its new quarters, 1,200,000 marks ($300,000) will be spent for its construction.

The whole plan of the new institution is on a magnificent scale. Government regulation of universities has its disadvantages, but where the best interests of education are consulted, as they seem to be here, results may be accomplished which private effort could not attempt. Thanks to the farseeing liberality and generous interest of the government, though calls are made on it from all sides, Berlin is likely to retain the place she has held for the last thirty years as a leader in education, and especially in medicine. With opportunities such as will be afforded in the new clinics and laboratories, still more may be expected of her in the first half of the Twentieth Century, than has been the case in the latter half of the Nineteenth.

One item in the budget of expenses for the Institute of Infectious Diseases here in Berlin for the year 1898 is especially interesting. Four thousand marks ($1000) is appropriated for the establishment, in connection with the Institute, of an experimental station for the treatment of rabies after the method of Pasteur. As yet the work is to be only tentative, it is said, but the change of front after the decided opposition that Pasteur's treatment has always met in Berlin, especially at the hands of Professor Koch and his school, makes the establishment of such a department in the Institute of which he is director a noteworthy and significant departure.

There has been no little uneasiness in many cities of Germany of late over reported cases of hydrophobia. From Hamburg and Dresden, as well as from about Berlin itself, such reports seemed not absolutely without foundation. From Königsberg, Breslau, and other places near the Russian frontier, came reports of cases, in which there could be no doubt that genuine lyssa was at work.

The German medical men who visited the International Medical Congress at Moscow were deeply impressed with the regard the Russians have for the Pasteur method of treating this disease. Their statistics showing its efficacy were freely distributed during the sessions of two or three of the sections. The Rabies Department of the Imperial Institute of Experimental Medicine of St. Petersburg was a striking object lesson. This institution is magnificently arranged, on a scale only second to that of the Pasteur Institute in Paris, if even this much is to be allowed.

Their results of treatment have been most satisfactory, and yet Russia is the hotbed of the most virulent form of rabies, from which probably most of the rabies of Europe comes. The wolves of the Steppes are often infected and give the disease to other animals. At times they attack men too, and their tendency to spring for the face and neck results in the most serious form of rabies. The virus is rapidly absorbed in large quantities, owing to the rich lymphatics of these parts; while the proximity of the point of infection to the nervous centers, in which by preference the virus localizes and reproduces itself, inevitably makes the infection extremely severe. The prognosis of head rabies, that is, the disease developing after a bite in the head region, is universally acknowledged to be particularly bad—yet it is with this class of cases that the tests in Russia were made.

Russian statistics on most things medical, as well as Russian medical and surgical opinions generally, will count for much more in the medical world since the profession has had a chance to see for itself the thoroughly scientific quality of the work being done there. So it has been in this case. Now that Berlin has fallen into line we can confidently look for the establishment of Pasteur departments in most of the medical universities of Germany. The end of the opposition to Pasteur's method is at hand. It is probable that this will lead to a great many changes in opinions in America too, for Americans generally have taken their cue in the matter from the Germans rather than from the English. In England the best opinion has long since declared in favor of the treatment, and in the English Army, in the colonies at least, the bite of an animal thought by a physician or a veterinarian to have rabies, must be followed by the Pasteur treatment, if the affected individual is to retain his connection with the army.

Three new medical journals have seen the light in Germany within the last couple of months. It is an index of the immense number of medical journals that already exist over here, that practically all three of them are to be devoted to the reviewing and abstracting of other medical journals. The *Dermatologisches Centralblatt*, edited by Dr. Max Joseph here in Berlin is one. *The Medicine of the Present*, a sort of medical *Review of Reviews*, also to be issued here in Berlin, is another; while the third, *The Centralblatt für die Grenzgebiete der Medicin und Chirurgie* (Review of the Borderland Lying Between Medicine and Surgery), though edited by Dr. Hermann Schlesinger of Vienna, is published by Fischer of Jena, and is evidently intended to draw subscribers from all over Germany. It is to be a supplementary journal to the *Mittheilungen aus der Grenzgebiete*, etc. (Communications from the Borderland, etc.), edited by Professor Naunyn of Strassburg, and Mikulicz of Breslau, and which, though but a year or two old, is regarded as one of the standard medical journals here in Germany.

When so many *Reviews of Reviews* can find a place, it is no wonder that the disaffection among medical men, as to the volume of periodic literature that is being poured from the press, is on the increase. *Schmidt's Jahrbücher* reviews 170 important contributions to the literature of tabes which have appeared in the course of the last year. Some of them are volumes, many of them almost monographs. It is evident that for the practitioners, a still further degree of potency in the concentration of his medical literature will have to come, and we will ultimately have a *Review of the Reviews of Medical Reviews*.

Recently there have been some interesting contributions to the question of the means of deciding, with some assurance, whether people found dead, seemingly from exposure to cold, have really died from freezing or not. The well-known rose color of the cutaneous surface, which comes on as the result of cold, which paralyzes especially the peripheral vasomotor nerves just before death, is not always present, and may sometimes occur under other conditions. The recent study of that little-known condition, paroxysmal hemoglobinuria, seems to have supplied a new sign of valuable significance. In certain people whose red blood-cells are not quite normal, a great many of them perish when exposed to even slight cold, and hemoglobin appears in the urine. In even perfectly normal individuals, when exposed too long to severe cold, a certain amount of hemoglobin appears in the urine; so that in people frozen to death, it is claimed, this substance will always be found.

TRANSACTIONS OF FOREIGN SOCIETIES.

Paris.

A THEORY OF GRAVES' DISEASE—PROTARGOL, A NEW SILVER SALT FOR USE IN THE EYE—GASTRIC HEMORRHAGE—BLOOD-LETTING, EMETICS, AND BLISTERS—PERFORATING ULCER OF THE DUODENUM—HOLLOW RENAL CALCULUS—SURGICAL TREATMENT OF ULCER OF THE STOMACH—OPERATION IN UNUNITED FRACTURES—DANGERS OF PICRIC-ACID TREATMENT OF BURNS—ORCHITIS TREATED BY REFRIGERATION.

AT the session of the Academy of Medicine, held January 11th, CORNIL spoke of *a theory of Graves' disease* which presupposes that the general condition which underlies this affection is an arthritism, and that the immediate cause is a thyroid insufficiency. In his opinion there are other conditions capable of preparing the organism for the advent of this disease. Infectious diseases which favor auto-intoxications may produce the conditions favoring the development of exophthalmic-goiter prebasedowic states. In other words, in Basedow's disease there are two intoxications of different origin, one superimposed upon the other. The first is a diathetic intoxication whose principal localization is in the thyroid gland. The second, a result of the first, is the thyroid intoxication properly so-called. In accordance with this theory, treatment should be divided into two parts: the treatment of the general disease, and treatment of a symptomatic nature. The general treatment is hygienic. Symptomatic treatment consists in faradization of the carotid region. If this is frequently repeated there will rapidly follow an improvement in the condition of the patient practically equal to a cure.

DARIER mentioned the use of *a new silver salt in eye troubles—protargol*, which is a combination of protein and silver. This substance is not at all irritating, and besides its bactericidal property it also has the power of penetration, and presents the advantage of not being precipitated in solutions by albuminous material, by sulphids, or by alkalies.

At the meeting of January 18th, DIEULAFOY described *two cases of gastric hemorrhage* so great that in both life was endangered. One of these patients was successfully operated upon, and the blood was found to come from a very superficial ulceration, so slight that it was discovered with difficulty. The lesion was sutured, and there was no return of the hemorrhage. At the autopsy of the patient who was not operated upon, an exactly similar condition of affairs was found. As neither of these erosions had extended beyond the external layer of the mucous membrane, they could not properly be considered as "simple ulcers of the stomach;" though it is possible that they represent the initial stage of that disease. If gastric hemorrhage is slight, one may content himself with medical remedies to control it; but in all hemorrhage which threatens life, recourse should be had to a surgical operation.

HAYEM expressed himself as astonished that any one should counsel operation in these cases, as many patients recover after extensive hemorrhage, under a treatment consisting of absolute rest in bed and a milk diet; to which injection of salt solution may sometimes be added with benefit.

At the session of January 25th, DUPLAY insisted upon the advantage of intravenous injections of large quantities (three pints) of artificial serum in surgical operations accompanied by severe hemorrhage. By this procedure he was able to save a patient upon whom he operated for gastric hemorrhage. In order to find the ulcer, which was upon the posterior surface of the stomach, the entire organ was inverted through an incision in its anterior wall. Marion has reported six similar operations in foreign countries with three deaths from collapse, two of them occurring within a few hours after operation. It is at least possible that these patients might have been saved by injections of saline solution. Gastro-enterostomy offers little hope of controlling the hemorrhage, and is not the operation to be chosen in these cases. The stomach should be widely opened and the ulcer sutured, or if need be, excised.

ROBIN read a paper upon *blood-letting, emetics, and blisters*, and advocated a return to their use. There can be no doubt he said that blood-letting increases respiratory exchanges and determines a superactivity of all the phenomena of nutrition. Emetics have a most powerful action upon the capacity and aeration of the lungs, upon the formation of carbonic-acid gas, and the absorption of oxygen. There is, therefore, a chemic as well as a mechanical reason to justify the use of emetics, especially in the treatment of bronchial affections. Repeated examination of patients treated by blisters has shown that the absorption of oxygen is increased by their use. This is apparently due to the fact that in a given time more air is drawn into the lungs.

At the session of the Surgical Society, held January 5th, SCHWARTZ referred to four cases of *perforating ulcer of the duodenum*, in three of which surgical relief was attempted. Unfortunately all four patients died. The diagnosis of peritonitis due to perforation of duodenal ulcers is often extremely difficult. The most likely errors are those of intestinal obstruction and peritonitis due to appendicitis. In a recent collection of twenty-three cases, it is noticed that seventeen mistakes of this character were made in diagnosis. The presence of absolute constipation and the absence of gas, as a result of paresis of the intestines, exists in cases of peritoneal septicemia, and the surgeon who has made a diagnosis of intestinal occulsion often closes the abdomen without having found anything whatever, and only at the autopsy is the condition revealed. The results of operation are not brilliant. In the twenty-three patients referred to, only three were cured. It is to be noted, however, that only five of these operations were performed in the first twenty-fours after the outset of symptoms, two of the cures which resulted being among these five cases.

ROUTIER and HARTMANN mentioned instances in which they had failed to find the seat of the trouble, but had drained the abdomen. In both cases there was temporary improvement, life being prolonged for some days, but a permanent cure did not result.

TUFFIER reported a rare form of *hollow calculus of the kidney* found at autopsy upon the body of a man aged sixty-three years. Sections of the calculus showed that the inner layers were the most recent. Such a calculus apparently begins in an incrustation of the lining of the pelvis of the kidney.

At the session of January 12th, CHAPUT spoke of the *surgical treatment of ulcer of the stomach*. He mentioned five instances in which he had operated for ulcer of the stomach, with four recoveries. Two of the ulcers were of a carcinomatous nature. Twice he performed a gastro-enterostomy, twice a gastro-enterostomy combined with an entero-anastomosis, and once a pylorectomy. The one fatal case was complicated with an abscess of the pancreas. Chaput considered intestinal anastomosis an indispensible accompaniment of gastro-enterostomy. He preferred the retrocolic method.

PICQUE mentioned the value of *Hueter's sign* in deciding upon operation in *ununited fracture*. This sign is the lack of transmission of osseous vibration, noticeable when there is interposition of muscular fissues between the ends of the fractioned bone. BERGER said that one ought not to wait more than fifteen days in such cases, and that if extension for that length of time does not result in union, operation is indicated. HENNEQUIN mentioned the fact that in very oblique fractures there might be absence of crepitus, without muscular interposition. The same might be true in transverse fractures, when periosteum had slipped in between the bones.

At the session of January 19th, WALTHER spoke of the *treatment of burns by picric acid*. It is too little known that this remedy may produce in children symptoms of acute poisoning; moreover, it frequently causes so much pain that its use has to be abandoned.

BRUN had seen a child of eighteen months die with vomiting, diarrhea, and a yellow color of the skin, which followed the treatment of burns of the leg with picric acid.

REYNIER said that picric acid may be used with benefit in superficial burns, as it often instantly relieves the pain. In deep burns, however, its use is contraindicated.

At the session of the Therapeutical Society, January 12th, DU CASTEL stated stated that the instances in which it is *necessary to treat in bed patients suffering from orchitis* are very rare. He further mentioned the fact that an antiphlogistic treatment of this affection is both useless and dangerous. As long ago as 1888, Diday showed that the application of ice gave great relief. Acting on this suggestion, Du Castel makes a superficial application of chlorid of methyl to the scrotum on the affected side, covers it with a light layer of cotton, and allows the patient to go about wearing a suspensory bandage. Refrigeration may also be performed with chlorid of ethyl if the chlorid of methyl is not obtainable. This treatment has given good results, not only in uncomplicated cases, but also in those in which there is an associated inflammation of the tunica vaginalis. There are certain rebellious cases which will not respond to any remedies, but they, too, do as well under this method of treatment as under any other.

SOCIETY PROCEEDINGS.

NORTHWESTERN MEDICAL AND SURGICAL SOCIETY OF NEW YORK.

Stated Meeting, Held January 19, 1898.

THE President, L. DUNCAN BULKLEY, M.D., in the Chair.

DR. JOSEPH COLLINS read the paper of the evening, entitled

THE TREATMENT OF DELIRIUM. (See page 257.)

DISCUSSION.

DR. ROBERT A. MURRAY: There is one point upon which the author has not touched, and that is the difference in patients in their liability or non-liability to delirium. That some persons have a tendency to delirium is as well known as is the fact that some are more susceptible to the action of mydriatics and narcotics than are others. This is one of the things which most strikes the physician, especially in the treatment of children. The author's classification is certainly very good as a basis for therapy. In regard to baths, the warm bath has a better effect in most cases than the cold. Many of these patients, particularly women, are very restless, and a warm bath seems to better quiet the nervousness. The point which the author has made with reference to the proportionate relation of fever to delirium is well taken; but there is, however, a delirium which is dependent upon fever and which disappears when the temperature goes down. What has been said against the use of bromids in delirium is also good; for most physicians who occasionally see such cases in general practice seem to think that depressants are indicated, especially in alcoholic delirium. The treatment employed by the late Dr. Alonzo Clark, who gave the latter class of patients plenty of infusion of wormwood, put them in a padded cell, and watched the pulse, was not far out of the way. Much may be accomplished without the use of hypnotics, although necessity sometimes compels their administration. In such cases sulfonal is better than trional. In the delirium of pneumonia phenacetin with caffein and codein has a good effect. The author's mention of the delirium of chorea brings to mind the delirium of rheumatism; for there is a delirium of rheumatism, and it very much resembles that which occurs in uremia. In these cases, when the temperature is high, the cool bath gives excellent results. There is also a delirium which is due to pain. As a rule, however, delirium is caused by poisoning due to the retention in the system of effete matter or to the entrance of extraneous poison.

DR. B. F. CURTIS: The paper is so exhaustive that it leaves but little to be added, except perhaps from a surgical standpoint. The treatment of surgical delirium is generally a rather simple affair. It is usually due to septic infection and its accompanying fever, and is treated by the removal of the cause—sepsis. In the asthenic and typhoid forms of delirium treatment is of but little avail. Another form is that due to intoxication by iodoform, and it is hardly necessary to say that great care should be exercised in the use of this drug. In cases in which there is an extensive wound which has been dressed with iodoform, and delirium occurs, the dressing should be immediately removed. It is especially necessary to be on the watch for these symptoms in cases in which the patient is old.

This form of delirium is particularly likely to be manifested at night or when there is any rise of temperature. In such cases the mental state may remain perturbed and the patient practically insane for a time, and perhaps permanently so. In a case recently seen, that of a man sixty years of age, who had been operated upon for a very extensive tumor of the jaw, iodoform poisoning developed, and although every other condition cleared up, the dementia remained. As a rule, however, the delirium of senility is the easiest of all to treat. In surgical cases in the aged, if the patient is in fair health, the mind will generally remain clear if the bed is left as soon as possible and if nutrition is maintained. Stimulants are indicated, especially milk punches, which should be given at night during the fasting hours. In jaw cases, and these are often in old people, it is very necessary to get the patients out of bed as soon as possible. This may be done on the third or fourth day, even after removal of the upper jaw, unless there is much exhaustion from hemorrhage.

In regard to the delirium accompanying head injuries, I recently operated upon a patient for epilepsy in whom there was a cystic clot in the brain. The skull had been fractured five years before, and had been trephined at that time, a considerable amount of bone being removed leaving a gap in the skull the size of a silver quarter. The patient had also lost a good deal of brain substance, and there was present a left hemiplegia, which dated from the time of injury. Epilepsy had slowly developed, the spasms beginning on the left side, chiefly in the arm. Operation showed that the superficial part of the brain, just below the fissure of Rolando, was converted into loose cellular tissue containing serum in small cystic cavities, and the epilepsy had apparently been caused by its presence. Dr. Hammond, who was present at the operation, thought it would be best to remove all this cicatricial tissue, and this was done. The patient made a good recovery from the operation, although during the first twenty-four hours he had three very severe epileptic attacks. He was given sodium bromid, gr. xxv, three times daily. On the second day after the operation the temperature rose to 101° F., although the condition of the wound was aseptic. The temperature came rapidly down, and the drainage-tube was removed. About a week after the operation he began to act strangely, being excited and difficult to control, and the temperature began to rise. He complained of a great deal of headache and of pain in the paralyzed side. The paralysis had not been increased by the operation, which did not, however, involve any of the motor centers. During the following two weeks the condition became worse, and the temperature was so high that I determined to reopen the wound. This was done, the incision being made to the depth of about an inch, and a small quantity (about half a dram) of broken-down tissue evacuated and a drainage-tube introduced. The temperature then went down and the patient became more manageable. The scalp has since fallen in where the bone was removed.

The most interesting feature in this case is that the temperature and the delirium did not seem to go together. The delirium was apparently an independent condition. It is also difficult to account for the temperature with the low degree of infection present; yet this would seem to have been the cause of the rise of temperature, for when the wound was reopened there was a cessation of the symptoms. In my experience, head injuries in which there is delirium are always accompanied by a septic condition. The temperature in these cases is a very poor guide to the presence of a septic condition, however.

DR. G. M. HAMMOND: I am very much pleased with Dr. Collins' paper. I do not think any of us will take issue with him in the main conclusions which he has reached. The principal thing is to induce sleep and maintain nutrition. I would like, however, to say a word of caution in regard to the use of sulfonal in these cases. Large quantities of it are required to produce sleep, and, if there is any degeneracy of the cardiac muscle, a serious result is apt to follow. Particularly is this likely to be the case in senile patients, in Bright's disease, and in typhoid fever. In a case of alcoholism I once gave 40 grains of sulfonal, and in thirty minutes the patient was in a state of collapse, and it was with difficulty that he was revived. I have also used chloral a number of times, particularly in alcoholic cases, and have never observed any unpleasant effects. I much prefer it to the other hypnotics. One point which the author mentioned but did not sufficiently emphasize is that these remedies are not given to patients to cure them, but to keep them quiet. This is sometimes necessary, although I strongly deprecate the practice of giving hypnotics to the nurse to be given to the patient as she may think necessary. I have known a nurse to give a patient as much as 1/15 of a grain of hyoscyamin to induce rest, thus rendering the patient unconscious for hours. This is a very dangerous practice, and, of course, should be depreciated.

I think I can agree with the previous speakers in regard to the use of the hot bath, for I have seen many cases in which it seemed preferable to the cold. It is much more grateful to the patient, particularly in rheumatic cases. The cold bath is probably more efficacious in a typhoid condition.

DR. S. H. DESSAU: I certainly concur in what has been said by the author. The paper is a most instructive one to the general practitioner, and the subject of classification has been handled in a masterly manner. The only point upon which I can add anything is that in regard to the delirium of pneumonia. The details which the author has given us in regard to this show that the most serious form occurs in the streptococcic variety of pneumonia. I have found that in a certain number of cases occurring in children delirium occurs at the onset of the affection, especially when the apex of the lung is involved. In regard to the use of baths or the cold pack in the treatment of delirium of scarlet fever, this treatment has been approved by those who have had a wide experience in these cases. The temperature and the delirium seem to be so closely associated that it is difficult to think that the one is not dependent upon the other, although the author claims that the two conditions are entirely independent.

I have certainly been enlightened in regard to primary delirium due to parenchymatous encephalitis. Some years ago, before the present method of treating delirium was in vogue, I was called to see a robust young man who was in a most violent delirium. He had not been long in this condition, nor had he been using alcoholic liquors to excess. The temperature was 105° F. At that time veratrum viride was being used a great deal, and I thought I would try it. A young medical student living in the same house agreed to take care of the patient, and I gave him the remedy; to be guided in its administration entirely by the condition of the pulse, which was very full, bounding, and beating at the rate of 120 or 130 per minute. I left directions that the patient should be given a drop of the tincture of veratrum viride every hour until the pulse was brought down to 80. He was so violent that it required three men to hold him in bed. The treatment was carried out very carefully, and the next morning when I called he was asleep. Nothing was given but the veratrum viride, and it brought down the pulse and temperature and stopped the delirium.

DR. R. C. M. PAGE: In regard to the delirium of typhoid fever and pneumonia, it has been claimed by Bouchard, Epine, and others, that it is caused by impaired digestion, followed by the formation of ptomains and a corresponding auto-intoxication. It seems to me that it is more dependent upon a weak heart and a diminished volume of blood with anemia of the brain. Many of these cases are relieved by proper stimulation, although I do not think that this stimulation acts as an antidote to the ptomain poison, but rather keeps up the heart and nourishes the brain beyond the point at which delirium is produced.

DR. J. RIDDLE GOFFE: The author has included the diseases and pathologic conditions in which delirium occurs in a masterly sweep which we can but admire. It is rather unusual for a symptom to be taken as the chief topic of a discussion; still, the interest which has been aroused by the subject in its various phases justifies the importance which has been given to it. My experience with delirium has been almost exclusively confined to puerperal and surgical cases, and treatment has been stimulation of the heart and attention to the bowels. In septic conditions following laparotomy the treatment has been the same. I have quite extensively used phenacetin, combined with codein and alcohol, in these cases, and with good results. I have had three cases in which iodoform poisoning occurred, accompanied by a low, muttering delirium. I have employed no special treatment except to prevent further absorption. One of the cases, however, fell a victim several weeks later to the most aggravated attack of jaundice I ever saw. It is, of course, a question whether this could in any way be attributed to the iodoform poisoning.

DR. SIMON BARUCH: I regret that I did not hear all of the paper. I may say, however, that I am in accord with much the author has said, and especially would I emphasize the fact which he feared would not be accepted by the general practitioner, *i.e.*, the frequent lack of relationship between hyperpyrexia and delirium. There is no doubt in my mind that the two are usually independent of each other, especially in typhoid fever. The best proof of this is that at present I never see delirium in this disease in private practice, because I have the patient bathed by the Brand method from the fourth or fifth day—in suspicious cases—even before the diagnosis is made, whereas fifteen or twenty years ago, before I began bathing my patients, delirium was constantly a symptom, and I often find it present in hospital cases which are first seen late in the course of the disease. It has been claimed that the cold bath prevents delirium by reducing the temperature. I have always combated the boasted antithermic agency of the cold bath. While reduction of temperature is incidently produced by it, it is the best agent we can employ because it counteracts the manifestations of toxemia, improves the impaired action of the heart, and is, therefore, the most reliable cardiac tonic we have when properly used. It reduces the temperature by favoring oxidation and elimination of toxic products, which are the essential factors in causing delirium, and enhances digestion and appetite. I cannot agree with the author that the delirium which occurs in the later stages of typhoid is due to exhaustion. In most cases I think it is the result of sepsis from local infection.

In the delirium occurring in the early stages of scarlet fever (sometimes without much rise of temperature) the best way to give the bath is to submerge the patient, then repeatedly and rapidly remove him from the bath, or a child may be placed in an empty tub, or one in which there is a little warm water, and one or more affusions over the back, chest, and head may be given, followed by very gentle rubbing, after which the child may be put to bed. This may be repeated every two hours; or a full bath at 85° F. reduced to 70° F. may be given for a few minutes. The same treatment can be employed with advantage in typhoid fever when the temperature is below 102° F., in cases in which there is delirium.

In delirium tremens I think powerful hypnotics and anodynes are contraindicated; hence, I always avoid them. In such cases attention to nutrition is the principal indication.

DR. COLLINS, in closing: The points which have been raised, with the exception of that made by Dr. Jacobus, are well taken. Dr. Curtis said that when delirium occurs after an operation upon the cranium, he feels sure that there is septic infection. I presume this conclusion is based upon personal experience. I do not think that in many of the cases in which there is delirium following surgical operations that it is necessarily dependent upon the temperature.

I am much gratified by Dr. Amidon's remarks, but perhaps I shall be allowed to say that I am not so wedded to the use of sulfonal and trional that I cannot be divorced from them. They are agents which are less apt to do harm in the hands of the general practitioner than is chloral. Personally, I have had no disagreeable experience with chloral, but I know that the effect of its repeated use is hemolytic. It very rapidly destroys the red blood-corpuscles and produces profound anemia.

As to Dr. Jacobus' statement in regard to sunstroke, it should be said that in some cases of insolation there is no rise of temperature. Sunstroke has been proved to be dependent upon an acute intoxication, probably autotoxic, which causes in turn a parenchymatous encephalitis. I have now under treatment two cases of disseminated sclerosis which began last August as cases of sunstroke. In other words, the lesion in the beginning was acute disseminated encephalitis, the foci of which have undergone transformation into sclerosis. Van Gieson has shown that in some instances, if not in all, sunstroke is an acute toxemia. The poison acts upon the heat centers and produces fever. It acts upon the intellectual areas to produce delirium. It is faulty logic to say that the delirium is dependent upon the fever. Dr. Fruitnight has cited some examples of the widespread and deep-seated impression that flightiness is due to to febrility, but I agree with him in denying it.

In regard to delirium tremens, it has seemed to me that physical restraint contributes to the great mortality. The most potent way of producing alcoholic pneumonia is by the use of the captive-sheet made fast across the patient's chest. I place two attendants in charge of such patients, and order ⅙-grain calomel triturates every hour with a view to clearing out the intestinal tract. I do not often use sedatives, and can only repeat what has been said in the paper that it is a pernicious habit to give chloral and the bromids as a routine practice, and follow it up by digitalis to counteract the depressant effect which they produce. When the alimentary tract is in a condition to receive food and absorb it, recovery will ensue if attention is directed to alimentation alone. Naturally, I do not mean to say that oftentimes chloral and the bromids are not the most useful measures at our command, but they should be given cautiously. I am very much opposed to the hot bath in delirium tremens, for I have seen much depression and even collapse follow in cases in which there was an asthenic condition. In such cases the warm pack is better, for it is not followed by a depressant effect.

I have been gratified to hear Dr. Baruch's remarks, but I cannot agree with him in what he has said about typhoid fever, although I am well aware that to disagree with him on any point connected with the treatment of this disease must seem presumptuous. I believe that at the end of the third week of typhoid fever there is an asthenic general condition and an immune state of the blood which does not lend itself to the further absorption of toxic products, whether septic or pathogenic. I believe, moreover, that the clinical manifestations are in entire accord with this statement. There are no evidences of infection at this stage, and I believe that the delirium which occurs is the delirium of exhaustion.

HARVARD MEDICAL SOCIETY OF NEW YORK.

Stated Meeting, Held December 18, 1897.

THE President, JOHN WINTERS BRANNAN, M.D., in the Chair.

DR. JOSEPH A. KENEFICK read the paper of the evening, entitled

SOME MANIFESTATIONS OF SYPHILIS IN THE UPPER RESPIRATORY TRACT. (See page 266.)

DISCUSSION.

DR. EUGENE FULLER: The author has said that late manifestations of syphilis of the respiratory tract are especially liable to occur in those patients who have not received careful treatment during the early stages of the disease, and this is true, still there are cases in which individuals have taken extremely good care of themselves and yet have had very troublesome late manifestations of syphilis. I have in mind a man whom I saw for the first time seven years ago, and who, during five years, religiously followed the treatment ordered, but he had on two occasions relapsing gummatous lesions which required the most heroic treatment.

In regard to the removal of bone in cases of syphilis of the air passages, I understood the author to say that he would be conservative in this particular, especially in cases in which there is necrosis of the turbinates, etc. I fully agree with him in this. It is much the better treatment not to interfere with bony structures. The diseased bone will come away of itself if left alone, and in this way there will result less loss of tissue than if operation were attempted. A patient of mine with necrosis of the jaw has been very persistent in his request that an operation be performed. This, however, I refused to do, and now the bone has become sequestrated and only a small piece of it is coming away.

The subject of syphilis in connection with disease of the kidney is most interesting, but it is a question whether the mercury does the damage to the kidney or whether it is caused by the early syphilis. It has practically been decided that the latter theory is correct.

As far as stomatitis is concerned, it is best to persist in the administration of the mercury, and at the same time keep the mouth as clean as possible. For the latter purpose peroxid of hydrogen is very efficient as a mouth-wash.

DR. HOWARD LILIENTHAL: I have been particularly interested in the statement made by the author that the fact that a lesion rapidly resolves under antisyphilitic treatment does not necessarily prove that it is a syphilitic lesion. This is a point not often taken. In regard to operative treatment, I think that in cases in which there is circumscribed ulceration about the tongue, for instance, which does not respond to antisyphilitic treatment, operative measures should be considered, and enough of the ulcer removed to permit microscopic examination.

Stomatitis should always be forestalled by the most rigorous care of the mouth and gums. I direct the patient to use a tooth-brush and a mouth-wash at least every three hours, and as a result I have not found it necessary to discontinue the treatment on account of stomatitis in cases in which this rule has been carried out. I have, however, observed cases in which salivation has occurred from neglect of the mouth, or in which the patient has been taking mercury on his own responsibility. In such cases the use of the remedy must be discontinued or the patient's general health will suffer.

DR. F. R. STURGIS: The author has spoken of the late appearance of secondary lesions. It is well to bear in mind that in the text-books the division of syphilis into stages is very misleading. Such secondary lesions as mucous patches, chronic and stubborn to treatment, often appear several years after the initial symptoms, and in some cases there is complete destruction of the hard and soft palates even during the first six months of the disease. This was the case in a patient of mine who was tuberculous, and who took the iodids very badly. His lesions were severe, and from the first were attended by ulceration. He died within a year. Late lesions are usually attended by destructive breaking down. The lesions of the nervous system which occur in the early stages are not, as a rule, as severe as when they appear late, nor are they as rebellious to treatment.

As to the question of whether treatment will prevent the development of late symptoms, I agree with Dr. Fuller, and believe that the best safe-guard is thorough treatment, although this does not always have the desired effect. It is here that the question of intermittent treatment must be considered. Mercury, when first given, acts as a stimulant and later as a depressant; if it is administered during a long period, the patient loses flesh and the red blood-corpuscles diminish in number. These symptoms are an indication for stopping the treatment. I believe, however, that a thorough course of mercury or iodid will usually place the patient in the best condition to withstand the late symptoms.

With regard to the kidneys, I also agree with Dr. Fuller. I am loath to believe that mercury properly administered ever produces disease of the kidneys. When lesions of this kind occur I believe that they are due to the syphilis and not to the mercury.

So far as the relative merits of mercury and iodid are concerned, I regard mercury as the right bower and the iodids as the left. The latter are useful on account of their rapid action in checking ulceration. In the early lesions the iodids are not of much service except as a tonic. I would confine the use of the iodids to those cases in which rapid therapeutic effect is desired, when there is loss of tissue, and especially in cases of syphilis of the nervous system. In these it should be given to the point of tolerance—until toxic effects are produced or the symptoms checked.

I also believe that the less we interfere surgically with a syphilitic lesion the better.

I am convinced that many cases of lupus reported as cured by the iodids are late manifestations of syphilis. Lupus invades cartilage and not bone; therefore, when there is ulceration of bone, the disease is syphilis. Given a lesion the nature of which is doubtful, and which is relieved by the iodids, I should be inclined to believe it syphilitic.

DR. CHARLES L. GIBSON: I would like to emphasize very strongly what Dr. Lilienthal has said in regard to the care of the mouth during the administration of mercury. I have always considered most severe those cases in which there are lesions of the upper air-passages. Patients presenting these lesions do not tolerate treatment well, consequently its effect is less marked. In some instances the hypodermic method of administering mercury is indicated. This method is especially applicable in the more severe cases.

In regard to the treatment of syphilitic bone lesions, I am not very familiar with such manifestations in the upper air-passages, but in regard to syphilis of the bones elsewhere in the body, I think that constitutional treatment is very limited in its effect. In such cases the treatment should be pushed as far as possible, and, when it is noticed that there is no further improvement, operation should be considered. I have had several cases in which operation has produced a wonderful effect after constitutional treatment had ceased to be of benefit.

DR. STURGIS: It has been noticed at the City Hospital that on Saturday and Sunday the mouths of syphilitic patients are always more tender, and I am convinced that this is due to the fact that they eat salt fish on Friday. The mouth symptoms are always more marked in salt-eaters. I am inclined to think that the salt is acted upon by the mercury and forms a bichlorid of this metal.

In regard to the treatment of bone lesions, it should always be remembered that the necrosis extends to the original limits of the ostitis, whether the process is located in the nose or elsewhere. My experience has been that interference aggravates the affection, so I am exceedingly cautious about meddling with necrosed bone in syphilitic subjects.

DR. FULLER: In regard to the question of the treatment of syphilitic bone-lesions, I do not think that the rule of non-interference holds good in cases in which the leg is involved. It has been said that these bone-lesions should be left alone and that repair will go on when the syphilitic element has been eliminated. When the tibia or fibula is involved, however, I think that the blood pressure caused by the patient walking about will prevent repair even when the syphilitic element has disappeared.

The question of the hypodermic injection of mercury is a very interesting one. I have employed for this purpose a solution of 1½ grains of salicylate of mercury to 30 minims of benzoinol. The injection should be made into the buttock, and care should be exercised in order to avoid introducing bubbles of air, otherwise severe pain will result. The first injection is apt to be more painful than subsequent ones. This treatment I have noticed on rare occasions to be followed by a fit of coughing which resembles the paroxysms of whooping-cough. Occasionally a mercurial diarrhea will result. A strong mercurial odor of the breath will be noticed in cases in which the toleration point of the drug has been reached. This latter sign is a good test as regards further hypodermic medication, as such treatment should not be repeated while this odor persists.

DR. KENEFICK: In regard to the effect of mercury upon the kidneys, it is important that precautions be taken in every case to avoid overtaxing these organs.

One of the things to be considered in dealing with syphilis of the bone is the fact that the necrotic process begins at the point of bony and cartilaginous union. I quite agree with Dr. Fuller in regard to the advisibility of non-interference with bone-lesions, except under certain conditions. In cases in which there is prolonged suppuration, in those especially accompanied by the many disagreeable features due to the presence of dead bone, the patient will often be glad to submit to operation.

REVIEWS.

THE ORIGIN OF DISEASE. By ARTHUR V. MEIGS, M.D., Physician to the Pennsylvania Hospital. Pp. 229. Philadelphia: J. B. Lippincott Company, 1897.

THIS work, which is devoted especially to disease resulting from intrinsic as opposed to extrinsic causes, is based upon various papers published by the author during recent years, later elaborated and brought together in a volume which appeals to every thoughtful physician. When we read in the preface that "specialism therefore has gone sufficiently far, if not already too far, in medicine, and it is time that something be done to connect the various disjointed threads of knowledge, the true value of which can never be known until they are woven into a complete whole," we appreciate the effort which he has made to bring nearer together pathology and clinical medicine, and congratulate him upon his successful result.

After chapters devoted to an introduction, diseases of age, and origin of disease, there follow those presenting various conditions found in the blood-vessels, heart, lungs, liver, spleen, stomach, intestines, kidneys, and spinal cord. Not only is the text describing these excellent, but 137 original illustrations, drawn to scale and etched directly from the reflection by the camera lucida, give an accurate and at the same time vivid presentation of the tissues under consideration. No adequate synopsis of this book can be given within the compass of a review, but this much may be said: the course of disease is not to be sought for in a single organ, but rather in the involvement of many organs and tissues; many changes usually located in tissues are really dependent upon changes in blood-vessels; the essential condition in many apparently diverse pathologic results is practically one and the same; and finally the old terms, for example, Bright's disease, do not satisfy the present concept of the advanced internalist.

So while we are advancing in knowledge and finding that a broad interpretation of the results of microscopic research as given by the clinician adds to the sense of security with which he reaches his diagnosis, it is perfectly evident that this book will afford little satisfaction to those whose field of view is bounded by the edge of a cover-glass. As an example: "So far as concerns human beings, there is no existing evidence, either clinical or experimental, which can, when judicially examined, be considered to show that consumption is infectious" (p. 28). Again: "Since it has been proven that cases of consumption do result from inflammation, and since at the same time it has not been scientifically demonstrated that the bacillus tuberculosis ever is its cause in human beings, but only that the bacillus is present in the altered tissues of persons suffering with the disease, it is much more logical to believe that consumption is only the result of ill-ordered growth and disintegration of the natural component parts of the organism" (p. 29). To this the pseudo-scientific hirelings of health boards will dissent and professional alarmists will continue to disturb the public for their own private ends. Among practical matters we may cite that compensatory hypertrophy of the heart, as ordinarily described and understood, has no existence; such hearts are degenerated and weakened (p. 84). Amyloid deposit is only a form of fibrous tissue in which there are few nuclei and great quantities of structureless substance (p. 150). The so-called new bile-ducts, the formation of which is the most pronounced feature of Charcot's hypertrophic cirrhosis of the liver, are not bile-ducts, but an early stage of cystic disease (pp. 109, 110). The three remaining chapters treat of the diagnosis, prognosis, and treatment of chronic disease, and are suggestive rather than specific, as, indeed, their brevity necessitates. In the last a change of the habit of the body, as the author expresses it, is believed to be of the most importance. We have read this book with unusual interest because it is instructive throughout, not in any narrow hemmed-in field, but in the broad domain of internal medicine. It bears intrinsic evidence that it is the work of an educated and accomplished physician, who is not only a student and careful observer, but a philosopher as well. The single criticism which we would make is in reference to "fragmentation" of heart muscle (p 80), concerning which some recent work might have been reviewed. The dedication of this book is to Bright, Gull, and Sutton, who have added so much to knowledge in laying foundations upon which others have raised a substantial superstructure. Of this the author has given us a satisfactory and comprehensive view in a volume which is a credit to American medicine.

GENITO-URINARY SURGERY AND VENEREAL DISEASES. By J. WILLIAM WHITE, M.D., Professor of Clinical Surgery, University of Pennsylvania, and EDWARD MARTIN, M.D., Clinical Professor of Genito-Urinary Diseases, University of Pennsylvania. Two hundred and forty-three engravings and seven colored plates. Philadelphia: Lippincott & Co.

THIS work, which consists of over 1000 pages, is devoted to venereal diseases, syphilis, and the diseases of the genito-urinary and sexual organs. The authors have endeavored to cover a very large field, and in making such an attempt have omitted much in the way of detail and description that is of great value to the physician and student as well. In several instances, anatomic and pathologic considerations are too briefly dealt with, and the omission of foot-notes, containing useful references and giving due credit to the authorities quoted in the text, is a great mistake in a book of such pretensions. The views expressed throughout the work in regard to this class of diseases are, with certain exceptions, in accord with those held by many authorities. We regret to see much diffuseness of statement and want of lucidity, as an example of which the following astonishing assertion is made: "In chronic anterior urethritis the urethrometers or acorn bougies will show in old cases certain points of lessened dilatability. There will be no other symptoms, while in chronic posterior urethritis there are often tenesmus, prostatorrhea, frequent micturition, spermatorrhea, sexual irritation, increased desire, frequent pollutions, precipitate, often painful ejaculation, feeble erection, impotence, and neurasthenia." Such a conglomeration of varied symptoms as the above, strung together without any attempt at explanation or classification, is wholly unwarranted in a work which professes to be authoritative and scientific. In speaking of the treatment of chronic anterior urethritis, the authors say that "usually the meatus is found to be narrowed," and they advise meatotomy and the passage of full-sized sounds every few days. Such a broad statement as this, made without reserve, is highly dangerous, and if followed as routine treatment will lead to much discomfort and misery for the patient. Meatotomy is a valuable operation in selected cases, but its routine performance must be condemned as bad surgery. In describing external urethrotomy Souley's operation is not mentioned, and although his tunnel catheters, sounds, and filiforms are described and depicted, he is not even credited for their invention; this is an unfortunate omission, considering Souley's valuable contributions to genito-urinary surgery. Three lines are devoted to the treatment of stricture by electrolysis, and the work of Professor Fort of Paris is not even mentioned. Oversight of this kind renders the work of little value as a book of reference. Gonorrheal rheumatism has barely three pages allotted to it, and in speaking of its treatment no mention whatever is made of local urethral medication. This subject, therefore, cannot be considered up to date, and will not be of any aid to the physician who is treating such cases. In the treatment of chancroid, cauterization is given too prominent a place; the authors mention other methods, but say that "immediate and complete destruction of the chancroidal ulcer is the safest routine treatment," and recommend the actual cautery as the best instrument for the purpose. Such painful and routine treatment is not usually indicated in these days of antiseptic dressings and irrigations. Six very unsatisfactory chapters are devoted to syphilis, which is described at length, but it seems strange that the authors did not use their own cases to illustrate the text, as so many of the cuts they have employed, the colored ones especially, are far from good. Many of the chapters on genito-urinary surgery are very good, and one regrets that the authors did not confine their work to these subjects instead of padding it with desultory descriptions of syphilis and venereal diseases. The book is well gotten up, being clearly printed on good paper, but the illustrations are not, as a rule, up to the standard.

THERAPEUTIC HINTS.

For Pruritus Ani.—

℞ Sod. hyposulph. . . . . . ℥ i
Ac. carbolici . . . . . . ʒ i ℈ i
Glycerini . . . . . . ʒ v
Aquæ dest. . . . q. s. ad. O i.
M. Sig. Apply on compresses to the anus.

For Favus of the Nail.—LEISTIKOW advises spraying the part with an ethereal solution of pyrogallol, and the subsequent application of the following mixture:

℞ Pyrogallol . . . . . gr. xxiv
β naphthol . . . . . gr. xxxii
Hydrarg. ammon. . . . . gr. xv
Tinct. guaiaci . . . . . ℥ i.
M. Sig. External use. Apply by means of a brush.

For Herpes Labialis.—Tincture of capsicum is highly recommended as an efficient early application.

To Remove Freckles.—

℞ Nitrobenzene . . . . . gr. xv
Naphthalin . . . . . gr. lxxx
Milk of almonds . . . . . ℥ v.
M. Sig. External use.

For Sciatica.—

℞ Sol. nitroglycerin (1 per cent.) . . ʒ ss
Tinct. capsici . . . . . ʒ iss
Aq. menth. pip. . . . . . ʒ iii.
M. Sig. Five drops three times daily in a small quantity of water; then increase to ten drops three times daily.—*Troussevitch.*

For Irritable Bladder.—

℞ Salol
Tinct. hyoscyami } aa . . . ʒ ii
Inf. buchu. . . . q. s. ad. ℥ vi.
M. Sig. One tablespoonful three times daily.

For Follicular Tonsillitis.—

℞ Creosote . . . . . . gtt. viii
Tinct. myrrhæ
Glycerini } aa . . . ℥ ii
Aq. . . . . q. s. ad. ℥ viii.
M. Sig. To be used as a gargle every two hours.

For Seborrhea of the Scalp.—

℞ Captol
Chloralis hydratis
Acidi tartarici } aa . . . gr. xv
Ol. ricini . . . . . . m. viii
Spiritus . . . . . . ℥ iii
Ol. rosæ . . . . . . q. s.
M. Sig. Rub lightly into the scalp with the hand.—*Eichhoff.*

THE MEDICAL NEWS.

A WEEKLY JOURNAL OF MEDICAL SCIENCE.

VOL. LXXII. NEW YORK, SATURDAY, MARCH 5, 1898. NO. 10.

ORIGINAL ARTICLES.

NOTES ON APPENDICITIS, WITH REPORT OF INTERESTING CASES.

BY JOSEPH D. BRYANT, M.D.,
OF NEW YORK;
PROFESSOR OF THE PRACTICE OF SURGERY AND OF OPERATIVE AND CLINICAL SURGERY IN THE BELLEVUE HOSPITAL MEDICAL COLLEGE.

THE uncertainty of things at their best, emphasized by the fact that the hidden manifestations of disease so seldom present harmonious and easily comprehended features, even to those of much experience, leads me to sketch a limited number of unusual cases of appendicitis. While I am not disposed to question the assertion of those who say that appendicitis can be diagnosed with reliable certainty, still I do express the opinion that often its non-existence cannot be known without the aid of operation, and sometimes not even then, until determined by microscopic examination. At first, attention is directed to a class of cases of chronic appendicitis, characterized by abundant and often enormous fibrinous exudation. Five only of this class of cases will be cited now; those that are most indelibly fixed in my mind.

A few years ago a patient was referred to me with a history of repeated attacks of acute pain in the right side of the abdomen, attended with rapid increase of temperature, inguinal tenderness, and the presence of a tumor at the point mentioned. At the time of observation a large, irregular, and immovable tumor was present in the iliac fossa, characterized by moderate tenderness and marked induration. The tumor had been present for several months, and had increased in size and tenderness after each succeeding acute attack, slowly resuming, however, somewhat smaller dimensions during the intervals. Chronic appendicitis had been suspected, in which I concurred, and an operation was advised in the event of another attack. Subsequently the operation was performed by Dr. Mitchell of Providence, and a large mass of induration was found below the cecum, into which an opening was made in the unsuccessful search for the appendix. Finally, the wound was lightly packed with gauze. It rapidly healed, and the induration entirely disappeared. No further trouble occurred during the year or so that the patient remained under the observation of Dr. Mitchell.

The second case of this nature coming to my notice was treated by me in the search for the appendix in a similar manner, and with similar results in all respects.

In the third case, not only was there an enormous amount of long-standing induration, but also local and constitutional evidences of recent suppuration. A free incision was made into the abscess, pus evacuated, and the abscess cavity lightly packed with gauze. It was advised in this case, for good reasons, that the appendix be removed by an independent operation as soon as the induration had disappeared, which was accordingly done with entire success.

The most interesting case of this series came under observation last winter. The patient was a male, an artisan, about thirty years of age, who had a fair physique, and had enjoyed good health aside from the affection under consideration. He did not present a history of specific disease. About six months previously the patient had undergone an exploratory operation upon a large, indurated tumor of uncertain character, located in the right inguinal region. It was thought that it might contain an appendical abscess. On exposure of the tumor it was regarded as an inoperable sarcoma of the cecum, and the wound was closed. Although the tumor diminished somewhat in size after operation, the idea of malignancy was not relinquished.

At first I had no disposition to question the diagnosis, or the opinions of the surgeons to whom the case was submitted for examination. However, it was later noticed that the ice-bag, which was applied to relieve pain, caused a flattening of the growth, as though it were of a doughy nature. The mass filled the right iliac fossa and markedly encroached upon the region of the cecum. It was noticed, too, after a few days, that the size and tenderness of the tumor varied from time to time, in unison with the temperature fluctuations, and especially was this true when there had been much pain at the seat of the growth. These incidents, together with the past history, and the fact that the tumor had diminished in size after the first operation and was no larger now than at that time, caused me to exclude malignant disease as an element in the diagnosis, and to express a positive belief that the case was one of chronic fibrinous appendicitis.

An incision made along the line of the previous operation freely and promptly exposed the tumor. It involved the lower half of the cecum and extended down nearly to Poupart's ligament, filling almost the entire iliac fossa. The tumor was hard and immovable. It was puzzling at first to fix upon a plan of exploration of the growth, as one did not care to incise it, fearing to cut the cecum. The fibrous band of the colon, commonly leading to the origin of the appendix, disappeared in the indurated mass, which could not be separated from the cecum without tearing away the serous covering, and thus laying a foundation for sloughing of the wall of that viscus.

After a little hesitation the sharp end of an ordinary periosteotome was introduced into the growth, in the line of the fibrous band before noted, and the growth pried open, thus dividing it into two parts of about equal size united below by the deeper tissues. At the line of separation the base of the appendix was seen extending indefinitely downward and inward into the mass. By the careful use of scissors and the patient application of the grooved director a complete appendix, about four inches in length and very much thinned at the lower end, was withdrawn from the indurated mass. No other evidences of inflammatory action than thickening of the appendix and moderate circumscribed congestion of the contiguous peritoneum were found outside of the appendix, save the mass already mentioned. The appendix was removed, the main portion of the wound closed, and gauze drainage established. The patient made an uneventful and complete recovery, and when last heard from was entirely well. The appendix was microscopically examined by Dr. Dunham and pronounced to be chronically inflamed throughout its entire structure, with muco-pus at the end, confined by the thinned walls of the appendix and a stricture of the lumen above.

The fifth case of this number came under my notice in Bellevue Hospital during the spring of 1897. A sturdy young man of good history was referred to my care, suffering from chronic appendicitis attended with fibroplastic induration. The tumor was well marked, somewhat tender, and the temperature fluctuated in accord with the occasional pains in the growth. Believing the case to be one of fibroplastic appendicitis, and not attended with immediate danger, it was decided to study its peculiarities for a few days before operation, with the entire and glad consent of the patient. For three days the temperature fluctuated from 100° to 102° F., *per rectum*, when there was a sudden chill, followed by sweating and a high temperature. On the following day the symptoms resumed the moderate trend which characterized the period before the chill. The next day a repetition of the same phenomena ensued. It was then ascertained that the patient had been at a comparatively recent date attacked by chills and fever. Quinin in suitable doses promptly reduced the temperature to 100° F., and the tumor began to rapidly disappear.

All of the previous symptoms nearly but not entirely disappeared. However, the patient desired that the appendix be removed, in which sentiment I fully concurred, and he was, accordingly, at once operated upon. No induration was found, and the appendix was intact, but contained an enterolith the size of a bean, lodged near the middle and bathed in mucopurulent fluid, a fact which I suspected because of the lingering tenderness and the trifling increase in temperature which had continued to characterize the case. The patient made a prompt and uneventful recovery.

It seems to me that the outcome of these cases suggests the following: (1) That an enormous deposit of lymph may be the only product of some forms of appendicitis. (2) That even though repeated attacks occur, suppuration is not a common complication of this condition. (3) That free incision of the mass attended by light packing with gauze, is followed by rapid absorption of the induration, and often by cure. (4) That suppuration may occur; therefore, the appendix should be at once removed, if practicable; if not, as soon thereafter as possible. (5) That chronic inflammation of the appendix, with fluctuation of a mild degree, provokes a response of apparently similar nature in the surrounding fibrinous mass. (6) That fibrinous induration due to chronic appendicitis, may be mistaken for sarcoma of the cecum.[1] (7) That the influence of malaria may stimulate the fibrinous variety of chronic appendicitis, and that possibly the symptoms may be dispelled by the use of quinin.

The remaining cases to which I shall refer are miscellaneous, and each in itself is pregnant with meaning.

A little more than a year ago a young man suffering from all of the marked symptoms of appendicitis was seen in consultation. It was noted that he had already gone through not less than two similar attacks; one some six years before, from which he was relieved by the opening of a large abscess. The second attack occurred some four years later, at which time he was taken to a private hospital, and his appendix was said to have been removed by the surgeon in charge.

In view of the history, and also of the fact that

[1] The last fact is still further strongly emphasized by the knowledge of another case which came to my attention at a medical meeting not long since, in which a surgeon, competent, eminent, and candid, acknowledged that he had recently removed the cecum for supposed sarcoma, only to find on careful examination of the specimen that it was a case of fibrinous induration caused by a chronic appendicitis. It is proper to say, I think, in this connection, that this patient also made a prompt recovery.

the patient was then improving, it was deemed inexpedient to operate. Therefore, the patient was admonished that should another attack occur, an explorative operation should be performed. He recovered from this attack, but soon experienced a second one, although not so severe as the first. He came under my charge during the abatement of the recurring attack, at which time there was no difficulty in finding and removing a complete appendix about three inches in length.

About six months ago I was requested to see in consultation a case of appendicitis in a young man of sturdy frame and active occupation. The illness began two days previously and was characterized by the usual though rather mild symptoms. At the time of my first visit there was tenderness, without tumor or tension; pain on deep inspiration; axillary temperature, 99° F.; pulse, 90. However, the symptoms had ameliorated since the day before. The patient objected to operation and was assured that there was no urgent necessity for interference. At the last moment it was suggested that the temperature be taken by the bowel, and 101.5° F. was registered. Careful observation of the condition was advised, and it was also recommended that in case the symptoms continued, the patient should be at once operated upon.

On the following morning the symptoms had increased in severity, and at nine o'clock the patient was admitted to St. Vincent's Hospital. The pulse was 99; temperature, 99° F.; tenderness and tension slight, and an entire absence of appreciable tumor. However, the patient was anxious, and vehemently urged an operation. Slight capillary paresis was noted, and an indefinite sense of nausea was present. For reasons unnecessary to mention, operation could not be performed during the next four hours. Nevertheless, it was done as promptly as possible, and at the time the pulse had arisen to 120 and the temperature to 104° F.

A dusky surface of the body at this time was plainly evident, and the patient's anxiety had markedly increased. Operation revealed the presence of a gangrenous appendix 4½ inches long, extending upward at the outer aspect of the ascending colon nearly to the hepatic flexure. The appendix was removed with some difficulty on account of its great length and the existence of firm adhesions at its upper end. On removal, the middle half was found to be completely gangrenous, but in no place had perforation occurred. Several small fecal concretions bathed in mucopurulent fluid were freely movable in its lumen. A grayish, offensive, and watery fluid was present around the site of the organ; little evidence of limiting adhesions was found. The wound was cleansed, dressed lightly with gauze, and the patient put to bed. In spite of all effort he died within twenty-four hours from the effects of the profound sepsis established prior to the operation.

This case illustrates several interesting and somewhat unusual features: (1) The marked length and unusual situation of the appendix is especially worthy of comment. In this case the appendix passed upward over the cecum to a position at the outer side of this viscus. The appendix is placed along the outer side of the colon and extends upward in about one in eighty instances in the male, and somewhat more frequently in the female. In about half the autopsies in males the appendix is found to be from four to six inches in length. (2) The unusual extent of the gangrene of the appendix at the time of operation indicated with absolute certainty the presence of gangrene at the time of the first visit. At all events, the history of the case at that time—less than twenty-four hours before—did not suggest the acuteness of the impending danger.

In appendicitis a comparatively rapid pulse with a low temperature is an ominous manifestation. The character of the pulse is of greater significance in these cases at the outset than is that of the temperature. The presence of an accelerated pulse with a rationally increased temperature at the outset need not be regarded as unfavorable. However, symptoms, like false friends, no matter how closely watched and discreetly treated, too often cause unexpected discomfiture.

The second of the miscellaneous cases is one which illustrates the outcome of successful surgical action on apparently mistaken hypotheses in a hysteric patient.

A female, about thirty-five years of age, with a distinctly hysteric tendency, was referred to me for diagnosis and treatment. The recital of her past history revealed the fact that she had suffered from persistent and annoying pain in the pelvic, right inguinal, and lumbar regions for a long time, for the relief of which the left ovary had been removed and right nephrorrhaphy practised some time before. Inasmuch as there remained only the appendix, uterus, and the right ovary, my attention was directed to their condition.

No evidence of ovarian, uterine, or broad-ligament disease could be found, a fact which was verified by the late Professor William T. Lusk. However, careful palpation disclosed the seat of the appendix, its extent, apparently increased size, and the presence, on moderate pressure, of the pain which had characterized her affliction. In fact, she exclaimed: "That is the same kind of pain I have had all the time."

It is hardly necessary to add that the appendix was removed. The patient made a prompt and satisfactory recovery so far as the surgical end of the affair was concerned, but the pain continued the same as before. Dr. Dunham examined the appendix, and reported the presence of a mild chronic inflammation of the walls and beginning gangrene of the lining membrane near the middle and at the seat of a small enterolith. Certainly, the justification of the removal is witnessed by the lesions found, irrespective of the operative outcome of the case.

At least one striking conclusion may be drawn from this case: the possibility of the presence of a gangrenous process in a chronically inflamed appendix, with no suggestive manifestations of its presence except the apparently increased size of the organ in question, and a pain on pressure which was not relieved by the removal of the appendix. Had the pain been absent, I doubt if the increased size of the appendix would have attracted attention. Since the removal of the organ the patient has submitted to removal of the right ovary, and is still anxious for further effort to relieve the pain which yet torments her.

Early last spring the late Professor Lusk requested me to see with him a lady who was suffering from a second attack of appendicitis. As the symptoms had much improved, delay, with the view of removal of the appendix in the interval, was agreed upon. About four weeks afterward he hastily summoned me again on account of another attack. The temperature was 103° F.; pulse, 110; local tenderness without tension or tympany was present. As it was then late it was thought better to await the developments of the early morning hours than to operate at that time. The violence of the symptoms increased, however, so that by the time the operation was performed (the following day) the temperature was 104.5° F., and the pulse 130. Increased pain, beginning tension and tympany were then present. The appendix was easily found, but removed with some difficulty, as from an old adhesion its extremity was adherent to the brim of the pelvis. At the middle of the organ there was found an enterolith the size of a kernel of corn, bathed in a thin mucopurulent, sanguinolent fluid. The temperature and pulse were nearly normal on the following day, and the patient made an uneventful recovery.

This case seems to me to illustrate the prompt and high degree of febrile action which may sometimes result from infection in appendicitis in the absence of even approaching perforation.

During the summer of 1896 a young, robust, though nervous young woman, came to my notice, complaining of moderate pain and limited tenderness on deep pressure at the seat of the appendix. The pulse was normal, but the temperature was slightly and continuously elevated. She had suffered thus for some time, and was regarded by her physician as having a mild form of chronic appendicitis. After observing her a few days it was advised that the appendix be removed, which counsel she gracefully declined, and soon, when somewhat improved, passed from my observation.

The following year I was again called to her bedside, and found her presenting in every respect the symptoms of the year before. During the interval she had experienced two or three light attacks. On this occasion she was anxious for a prompt operation. At this time the point of tenderness was well marked, and the presence of a small, tender tumor, the size of the first phalanx of the index-finger, could be easily determined on deep pressure. Operation was promptly performed, and the most careful scrutiny failed to disclose the evidence of the least inflammation, or even the presence of an appendix. She made a prompt recovery, and has not suffered in a similar manner since that time.

This case is of special anatomic as well as pathologic importance, for the following reasons: (1) the absence of the appendix, which, according to Ferguson, was found absent about once in 200 careful dissections. In 131 autopsies observed by Dr. Herman Biggs, at my request, some years ago, the shortest appendix was a quarter of an inch in length and in no instance was it absent. (2) A small tumor was found in the posterior wall of the cecum, in the line of the common origin of the appendix. This growth was the deep-seated tender point which was mistaken for a diseased appendix.

In conclusion, it seems to me that these cases, briefly depicted, illustrate respectively and in no uncertain manner, the fruition of discreet anticipation and the frost of unexpected fallacy.

SENILE EPILEPSY, WITH REPORT OF FOUR CASES.[1]

By CHARLES LEWIS ALLEN, M.D.,
OF WASHINGTON, D. C.;
LECTURER ON NERVOUS DISEASES IN THE GEORGETOWN UNIVERSITY.

WHILE epilepsy may begin at any age, in the great majority of instances the first attack occurs during early life. Gowers in an analysis of 1450 cases of epilepsy found that in seventy-five per cent. of them the disease began before the age of twenty. Between the age of twenty and thirty the percentage was 15.7, while from this time on it rapidly diminished until after the age of sixty years it was but one-third of

[1] Read at a meeting of the Medical Society of the District of Columbia, October 8, 1897.

one per cent. Other authors assert that in old age—after the sixtieth year—there is again a somewhat increased liability to the disease. It is certain that while not common there are cases in which attacks more or less typically epileptic come on in people of fifty-five years or over, who have never had such seizures before and in whom there is no evidence of gross brain lesion, of any source of reflex irritation, or of any intoxication capable of causing the attacks in question. By some authors all cases of epilepsy beginning after the thirtieth year are classed as "late epilepsy." When the disease appears first during old age it seems to differ somewhat from that which makes its advent during the prime of life. Since it is to the discussion of the epilepsy of old age that this paper is devoted, only cases in which the first paroxysm occurred after the fifty-fifth year, and in which the causal agents mentioned above are not present, will be considered.

Senile epilepsy was not unknown to the older writers, though its literature belongs in the main to recent years. Cases were described by Heberden, Trousseau, Maisonneuve, Herpin, Devay, Portal, and others, but the earliest monograph on the subject is the thesis of Jabot, published in 1890. He collected and analyzed fourteen cases from different sources and adds two observations of his own. Since then there have been a number of contributions to the subject, and senile epilepsy seems now fairly well established as a special variety of the disease. In the etiology of this form of the affection neurotic heredity may play a rôle, but it is a much less important factor than in early life. Indeed, it seems unlikely that a person having any strong hereditary predisposition would go throngh the period of greatest stress without developing the disease and should then be attacked by it in old age. It is to be remarked, however, that while ordinarily epilepsy is manifested about the time of puberty, when the nervous system is developing very rapidly and its cells are consequently in a state of unstable equilibrium, old age is a period in which degenerative changes are taking place and instability of nerve-cells is again a feature of body activity.

Syphilis and the abuse of alcohol may exert a causative influence in old age as at any other period of life, but the cases in which the attacks are the direct result of either of these agents are hardly to be considered as true epilepsy at any period of life. The same remarks apply to trauma, gross brain disease, and intoxications. Observations so far do not enable us to assign to senile epilepsy a course and symptoms differing in any marked degree from the epilepsy of earlier life. The seizure may come on suddenly or there may be prodromal symptoms such as dulness, buzzing in the ears, dim vision, or even local spasms. There may or may not be an aura. When the latter symptom has been noted it has generally been some sensation arising from the epigastric or precordial region. The attack may be one of *grand mal*, of *petit mal*, or an "absence" of any one of the changed mental states which constitute the epileptic equivalent. As to which form is most frequent, the experience of different observers is somewhat at variance. A study of the reported cases, however, and my own experience as far as it goes, leads me to think that while a convulsion followed by coma is perhaps the most usual form, the attack is apt to be atypical, the convulsion being but slight or entirely wanting—often only a short tonic spasm occurring—while the coma is quite profound, resembling closely the coma of apoplexy, and as this is the stage which the physician is most likely to observe, the latter disease is apt to be diagnosed, until the rapid recovery of the patient makes evident the true nature of the case. In fact the older physicians described the attacks as apoplectiform or pseudo-apoplexy.

The seizures do not generally occur with great frequency, seldom oftener than once or twice a month, perhaps only once or twice a year. They come on more frequently at night than during the day. There may or may not be tongue-biting. Involuntary discharge of urine is common. Vertigo, attacks of *petit mal*, and "absences," as well as slight localized spasms, are frequent, often antedating by some time the more severe attacks. After an attack of *grand mal* the patient may be in a dazed condition for several hours or days. Mental failure is common in the subjects of senile epilepsy, but it does not differ specially from that usual in old people, nor is the insanity which is sometimes present different from senile insanity in general.

The following cases have been observed by the writer during the past year:

CASE I.—Mrs. M., aged seventy-four years; family history negative. She never had convulsions or any other nervous disease during her earlier life; had always led a quiet regular existence, and, until recently, had enjoyed good health. During some years she had digestive disturbances, and her nutrition had suffered somewhat. For several months previous to coming under my observation she had attacks, coming on about every two or three weeks, and presenting the following characteristics: She is noticed to be wandering about in a dazed condition. When spoken to she answers, but somewhat incoherently, talks about things and people having no connection with the time and place, and is entirely unable to locate herself. Upon being persuaded to lie down and to take a little stimulant she gradually recovers, and has absolutely no recollection of what has occurred. These attacks are very apt to come on after some exertion such as mounting the stairs or straining at stool. She has also occasional attacks of giddiness but has never had convulsive movements of any sort. Examination showed a medium-sized and rather feeble woman. There was some tremor of the hands, rather coarse in character and not increased on movement; slight tremor of the tongue; no facial paresis; pupils equal and reacted to light and for accommodation. The movements of the hands and gait were normal; no ataxia; reflexes normal; no sensory disturbance; heart dulness of normal area. Heart action rather feeble; no bruit, but slight prolongation of the first sound. Arteries about the head somewhat hard and thickened; radial arteries normal. The urinary examination was negative.

She was given strychnin and cod-liver oil, and was directed to pay special attention to keeping her bowels open. During the spring she improved and in the summer was able to go for some time to the seashore. She is now (November) somewhat improved in nutrition, and since the beginning of the summer has not had more than three or four attacks. While there have been no convulsive phenomena, the attacks have all the characteristics of the epileptic equivalent, and should doubtless be considered as such.

CASE II.—Cornelius B., aged about seventy-five years, negro; knew nothing of his family history, and denied both syphilis and the abuse of alcohol. He had been married twice, and had had a number of children, all but one of whom died young. He enjoyed good health until seven or eight years ago when he had an attack of erysipelas, but on what part of the body he can not remember. Since then he has had fits on an average of about twice a month, though no accurate account of them has been kept. He feels a dulness and heaviness in the head for some time before the fit, but there is no aura. The attack is one of typical *grand mal*, consisting of tonic, then clonic spasms, followed by sleeping and dulness for some time, and he occasionally bites his tongue. The attacks occur most frequently at night, seldom by day. Examination showed him to be tall, well built, and very black. He presented marked arcus senilis. Examination of the lungs was negative; heart action rather weak; apex beat neither visible nor palpable; heart sounds clear; no bruit; area of cardiac dulness rather less than normal. Arteries, carotid and femoral, normal; brachial, radial, facial, and temporal, hard and thickened; pulse, 84 and regular. Liver dulness slightly less than normal, otherwise examination of abdominal organs was negative. Pupils small, did not react to light, but reacted for accommodation; no paresis or paralysis of any muscles; no sensory disturbances. Slight tremor of the hands; speech normal; reflexes normal; no trouble with bladder or rectum.

Since the patient was first seen he has continued to have hard fits about one or twice a month. The ward attendant, a fairly intelligent person, describes them as typical *grand mal*, and says they almost always occur at night, sometimes two or three in succession. At this time the patient looked older and more feeble, and the arteriosclerosis had progressed somewhat, but otherwise there was no change in the condition. He took bromids during the summer, but the attacks did not seem to have been to any extent controlled by the medication.

CASE III.—Mrs. G., aged seventy-four years; family history negative. The patient had led a stormy life, with much worry and hard work. She had possessed great intelligence, and had been very industrious, was always temperate, and had usually enjoyed good health until the beginning of her present trouble. There is no history of epilepsy or other nervous disease in earlier life. About thirteen years ago she was noticed to be failing mentally, but kept on for some time with her work as a music-teacher. At first she was melancholy, with occasional periods of excitement, but has never been suicidal or homicidal. For the last three years she has been demented and at times very restless and noisy. During August, 1896, immediately after coming from the closet, she suddenly fell on the floor in a tonic spasm. Her head was drawn to the left, limbs rigid, and her arms were extended over her head. There was no frothing at the mouth or tongue-biting. The convulsions lasted two or three minutes, and were followed by three hours of unconsciousness (deep sleep?), from which she was aroused by the entrance of a physician, spoke at once, and showed no paralysis. During May, 1897, she had another fit, coming on under similar circumstances, and in all respects like the first, except that it was not so severe.

The patient was a small, feeble old woman. There was no paralysis or alteration of gait or reflexes; no tremor. The lungs were normal; cardiac dulness of normal extent; heart sounds normal; no murmur. The pulse was seventy-five per minute and regular; tension increased. Arteries, especially those about the head, showed arteriosclerosis. Examination of the abdominal organs was negative, as was also that of the urine.

September 21st she had another fit similar in all respects to the previous attacks. Her daughter, whom I requested to particularly observe the character of her pulse should she have another attack, reported that it did not seem abnormal. October 10th, she fell into a state of unconsciousness which continued thirty-six hours, after which she recovered without any trace of paralysis. I was able to see her but a few times, and treatment was irregular and unsatisfactory.

CASE IV.—John D., exact age could not be ascertained, apparently between seventy and seventy-five years; lawyer. Admitted to hospital August 17, 1897 His family history was unknown. He was said to have had a convulsion seventeen years ago; no history of injury. Since then his mind has been weak and he has not done any work. He has been restless and confused, has had delusions of persecution and has threatened his friends. August 20th, he had a fit and fell to the floor, but soon recovered consciousness. The exact nature of the attack could no be learned. September 7th he had an attack of *petit mal*.

Examination showed him to be a medium-sized, rather poorly nourished man. His pupils were equal, medium-sized, reacted to light and for accommodation. The tongue, when protruded, did not deviate from the middle line, and was without tremor. There was no paresis or sensory disturbance; speech good; reflexes normal; heart of normal size; first sound slightly prolonged, but there was no murmur. There was some thickening and stiffness of the arteries, especially of those about the head. Urinary examination negative. Mentally the patient was very weak. He was quite suspicious, and had delusions of persecution.

Cases of apoplectiform or epileptiform attacks occurring in old people, in which recovery is rapid and without paralysis, were known to the older writers, and were by them ascribed to cerebral congestion. Trousseau depicts such cases, and says that while he formerly regarded them as apoplectiform and congestive he later learned to look upon them as epileptic. In most of these cases it may be noted that there was disease of the heart or vessels. In the first half of this century Adams and Stokes published observations of cases in which coma and convulsions with extremely slow pulse had occurred in persons usually in advanced life, and in whom disease of the heart and arteries, generally fatty degeneration and atheroma, was found.

New observations have been recorded from time to time, and late writers have sought to establish the existence of a distinct disease, or better, perhaps, a symptom-complex, characterized by slow pulse and epileptiform or apoplectiform attacks, the anatomic basis of which is a sclerosis of the arteries of the medulla and pons with degeneration of the heart-muscle, and to which they give the name "cardio-bulbar-sclerosis," or after the authors referred to above, the "Stokes-Adams disease." The association of epilepsy with cardiac disease has been specially brought out in an admirable article by Lemoine. He describes three cases in which the epileptic attacks seemed directly due to valvular lesions, and divides the cases of heart epilepsy into two classes, due respectively to cerebral congestion and to cerebral anemia, the first having mainly mitral, the second aortic lesions. His cases, however, were all in young people. That acute anemia of the brain can produce epileptiform convulsions was long ago shown by the classic experiment of Kussmaul and Tenner. Now we well know that in arteriosclerosis the arteries are thickened and stiff and their lumina more or less encroached upon; hence, even a slight contraction of the muscular coat may have quite a powerful effect upon the blood-supply, especially in the brain. It seems likely that the vertigo, temporary numbness of extremities, and occasional local spasms, observed in the subjects of arteriosclerosis are due to local anemia produced in this way. Nerve-cells whose nutrition is disturbed become irritable, and the cells of the cortex may readily suffer when the arteries which supply this region are diseased. While the epileptic attack generally begins with a discharge of energy from the cells of the cortex, the researches of Nothnagel, Zichen, Bechterew, and others, seem to show that the tonic spasm at least may have its origin in the medulla and that from an irritation starting in this region the cortical cells may be secondarily affected. Again, by failure of the blood-supply to the medulla the vasomator center may be irritated and the cortical circulation may be secondarily influenced; so there may be either direct or secondary action upon the cortical cells.

Arterial sclerosis is specially a disease of old age. It has been present in greater or less degree in all the cases of senile epilepsy which have came to autopsy and has generally been accompanied by degeneration of the myocardium. This fact is especially insisted upon by Mahnert, who urges the necessity for separating this class of cases from heart epilepsy in general and grouping them together under the name of "senile arteriosclerotic epilepsy." While we may not always be able to determine the presence of any considerable degree of arteriosclerosis by surface examination, the location of the changes is very capricious, and we can by no means assume on that account that the arteries of the brain are healthy. An experience bearing directly upon the subject is furnished by Naunyn, who reports three cases of senile epilepsy, one with autopsy, and in all of which there was arteriosclerosis. By firm compression of the carotid arteries of these patients, the pulse could be brought down from 80 to 40 per minute, and an attack, varying from slight giddiness and muscular twitching to a full convulsion, could be produced. He then tried the same maneuver upon other people not the subjects of epilepsy, and found that while in young and healthy individuals no effect is produced, those having even a moderate degree of arteriosclerosis, experience unpleasant sensations in the head, as well as pallor, vertigo, and slight muscular twitchings. His experience coincides with that of Concato, Kussmaul, and Tenner. This result of carotid compression, known generally as "Griessinger's symptom," was formerly thought to indicate thrombosis of the basilar artery, but this has been found to be incorrect. In one of Naunyn's cases in which it was present, the basilar and vertebral arteries were healthy, while the carotids and sylvians were thickened and of diminished caliber.

Naunyn, however, gives warning of the danger of the procedure mentioned above, as one of his patients, after the pulse had been reduced from 96 to 40 per minute and a convulsion had been produced, stopped breathing, and artificial respiration was necessary to save life. In some of the cases of senile epilepsy which have come to autopsy foci of softening have been found in different portions of the brain, but it seems most likely that they have not been responsible for the production of the attacks, but have developed within the last few months of life, as they could hardly have existed for the number of years during which the fits were occurring without having given rise to some other symptom.

From the foregoing it seems likely that senile epilepsy, if not identical with, at least bears a close relation to the "Stokes-Adams disease," and has a similar pathology. It is evident also that it should hardly be termed an idiopathic epilepsy, but that it belongs rather to the ever-growing class of symptomatic epilepsies. When we consider, however, that of the great number of people having arteriosclerosis so few develop epilepsy, the arterial theory does not seem entirely sufficient to alone account for all cases, and we are constrained to survey the field for other factors. Of course, in different cases there may be different arteries affected, and the changes produced in the brain may vary in their location, but this is not an entirely satisfactory explanation. While neurotic constitution—hereditary or acquired—may play a rôle, it is not as important as in early life. A theory which is held by many with regard to epilepsy at any age is that the exciting cause of the attacks is the presence in the blood of some toxic substance produced in the body by disturbed metabolism, an auto-intoxication. Examples of such poisons are uric acid and kreatinin, and by the injection of the latter into the circulation convulsions have been produced in animals. All are familiar with the fact that in epileptics the fits are increased in number by constipation and excessive intestinal fermentation.

Haig insists that the excessive production or diminished excretion of uric acid is, in many instances at least, the exciting cause of the epileptic seizure. The subjects of arteriosclerosis are often of a uric-acid diathesis, and usually suffer from indigestion and fermentation, so, in them, auto-intoxication may readily occur. Hence, we must conclude that while disease of the heart and arteries and consequent disturbance of brain nutrition are probably the prime causes in the production of senile epilepsy, other influences, such as age, neurotic constitution, auto-intoxication, and reflex disturbances may play a rôle, and at times an important one.

The diagnosis is to be made by the exclusion of gross brain disease and intoxications, and after a careful examination this is not usually difficult. If the patient is seen for the first time during an attack there may be a question as to whether it is apoplectic or epileptic, and time alone may make the diagnosis clear. Epilepsy differs from ordinary syncope by its sudden onset, the convulsive movements, the complete loss of consciousness, and the absolute lack of recollection of the attack on the part of the patient. The minor attacks and "absences" may offer more difficulty, but a careful study of the case will generally make evident its nature even when severe attacks are not present.

That the prognosis is unfavorable is evident from the nature of the case, as arteriosclerosis is an incurable disease, and the fits constitute a direct menace to life. However, years may elapse before the fatal issue, and by suitable treatment a good deal may be done to favorably influence the course of the affection and to prolong life. As arteriosclerosis is practically always present a dietetic and hygienic régime suited to this disease should be insisted upon, and the appropriate medicinal treatment should be applied. The limits of this paper, however, do not permit of a detailed description of the management of arteriosclerosis and its results, and with it, probably all are familiar. The occurrence of the fits does not seem to be influenced by the use of bromids to anything like the same extent as in early life, In the cases of cardiac epilepsy reported by Lemoine, bromids were without effect, while by the use of the cardiac tonics, notably digitalis, the fits were very much diminished in number. Naunyn and others have had a similar experience in senile epilepsy. In arteriosclerosis, however, though digitalis is sometimes indicated when there is great failure of compensation, with edema, etc., it has the disadvantage of increasing the arterial tension, so for constant use strychnin and caffein will be found the better heart tonics. When the pulse tension is high, they may well be combined with nitroglycerin or with sodium nitrite. Mahnert suggests the combination of caffein and bromids in an effervescent drink. If causal agents other than arteriosclerosis are found they should be removed if possible. In any event attention should be paid to the digestive and excretive functions, and an effort should be made to combat anemia, if present, to regulate the circulation, and to improve bodily nutrition.

Gladstone to Undergo an Operation.—The laryngologists and rhinologists are again in evidence, and about to display their skill in an operation upon Mr. Gladstone to relieve the pain caused by necrosis of some of the bony structures of the nose.

PNEUMONIA IN PRIVATE PRACTICE.

BY M. HOWARD FUSSELL, M.D.,
OF PHILADELPHIA.

THE purpose of this paper is not the presentation of any new or startling discoveries in regard to the pathology and treatment of pneumonia, but rather the expression of the writer's opinion that it is worth while to record a series of fairly careful observations of this disease, as it occurs in private practice, in contrast to its somewhat different manifestations in hospitals.

TABLE I.

Number of Cases.	Ages.	Deaths.	Mortality. (Per cent.)
8	1 year or under.	5	62.5
11	2 years.	0	0
21	3 "	5	23.3
10	4 "	2	20.
5	5 "	0	0
9	6 "	0	0
5	7 "	0	0
3	8 "	0	0
1	9 "	0	0
9	10 to 20 years.	0	0
18	21 to 30 "	2	11.1
8	31 to 40 "	2	25.
13	41 to 50 "	3	23.
11	51 to 60 "	3	27.
2	60 years or over.	0	0
134		22	16.4

In a series of cases of pneumonia Wells found the mortality to be 18.1 per cent.; thus it will be seen that the mortality in the 134 cases observed by me (16.4 per cent.) closely approximates that of Wells. Professor Osler has made the statement that pneumonia is one of the most fatal of the acute diseases, a statement amply borne out by my own as well as by the experience of others.

As will be seen by reference to the table, two cases occurred in patients over sixty years of age, neither resulting fatally; both were remarkable instances of recovery in spite of the presence of very extensive lesions, and as such are worthy of record:

CASE CXXXII.—A woman, aged seventy-two years, with marked mitral regurgitation—fully compensated. She was suddenly seized with a chill, pain in the right side, and high fever. On my first visit I detected signs of beginning consolidation, which finally involved the entire right lung. The disease ran an ordinary course, during which the heart never faltered, and ended by crisis on the seventh day. This occurred ten years ago and the woman is still alive, although it should be noted that she has never regained her previous good health.

CASE CXXXIII.—A woman, aged eighty-six years; as in the previous case there was present an advanced organic disease of the heart. She was suddenly seized with fever, which continued three or four days. Examination revealed consolidation of the base of the right lung. Before her death, which occurred eight weeks later, the lung condition entirely cleared, the fatal termination finally resulting from failing compensation.

It would appear from the table that in ordinary practice more than one-half the total number of cases occur previous to the tenth year of life, and the highest mortality is observed in infants less than one year old. Between the ages of five and twenty-one years there were no deaths in a total of thirty-two cases.

Causes of Death.—In 4 cases in which a fatal termination occurred, a history of chronic alcoholism was presented; 3 of these were in patients over forty-five years of age in whom cardiac and circulatory changes were marked. In 3 cases advanced cardiac disease was a concomitant. One patient collapsed and died within twenty-four hours after being told by a friend, on the fourth day of the disease, that she was "very" ill. Two cases occurred in pregnant women, both of whom aborted and died within a few hours. One case was in an exceedingly obese individual, such a one as is likely to die during any severe illness; death resulted on the fourth day. One patient was up and about the house when general collateral edema developed, and death resulted within a few hours. Six cases occurred in apparently healthy children, who succumbed to the disease without any contributory influence. Five fatal cases were in infants under one year of age.

Sex.—Sixty cases were in males, with 13 deaths—a mortality of 20.1 per cent.; 74 were in females, with 10 deaths—a mortality of 13.7 per cent.

Family and Personal History.—In all cases the family history was apparently negative; the same may be said of the personal history.

Contagion.—I observed 4 cases in one house in consultation, none of which are included in the table. The father was the first to be attacked, and in three other members of the family the disease subsequently developed at intervals of about one week. Four of my cases were each followed by a second in the same house. In none of these did there seem to be anything about the premises to suggest a common cause. However, 4 or 5 cases in a series of 133 is not a large number, granting the disease to be truly contagious, and the four mentioned may not have had any etiologic connection. In all the remaining cases there was the freest sort of communication between the patient and other members of the family. Often, a child was ill in a room where two or three others were compelled to sleep; none of these, however, developed pneumonia. There is then, in these cases, absolutely no proof of the contagiousness of pneumonia—at least by the ordinary means of transmission.

Complications.—Whooping-cough was apparently a contributing cause in 4 cases; measles in 2; alcoholism in 7, and, as said before, 4 of these terminated fatally. Five patients were the subjects of valvular disease of the heart, and 2 of these died.

Three women were pregnant, all of whom aborted, and 2 died.

There was one patient, the subject of diabetes, a woman aged forty years, and one, a child of seven years, of nephritis, both of whom recovered.

Duration.—The duration of the disease, from the first manifestation to the crisis, varied from one to fifteen days. In 16, the crisis occurred on the fourth day, on the fifth day in 11, on the sixth day in 8, on the eighth day in 9, and on the ninth day in 12 cases.

Seat of the Lesion.—The base of the right lung was affected in 27 cases, resulting in 5 deaths; the right apex in 27 cases, resulting in 3 deaths; the left base in 47, with 6 deaths; the left apex in 4, with no deaths; the entire right lung in 15, with 4 deaths; the entire left lung in 5, with no deaths, and both lungs were affected in 10 cases, with 6 deaths. Without reference to any other condition it may be said that the greater the amount of lung tissue involved, the greater the mortality will be.

Special Symptoms.—Signs of meningitis occurred in five cases, all in children under five years of age. In two of these the apex alone was affected, in two the base, and in one the entire lung. The symptoms consisted in severe delirium, opisthotonos, strabismus, and convulsions. Indeed, in some instances, the symptoms were so severe that a diagnosis of tuberculous meningitis was made, as an example of which Case XIV. may be cited: A child two years old, already ill with whooping-cough, suddenly developed a very high fever. On examination the apex of the right lung was found consolidated. On the third day the child had a convulsion, followed by marked strabismus, entire loss of sight, opisthotonos, and muscular twitchings, with the thumbs drawn into the palms. Considering the history of whooping-cough, with the very limited consolidation at the apex, it was decided that the child had meningitis of tuberculous origin. On the tenth day, however, crisis occurred, following which the signs of meningitis gradually disappeared. The child is now—five years after the attack—a strong, vigorous boy.

Signs of meningitis in pneumonia are well known, and are usually spoken of as occurring with lesions of the apex. In two of these cases, however, the base was affected. The lesson to be learned from the case just cited is that even in the face of most positive symptoms, meningeal signs accompanying pneumonia may usually be considered as symptomatic.

Irregular Temperature.—In several of my cases the temperature was so markedly irregular, actually intermittent, and the physical signs were so delayed that a diagnosis was not made for a period of three or four days. This was especially noted in the following case in which a fatal termination occurred: The boy, aged six years, was said to have fever. I saw him first during the morning, at which time the temperature was 98.8° F. The next morning I found him out of bed and running about the house. He presented a normal temperature and absolutely no symptoms, but a history of having had fever the previous evening. The next morning there was slight fever and some cough. From this time on the temperature became higher, marked physical signs developed at the right apex, consolidation rapidly spread throughout the entire lung, and the patient died on the tenth day.

Early Physical Signs.—The physical signs of an advanced consolidation are too well known to require mention. It has seemed to me, however, that the very first signs of approaching consolidation are dulness on percussion and weakening of the breath sounds over the affected area. These signs are far more constant than the famed crepitant râle, which when present, while a sign of beginning consolidation, is far too often absent to be of any great diagnostic value.

Signs of Crisis.—In a number of my cases I have observed the occurrence of a few fine râles of beginning resolution just before the crisis, from which I have been able to state correctly in a number of instances that the crisis would probably occur within a few hours.

Appearance of the Tongue.—In these days of exact diagnosis it may seem out of date to refer to the tongue of pneumonia, but the thickly coated, white tongue, with papillæ only less prominent than in the first stage of scarlet fever, with a red tip and edges, is often the first sign which marks the occurrence of pneumonia.

Fear of Falling.—This is another most characteristic symptom of pneumonia in children. During the first few hours or even days of illness, before the physical signs are evident, a child will have constantly high fever, and will lie still if undisturbed, but the moment it is lifted, it clutches at the nurse and manifests great fear of falling. This symptom has become to me almost pathognomonic in children.

Pain in the Abdomen.—Children constantly place their hands over the abdomen and say they have stomach-ache when questioned as to whether or not they have pain. I once made a post-mortem examination in a case in which the child had been unmanageable, physical diagnosis impossible, and in which the only symptoms were irregular fever and abdominal pain, with much distention. A diagnosis of enteritis had been made. The autopsy showed a consolidated lung with empyema. I recently saw a case of complete consolidation in a child of six years in which the only symptoms were abdominal pain and a temperature of 100° to 102° F. This pain, of necessity, originates in the irritated intercostal nerves at the site of the inflamed pleura. Its cause is the same as that which gives rise to the expiratory moan.

Physical Sounds.—It is a notorious fact that the physical signs of pneumonia in children are anomalous. They may be almost indefinitely delayed or finally appear when the child is almost convalescent, and the same is occasionally true in the case of adults. In Case LXXVII., that of a girl, thirteen years old, there were no definite physical signs until the fourth day, when they suddenly appeared. In Case XCII., a man, twenty-six years old, the physical signs did not appear until the fourth day, and the symptoms and history were suggestive of typhoid fever. Only careful repeated examination established a diagnosis of pneumonia.

Complications.—Nephritis occurred in two cases, in both of which there was complete recovery, casts and albumin disappearing from the urine about a week after the crisis. In neither case did the kidney affection give rise to symptoms, and in neither was treatment directed to this condition. In one case, a child, aged six years, empyema followed a rather severe attack of pneumonia; recovery was complete after tapping and drainage. Delayed resolution characterized three cases, in none of which was tuberculosis a sequel.

Prognosis.—In an acute disease having a mortality of eighteen per cent. the prognosis must necessarily be guarded; but given an individual, in private practice, between the ages of two and thirty years, with a sound heart, and possessing tissues not degenerated by the excessive use of intoxicants, one can with a good deal of confidence foretell recovery. Two important characteristics of pneumonia must, however, be remembered: the local lesion and the systemic poisoning. In many cases there are extensive lesions, and yet, aside from the discomfort attending the involvement of such an important structure as the lung, there is little suffering. On the other hand, in many cases in which the local lesion is comparatively insignificant the systemic poisoning is so severe that death often and suddenly occurs.

Treatment.—In a disease in which, in fully one-half of all cases, treatment is apparently ineffectual, and in which recovery is frequent even when treatment is not attempted, the cases not being seen by a physician, one must speak of the value of remedial measures with great diffidence, especially as regards drugs. I believe that much good may be accomplished by proper treatment, and that it is criminal to permit a patient with pneumonia to be wholly without treatment, but I also believe that the administration of drugs or the use of local applications have absolutely no effect upon the course of this disease. In my opinion proper treatment consists of rest and care of the heart. Rest is certainly the most essential point in treatment. In Case CXXIV., the patient was doing well; there was no sign of collapse. I saw her at 10 A.M., at which time the temperature was normal and the pulse slow and steady. She arose from her bed, walked around the room, and within two hours was dead from failure of the circulation.

I have just seen a case in consultation, not included in my list, in which resolution was progressing nicely. The temperature was normal. The patient had violent post-febrile delirium. The action of her heart, which had previously been good, became rapid and irregular. A few hours' rest, obtained by means of morphin, caused the heart's action to become regular, and the patient is now well on the way to recovery.

Rest should be as absolute as possible. The patient should not be allowed to rise to have a movement of the bowels, but should use the bed-pan. If delirium is present, a hypodermic injection of morphin should be given. I once acted as nurse for a noted homeopathic physician who could not be restrained in bed; he was maniacal, attempting to climb out of the window, etc. His pulse was very rapid. A hypodermic injection of ⅛-grain of morphin put him to sleep; his pulse fell to 100 and was for the time much improved in quality. A consultation of his homeopathic attendants resulted in detention in bed by physical force. The delirium continued, and the patient finally died.

The next most important part of treatment is care of the heart, in regard to which rest is, of course, the prophylactic measure. When, in spite of absolute rest, the heart begins to fail, strychnin, digitalis, and whisky must be used. Strychnin, given hypodermically, will frequently abort a threatened collapse and carry the heart over a critical period. It has been said that such treatment is not rational, because it is but a whip to the jaded horse. That it is a whip is true, but if the tired heart can be made to make an extra effort and pull the load over the last acclivity it may be all that is necessary to insure recovery. In all cases of impending heart-failure I give strychnin hypodermically in $\frac{1}{30}$-grain doses every three hours. Its value is well illustrated in Case CXIV., in which a man, aged forty-seven years, with double pneumonia and moderate fever, progressed nicely until the sixth day. The heart's action then became rapid and the respirations reached the extraordinary rate of seventy per minute. This condition continued from 7 A.M. until midnight. For some unknown reason strychnin had not been used, though oxygen, digitalis, and whisky had been employed to the fullest extent. At 8 P.M. a hypodermic injection of $\frac{1}{30}$-grain of strychnin was given, and was followed by some relief. It was repeated at 10 P.M. and also at midnight. By 2 A.M. the respirations had fallen to 50, and from this time on convalescence was rapid. Digitalis and whisky, I believe, are valuable agents in pneumonia, but in an emergency their action is not to be compared with that of strychnin.

Venesection.—I have never employed venesection in pneumonia. In one case it seemed to be demanded, but was refused. With aconite and veratrum viride I have had no experience, having always been afraid to use them.

External Applications.—In all my first cases of pneumonia a jacket poultice was employed. It was troublesome, unclean, and uncomfortable, and, except under certain conditions, was soon discarded. Where there is much pain, and consequent embarrassment of breathing, the application of a poultice which envelops the whole chest affords such immediate and striking relief that its use seems justified.

When pain is severe, a small hot poultice over the affected area will give relief. Cotton jackets I still use, but I must confess, knowing that they accomplish little or nothing except perhaps to quiet the minds of the patient and friends.

Cold.—A cold bath when the temperature is high gives the greatest relief, and under its influence a delirious patient will frequently go quietly to sleep. In Case XXXVII., in which the patient died with a temperature of 107° F., I believe the fatal termination might have been prevented by the application of cold.

Local applications of ice to the affected side are theoretically correct. They certainly relieve pain, but my own experience with them has not been encouraging. I *still* employ them when there is a tendency to hyperpyrexia.

The pain, which is frequently the most annoying symptom, can best be relieved by the application of ice, a poultice, by means of cups, and, last, by the administration of opiates.

Imperial Measles.—According to the daily papers, the Empress of Russia is suffering from a slight attack of measles.

THE EARLY DIAGNOSIS OF MALIGNANT UTERINE DISEASE.[1]

BY L. GRANT BALDWIN, M.D.,
OF NEW YORK;
GYNECOLOGIST TO ST. PETER'S HOSPITAL, BROOKLYN.

THE statement that malignant disease of the uterus is a frequent cause of death, will not, I am sure, be disputed, and likewise, I take it, it will not be denied that if seen sufficiently early, cancer affecting any part of the uterus is amenable to surgical treatment, and when such is applied according to the best modern methods, it offers, in many cases, brilliant chances of either saving or greatly prolonging life; *i.e.*, if a case is seen when the disease is confined to the uterine tissue itself, and before either the blood-vessels or lymphatics are involved, a complete hysterectomy will add to the days and comfort of the patient, if not effect a permanent cure. Unfortunately, however, the happy combination of circumstances which I have sketched does not usually obtain; quite the contrary, when the case first comes under observation the disease is discovered to have already progressed beyond those limits within which a hysterectomy may be performed, and in many cases not even a palliative scraping followed by cauterization offers any considerable chance of relief. Indeed, the infection is usually so far advanced that any interference will only serve to hasten its progress.

The hope that my efforts may be in a slight degree productive of a change which will bring these cases sooner under the care of the surgeon must be my excuse for asking attention to this subject.

Of the twenty-seven cases of cancer of the uterus observed by me during the past eighteen months in hospital and dispensary practice, twenty-four were beyond any operative treatment, and to only one patient could I offer hopes of permanent relief. The cases seen in private practice have made a decidedly better showing. In this respect I have no doubt that my experience is in line with that of my colleagues. There is a widespread tradition among both the members of the medical profession and the laity that at or near the menopause a woman is licensed to encounter all sorts of symptoms and conditions, which, occurring at any other period of life, would be considered abnormal and require the most rigid investigation as to causation, but when manifested at that time are regarded only as a part of the ills to which flesh is heir, and are thought by both family physician and patient as due to "change of life." Many may doubt the truth of this, but possibly it will strengthen the argument when I say that in all the cases given as having been seen during the past eigh-

[1] Read at a meeting of the Kings County Medical Association, January 11, 1898.

teen months such a belief was universally expressed, either quoted from the family doctor or stated on the patient's own authority. In many cases the physician consulted had not even suggested an examination after eliciting the gravest symptoms, and the patient had left with a prescription for ergot and a promise of recovery when the "change" was over.

The following is the history of a case which will serve as an example, and is, I promise you, no exaggeration colored for the occasion:

CASE I.—Mrs. J., aged forty-three years, a native of Ireland, married twenty-five years, and the mother of ten children, the youngest being seven years old. She had never had a miscarriage. She had been ailing eighteen months. She was well nourished, had not lost flesh, and looked the picture of health. Her only symptom up to three months before coming under observation had been gradually increasing menorrhagia and metrorrhagia; no dysmenorrhea, *no foul-smelling discharge*, and *no pain* between the menstrual periods. Up to this time she had not consulted a doctor, believing, as she said, that as soon as the change was over she would be all right. For the last three months she had suffered much from irritability of the bladder and painful defecation, and had seen two physicians who, she said, agreed with her opinion of the case. Examination revealed malignant disease of the uterus. The womb was absolutely fixed in the pelvis by extension of the disease to the broad ligaments, bladder, rectum, and vagina, and the condition was, of course, inoperable.

The symptoms of cancer of the uterus which I learned as a medical student, at least the ones which were prominently mentioned, were pain, loss of flesh, a cachexia, and a foul-smelling discharge, and to a great extent these are the symptoms especially noted in many of the text-books of a few years ago. It is true, minor symptoms are given, but stress was not laid upon them. I am convinced that I was not taught differently from many others from the fact that I constantly have these symptoms put forward in a consultation to prove, by their absence, that the case under consideration is not one of cancer; and especially is this true of pain and cachexia.

In my judgment, when a case presents any one of these signs or symptoms to any considerable extent it will matter but little whether or not a diagnosis is made, for the patient will have left behind the hope of successful treatment weeks if not not months before.

A natural inquiry is: Why are the effects of malignant disease of the uterus so different from those of the same disease in other organs; in the stomach for instance? My reply is that when the uterus is the organ attacked these grave symptoms are late in appearing. The uterus is not normally a highly sensitive organ. It is well known that the cervix may be cut or pricked to a considerable extent without causing very much pain, and in the development of a cancer of either the cervix or body of the uterus there is but little pain until such time as the new growth causes pressure on the great nerve trunks, involves the peritoneum, or effects by extension the bladder or rectum. The uterus having no connection with the chylopoietic viscera but slight inroads are made on the general health of the patient until adjacent organs or structures are infiltrated.

Some authorities attach especial importance to a foul-smelling vaginal discharge as diagnostic if not pathognomonic of cancer involving some part of the genital tract. That cancer of the uterus gives rise to a peculiar smell I do not for a minute believe. The odor comes from either sloughing tissue or decomposing discharge. Only recently I saw a sloughing fibroid which protruded from the cervix in which a diagnosis of cancer had been made from the odor. In many of my cases the general health was excellent, and yet the uterus was completely infiltrated with cancer. What, then, is there that should direct the attention of the physician to the uterus and that indicates a vaginal examination? The first step to an earlier diagnosis of this most terrible affection is education of the laity, with the end in view of destroying the idea that the menopause is an abnormal phenomenon, attendant upon which the sufferer is sure to nearly if not quite bleed to death every two to six weeks, for a period ranging from six months to as many years. I promise this is no exaggeration of what I have been told over and over again, and if any one doubts, to be convinced it will only be necessary for them to make some investigations on their own account. How this education is to be accomplished I cannot say; but for my own part I do not miss an opportunity of explaining the falsity of such conclusions.

The one sign of malignant disease of the uterus which should always be investigated, and especially so when it occurs at or near the menopause, *is hemorrhage*. We may say, I think, that in *all* cases in which the menstrual period becomes prolonged, the flow more profuse, or the interval shortened, the most rigid examination, no matter what the condition or age of the patient may be, is demanded. In all cases which I have observed bleeding has been the earliest symptom. This is probably more particularly so when the disease originates in the body of the uterus; as from the cavity of the organ comes the normal menstrual flow, it is natural to conclude that any new growth in this situation would cause a variation from the normal. It not infrequently happens that a woman will pass through the menopause without any untoward symptoms, and yet at a subsequent time be taken with a bloody discharge from the vagina. This is, of course, especially suspicious.

A well-marked case of this kind was seen by me last May, with Dr. J. W. Parrish:

CASE II.—Mrs. F., aged sixty-three, native and resident of Long Island, had a normal cessation of menstruation at the age of forty-eight. For about three months prior to her visit to Dr. Parrish she had noticed a slight show of blood at frequent intervals, becoming constant, but never profuse, in fact only a few drops during the twenty-four hours. There was *no odor* to the vaginal discharge.

Bimanual examination revealed a small uterus, but yet too large for one not functionating for nearly twenty years. The cervix was somewhat eroded, and blood could be seen oozing from the external os.

A curetting brought away some small particles from the cavity of the fundus which were proven by the aid of the microscope to be carcinomatous. Vaginal hysterectomy was performed. I examined her during December, 1897, and there is as yet, eight months after operation, absolutely no evidence of any return of the disease. In this case the symptoms began the longest time after the menopause I had ever observed, and she came under observation with the least possible delay.

In some cases the bleeding is caused by coition at a period earlier than that at which any derangement of the menstrual flow is noticed. This is especially true when the disease has its origin in the cervix.

Another comparatively early symptom is an intermenstrual, watery, irritating discharge, but not necessarily foul smelling. This, when the disease begins in the cervix, may precede any change in the amount or frequency of the catamenial flow, but, very generally, it soon becomes stained with blood. Of course, I do not intend to infer that malignant disease of the uterus will be found in all cases to be the cause of hemorrhage from the vagina, but I do say that in all cases a cause of the bleeding may be found and that it should be sought for and if possible removed. If it is proved to be a result of some benign condition so much the better for the patient.

In nearly all cases coming under observation at a period of the disease sufficiently early for total extirpation of the uterus, to offer any reasonable hope of a cure, will require for diagnostic purposes a preliminary scraping, and a microscopic examination of the material removed.

In conclusion let me say that the cessation of menstruation is a natural transition from the active to the quiescent state of the sexual life of the human female; as natural, indeed, as its inception at puberty. True it is that this is a critical time in a woman's life, but this fact only makes it more imperative that we, as physicians, should investigate symptoms occurring at this period, and not permit either ourselves or our patients to attribute them to that much abused condition—"change of life."

CLINICAL MEMORANDA.

TWO CASES OF MALARIAL FEVER.

BY ALDRED S. WARTHIN, M.D.,
OF ANN ARBOR, MICH.;
INSTRUCTOR IN PATHOLOGY IN THE UNIVERSITY OF MICHIGAN.

TWO very interesting cases of malaria came under my observation during the summer of last year which emphasize certain important clinical points in regard to this disease.

As house-physician in the Manitou Park Hotel, Torrington, Colorado, during my summer vacation, I was asked to see one of the guests, a young lady from St. Louis, who was having a very severe chill. The paroxysm being typically malarial, I at once made a microscopic examination of her blood and succeeded in finding the large pigmented forms of the malarial organism. Quinin was withheld, and on the second day afterward, two hours before the second chill, the organisms were found in large numbers. The diagnosis of tertian malarial fever being established, the patient was given the regular quinin treatment, and as a matter of course promptly recovered.

Three months before in St. Louis the patient had had an attack of what was diagnosed as typhoid fever by a homeopathic physician who gave her an irregular quinin treatment. Recovering within two weeks, she came to Colorado, and had been well up to the time of the second attack. The patient's description of her first illness corresponded precisely with that of malaria, and there is no doubt in my mind that that was the disease.

The second patient, a male, from the same locality, left the Mississippi Valley eight months before, after a severe attack of malaria which was diagnosed and treated as such and apparently entirely cured.

A typical malarial paroxysm occurring without premonition, the patient's blood was examined and the organisms found. He was left without quinin until the third chill—the disease being of the tertian form—and the organisms were found in abundance two hours before the expected paroxysms. This case was also promptly cured by the usual quinin treatment.

Manitou Park is a mountain valley about 7750 feet in altitude, covered with pine forest, of sandy soil, its only water being a clear trout stream. The climatic and telluric conditions are as opposed to those favoring malaria as one could well imagine. That the malarial organism is indigenous here can hardly be believed, and the cases must be looked upon as importations. The fact of previons attacks in malarial regions bears this out.

The cases, then, are interesting because of the long time elapsing after the first infection, the long residence in a non-malarious region without symptoms, and the sudden outbreak of the disease under such favorable climatic conditions.

Cases developing within the second season after return

from Africa have been noticed at Berlin; and Osler and Mannaberg also report cases of an incubation period extending from one season to the next. The development of the disease within short limits of time after leaving malarious regions are by no means rare.

It is evident that malarial organisms may remain quiescent in the body for a long period of time, and suddenly become active under the most favorable conditions of climate and altitude. These conditions apparently have no effect upon the development of the organism if the body has been previously infected.

One of these patients was thought to have "mountain-fever." While there is no doubt in my mind that the majority of cases classed under this head are typhoid, yet it is probable that some, if not a large number, may be imported cases of malaria. It is an exceedingly common thing for residents of the Mississippi Valley to come to Colorado to recuperate after an attack of malaria. Many of them have attacks of so-called "mountain-fever," and it s probable that some of these may be attacks of malaria as in my cases. I simply suggest this, hoping that future blood-examinations may settle the question in those cases of fever occurring in visitors to the State of Colorado.

Dr. Sewall of Denver (*Colorado Med. Jour.*, September, 1896) reports a case of remittent fever in which the malarial plasmodium was found by Dr. Crouch in a patient originally from Louisiana, but who had not been out of Colorado for five years. I did not have access to Dr. Sewall's paper until after writing the above and after my return to Ann Arbor. I find that he has preceded me in the suggestion that some cases of "mountain-fever" may be malaria, and in calling attention to the importance of a blood examination in this disease; my cases, therefore, lend support to his suggestion.

NOTES ON CASES OF SYPHILIS.

BY JAMES C. JOHNSTON, M.D.,
OF NEW YORK;
DERMATOLOGIST TO THE NEW YORK LYING-IN HOSPITAL; PHYSICIAN TO THE CLASS OF SKIN AND GENITO-URINARY DISEASES IN THE OUT-DOOR DEPARTMENT OF THE PRESBYTERIAN HOSPITAL.

Syphilis Vegetans.—This condition is generally believed to be a result of mixed infection. My case occurred in a German women, fifty-nine years of age, living with unhygienic surroundings, and her person being undescribably filthy. No history was obtainable, but she showed unmistakable syphilitic ulcers of the upper third of both legs. On the dorsum of the right foot, extending from the joint flexure to the end of the metatarsal bones, was a patch composed of smaller lesions partially fused at their bases. The original efflorescence had been an ulcer which, spreading peripherally, had taken on vegetative overgrowth, directly analogous to the process which converts pemphigus vulgaris into pemphigus vegetans. The patch had been in existence some months so that time had been ample for the cauliflower appearance of the vegetations to be obscured by a thin covering of newly formed epidermis. The excrescences, though fused at their bases as mentioned, were separate and distinct above, each being rounded to a slight eminence. The color, after thorough cleansing with green soap, was pink; there was no crusting and no ulceration. The borders of the patch gradually faded into the surrounding skin.

Antisyphilitic medication in these cases usually has no more effect than upon the "parasyphilides," affections which are not luetic in themselves, but flourish upon the syphilitic soil, of which the pigmentary syphilide and paresis (in most cases) will serve as examples. Surgical measures must, as a rule, be taken for the removal of the vegetations, such as curetting, excision, or the use of the cautery. Pressure applied by elastic bandages or plaster dressings has been used, but in this instance a good result was obtained by covering the patch with mercury plaster and by pushing the administration of iodid of potassium until the patient was taking 60 grains three times daily. The plaster should be removed, and it and the surface cleansed twice daily. A new piece is necessary only every second or third day.

Syphilitic Paronychia and Onychia.—Syphilitic paronychia occurs in three forms: (1) dry, (2) inflammatory, and (3) ulcerative. The clinical phenomena in the first two classes usually appear early in the course of the disease. The ulcerative case to be described began close to the end of the second year.

The man, a butcher by trade, had received little or no treatment since the disappearance of his early eruption. Following a slight injury there appeared at the border of the nail on the right middle finger, a hard, indolent papule, which soon ulcerated and spread along the groove and beneath the nail, raising it from its bed. When first seen, the crateriform ulceration was a quarter of an inch in diameter. The discharge from the sore was thin and ill-smelling. The ulcer was shallow and uneven, covered by unhealthy, apparently gangrenous granulations. The nail, loosened to the extent of one-half its width, had lost its luster, was deeply ridged longitudinally, and of a yellowish color. Nosophen was dusted over the surface, and when in combination with potassium iodid administered internally it had set up reparative action, it was replaced by mercury plaster. The latter restrains exuberant granulation in addition to its stimulative action. Recovery followed, complete, except for a slight deformity of the nail on the affected side.

This paronychia must be carefully distinguished from the simple, non-syphilitic and the diabetic varieties. Differentiation is often difficult. The therapeutic test is worthless. A curious fact, worthy of note in connection with these paronychial gummata, is that they are prone to occur at the site of an extragenital chancre of the finger, as is too often seen in medical men. The gumma differs very little from the primary lesion.

Syphilitic onychia also has three recognized forms: (1) the *onyxis craquelé* of Fournier, in which the nail is cracked and broken; (2) the form in which it is partially or entirely shed; (3) hypertrophic onychia. My cases belong to the second variety, and the one described will serve as a type.

The patient, a young woman, first visited the Presbyterian Hospital during June last whith a chancre of the lip, the result of kissing a syphilitic subject. It was followed by a rather severe form of the disease, the mouth lesions being particularly annoying. She was progressing fairly well with treatment by means of inunction, when, during October, my attention was accidentally drawn to the nails. Those of the thumb, middle, and little finger of the left hand, two of the right hand, and the nail of one great toe were affected. Involvement of the fingers is rather more common than the toes in these cases; of the latter, the great toe is most often attacked. The nails were marked with longitudinal furrows, were lusterless, yellowish, with a multiplicity of *flores unguium*. The lunulæ had disappeared, and in every one separation had taken place at the posterior border. The line of adhesion to the bed could be seen by pressing down the free end. After complete separation from the matrix the old nails continued to move forward leaving the bed bare between them and the new appendages, which were soon formed.

The new nails are ridged at first, but soon attain their proper shape. The process is slow but entirely painless. Inflammation is not present. The prognosis is good under treatment. Local measures are unnecessary if constitutional treatment is actively pursued. Between the time of the fading of the eruption and disappearance of the chancre, the patient was taking quarter-grain pills of mercury protoiodid, four times daily. On observing the onychia, they were discontinued and nightly inunctions of a dram of mercurial ointment were employed instead. The patient is progressing favorably.

Paresis Illustrating the Motor Type of the Disease. —In view of the claim, according to Fournier ("Les Affections Parasyphilitiques," p. 137, *et seq.*), that syphilis is an etiologic factor in sixty to eighty per cent. of all cases of paresis, the introduction of the subject here is as proper as any of those previously considered. The case in question is of peculiar interest because of the change observed by neurologists (Collins, *Post-Graduate*, January, 1898) in the character of the symptoms during the last few years. It points a warning, also, to syphilologists, to be careful in giving an opinion as to the ultimate outcome of syphilis even with proper treatment.

The patient is a man, aged thirty-five years. He gives a clear history of syphilis acquired ten years ago, for which he was under treatment (in good hands) for a year or more. The present illness began, according to his account, six months previous to my first examination, but it is likely that the insidious onset remained unnoticed for some little time. The first symptom noticed was difficulty in movement, interfering with his occupation; that which brought him to the clinic was incontinence of urine. He presented none of the mental phenomena formerly so common, no exaggeration of ideas as to his own importance, material circumstances, etc. Except for a certain slowness in comprehending and answering questions, his mentality appeared little changed. The motor symptoms were, on the contrary, thoroughly developed. His gait was paraplegic, the toes being dragged upon the ground, and it was almost impossible for him to accomplish the buttoning of his coat. His grip was feeble, slightly better in the right than in the left hand. The Romberg symptom was present, the knee-jerks exaggerated, and ankle-clonus marked. It was not practicable to have the eyes thoroughly examined, but the pupils were unequal, the left being larger, and they failed to react to light. The characteristic, slow, scanning speech of general paralysis and the difficulty in phonation were marked. Elision of consonants and lack of control of lip- and tongue-movements formed a close resemblance to the vocal effort of the inebriate. It was, in fact, difficult to determine whether the slowness in answering questions was due to difficulty in phonation or to impaired understanding. The patient stated that his attention had not been previously drawn to the changes in his speech. His digestion seemed good, and with incontinence of urine there was no lack of control of the sphincter ani. Iodid of potassium and tincture of belladonna were given in the hope of ameliorating, if only for a time, the distressing affection.

A CASE OF SPLENIC ANEMIA, OR SPLENIC PSEUDO-LEUKEMIA.

By HERBERT MAXON KING, M.D.,
OF GRAND RAPIDS, MICH.;
PHYSICIAN TO BUTTERWORTH HOSPITAL.

JANUARY 5, 1897, I was consulted by a young woman for the relief of pain in the throat which attended the act of swallowing. The patient was twenty-one years of age, unmarried, and was born in Sweden; she had been employed as a servant in the household of a small family for upward of six months, and occupied this position at the time of the examination. Some ten days before consulting me she had "taken cold," and had experienced pain upon swallowing food (both solid and liquid) ever since. She regarded this sore throat as a very trifling affair, and would not have consulted a physician except that her employers had insisted that she should do so. Her father was living and in good health. Her mother died at thirty-six years of age from consumption, and the maternal grandmother also died of consumption, while one sister had what in all probability (judging from description) was tuberculosis of the knee-joint. Upon examination the skin and mucosa were found markedly anemic. The pulse was 80, full and regular, and the temperature normal. Examination of both thoracic and abdominal viscera was negative, with the exception of the spleen, which was sufficiently enlarged to be easily palpable and was slightly sensitive to pressure. The nares and nasopharynx were normal, except for the anemic mucosa. The posterior wall of the middle pharynx was hyperesthetic and covered with a thin layer of viscid mucus. With the exception of the pale color of the mucous membrane, the larynx was also normal. At this time I considered the case one of mild pharyngitis complicating a depraved general condition. The patient was given iron, manganese, and quinin. Simple local treatment sufficed to relieve the pharyngeal symptoms.

I did not again see the patient until February 25th, when she came to my office (again at the request of her employers) complaining of pain in the left side, a general indisposition to work, loss of appetite, fatigue upon the slightest exertion, and a return of the pain on swallowing.

The appearance of the patient at this time was startling to say the least. Seven weeks before she had been anemic, but not more so than would be accounted for by many unimportant departures from the normal standard. Now, however, the skin was very sallow, and the lips, conjunctivæ, tongue, and nails were colorless. In fact, the whole appearance was at once indicative of the existence a very grave condition. Upon this occasion I made a much more exhaustive inquiry into the personal history of the patient, from whom I obtained the following, as having some possible etiologic bearing upon the case: When a very young child the glands at the angle of the jaw on the right side became enlarged and suppurated. The patient remembered little about them except that they were called "scrofulous sores," the cicatrices of which were quite conspicuous. At the age of ten years she had scarlatina, after which recovery was perfect. At seventeen years menstruation began, and the epochs have shown no irregularity since then except upon one occasion three years ago, when two or three months passed without menstruation. For the first year menstruation continued five to six days, when it fell to three or four days, and never continued more than three days after the patient was nineteen years old. Recently the periods had been still shorter, until at the last menstruation, February 15th, it continued but one day. She had had an inconsiderable leucorrhea during the past two years.

During March, 1896, the patient was sent to Butterworth Hospital, where she was treated for remittant malarial fever in Dr. Hugo Lupinski's service. Upon examination I found a slight edema of the face and lower extremities. Palpation of the abdominal viscera at once disclosed the presence of an enormously enlarged spleen. It had increased to double the size noted at the first examination, the splenic dulness beginning in the axillary line at the seventh rib and extending downward to the crest of the ilium and forward to the median line. On this account respiration was somewhat embarrassed, while the obstruction to the return circulation explained the edema. An anemic murmur over the somewhat displaced heart could be easily heard. The patient had lost in weight but was not emaciated. There was present, however, the severe anemia and a "lemon-yellow" color of the skin. The urine was practically normal, a specimen of which, obtained about this time, gave a specific gravity of 1017, was acid in reaction, and albumin, sugar peptones, and bile were absent; urea 6 grains to the ounce. A centrifuge precipitate gave only normal epithelial cells from the vagina, bladder, and possibly a few from the pelvis of the kidney; no casts or crystals, and a very small number of pus-cells, doubtless from the vagina. Repeated examination of the urine gave about the same result. Upon the several occasions of recording the temperature it was found to be 100° F. The pulse was small, wiry, and remained in the neighborhood of 100 per minute.

A careful examination of the patient's blood revealed the following condition:

Erythrocytes, 1,875,000 per cubic millimeter; leucocytes, 4685 per cubic millimeter; proportion, 1 to 400; hemoglobin, 35 per cent.; color index, .95 (approximately).

Qualitatively, the leucocytes were not far from normal, although eosinophiles were fewer than I have commonly found them. The red cells showed a somewhat greater departure from the normal, there being some poikilocytosis (not marked), while microcytes were more numerous. Aside from the presence of an occasional normoblast there were no nucleated red-cells. The results of the blood examination safely excluded the various forms of leukemia. The entire absence of leucocytosis made malignant disease (which would manifest itself in marked anemia) highly improbable. The high color index would exclude chlorosis, and the comparative absence of poikilocytosis and microcytosis would exclude pernicious anemia.

Thus the question of diagnosis was narrowed down to (1) secondary anemia from tuberculosis or malaria, and (2) to that comparatively rare form of disease recognized by Banti as splenic anemia or splenic pseudo-leukemia. After exhausting all available means, with negative results, I excluded tuberculosis, while repeated examination of the blood failed to discover the presence of any of the malarial organisms. By this process of exclusion, therefore, the diagnosis of splenic anemia, or splenic pseudoleukemia was made.

The blood was examined again March 4th, and March 16th, with the following results:

Date.	Erythrocytes. (Per c.mm.)	Leucocytes. (Per c.mm.)	Hemoglobin. (Per cent.)	Color index. (Approximately.)
March 4th.	2,500,000	Not counted.	23	.72
March 16th.	2,600,000	6500	22	.7

Qualitative changes found at these examinations were in brief, as follows: Poikilocytosis, slight; very few macrocytes and an occasional normoblast present; polychromataphilia quite marked. A number of myelocytes were found, as well as a relative excess of lymphocytes; adult cells rather below normal, while no eosinophiles were present.

From February 25th to March 16th, there was much pain in the left side, referable to the area of splenic dulness, as well as persistent edema of the face and lower extremities. Labored respiration upon slight exertion was marked, and the anemic murmur was clearly distinguishable. From the 10th to the 16th of March, there was some improvement in the general condition, but the prognosis remained necessarily grave. After March 16th, I did not again see the patient until May 1st. At this time I found an apparently improved condition, anemia being less marked, although still striking, and the "fatty" appearance of the eyeball had disappeared, as had the edema of the extremities. At this time the murmur was still distinct though not quite so loud.

Upon palpation I found the spleen reduced in size, the dulness at the widest point extending to the external border of the rectus and from the eighth rib to within one inch above the crest of the ilium.

In conclusion, I may say that though I should hesitate to give a prognosis in this case, still it is my belief that recovery is possible.

MEDICAL PROGRESS.

Fractures of the Lower End of the Radius.—KAHLEYSS (*Deut. Zeitschr. f. Chir.*, vol. xlv, p. 531), having examined and photographed with the aid of the Röntgen-rays forty-eight recent fractures of the lower end of the radius, is of the opinion that some of the widely accepted statements concerning this common injury are erroneous. Such fractures may be classed as follows: (1) Separation of the epiphysis, which occurs only in early childhood in a pure form, and in late childhood is invariably associated with fracture of the diaphysis; (2) incomplete fractures, which in the form of fissures are really far rarer than has been supposed; (3) complete fractures, which may or may not involve the whole thickness of the bone.

Fissures were found to give such slight symptoms that their diagnosis from contusions of the radius is very difficult without the aid of the Röntgen-rays. The possibility of palpating the edges of a fissure is ridiculed by the writer. Such cases are undoubtedly complete fractures. In the forty-eight cases examined a fissure was found but twice, and in both instances it was produced by a fall on the back of the hand.

Of the complete fractures, eighty-nine per cent. involved the whole thickness of the radius, while in eleven per cent. only the styloid process, or a part of the articular surface, was separated. In two-thirds of the complete fractures the break was a single fracture, and in one-third more than one fracture-line existed. Half of the single fracture-lines ran practically straight across the bone; half were oblique or (a few) irregular. In three-fourths of the cases in which more than one line of fracture existed the break was Y-shaped.

The distance of the line of fracture from the articular surface was given by Colles as 1.5 inches. Others have said that this distance is too great. The photographs showed it to be in most cases from one-half to one inch. In oblique fractures the line of break was from half an inch to an inch higher on the radial side of the bone than on the ulnar side. The radiocarpal joint was involved in forty-two per cent. of the cases.

Displacement of the lower fragment, contrary to the commonly accepted opinion, took place almost invariably upward, backward, and outward. Rotation of the fragment about its sagittal axis was very infrequent, but rotation about its frontal axis was often found. Another unexpected discovery was the frequent occurrence of fracture of the tip of the ulna. This was found to exist in no fewer than seventy-eight per cent. of all cases, and is, therefore, by far the commonest complication.

Kahleyss disputes the idea of Lecomte that fractures of the lower end of the radius are purely tearing fractures, due to strain on the bone from over-extension of the posterior carpal ligament. He agrees with Löbker that they may be caused in this manner; but he asserts, as does the latter, that they may also be caused by a direct blow on the lower end of the bone. The common cause of the typical oblique fracture, however, is a combination of these two forces, strain and blow.

A New Incision for Operation upon the Shoulder-Joint.—SENN (*Nashville Jour. Med. and Surg.*, January, 1898) has devised an incision for operations upon the shoulder-joint which he believes is an improvement upon any yet proposed. The scar resulting from the operation is well protected by the prominence formed by the acromion, and at the same time the incision allows free access to every part of the shoulder-joint and its immediate vicinity. The external incision is made so as to form an oval cutaneous flap which is turned upward, exposing the upper half of the deltoid muscle. It is commenced over the coracoid process, and is carried downward and outward in a gentle curve as far as the middle of the deltoid muscle, when it is continued in a similar curve upward and backward as far as the posterior border of the axillary space on the same level as that at which it was commenced, that is, a point opposite the coracoid. The semilunar flap is next dissected up as far as the base of the acromion process and then reflected back. The acromion process is detached with a saw and turned downward with the deltoid muscle attached. The capsule of the joint is now freely exposed. If the operation is for an irreducible dislocation, the head of the humerus may now be easily found and replaced; if it is performed in order to remove diseased tissue, the joint may be opened and its interior subjected to careful examination. It is rarely necessary to drill the bone for the placing of the sutures as a catgut suture of the periosteum is sufficient. The divided portion of the deltoid muscle is sutured separately with catgut, and the cutaneous flap is brought down in position and sutured in the usual manner. After the operation has been performed for disease of the shoulder-joint drainage is necessary for two or three days. In aseptic cases primary union should be obtained.

Complete Hysterectomy.—CHALOT (*Centralbl. f. Gyne.*, November 13, 1897) has attempted to find a method of hysterectomy which will be far more radical than the usual methods of removal, either through the vagina or through an abdominal incision. The necessary points of a perfect operation are: (1) removal of the diseased tissues in one mass by an incision wide of the new growth; (2) careful excision of all affected glands. According to the writer, these principles can only be carried out by means of a celiotomy with the patient in the Trendelenburg position, the removal of the uterus being preceded by ligation and division of the internal iliac arteries, and by transplantation of the ureters. The transplantation of the ureters may, if more convenient, follow the excision of the uterus. Either the rectum, or, in some cases, the bladder, may serve as the receptacle of the urine. These four steps of the operation constitute a new method of hysterectomy, called by the inventor, "ultra-uretera hysterectomy."

THE MEDICAL NEWS.

A WEEKLY JOURNAL

OF MEDICAL SCIENCE.

COMMUNICATIONS are invited from all parts of the world. Original articles contributed *exclusively* to THE MEDICAL NEWS will after publication be liberally paid for (accounts being rendered quarterly), or 250 reprints will be furnished in place of other remuneration. When necessary to elucidate the text, illustrations will be engraved from drawings or photographs furnished by the author. Manuscripts should be typewritten.

Address the Editor: J. RIDDLE GOFFE, M.D.,
No. 111 FIFTH AVENUE (corner of 18th St.), NEW YORK.

Subscription Price, including postage in U. S. and Canada.

PER ANNUM IN ADVANCE	$4.00
SINGLE COPIES	.10
WITH THE AMERICAN JOURNAL OF THE MEDICAL SCIENCES, PER ANNUM	7.50

Subscriptions may begin at any date. The safest mode of remittance is by bank check or postal money order, drawn to the order of the undersigned. When neither is accessible, remittances may be made, at the risk of the publishers, by forwarding in *registered* letters.

LEA BROTHERS & CO.,
No. 111 FIFTH AVENUE (corner of 18th St.), NEW YORK,
AND NOS. 706, 708 & 710 SANSOM ST., PHILADELPHIA.

SATURDAY, MARCH 5, 1898.

THE LATEST FACTS ABOUT PHAGOCYTOSIS.

AFTER the investigations of Buchner had proved beyond a doubt that both blood and blood-serum possess the power to destroy bacteria, the question of the exact nature and the origin of the substance to which the blood owed this attribute was still an open one. Buchner, Hahn, and Denys assumed the existence of an albuminous substance which they called "alexin." This they thought came from the polynuclear leucocytes, and believed that in it lay the bactericidal power of the blood. This theory enhanced the importance of the blood-serum and the lymph, and was apparently in sharp contrast to that of Metchnikoff, who asserted that the leucocytes took the bacteria into their protoplasm, swallowed them, as it were, and digested them, thus protecting the body from their pernicious influence. When it came to be recognized that alexin might come from the leucocytes, the opposition to this phagocytic theory of Metchnikoff was not so pronounced as formerly. For it was easy to suppose that the bactericidal substance which was derived from a leucocyte might be active while yet in the body of the cell. On the other hand, it is equally supposable that alexin may be produced only outside the body of the leucocyte—perhaps by its death.

This question is not yet satisfactorily settled, and several investigators have been working for its solution. Recently Schattenfroh published at length the results of a long series of experiments which he had conducted along this line. His conclusions are as follows: (1) The leucocytes of rabbits and guinea-pigs contain a bactericidal substance—at least such a substance is set free when they are destroyed. (2) The bactericidal power of this substance is not destroyed by drying the cells, nor by keeping them at a temperature of 60°C. (140° F.) for half an hour. It is lost if the leucocytes are kept at 80° to 85° C. (176° to 185° F.) for a half hour. (3) By macerating leucocytes for a short time in warm normal salt solution, or for a long time in cold normal salt solution, an extract free from leucocytes is obtained, which possesses a bactericidal power of varying toxicity for different kinds of bacteria. (4) The bactericidal power of blood and that of such leucocytic fluid are not always parallel. Nevertheless it does not necessarily follow that they are not due to the same substance. (5) Leucocytes contain, besides the bactericidal substance referred to, another body which acts in an antagonistic manner.

Lowit, by tying the aorta, was able to reduce the number of leucocytes in the blood circulating through the head and lungs. He found that when their number was less than 800 to the cubic millimeter, the bactericidal power of the blood was greatly reduced or even absent. As the polynuclear leucocytes disappeared more rapidly he concluded that they are especially potent in bactericidal power.

Jacob has found that by the use of protalbumose he can produce hyperleucocytosis, and that the blood or serum from an animal which has been thus treated, will, if injected into the circulation of another animal, enable it to withstand an otherwise fatal dose of pneumococcic infection. He hopes, therefore, to be able to exert a favorable influence upon infectious diseases by inducing an artificial hyperleucocytosis in the individual. These are some of the results of recent research in this interesting field.

THE BRUSH BILL AMENDED.

THE editor of the MEDICAL NEWS has been favored with a personal letter from Dr. Brush, the author of the bill modifying the powers of the Board of Health, in which he assures the editor that practically all of the suggestions made in the editorial columns of the MEDICAL NEWS of February 19th, an advance copy of which had been sent to him, have been accepted and the bill already modified in accordance therewith: The president of the Police Board is restored to membership in the Board of Health; the term of service remains six years instead of four; the office of president of the board may be filled by a physician as well as a layman, and the Mayor shall designate one of the commissioners appointed by him to be the president; the board is empowered to prepare and to preserve vaccine lymph and to produce diphtheria antitoxin and other antitoxins for the use of the department; the board is not restrained from placing pulmonary tuberculosis among the contagious diseases, nor from enforcing the regulations concerning tuberculosis recently promulgated by it.

If restraining the board from the sale of its products shall so cripple its financial resources as to curtail the lines of research which have been prosecuted with such great success, it will become the duty of the profession to see to it that necessary appropriation of the public moneys shall be forthcoming. The acknowledgment by the superintendent of the Institut Pasteur, accorded the workers in the laboratories of the Board of Health, as presented in another column, is a source of gratification, not only to the medical profession of this city but also to the entire community, and reflects credit upon those who have had the foresight to anticipate the possibility, and provide for the accomplishment, of such results.

THE REMARKABLE SUCCESS OF THE NEW YORK BOARD OF HEALTH IN PRODUCING DIPHTHERIA ANTITOXIN.

IN the MEDICAL NEWS of February 12th it was stated editorially, on the authority of the superintendent of the laboratories of the New York Board of Health, that the laboratories of this department had surpassed all others in producing a high-grade diphtheria antitoxin, and that the virulent cultures of the diphtheria bacillus from which these antitoxins were obtained had been sought by the biologic laboratories of England, France, and Germany. While no one has ventured to deny this statement publicly, it has been scoffed at in private by enemies of the department as an idle boast. It is gratifying, therefore, to find this statement confirmed and the obligation of the Institut Pasteur recognized in an article by L. Martin, chief of the laboratory of the Institut Pasteur in the January number of the *Annales de l'Institut Pasteur.*

The author gives the results of a long series of investigations in which he has carefully gone over the recent work of Park and Williams of the laboratory of the New York Board of Health (*Journal of Experimental Medicine*, vol. i, No. 1) and of Spronck (*Annales de l'Institut Pasteur*, 1895). His conclusions coincide with those of Park and Williams in all important respects. With the diphtheria bacillus sent to him by them he was able, by following their methods, to produce a toxin ten times as strong as any he had formerly obtained. He has been able to obtain no bacillus from cases of diphtheria in Paris which approaches in toxicity the one sent him from New York, and with the stronger toxin from the American bacillus Martin has been able to produce in his horses an antitoxin triple the strength formerly obtained. He finds that the bacilli grown in bouillon under a current of air, as advised by Roux and Yersin, produce toxin more quickly than when grown in the ordinary wide-mouth flasks. The increased rapidity of the production of the toxin is not sufficient, however, to compensate for the difficulties encountered in carrying out the process.

Although with ordinary nutrient bouillon rendered sufficiently alkalin Martin found strong toxin produced in the cultures with a fair degree of regularity, nevertheless, still better results could be produced with a bouillon so prepared that it contained no substances capable of producing an acid fermentation with the diphtheria bacillus. This he obtained by a special process from the pig's stomach.

Martin records the interesting fact that a diphtheria bacillus which, when injected into a rabbit, shows no virulence, may, nevertheless, produce in bouillon a strong toxin. He presents many additional points which are of interest to bacteriologists, especially those interested in the production of antitoxin.

In this article by Louis Martin there are several statements which have a bearing on the value of experimental work by public laboratories in subjects which naturally come most directly under their supervision. He states: "It is certain that with the work of Park and Williams a great advance has been accomplished in the production of diphtheria toxin. Previous to their work toxins fatal in doses of 1/10 to 1/30 of a c.cm. had been produced, but they have obtained toxins of which 1/100 to 1/200 c.cm. is the fatal dose. The serums up to the time that I obtained the stronger toxins were of 100 units strength; now after their employment they are of 200 and 300 units strength."

Again: "It is to be hoped that serums of still greater strength will be obtained in the future from the increased activity of the toxins. This will render more easy and certain the serum treatment and permit the mortality of diphtheria to be diminished still further."

Inquiry at the research laboratory of the New York City Health Department reveals the fact that this exceedingly virulent diphtheria bacillus referred to, has been sent, free of charge, to nearly all the laboratories, both public and private, in this country, and also to England, France, and Germany.

Thus the advance accomplished at the New York laboratory in the methods of producing toxin and the bacillus there developed have markedly helped in giving to all physicians, from whatever source they may obtain it, an antitoxin of greater strength than ever before.

It should be remembered by those who feel so strongly that the sale of its surplus of antitoxin by the Board of Health of New York is a wrong to private capital, that all the money thus obtained is spent in experimental work, that it cannot be obtained otherwise, and that the results of this work are freely and entirely given out so that all may make use of them. It is only by having a number of such laboratories freely helping each other and freely giving out their information to physicians that rapid advance is possible.

THE DISPENSARY BILL.

THE advocates and opponents of the bill regarding the management of dispensaries in New York State have been given a hearing before the Senate committee to which it had been referred. A remarkable feature of the argument of one opponent of the bill, who is president of one of the large dispensaries of New York City, was the statement that the underlying motive which inspires this legislation is the desire of the medical profession to increase their incomes.

The spiteful peroration with which this gentleman closed his harangue is not indicative of that cheerful and willing spirit of reform which he insisted earlier in his address characterizes the managers of all dispensaries. He said: "If this act is to go through, by all means change its title. Write it plainly: An act to prevent medical treatment at moderate rates and to permit unlimited charges by physicians. In a word, gentleman, make it an act to create a medical trust." Right here it might be well to call the attention of the wealthy managers of dispensaries to the possibility of the fact that in the sharp rivalry of the different dispensaries to increase their business, they lose sight of the primary object of the dispensary, and judge of the success of their work by the increased number of persons they have induced to seek aid at their hands. The business principle that "the larger the business the more successful the undertaking" does not hold good in charity work. The extension of the principles of paternal government, and the debauchery of the moral sense of personal responsibility in the recipients of charity—and this is what the dispensaries of New York are doing—is not a benefit to the community, but a curse.

Anent this subject the current number of the *Philadelphia Medical Journal* says: "Legal advice, groceries, clothes, and housing are as necessary to our Lord Demos as medical advice and drugs. Why then should not lawyers, store-keepers, farmers, and artisans give from one-fourth to one-half of their time and labor in free service to their fellows? The medical men have thus given of their time and lives—and what is their reward? A profession divided against itself and half of the outside world living like a parasite upon its powerless host. The idea is growing fast in the parasite's cunning mind that by playing the two factions of the profession against each other he can feed on unmolested. Astute politicians are availing themselves of this, and leading us at a rapid pace down the smooth *decensus averni* of socialistic depravity. It is clearly high time that we should turn about and painfully return to honor and self-respect, and in doing so show the world how to regain the same qualities. This is not a case of Profession *vs.* The People—but it is a case of the people against itself."

ECHOES AND NEWS.

A New Disease in the Klondike.—It is said that cerebro-spinal meningitis is epidemic among the gold-seekers in Alaska. The disease is rapidly fatal.

Water Purification by Electricity.—An association has been formed in Paris to exploit the new method of purifying water by means of electricity. This process has been endorsed by Drs. Tyndal and Roux.

Resignation of Professor Esmarch.—Professor Esmarch of the University of Keil is about to resign the chair of surgery, which he has occupied since 1857. Professor Esmarch is seventy-five years of age.

New York Will Pay for Tuberculous Cattle Destroyed.—The bill authorizing the Board of Health of New York City to pay for cattle destroyed because of tuberculosis has been passed by both branches of the Legislature.

Bombay Hospital Destroyed by Fire.—One of the plague hospitals at Bombay was destroyed by fire on February 19th. Twelve European and eighty-four native patients were saved. Three patients died from shock.

Soldiers Vaccinated.—All the soldiers at Fort Ethan Allen, at Essex Junction, Vermont, have been ordered to be vaccinated at once on account of the possibility of being ordered to Cuba where smallpox is prevalent.

A Correction.—In Dr. Gallant's article on "Inguinal Hernia," which appeared in the MEDICAL NEWS of last week, acknowledgment should have been made for the illustration, which was obtained through the courtesy of *Mathew's Medical Quarterly*.

Faithfulness of Surgeon Honeberger.—The day-book of the chief medical officer of the cruiser "Maine" has been recovered from the wreck. It bears witness to the methodical habits of Surgeon Honeberger, for the record was brought up to the last moment before the wreck of the ship.

Vigilance at Quarantine.—A vessel has just arrived and is being detained at quarantine in Pensacola, Florida, from Para, Brazil, bringing the report that while the vessel was at Para the captain's daughter and six of the crew were attacked with yellow fever and sent to the hospital at that place where they all died.

The Senn Medal.—Those members of the American Medical Association who intend to compete for the medal offered by Dr. Nicholas Senn for the best essay on some surgical subject are requested to forward the typewritten copies of contributions to J. McFadden Gaston, M.D., Atlanta, Ga., immediately.

New York Climate too Severe for Eskimos.—One of the band of Eskimo which accompanied Lieutenant Peary's expedition on its return from the North, recently died of pneumonia at Bellevue Hospital. All of the party have suffered from colds of varying severity, and at one time four of them were under treatment for this disease.

Degeneracy in Russia.—The Russian *Novoye Vremya* complains of the degeneracy of the present inhabitants of the great Empire and attributes it to the lack of proper nourishment. It declares that the lower class have one-third less to eat than their grandparents had and they are proportionately suffering from the lack of other essentials of life.

American Neurological Association.—The Council announces that the Twenty-four Annual Meeting of the Association will be held in New York at the Academy of Medicine on Thursday, Friday, and Saturday, May 26, 27, and 28, 1898. There will be two sessions daily, one from 10 A.M. to 12.30 P.M., the other from 2 P.M. to 4.30 P.M.

Bill to Prohibit the Practice of Faith-Cure.—A bill is in preparation which so amends the New York health laws with regard to the practice of the healing art as to prevent practice by persons who profess to cure by mental processes alone. The direct antithesis of this measure has appeared in the form of a bill incorporating osteopaths. The article called eternal vigilance was never in greater demand.

Important Work of the United States Department of Agriculture.—The United States Senate has authorized the immediate publication of a second edition of Bulletin 19 of the Bureau of Animal Industry on "The Inspection of Meats for Animal Parasites." This bulletin was issued on February 8, 1898, and has been in such demand that at present it is impossible to obtain a copy. Physicians desiring copies of the second edition should address their Congressmen or Senators.

Removal of the Stomach.—A correspondent writes to the *Medical Press and Circular* (London) stating that Dr. Schlatter's recent removal of the stomach is not the first case of the kind on record, for the operation had already been performed by Professor Maydl. The patient survived and was alive and well six years after the operation. The case is reported in full in the *Wien. Med. Woch.*, August 26, 1896, and is briefly mentioned in the *British Medical Journal*, Epitome, ii, No. 323, 1896.

The Post-Graduate Must Reinstate Professor Kelsey.—Professor Charles B. Kelsey has received from the Supreme Court a peremptory writ of mandamus directing the Board of Directors of the New York Post-Graduate Medical School and Hospital to reinstate him as a professor of that institution. Dr. Kelsey was dismissed without a hearing by a majority vote at a meeting of the board which was not attended by all the members. The Court decided that this was illegal, as it requires a majority of the entire board to dismiss a member of the faculty.

Home for the Treatment of Incipient Tuberculosis.—The Working Girls' Vacation Society of New York City has established at Santa Clara, Franklin County, N. Y., a vacation house for the treatment of incipient cases of pulmonary tuberculosis, occurring in unmarried working girls. There is a resident woman physician, and a complete equipment for the modern management of this class of cases. The altitude is about 1700 feet. The price per week is $7, which covers all expenses except laundry. All persons applying for admission should be referred to the medical director of the Society at 222 West Thirty-eighth street, New York City.

Pasteur Institute at Constantinople.—The bacteriologic laboratory which was founded by Pasteur at Constantinople by request of the Sultan has recently re-opened its doors after a long period of idleness due to the incompetency and carelessness of the State officials and to lack of funds. The French *chargé d'affaires* protested, as did the Imperial Society of Medicine, and in this way the attention of the Sultan was drawn to the precarious state of an institution in which he had taken the greatest interest. It is probable that the work of the institution will be greatly developed, for orders have been given that the director of the institute shall want for nothing.

Osteopathy in the State Legislature.—There is some consolation in the reflection that only about one-tenth of all the bills introduced in the State Legislature are enacted into law. A bill known as Assemby Bill No. 939, entitled "An Act Regulating and Legalizing the Practice of Osteopathy in the State of New York," has recently been introduced at Albany by Mr. Raplee. A similar bill was introduced this winter in the Legislature of Illinois, but it met with such a torrent of protest from the medical profession that it was promptly defeated. A few hundred letters of remonstrance addressed to Mr. Rapiee, the author of the present bill, would probably consign this measure to a worthy fate.

Dr. McGraw of Detroit Sued for Malpractice.—A patient of Dr. Theodore A. McGraw recently brought suit against the Doctor in the Wayne Circuit Court for $5000 damages for malpractice. The plaintiff averred that during May last he was suffering from acute pain in the right leg caused by osteitis of the tibia, and employed the Doctor to operate upon it and remove the diseased portions of bone; that the surgeon made a mistake and operated upon the tibia of the left leg. These facts are true except as to the "mistake." After the patient had been anesthetized, the doctor found that both legs were similarly affected. He asked which one he was to operate upon, and the patient's father replied that it was the left leg. The surgeon acted upon the decision of the father and operated upon the left tibia. The judge decided that the Doctor had a right to rely upon the decision of the father of the plaintiff in this matter, and directed the jury to find a verdict for the defendant.

The Cause of Yellow Fever.—In our Berlin letter of this week it will be noted that the trend of German medical thought does not seem inclined to accept as final Sanarelli's declarations as to his discovery of the bacillus of yellow fever. Our foreign correspondent mentions German conservatism as a reason for this skeptical way of regarding Sanarelli's alleged discovery. It is indeed lamentable that the Germans are not as ready to employ their almost wonderful critical acumen in the discussion of "German discoveries" as they are those of France, Italy, and even those of benighted America. As an example we might mention Pasteur's work on rabies, which, we learn, they are only beginning to recognize as having something "in it." Bacteriologic science has not as yet accepted Sanarelli's discovery as the proven cause of yellow fever, but at the same time we see no good reason for deserting Sanarelli for a yeast and mold—the latter having been put forward as the possible etiologic factor of yellow fever.

Resolution.—The following resolution, offered by Dr. J. H. Burtenshaw, was passed, with but one dissenting vote, by the Medical Society of the County of New York at a very largely attended meeting held February 28th: "*Resolved*, That the Medical Society of the County of New York reaffirms its indorsement of the bill to amend the State Charities Law, relating to the Licensing and Regulation of Dispensaries by the State Board of Charities, now before the Legislature of the State, and that it urges the immediate passage of the bill in its present form. *Resolved*, That this resolution be signed by the president and secretary of this society, and that copies be forwarded to the Lieutenant-Governor, the Speaker of the Assembly, and the chairmen of the Committees on Public Health of the Senate and Assembly." This action clearly demonstrates the position taken by the largest medical society in the State with regard to the Dispensary Bill, and should once and for all put an end to the unreliable statements which have been spread broadcast of late regarding the sentiment of the profession in New York City in opposition to the measure. Similar action has been taken also during the past week by the Medical Society of the County of Kings, the New York County Medical Association, the New York Medical League, and the Committee of the New York State Medical Association.

Bulletin of the Chicago Health Department.—For nearly two years the Department of Health of Chicago has been investigating the claims made for formaldehyd as a disinfectant, with especial reference to its value for household or domestic disinfection. The results have been so satisfactory and the remarkable bactericidal properties of formic aldehyd have received confirmation in such a practical manner through the experiments made that at the suggestion of Dr. Reilly, assistant commissioner, an inexpensive vaporizer has been devised for use in the room occupied by a diphtheria patient. This vaporizer consists of a shallow cup supported over an ordinary cheap lamp, such as is made to burn kerosene. Methyl alcohol is used for the flame. The cup is nearly filled with a solution consisting of about one part of a forty-per-cent. formalin solution and five parts of boiling water. The flame is so adjusted as to keep the solution just at the boiling-point. The device in use costs less than 20 cents. Twenty-one deaths from influenza occurred in Chicago during the month of January, 1898, as against a total of fifteen for the entire year of 1897. The epidemic of influenza was the chief factor in increasing the total number of deaths from 21,897 in 1890 to 27,754 in 1891—an increase of more than one-fifth. A return of the disease is very much feared. The health commissioner has called attention to the fact that influenza is a germ disease and, therefore, contagious. He advises that people "keep out of the way of contagion," by which is meant, among other things, avoiding close contact with one suffering from the disease, not sleeping in the same room, much less in the same bed, with such a sufferer, and not using any article or utensil in common with him.

Obituary.—Dr. Edward C. Seguin died of cirrhosis of the liver on February 19th at his home in New York City. Dr. Seguin was born in Paris, France, in 1843. He was the only child of Dr. Edouard O. Seguin, who, with his family, came to the United States in 1850 and settled in Cleveland, Ohio. In 1861, then residing at Mount Vernon, N. Y., young Seguin began the study of medicine with his father, attended three courses of lectures at the College of Physicians and Surgeons, New York, and was graduated in 1864. Meanwhile Dr. Seguin had entered the medical department of the army. He was appointed a medical cadet in the regular army and served two years, until August, 1864. Later he was assigned to duty at Forts Craig and Seldon, New Mexico. During the winter of 1869–70 Dr. Seguin studied in Paris under Brown-Séquard, Charcot, Ranvier, and Cornil, and has since made the treatment of nervous diseases a specialty. In 1871 he became a member of the Faculty of the College of Physicians and Surgeons, and lectured in this institution on diseases of the spinal cord and on insanity from 1871 to 1885. In 1873 he founded the clinic for nervous diseases. He was one of the founders of the American Neurological Association and of the New York Neurological Society. He was also a member of the New York Pathological Society and of many medical societies of this country and of Europe. In 1894 his health began to fail, and he gave up professional work in July, 1896. To the New York Academy of Medicine Dr. Seguin bequeathed an oil painting of his father, Dr. Edward Onesimus Seguin; an autograph letter from Pope Pius IX., dated December 16, 1847, in which his Holiness compliments Dr. E. O. Seguin for his work in ameliorating the condition of imbecile children; a bronze medallion of Charcot, which was presented to him by the renowned French master, and a large portrait of Brown-Séquard. To the Academy he also left the greater part of his library. All his instruments and appliances for the study of the nervous system, all his pathologic specimens and part of his library, he gives to the pathologic laboratory of the Alumni Association of the College of Physicians and Surgeons, to be set apart and specially catalogued, and not to be permitted to leave the laboratory. If the association will not accept the charge and the conditions, the bequest is to go to the Academy of Medicine under the same conditions.—Dr. Charles Jasper Bickham recently died of heart disease at his residence in New Orleans, La., in his sixty-eighth year. Dr. Bickham was born near Covington, La., in 1830, and was the son of a prominent planter. He was educated at an institution in Texas, which subsequently became the Southwestern University. After four-years' study he received the degree of Master of Arts. He graduated in medicine in 1856, and was soon after appointed Assistant House Surgeon at Charity Hospital, New Orleans, which position he filled with distinction until 1859. Dr. Bickham was demonstrator of anatomy in the Louisiana Medical College from 1867 to 1872. In 1894 he was appointed a member of the Board of Health, and served until 1896, when he resigned on account of ill health.—Surgeon Thomas B. Bailey, Passed Assistant Surgeon of the United States Navy, was found dead in his room at a hotel in Washington, D. C., February 24th. He left a letter providing for the distribution of his effects and expressing the fear that he was about to die from heart disease. He had just returned from a tour of duty in China, and had been appointed to duty at the Washington Navy Yard.—Dr. John P. Maynard died at the age of sixty-two years at his home in Dedham, Mass., February 26th. He was born in Boston, and was a graduate of Yale College and the Harvard Medical School. Dr. Maynard was the discoverer of collodion, and suggested its application in surgery.

CORRESPONDENCE.

MIDWIVES.

To the Editor of the MEDICAL NEWS.

DEAR SIR: Dr. Henry J. Garrigues' article on "Midwives," in your issue of February 19th, page 232, is strangely inaccurate in the opening paragraph. I was the author of the bill mentioned by Dr. Garrigues, and before reading it at a meeting of the Medical Society of the County of New York I consulted the president of the society, Dr. S. O. Van der Poel, and Drs. Abraham Jacobi, Paul F. Mundé, Allen S. Church, Alfred L. Loomis, Cornelius R. Agnew, John L. Campbell, and others, all of whom were in favor of the bill. The bill in question proposed the establishment of a school of midwifery in connection with a maternity hospital, where the pupils would receive instruction in anatomy, physiology, and obstetrics under the best professors, and, before being graduated, be obliged to attend cases of obstetrics under the supervision of competent physicians, and then receive instruction in asepsis, antisepsis, and hygiene.

It was intended that this school should be entirely under the control of medical men. The board of managers (medical men) were to appoint the professors and to have general supervision of the school and hospital. I read the bill at a stated meeting of the Medical Society of the County of New York during the administration of Dr. S. O. Van der Poel. After a short discussion it was referred to the Commitia Minora of the Society, and the next stated meeting was appointed for its discussion. The Commitia Minora reported adversely upon the bill, and after a long and somewhat heated discussion, in which Drs. Jacobi, Mundé, Church, and others, spoke in favor of the proposed measure and many professors of medical colleges against it, the society voted in the negative.

Before submitting my bill to the judgment of the Society, I had stated that if the Society did not approve I would do nothing more about it. The Society disapproved, and I locked the bill in my desk. It was never sent to Albany; it was killed in the County Medical Society. Queerly enough, the great objection brought against my bill was that graduates of the proposed school would be better instructed in obstetrics than those of the regular medical colleges.

With regard to any other bill introduced in the State Legislature, I know nothing.

PALMER C. COLE, M.D.

254 WEST FORTY-SECOND STREET,
NEW YORK, February 27, 1898.

"CHARITY ABUSES IN MICHIGAN."

To the Editor of the MEDICAL NEWS.

DEAR SIR: Under the above heading in your issue of February 19th will be found the following: "In Michigan the abuse referred to seems especially rife in the free dispensary of the University Hospital at Ann Arbor, and it is against this institution that criticism is particularly leveled." The above statement is in part false, and, I suppose, in part true. The statement that charity abuse is especially rife in the University Hospital at Ann Arbor is false. The other part of the statement, that criticism is particularly leveled at this institution, may be true. The facts in the matter are, briefly, these:

In 1883 the Board of Regents of the University of Michigan made a by-law excluding from the University Hospital all people who were able to pay for medical services. This by-law has been, and is, enforced. Some months ago, a well-to-do individual appeared at the hospital and demanded admission on the ground that he was a taxpayer and contributed to the support of the institution. His request was refused. He appealed to the Board of Regents. The Board laid his protest upon the table, and the old rule remains in force. Abuse of public charity in the hospital at the University of Michigan has never been great.

Respectfully,

VICTOR C. VAUGHAN, M.D.

ANN ARBOR, February 24, 1898.

THE DISPENSARY BILL: A REPLY TO DR. VAN FLEET.

To the Editor of the MEDICAL NEWS.

DEAR SIR: I ask the courtesy of the use of your columns in order to reply to certain of the statements contained in Dr. Frank Van Fleet's letter on the subject of the Dispensary Bill, printed in the MEDICAL NEWS for February 19th.

The so-called Joint-Committee Dispensary Bill, now before the Legislature of the State, embodies the result of many months of careful investigation by the committee having it in charge. It has been approved by the representatives of the great medical schools who were designated by the faculties of these schools to serve on the several committees, and has received the unqualified indorsement of the Medical Society of the County of New York, Medical Society of the County of Kings, Medical Society of the County of Queens, Medical Society of the County of Richmond, New York State Medical Association, New York County Medical Association, New York Medical League, New York Society for Advancing the Practice of Medicine, Kings County Medical Association, Brooklyn Medical Society, Brooklyn Medical Association, and the Long Island Medical Society, all incorporated bodies, and representing a membership of more than 5,000 reputable physicians of the State. It certainly is to be sincerely regretted that, according to Dr. Van Fleet's letter, the bill has not called forth the hearty support of the Committee on Legislation of the Medical Society of the State of New York, composed of *three* members!

The Medical Society of the State of New York, at its recent annual meeting at Albany, took no official action whatever in favor of, or against, the bill. The delegates to the Society from the county medical societies of New York, Kings, Queens, and Richmond were specifically instructed by unanimous vote of their several societies to vote in favor of indorsement of the bill, and there can be no doubt that it would have been so indorsed by the State Society had it not been decided at an informal conference of certain of the members that its consideration would interfere with the scientific work laid out for the meeting. Official confirmation of the fact that the bill was not acted upon during the meeting is contained in the subjoined copy of a letter recently received from the Secretary of the State Medical Society:

ALBANY, N. Y., February 12, 1898.

DEAR DOCTOR: In reply to your letter of inquiry just at hand as to whether the matter of the so-called Dispensary Bill was brought before the Medical Society of the State of New York at its recent meeting, I would say that it did not come up in any way whatever; it never was referred to in any way throughout the entire session. The Anniversary Address contained some reference to the topic of free dispensaries, but no action was called for or taken on it.

Yours very sincerely,

F. C. CURTIS,
Secretary.

17 WASHINGTON AVENUE.

The By-Laws of the State Medical Society (page 17) specify the duties of its Committee on Legislation as follows, the italics being my own:

There shall be a standing Committee on Legislation, consisting of three members, the duty of which shall be to watch the course of State legislation on medical subjects, and *to take charge of such matters pertaining to medical legislation as shall be referred to it by this Society.*

In spite of the fact that no official action was taken by the Society in connection with the Dispensary Bill, and that, in consequence, the bill was not referred to the Society's Committee on Legislation, the Chairman of that Committee, Dr. Van Fleet, has issued letters to the lay and medical press, as well as to many members of the profession at large, attacking the bill. To these letters, in addition to his name, he has appended his official title, and the impression is thus conveyed that their issuance has been authorized by the State Medical Society, and that they officially reflect the opinion of its members. On the contrary, these communications from the Chairman of the State's Society's Legislative Committee do *not* represent the opinion of the Society, their publication was *not* authorized, and the only inference that can be drawn is that they were published over the gentleman's official title with plain intent to mislead public opinion.

Dr. Van Fleet says in his letter to the MEDICAL NEWS: "You are mistaken if you think the Chairman of the Legislative Committee of the Medical Society of the State of New York is the only person opposed to the measure under consideration, for my action is indorsed by the whole committe, by the officers of the State Society, and by the majority of the medical men of the State." By the whole committee—of *three* members, of which Dr. Van Fleet is one! By the officers of the State Society—*four* in number! By the majority of the medical men of the State! The latter is a modest assertion, but Dr. Van Fleet fails to offer proof of its accuracy. Apparently the publicly recorded indorsement of the Bill by twelve of the largest and most influential medical societies of the United States carries no weight with this gentleman in comparison with the opinion of the solitary seven. "It is safe to say that not one-fourth of the profession of the City of New York would indorse this bill if its true character were known." Dr. Van Fleet probably does not know, which is very unfortunate, that during the past week, after plenty of time for mature reflection, five of the societies which originally indorsed the bill unanimously reaffirmed their indorsement, and in no uncertain tone either, one being the Medical Society of the County of New York, of which Dr. Van Fleet is a member.

Every argument brought forward by Dr. Van Fleet is amply refuted by the reports of the State Board of Charities for the years 1896 and 1897, and by those to the Medical Society of the County of New York of its Committee on the Abuse of Medical Charity, transmitted May 24 and December 27, 1897. The simple truth of the matter is that the Boards of Trustees of a majority of the large dispensaries located in this city, and certain physicians officially connected with these institutions, though well aware of the enormous amount of medical charity abuse which exists, have no desire to correct or control it. Their reasons for this are sufficiently obvious and need not be discussed at this time. The gross mismanagement of dispensaries in the City of New York has been a public scandal during the past twenty years, and yet in but one or two isolated instances has an attempt been made by the officials in charge to reform the abuses. It is only now, when a conscientious and determined effort is being made by the great medical societies to have all dispensaries placed on a plane with other incorporated institutions, and thus answerable to the proper authorities for the employment of appropriations and trust funds confided to their charge, and to make them subject to rules and regulations which will exclude the hordes of unworthy well-to-do applicants from the benefits of free treatment, that the cry is raised that if additional power is conferred upon the State Board of Charities every dispensary will be forced to suspend its operations, and great suffering will be entailed, in consequence, upon the deserving poor.

It is not the wish of those active in the present movement that even *one* dispensary now existing shall be closed, provided it treats only those applicants worthy of receiving free medical and surgical aid. There is no charity so beneficent, so far-reaching, or so freely bestowed as true medical charity, and so long as illness and misery exist just so long will the poor be welcomed to the institutions organized to alleviate their distress, and so long will doctors gladly minister to them. It is because thousands and tens of thousands of unworthy persons are treated at these free dispensaries every year without the slightest effort being made to investigate their claims of poverty that reform in management is demanded. The State Board of Charities is a constitutional body appointed by the Governor and confirmed by the Senate. During the past thirty-one years, or since its original institution, all matters under its jurisdiction have been managed intelligently, discretely, and with complete fairness. If the present Bill becomes a law it is the intention of the board to hold public meetings to which all interested in the subject of improvement of dispensaries will be invited, and suggestions as to the formulation of proper rules and regulations will be received and acted upon.

In conclusion permit me to say that in spite of the assertions of the Chairman of the Legislative Committee of the Medical Society of the State of New York and his committee of two, it is perfectly safe to assert that fully ninety-seven per cent. of the physicians of the City and State of New York favor the passage of the Dispensary Bill, and that the committee having it in charge will continue to receive the same cordial and hearty support which has been freely offered it since its labors began nearly two years ago.

Very truly yours,

JAMES HAWLEY BURTENSHAW,

Chairman of the late Committee of the Medical Society of the County of New York on the Abuse of Medical Charity.

128 WEST EIGHTY-SECOND STREET,
NEW YORK, February 28, 1898.

OUR BERLIN LETTER.

[From our Special Correspondent.]

THE MEDICO-LEGAL STATUS OF A HERMAPHRODITE, AND THE QUESTION OF SEX IN SUCH CASES—A BERLIN METHOD FOR THE SUPPRESSION OF QUACKERY—THE ETIOLOGY OF YELLOW FEVER AND YEASTS AND MOLDS—ALGIERS AS A WINTER-RESORT.

BERLIN, February 24, 1898.

APROPOS of the presentation before the last meeting of the Berlin Medical Society of a very perfect specimen of the genus hermaphrodite, who is on exhibition at one of the museums here, there was a discussion by some of the leaders of medical thought on the determination of sex in such cases. It is usual for the general public to think that a doctor can settle this question without difficulty. Experience, however, has shown that there can be few more tangled Gordian knots presented for unravelment than this same question of the determination of sex in certain doubtful cases.

Among others Virchow, who had made a careful examination in this case, said that he was free to confess that he could not tell to which sex the individual belonged. Even when such cases come to autopsy it is extremely difficult to decide whether the sexual organs found are ovaries or testicles, and, of course, on these organs depends the essential distinction of sex. Not alone is it difficult to decide macroscopically, which can easily be imagined from certain gross similarities of the organs, but even microscopically it is not always easy to find distinctive sex elements with absolute assurance.

The organs are most often ovaries in such cases, but the anomalous development which has affected the rest of the urogenital system usually has had its effect on them too. Much more connective tissue than is normal is present, and in the midst of this luxuriant connective tissue often the most patient search is required to reveal the presence of sexual elements. Often, too, there would seem to be even in the ovaries or testicles themselves a certain dubiousness of structure—an amphoteric condition—as if Nature herself had not quite decided which sex was to result. Perfect sexual elements of both kinds are not to be found, but there seems to be embryonic rudiments of both in an arrested early stage of development.

Professor Landau discussed the question from the practical standpoint of a man, who, within the last year, has been called upon to decide for legal purposes the question of sex in a dubious case. He very candidly said that lawyers and judges generally share the lay opinion as to the doctor's, and especially the gynecologist's, perfect capability of deciding this question, in which opinion they are, of course, often completely at fault. The ordinary external examination may be utterly deceptive, and the combined internal and external examination may give absolutely no sure grounds upon which to determine the question of sex. One may have under one's fingers the essential sexual organs, and yet be able to tell nothing about them. "Even if we have the opportunity," he adds, "to perform an operation and so obtain microscopic specimens, we still may not be able to decide the question, and no less an authority than Professor Virchow supports us in this conservative opinion."

In these doubtful cases, according to Professor Landau, the following practical rules are the best guide: The parent must decide, in very doubtful cases, what sex will be most convenient in rearing the child. The individual must decide for him or herself at the age of eighteen years whether he or she is to continue to be considered as belonging to that sex or not, and act accordingly. There is no country in Europe, except Russia, in which such a procedure would be contrary to law. In Russia the individual would have no legal status if he or she decided to belong to a sex different from that in which their declaration of birth was made.

In the case in which Professor Landau's opinion was asked, the individual had been brought up as a girl. At the age of four years the supposedly enlarged clitoris, at the base of which the urethra opened, was removed, because its development was looked upon as pathologic. At the age of eighteen years, however, the individual decided that he was a male. His voice, his beard, his general external appearance, and, above all, his sexual feelings were those of a man. Owing to the occasional occurrence of sexual perversion, this last is not absolutely decisive in the matter, yet in very doubtful cases it is the most trustworthy factor.

The external appearances, beard, voice, form, etc., may be deceptive, as they were in the case presented before the Society. She dresses in trousers and coat, wears a beard, and in general looks like a man of low stature. Her hips and buttocks are distinctively feminine, however, and her sexual inclinations are toward men. She claims that the sexual organ on one side is a testicle, while that on the other side is an ovary. Her opinion would have been laughed at, only that a Röntgen-ray photograph of her pelvis (which is characteristically feminine) and her femora brought out a remarkable fact. One of her femora was masculine, the other feminine in type, *i. e.:* one had the obtuse angle between the neck and shaft of the femur usually noticed in men; the other the almost right angle found normally in women. This is, perhaps, the first time that this fact has been noted in such a case, and is but another proof of the profoundly fundamental nature of the disturbance of development of the normal sexual being which underlies the hermaphroditic condition.

Some time ago a prominent German medical journal published the results of its investigation of Count Matter's so-called electrohomeopathic treatment, a much advertised method of treating all the ills to which flesh is heir, and a few others besides. Needless to say it was pronounced a humbug.

The investigation was a serious one. With us in America, however, beyond the publication of its results in a few medical journals, bringing to medical men a knowledge they might easily be presumed to have beforehand, nothing would be hoped for from it. Here the Police Commission took official cognizance of it, and formally announced in a circular which must be displayed in all drug-stores, that "the treatment in question has nothing to do with Hahnemann or his disciples, and is to be considered utterly worthless." The effect of such a circular is obvious. It is the proper method of treating a fraud. If in other matters police authority steps in to prevent swindling, *i. e.:* the pretence of selling something which is not delivered to the purchaser, why not in this also? Perhaps it is only in matters concerning the health of the people that deceit in buying or selling is not cheating.

The announcement of the discovery of the yellow-fever germ naturally attracted a good deal of attention here. Generally, however, opinions as to the absolute accuracy of the supposed discovery have not that air of certain assurance with which the announcement was welcomed in other quarters. While honors of various kinds have flowed in upon Professor Sanarelli from the French, and especially from his Italian compatriots, very little has been said of his work in Germany. Of course, one obvious reason for this is that Germany, as a nation, is very little interested in yellow fever; another and very important reason is, however, that further confirmation will have to be forthcoming before German conservatism will accept the discovery as final. It has been pointed out here that during the course of yellow fever many of the intestinal bacteria take on special characteristics; the bacterium coli, for instance, becomes especially virulent and even more proteiform, if possible, than before. The possibility of one of its varieties being considered specific for the disease, even after careful investigation, is not easy to eliminate. As the disease itself does not spread to animals, manifestations of pathologic conditions produced in animals can have very little weight. In animals the characteristic course of the disease is not reproduced, and so one of Koch's great criteria falls to the ground. One manifestation of the uncertain state of German opinion in the matter is the publication last week in a prominent medical journal here of an article from Rio de Janeiro in which a yeast and a mold are described as occurring in twenty-five bodies of yellow-fever patients, though not to be found in other bodies examined at the same time. While it would seem probable that there is in these cases some fault in the technic, recent work on pathogenic yeasts and molds shows that the possibility of human infection from these sources cannot be entirely eliminated.

Professor Fränkel, the distinguished laryngologist here, and director of the throat and nose department in the Charité, has just spent some time in Algiers. His recent report to the Society for Internal Medicine as to its extremely favorable climate and condition for a winter-resort attracted a great deal of attention. The climate of Algiers is warmer than that of the Riviera—as snow and frost are unknown, and there is less dust than in the cities along the northern shore of the Mediterranean, though it is confessed that occasional dust storms and frequent inconvenience from this source are disadvantages of the place. In Algiers itself the climate is moist as well as warm, and one is scarcely ever without sensible perspiration. At Biskra, only a few hours inland, it is so dry that one never perspires sensibly. Moisture on the skin is carried off at once in the air, which has very little humidity. There is then, within a short distance of each other, the two varieties of climate in regard to which it is so difficult to decide in any individual case of tuberculosis; whether the one or the other will be of benefit. Many consumptives improve in an extremely dry climate, but it is equally true that many do not; on the contrary, the condition is made worse. One has in Algiers a good opportunity to allow the patient to select for himself the place which seems to suit him best without the necessity of traveling a long distance.

In recent years some excellent arrangements, according to Professor Fränkel, for the care of patients have been made. There is not, moreover, the temptation to abuse his strength that some of the social obligations of the Riviera involve. As Algiers is also French territory, German opinion with regard to it is not dictated by the wish to avoid sending patients to France.

TRANSACTIONS OF FOREIGN SOCIETIES.

Berlin.

BRONCHIECTASIS IN A VERY YOUNG CHILD—COMPENSATORY-EXERCISE THERAPY OF TABES.

AT a meeting of the Medical Society, January 5th, VIRCHOW and HEUBNER exhibited a case of *bronchiectasis in a very young child.* The child came from a family in which disease of the lungs was common. As an infant it had had a severe intestinal catarrh, and often suffered from bronchitis. After an attack of pneumonia there developed a well-marked bronchiectasis, especially of the left side. The sputum was repeatedly examined for tubercle bacilli, but none were found. After this condition had continued several months the child developed measles, and upon recovery from this tubercle bacilli were found in the sputum. A fatal termination followed within a short time. Examination of the lungs showed a long-standing and well-marked bronchiectasis, the left lung being almost wholly destroyed and containing numerous cavities. There was, as well, tuberculosis, evidently of short duration, as none of the lesions were far advanced and none of the cavities were of an ulcerative character. Heubner again mentioned his belief that bronchiectasis frequently follows whooping-cough and measles in young children, and that if the child recovers from the respiratory disease, the bronchiectasis, if of a slight degree, may entirely disappear. He raised the question whether bronchiectasis in adults may not in most cases be traced to some such trouble in childhood.

VIRCHOW said that the case was particularly interesting to him as showing the very large amount of tissue which might be involved in the affection under consideration. In the left lung scarcely a trace of the parenchyma remained. In true bronchiectatic cavities, such as those presented in this case, the epithelium may be recognized even to the ends of the tubes.

BAGINSKY said that the occurrence of bronchiectasis in children is undoubtedly more frequent than is usually supposed. Whooping-cough is especially likely to be followed by this disease, although it may result from any form of chronic bronchitis or bronchopneumonia. He also mentioned an instance in his own practice in which a boy contracted whooping-cough at the age of four years. The disease was followed by a chronic catarrh of the bronchi, and this in turn gave rise to bronchiectasis. At the age of ten years the child developed tuberculous peritonitis and died.

At the Union for Internal Medicine, January 3d, EULENBURG spoke of *compensatory-exercise therapy in tabes,* as proposed by Fränkel. He disputed the claim, advanced by Jacob, that special apparatus is necessary to obtain good results, claiming that materials found in every house are quite sufficient.

ZABLUDOWSKY, while not disputing the advantages of this method of treatment, said that certain cases are too severe to expect good results from it alone, but that massage and exercise therapy should be combined. If this plan is systematically carried out with proper intervals of rest, even in the most desperate cases there is a steady gain.

GOLDSCHEIDER said that the principle underlying this treatment is so simple that it could readily be applied by any physician, which, for the patient, is a far better plan than handing the treatment over to a specialist. He, too, objected to the use of complicated apparatus, which, he said, was not in the least necessary.

VON LEYDEN said that by means of this mode of treatment the therapy of diseases of the spinal cord had been lifted out of the rut in which it had been so many years. He said that the theory that tabes is a syphilitic disease has never been proved, and that the good results which sometimes follow the use of mercury are accidental. Exercise therapy, on the other hand, marks a distinct advance in treatment. The exercises reach the whole disease. While a special apparatus is not necessary, still treatment with such apparatus is found to be more exact, and the results will, in consequence, be somewhat better with than without it.

KANN-ŒYNHAUSEN said that there was no record that massage alone, or Swedish movements, had ever proved beneficial in a case of tabes. Swedish movements are directed toward the muscles, while the exercise therapy, recommended by Fränkel, is an exercise of the nerves. A tabetic person can exercise his muscles for a long time without becoming tired, while the exercises toward a definite end, as recommended in this treatment, soon weary him, thus showing the difference between the two. An apparatus does good in keeping up the interest of the patient in his treatment.

JASTROWITZ said that in this connection the influence of suggestion should not be forgotten, and, again, it is interesting to note that tabetic patients, who have become maniacal, have almost entirely lost their ataxia.

London.

ADHERENT PERICARDIUM—OBSTRUCTION OF LABOR BY OVARIAN TUMORS IN THE PELVIS.

At a meeting of the Medical Society, held January 10th, BROADBENT discussed *adherent pericardium*. An absolute diagnosis of this condition can rarely ever be made; for the symptoms are merely those of embarrassment and dilatation of the heart such as occur in all forms of cardiac disease. The physical signs upon which most weight can be placed are as follows: (1) arrest of the normal respiratory movement seen in the epigastrium; (2) imperfect descent of the apex beat during inspiration; (3) absence of shifting of the apex beat with changes in the position of the patient. However, none of these signs necessarily implies the presence of adherent pericardium. Pulsus paradoxus and pulsation of the veins have been described as frequent symptoms, but Broadbent has rarely observed them. In one case there was pulsation of a vein in the anterior chest-wall, due to the fact that the internal mammary artery had been caught by adhesions so that the blood could pass through it only when the heart was in a state of systole.

DOUGLAS-POWELL said that such cases should be divided into two groups: those in which merely the opposing surfaces of the pericardium are adherent, and those in which the external surface of the pericardium is adherent to the mediastinal tissues. In the latter, the action of the heart is interferred with to a greater extent, since it is working in a tough, fibrous, and adherent casing. In these cases the stress falls chiefly on the right side of the heart, which faces the unyielding anterior wall of the thorax. In a case recently under his observation, occurring in a girl ten years old, there had been a double-mitral-murmur, great hypertrophy, systolic depression of the first, second, and third intercostal spaces near the sternum, and systolic depression of the fifth, sixth, and seventh intercostal spaces outside the left nipple line, and a long thrusting apex beat which did not shift with respiration or with change of position. At the autopsy, both internal and external pericardial adhesions were proved to be present. Retraction at the apex, pulsus paradoxus, and epigastric pulsation, were all absent.

EWART said that simple bands of adhesion about the apex had little clinical significance, and it is probable that a universal adhesion of the pericardial membrane, without thickening, does not seriously hamper the cardiac movements. He disagreed with Douglas-Powell that the right side of the heart suffers more than the left from the presence of pericardial adhesions, and maintained that the left heart, because of its normally greater mobility, is the portion that is chiefly affected.

LEES said that in cases in which there is cardiac disease the effect of the adhesion is to fix and render permanent the dilatation which is part of the original inflammation of the heart. He had noticed a sudden dilatation of the heart during a first attack of rheumatism in children and young adults. If pericarditis occurs it fixes and renders permanent this dilatation.

In closing, BROADBENT stated that clinical observation clearly shows that the right ventricle is more embarrassed by adhesions than the left.

At a session on January 5th, the Obstetrical Society discussed the *obstruction of labor by ovarian tumors in the pelvis*. SPENCER thought that if possible such growths should be pushed up out of the pelvis before the beginning of labor. Version, forceps, craniotomy, and incision or tapping of the tumor, should be rejected on account of their danger, and the abdominal operation is preferable to the vaginal for the removal of these tumors.

HERMAN said that a procedure described by Fritsch deserves fuller consideration. This consists in making an incision into the tumor through the vagina, and then stitching the margins of the opening together so that the cyst contents may escape extraperitoneally. In this manner the danger of tapping is avoided.

PLAYFAIR said that he had been able to collect 183 cases, which show that this complication of labor is not so extremely rare. While admitting that ovariotomy is the best course to pursue, this, of course, depends somewhat on the experience of the surgeon, and also upon suitable nursing. If these conditions cannot be fulfilled, and it is impossible to push the tumor up out of the way, vaginal puncture should be performed. The mortality in cases in which puncture has been performed is only eighteen per cent.

SOCIETY PROCEEDINGS.

KINGS COUNTY MEDICAL ASSOCIATION.

Stated Meeting, Held January 11, 1898.

THE President, J. C. BIERWIRTH, M.D., in the Chair.

DR. L. GRANT BALDWIN read a paper on

THE EARLY DIAGNOSIS OF MALIGNANT UTERINE DISEASE. (See page 300.)

DISCUSSION.

DR. HENRY C. COE: I felt very much complimented to be invited here this evening, and it occurred to me as I was crossing the bridge that the circumstances under which I came were quite different from those which have attended my former visits, and that I was no longer coming to another city, but simply to another part of the same great metropolis. This municipal union implies that the relations which will exist between us and our professional brethren in Brooklyn in the future will be even more friendly and intimate than they have been in the past.

The subject which the Doctor has so ably introduced is one of peculiar interest to me; in fact, I have been interested in it from the very first time I ever had anything to do with malignant disease. Every year the importance of the subject is more deeply impressed upon me. When we consider the fact that even the best German operators acknowledge that only twenty-five per cent. of the cases which come under their observation are in a condition for radical operation, and that gynecologists of wide experience in this country have made the statement that perhaps only ten or fifteen per cent. of such cases were operable when referred to them, it occurs to us that there must be something wrong—that there must be some reason why surgeons are not able to see a larger number of patients while the disease is still in the operable stage. Of course, as the Doctor said in his paper, a good deal depends upon the imperfect education of the laity in regard to the initial symptoms of malignant disease. Women are exceedingly loath to consult a physician, especially unmarried women who have passed the menopause and have never had any previous pelvic disease. They delay visiting their family physician even when they have marked hemorrhages. Many cases have come under my observation in which it was clear from the history that cancer had developed and that the symptoms had been concealed or disregarded for months until the time for successful interference had long since passed. As the author rightly said, the education of the laity is the first step in increasing the number of operable cases.

I am impressed with the great sameness in the history of cases of chronic carcinoma. Few of the unfortunates report their initial symptoms to their physician, or if they do, the doctor is easily persuaded that such are the ordinary phenomena of the menopause; and the disease is allowed to go on from month to month, and even from year to year, until finally an examination is made and it is found to be too late to do anything. It seems to me that the surgeon cannot be expected to accept all the responsibility in these cases. Of course he is not obliged to operate, but these patients are brought to him sometimes in the most advanced stage, with the expectation, or firm belief, that he is going to do a radical operation, and, contrary to his better judgment, he is led to attempt such an operation when he ought to let the patient alone. The contraindications to hysterectomy are becoming more strictly defined every year. I recently read an article by Olshausen in which he said that he would not attempt a radical operation in a case in which the disease was not absolutely confined to the uterus; but we rarely see cases in this stage.

Cases of carcinoma of the uterus are naturally divided into two distinct classes: those in which the disease involves the cervix, and those in which it develops in the body of the organ, and clinically there is a great difference between the two. I believe that patients with carcinoma of the body of the uterus are much more apt to reach the surgeon early than are those in whom the disease affects the cervix, because the former nearly always develops *after* the menopause, the hemorrhage is more significant, and the patient applies earlier for aid. The diagnosis is all-important, and we must rely to a certain extent on the microscope, but in this we are often disappointed. For example, in a patient with a typical hemorrhage, a portion of brain-like material removed with the curette is reported by the pathologist to be non-malignant, and yet we feel from the history of the case and from the condition of the patient that a radical operation is indicated. Under these circumstances the surgeon is naturally placed in a very disagreeable position. He is expected to give a positive opinion, and having once advised a radical operation, he must abide by his decision. I have more than once, after removing a uterus under such circumstances, opened it and felt immensely relieved to find my diagnosis confirmed; I am free to add that it has not always been confirmed. On one or two occasions I have been mistaken, not finding malignant disease at all; but I have often thought that if I were placed in a similar position in regard to a member of my own family, if the symptoms pointed to probable malignant disease of the body of the uterus, and there was a painful doubt whether such disease was present or not, I would prefer to have the patient undergo the risk of a radical operation rather than to remain in uncertainty for months, and possibly when the operation was done to find it was performed too late. I assume, of course, that all the ordinary means of settling the diagnosis have been exhausted. Apropos of menorrhagia as an initial symptom of carcinoma of the cervix in young women, to which reference has been made, I would emphasize the importance of this symptom following the normal puerpery. I have in several cases seen the disease advance rapidly in puerperal women. It doubtless developed during pregnancy, but gave rise to no symptoms, but soon after labor there were hemorrhages which were ascribed to an increase in the lochial flow. When the periods returned they were unusually profuse, and an examination showed that the disease had made rapid progress, although the labor had been normal. So, we must always remember that during and after the puerperal month a profuse flow is always an indication for examination.

The reader of the paper has properly laid stress upon the fact that pain, cachexia, and foul discharge are the symptoms, not of incipient, but of inoperable, malignant disease. This is a most important point. If we wait until these symptoms appear, in the majority of cases we have waited until any operation is of little value.

Nowadays, the only test of the success of an operation for malignant disease is freedom from recurrence. We have passed the stage when mere recovery from the operation is considered success in surgery. This was the case a few years ago, but now a recurrence within a year is a reproach to the surgeon, and shows that either his diagnosis was not exact, or that his technic was imperfect. The day is coming when operations for malignant disease will be judged entirely by this test, and you will see that this will tend to limit hysterectomy for cancer of the uterus to a comparatively small class of cases.

It is often difficult to distinguish an old case of laceration of the cervix with marked erosion from one of epithelioma; indeed, the microscope shows that many of the former are just on the border line between benign and malignant disease. In these cases I always amputate the cervix, because I believe it is a prophylactic measure, and that by a thorough operation at this stage we may prevent serious trouble at a later date. In such a case I do not excise a piece of tissue for examination. Here, it seems to me, is a valuable application of the operation devised by our esteemed fellow-townsman, Dr. Byrne. It is gratifying to think that Dr. Byrne in his old age has succeeded in establishing his just claims after so many years of successful work. Some of the most successful operators are seriously considering the propriety of abandoning hysterectomy for carcinoma of the cervix except in the incipient stage, and these are just the cases in which the best results are obtained by the use of the galvanocautery. So here is a valuable application of this method—in case of doubt, amputate with the galvanocautery.

I recently called attention to the great difficulty of making a pathologic diagnosis in many of these cases, and also to the fact that we are sometimes a little hard on the pathologist. We scrape out a little tissue the size of a pin-head and expect him to tell us exactly what the condition is. When we submit a specimen to the pathologist we should send a complete history of the case, not telling him what diagnosis we wish to have established, but at least giving him some clew as to the suspicion which we entertain, and then let him confirm or disprove our diagnosis, as his subsequent studies may determine. But we should remember that we cannot entirely depend upon his report. I was assisting a prominent gynecologist not long since in an operation for removal of the uterus in a doubtful case, which fortunately turned out to be malignant adenoma. The pathologist's opinion was rather amusing. The patient was about sixty-five years old, but the pathologist reported that a fragment of tissue expelled from the uterus contained chorionic villi! A thorough examination of a suspected case cannot be made in one's office. I doubt if any one is capable of giving a trustworthy opinion (especially with regard to the advisability of a radical operation) without making such an examination under anesthesia. This applies particularly to a case of possible disease of the corpus uteri. Dilate the canal, explore the uterine cavity, remove a fragment with the curette for examination, determine the mobility of the uterus and the presence or absence of metastatic deposits—in fact, omit no means of determining the true condition. To see a patient in one's office, to hastily diagnose the case and appoint a day for a radical operation—such a practice will sooner or later lead to serious error, if not to loss of reputation. I could cite a number of instances in which some curious mistakes have been made. I saw a uterus removed when the supposed carcinoma was simply a piece of sponge which had been in the vagina for several months. I have, as a pathologist, examined several specimens in which there was no trace of carcinoma, and have seen uteri removed for a sloughing fibroid and for various conditions not malignant disease. These mistakes would seldom be made if the patients were thoroughly examined more than once before operation. The diagnosis is so difficult and so important that we ought to exhaust every possible means before we arrive at a positive conclusion.

DR. LEIGHTON: Mr. President, my own personal experience has been that the family physician is not consulted until the case has progressed to a stage at which operation cannot be considered. Such patients are very apt to keep their symptoms to themselves, or possibly ask a neighbor or a woman friend about them. There seems to be the same disposition, I think, in regard to cancer of the breast. For some unknown reason patients are often disposed to keep the knowledge of its existence from the family physician as well as from the surgeon.

THE PRESIDENT: I would like to ask Dr. Baldwin if there is, in the early appearance of epithelioma of the cervix, anything characteristic which enables us to distinguish clinically a case of early epithelioma of the cervix from one of benign granulation; and, also, if these benign cases, of which I have seen a great many, have any special tendency to become malignant.

There can be no doubt in my mind as to the very grave importance of the subject as Dr. Baldwin has presented it. The cure of a case of carcinoma of the uterus, in my very limited experience, depends entirely upon early diagnosis. I think the paper is extremely timely and important as calling attention to the difficulties of diagnosis and the errors which are continually committed by both the physician and the people themselves regarding cases of cancer of the uterus, and especially in reference to the early diagnosis of this dread affection.

DR. BALDWIN: There may be a different odor to a sloughing malignant tissue than there is to sloughing fibroid tissue; I have never been able to determine the difference, and I fail to see why there should be any. An odor is not present in malignant disease until sloughing occurs, and the same is true of a fibroid growth, and I doubt if in either there would be an odor very different from that of decomposing steak under the same conditions.

As to the eroded cervix—whether cancer is a sequel of benign disease of this part of the uterus: In Dr. Emmett's statistics of malignant disease of the cervix, in the vast majority of cases there had been lacerations of the cervix, and I presume more or less erosion as well, and this has also been the experience of Dr. Byrne. In almost all cases the patients have borne children. Few of Dr. Byrne's cases were in single women, but the vast majority were in those who had borne children and sustained lacerations of the cervix.

I can hardly agree with Dr. Leighton that cancer of the breast is as late in coming under the care of the surgeon as cancer of the uterus. In my experience, a woman with a lump in her breast is very likely to seek advice; she worries about it, and while it is true that many conceal the affection, still I think in the greater proportion of cases cancer of the breast receives attention earlier than cancer of the uterus.

I think there is nothing in the granulations of an eroded cervix that is significant, but, of course, in some the appearance is that of malignant disease, and these are just the cases in which amputation of the cervix should be performed, as Dr. Coe has suggested.

REVIEWS.

MANHATTAN EYE AND EAR HOSPITAL REPORTS. Vol. iv. New York: The Knickerbocker Press, 1897.

THIS, the fourth number of the annual reports, is especially noticeable for the excellent articles on otologic and rhinologic subjects. Among them the papers on "Hysteric Deafness," by Dr. F. Pierce Hoover, "Disease of the Internal Ear," by Dr. T. J. Harris, and "Deflection of the Septum," deserve particular attention. Among the papers of ophthalmologic importance we notice "Asthenopia as a Forerunner of Neurasthenia," by Dr. D. B. St. John Roosa, and "Myopia Following Iridectomy," by Edgar T. Thompson, M.D. The volume concludes with a summary of cases treated and operations performed during the year.

ESSENTIALS OF BACTERIOLOGY. Being a Concise and Systematic Introduction to the Study of Micro-organisms for the Use of Students and Practitioners. By M. V. BALL, M.D., Bacteriologist to St. Agnes' Hospital, Philadelphia. Third edition, revised. Philadelphia: W. B. Saunders, 1897.

THIS little book, one of Saunders' Question Compends, is a very valuable one of its kind. The subject-matter is necessarily condensed, but the general arrangement of the material, the clear and concise modes of expression, and the rejection of all useless details, have produced a book which embraces most of the essential facts relating to bacteriology and laboratory technic.

In remarkably few words the author covers the ground of the classification, growth, methods of examination, staining, methods of culture, and appearances of bacteria. The commoner forms of non-pathogenic and pathogenic bacteria are then briefly described, and in an appendix the yeasts and molds, together with hints for the examination of air and water, receive consideration. The illustrations are ample, and for the most part, good; but the proofreading has not been careful.

In this book physicians and students will find an excellent means of acquainting themselves in a short time with the subject of bacteriology.

THERAPEUTIC HINTS.

Validol is a new remedy recommended by SCHWERENSKI in epilepsy and hysteria. It is a chemic combination of tincture of valerian and menthol containing an excess of the latter. The amount of menthol incorporated should be thirty per cent. The dose of the compound is from 10 to 15 drops, administered on sugar or in sweet wine. It excites gastric secretion, prevents fermentation and meteorism, while retaining full analgesic and antihysteric powers.

For Tapeworm.—LASS calls attention to the black oxid of copper as a non-toxic and efficient teniafuge. During the treatment acid foods and drinks should be avoided. For adults the remedy may be administered as follows:

℞ Cupri oxid. . . . . . . ʒ iss
Cretæ præp. . . . . . ʒ ss
Boli albæ . . . . . . ʒ iii
Glycerini . . . . . . ʒ iiss.

M. Ft. pil. No. CXX. Sig. Two pills four times daily during the first week, and three pills four times daily during the second week, at the end of which a dose of castor oil should be given.

For children the following is recommended:

℞ Cupri oxid. . . . . . gr. lxxx
Cretæ præp. } aa . . . . gr. xv
Magnes. carb. }
Tragacanthæ . . . . . ʒ iiss
Glycerini . . . . . . m. lxxx
Sacchari . . . . . . ʒ x
Aquæ . . . . . . q. s.

M. Ft. past. No. L. Sig. Two to three pastilles daily.

A Palatable Emulsion of Castor Oil.—

℞ Pulv. acaciæ . . . . . ʒ iv
Ol. ricini . . . . . . ℥ i
Elix. saccharini . . . . . m. xx
Ol. amygdalæ amaræ . . . . m. i
Ol. caryophylli . . . . . m. ii
Aq. dest. . . . . q. s. ad. ℥ ii.

M. Dissolve the gum in sufficient water, add the oil gradually, and finally the flavoring agents.

For Malignant Pustule.—It is recommended to inject subcutaneously from ten to twenty minims of the following solution, and to cover the affected area with sublimate compresses:

℞ Hydrarg. bicyanid . . . . 1 part
Aq. dest. . . . . . 100 parts
Cocain salicyl. . . . . q. s.

M. Sig. For hypodermic use.

THE MEDICAL NEWS.

A WEEKLY JOURNAL OF MEDICAL SCIENCE.

VOL. LXXII. NEW YORK, SATURDAY, MARCH 12, 1898. NO. 11.

ORIGINAL ARTICLES.

SOME INSTRUCTIVE CASES OF APPENDICITIS.[1]

BY H. A. HARE, M.D.,
OF PHILADELPHIA;
PROFESSOR OF THERAPEUTICS IN THE JEFFERSON MEDICAL COLLEGE; PHYSICIAN TO THE JEFFERSON HOSPITAL.

IN this brief paper I desire to call attention to several cases of appendicitis which, it seems to me, possess more than ordinary interest:

CASE I.—Male, nineteen years of age, came under my care for a sharp attack of pain in the abdomen, which was not referred to the region of the appendix, but was said to be half way between the ensiform cartilage and the navel. The patient presented the history of no less than nine such attacks during the previous six months, some of them so severe that the hypodermic use of morphin was necessary. In none of them was the pain appendicular in character. As soon as the abdomen was exposed it was seen that there was a swelling of considerable size in the right inguinal region. On palpation this swelling proved to be only slightly tender, but very hard and resisting. Even when the somewhat rigid abdominal wall over it was relaxed the mass remained hard and brawny under my fingers, and was so large, and dipped down so deeply, that its extent could not be accurately determined. The possibility of malignant growth seemed to be excluded by the age of the patient, the unimpaired general vitality, and the history of the attacks, which were usually associated with some nausea and vomiting, and the general typical symptoms of appendicitis. The diagnosis was recurrent appendicitis with great thickening and deposit of inflammatory exudate about the appendix, and perhaps about the entire caput coli.

In other words, the patient had had acute appendicitis several times, with surrounding exudation and a chronic inflammatory process between the attacks. The large mass of exudate made it evident that an operation during the acute process would not only be difficult but possibly fatal as well, and, therefore, nothing was said to the patient about operative interference. After recovery from the last attack the patient refused operation, but after being impressed with the fact that nine attacks within six months indicated the speedy development of others, and that in any one of these a fatal result might ensue, and, on the concurrent advice of one of our most able surgeons, he at last gave a reluctant consent to the operation.

He was operated upon during the period of quiescence, and the appendix was found greatly enlarged, thickened, and surrounded by a mass of exudate. It was removed with some difficulty, but with no serious damage to surrounding tissues. The operation was well borne, but within twenty-four hours nausea, followed by stercoraceous vomiting, ensued, and the patient speedily died. There were no other signs of obstruction, and collapse came on so quickly that nothing could be done for his relief. I still think my advice was theoretically good, but practically the man would have lived longer if he had not consented to the operation.

CASE II.—This case is in some respects the opposite of the one just reported. A man aged fifty-five years, had had at intervals of six months two attacks of violent abdominal pain and all the other symptoms of acute appendicitis. The last attack occurred two months before I saw him, when he came from a Western city for advice as to operation. At my request he was examined, in consultation, by two surgeons of high repute, who found some tenderness but no marked induration. As he was forced by his employment to be constantly traveling through small towns he feared an attack when away from home and competent skill, and, while naturally not desirous of operation, was willing to have it performed if it was thought that recurrences were probable. One surgeon advised operation as a prophylactic and curative measure, the other and myself agreed that it would not be necessary. This was four years ago, and there has been no sign of a third attack, the patient being at present perfectly well.

CASE III.—A man, aged thirty-eight years, who, six months before I saw him, began to have severe pain in the right inguinal region. Usually he had a paroxysm of pain about every week, and sometimes more frequently. The pain was sharply localized, and at McBurney's point there was great sensitiveness, although when the examination was made there had been no attack of pain for a week. The patient had lost ten pounds in weight since the attacks began, but his appetite was good, although he was constipated. He was treated by absolute rest, a careful diet, and regulation of the bowels. He did not have an attack during nine days previous to leaving my care. The tenderness disappeared, as did the patient, so the subsequent history cannot be reported, but in the light of the first and second cases I am glad I did not urge operation. An interesting point in this case was an entire absence of fever during the attack which the patient had while under my care.

CASE IV.—A woman, aged forty-eight years, was seized in the middle of the night with agonizing abdominal pain situated in the epigastric and left inguinal regions, or between the latter and the median line. I

[1] Read at a meeting of the Philadelphia County Medical Society, March 9, 1898.

saw her eight hours after the pain began, and found her still suffering greatly, but without agony. She had all the classic symptoms of appendicitis: vomiting, pain, and exquisite tenderness over the appendix. The pain was so diffused that it was hard to tell exactly where it was most severe. The abdomen was scaphoid-shaped and somewhat rigid. The appendicitis was so acute that I did not dare to advise against an operation, and the weather so hot and the patient so feeble that I much feared the results of surgical interference. A well-known surgeon suggested operation, and then, as I did not like to oppose my views to his, I called in a medical consultant who agreed that while an operation was strongly indicated by the local condition, the hot weather and feebleness of the patient were greater dangers than the affection itself, especially when added to the effects of operative interference. Operation was not performed, the patient received local and general treatment and recovered in about three weeks. This occurred during June, 1895. Since then there has been no return of the trouble, and for a third time I am glad the knife was not used.

CASE V.—A woman, aged thirty-three years, who, between January 1st and May 15th, had four attacks of appendicitis, each of greater severity than its predecessor. An operation during each attack had been refused, and also between the attacks. When the attack in May occurred, the case was so evidently an operative one that operation was insisted upon and was at once performed.

The operation revealed an abscess at the tip of the appendix, containing about one dram of pus. The abscess was ruptured during removal of the appendix. The wound was, however, carefully cleansed and all pus apparently removed. The patient then progressed favorably for two weeks. The wound healed by first intention and all seemed well, though there was no gain in strength. At this time the temperature gradually began to rise and to be more and more marked, so that the chart resembled that of intermittent malarial infection. The old wound showed no sign of infection, the blood no evidence of malaria, and there was no history of malaria. The wound was then opened, found healthy, and again closed. There was still fever and persistent loss of weight. Finally, the wound was opened a second time, on this occasion down to the site of the appendix, and still everything was apparently normal. The fever persisted, though sweats and chills were absent. Six weeks after the operation, the patient was seized with severe pain in the abdomen, the temperature suddenly became accentuated, and she became partially collapsed. An examination of the abdomen now revealed for the first time a marked swelling in the right inguinal region as well as pronounced evidences of peritonitis. An operation was advised as the only resource, but after the belly was incised the patient so nearly died on the table that it had to be given up. Death occurred two days later, and at the post-mortem a large abscess of the right ovary and tube was found from which general peritonitis had resulted. Infection of these parts had evidently occurred from the ruptured appendix, as the woman was unmarried and a virgin. The delay of operation in this case till the abscess was ready to rupture on the slightest touch, ultimately caused the death of the patient.

CASE VI.—Male, aged forty years, very stout, and of large frame. The patient was seized in the night with excruciating pain in the groin and throughout the whole abdomen. When seen by me, six hours later, the abdomen was already swollen and rigid. The pulse was rapid, but otherwise good. The abdomen was exquisitely tender. Operation was insisted upon, and was performed within an hour. The appendix was found gangrenous at its tip. He promptly recovered, and the operative interference without doubt saved his life.

CASE VII.—December 26, 1896, I was called to see R. L., male, aged ten years. I found him suffering from a moderate degree of pain which was situated in the right iliac region. He was in bed, had a coated tongue, and a temperature of 101.5° F. The history was that he had been taken during the night with several paroxysms of fairly severe pain, and had had several that morning. A week before, upon going to bed, he had had some nausea and gastric disturbance, probably due to intemperance in diet. Close questioning revealed the fact that during that week he had also had considerable pain in the bowels, although by no means so severe as at the time he was first seen by me. Not only was there marked tenderness over McBurney's point, but as I have frequently noticed in such cases, the patient complained of a good deal of pain in the neighborhood of the transverse colon. Placing a hand under the flank, or in other words, behind the appendix, seemed to reach the most tender spot. That evening I asked his relative, Dr. Howard A. Kelly, to see him in consultation, and it was decided that the best thing to do was to insist upon perfect rest, a liquid diet, and no medicine.

On the following day the pain was about the same, as was also the rigidity of the abdominal walls. As he had been freely purged on the 25th by means of citrate of magnesia and cascara sagrada it was thought wise not to administer any purgatives at this time. On the morning of the 28th the swelling and tenderness in the right iliac region was increased, and the pain was stated by the child to be much more severe. Another consultation with Dr. Kelly was requested, and he decided that it would be advisable to freely administer Rochelle salts. This was done, but after the third dose of a teaspoonful, vomiting occurred. Castor oil was then substituted, and two hours later resulted in two free movements of the bowels. The temperature during the 27th and 28th was about 99° F., both morning and evening. On the morning of the 29th, the pain seemed to be slightly relieved for a time, but the tenderness on palpation was quite as marked as ever, and the boy stated that the pain was returning as the hours passed by.

It was determined that it would be wise to interfere surgically, and an operation was performed on that day (Tuesday) by Dr. Kelly, assisted by Dr. C. P. Noble and two of Dr. Kelly's assistants from Baltimore. The appendix was found markedly inflamed, but it did not contain pus. There was a slight peritoneal hyperemia all around the neighborhood of the appendix. The boy did very well after the operation; his temperature did not rise above 99.5° F.; vomiting was very slight, and the case progressed favorably for a period of ten days. On Monday, January 10th, the patient was seized, however, with violent pain in the abdomen. On examination the abdomen was found to be neither scaphoid-shaped nor swollen, although it was tympanitic on percussion. Pain was excessively severe, and seemed to have its greatest point of intensity in a line drawn between the nipple and the anterior superior spine of the ilium to the right of the umbilicus. At this point it was thought, on careful examination, that there was increased resistance. The pain continued during twenty-four hours, notwithstanding the administration of $\frac{1}{16}$-grain of morphin, which gave relief only for a short time. The temperature remained about normal.

The next day, however, retching and vomiting became prominent symptoms, and, although not constant, occurred with sufficient frequency to be considered a grave indication. He had been unable to pass anything from the bowels from the time the attack began, though no food had been given him which could in any way have produced intestinal complications. Repeated rectal injections failed to have any result, except on one occasion, when a slight quantity of gas was passed. In view of his grave condition it was decided, two days later (Tuesday the 12th), that something must be done for his relief, and, after consultation between Dr. Edward Martin, Dr. Kelly, and myself, it was decided that the boy should be etherized, inverted, and that copious intestinal irrigation should be resorted to. At this time the boy was vomiting small quantities of liquid of a coffee-ground or grumous appearance, mixed with streaks of bright-colored blood, and there was marked abdominal distention. One and a half quarts of warm saline solution having been injected into the bowel without reducing the obstruction, the boy was placed upon the operating-table. After the injected liquid had been drained out by means of a rectal tube, Dr. Kelly opened the abdomen half-way between the umbilicus and his earlier incision for appendicitis. A small quantity of liquid was found in the abdominal cavity, there was evidence of slight peritonitis, and two large knuckles of gut were found adherent to the abdominal wall, producing intestinal obstruction by preventing peristaltic movement. The bands of adhesions were broken up, the wound was closed, and the child put back to bed in fairly good condition considering the gravity of the case. Twenty-four hours after the operation the bowels moved freely, and a considerable quantity of fecal matter was passed.

The patient made a good recovery from the operation, and was kept on a strict liquid diet for a period of four or five days. His temperature during this period never being febrile, but he suffered from time to time from more or less violent attacks of abdominal pain. His condition, however, steadily improved until Tuesday, February 2d, when I called at 4.30 A.M., because he was suffering from violent pain which was not relieved by a hypodermic of morphia given at 6 P.M. the previous evening. I found him with excruciating abdominal pain, a tense and rigid abdomen, and some slight nausea. The boy had not had a movement since the previous morning. Morphin ($\frac{1}{16}$-grain) was given hypodermically, and though repeated at 9 A.M. the next morning, did not afford material relief. I immediately telegraphed for Dr. Kelly, and, after a careful examination, it was decided that he had about one and a half quarts of liquid in his abdominal cavity, and that there were evidences of adhesions obstructing the intestines. In view of the gravity of a third operation it was decided by Dr. Kelly, Dr. Martin, and myself to take the risk of waiting twenty-four hours. At the end of that time, the various rectal injections having failed, another one was given with the result that he passed a large amount of fecal matter, following which the pain subsided. Convalescence was established, and the boy was considered cured, Friday, February 19th, although at that time there was still present, as there had been from his first getting up, February 10th, slight impairment of power in the lower extremities (partial paraplegia).

These cases, which are taken as types from a larger series, illustrate the fact that the physician assumes a grave responsibility if he urges an operation, perhaps as grave as if he opposes it; that he cannot afford to leave a decision as to the wisdom of operation entirely to his surgical colleague, and, finally, that patients with appendicitis often recover and remain well, or, in other words, in all cases an operation is not necessary, either for immediate relief or for the prevention of other attacks. On the other hand, there are cases which are so fulminating in character that an hour's delay is dangerous, and I am inclined to believe that in cases with early fixation of the body and abdominal muscles and without much temperature disturbance, operation is more necessary than in those in which the pain is greater, more continuous, and more severe on pressure.

COMPOUND FRACTURES INVOLVING THE ANKLE-JOINT.

BY C. C. WORDEN, M.D.,
OF NASHVILLE, TENN.

IN the consideration of this subject the ordinary classification of injuries to the ankle-joint will be adopted; for the reason that any simple fracture may become compound in a proportion varying directly with the quality of the injuring force. It is impossible, however, to determine exactly which bones are invariably involved in such injuries, or the manner in which they are broken, since there may be a fracture of any or all of the three bones forming the joint, the lines of fracture varying with the quality, quantity, and direction of the violence producing the injury. In addition, it will be necessary to include in the classification such bones as serve to maintain the integrity of the joint, though not directly contributing to its formation. The subject, then, must embrace such compound fractures as involve the tibia, fibula, whether malleolar or supramalleolar, astragalus, and the os calcis, when the latter shares the injury with the foregoing. Fractures of the tibia or fibula, alone or together, above the malleoli, as a general rule do not involve the joint, even when they are compound. The exceptions are noticed in cases in which the lacerations are prolonged into the joint, either from severe lacerating or continued force, which, after causing the fracture, continues to act. As an example of such force may be mentioned an injury to the ankle from being caught between two objects, the one stationary and the other in motion.

Injuries Caused by Eversions of the Foot.—A classic Pott's fracture when compound will usually show the laceration high above the malleolus and opposite the site of the break in the fibula; but cases are frequently observed in which the laceration occurs opposite the internal malleolus. In such an instance the eversion of the foot is extreme and the fractured inner malleolus generally presents in the wound. In these injuries the unyielding internal lateral ligament carries downward the tip of the malleolus, the synovial sac is opened and the joint exposed. The obliteration of the mortise permits an inward dislocation of the astragalus which follows the outward displacement of the foot. The same force may cause a fracture of the outer articular border of the tibia, or a laceration of the tibiofibular, or interosseous ligament, and a consequent dislocation of the tibia inward. In these instances we may expect to find a laceration of the anterior fasciculus of the external lateral ligament, the reason for this being that the astragalus partakes of the outward deviation of the foot and swings inward while the lower fragment of the fibula is carried outward. This allows partial luxation of the astragalus inward. The degree of the luxation depends upon the severity of the injury.

Fracture of the inner malleolus alone, when compound, may or may not be accompanied by dislocation of neighboring bones. The chances are that partial dislocation will occur if the fracturing force be violent, for the reason that the line of fracture through the malleolus is usually transverse, or nearly so, and sufficiently high up to destroy the inner side of the mortise and allow the joint-fluid to escape. When the external lateral ligament yields the degree of luxation may be extreme, the superior articular surface presenting inward. This is facilitated by a fracture through the lesser process of the os calcis.

As a result of forcible eversion of the foot the external malleolus may be fractured and compounded at the site of the fracture, below and posterior to it, or near the internal malleolus. It will usually be found in such cases that the foot has not only been everted but carried bodily outward as well. The astragalus glides outward from its socket with little or no obstruction, and is largely instrumental in causing the compounding of the fracture. A fracture of the lesser process of the os calcis may complicate such extensive injuries, and it is usually accompanied by marked deformity. In the study of injuries of this nature there must be borne in mind the liability of involvement of the blood-vessels, nerves, tendons, and soft parts generally.

Fractures Caused by Inversion of the Foot. — Compound injuries resulting from this cause are more common than elsewhere about the joint because of the more exposed position of the fibular surface and the greater frequency with which the foot encounters inward displacement. Since any fracture of the ankle may by chance become compound it will be well to consider such injuries as commonly occur in this region. The arrangement of the fibers of the external lateral ligament predisposes to two varieties of injury. Either there will be a transverse fracture of the outer malleolus at the tip or base, more commonly the latter, or a fracture of the sustentaculum tali, or of both. By reason of direct pressure of the astragalus upon the inner malleolus the latter is often broken. The forcible eversion of the astragalus brings pressure to bear upon the deltoid ligament, the inner malleolus, and the lesser process of the calcaneum. If this powerful ligament refuses to yield the result will be a vertical line of fracture through the lesser process unless the inner malleolus yields first. The astragalus itself may be broken, particularly when the breaking force is vertically and laterally applied. The line may run transversely and include merely the tibiofibular articular surfaces, or may run vertically and from before backward anterior to the tibial articular facet. When the injury is severe the following may be presented: The laceration on the outer aspect of the ankle widely gaps, revealing the tibial articular facet of the astragalus which lies upon its side. The foot may be straight or strongly inverted, depending upon the amount of damage to the calcaneum and the calcaneo-astragaloid ligament. The tibia may show a line of fracture running transversely less than a centimeter above its articular surface, and in this respect differing from a supracondyloid fracture. The fibula usually breaks at a point about an inch lower than in Pott's fracture, and shows a transverse line of fracture or even multiple lines.

Fractures Due to Crushing Injuries. — Under this division may be classed such severe compound fractures as result from severe crushes and falls upon the feet. The damage to the joint and soft parts is extensive and usually amounts to disintegration of the former. The articular surfaces of the tibia, fibula, calcaneum, and astragalus are commonly ground in pieces, the periosteum badly torn, and the soft parts pulpified. It would be useless to attempt any classification of such injuries. The amount and variety of damage is, of course, variable.

The *symptoms* of compound fracture involving the ankle-joint are those of simple fracture, modified, however, by the damage to the soft parts.

The *diagnosis* depends upon the symptoms and physical signs, and is facilitated in a ratio variable with the extent of the compounding.

In the *treatment* of such injuries the surgeon has no set rules to follow. Each injury is a law unto itself. Each patient rightly may demand two-fold efforts: those directed toward maintenance of the best general condition, and those which aim to preserve the joint. The former may demand the abandonment of the latter. In general the treatment may be said to consist of reduction of the fractures or dislocations and in cleansing the joint and closing the wound under strictest aseptic rules, and lastly, immobilization of the affected part by some suitable devise. When reduction is easily accomplished and there is little tendency to subsequent displacement, any unnecessary manipulations or interference with the wound should be rigidly interdicted. The exception are those cases in which the joint is full of macroscopic particles of dirt, filth, pieces of stocking, etc. It is wise to let the joint alone when evideuces of contamination are wanting.

In cases in which the deformity is not easily corrected and in which it is difficult to maintain the fragments in position, as, for instance, when the astragalus has turned upon its side, it is perfectly allowable to manipulate the parts through the laceration. When the wound is merely a puncture it is better to further incise and carefully inspect the field of injury. By so doing the deformity is better corrected and the prognosis is not altered. In this connection there appears a class of cases that demands a similar procedure: When the injury has caused an irreducible deformity and extensive mangling of the soft parts, without actual compounding, the joint and tissues will be found full of blood. It will become evident that on account of the damage the pressure from within will not allow the skin to recover its vitality and thus will cause it to slough. By rendering the injury compound the deformity may be remedied and the hemorrhage checked. Failure to properly reduce recent deformity will call for subsequent consideration of various operative measures, including actual resection of the joint. When the articular surfaces about the joint are badly shattered, resection at the time of injury, or later, will yield good results; under such circumstances ankylosis is, of course, expected.

As to the question of amputation: It is always better to preserve the foot, if possible, unless by so doing the patient's chances of recovery are lessened. If the patient be in good general health, and the circulation beyond the site of injury can be maintained, it is best to try and save the foot. A plaster dressing to the leg and foot, with fenestræ or interruptions where necessary, and suspension of the limb will meet the requirements in the vast majority of cases. Anterior and posterior splints of iron embedded in the plaster and arched over the fenestræ or interruptions will afford better support and greater rigidity to the part.

CASE I. — F. S., Swede, forty-five years of age, an iron miner, of large and powerful frame, and in rugged health. July 12, 1897, while he was riding on an ore-dump the car jumped the track and jammed his ankle between the axle and a pile of rails lying by the tramway. The man was brought to the hospital and anesthetized. Examination showed the following condition: On the outer aspect of the leg and foot was an irregular laceration of the skin and soft parts, four inches in length, extending from a point one inch above the malleolus, across it, downward and forward. The external and anterior fibers of the external lateral ligament were torn across. The fibula was broken transversely immediately above the malleolus. The astragalus was luxated forward and outward sufficiently to show nearly all its superior articular surface. The interosseus ligament was intact. The malleolus was in relation to the astragalus, the anterior and posterior ligaments having yielded. The foot was decidedly inverted. The tibia and deltoid ligaments were not damaged. Hemorrhage was slight. The wound and joint were full of pieces of yarn, shreads of leather, and hematite. The foot, and the astragalus with it, were easily replaced in a normal position, and the outer malleolus carried into its proper relation. There was little or no tendency to subsequent displacement.

The laceration was closed with interrupted silkworm-gut sutures. The foot and leg, from toes to knee, were encased in plaster over a stout anterior splint of iron. In this dressing large fenestræ were left over the site of the wound. The wound was antiseptically dressed. Three days later a few of the stitches below the malleolus and in the middle portion of the laceration were removed to facilitate the discharge of a small quantity of pus, the presence of which the thermometer had indicated. Subsequently the reopened wound healed by granulation. The upper and lower sutures held and secured primary union. At the end of six weeks the dressing was removed. The foot was in excellent position and the wound entirely closed. The motions of the joint were not less than would be expected from such a period of enforced rest. The patient walked without crutches on November 1st, and returned to work one month later. There was at that time no impairment of motion, nor was there the slightest limp. The only evidence of injury was the cicatrix of the laceration.

CASE II.—L. O., Swede, thirty-eight years of age, and by occupation a carpenter. The patient had pulmonary tuberculosis. Bacilli in great numbers were first demonstrated to be present in the sputum during March, 1897. His wife was then in an advanced stage of the same disease. June 24, 1897, the patient was building a cellar-way at the hospital. He attempted to walk across the top of the opening on a board one-half inch in thickness. The plank gave way letting him fall a distance of eight feet, striking the outer half of the plantar surface of his right foot on the edge of the bottom step in such a way as to cause strong abduction. He was immediately carried into the hospital and anesthetized.

Examination showed the following injury: The foot was everted to an angle of eighty degrees with the shaft of the leg. The laceration was long and irregular, running downward and forward just beneath the internal malleolus. The tibia protruded about three inches and showed a transverse fracture one centimeter above the articular surface. The shaft was not injured. The astragalus was badly shattered, being broken vertically and transversely into several fragments. A vertical line of fracture traversed the lesser process of the calcaneum. The interosseus ligament and the external lateral ligament appeared to be intact. The fibula was comminuted. There was a transverse supramalleolar fracture, and also lines of fracture running through the malleolus forward and inward and forward and downward. Hemorrhage was not severe. In order to manipulate the fragments of the astragalus it was necessary to enlarge the laceration. None of the fragments seemed to be entirely detached. They were replaced with some difficulty. The foot was brought into proper relation to the leg and the articular surface of the astragalus, that is, what remained of it, placed in apposition with that of the tibia. The comminuted external malleolus was pressed and molded into a good position against the astragalus. The circulation in the foot was good, the anterior and posterior tibial arteries having escaped injury. A rubber drainage-tube was placed in the central portion of the laceration, and another was introduced through a counter-opening made just anterior and below the tip of the external malleolus. The laceration was then sutured above and below the tube. The foot and leg were encased in a plaster dressing over anterior and posterior iron splints, leaving an interruption at the ankle. The limb was suspended and swung clear of the bed. On the third day the tubes were removed. Considerable foul pus had found its way out of the wound. This discharge continued uninterruptedly. Some fragments of the astragalus necrosed, and a probe detected softening of almost the entire bone, and also of the articular surface of the tibia. By August 1st the counter-opening had closed, but the sloughing of the necrosed fragments continued through the original laceration. By the end of the month the discharge had greatly diminished. The sinus persisted and was about an inch in depth. The patient's general condition was not seriously impaired.

At the present time the patient is about on crutches, and he rests a fair amount of weight upon the foot. He complains of pain, but indicates it well forward in the tarsus, the usual situation of pain after long immobilization of the foot. The sinus persists, and is three-quarters of an inch in depth. The discharge is thin and scanty. There is a limited yet fair amount of motion. The patient's general health does not improve. Tubercle bacilli in great numbers are present in the sputum. It will be safe to assert that the patient will not survive sufficiently long to ever have the use of a sound though perhaps ankylosed joint. The accident occurred in the region of Lake Superior, where the summer is brief and the winters trying to persons of rugged health, and disastrous to those with tuberculous tendencies. It seems to me that it would have been better surgery in this particular case to have amputated the foot and spared the patient the tedious months of suppuration during which he was confined to his room. The chances for ultimate use of the foot are nil, and the shock following amputation would not in all probability have exceeded that of the original injury. Crutches were inevitable in any case, yet their earlier use, following amputation and the patient's increased out-door activity during the most favorable season of the year would have contributed much to his well-being. This is particularly true since he was in an early stage of consumption at the time of the accident.

CASE III.—E. P., a Finn, of temperate habits, and in robust health, twenty-eight years of age. His occupation was gold-mining. November 23, 1897, his left ankle was caught under a "fall of ground." Examination should a long, jagged laceration through the skin and soft parts on the outer aspect of the left ankle. There was slight inward displacement and rotation of the foot. The articular surfaces of the tibia and fibula were crushed and pulverized. The astragalus and sustentaculum tali had met a similar fate. The wound and joint were ground full of dirt. The soft parts all about the ankle and well forward on the foot were badly crushed. Pulsation of either the anterior or posterior tibial artery could not be detected. Hemorrhage was free, but not severe. The patient rode five miles to the hospital in an open sleigh. As he was suffering from shock and cold he was immediately put to bed, warmth and stimulants exhibited, a temporary dressing applied to the injured limb, and every effort made to arouse the circulation in the foot. It soon became evident that the part was dead. Accordingly, on the following morning, an amputation was performed at the lower third of the leg. Had the integrity of the circulation been maintained there would have been an attempt to favor the man's condition by the following operative measures. The loose fragments of the tibia and fibula would have been removed and both bones sawed transversely through immediately above the uneven line of fracture. The astragalus would have also been removed, and the superior articular surface of the calcaneum sawed or chiseled off transversely. The tibia and fibula would have been wired together, the foot carried up, and the os calcis wired to both the tibia and fibula. Ankylosis would have been the object sought.

The man made an excellent recovery following the amputation, and at the present time goes about with the aid of an artificial limb.

MASTOIDITIS.

By WM. C. BANE, M.D., OF DENVER, COL.

Diagnosis.—Mastoiditis is seldom a primary affection, being usually a complication of otitis media. It is characterized by pain and tenderness in the mastoid, at first slight, but rapidly becoming both severe and persistent, especially at night, disturbing or preventing sleep. The pain may radiate to the temporal, occipital, or supra-orbital regions. Tenderness on pressure or on percussion of the mastoid, over the antrum, the tip, or both, will be complained of if the inflammation has continued for a few days. In exerting pressure it is necessary to avoid the auricle, in view of the fact that the pain excited in the inflamed canal or middle ear may be misleading. In some persons the tip of the mastoid is normally quite tender. Edema back of the ear may or may not be present, even though the interior of the mastoid be necrotic. However, there is usually more or less infiltration of the tissues over the mastoid in the acute and sub-acute forms of mastoiditis.

With periostitis, there is tenderness, redness, and swelling over the mastoid. Fluctuation is indicative of the presence of a subperiosteal abscess, in which case there is usually displacement of the auricle. Inflammation originating in the external canal may extend to the periosteal covering of the mastoid and finally result in the formation of an abscess. In young subjects it may pursue such a course from the middle ear without perforating the cortex, having found exit through the Rivinian segment.[1] In children, in whom the cortex is quite thin, perforation may occur within a day or two after the pneumatic cells have been invaded. The abscess occasionally ruptures through the internal surface of the mastoid, and thus pus enters the tissues beneath the sternocleidomastoid muscle. This was true of a case which I observed a few years ago. The local temperature, according to Politzer,[2] will frequently be elevated above that of the healthy mastoid. Body temperature is an uncertain guide. During the acute stage it may vary from normal to 103° F. When the more acute stage is over the temperature may be normal even though the destructive process still continues. When the temperature fluctuates, rising and falling suddenly several times within twenty-four hours, it is indicative of involvement of the lateral sinus. The pulse under such circumstances is rapid, small, and thready.[3]

Abscess of the mastoid complicating acute otitis media is usually located in the middle and lower portions of this bony process contiguous to the cortex. Politzer's observations have led him to believe that the mastoid abscess is isolated and almost without exception has no communication with the antrum.

In most cases of mastoiditis originating during the course of an otitis media it will be observed that the posterior-superior wall of the meatus, near the drum membrane, is bulging and tender. When the canal is thus depressed in a case of otitis media purulenta, and in which there is a history of pain and tenderness in the mastoid, and perhaps a variation in the local and general temperature, a diagnosis of mastoiditis is justifiable. The bulging of the posterior-superior wall of the canal, like the pain in the mastoid, is not always present. In January of the present year I operated in two cases of mastoiditis, in neither of which was there a bulging of posterior-superior wall, nor the typical pain of mastoiditis, and yet in both the mastoids were diseased. In one I exposed half an inch of the lateral sinus before all the necrotic tissue was removed.

Prognosis.—Mastoiditis is a grave malady, though when it complicates acute otitis media, if promptly treated, the prognosis is generally favorable. During the exanthemata, however, its progress is rapid and destructive, and efforts to check it are not usually successful. When mastoiditis develops during the course of chronic otitis media the outlook is grave, especially when there is a history of previons attacks of a subacute character. The inflam-

[1] Dench, "Diseases of the Ear," page 447.
[2] Politzer, "Diseases of the Ear," third ed., page 491.
[3] Macewen, "Diseases of the Brain and Spinal Cord," page 237.

mation of the ear which so frequently develops during an attack of influenza is usually severe, and often extends to the mastoid.

When the discharge in otitis media and mastoiditis does not find free exit through a perforated membrane, the pus may find its way through the mastoid cortex, outwardly, anteriorally, or even into the digastric fossa. It may enter the middle fossa of the brain through the roof of the antrum or tympanic vault, or possibly the region of the lateral sinus.

In a few cases of mastoiditis recovery occurs without an operation, yet in order to prevent bone destruction and brain complications vigorous abortive treatment is necessary. Delay may result in brain abscess, sinus thrombosis, phlebitis, or meningitis.

On March 20th, of last year, I saw two cases of lepto-meningitis which had resulted from otitis media. In both, the disease had invaded the brain through the tympanic vault. One case was in a strong, muscular man, about middle age, whom I saw in consultation. He was in a semi-comatose condition. A history of long standing otorrhea was obtained. An operation was performed within a few hours, and revealed the existence of extensive caries of the mastoid and middle ear, with a perforation through the tympanic vault. The prognosis was, of course, very unfavorable, and the man died within twenty-four hours. At the post-mortem evideuces of extensive meningitis were found.

The second case was in a robust young man, who several weeks before had had an attack of otitis media, which, under treatment, had subsided. Shortly after, and following exposure, there occurred a second and subacute attack of the same affection. This was followed by brain symptoms. The mastoid was opened by a colleague, but the operation did not result in finding any evidence of disease. Symptoms of meningitis developed. At the autopsy a purulent meningitis (limited to the posterior fossa) was found, the pyogenic material having entered the brain cavity through the vault of the tympanum.

Treatment.—When a case of mastoiditis comes under observation at an early stage abortive treatment should be tried. This consists of rest in bed, light diet, and free evacuation of the bowels obtained by the administration of calomel and a saline. If the drum membrane is congested and bulging it should be freely incised through its posterior-superior portion. The incision should also extend for a short distance along the posterior-superior wall of the canal to allow free drainage from the middle ear and attic, as well as depletion of the wall adjacent to the antrum. When a perforation exists it may be necessary to enlarge it in order to provide free drainage. The ear should be irrigated with a hot antiseptic solution several times daily. Cold, applied by means of the Leiter coil, or Bishop ice-bag, is a valuable aid in checking the inflammation, and should be continuously employed during twenty-four to forty-eight hours.

Dench[1] mentions a diagnostic point in the application of cold, in that if the pain is neuralgic, it will be increased by cold, but if due to inflammation, it will be diminished. Local blood-letting by means of either the Swedish or artificial leeches will render valuable service in plethoric subjects.

Following this treatment there may be an apparent improvement in the symptoms; but if, on reexamination, it is found that the tumefaction and tenderness still continue, surgical measures should be at once instituted. Dench states that "this experience has so often fallen to my lot that I never continue the effort to abort the attack for more than forty-eight hours, feeling certain, if marked improvement has not occurred in this time, that operative treatment will be subsequently necessary." The pain may be modified by the administration of codein and acetanilid; the latter, of course, also reduces the temperature. When general headache exists, the ice poultice, consisting of bran and pounded ice, will render valuable service. If abortive measures fail after two- or three-days' trial, longer delay is unwise, especially if the mastoiditis has developed during the course of a chronic otitis media.

In mastoiditis complicating acute otitis media it is safe to continue the treatment a longer time before instituting operative measures, as in such cases the abortive treatment often gives relief.

Operation.—When a subperiosteal abscess has formed it should be evacuated by an incision about three-eighths of an inch back of the auricle and parallel with it. Should there be a fistulous opening in the bone it will be necessary to proceed as in a regular mastoid operation. When an operation is to be performed, the head, for a distance of three inches from the auricle, should be shaved, and cleansed with soap and water, with ether, and then with a 1-to-1000 solution of bichlorid of mercury. At this day it is not necessary to emphasize the necessity of careful asepsis and antisepsis, the details of which may be safely left to the judgment of the operator. Before the operation the patient's bowels should be moved, and no food given during the previous six hours. The necessary instruments consist of scalpel, periosteum elevator, artery forceps, retractor (Allport's being one of the best), chisels, mallet, curettes, spoons, gouges, probes, scissors, and rongeur forceps. The head should be covered with sterilized towels, leaving exposed the region to be operated upon.

The exact method of procedure cannot be known

[1] Dench, "Diseases of the Ear," page 450.

in advance of the operation. The incision down to the bone should be made from the tip of the mastoid to a level with the upper attachment of the auricle, about three-eighths of an inch from the posterior attachment of the latter. The periosteum should then be elevated, and the retractor placed in position. If no fistulous opening is observed in the bone, an opening should be made with the chisel over the antrum. The opening should be made close to the posterior bony wall of the meatus, and not above its upper margin.

After entering the cortex, if the interior is found to be necrotic or soft, the narrow rongeur forceps can be used to remove this portion of the bone, after which the interior, or all unhealthy tissue, may be removed with a sharp spoon. If it is desirable to excise the posterior canal-wall, it can be very conveniently accomplished with the narrow rongeur forceps (Bacon's) and chisel. All the diseased tissue must be removed, even though in doing so it becomes necessary to expose the lateral sinus and facial nerve. Great care is necessary to avoid wounding the facial vein or nerve.

It is very important that the operator be familiar with the anatomy of the parts, as well as to know that in no two cases will the mastoid be found of the same shape, density, or thickness.

During the operation frequent drying of the wound with sterilized gauze is necessary, to permit observation of the depth of the wound and determination of the condition of the tissues. After removing all dead and diseased tissue the wound should be freely irrigated with salt or bichlorid solution. The upper part of the flesh-wound may be closed with stitches, down to the upper part of the cavity in the bone, after which it should be loosely packed with sterilized or iodoform gauze. Between the edges of the flesh-wound only a thin layer of gauze is required; thus the parts will earlier assume their normal position. Next, over the whole operative area, should be placed several layers of sterilized gauze, and then a layer of cotton, all of which is held in place by a gauze bandage.

It is not necessary to change the first dressing for four or five days, unless the wound becomes painful, or the temperature rises above 100° or 101° F. Subsequently, the dressing should be changed every two or three days. The wound should be allowed to heal from the bottom, and if healthy granulations are slow in forming, they may be stimulated by a mixture of balsam of Peru, iodoform, and guaiacol.

The wound may be allowed to close, in some cases, within two or three weeks, while in others it becomes necessary to keep it open for two or three months. The operation itself is not dangerous when properly performed; the danger lies in not instituting operative procedures early enough, before brain complications occur.

THE EPIDEMIC OF DENGUE AT HOUSTON, TEXAS; CLINICAL REPORT OF CASES.

By I. B. DIAMOND, M.D.,
OF HOUSTON, TEXAS.

DURING the epidemic of so-called dengue fever which prevailed extensively here and elsewhere throughout Texas last summer, different opinions were expressed as to the true nature of the disease. A number of the symptoms appeared analogous to those observed in yellow fever, so that a differential diagnosis between the two affections was often difficult. A number of such cases, which I deem worthy of publication, came under my observation.

Out of 71 cases, observed and treated, 23 were in children; to these latter I will refer later. In the majority of cases the onset was sudden. In many, a severe chill marked the beginning of the attack, and it was not uncommon to observe a succession of chills one after the other. The chill was soon followed by backache, pains in the head, bones, joints, and muscles, and also by loss of appetite, nausea, and vomiting. Nausea was constantly present in the majority of cases. The tongue was coated white, and frequently redness around the edges was observed. The bowels, as a rule, were constipated and difficult to move by medication. The face was flushed, skin dry, and conjunctivæ injected. The elevation of temperature was gradual, and during the course of the affection ranged between 103° and 106° F., and the pulse 100 to 120 per minute.

In the majority of the cases it was noticed that the pulse gradually became slow on the second and third day, frequently as low as 50 beats per minute, while the temperature remained as high as 103° F., or even higher. This want of correlation between pulse and temperature was a marked feature in my cases. The urine in many cases was of light color, and micturition frequent and painful; while in others it was high colored and diminished in quantity. Albumin was present in a few cases. Unfortunately, no systematic examination of the urine was made. While albumin was sometimes absent on one occasion, it would not infrequently be found on subsequent examination. During the thirty-six to seventy-two hours following the onset of the affection the pains constantly increased in severity, especially those in the head and back. The pains were described by many patients as tearing and crushing. At this stage the patients felt very uncomfortable, became exceedingly restless, and unable to sleep. Slight delirium was noticed in a few cases. Cold feet and chilliness were often complained of during the fever. After the disease reached its height, usually on the third day, the fever began to abate and the pains to subside, leaving the patient in a prostrated condition. In a number of my cases an eruption soon appeared, followed again by a second paroxysm, with pain, fever, etc. Itching was often present, associated with a tense and hot skin, especially of the palms of the hands and soles of the feet. The eruption, as a rule, was punctiform, deep red in color, and the size of a pin-head. In a few instances it was more or less diffuse, and in one case it had the typical appearance of urticaria. The eruption continued but a few days, when convalescence, often protracted, began. Nearly all cases resulted in recovery. Extreme debility, mental and nervous exhaustion, were marked in the majority of my cases. Weakness and pains in the lumbar region, which became aggravated on walking, were frequently complained of during convalescence. Appetite soon returned, and in many it even became ravenous. A peculiar and bitter taste in the mouth, especially on taking food, was often complained of, and this symptom usually continued some time. Cramping pains in the abdomen, described as colicky in character, and continuing for several weeks, were also complained of by many patients.

An icteroid hue of the face and conjunctivæ during convalescence was noticed in a number of my cases. In several cases minute hemorrhages, which gradually disappeared, were observed in the conjunctivæ. In six cases vomiting was a prominent symptom, and continued throughout the course of the affection. In these cases weakness was marked, pulse slow, tongue red and dry. In one, that of a woman aged fifty years, gastric hemorrhage occurred on the second day. The blood was mixed with the vomit. The matter from the stomach usually consisted of bile and mucus. Nothing was retained by these patients for any length of time.

Pains in the abdomen were often a prominent symptom. In some it was referred to the pit of the stomach, in others, to the region of the appendix. In one case, that of a young married woman, the pain was referred to the region of the gall-bladder; in another, in a young man, there was constant pain in the left inguinal region, radiating down the left leg. Another feature in this case was complete obstruction of the bowels during six days; the patient vomited considerably, his temperature ranged between 100° and 104° F., and the pulse from 80 to 100 per minute. During this time he complained of severe frontal headache. I may state that medication and enemata were employed without avail. The constant application of ice was resorted to with good results. It was used in all cases in which pain in the abdomen was constantly present.

In two of my cases marked jaundice was present throughout the attack. Menstruation occurred in a young woman during her illness; it had more the character of a hemorrhage than of menstruation. The discharge was dark red, almost black in color, and continued several days. This was also accompanied by pain in the lower part of the abdomen.

Relapses followed in seven of my cases after an interval of from one to five weeks. The relapse was usually more severe than the primary attack, as is illustrated by the following case:

Mrs. N., white, aged twenty-eight years, the mother of three children, and at the time of the attack in the ninth month of gestation. She had recently recovered from a mild attack of the disease under consideration. On November 2d, twelve days later, she was taken with a severe chill, which was repeated several times during the night. The first chill was followed by cephalalgia, backache, and severe pains in the abdomen. The tongue was coated and red around the edges; nausea and vomiting were present, as well as constipation; temperature, 105° F.; pulse, 110. The face was flushed and the eyes injected. These symptoms continued until the third day, November 5th. During the night of the fifth she became delirious; temperature, 106° F.; pulse, 110. There was sordes of the lips, and the tongue was swollen and red. The pains increased in severity. Fetal movements had not been observed for several days, which, of course, indicated the occurrence of fetal death. On the following morning she was taken with true labor pains, and after several hours gave birth to a dead child. Undoubtedly the fetus died either as a result of the high maternal temperature or from infection, transmitted from the mother, as the infant was not cyanosed when born. The mother had fever for several days following parturition; temperature ranging from 101° to 104° F.; pulse about normal. On the following day she had a moderate hemorrhage from the nose which lasted several hours. The tongue continued red and dry. Diarrhea followed and lasted during the next three days, the patient having from ten to twenty evacuations daily. She gradually improved after the ninth day, and finally recovered.

In one of my cases there were marked renal symptoms and general dropsy. The urine was dark and smoky, and loaded with albumin and cast, as well as blood-corpuscles in different stages of degeneration.

In children the disease ran a comparatively mild course. In twelve a distinct rash was present. The youngest child attacked, in whom the rash was also present, was an infant three weeks old. The mother, as well as the other members of the family, had the disease during the same week, so this was undoubtedly a true case of dengue. In two children the affection was at first mistaken for measles, and in another for scarlatina. The rash usually appeared earlier than in adults. Constitutional disturbances was not so marked as in older patients. Chilly sensations were occasionally present. The fever was usually slight. Headache was constantly present. The face was flushed and conjunctivæ injected. The tongue was coated, appetite lost, and vomiting was an occasional symptom. As in adults, the bowels, as a rule, were constipated. The children were restless, and preferred to walk about during the illness.

In four cases an icteroid hue of the face and conjunctiva was observed, and in two there was marked jaundice. In these cases the attack was more severe. Pains in the abdomen were usually complained of. In children the disease was first manifested by the occurrence of a chill, following which the temperature ranged from 100° to 103° F.; pulse 100 to 120. A general hyperesthesia of the skin was also noticed. When touched the child would cry out as though in pain. In three cases the attack resembled typhoid fever, and continued over two weeks. Swelling and redness of the right knee and ankle developed in a boy of twelve years of age during the attack, and continued five days. This is the only instance in which this symptom was observed, although it has been described as one of the features of dengue.

The treatment was entirely symptomatic. In many instances treatment was not necessary. The bowels were usually moved by means of small doses of calomel, followed by a saline. Quinin was at first administered, but its use was soon abandoned. The main treatment was directed to the relief of pain and the reduction of temperature. For this purpose codein, in combination with acetanilid and caffein citrate, often sufficed. Occasionally morphin was necessary. Applications of ice proved very valuable in causing a reduction of fever and for the relief of the pains in the abdomen and head. For sleeplessness, bromids were given, but often with but little effect. In such cases whisky had a favorable action, and was freely given. For the nausea and vomiting small doses of creosote proved beneficial, while in more severe cases the hypodermic administration of morphin became necessary. During convalescence strychnia and preparations of phosphorus for the nervous prostration proved very helpful.

The Cuvier Prize Awarded to Professor Marsh.—The Cuvier prize of the Academy of Sciences, Paris, value 1500 francs, has been awarded to Professor Marsh of Yale University. This prize is awarded every three years for the most noteworthy work on geology or on the animal kingdom.

FOREIGN BODIES IN THE CORNEA.

BY EDWARD JACKSON, M.D.,
OF PHILADELPHIA;
PROFESSOR OF DISEASES OF THE EYE IN THE PHILADELPHIA POLYCLINIC; SURGEON TO WILLS' EYE HOSPITAL.

A PATIENT'S statement that there is a foreign body in the eye is not altogether reliable, for the presence of inflammation, swollen conjunctival veins or papillæ, or an abrasion of the conjunctiva, may all give rise to the same sensation. Even when a foreign body has previously been present the resulting injury to the cornea or conjunctiva may cause a similar sensation, though the removal of the invading material has already been effected. On the other hand, should such a body be so deeply embedded in the cornea that it does not give rise to irritation of the conjunctiva, it may remain for several hours or even days without causing any discomfort whatever, and the circumstances under which it gained entrance may be quite forgotten. The symptoms of inflammation come on gradually, and the distinctive sensation of a foreign body may be absent; so that either a positive or negative history may be equally misleading.

Hyperemia, when present, is very suggestive of a foreign body in the cornea, though it will usually require some hours or even days for its development. It is always partly pericorneal. If the foreign body is located near the center of the cornea the pink discoloration will extend around the entire limbus, if it is located near the margin the hyperemia will be greatest in the adjoining portion of the limbus. On the other hand, if the foreign substance is embedded in the conjunctiva or lid the redness will be irregularly distributed.

The diagnosis, however, rests upon the results of careful inspection. For this purpose either oblique illumination with a lens or diffuse daylight is necessary. In the use of the first the cornea should be strongly illuminated, the condensing lens being so held as to concentrate the light upon it, and the eye should be viewed from different points. A foreign substance of dark color may be best detected against the iris, while one which is light in color will be most easily found when it is strongly illuminated and seen against the dark background of the pupil. With inspection by direct daylight, the surgeon's eye should be so placed that it will receive the reflected light from different parts of the cornea. An irregularity in the corneal surface, such as is caused by an abrasion or the presence of a foreign substance, will cause a corresponding irregularity in the reflection. Slight irregularities of the corneal surface may, however, be filled with mucus, thus concealing any body which may be present. To prevent this the cornea should be wiped with absorbent cotton.

A substance embedded in the cornea may also be detected by means of the ophthalmoscopic mirror, a strong convex lens being placed behind it. Thus, on viewing the cornea from different directions, the foreign body will in some position be brought in front of the illuminated pupil and will appear black against the red background.

When a body is allowed to remain in the cornea, the resulting inflammation gradually increases and suppuration usually occurs. By this process the invading substance is loosened and either rubbed off by the lids or washed away by the lacrimal secretion, after which the ulcer slowly heals. In a few cases there seems to be an active proliferation of tissue, mostly epithelial, which covers the foreign body. In this way it may be retained and be the cause of an inflammation which may continue weeks or months. In such a case the tissue covering the foreign substance appears dry and white, and to it runs a sharply defined area of conjunctival or subconjunctival hyperemia, resembling that which is typical of a fascicular keratitis. A series of cases in which foreign bodies were thus retained in the cornea for periods varying from three weeks to eighteen months have been reported by the writer (*Brit. Med. Jour.*, June 8, 1897). Extremely minute foreign bodies, so retained, gradually making their way with the lymph currents toward the center of the cornea, are by some authorities regarded as the cause of pterygium.

It is hardly necessary to say that treatment implies the prompt removal of the cause of the trouble, with the single exception of powder stains or "grains" in the cornea, which have been present long enough to have become somewhat disintegrated and to have ceased to be a cause of irritation or inflammation. Any damaged corneal tissue should also be removed; for if left to come away of itself it will result in a delay in the healing process. Thorough treatment also implies removal of the brown stain which sometimes surrounds a foreign body in the cornea. I have never observed a case in which the presence of such stained tissue was permantly tolerated.

Removal of the foreign substance is usually accomplished with the aid of a spud. Varying forms of this instrument have slight advantages in different cases. The instrument which seems to me most generally useful is straight with a rather small or pointed end, not sharp, but still more nearly approximating a point than many of the spuds to be found in the shops. This instrument should not be used as a scraper, and removal of the foreign body will not be facilitated by sudden "digs" made with it. It should be carefully and accurately placed in contact with the cornea, by the side of the body to be removed, and then pressed rather firmly into the tissue until, by a wedge-like action, the body is forced out, the spud passing under it. To easily accomplish this it is necessary that the surgeon's hand and the patient's eye be as steady as possible.

Previous to attempting removal the eye should be thoroughly anesthetized by means of one or two instillations of a four-per-cent. solution of cocain, or a one-per-cent. solution of holocain. Meanwhile, the patient should be accustomed to the presence of the fingers and the instrument before the eye by touching the organ in question with the fingers and by moving these close in front of it until it is demonstrated that there really is nothing to fear. The patient should be urged to look at some object steadily, regardless of what is being done to the eye.

When the particle to be removed is a splinter of wood or a piece of grass or grain more or less firmly embedded, it may be necessary to deal with it much as one deals with a splinter embedded in the skin. A small needle or the point of a Graefe knife should be passed down alongside the splinter, to its end if possible, and then made to cut outward, so as to provide a free opening. The spud may now be used to turn out the foreign body in the ordinary way.

"Powder grains" in the cornea during the early stage of irritation and inflammation should be removed by means of the galvanocautery. Such particles are not actually "grains," but bits of charcoal diffused through the corneal tissue; and they can only be removed by destruction of the tissue involved. Any attempt at their removal with needles or knives favors the extension of infection and inflammation.

When a foreign body is deeply embedded in the cornea and extends through into the anterior chamber, its removal is a more serious matter. In such cases it is usually found that the escape of aqueous humor has left the eyeball comparatively soft, and allows the iris and lens to fall forward and perhaps to come in contact with the foreign body. In such cases early removal is particularly important. Until the time of operation the eye should be kept perfectly quiet, so that an opportunity is furnished for the accumulation of aqueous humor and restoration of the anterior chamber. The eye should, of course, be anesthetized by means of a strong solution of cocain. A broad needle, not lance-shaped or like the keratome, but one gradually tapering to a width of three millimeters at a distance of eight to ten millimeters from the point, should be thrust through the cornea near the foreign body, so as to pass beneath it, and the point made to engage again in the cornea, but not to entirely perforate it. Having the needle passed back of the foreign body, so as to prevent it from being pushed into the anterior chamber or from injuring the iris or lens, removal of the body may be easily accomplished.

In all these manipulations some sort of a magnifier will prove of great assistance. The binocular magnifier, described by me in the *Archives of Ophthalmology* for April, 1897, is the most satisfactory; it gives the greatest enlargement compatible with sufficient working space between the lens and the eye, and offers the benefit of binocular vision without any excessive strain of convergence.

ARTERIOSCLEROSIS AS A CAUSE OF KIDNEY DISEASE.

BY EVERETT J. BROWN, M.D.,
OF DECATUR, ILL.

MOST observers now agree that the kidney changes accompanying a general arteriosclerosis are secondary to the constitutional affection. On the other hand, there are writers who still hold to the theory that all sclerotic changes in the blood-vessels follow a primary fibrous change in the kidneys; that in most cases of general arteriosclerosis the most serious pathologic results are manifested in the kidneys, heart, brain, and liver. Bright himself noticed that chronic renal disease was often associated with hypertrophy of the left ventricle, and all subsequent investigators have confirmed his observations. Grainger Stewart found cardiac hypertrophy in forty-six per cent. of the cases of granular contracted kidney; Loomis, in sixty per cent; Dickinson, in seventy-four per cent., and Galabin in eighty per cent.[1]

Strumpell is inclined to regard the effect of a general arteriosclerosis upon the kidneys as more important than the changes induced by it in the heart and brain, and he only mentions the "granulated" senile kidney as being largely due to atheroma of the renal arteries. In writing of the etiology of arteriosclerosis, he classes nephritis with excessive use of alcohol, syphilis, rheumatism, gout, and lead-poisoning as the cause of the affection in question. Regardless of whether the kidney lesion is primary or secondary, there is no doubt that renal symptoms occur in the majority of cases of general arterial sclerosis. In nearly all autopsies, according to Osler, in which this disease is found there are also evidences of kidney degeneration—either a diffuse or localized sclerosis of the interstitial tissue. It is seen in a typical manner in the senile form of nephritis, and it not infrequently develops earlier in life as a result of chronic diffuse nephritis. Osler further states that it is difficult to decide clinically whether the arterial or the renal disease is the primary affection.

The degeneration which occurs in the general arterial system is also found in the arteries of the kidneys, and in all cases there is an excess of fibrous tissue. Gall and Sutton noticed the predominance of the fibrous change in the external coat of the arteries, in the form of a fibroid hyperplasia, which they call a "hyalin fibroid transformation." The internal coat was also sometimes markedly thickened, and the muscular coat showed a relative increase in thickness, though in some parts the latter was wasted and degenerated. In forty post-mortem examinations in cases of chronic renal disease, Loomis found, as regards the systemic and renal arteries, that the external coat was thickened in many cases; it alone was diseased in twelve instances, and the muscular coat was thickened in five. In twenty-one cases in which the kidneys were involved this fibrosis could not be distinguished from that of the neighboring interstitial tissue or from that about the glomeruli. From this it is seen that the morbid changes are external to the arteries as well as in their walls.[1]

In regard to the effects of chronic renal disease on the heart and blood-vessels, Dickinson says:[2] "There occurs a hypertrophy of the cardio-arterial system which is unusual from its origin to its termination, and comprises not only the ventricles and arterioles, but affects also the intermediate arteries of every size." He has further shown from post-mortem evidence that the arteriosclerosis is more constant than cardiac hypertrophy in relation to chronic renal disease; on the other hand, in some cases of renal involvement the arteries are perfectly normal while the cardiac disease is marked.

The presence of renal disease may be suspected in every case in which the four pathognomonic signs of general arteriosclerosis are present. These signs are: Increased arterial tension, palpable thickening of the arteries, hypertrophy of the left ventricle, and accentuated aortic sound. Even before direct evidence of disease of the kidneys is presented its existence may be suspected whenever a forcible heaving of the left ventricle and increased tension of the blood-vessels are noticed.[3] On the other hand, in many cases of arteriosclerosis there are few symptoms except those of the renal disease.

In a typical case of general arteriosclerosis with involvement of the kidneys the symptoms are somewhat as follows: The patient is a man, over forty years of age, who presents a history of having always enjoyed robust health. His appetite is good, often excessive, and his diet has consisted largely of meat and other highly nitrogenous foods. His occupation is such as to give him little opportunity for physical exercise, and his inclinations in this direc-

[1] Sanson, "Twentieth Century Practice of Medicine," vol. iv.

[1] Sanson, "Twentieth Century Practice of Medicine," vol. iv.
[2] *Lancet*, July 20, 1895.
[3] Sanson, *loc. cit.*

tion are slight. He has a healthy appearance, possibly a florid complexion, and on slight exertion becomes short of breath. He has some dyspepsia, headache, or maybe a recurring bronchorrhea. At night he finds it necessary to rise twice or oftener to void his urine, which is pale and increased in quantity, but quite clear and free from sediment. The specific gravity of the urine is low—1012 to 1018—and there is a diminished amount of urea and and a small amount—often a mere trace—of albumin. Microscopic examination reveals the presence of a few small hyalin casts. The pulse is full, hard, and easily compressed, and the artery is palpable between beats, and even when it is firmly compressed with the finger its outline can still be felt below the point of pressure. At the aortic interspace the second sound of the heart is distinctly accentuated, and at the apex the pulsation is abnormally strong, and is noticed lower down and to the left, showing the presence of cardiac hypertrophy.

Such a case as has just been outlined requires years for its development, and evidences a constant progression toward death, either from uremia or one of the concomitants of the accompanying arteriosclerosis, such as apoplexy from a ruptured cerebral vessel, an embolus, rupture of a thoracic aneurism, gangrene from an obliterating endarteritis, or a moist gangrene from embolic occlusion of the large artery of an extremity.

In treating old men and women for the various pathologic accompaniments of senility, all physicians have noticed that although the urine of such patients, after frequent examinations, shows nothing abnormal except, perhaps, a low specific gravity and polyuria, yet just before death they develop symptoms of uremic poisoning and suppression of urine, and when the kidneys are examined post-mortem they are found to be contracted. The nephritis of arteriosclerosis is a much more common disease than is usually supposed, and the clinical picture is not always as pronounced as my description of a typical case would imply. The morbid picture is often composed of a series of vague and indefinite symptoms which are difficult of interpretation. The changes in the heart and circulation often produce subjective symptoms referable to the kidneys long before any are noticed by the physician. A life-insurance examination may perhaps reveal an unsuspected nephritis. Disturbances of vision lead many such patients to consult an oculist, who is the first to discover changes in the fundus of the eye pointing to a kidney lesion, an indication which is confirmed by a subsequent analysis of the urine.

The prognosis depends upon the age of the patient, the etiologic factors in the disease, and especially upon the stage of the process affecting the renal tissues. Mahomed[1] describes a pre-albuminuric stage of Bright's disease, to be detected by the increased arterial tension before the commencement of any kidney change or the appearance of albumin in the urine. By carefully observing the degree of tension of the radial artery, much valuable information in regard to the progress or arrest of the disease may be obtained, for with the diminution of dropsy and albumin the artery will be found more compressible, while with the increase of arterial tension there will be an increase of albumin, increased hypertrophy of the left ventricle, increased edema, retinal hemorrhages, and uremic symptoms. As the kidney lesion is only one of several morbid elements in this disease, the prognosis depends much upon the ability of the other organs to continne the performance of their functions. Many cases terminate with a predominance of nephritic symptoms, such as dropsy and uremia, while others present a perfect clinical picture of chronic valvular heart disease with a loud blowing murmur at the apex, which may deceive the practitioner. Other patients die from cerebral hemorrhage, sudden rupture of a thoracic aneurism, or from gangrene of the extremities. In some cases a severe bronchitis with marked emphysema develops, and often in the senile form of the disease the cause of death is ascribed to "old age," not only by the laity, but by physicians as well.

The following cases illustrate two forms of general arteriosclerosis, in one of which there was a predominance of renal symptoms, and in the other prominent renal manifestations, with a fatal termination, immediately due to circulatory changes.

CASE I.—H. B., farmer, aged forty-nine years. December 22, 1896, examination showed the presence of general arteriosclerosis. The pulsation of the temporal and radial arteries was very forcible, and the vessels themselves were very tense and easily palpable. The area of heart-dulness was increased, and the apex beat was in the seventh interspace. There was general edema, especially marked in the feet, and some dyspnea and insomnia. Constantly recurring headache had been a feature of this case for several years. At this time he was still able to continue at his daily work. He arose three or four times every night to urinate. The result of the analysis of the urine was as follows: Color, pale yellow; total quantity, 75 ounces; reaction, acid; specific gravity, 1018; albumin, three-fourths volume. The microscope showed the presence of many large and small granular and hyalin casts. Sugar was not present. By means of a proper diet and the free administration of eliminants the dropsy was much improved.

[1] Mahomed, *Medico-Chirurgical Trans.*, p. 197, 1874.

CASE II.—Mrs. A. S., farmer's wife, aged forty-seven years, was in the midst of the climacteric. At the time of examination she menstruated every three or four months. She complained of universal pains, frequent headache, and palpitation of the heart. There was some swelling of face and extremities, much dyspnea on slight exertion, bronchitis, pain after eating and flatulence. Physical examination showed a systolic murmur at the apex, and increased area of heart-dulness. The apex beat was to the left of the nipple line. The palpable arteries were tense and cord-like, but not tortuous. The specific gravity of the urine was 1018. There was present considerable albumin, but no sugar. Patient was kept under observation four years, and by means of digitalis, tonics, and eliminants she was made more comfortable. Much of the edema and dyspnea disappeared. Finally, however, she was seized with a sudden pain in the left leg, the left foot became cold, the tibial arteries ceased to beat, and death occurred within a few days from moist gangrene due to the lodgment of an embolus at the bifurcation of the popliteal artery.

NEW INSTRUMENT.

FORMALDEHYD DISINFECTION.

BY JACOB R. JOHNS, M.D.,
OF PHILADELPHIA.

THE difficulty attending the application of formic aldehyd to general disinfection has led to the devising of a score or more lamps and generators supposed to meet the indications. Many of these, because utterly devoid of merit, have never come into prominence, while others, which possess some value and a more or less restricted field of usefulness, are quite well known. No less than seven different forms of apparatus were exhibited at the last meeting of the American Public Health Association in Philadelphia. The difficulty appears to lie in the liberation of the gas in its most active form in sufficient volume and with sufficient rapidity to overcome all unavoidable loss through holes and crevices, and thus do the work thoroughly.

Three methods requiring different apparatus are in vogue. In the first and oldest, the gas is generated directly from wood alcohol upon the principle of retarded combustion; in the second, it is liberated from pastilles of paraformaldehyd exposed to the action of flame, and in the third, the gas is derived from an aqueous solution of known strength. In the first two classes the apparatus must be confined in the closed apartment which is being disinfected, where it is a source both of danger and uncertainty of action.

If lamps burning wood alcohol are used, the operator can never know what per cent. of alcohol is completely consumed and what is changed to available formaldehyd gas. The volume of gas generated is always uncertain, and never large even when the apparatus is operated by an experienced chemist. In the effort to obtain sufficiently large volumes of gas during the same period of exposure the second and third methods have been devised. In the third method a new difficulty was encountered, that arising from polymerization, which promptly arrests the process.

The failure of the last process mentioned led Trillat and others to devise a means for generating the gas under pressure. This requires an extremely bulky apparatus and introduces a new element of danger, that from explosion. The latter element and the fact that polymers are formed led to the employment of the polymerized product in pastilles, which, while it gives better satisfaction than is obtained from alcohol lamps, affords but little gain in either the volume of gas or the rapidity of elimination.

Another method, intended to overcome all the foregoing difficulties, is that used in the apparatus here shown. (Fig. 1.) The method is both simple and novel. The apparatus consists of a copper coil placed over a Swiss heating lamp and beneath a receiver in which is placed commercial formaldehyd, an equeous solution containing forty per cent. of formic aldehyd gas, and ten per cent. of methyl alcohol to make the solution permanent. A small valve protects the opening from the receiver into the coil. When the latter is red hot the valve is opened to admit a small stream of the formaldehyd solution into the coil. Instantly it is vaporized, and the vapor containing the free gas is heated to upward of 1000° F. as it passes through the coil and a short hose through the key-hole, or other suitable opening, into the room to be disinfected. The apparatus is always on the outside of the apartment being disinfected, and under constant observation. The process does not permit of the formation of polymers, nor present the least danger of explosion, since the gas is not generated under pressure. It is especially adapted to apartment disinfection. With such an apparatus one man can easily disinfect upward of twenty apartments per day.

FIG. 1.

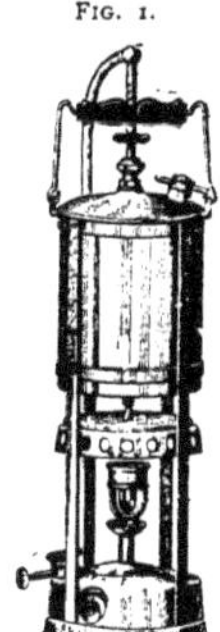

Formaldehyd generator.

This method was introduced by the Sanitary Construction Company of New York, and the apparatus is made by the H. K. Mulford Co. of Philadelphia.

MEDICAL PROGRESS.

The Parasites of Malarial Fever.—THAYE· (*Yale Med. Jour.*, January, 1898) gives the results of careful observations made in 1719 cases of malarial fever. He finds three distinct parasites; the tertian, the quartan, and the estivo-autumnal. No transitional forms have ever been observed.

The tertian parasite, in its earliest stages, is a small body lying within the red blood-corpuscle. It is possessed of active ameboid movements, but on account of its lack of color is observed with difficulty. However, it is readily detected by the practised eye, even in fresh unstained specimens. As the parasite grows it accumulates fine pigment granules which at the end of thirty-six hours have gathered together at one point, usually the center of the organism. The parasite next undergoes sporulation, and is separated into its central pigment clump and a surrounding mass of small, round, hyalin bodies, which are complete young parasites ready to attack fresh red blood-corpuscles. The life history of a parasite occupies forty-eight hours, and sporulation takes place in all the parasites at the same time, thus producing the febrile paroxysm in the patient.

The quartan parasite, in its early stages, greatly resembles the tertian, though its ameboid movement is weaker. As it grows the pigment granules are larger and darker than those of the tertain, and are inclined to gather in the periphery. Sporulation proceeds along symmetric lines, the parasite dividing into from six to twelve regularly arranged radial leaflets. The cycle of development requires seventy-two hours.

In both tertian and quartan infections more than one group of parasites may be present in a patient, giving, in double tertian and triple quartan infections, a chill every day. In double quartan infections there will be a chill upon two successive days and none upon the third.

The estivo-autumnal parasite is associated with fever which is more or less irregular. This form is rarely found in the milder malarious districts. The parasite is a biconcave disc with a well-marked central depression, so that it may appear like a ring. It is smaller than the tertian and quartan parasites and materially differs from them in the fact that it is usually found in the circulation only in its earlier stages of development. The later stages of development may be observed in blood aspirated from the spleen. This procedure is not without danger and should be carried out with the strictest aseptic precautions. After a certain length of time, varying from five days to two weeks, there appear in the circulation crescentic bodies with sharp refractive outlines containing pigment. If these are closely watched filaments may sometimes be observed to burst out from the parent cell and sometimes to break away from it to rush off alone across the field of vision. In the estivo-autumnal parasite sporulation does not occur in groups and hence the irregularity or continuousness of the fever.

The existence of these three distinct types of parasites has been proved not only by clinical observation, but further by careful inoculation experiments. Fresh blood from an infected patient, if introduced under the skin of a healthy man will invariably reproduce the same type of fever. There are still many questions in connection with this subject which cannot be definitely answered. Why should the process of sporulation cause fever? This is presumably because some toxic substance is set free from the parasite itself. The significance of the flagella has also puzzled observers. Recently MacCallum observed the penetration of a free flagellum into one of the non-flaggelate parasites. This observation strongly supports the idea previously advanced that flagellation and fertilization are intimately associated processes. At any rate, the old idea that flagellation is a degenerative process seems absolutely untenable.

As to modes of infection, there are at present considered to be three, *viz.*: by air, water, and by the bites of insects, especially the mosquito. The last is at present most popular. At the close of this most interesting article Thayer insisted upon the importance of the discovery of the parasite in the blood as the only diagnostic sign of malarial infection; a sign in many ways parallel to the demonstration of the tubercle bacillus in phthisis, or the Klebs-Löffler bacillus in diphtheria.

Results of Postural Drainage.—BURRAGE (*Annals of Gyne. and Pediat.*, January, 1898) has of late employed the postural method of draining the peritoneal cavity after abdominal operations, described by Clark in the *Johns Hopkins Hospital Bulletin* of April, 1897. This method consists in flushing the peritoneal cavity with sterile salt solution, wiping it dry with gauze, and then introducing from one to two pints of sterile salt solution. The abdomen is then closed and the foot of the bed raised eighteen inches, thus favoring a flow of fluid from the pelvis to the diaphragm, where absorption of liquids contained in this great lymph-sac proceeds with the greatest rapidity. By the use of this method it is possible in many cases to close the abdomen under circumstances in which drainage is usually considered necessary. Clark said, in fact, "the greatest safety lies in closing the abdomen without drainage except in cases of purulent peritonitis, or in operations in which there has been extensive suturing of the intestines, and also in a few other rare conditions."

The twenty-seven patients which Burrage mentions as having been treated by this method all recovered, although in this respect the new treatment did not differ much in result from that previously used in the same hospital in 167 celiotomies performed during the last eighteen months, in only one of which was there a fatal termination. In the new method it is well to keep the foot of the bed elevated at least thirty-six hours. The salt solution increases the amount of urine and diminishes thirst. Vomiting is facilitated by elevation of the foot of the bed. Swallowing is rendered more difficult, but is still easily possible if slowly performed. There is less nausea and less abdominal distention and pain. In two very fat women there was some embarrassment of respiration. The writer expressed himself as well satisfied with the new treatment, which he considers a distinct advance in abdominal surgery.

THE MEDICAL NEWS.

A WEEKLY JOURNAL

OF MEDICAL SCIENCE.

COMMUNICATIONS are invited from all parts of the world. Original articles contributed *exclusively* to THE MEDICAL NEWS will after publication be liberally paid for (accounts being rendered quarterly), or 250 reprints will be furnished in place of other remuneration. When necessary to elucidate the text, illustrations will be engraved from drawings or photographs furnished by the author. Manuscripts should be typewritten.

Address the Editor: J. RIDDLE GOFFE, M.D., No. 111 FIFTH AVENUE (corner of 18th St.), NEW YORK.

Subscription Price, including postage in U. S. and Canada.

PER ANNUM IN ADVANCE	$4.00
SINGLE COPIES	.10
WITH THE AMERICAN JOURNAL OF THE MEDICAL SCIENCES, PER ANNUM	7.50

Subscriptions may begin at any date. The safest mode of remittance is by bank check or postal money order, drawn to the order of the undersigned. When neither is accessible, remittances may be made, at the risk of the publishers, by forwarding in *registered* letters.

LEA BROTHERS & CO.,
No. 111 FIFTH AVENUE (corner of 18th St.), NEW YORK, AND NOS. 706, 708 & 710 SANSOM ST., PHILADELPHIA.

SATURDAY, MARCH 12, 1898.

THE BACTERIOLOGY OF RHEUMATISM.

ABOUT ten years ago it was announced by Bordas that he had discovered the micro-organism of acute articular rheumatism, and attention was called to his claims by an editorial in the MEDICAL NEWS. He asserted that the organism which he had isolated possessed certain definite bacteriologic characteristics, and that if it was injected into the body of the lower animals they immediately suffered from inflammatory joint affections, which in every way resembled those commonly seen in acute articular rheumatism. It was also stated that this micro-organism, which Bordas asserted was the cause of acute articular rheumatism, was peculiarly susceptible to salicylic acid, and so it was pointed out, if we could believe in this research, that the explanation of the value of salicylic acid in acute articular rheumatism had at last been discovered.

Whatever promise, however, was held out by this research was taken away from us by the failure of other investigators to confirm its results, and while the profession has become, with each succeeding year, more and more convinced of the fact that acute articular rheumatism is distinctly an acute infectious disease, definite statements as to the character of the infecting micro-organism have not been forthcoming. In this connection, therefore, a more recent research (*Société de Biologie,* July, 1891) which was published by Dr. Achalme of Paris, is of considerable interest. He claimed to have demonstrated a bacillus which he obtained in patients suffering from acute rheumatism, and he described various means of differentiating it from other micro-organisms of similar appearance.

Since this paper was published, Riva, Cheosteh, Michaelis, and Triboulet and Coyon have carried the investigation still further, and the latter claim that an elongated coccus found in pairs, or grouped in chains at times, is responsible for the malady. It is an anaerobic organism, easily cultivated in bouillon or ascitic fluid and is easily stained by thionin, but it is not discolored by the Gram method. These investigators assert that this is the real organism of rheumatic fever, and that the bacillus of Achalme is found as a complicating infection in certain cases. Unfortunately, as we see so often among other researches in the early stages of our knowledge concerning infectious maladies, these investigations of Triboulet and Coyon have in turn been criticised by other bacteriologists, who assert that certain staphylococci, which are in every way comparable with the coccus which it is claimed is the cause of acute articular rheumatism, are found in rheumatic cases, and Singer of Vienna has asserted that acute rheumatism is only a form of acute septicemia without a specific microbe. Whatever may be the truth of the claims put forward by these various investigators, practising physicians must watch with interest any conclusions arrived at in regard to the bacteriology of a malady which is a millstone about the neck of scientific medicine.

THE DETERMINATION OF SEX.

IT is not improbable that Professor Schenk, of Vienna, would gladly recall the idle words anent the influencing of sex by giving certain dietaries to the parents, if he knew the kind of company that his ridiculous so-called discovery was to lead him into. Not that he ever said one-tenth of all that has been attributed to him, but it matters not how little escaped his lips, he said far too much. It contributed to the destruction of his scientific reputation; the public press has done the rest. The immediate result of the propaganda, much more serious than the smirching of the Herr Professor's reputation, has been the development and uprising of "Sex-regulators" all over the country. It is not surprising that the Nutmeg State should furnish a number of them. Its inhabitants have made a record for themselves concerning their shrewdness which has come thundering down to posterity. According to the *Sun*, a Danbury physician declares that not only can he tell the sex of an unborn child, but that he knows the secret whereby it is possible for human beings to produce male or female at will. Oh, enviable Danbury physician! If you are truthfully and accurately reported, please let the male child come often enough to balance the awful disproportion now existing between the adult sexes in your own State; and please, furthermore, after the accomplishment of this worthy work, for which woman, particularly spinster woman, will rise up and call you blessed, transfer your presence and remain sufficiently long in New Hampshire to allow the evidence of your power, mysterious and concealed in the intricate recesses of your concept center, to show itself sufficiently to at least encourage the forlorn maidens of that deserving State. For ourselves and the West we ask nothing. We are deeply cognizant that the steamship companies are supplying a demand for husbands in "wooly" sections of our country, by dumping in the refuse of semi-civilized Europe, and that they will continue to do so until restrained by Congress, or until they have exhausted the pauper and criminal supply of the Old World, the degenerate Old World. We know, moreover, that the decadent imported male cannot withstand the rigors of the New England climate, and that, therefore, the discouraging disproportion of females there cannot be remedied in this way. Not that there are too many females in New England, there never can be too many. They are only proportionately too many, and it is this that we ask the doctor with the secret to set right. We confess to a fear that our petition will be of no avail because the concluding sentence of the report which we quote from the *Sun* is portentous, to say the least. It reads: "The doctor is willing to impart his knowledge to families of which he is the regular physician." Let those who are tired of the sameness of sex in their progeny enroll themselves at once, for this physician will soon be the apotheosis of the family doctor and the most conspicuous type of "the busy practitioner."

THE MARINE HOSPITAL SERVICE AND THE ALABAMA SMALLPOX EPIDEMIC.

DURING the closing days of last year, the Mayor of Birmingham, seconded by State Health-officer Sanders, with the approval of the Governor of Alabama, requested Surgeon-General Wyman of the Marine Hospital Service to aid the local authorities in suppressing an epidemic of smallpox in Birmingham, Alabama. Accordingly, on December 31st, Passed Assistant Surgeon G. M. Magruder, who has had extended experience in dealing with this disease, and who managed in behalf of the Government the colony of negroes who were returning to the United States from Mexico in 1895, and among whom smallpox had broken out at Eagle Pass, Texas, was placed in charge of the undertaking. Dr. Magruder reached Birmingham January 4th, and immediately began a systematic campaign against this widespread epidemic, for it was not confined to Birmingham, but had spread into many of the adjacent counties. It had existed in Birmingham since the middle of July, and the total number of cases recorded to the close of 1897 was 406, out of which number there had been but 15 deaths. The general character of the epidemic had been mild, and the disease confined mostly to the negro population. Indeed, so mild had it been that but little attention was paid to it by the local authorities, and cases in full bloom were occasionally found in persons walking about the public streets. It was not regarded by the class affected as smallpox, but by them was called "African itch."

It appears that there are but few local health organizations in Alabama, and the execution of such laws as relate to protection of the public health is confined to judges of probate for the various districts. During this outbreak no attempts at general vaccination had been made, no restrictions placed upon persons suffering from the disease, and in the outlying counties no effort made to isolate them. As a result, in one county, Lownds, for example, the officials estimated the number of cases which had occurred at from 2000 to 2500, but it was admitted to be a mere generalization without the basis of recorded cases. Facilities for vaccination were provided by the purchase of vaccine by the authorities, who distributed it among local physicians. The lack, however, of any systematic control of cases resulted in continued spread of the disease, until the authorities had expended all the money available for prophylactic measures, and when at the end of their resources made application, as above stated, for Federal aid in suppressing the epidemic.

Dr. Magruder immediately organized a corps of thirty assistants, and with an ample supply of vaccine virus, began on January 9th, a house-to-house inspection in Birmingham, vaccinating every person when such action was indicated. This course of procedure was immediately adopted, upon the acceptance by the authorities of Birmingham and Jefferson County of aid from the Government. A lazaretto was established upon a military basis, and communication between it and the town was rendered impossible. From January 9th to January 26th, inclusive, 14,751 houses and 58,812 persons were inspected, of the latter 25,042 were vaccinated; 144 houses were disinfected. This work was so efficiently done that the number of cases occurring in Birmingham and other localities in Jefferson County was reduced from seventy per week, as reported on January 15th, to eighteen per week as reported on February 5th. Two house-to-house inspections were made in Birmingham, and a third partial one followed.

It is to be noted that the smallpox exists in the mining districts of Kentucky and Tennessee, and the origin of the epidemic in both States was undoubtedly due to the migration of the negroes employed in the mines of Alabama to similar localities in the two States mentioned.

Information has been received of the prevalence of the disease in at least twenty-five localities in Alabama. The attention of the State health-officer has been called to these facts, but it is said that he has no State funds with which to meet the emergency. It is obviously the duty of each locality to protect itself from the spread of this well-understood epidemic disease; whatever action is taken by the Marine Hospital Service is with a view to prevent its spread to adjoining States. Dr. Magruder, with two or three officers of the Service, acting on orders from Surgeon-General Wyman, is visiting in succession the infected localities and instructing the local authorities how to act. In several instances he has induced the county and town officials to bestir themselves and raise the necessary funds, which it would seem the State health-officer should have done. Expenditures for vaccine and inspection service have been assumed by the general Government only when all other means of meeting them have failed, and only as a part of interstate quarantine procedures.

FAIR CRITICISM AND COMMON SENSE.

THERE is no danger of any misunderstanding among the readers of the MEDICAL NEWS as to its position upon the question of the contagiousness of pulmonary tuberculosis and the importance of placing that disease among those requiring hygienic control. Nor can the strained, artificial efforts of the *Philadelphia Medical Journal* avail to place the MEDICAL NEWS in a false light upon this subject. The readers of the former journal, as well as those of the MEDICAL NEWS, like fair play and honest criticism, and when a contemporary sneaks in at the back door, snatches a sentence from its legitimate connections in a book review, and sets it up as the complete embodiment of editorial creed upon a grave pathologic and hygienic question, some other motive is apt to be ascribed to the act than an honest seeking after truth or the promotion of ordinary ethics. The motive is not far to seek, and the method is not such as becomes honorable criticism.

The medical profession that has read or that may read the quoted sentence as used by the reviewer in discussing the excellencies of Dr. Meigs' volume on the "Origin of Disease" (MEDICAL NEWS, February 26, 1898, p. 287) will not consider itself besmirched by epithets or saddled with false motives. A little common sense is all that is necessary to keep the judgment clear on those points, and he errs grievously who denies the medical profession its share of that commodity—as our contemporary apparently does.

ECHOES AND NEWS.

Cameron Prize Awarded.—The Cameron prize of the University of Edinburgh has been awarded to Professor T. R. Fraser for his researches in practical therapeutics.

Measles on English Warship.—An extensive epidemic of measles is prevailing among the cadets on board the English training-ship "Britannia" at Dartmouth, England.

"Black Blister" in India.—According to the daily papers, an epidemic of "black blister" has broken out in the State of Hyderabad, and fifty deaths are occurring daily.

A Donation to the Pasteur Institute.—The Pasteur Institute of Paris has received a donation of 50,000 francs from Madame Emile Durand, to be used to promote the study of tuberculosis.

For the Neuralgia of Herpes Zoster.—The pain of both the prodromal and the post-eruptive stages is said to be relieved by the administration of lactophenin in 20-grain doses three times daily.

Dispensary Bill Favorably Reported.—The Senate Committee on Public Health has reported favorably the dispensary bill for New York City, which is designed to prevent the abuse of charity at such institutions.

Biography of Ernest Hart.—The widow of the late Ernest Hart is collecting the correspondence of her husband, together with information bearing upon his public work, to be used in preparing a biography of this distinguished man.

Medical Students in New York.—The recently issued annual report of the Board of Regents of the State of New York shows that there are 4025 students of medicine in the State, an increase of 150 over last year, and a gain of 605 within three years.

Dissecting in Paris.—According to the *Gazette des Hôpitaux* (Paris) there is a great scarcity of dissecting material in the medical schools of the French capital—less than half a body for each of the 1573 students who have been dissecting there this winter.

The Tarnier Prize.—By the will of the late Professor Tarnier a yearly income of 5000 francs is left to the Paris Academy of Medicine. Of this, 3000 francs is to form a prize to be known as the Prix Tarnier, which is to be awarded each year for the best work in obstetrics and gynecology.

New York Medical College and Hospital for Women.—Plans have been filed for a building to be erected on the north side of One Hundred and First Street, near Manhattan Avenue, for the New York Medical College and Hospital for Women. The building will be three stories in height, and will cost $28,000.

Retirement of Dr. Playfair.—Dr. W. S. Playfair will soon retire from the duties of the chair of Obstetric Medicine and the Diseases of Women at King's College, London, as he has reached the age limit. Dr. Playfair has been connected with King's College and King's College Hospital for the past thirty-five years.

Smallpox in Greenfield, Mass.—Several cases of smallpox have been reported in Greenfield, Mass., and fears are entertained that the disease will become epidemic. A joint meeting of the board of health, selectmen, and physicians of the town has been held to decide upon measures for stamping out the disease.

Disinfection with a Vengeance.—It is announced by the publishers of a daily paper in an English town in which smallpox is epidemic, that each copy of the paper "is impregnated with a vaporous disinfectant which not only sterilizes the journal, but converts it into a factor for the widespread distribution of disinfecting influence."

Memorial to Two Naturalists.—A brass tablet has been placed in the biological laboratory of Johns Hopkins University in memory of James Ellis Humphrey, associate professor of botany in that university, and Franklin Story Conant, Bruce Fellow of the university, both of whom died in Jamaica last summer, where they were engaged in making botanic studies.

Klondyke Doctors Must Pass Examination.—According to the *Medical Sentinel*, medical men, who are planning to go to Klondyke in the hope of making a fortune by the practice of their profession, will find that they will not be permitted to practise unless they have passed an examination before the Board of Medical Examiners of the Northwest Territory at Calgary, of which Dr. Britt of Banff, N. W. Territory, is Registrar.

Serum Treatment of Burns.—Tomasoli, an Italian dermatologist, is treating extensive burns by daily injections of an artificial serum composed of a solution of sodium chlorid and sodium bicarbonate with the most excellent results. In an article in the *Monatsschrift für practische Dermatologie*, Tomasoli states that serum from a scalded dog will kill a well one if injected into his veins, but that the fatal result can be prevented by an injection of the artificial serum just described.

State Hospital for Consumptives.—The Senate Committee on Public Health, to which was referred the resolution relating to the establishment of a State hospital in the Adirondack Mountains, New York, for the treatment of pulmonary tuberculosis, has recommended that a joint committee of five, two from the Senate and three from the Assembly, be appointed by the Legislature to make further investigation of this subject; that $1000 be appropriated to meet any necessary expenses of such investigation, and that the committee report its conclusions and recommendations to the next Legislature.

New York Sanitary Code.—A general amendment to the New York Charter, relative to the public health, was recently introduced into the Legislature. It provides that new provisions, amendments, or additions to the sanitary code shall be proposed by the Board of Health and submitted to the Council of the City of New York. Within thirty days the Council shall take a vote upon the adoption of said provisions, and, if adopted by a majority, they shall become law. The present sanitary code shall be submitted, within sixty days after the passage of this act, for adoption or rejection by said Council.

Hospital for Ruptured and Crippled Must Sue City for Funds.—Comptroller Coler is withholding the appropriation of $26,250 made by the Board of Apportionment to the New York Hospital for Ruptured and Crippled upon the ground that the institution has been overpaid $59,169.80

by the city for the board and care of pay-patients. Edward W. Sheldon, counsel for the hospital, contends that the fact that the city paid $150 a year for each of these patients should not debar the hospital from receiving some money from them inasmuch as it costs the institution $250 a year to care for each. Comptroller Coler refuses to pay over the money, and has advised the hospital to bring a friendly suit against the city, saying that the hospital has a right to the money set aside for its use unless the city should show a counter-claim based on the report of the Commissioners of Accounts.

President of Health Board Resigns.—Nathan Straus, president of the New York City Board of Health, sent his resignation to the Mayor on the third inst. In less than an hour Colonel M. C. Murphy was sworn in to fill the vacancy. Mr. Straus, who is interested in a number of business enterprises, pleaded in his letter of resignation that his private business required so much of his time that he found it impossible to continue longer in the service of the city. It is hinted, however, that Mr. Straus' resignation is due to the refusal of the Board of Estimate and Apportionment to allow him sufficient funds to carry on the work of the department according to the accustomed standard. Colonel Murphy was born in Limerick, Ireland, in 1841, and has lived in this country since he was seven years old. He was educated at the public schools, and afterward worked in the composing-room of a daily paper in New York City until the breaking out of the Civil War, through which he served. He was elected to the Legislature in 1866, and for fourteen years represented the lower district of the city in either the Senate or the Assembly.

A New Building for the New York Skin and Cancer Hospital.—On March 5th the New York Skin and Cancer Hospital dedicated and opened for occupancy its new building at the corner of Second Avenue and Nineteenth Street. Addresses were made, there was music, and tea was served by the women of the reception committee. The building is devoted exclusively to cancer and diseases of the skin. The new hospital easily provides seating capacity and treatment-rooms for more than one hundred in its dispensary, and the wards and private rooms are large enough to contain forty-two beds, and at the same time accommodations for the staff and employees. It is the only hospital in the country devoted exclusively to cancer and skin diseases. The new operating-room is spacious and well-lighted, and connected with it are an etherizing-room, an instrument-room, wash-room, and doctors' dressing-room. There is also a well-equipped microscope-room for study, and arrangements for photography. The bath system has an especial value for this hospital. The new building has an equipment of baths unique even among all the luxuriously fitted up and recently built hospitals in the country. Russian and medicated baths, constructed on the best models for cleanliness and efficiency, have been put in to supplement the ordinary baths, and the bath-rooms and appurtenances look particularly pure and inviting, being fitted up in marble, mosaic, and white enameled iron.

The Patent on Antipyrin Expires in July.—In July of this year the antipyrin patent, held by the Hochst colorworks, will expire by limitation, it having run its course of fifteen years—the span of life allowed to a German patent. During these fifteen years the monopolists have sold the drug at about $12.50 a pound, but it will, of course, fall considerable in price the moment the manufacture and sale are permitted to competitors. It is anticipated that the price will shortly fall to at least half its present standard, when the usual convention of the principal competitors will probably be called and the inevitable trust formed, leading to a consequent rise in price. It is rumored that a number of chemical works are busy with the manufacture of antipyrin, so as to be prepared with it immediately upon the expiration of the patent.

A New Measure.—A measure which forbids the general distribution of pamphlets, circulars, and other advertisements in which symptoms of diseases are described, is now pending before the Ohio Legislature.

Chloroform Anesthesia by Gaslight.—An unusual accident recently happened in the Catholic Hospital at Herne, in Westphalia. A man who had been shot in the abdomen was brought to the hospital at night and immediately operated upon by gaslight. The operation was very difficult, and the chloroform narcosis was kept up for four hours. As a result of the decomposition of the chloroform by the gaslight, producing powerful chlorinated vapors, two of the surgeons and several of the Sisters of Mercy were overcome, and one of the latter has since died.

Paris Hospitals and the X-Ray.—The Municipal Council of Paris is considering a proposition for the establishment of a radiographic service in each of the hospitals under the control of the Assistance Publique, the service to be under the direction of the medical staff of the hospitals.

Insufficient Hospital Accommodation in Paris.—According to the *British Medical Journal*, the Assistance Publique can dispose of only 7529 beds in the various hospitals. On an average 1200 beds are vacant yearly, for which there are 8200 applicants in a suitable state for admission. M. Lampere, a member of the Municipal Council, advocates the establishment in the environs of Paris of a hospital with 6000 beds, all of which are to be placed at the disposal of the Assistance Publique.

The French Congress of Alienists and Neurologists.—The Congress of the French Alienists and Neurologists will be held at Angers on August 1st and the following days. The questions proposed for discussion are as follows: (1) Post-Operative Psychical Disturbances; (2) The Part Played by Arteritis in the Pathology of the Nervous System; (3) Transient Delirium from the Medico-Legal Point of View.

The X-Ray and a Suit for Damages.—Dr. Frank Boyd of Paducah, Ky., was recently sued by a patient for $10,000 damages on account of a severe dermatitis which followed an X-ray examination. The plaintiff claimed that the apparatus was carelessly employed, but a verdict was given for the defendant.

Medical Examining Board of the United States Army.—A board of medical officers to consist of Colonel Dallas Bache, Assistant Surgeon-General; Major Walter Reed, Surgeon; Major James C. Merrill, Surgeon; Captain William H. Arthur, Assistant Surgeon, and First Lieutenant Alexander N. Stark, Assistant Surgeon, is constituted to meet at the Army Medical Museum Building, Washington, D. C., on Monday, May 2, 1898, at 10 o'clock A.M., for the examination of candidates for admission to the Medical Corps of the army.

A Preventive of Seasickness.—A compressing belt which it is claimed will prevent seasickness, even in those most easily affected, is being patented by Galliano of Turin.

Fiske Fund Prize Essay.—The trustees of the Fiske Fund, at the annual meeting of the Rhode Island Medical Society, held June 3 1897, announced that they propose the following subject for the year 1898: "The Neuron Theory, as Related to Brain and Nerve Diseases, in the Light of the Most Recent Investigations." To the best essay upon this subject worthy of a premium they offer the sum of $350. Further information may be obtained of the secretary of the trustees, George L. Collins, M.D., 223 Benefit street, Providence, R. I.

Popularity of Glass Eyes.—According to a German authority the astonishingly large number of 2,000,000 glass eyes are made every year in Germany and Switzerland, while one French house manufactures 300,000 of them annually.

Water-supply of Mobile, Ala.—Dr. George A. Ketchum of Mobile, dean of the faculty of the Medical College of Alabama, professor of medicine, has a lasting memorial for his long professional career in the Gulf City's waterworks. To his energy and perseverance also is due the magnificent water-supply of the city. The water is brought from a distance of twelve miles, is pure, bright, and sparkling, and comes with satisfactory pressure. It is realized to-day that no one thing is more important for the health and welfare of a community than a good supply of agreeable and safe potable water. Dr. Ketchum has given such to Mobile, and that alone is a grander monument than stone or bronze could furnish.

CORRESPONDENCE.

OUR PHILADELPHIA LETTER.

[From our Special Correspondent.]

GLIA AND GLIOMATOSIS—BLOOD FINDINGS IN DISEASES OF THE CARDIOVASCULAR SYSTEM—AN INSTANCE OF LABORATORY INFECTION—STUDENT'S INFIRMARY AT THE UNIVERSITY HOSPITAL—NEW SCHOLARSHIPS AT THE JEFFERSON MEDICAL COLLEGE—DR. WILLIAM PEPPER—THE DECLINE OF THE TYPHOID OUTBREAK.

PHILADELPHIA, March 5, 1898.

SIMON FLEXNER, of Johns Hopkins University, during the course of some remarks on glia and gliomatosis, at the last meeting of the Philadelphia Neurological Society, expressed the opinion that the neuroglia, unlike other connective tissues, is probably derived from the ectoderm—a generally accepted view at the present time. He divided glia tissue into two types—embryonal and adult; three varieties of cells are recognized: ependyma-cells, astrocytes, and astroblasts; glia fibers are now known to be separate, and not extensions from the protoplasm of cells, as formerly believed. Speaking of the different types of glioma, Flexner remarked that this growth is now known to be wholly distinct from sarcoma, and that the type of the tumor is dependent upon the type of cells which predominate in it. One variety contains a majority of astroblasts; another variety is chiefly made of astrocytes, and a third variety is composed mostly of ependyma-cells. Rapidly growing tumors show no differentiation between the cells and the fibers, and correspond to the embryonic type; while to the adult type belong those tumors of slower growth which show a differentiation between the fibers and the cells. Gliomatosis was considered in the light of a fault in development, and the relationship between gliomatosis and syringomyelia was thought possible of demonstration by future investigators.

Stengel, at the last meeting of the Pathological Society of Philadelphia, gave an interesting summary of the blood-findings in diseases of the cardiovascular system. These diseases he classed as inflammatory, degenerative, and mechanical. In the inflammatory type the chief characteristics of the blood consist in a variable degree of leucocytosis, reduction in the number of erythrocytes per cubic millimeter, and in the inconstant presence of certain pathogenic micro-organisms. The speaker mentioned, in passing, two instances of a very high percentage of polymorphous neutrophiles in leococytosis—the percentage of these cells in one instance constituting no less than ninety-nine per cent. of the total leucocytes, and in the second instance, 98.5 per cent. In the degenerative type, particularly when there is an accompanying atheroma, the blood examination may reveal the presence of small bits of foreign matter, and of oil-droplets. Concerning the mechanical type, important changes due to inspissation and dilution of the blood are found; very high counts are sometimes present, due to an increased viscosity of the blood and to peripheral stasis. Mitral lesions frequently produce counts of from five to seven million erythrocytes to the cubic millimeter, but a normal or subnormal count is more common in aortic disease.

The infection of bacteriologists while working with virulent cultures is so rare, in spite of the risks sometimes taken, that an instance of genuine self-infection with the Klebs-Löffler bacillus, reported by Riesman in the current number of the *Philadelphia Medical Journal*, is of no little interest. Briefly, the instance reported is as follows: A well-known Philadelphia bacteriologist, while transplanting with a pipet measured quantities of virulent cultures of diphtheria from one flask to another, accidently received some of the culture directly into the back of his mouth; he spat out the mouthful of culture, and, without even rinsing his mouth with water, continued his work for the day. Two days later he noticed a white patch on both tonsils, from which cultures were then made, and a pure growth of the diphtheria bacillus obtained. Four thousand units of diphtheria antitoxin were then injected, 2000 during the morning, and a like quantity during the afternoon; and the next day 2000 units additional were given, with the final result that the membranous patches became smaller, and disappeared on the fifth day. During the appearance of the membrane there were no marked subjective symptoms. Notwithstanding local application of hydrogen dioxid and other antiseptic agents after the fifth day of the infection, cultures from the surfaces of the tonsils continued to show the presence of diphtheria bacilli for a period of almost three weeks after the total disappearance of all local signs. The incident, apart from its interest as an unusual occurrence, is of some value in determining the period of incubation of diphtheria, which in this case was certainly not more than forty-eight hours, nor less than forty hours. However, the value attached to this point must be more or less modified by the circumstances surrounding the infection, particularly the exceptional virulence of the culture and the quantity and the purity of the infecting agent—all of which conditions would tend to produce evidences of infection more quickly than had the exposure been an ordinary one.

The Provost of the University of Pennsylvania has announced that the various classes of that institution have united to contribute to a fund to provide a special ward in the University Hospital for the exclusive use of the students of the University, who may require hospital care in time of illness or disability. The ward will be known as the "Student's Infirmary," and will be fitted up as soon as the requisite funds for the purpose have been collected.

By the will of the late Dr. Francis W. Shain, who died in Jersey City in 1896, two scholarships, to be known by the donor's name, are to be established in the Jefferson Medical College. These scholarships are to be awarded by competitive examination in the English branches to graduates of the public schools of this city. The sum of $3000 is also left to the Jefferson trustees, the interest of which is to constitute three annual prizes to be awarded to the graduates passing the best examinations in practice of medicine, in surgery, and in physiology, respectively.

Dr. William Pepper, who has been spending several weeks in the South, is expected back next week. The indisposition from which he suffered has been wholly removed by his enforced rest, and he will enter upon his professional duties immediately upon his return.

There has been a decided decrease in the number of new cases of enteric fever during the past two weeks, so much so that hopes are now entertained that the present outbreak has about run its course, and that the city will now settle down to its "normal" number of weekly cases—normal for Philadelphia, but abnormal, decidedly so, for other communities. During the week of March 5th 122 new cases of typhoid were reported to the Philadelphia Board of Health, during which period 17 deaths occurred from this cause. For the week ending February 26th, 141 cases, with 21 deaths were reported. Meanwhile, Councils wrangle over what is popularly known as the "water-snake" bill, or the proposition made by a syndicate to furnish the city at prohibitive terms with a supply of filtered water. The "snake" will probably have been killed by the time these lines are in print, for although it passed with a rush through one branch of Councils, the career of this most extraordinary measure was blocked by some of the more honest members of the other branch. At all events the mayor is pledged to veto the steal should it manage to receive a majority of votes in both branches of Councils. Diphtheria is again on the increase, and measles is everywhere. Of diphtheria, 86 new cases, with 26 deaths were reported this week, as compared with 71 cases and 17 deaths last week. There were 41 new cases of scarlet fever this week, with 2 deaths, against 45 cases, with a single death, last week. And in spite of infection of every sort, in all quarters, Philadelphia may call herself a healthy city, as evidenced by the death-rate reported for last year, recently noted in these columns.

OUR BERLIN LETTER.

[From our Special Correspondent.]

THE EMPEROR'S BIRTHDAY—REACTION AGAINST ANIMAL EXPERIMENTATION BY CLINICIANS—DRINKING-WATER AND THE PRESERVATION OF THE TEETH—THE PASSING OF LANDRY'S PARALYSIS.

BERLIN, March 2, 1898.

ON January 27th Berlin celebrated the Kaiser's thirty-ninth birthday in most loyal fashion. The crowds who gathered near the palace at all times during the day, but especially in the evening, to catch a glimpse of him, were an evident sign of the high esteem in which he is held by most Germans. It has become the fashion for the foreign press generally to belittle him, to point out his overweening vanity, his thorough self-conceit, and his absorption in his own interests and in those of his family. Most of us foreigners who come here have such impressions. Medical men are apt to know something of certain physical defects of the emperor, and to consider them but signs of an organic degeneracy underlying his mental peculiarities. It is quite the fad for the American and English political press to talk in this strain.

I cannot help but think that most of us change our minds when we have learned to appreciate his actions a little better. Instead of absorption in self, one learns to see in him a lively interest in everything that interests the great German nation. He thinks so much of German language, literature, and science, that any personal inconvenience to which he may be put for the encouragement of these seems to count as nothing to him. Medical men who observed his graciousness at the reception to the members of the Leprosy Conference must have been impressed with his lively interest in anything that might protect his people or redound to the glory of German science.

He knew enough of the subject to talk pleasantly, yet interestingly and interestedly, with the representatives of the various nations. He had the tact to spend a notably longer time with the French representatives than with others. He won everybody by his uncondescending graciousness. There is a personal magnetism about the man which makes those who come in contact with him almost involuntarily do him honor. He went down to Hungary not long ago, where, as a rule, Germans are cordially hated, and completely won the youth of the Hungarian University. The relations between the countries have taken on quite another aspect since. He has not consented to occupy the place of innocuous retirement that somehow it has come to be thought the ruler of a constitutional monarchy should occupy. He has felt the responsibility of the duties devolving upon him, and has endeavored to show his interest in the vital processes going on in his empire. Duty seems ever to have been a precious word to him, as he has been a model husband and father. His duties as head of the state have involved his public assumption of faculties of state that seemed to thrust him too much into the foreground. He is the head, however, of one of the best-governed countries in the world, and his manifold interests are furthering its development in wonderful ways. Millions are spent on the army and navy, but millions too for the University and a new Charité.

Much more might be said, but at least this must be added: a medical man who has studied a little closely the evident purpose of the emperor to be what he is supposed to be—a ruler of his people—cannot but protest against certain utterly false views in regard to him which seem to prevail among foreign medical men. He is a German of the Germans, but, instead of the weak-minded prince with delusions of grandeur that an English press, jealous, perhaps, because their male rulers for a century have been anything but presentable, would picture to us, he is an eminently sane, thoroughly responsible monarch, from whom every, even the slightest, interest of his empire claims attention.

In certain quarters here in Europe a reaction against animal experimentation is evidently setting in. This department of biology has its place, but that place is evidently not the laboratory of the clinical professor of medicine, nor always of surgery, either. In the hands of the physiologist, animal experimentation has led to some of the great discoveries, but only when a thorough knowledge of comparative physiology enabled the experimenter to properly appreciate how much the results of experiments on animals could be applied to human beings, and how much was utterly inapplicable. Even in the hands of professed physiologists it has been the source of a good deal of error, because it was often unwarrantably assumed that observations made on animals would hold good in men.

In the recent rapid progress of medicine the quest for the new has led workers in all departments into the apparently rich field of animal experimentation. Discoveries of drug effects seemed easy, and organic changes of the most varied kinds were artificially produced, and then their mode of origin suggested as the explanation of analogous processes in human beings. With usually no knowledge of comparative physiology to guide them, and too often the spirit of acquiring cheap notoriety to urge them to publication, it is no wonder that animal experimentation, except under proper safeguards, is coming into disrepute. This state of affairs is unfortunate, because it constitutes the best argument of the antivivisectionists, though the abuses which have crept in can in no way lessen the value of the great discoveries which physiologists have made by the proper use of vivisection.

Professor Von Jaksch, in his latest work on "Intoxications," in Nothnagel's Series, takes care to say that none of his conclusions are founded on observations made on animals, and within this last month or two I have heard at least three university medical professors decry the invasion by animal experimentation of so-called clinical medicine. A prominent journal of "Clinical Medicine" (*sic*) here in Germany, within the last couple of months published an ordinary-sized number of 150 pages, containing three articles with the following titles: "Physical and Chemical Examinations of the Osmotic Pressure of Animal Fluids," "The Law of the Excentric Position of the Long Tracts in the Spinal Cord," and "The Effects of Thyroid Preparations on the Animal Organism." If at some future day such a journal is to be taken as an index of the interests of clinicians in our day, verily, it will be thought that the rich field of clinical, *i. e.*, bed-side observation, had been abandoned for the fantastic theorizing or seductive illusions of animal experimentation.

Dr. Röse of Munich found in examining recruits that the state of preservation of the teeth seemed to depend to a great extent on the salts in solution in the drinking-water of the part of the country from which they came. Most of the recruits who came for examination were from the country districts, so that a good many of the factors that lead to early decay of the teeth in cities—the sudden change from hot to artifically cold foods and drinks, from the very sweet to the very acid, and, in general, the excessive consumption of sweets and acids could be eliminated. He thought that under these circumstances he could set it down as a general law that, the harder the water of a district, *i. e.*, the more calcium and magnesium salts it contains in solution the better the teeth of the inhabitants; while, on the contrary, the softer the water, *i. e.*, the more free from these salts, the worse the teeth. Dr. Röse thought that he could tell from the color of the inhabitants' teeth how much lime there was in the water of the neighborhood they lived in.

This generalization was not readily accepted. It was pointed out that too few observations had been made to admit of any widely applicable conclusion. There comes now from Sweden a rather startling confirmation of it. Swedish dentists, from the statistics of some 2000 patients from all over the country, collected by Förberg, agree that the rule is a true one, and that the preservation of the teeth depends on the lime salts in the drinking-water. If so, it is probable that other bony structures are subject to the same influence, in which case observation may lead to some important influences as to fracture idiosyncrasies and certain other conditions of the bony skeleton of which little is known.

Landry's paralysis, acute ascending paralysis as it has also been known, is at present, it would seem, in an eclipse. Whether it will ever emerge from the darkness again remains to be seen. Neurologists and clinicians all speak of it in a very dubious way, and many of them deny its independent existence. The symptom complex under which it masqueraded for a time is now known to belong more properly to a peripheral neuritis, beginning at the ends of the extremities and gradually invading larger and larger nerve trunks. It is said that all the cases of so-called Landry's paralysis may be included under this head, and cases of the disease in which the peripheral nerves were examined always showed neuritic changes. As to the other pathologic alterations found in the nervous system after death from the disease, they are too varied, too little connected with one another, and too often contradictory of one another to furnish a genuine pathologic basis for an independent disease.

TRANSACTIONS OF FOREIGN SOCIETIES.

Paris.

PREVENTION OF DEATH FROM AIR-EMBOLISM — MARKED LEUCOCYTOSIS IN INFANTILE PERTUSSIS—THE BACILLUS OF RHEUMATISM—RESTITUTION OF THE MUCOUS MEMBRANE OF THE URETER AND BLADDER—ANGINA DUE TO STREPTOCOCCIC INFECTION AND FOLLOWED BY POPLITEAL PHLEBITIS.

AT the session of the Biological Society, January 22d, BEGOUIN spoke of the *asphyxia which follows the introduction of air into the jugular vein*, and of the means which may be employed to prevent death under such circumstances. Death is due to the accumulation of air in the right ventricle, and in rabbits and dogs artificially asphyxiated by air blown into their veins, Begouin was successful in saving life by puncturing the right ventricle with a fine, hollow needle, and aspirating the contained air. He believes that the same treatment will be followed by success in operative accidents of this character.

MEUNIER called attention to the very *marked degree of leucocytosis which exists in infantile whooping-cough*, a degree far in excess of that which accompanies other respiratory troubles. This leucocytosis appears early, before the characteristic spasms of coughing come on. The maximum, according to the blood-count in several cases, averages 30,000 white cells per cubic millimeter. The increase in white globules depends upon the lymphocytes, so that the proportion between them and the polynucleated leucocytes is inverted. Intermediate forms and eosinophiles are only slightly altered in number. This variation in the constitution of the blood is difficult to explain. It may perhaps be due to the extreme congestion of the bronchial and tracheal glands which occurs in whooping-cough.

At the session of January 29th, TRIBOULET showed the heart of a rabbit which died twenty days after inoculation with a culture of *coccobacilli obtained from the blood of a patient suffering from acute articular rheumatism*. This rabbit's heart showed typical lesions of rheumatic endocarditis, and in the veins of the mitral valve were found diplococci. There was, moreover, a thickening of the pericardial and pleural membranes, though the serous membranes of the abdomen and of the joints were absolutely unaffected. Pure cultures of coccobacilli were obtained from the blood and principal organs. Although these organisms have been found in the blood of several rheumatic patients their rôle in this disease is not absolutely determined, and the rabbit in question cannot properly be said to have had rheumatism, inasmuch as the joints were not affected.

APERT placed small quantities of blood from two patients suffering with chorea and endocarditis in tubes of anaerobic milk. One culture remained sterile; in the other, a diplococcus developed similar to that described as occurring in rheumatism.

At the Academy of Medicine, February 1st, CORNIL read a paper upon the *restitution of the mucous membrane of the ureter and bladder* after experimental incisions made in dogs. In the first animals experimented upon a ligature was placed upon the ureter, with a fistula above it, and the bladder was sutured so as to divide it into a right and left portion. The lower portion of the ureter and one-half of the bladder were thus kept free from contact with the urine. Incisions in these portions of the bladder and ureter healed perfectly even though left without suture. In another dog the upper portion of the bladder was removed, and the large omentum stitched to the cut edges so as to complete the walls of the viscus. It united without difficulty besides forming anteriorly very close adhesions to the abdominal wall, thus in a measure restoring the portion of the bladder which had been removed.

At the Medical Society of the Hospitals, January 28th, TROISIER mentioned a case of *angina due to streptococci* in a young man. A week after recovery he was seized with pain in the right leg, and again entered the hospital. He presented the symptoms of *phlebitis in the popliteal region*. This complication disappeared within about two weeks. It was concluded that an infection from the tonsil had entered the blood and set up this phlebitis. A culture made from the blood on the third day after the appearance of phlebitic symptoms remained sterile. This was, however, rather late in the course of the disease to expect to find organisms in the blood, and, moreover, streptococci are demonstrated in the blood with difficulty, even in cases of severe infection.

Vienna.

REMOVAL OF SYPHILITIC GUMMA OF THE BRAIN—RUPTURE OF THE BICEPS TENDON—BRONCHITIS WITH CONCRETIONS—USE OF LEAD PLATES TO FACILITATE THE LOCATION OF FOREIGN BODIES IN THE HEAD BY MEANS OF ROENTGEN-RAYS—ATYPICAL FORMS OF ACUTE RHEUMATISM—A CASE OF CHRONIC TETANUS—A DISCUSSION ON CHLOROSIS.

At the session of the Imperial Royal Society of Physicians of January 21st, SCHLESINGER described a case of *gumma of the cortex of the brain which had been successfully removed.* The patient had been subjected to energetic treatment with mercury and the iodids, but, nevertheless, pain and paralysis increased, and operation was, therefore, determined upon. Before operation there was paresthesia of the right side of the tongue, of the right cheek, and finally of the right upper, and later of the right lower extremity. The tumor was found to be situated partly in the anterior central, and partly in the posterior central convolution, and had a diameter of more than one inch. It was caseous and was removed without much difficulty, leaving a cavity about one-half inch in depth. The paralysis rapidly disappeared and the ability to speak was almost wholly regained within ten weeks. Schlesinger thinks that an operation of this character is indicated in those patients in whom the lesion is cortical and circumscribed, and whose symptoms are increasing in spite of antisyphilitic treatment.

At the session of January 28th, VON HOFMANN presented a male patient aged twenty-eight years who *ruptured the long biceps tendon* a year and a half previously without any serious loss of function. The typical symptoms of rupture were present, *viz.*, a depression above the belly of the biceps, an unusually marked swelling of the latter, which was also abnormally near the ulna.

MAGER exhibited a woman who, after recovery from a severe attack of pneumonia, suffered from *violent attacks of coughing*, lasting for hours, and associated *with expectoration of small concretions* covered with mucus and occasional specks of blood. Altogether about thirty such concretions had been coughed up. They consisted of calcium phosphate and calcium and magnesium carbonate. Tubercle bacilli had never been found in the sputum and the physical examination of the lungs was negative.

STOCKL described two cases in which *foreign bodies* in the head were *located with exactness by the use of the Röntgen-rays facilitated by covering portions of the head with lead plates* in order to bring out more sharply the density of the different shadows.

SINGER spoke at the session of the Medical Club of January 19th, upon *atypical forms of acute rheumatic arthritis.* Typical rheumatism is characterized by swelling of the joints and disorders of the skin, heart, and of the serous membranes, which are favorably influenced by salicylates. In 1885, Immermann called attention to certain cases of neuralgia of the trigeminus beginning with fever and accompanied with swelling of the joints and heart symptoms and which were favorably influenced by salicylates. Edlefsen called this an embryonic form of polyarthritis, and to-day we include in it certain cases of sciatica. That chorea is to be classed among the atypical forms of rheumatism is shown by the symptoms in the joints and endocardium as well as by certain bacteriologic discoveries. Moreover, polyneuritis has much in common with polyarthritis, which it often follows. The post-rheumatic muscular atrophies which owe their existence to polyneuritis must also be included in this classification. Herpes labialis and herpes zoster may also be considered, as atypical manifestations of rheumatism. Therefore the joint symptoms should be regarded as the most striking rather than the most universal manifestations of rheumatism. The most reliable symptom is fever, which is common to all forms and often extends beyond the period in which there are symptoms in the joints. The etiology of the disease lies in an infection of the blood.

PINS thought Singer went too far in describing rheumatism as an infection of the blood. The fever could be explained by an inflammation of the vessels of some particular organ.

At the session of January 26th, PINELES described *a case of chronic tetanus.* Twenty years ago the patient, at that time a girl of seventeen years, passed through a severe attack of typhoid fever which terminated in painful contractions, taking the form of tetanus. Every year since that time the tetanus recurred during the months of January, February, or March. During the last fourteen years there had been a disturbance of the stomach and intestines, manifesting itself at different periods of the year, often in the form of a persistent diarrhea. The tetanic symptoms, however, occurred during the months mentioned.

At the session of the College of Doctors of Medicine, January 24th, KAHANE read a paper upon *chlorosis.* He denied that there is any real specific for this disease, and asserted that iron is contraindicated in many cases. Iron, according to this author, acts not by supplying the deficiency of this metal in the blood, but by circulating in the blood in minute particles and irritating those organs which make blood. Recently it has been claimed that arsenic, corrosive sublimate, and phosphorus act in a similar manner. In the treatment of chlorosis stress is chiefly to be laid upon diet and hygiene. Beefsteak and red wine by no means fulfil all the indications for treatment. Rest in bed is very important. The physician should not compel the patient to eat much meat if this food is distasteful. Bavarian beer is extremely beneficial in chlorosis and is usually eagerly taken.

SOCIETY PROCEEDINGS.

NEW YORK ACADEMY OF MEDICINE.—SECTION ON ORTHOPEDIC SURGERY.

Stated Meeting, Held before the Academy, Thursday, February 18, 1898.

THE President, E. G. JANEWAY, M.D., in the Chair.

DR. T. HALSTED MYERS read the paper of the evening, entitled

NON-TUBERCULAR INFLAMMATIONS OF THE SPINE; SYPHILITIC, RHEUMATIC, MALIGNANT, GONORRHEAL, TYPHOID, INFECTIOUS, TRAUMATIC.

The author said that since the discovery of the bacillus of tuberculosis the tendency has been to ascribe to this disease the ever-increasing number of inflammatory lesions of the spine, and to consider tuberculous quite a number of kyphoses which are the result of syphilis, malignant, or infectious disease, or traumatism.

Syphilitic lesions of the vertebræ are comparatively

rare, although quite a number of cases have been reported by such authorities as Fournier, Virchow, Michel, Gross, Astley Cooper, and others, in which syphilitic lesions were found in every part of the spinal column. The cervical region is apparently the part most frequently attacked. The diagnosis presents many difficulties.

Of the rheumatic inflammations of the spine, rhematoid arthritis is the most common. This affects the bones as well as the joint structures. It is a chronic progressive disease, and is never accompanied by suppuration. Massage, suspension, and bracing are indicated, in addition to antirheumatic constitutional treatment.

Malignant disease of the vertebræ is rare, and often the diagnosis is not made until after death. Sarcoma and carcinoma appear in about equal frequency, and are generally metastatic, although both may be primary. In the latter the diagnosis is especially difficult. Pain is a prominent symptom. Motor paralysis is not always present. Affections of the spine due to gonorrhea are extremely rare. In a series of 119 cases of gonorrheal rheumatism there was no involvement of the spine in any. In 116 cases reported by Nolan, two were found in which there was arthritis of the vertebræ; in these there was also involvement of other joints.

Typhoid spine is supposed to be an inflammation of the periosteum or fibrous structures of the spine, which begins soon after the fever has subsided. The condition is not at all uncommon. The typhoid bacillus has been found in the inflammatory foci as long as seven years after the beginning of the disease.

Infectious inflammation not infrequently attacks the spine after scarlet fever, measles, tonsillitis, etc., probably by direct transmission from the throat lesions. The lesion consists of a periosteitis or an arthritis of the vertebral articulations.

Traumatic inflammation of the spinal column often stimulates Pott's disease. Fractures of the vertebræ should be carefully protected for a long period in order to prevent deformity and paralysis, and to relieve pain and disability.

DISCUSSION.

DR. C. C. RANSOM: Although it is customary in speaking of rheumatic and gouty diseases of the spine to include rheumatoid arthritis in the same category, this affection is so different in its morbid anatomy, prognosis, and treatment that it seems to me best to describe it separately.

Affections of the spine due to rheumatism and gout are of comparatively rare occurrence, and are seldom seen unassociated with involvement of some of the other joints. In nearly 1000 cases of rheumatism and gout treated at Richfield Springs, I have notes of only three or four in which the intervertebral joints alone were involved. The lower dorsal and upper cervical regions are the seat of the disease, which is usually of the subacute or chronic type, and differs in no respect from that which affects other joints. We frequently see individuals predisposed to rheumatism or gout who more or less suddenly develop pain and tenderness in these regions with a varying degree of stiffness and rigidity. A careful examination, however, discloses the fact that the affection is muscular and not arthritic, and the process is, as a rule, of much shorter duration. The tenderness in the true arthritic cases is elicited only on deep pressure, and the pain on movement, while usually quite severe at first in both affections, will disappear more rapidly on continued movement in the muscular type of the disease. In protracted cases of the joint affection a considerable deformity will sometimes occur, with complete immobility due to contracture. This can be almost entirely overcome, especially in young subjects, by judicious exercise and proper treatment. Changes in the cartilaginous or osseous structures of the joints are exceedingly rare, and it is only in very exceptional cases, and in patients of advanced years, that permanent changes in the ligaments—the so-called "fibrous anchylosis"—occurs.

Not much difficulty should be experienced in making the diagnosis of rheumatism or gout of the spine. From muscular rheumatism, the chronicity of the trouble, and usually the involvement of other joints, together with the deep-seated tenderness, will suffice for purposes of differentiation. From rheumatoid arthritis, the absence of deposit above the articulations, together with the characteristic deformities of the other affected joints in this disease, and the accompanying atrophy, will aid in making the diagnosis. The absence of tenderness on vertical pressure, as the jarring in walking, etc., is sufficient to distinguish it from spinal caries.

In the treatment of these cases the general methods usually employed in rheumatism and gout will be found to give good results. Specific remedies, such as the salicylates, iodid of potassium, and colchium, may be used in the more active stage of the disease for the relief of pain and some of the more distressing symptoms, but to cure the affection dependence must be placed upon general tonic and hygienic treatment, which latter will include hydrotherapy, properly conducted exercise, and massage. Of the tonics, iron, arsenic, and the hypophosphites are of the greatest value, and in my experience it is only in very exceptional cases that these remedies do not do good. Of hydrotherapeutic measures, general baths of natural mineral waters, followed or combined with the local douche over the spine, or alternating hot and cold water with varying pressure, will be found of great service. In all cases properly conducted massage is of benefit. This should begin with light movements over the painful area, working outward from the spinous processes, and followed by vibratory movements and passive motion. As soon as the pain on motion has sufficiently subsided to permit active movements, these should be instituted, and a proper form of active exercise prescribed and regularly carried out. In matters of diet the same rules should be followed as in all cases of gout and rheumatism, bearing in mind the fact that in matters dietetic every individual is a law unto himself.

Rheumatoid arthritis affecting the spine is of much more frequent occurrence than the foregoing, and more serious as to its depressing influences and unresponsiveness to treatment. In elderly men, especially, it is not uncommon to find this disease affecting the intervertebral joints alone, and most cases of senile kyphosis are probably due to this affection. In younger individuals the involvement of the spine is almost always an accompaniment of the disease in other joints, and, indeed, this articular tendency is one of the characteristic and distinctive features of the disease. It may begin with more or less pain in the joints following exposure to cold or wet, and in these cases it very much resembles an attack of subacute rheumatism, but, as a rule, the onset is very gradual. The upper cervical and lumbar intervertebral joints are the ones usually affected, although the disease may appear in any region and involve the entire spinal column.

In rheumatoid arthritis structural changes takes place in the affected joints from the very onset of the disease. As a result of the bone changes and curvatures the entire column becomes shortened and the surrounding muscles atrophy. Except in the early stages of the disease, the diagnosis presents no difficulties. In the beginning it may be confounded with chronic rheumatism, but the involvement of other joints, and the beginning deformity and muscular atrophy, are sufficiently distinctive. The disease rarely tends to shorten life, except in severe cases in which great deformity may give rise to pressure upon the cord. There is very little to offer in the way of treatment. The progress of the disease must be checked if possible. The classic remedies used in rheumatism and gout have little if any effect, and with the exception of iodid of potassium, they are, in my opinion, more apt to do harm than good. Above all other drugs, the tonics, such as iron, arsenic, phosphorus, and the hypophosphites, will be found of value. The diet should be simple, but very nourishing. Hydrotherapy is of value for its general effect. Massage is also beneficial in restoring healthy activity of the tissues, but it should be used with great care and only upon the muscular tissues, the joints being left alone.

Dr. V. P. Gibney: Malignant disease of the vertebræ is a condition very interesting to both the specialist and general practitioner because of the peculiarity of the symptoms presented and the difficulty in making the diagnosis. Dr. Myers has said that the latter is usually made by autopsy. I think this is going too far, for in many cases the diagnosis may be made before death. The severity of the symptoms is so great and the pain in some regions so acute and persistent that their significance is often recognized. Malignant disease should be suspected if a cicatrix is found in the mammary region, giving evidence of a previous amputation of the breast—a fact which is often concealed by the patient. Carcinomatous disease of the vertebræ presents much the same features as sarcoma. The deformity is very slight. The severe pain in these cases may be referred to the terminal branches of the nerves. Treatment nearly always fails to give relief.

There is one other condition of the spine which the author has not mentioned, and that is spinal irritation. This is a common disorder, and there is often present an irregularity of the spine which is apt to lead one to believe that the condition is one of caries. Tenderness over the spinous processes will be present, however, and this is rare in Pott's disease, especially in children.

We are not apt to look for tuberculous disease of the spine in adults, although it may occur. I have sometimes thought that the diagnosis might be determined by the employment of tuberculin, though few investigations have been made in this direction.

Dr. W. R. Townsend: I wish to call attention to the fact that these non-tuberculous affections of the spine are rare as compared with those of tuberculous origin. It has been said that but three examples of infected spine have been found in a series of one thousand cases. My experience bears out this statement. Syphilitic disease of the spine is rare. When it does exist, the disease is generally inherited. In rheumatic diseases of the spine the character of the kyphosis will usually determine the diagnosis, for there is not apt to be a distinct projection or much destruction of bone.

Dr. Samuel Lloyd: In regard to traumatic conditions of the spine there are two which may readily be mistaken for tuberculous disease. The first is that in which injury has resulted in tearing of the spinal muscles, hemorrhage, and possibly infection at a later date. Some years ago I saw a child in which this condition existed. There was a history of injury followed by comparatively rapid interference with the motions of the spine, paralysis below the point of injury, anesthesia, and rectal and bladder symptoms. The trouble was supposed to be due to compression, but in a short time inflammatory symptoms developed, the rigidity extended up the spinal column, and the case presented the picture of tuberculous spine. Operation was performed, and an ordinary abscess was found in which there was a blood-clot that had caused pressure on the spinal cord. The child recovered.

The other condition which simulates tuberculous disease of the spine is partial dislocation or fracture of the vertebræ caused by a heavy body falling upon the spine. I saw such a case in which this condition was mistaken for tuberculous disease and treated as such. An injury had been received, but it was thought to be a sprain which resulted in a tuberculous process. The patient improved somewhat under treatment, but later received another injury of the spine and became paralyzed. I was able to make out a partial dislocation of the eleventh dorsal vertebra which formed the apex of a kyphosis. I advised against operation and the man died with the usual symptoms of exhaustion following destruction of the spinal cord. Autopsy showed that there was an old unrecognized dislocation and that the inflammatory material thrown out at the time of the first injury had been torn apart by the second, thus allowing still greater dislocation of the bone. In such cases the diagnosis depends upon whether or not crepitus can be obtained. It is difficult to determine whether there is only rupture of the ligaments or whether partial dislocation or fracture has occurred, especially when symptoms of compression do not at once follow the injury. I remember seeing such a case at Randall's Island Hospital. The patient left the hospital at the end of ten days, wearing a support, because it was thought that he had sustained nothing more than a sprain. Within a month he became entirely paralyzed and a distinct callus had formed at the site of the injury.

DR. R. H. SAYRE: The non-tuberculous inflammations of the spine with an anteroposterior curvature, which, associated with rickets, occur in small children, should not be overlooked. These inflammations of the joints which complicate rickets are too often attributed to tuberculosis. I have seen a number of such cases in which there was marked anteroposterior curvature of the spine and in which the symptoms presented were those of Pott's disease.

I do not think Dr. Myers mentioned the possibility of confounding erosion from aneurism with Pott's disease. I have seen two or three cases in which this occurred. There are several cases on record in which too violent suspension, the kyphosis being unsupported, was followed by death from rupture of an aneurism.

In making the differential diagnosis of syphillis of the spine the presence of multiple neuritis would be in favor of syphillis. I have seen only one such case, though in it there was a distinct syphilitic history as well as other characteristic symptoms of specific disease.

I have seen one or two cases of obscure disease of the spine in which various diagnosis were made. In one there was marked limitation of motion and decided pain. Later the inflammation involved the entire spinal column, which finally became absolutely rigid. The stiffness also involved the ribs at their articulations with the spine to such an extent that respiration was seriously interfered with. The patient somewhat improved under gentle massage.

DR. B. F. CURTIS: The author has referred to malignant disease of the spine occurring secondarily to cancerous disease of the breast. I recall a case in which the right breast had been amputated a year previously for a growth the exact character of which was uncertain. Five months before the patient was admitted to the hospital she began to have pain in the back and in the right side of the chest. Examination showed practically nothing; all the organs seemed normal; there was no recurrence in the breast, and the pain was supposed to be due to neuralgia or rheumatism. Later the reflexes disappeared; the prick of a pin could not be felt below the umbilicus; there was retention of urine and involuntary discharge of feces, and, finally, complete paralysis. The pain in the back still continued, and a kyphosis developed in the mid-dorsal region. The patient was examined by a number of medical men whose diagnoses varied from secondary deposit to Pott's disease. Operation was urged, and rather against my own judgment I was induced to do a laminectomy. I found the cord slightly compressed and congested at the point of kyphosis. The sixth dorsal vertebra was softened and pressed somewhat on the anterior surface of the spinal cord. There was, however, no marked thinning of the cord at this point, and nothing to account for the severity of the symptoms. The wound healed by primary union, but the operation did not relieve the symptoms. Early in the treatment a large bed-sore developed on the sacrum, which finally became necrotic, and the patient died of sepsis on the sixteenth day after the operation.

DR. GEORGE R. ELLIOTT: While it is evident that the author of the paper wishes to avoid the strictly neurologic element in traumatic spine, I do not think it has been made sufficiently clear just what he means by the latter. I infer from his carefully prepared cases that he means spinal injuries which produce true organic lesions, and the discussion seems to bear this out. The lesson we are taught as a result of autopsies is that true organic lesions of the spinal column and cord following traumatism are not common. Lesions are diagnosticated and nothing found. The point I especially wish to make is the value of being able to differentiate the traumatic spine with a lesion from the so-called railway spine or spinal neurosis which it is not the province of this Section to discuss. When there is a distinct lesion, such as fracture of the vertebræ, laceration of ligamentous structures, extradural hemorrhage, etc. (the cord itself almost invariably escaping), there is presented a clean-cut symptom complex in the form of possible bony change, true atrophy of muscle (usually localized), true motor paralysis, distinct electric degenerative reaction, and clearly demonstrable objective symptoms which are especially valuable from a medico-legal standpoint. Recently, a patient of mine recovered damages for a spinal injury. There was atrophy of the leg to the extent of one inch, degenerative electric reaction, partial true motor paralysis of the legs, disturbances of the bladder, some external evidence of bone injury, pointing clearly to actual organic lesion of the ligamentous structures and bone, with the secondary inflammation extending to the cord. In addition to the organic changes the patient had the neurotic picture —the neurosis engrafted upon it—which alone, as we know, admits of endless neurologic speculation. Hence, I wish to repeat that the importance of searching for evidence of actual destruction due to traumatism, and the ability to demonstrate it cannot be overestimated.

DR. C. N. DOWD: Malignant disease of the breast is often followed by a recurrence in the spine. Some years ago I reported twenty-nine cases of amputation of the breast for malignant disease, and in five of these there followed distinct symptoms of carcinomatous disease of the spine. The diagnosis was not proved by autopsy, but the clinical symptoms left little doubt as to the nature of the trouble.

DR. A. B. JUDSON: In non-tuberculous disease of the spine the diagnosis is of the greatest importance. A review of the symptoms reveals many which are absent in Pott's disease, and we are thus enabled to exclude it. A diagnostic point is to be found in the fact that in non-tuberculous inflammations the symptoms are prompt in onset instead of being insidious.

DR. E. G. JANEWAY: I have seen a number of cases or carcinomatous disease of the spine. Primary malignant disease of the spinal column is rare, but its appearance secondary to the existence of the disease in the breast or elsewhere is quite common. Severe pain in the back in a patient who has had cancer can generally be attributed to malignant deposit in the spine. The diagnosis of primary new growth is more difficult, but it can usually be made by careful observation of the case. Protracted pain in the spinal column is either due to new growth, inflammatory disease, or to aneurism. One case which I recall was that of a woman who had been shot in the mouth with a blank cartridge. Stiffness of the neck and spinal paralysis developed, and the autopsy showed inflammation running down the vertebral notches, with secondary inflammation of the cord. I once saw a boy who had been kicked and who was suffering from what was supposed to be spinal meningitis. Autopsy showed necrosis of the sacrum, with the exudate outside of the dura mater but extending along the roots of the nerves.

The point brought out by Dr. Sayre in regard to aneurism is a good one. I have seen several such cases which were supposed to be tuberculous.

If is often difficult to make a correct diagnosis in the cases of spinal inflammation: for instance, in those instances in which the patient is tuberculous and presents a history of syphilis. The only way to make the differential diagnosis is to go over all the points of each disease and exclude as many as possible, not forgetting the possibility of two diseases being present in the same individual.

DR. MYERS, in closing: The differential diagnosis between syphilitic and tuberculous disease of the spine is very difficult. In the case I referred to in the paper, there was a family history which indicated syphilis, and the strong, healthy appearance of the child made me exclude tuberculosis. The patient improved under the administration of iodids and mercury.

In the cases of malignant disease which I have seen, pain has been very severe up to the time when the paraplegia became complete. Dr. Shaffer has said that he looks upon severe pain before the appearance of motor symptoms as rather diagnostic of malignant disease.

REVIEWS.

A TEXT-BOOK OF THE PRACTICE OF MEDICINE. By JAMES M. ANDERS, M.D., LL.D., Professor of the Practice of Medicine in the Medico-Chirurgical College, Philadelphia; Attending Physician to the Medico-Chirurgical and Samaritan Hospitals. Illustrated. Philadelphia: W. B. Saunders, 1898.

IT would seem that there had been a surfeit of text-books on the practice of medicine of late. Almost every teacher has within the past two years made public his methods and beliefs in the shape of a book. If all were as thorough and as complete, however, as the one under consideration, there would not, and could not be, too many. It is a work thoroughly scientific, modern in every sense, embodying and expressing Professor Anders' views, which are those of the best men in the profession.

There are some peculiar points of classification to which attention should be directed. Acute and subacute articular rheumatism are placed under the infectious diseases, and tuberculosis as well. Dr. Anders follows recent German thought, however, in considering chronic articular rheumatism different in its etiologic nature from the acute variety, and hence includes it under the group of infectious diseases of unknown etiology. The other diseases embraced in this group are muscular rheumatism, Weil's disease, Schlammfieber, and Malta fever. Mainly nervous diseases, the choreas, migraine, epilepsy, tetany, hysteria, etc., are included under Anders' classification of diseases of unknown pathology, while under the diseases of the muscles he describes the various atrophies and dystrophies. These peculiarities of classification do not mar the work in any way, expressing, as they do, the author's own views.

A very valuable feature of the work is the care taken in making the diagnosis of disease clear. Throughout the book are placed fifty-six tables of differential diagnosis, which are made with great care, and which cannot fail to be helpful to the student and practitioner. It is very evident that the hardest kind of work and the utmost watchfulness are responsible for the general excellent tone of the book. The latest bacteriologic facts and clinical investigations are to be found in its pages. Omissions are exceedingly rare. Of important ones, we have noted only that under the treatment of hemophilia the application of normal human blood to the bleeding surface is not mentioned. This is but trifling, it is true, yet it shows how quite perfect the book must be in every other respect. The spelling and terminology are those of modern lexicographers.

The book is handsomely printed on heavy paper, and the illustrations are numerous, beautiful, and instructive. They include Röntgen-ray photographs, some admirable charts of the anatomy of the nervous system, and Thayer and Hewetson's plates of the malarial parasites. The book can be unreservedly commended to student and practitioner as a safe, full compendium of the knowledge of internal medicine of the present day.

LECTURES ON APHASIA. By DR. BYROM BRAMWELL. Reprinted from the *Edinburgh Medical Journal*, July to December, 1897.

THIS brochure consists of a series of lectures which originally appeared in the *Edinburgh Medical Journal*, and which embody a number of interesting cases of aphasia that appeared in the *Lancet* during 1897. The author has put the profession under obligations by gathering between two covers his important contribution to a difficult and fascinating subject, and thus adding to its accessibility. The author is well known to his medical brethren on this side of the water, not alone because of his monumental "Atlas of Medicine" and "Diseases of the Spinal Cord," but by his contributions to many other subjects in pathology and internal medicine which his writings have illuminated. His reputation as a close observer and profound thinker will be enhanced by these lectures, which, in the opinion of the reviewer, are among the most important contributions to the subject of aphasia in the English language since the appearance of the Ross lectures, which were published in the *Manchester Chronicle* about ten years ago. Bramwell follows the teachings of Dejernie in his description of the zone of language, inasmuch as he does not regard a graphic motor center as a component of the speech area, but as a subdivision of the Rolandic cortical area to which is allocated the central representation of complex coordinated movements which are subservient to and executive of impulses starting from the speech area. Moreover, he is not a believer in the autonomous activity of the individual speech centers, the auditory, the visual, and the articulatory, but contends that finished speech is the result of the harmonious activity of these three centers, while admitting naturally that the primary revival of the word, and, indeed, the monitorship, may be assumed in different individuals by one of these centers.

This is an important advance in the conception of aphasia, and a more general recognition of it will, we believe, do much to make an understanding of the complexities of the symptom more ready.

Another very important stand taken by the author in these lectures is in reference to the unconscious education which the hemisphere opposite to that which contains the "executive" zone of language receives, and which unconscious education may prepare it for the assumption of executive function when the area intended autogenetically and phylogenetically for the speech area is destroyed as the seat of a lesion. This subject is of great importance when one is confronted with the problem of re-educating the aphasic patient.

The different varieties of aphasia are discussed in an exhaustive and lucid manner in the first few lectures, while the last lecture is devoted to an attempt at explanation of the process of education of the different speech centers, with a discussion of the mental idea of movement or action and a consideration of internal speech and thought. To him who has not thoroughly familiarized himself with the hall-marks of this most important symptom, the first lectures will most appeal, for it will be apparent to the casual and to the close reader that he must needs look far to find a more straightforward, yet withal comprehensive, presentation of the subject than in these pages.

Those who have labored with the subject of aphasia to begin to comprehend its intricacies will find in the closing chapter much that is worthy of their careful consideration. The point of view is particularly a personal one, and every student of language will look forward with pleasurable anticipation to its further elaboration in the future by the author.

CUTANEOUS MEDICINE: A SYSTEMATIC TREATISE ON THE DISEASES OF THE SKIN. By LOUIS A. DUHRING, M.D., Professor of Diseases of the Skin in the University of Pennsylvania. Author of "A Practical Treatise on Diseases of the Skin," and "Atlas of Skin Diseases." Part II.: Classification—Anemias, Hyperemias, Inflammations. Illustrated. Philadelphia: J. B. Lippincott Company, 1898.

THE high standard of this exhaustive work on diseases of the skin is maintained in the present volume, which will be received with the utmost satisfaction by the medical profession. The author has modified his earlier classification of skin diseases, chiefly in the omission of an etiologic class. The present plan consists of anemias, hyperemias, inflammations, hemorrhages, hypertrophies, atrophies, new formations, anomalies of secretion of the glands, and neuroses. Strange to say, the diseases due to parasites are included under inflammations. The anemias are disposed of in three and the hyperemias in twelve pages, the balance of the book being devoted to inflammations, eczema being the chief disease described, and occupying over one hundred pages. As regards the mycotic nature of eczema, Duhring considers it more than likely that the bacteria present are adventitious and secondary, and he is of the opinion that the views of Unna and others on the subject have not been sufficiently substantiated to warrant the microbic origin of this disease as positive. There still seems to be much difficulty in defining eczema seborrhoïcum as described by Unna, and the author claims that in typical cases this disease "may be looked upon either as a form of eczema complicated with seborrhea or as a seborrhea upon which eczema has supervened." The pathology of eczema receives adequate attention, and the section devoted to its treatment is handled in a most comprehensive and exhaustive manner, all the more recent observations and practical discoveries being touched upon.

A lengthy and elaborate chapter is devoted to dermatitis herpetiformis, and the characteristic features of this disease are discussed in a satisfactory manner. From beginning to end the book is written in the usual pleasant style of the author, and throughout it abounds in those original observations which show conclusively the result of vast experience.

The work contains many full-page illustrations, made mostly from photographs. Only the highest praise can be bestowed upon this feature of the book, and we much prefer these illustrations to many of the colored lithographs recently noted in works on the skin, though in some instances the value of chromolithographs should not be underestimated. Many of the fine histologic drawings made by Gilchrist have been introduced, and serve to illustrate the text in an admirable manner.

As a whole, the book is eminently satisfactory and thoroughly in accord with recent teachings on diseases of the skin, and we take great pleasure in commending it to all interested in the subject.

A MANUAL OF OBSTETRICS. By A. F. A. KING, A.M., M.D., Professor of Obstetrics and Diseases of Women and Children in the Medical Department of the Columbian University and in the University of Vermont. Seventh edition. Philadelphia and New York: Lea Brothers & Co., 1898.

IT must indeed be gratifying to the author of this manual of obstetrics to find edition after edition of his popular work called for; and this, too, despite the fact that within recent years several new manuals upon this subject have made their appearance. The present edition is even better than its predecessors. Throughout the work the life-saving value of aseptic midwifery is insisted upon, and in his concluding remarks on puerperal septicemia the author lays particular stress upon prophylaxis as superior to anything that may be done once sepsis has supervened. This chapter has been entirely rewritten and is absolutely modern, including an excellent discussion of the serum-therapeutics of puerperal sepsis. The chapter on extra-uterine pregnancy is particularly good, and surgical treatment of the affection is correctly insisted upon as the best. The whole work bears evidence of careful revision and is thoroughly up to date. As it always has been, so it is now, one of the safest primers of obstetrics which can be placed in the student's hands. It is thoroughly practical, concise, and modern. The publisher's work is above criticism.

MEDICAL REPORT OF THE SOCIETY OF THE LYING-IN HOSPITAL OF THE CITY OF NEW YORK. New York: D. Appleton & Co., 1897.

THIS report corresponds to our notion of what a hospital report should be. From cover to cover it is full of good things and shows unmistakably what the Lying-in Hospital is doing. That its work is scientific and, at the same time, beneficent, the perusal of this report conclusively shows. Since its foundation in 1890, 10.233 patients have been delivered by the students and instructors, with a total of 43 deaths, a record of which any institution might be proud, and when it is recalled that the vast majority of the cases treated by the hospital occur in tenement-houses, the death-rate is remarkably low.

The report contains several interesting monographs, the work being based on the service of the Hospital. Some of them are "The Premature Interruption of Pregnancy," by Clifton Edgar; "Asepsis, Morbidity, and Mortality," by Samuel W. Lambert; "Deformed Pelves," by Austin Flint, Jr.; "Placenta Previa," by George R. White; "Fractures in the New-born," by Churchill Carmalt, and the reports of the curator, orthopedic surgeon, embryologist, pathologist, and bacteriologist. The report of the embryologist, Professor George T. Huntington, consists of a "Contribution to the Topographical Anatomy of the Thorax in the Fetus at Term and in the New-born Child," and is an especially thorough and valuable scientific article. Lack of space forbids our entering into further detail concerning many vexed and interesting obstetric questions which are here discussed. The report is unique among hospital records, and should be carefully studied by every thoughtful student of obstetrics.

CENTRALBLATT FUR DIE GRENGEGEBIETE DER MEDIZIN UND CHIRURGIE. Herausgegeben von DR. HERMANN SCHLESINGER, Privat-docent an der Universität in Wien. Vol. I., No. 1. Jena: Gustav Fischer.

THIS new *Centralblatt*, under the editorship of Dr. Hermann Schlesinger, aims to supplement the journal published by the same house dealing with topics that lie in the borderland of medicine and surgery. The object of this monthly will be to sift the literature on topics coming within its range and to present it in the form of abstracts. As the editors point out, the literature of medicine has grown so enormously in recent years, that no one man can keep fully abreast of it. He hopes that this journal may aid the general practitioner, the medical consultant, and the surgeon in their reading.

The first number contains two monographs, one on the recent advances made in the study of brain abscesses of otitic origin, the other on the pathology and treatment of floating kidney. Both have appended voluminous bibliographies. The remainder of the volume is taken up by abstracts, the general nature of which will be indicated by the mention of a few of the titles: "A case of meningitis and epidural abscess with the presence of the influenza bacillus"; "Formation of renal calculi following a fall on the back"; "On tuberculosis of the kidneys"; "The limits of nephrectomy"; "The diagnostic value of catheterization of the ureters as it influences renal surgery." The new *Centralblatt* will, we hope, meet the same favor as its predecessors.

THERAPEUTIC HINTS.

For Chlorosis.—

℞ Ferri et potassii tartrat. . . . . ʒ ii
Liq. potass. arsenitis . . . . ʒ i
Aq. dest. . . . . ʒ iii.

M. Sig. Five to ten drops in a little wine three times daily before meals.—*Casale.*

Metallic Iodin in Syphilis.—BONVEYRON states that he has succeeded by the administration of large doses of metallic iodin in effecting rapid cures in very severe cases when other modes of treatment had failed. These cases presented pulmonary, cerebral, and bone lesions. He prescribed as follows:

℞ Iodi pur. . . . . gr. xv
Potass. iodidi q. s. ad. solut.
Glycerini . . . . . . ʒ iiss
Ac. citrici . . . . . . ʒ iiiss
Syr. simpl. . . . . q. s. ad. Oii.

M. Sig. Two tablespoonfuls daily, increasing by one tablespoonful daily until nine are taken each day.

For the Application of Collodion and Salves in Ophthalmology the use of a glass stirrer, with smoothly rounded tip, is suggested. This is easily cleaned and sterilized, and with it there is no danger of accidental injury to the eye.

For Acute Colic, the result of indiscretion in diet, the following is recommended:

℞ Chloroformi . . . . . . ʒ iss
Tinct. opii deodorat. . . . . ʒ i
Camphoræ . . . . gr. xv
Ol. cajaputi . . . . . . ʒ i
Aquæ . . . . ℥ ii.

M. Sig. One teaspoonful every hour or two.

For Chronic Diarrhea.—

℞ Cupri sulphat. } āā . . gr. i
Morphinæ sulphat. }
Quininæ sulphat. . . . . gr. xxiv.

M. Ft. pil. No. XII. Sig. One pill three times daily.

THE MEDICAL NEWS.

A WEEKLY JOURNAL OF MEDICAL SCIENCE.

VOL. LXXII. NEW YORK, SATURDAY, MARCH 19, 1898. NO. 12.

ORIGINAL ARTICLES.

INTUBATION IN DIPHTHERIA.[1]

BY W. K. SIMPSON, M.D.,
OF NEW YORK;
SURGEON TO THE NEW YORK EYE AND EAR INFIRMARY; INSTRUCTOR IN DISEASES OF THE NOSE AND THROAT IN THE COLLEGE OF PHYSICIANS AND SURGEONS (COLUMBIA UNIVERSITY).

IT can be said with truth that the advent of intubation for the relief of diphtheritic croup undoubtedly marked one of the greatest achievements of modern medicine, and, in connection with the present antitoxic treatment of diphtheria, has most materially lessened its mortality and robbed of its horrors one of our most fatal diseases. This can be appreciated if we consider for a moment the status of tracheotomy in its relation to croup before the days of intubation, and we cannot do better than quote the words of Dr. O'Dwyer in answering the question, "What led to the first experiment in intubation?" "Complete failure with tracheotomy in the New York Foundling Hospital, extending over a period of several years."[2]

Notwithstanding that in a certain percentage of cases of tracheotomy under the most favorable conditions recovery ensued, the horrors and difficulties incident to operation in young children, the added surgical wound, with the chances of increased infection, the skilled and laborious attention necessary in the after-treatment, and, above all, the great fatality, caused an abhorrence alike on the part of both parent and physician—to the extent that the latter gladly delayed surgical interference as long as possible, and in many quarters the operation was practically abandoned and the little ones allowed to die after the gamut of non-surgical methods had been run. I have often thought that the delay due to this great dread of tracheotomy was itself largely accountable for the fatality attending its performauce; for it was a brave surgeon who would tracheotomize in the earliest stages of laryngeal croup. It is fair to suppose that had this dread not existed and had the operation commonly been performed at an earlier stage the results would have been better. No wonder is it then that a thinking mind in constant association with diphtheritic croup and its deplorable results set about the institution of some other means for its relief; that such means were successfully put in practice, and that the unremitting paticnce and toil of the inventor were finally rewarded experience has fully demonstrated.

[1] Read at a meeting of the New York Academy of Medicine, under the auspices of the Section on Laryngology and Rhinology, March 3, 1898.

[2] O'Dwyer, "The Evolution of Intubation."

The real battle of intubation was waged and its glories won before the days of antitoxin, and had the percentage of recoveries been even less than that furnished by tracheotomy, it must not be forgotten that the simpler nature of intubation permitted its performance in hundreds of instances in which either the parents or physician would have objected to or even refused tracheotomy, thus in intubation furnishing an opportunity of at least attempting to save life, which would have been forever denied through tracheotomy. This is, doubtless, the individual experience of those who have intubated to any extent, and it receives further confirmation from the collective investigation of the American Pediatric Society,[1] in the report of which it is stated that out of 657 cases in which operation was performed there were 637 intubations and 20 tracheotomies. This is a point which has not been sufficiently emphasized in considering the great value of the former operation.

No new operation to supplant a well-grounded procedure can thrive without passing through the crucible of criticism and thorough testing, and intubation has been no exception to this rule; received, at first, both here and abroad with its measure of opposition and doubt, it may be safely said that they have been overcome, and that, in this country at least, it has rendered tracheotomy practically obsolete as a primary operation. It may always be taken for granted, in a case of general or pseudo-diphtheria, that the onset of laryngeal symptoms, *i. e.*, croupy cough, loss of voice, and impaired breathing, indicates laryngeal extension of the disease, and this at once raises the question when to intubate, and let me say here, parenthetically, that my subsequent remarks will entirely consist in a consideration of intubation and its relations to the antitoxic treatment.

The question of when to operate is always of vital importance, and especially so if for any reason antitoxin is not employed. We can recall the various opinions which have been held on this point, ranging from intubating at the very beginning of the manifestation of croupy symptoms to waiting for the

[1] "Report of the American Pediatric Society," 1896–7.

more positive condition of progression marked by recession of the extraneous muscles of respiration and signs of cyanosis.

It has been well proven by the report of the American Pediatric Society already referred to, that in sixty per cent. of the cases of laryngeal diphtheria intubation is not required, if reliable antitoxin has been properly administered at an early stage of the disease. If, however, croupy symptoms supervene and progress, the use of the antitoxin should be continued, the dosage being based upon the age of the child and the amount previously given, and at the same time the croupy symptoms should be watched, remembering that it sometimes requires twenty-four hours for the full effect of the antitoxin to be manifested; this is especially important if the symptoms of laryngeal stenosis are the first indications of the presence of diphtheria. In either event, and here the initial dose of antitoxin should be a full one, in the interval while waiting for the antitoxin effect, if the symptoms of stenosis are progressive, intubation should be immediately performed; *never*, in any instance, is it justifiable to await the approach of the severer symptoms of stenosis. After intubation the use of antitoxin should be continued on the principles already given, to be discontinued as the membrane shows a marked tendency to exfoliate, and the respiratory symptoms a tendency to disappear, and as the other general conditions, especially the pulse and temperature, resume a more normal condition.

HOW LONG SHALL THE TUBE REMAIN IN THE LARYNX?

In pre-antitoxin days the average period during which the tube was allowed to remain in the larynx was from six to seven full days. Under the present mode of combined treatment the time may be somewhat shorter, varying in different experiences from three to five days. The usual time at the Willard Parker Hospital is at present four days, and at the New York Foundling Hospital three days. Personally, in private practice, I prefer to leave the tube in the larynx during five full days if there are no indications for removing it, on the general principle of avoiding unnecessary reintroductions.

In hospital practice, where assistance is always at hand in case of emergency, there is less danger in leaving the tube in a shorter time; for, should occasion arise, it can be at once replaced. Verbal reports from the institutions mentioned do not show any comparative increase of the necessity for reintroductions between the older and the present methods of combined treatment. The duration of the disease has been so shortened by our present treatment that undoubtedly in many cases the tube may be removed earlier without the necessity of reintroduction.

The principal indications for removing the tube previous to its final removal are severe discomfort or pain from pressure, especially if the pain be radiating in character, thus indicating the occurrence of ulceration, severe attacks of coughing, and sudden stenosis due to the lodgment of membrane in the lumen of the tube. This last-named condition is, perhaps, more likely to arise earlier under the antitoxin treatment on account of the earlier exfoliation of the membrane. In some instances, however, if the membrane be sufficiently loosened to block up the tube, the latter will be coughed up with the membrane. This is especially the case with the present rubber tubes, especially if the tube does not fit too tightly. If under these circumstances the tube is expelled, its reintroduction may *not* be necessary, or at any rate, the necessity of reintroduction will, as a rule, be sufficiently delayed to permit reintroduction by the physician in charge.

In a very small percentage of cases of intubation, after the original cause of the stenosis has ceased to operate, there occurs a more or less permanent stenosis, necessitating almost constant use of the tube for a period of a few days to some months. These cases are classed under the head of "retained intubation tubes." The course and treatment of this condition is most elaborately set forth in a classic article by Dr. O'Dwyer, read before last years' meeting of the American Pediatric Society, to the report of which I refer the reader for a detailed exposition of the subject, though it requires further experience for its full elucidation, which will only come from a very careful study of the few cases that will occur from time to time.

Dr. O'Dwyer, in giving the cause and seat of this persistent stenosis, says: (1) "The cause of persistent stenosis following intubation in laryngeal diphtheria can be summed up in the single word, traumatism. Paralysis of the vocal cords may possibly furnish an occasional exception to the rule. (2) The injury to the larynx is done by a tube which does not fit properly. It may result either from an imperfectly constructed tube, or from a perfect one which is too large for the lumen of the larynx, although suitable to the age of the child, or from a tube that is perfect in fit and make if it is not cleaned at proper intervals. (3) The *seat* of the lesion which keeps up the stenosis is just below the vocal cords in the subglottic division of the larynx, or that portion bounded by the cricoid cartilage. Exceptions to this rule result from injury produced by the head of the tube on either side of the base of the epiglottis just above the ventricular bands."

Dr. O'Dwyer sums up the avoidance of its occurrence and its treatment when present in a full appreciation of its causes and the skilful use of tubes of proper size, shape, and construction, and the use of the hard rubber tube now in vogue, which can be worn indefinitely without the occurrence of the calcareous granules which appear on the metal tubes, and which may become a focus of ulceration; further, the rubber tubes at their impinging points do not produce the same degree of pressure as do the metal tubes.

TECHNIC OF THE OPERATION.

The patient should be held firmly upright on the left thigh of an assistant, whose legs are tightly closed on the patient's legs. The left arm of the assistant is thrown around the back of the patient, holding the left hand and arm of the latter, while with the right hand the assistant holds the patient's right hand. The right side of the patient is firmly held against the breast of the assistant, the left side of the patient being free. The second assistant stands back of the patient, holding the head firmly in a suspended position, and steadying the mouth gag with the left hand. There should be no twisting of the neck of the patient, who should be held perfectly straight. This cannot be too strongly emphasized, as it especially pertains to the successful introduction of the tube. The proper-sized tube having been chosen according to the scale, it should be threaded, always using braided silk of a size which will pass easily through the opening in the tube, and of a length which will permit of being looped over the patient's ear when the tube is in position, and so tied that the knot is always at a point farthest away from the tube.

The operator, standing or sitting in front and a little to the right of the patient, at a height which gives easy access to the mouth, the patient's mouth being well open and the gag on the left side, passes his left forefinger well down into the larnyx over the epiglottis until he feels the two small tips of the arytenoid cartilages, which indicate the posterior portion of the larynx. Then the introducing instrument is quickly passed down over the palmar tip of the left forefinger until the end of the tube engages in the larynx, gentle pressure being continued until the tube is well down in the larynx, when the left forefinger is transferred to the head of the tube and the obturator removed by liberating the sliding catch on the handle of the introducer. The left forefinger should remain gently pressing the head of the tube until the obturator is well out of the mouth. *Care* should be taken that the obturator is not removed in any way from the tube until the latter is well down in the larynx, thus avoiding any danger of stripping off or wounding the mucous membrane.

Successful introduction of the tube is almost immediately rewarded by relief from the difficult breathing, which becomes more and more marked as the minutes go by and the patient passes into a condition of rest which is in marked contrast to that which necessitated the operation. The means of knowing that the tube is properly placed in the larynx, are first, the relief in breathing, and second, the characteristic cough which immediately occurs and is of a moist metallic character produced by mucus and air passing through a metallic tube. This cough should always be looked for, and if not present should be provoked by the administration of a teaspoonful of diluted whisky or brandy. The character of the cough is peculiar and is far better appreciated by being heard than from any description. Oftentimes, in moribund cases, the cough may be delayed or be but feeble when it is heard. The cough is valuable in clearing the trachea of secretions, and as an indication of the firmness with which the tube is retained in the larynx.

Another way of determining whether or not the tube is in the larynx is by passing the left index-finger down into the esophagus and feeling the tube through the anterior wall of the former. This means is of great service if for any reason the breathing is not fully relieved and if it is desired to be positive as to the position of the tube. If, however, after the introduction of the tube the breathing is not relieved or becomes suddenly worse, the question of having pushed down with the tube some detached membrane is to be considered—this accident may happen, but as a matter of fact is very rare. If it were of frequent occurrence it would be a most serious objection to the operation. The reason of its infrequency is that the stenosis is not entirely due to a complete membranous cast of the larynx and trachea, through which the tube has to pass, but to lessening of the lumen of the larynx by infiltration of the submucous tissue. This can be easily observed in a cross-section of a larynx from a case of diphtheritic croup.

The accident mentioned is more likely to occur in late cases of croup in which the membrane has begun to exfoliate, and at any time when traumatism has been occasioned by the introduction of the tube. It is accompanied by excessive coughing and a flapping sound caused by the loosened membrane. If for this or any other reason the breathing is not relieved, the tube should be withdrawn by the string and the child encouraged to dislodge the loosened membrane by coughing, after which a second attempt at introduction should be made. It sometimes happens that pieces of detached membrane accompany the withdrawal of the tube. If it is reasonably certain that loose membrane is blocking the tube and is not readily expelled, a short cylindrical tube (foreign body tube) may be inserted. These tubes for a given age are much larger in caliber than the ordinary ones, and allow large masses of membrane to be expelled. Owing to their larger size they should not be left in the larynx more than a few hours on account of the pressure which they cause.

Another accident which may possibly occur is the introduction of the end of the tube into one of the ventricles of the larynx. This is obviated by using the present type of tubes, somewhat bulging on the end, which thus permits them to override the ventricles, and by keeping in the median line during introduction. Introduction of the tube into the esophagus will sometimes occur. This can be appreciated by failure to relieve the difficult breathing, and by attempts on the part of the patient either to expel the tube or by efforts to swallow. If the string is observed to be disappearing within the mouth, it is evident that the tube is in the esophagus, and it should be immediately withdrawn. This accident is an avoidable one and need not occur if the proper rules are followed. In the cases in which I have seen the tube swallowed it has been passed through the alimentary canal within from two to four days without any accident. The tube may be occasionally swallowed when coughed up by the patient.

The string should be permitted to remain in place, being passed over the left ear, until quiet breathing is restored, from fifteen minutes to half an hour, and should then be removed by cutting one side of the loop close to the mouth, taking hold of the long end, and withdrawing while the left forefinger is making gentle pressure down on the head of the tube. Never, under any circumstances, remove the string without making pressure on the head of the tube, as the string becomes twisted in the mouth and will be caught in the eyelet of the tube and the latter itself withdrawn unless the counter-pressure is made. Another very important precaution in regard to the string is that the person holding the child should never release the child's hands until the string is removed by the surgeon. Almost the first thing a child will do if the hands are released is to instinctively pull at the string, resulting, of course, in withdrawal of the tube.

It is the practice of some, in preparing the child, to tightly encase the arms and chest in a draw-sheet wrapped around tbe body. While this keeps the hands out of the way, it is open to the objection of too firmly constricting the chest, and in case of artificial respiration being necessary, much valuable time may be lost. Also, some operators prefer to introduce the tube while the patient is in the dorsal position. I have had no experience with this mode of procedure and cannot speak of its merits.

In extracting the tube the same precautions as to the position and management of the patient during introduction should be followed. The instrument for this purpose is called the extractor. Before being used, it is absolutely imperative that the thumb-screw on the under side of the instrument should be so set that the proximal jaw can open just sufficiently to exert the proper amount of pressure within the opening in the tube. If the jaws are open too widely there is great liability of lacerating the surrounding mucous membrane in ineffectual attempts at removal. It is good practice to test the degree of opening of the extractor on a tube of the same size as the one in the larynx. In extracting, the left forefinger should be passed down on the head of the tube until the opening is felt, and then the extractor, closed, is passed down until the point strikes the head of the tube and enters the opening in front of the tip of the finger. When in the opening in the tube, the jaws of the instrument are opened by thumb pressure on its handle, and the tube withdrawn, pressure being continuous until the extractor and tube are removed from the mouth. Never have the thumb on the lever until you feel sure that the end of the instrument is in the tube.

The operation for extracting is perhaps more difficult than that of introduction, as it requires a finer degree of touch to determine the opening in the head of the tube, and the difficulty is increased in proportion to the smallness of the tube. Modifications, from time to time, have been made in the head of the tube and in the extractor to facilitate removal, but the original procedure just described is the one almost universally employed. Extraction by pushing out the tube from below without any instrument may successfully be performed—if for any reason great difficulty is experienced in the application of the usual method—or in case of emergency when the tube must be removed by the nurse in absence of the surgeon. This is done by slightly inverting the patient, and, with mouth open, placing the thumb in the episternal notch and pushing the tube up in the mouth and grasping it with the fingers of the other hand or with a pair of ordinary forceps. This can be done by any one of ordinary intelligence in charge of the case, and is, under these circumstances, a most admirable method of extraction.

After removal of the tube the patient should not be left until there is sufficient evidence that the tube will not have to be replaced. A small dose of opiate may then be given to allay cough and irritation. Slight cough and hoarseness generally continue a few days to two weeks, especially the hoarseness, which, however, passes away without incident.

Feeding after intubation is best accomplished by having the child in an inclined position, the head being down. This is commonly called the "Casselberry" method. It is best performed by raising the foot of the bed, removing the pillow, and bringing the child to the edge of the bed on the side, and using for the purpose of feeding an ordinary duck-shaped feeding cup. This procedure prevents, in a great measure, fluids from entering the tube and the accompanying paroxysms of coughing. However, it is remarkable how some children, with a tube in the larynx, will readily learn to swallow in the ordinary upright position.

I consider it also very excellent practice to keep the patient in the feeding position during the entire period in which the tube remains in the larynx, in order to lessen the chances of secretions passing down through the tube, and thus, possibly, causing the development of pneumonia. The frequent removal of the tube for purposes of feeding has been advocated by some, but I think such a practice should be mentioned only to be condemned.

The food should be fluid or semi-solid, solid particles of food being avoided so as not to run the danger of large pieces being drawn into the tube. In case great difficulty is experienced in the use of the mode of feeding mentioned above, recourse may be had to alimentation through the esophageal catheter, passed either through the nose or through the mouth, or, as a last resort, rectal alimenation may be employed.

I think it most important to watch the respirations during the entire period of intubation, as bearing on the progress of the disease. If they continue about normal it is indicative of favorable progress; if they show a tendency to increased rapidity, it is indicative of extension of the membrane—fortunately, however, the latter does not occur as frequently as it did in pre-antitoxin days.

The prognosis of diphtheria under the present combined treatment is, I think, remarkably favorable, especially as compared with the results formerly obtained. A reference to this point in the report of the collective investigation of the American Pediatric Society[1] gives the mortality in cases operated upon by intubation, and in which antitoxin was administered, as 27.24 per cent. This is in strong contrast to the previous mortality which ranged from 69.5 per cent. to 75 per cent. I have no doubt but that the prognosis will continue to be even more favorable as there is gained a better understanding of the combined treatment.

In a very small number of cases it may become necessary to perform tracheotomy, in the event of failure of intubation, but when this has been done, the percentage of recoveries has been very small, and conditions have been found which could hardly be reached by either operation.

In contemplating the performance of intubation one should not rely entirely upon written description for his guidance, but should acquaint himself with the operation by practice on the cadaver. This is, I think, a *sine qua non*. The perfected tubes of the present time are made of hard rubber over metal. This, as I have said before, allows the tube to be retained longer without the occurrence of calcareous deposits. These tubes exert less pressure, and can be more easily expelled in case of plugging with membrane.

In conclusion, what can be more fitting than to dwell for a moment on the results of intubation and its teachings. In a word, it has given us a comparatively simple means of combating a fearful emergency; it has taught us exploration of the larynx by the finger; it has taught the mind and hand to work in quickest harmony; it has taught us alertness and deftness in meeting emergencies, and has opened up and created anew the treatment of the entire domain of laryngeal stenosis.

Let us then honor the memory of Dr. O'Dwyer since he left to humanity such a legacy.

[1] "Report of the American Pediatric Society," 1896-97.

INTUBATION IN ACUTE NON-DIPHTHERITIC STENOSIS OF THE LARYNX.[1]

BY CHARLES H. KNIGHT, M.D.,
OF NEW YORK.

IT is customary to consider intubation chiefly in connection with diphtheria and to lose sight of its utility in other fields, less important only because more restricted. In that division of the subject of intubation assigned to me in the present discussion much of interest may be found. My purpose is, however, to briefly enumerate some of the conditions in which intubation has been adopted, or in which it may be applicable, and to call to your attention certain points of special interest.

Edema of the glottis, as a result of injury, burns, or scalds; from swallowing corrosive liquids; from the inhalation of irritating vapors, and perhaps, occurring in the course of a phlegmonous laryngitis, or, as a symptomatic phenomenon, is a condition which often rapidly develops, and, of course, for its relief requires prompt interference. The classic mode of dealing with it, proposed by Lisfranc, namely, scarification, is associated with the name

[1] Read at a meeting of the New York Academy of Medicine, under the auspices of the Section on Laryngology and Rhinology, March 3, 1898.

of a distinguished surgeon of New York, the late Gurdon Buck, who, in an elaborate essay, graphically described this method of treatment and the relief from distressing symptoms afforded by its application. Yet, in a certain proportion of cases in which the tissue seems to be infiltrated by what has been termed a "solid edema," scarification does not suffice, the dyspnea is not relieved, and we are compelled to have recourse to tracheotomy, or to a very ancient method of successfully overcoming stenosis of the larynx, employed by McEwen and others, and that is, the passage of a catheter through the upper air track. Under these circumstances, and but for one obstacle, the ideal operation would be the introduction of an O'Dwyer tube. The area of edema may be so extensive that the tissues overhang and obstruct one or the other orifice of the tube. This is especially likely to happen in traumatic edema, and even in the idiopathic variety of the same affection the epiglottis may be so tumefied as to be the chief source of obstruction, though this may be met by combining scarification with intubation.

It is well known that the upper part of the larynx is usually the part most affected by edema, and this region is, of course, most accessible to the knife. Stenosis from swelling of the ventricular bands, or vocal bands, might be obviated by the use of the tube. Edema of the true cords is very rare. Gottstein quotes a case reported by Risch, which resulted fatally, both cords, as well as the vestibule of the larynx, being involved, and mentions having several times seen a single cord so affected as to resemble a long, narrow polypus. A case has been reported by Semon in which the process was limited to the true cords.

In a paper on "Intubation in the Adult, with Special Reference to Acute Stenosis of the Larynx," Casselberry of Chicago (*Trans. Am. Laryngolog. Asso.*, vol. xviii, p. 78, 1896) relates the history of two cases, one of probable subglottic edema or infiltration, and the other of edema of the glottis with secondary involvement of the lungs. The patient in the former case recovered after having worn a tube one week. The latter patient died during performance of tracheotomy, after failure of intubation. The second case is instructive as illustrating one obstacle to success in attempting to use the tube. The patient had a chronic spasm of the masseter muscles, which prevented opening the mouth sufficiently to permit the passage of the index-finger as a guide. Immediately after death in this case the jaws were forcibly separated, and the intubation-tube was easily introduced, at the same time the interesting fact being demonstrated that the edematous epiglottis did *not* overhang and occlude the upper orifice of the tube. This author believes that "pressure decubitus," urged by some as a contraindication to intubation in acute inflammatory edema, may be due to selection of too large a tube, and he therefore advises the use at first of the smallest adult tube. He lays down a number of rules as to the technic of intubation in adults, and among them recommends the performance of the operation under guidance of the laryngoscope in those patients accustomed to the presence of the mirror in the throat.

In the discussion of the foregoing paper Ingals expressed an opinion unfavorable to intubation in acute stenosis of the larynx in adults, although the cases he cites hardly seem to justify his conclusion.

Two cases of intubation for edema, one in a child of two years, have been recorded by W. F. Brook (*Jour. Laryngol. and Rhinol.*, vol. 8, p. 640, 1894). In the second case the passage of the tube was prevented by an enormously swollen epiglottis and the operator was about to tracheotomize when it was found that the obstruction had been relieved by laceration of the tissues during the efforts to pass the tube. The same author reports three cases of intubation for acute laryngitis in infants, and, in regard to these, remarks that in all tracheotomy must otherwise have been performed. No opposition to the operation was offered on the part of the relatives, and no difficulty was found in feeding the children; one, a four-months' old baby, taking the breast while the tube was in position. He expresses his intention to employ intubation under the following circumstances: (1) In spasm of the glottis from any cause; (2) In severe cases of laryngismus in infants; and (3) whenever the presence of a foreign body in the trachea is suspected.

In cases of the last-mentioned variety sudden and fatal spasm of the glottis may supervene even in the absence of positive evidence of the lodgment of a foreign body in the air-passage. Cases of this kind in which the foreign body is small enough to pass the lumen of the tube are included by Lefferts in his list of conditions amenable to intubation (*N. Y. Med. Jour.*, December 9, 1893).

A warm advocate of intubation is found in Feraud (Thèse de Lyon, 1898, *Jour. Laryngol. and Rhinol.*, No. 8, 1894), who maintains that it is adapted not only to the laryngeal complications of diphtheria, but to numerous forms of laryngeal stenosis, especially edema or inflammatory tumefaction. This condition is included in a list of those in which the operation is indicated by A. Rosenberg, who reports twelve cases, representing a variety of diseases thus treated (*Arch. für Laryngol. und Rhinol.*, 1893, B. I. H. 2).

The feasibility of intubation in edema of the larynx is not generally admitted. In fact, a recent writer affirms that in phlegmon of the larynx, owing to distortion of the parts, insertion of the tube would be extremely difficult, and, if put in place, its retention would be improbable. With strange inconsistency he then remarks that dyspnea is an *early* symptom, and is due to serous infiltration rather than to pus formation. The latter statement being undoubtedly correct it is hard to see why intubation should be any more difficult in this than in other forms of stenosis of the larynx. In view of the many advantages of intubation, so often recounted to us, it might be wise, the condition of the patient permitting, to give it a trial before resorting to the graver operation of opening the trachea.

Wounds and injuries of the larynx comprise a very interesting group of lesions. Obstruction to breathing may follow in consequence of the formation of a hematoma, or of emphysema, or as a result of the protrusion of a fragment of tissue into the air tract, and, in the case of fracture, a depressed portion of cartilage may occlude the larynx. So probable is the development of stenosis from one of the foregoing causes or from subsequent edema and swelling that many authorities advise preliminary tracheotomy even in the absence of urgent dyspnea. In the case of a depressed fracture of the larynx it has been proposed by Paras to support the fragment by inflating a rubber bag within the larynx after tracheotomy had been performed. Here the laryngeal tube would have the obvious advantage of supplying air to the lungs, as well as giving support to the fractured cartilages.

Spasm of the larynx in adults may occur in hysteria and as a result of irritation, without compression, of the pneumogastric or recurrent laryngeal nerves. It also occurs in ataxia, chorea, epilepsy, tetanus, and hydrophobia. Under these circumstances special treatment is rarely indicated. The majority of cases of hysteric origin will yield to a strong mental impression or to hypnotic suggestion. P. McBride mentions a case in which relief was afforded by an attempt at intubation. Paralysis of the abductor muscles of the larynx is a condition often difficult of differentiation from spasm of the adductors, and like the latter it may induce serious embarrassment of respiration, and should be equally mitigable by intubation.

Laryngismus stridulus, spasmodic croup, or subglottic laryngitis, usually yields to general and local medication. Although the symptoms are often most alarming the question of surgical intervention seldom arises. The number of fatal cases on record does not exceed six or eight, but even though the danger is comparatively slight, there are cases in which the laryngeal stenosis is very obstinate and persistent. Under such conditions may it not be judicious to relieve the distress of the patient and the relatives by such a simple procedure as the insertion of an O'Dwyer tube? In the *Journal of Laryngology*, vol. x, p. 183, 1896, a case of spasm of the glottis at the onset of an attack of measles is reported by Burgess. In this instance artificial respiration was continued during six hours. Intubation would have given relief in as many minutes.

My personal experience with intubation in spasm of the larynx is limited to a single case, of which the following is a brief history:

The patient was a lady of middle age, upon whom Dr. W. T. Bull had previously performed a thyroidectomy on account of a large bronchocele which was beginning to impede respiration by compressing the trachea. At this operation the vagus and its branches were not seen, and it is not supposed that they suffered any damage. The resulting cicatrix was pliable and nonadherent. Nevertheless, a few months after the removal of the thyroid tumor the patient began to have paroxysms of dyspnea, occurring at irregular intervals and without apparent cause. They increased in frequency and severity, and became so alarming, both to the patient and her friends, that it was proposed to intubate the larynx. At Dr. Bull's request I first introduced a medium-sized O'Dwyer tube, which passed in with ease, provoked no special irritation, and of course relieved the dyspnea. After wearing the tube several days the patient became so averse to permanent loss of voice that she insisted upon its withdrawal and the performance of a tracheotomy. At the time the patient was last heard from she was still wearing the trachea tube.

In conclusion, I would emphasize the value of intubation as an aid to tracheotomy. It has been extensively used for this purpose by Von Bokay, who claims no originality in the idea, but recommends it on the ground that the presence of the laryngeal tube permits one to open the trachea deliberately, thereby reducing the risks and complications attending a rapid operation (*Arch. für Kinderheilk.*, B. xxiii, H. 4 and 5).

Although it is not strictly within the scope of this paper, I would call your attention to an article by C. L. Green (*Brit. Med. Jour.*, ii, 1058, 1897), entitled "The Feasibility of Controlling Pernicious Vomiting by Means of Intubation of the Larynx with a Specially Adapted Tube, with a Reference to the Possible Relief of Otherwise Intractable Hiccough and Pertussis." Two cases of whooping-cough in which the asphyxia was relieved by intubation have been reported by Taub (*Pesth. Med. Chir. Presse*, No. 11, 1893).

No review of the subject of intubation may approach completeness without a word in eulogy of the conscientious care and patient industry with which O'Dwyer sought to perfect this procedure. Every technical detail had been minutely studied, nearly every objection had been met and overcome before he offered his conclusions to the world. A striking commentary on the success of his labors is found in the observation that almost every modification of his original method has proved to be a mutilation rather than an improvement. Painstaking thoroughness, persistent testing of his theory, and, finally, assured confidence in his results, characterized his work. A similar spirit in the investigation of other subjects related to medicine might ere long win for it the appellation of an "exact science."

Thus, I offer my feeble tribute to the scientific zeal, intelligence, and honesty of our lamented colleague.

INTUBATION IN CHRONIC STENOSIS OF THE LARYNX.[1]

BY D. BRYSON DELAVAN, M.D.,
OF NEW YORK.

IT is a rare thing in the history of any scientific invention that the originator of the idea has made the field covered by it entirely his own. Such, however, has been the achievement of Dr. O'Dwyer in the evolution of the method for relieving laryngeal stenosis by intubation. From his first demonstration down to his last critical reviews upon the subject he showed a complete mastery of it in all its mechanical details, its various practical applications, its pathologic relations, its possibilities of danger, and its vast capabilities for the relief of suffering. Indeed, the more one studies the history of intubation the more the fact impresses itself upon the mind that O'Dwyer not only created but perfected his art, standing always in the relation of teacher to his contemporaries, and rounding out the full completion of his career by leaving behind the consummation of a new era in surgery. The development of intubation may be studied to the best advantage, therefore, in the writings of O'Dwyer himself; for, notwithstanding the excellent work of others in this department, almost every suggestion made by them will be found to have been forestalled by him, and every minor detail of their technic of any value already placed on record or foreshadowed in his published reports.

If this statement be correct with regard to the use of intubation in acute conditions of the larynx, it is preeminently true in the application of the method to stenosis due to chronic causes. In no department of surgery have greater difficulties been more successfully met and overcome. The peculiar position, structure, and conformation of the larynx render the soft parts lining its interior particularly liable to injury from disease, while in the process of healing cicatrices are apt to form which are frequently very dense in character and almost sure, in the course of their contraction, to reduce the normal caliber of the organ. When this process of stenosis has exceeded certain limits and the patient is no longer able to inhale sufficient air to support life, or when the already narrowed opening becomes suddenly occluded by accident or intercurrent disease, the situation is, of course, most serious. Here, as in stenosis from other chronic causes, instant relief must be afforded either by tracheotomy or by some device by which the patency of the larynx may be restored. On the other hand, if dangerous symptoms are to be prevented, the patient must be treated before they appear, by some means which will dilate the narrowed region and thus keep it free.

Twelve years ago the great principle established by O'Dwyer, namely, that the larynx is capable of tolerating long-continued pressure from within, was applied by him to this particular class of cases. Before this time laryngeal stenosis had been treated by the rapid introduction and withdrawal of a dilator of one form or another, or, tracheotomy having been performed, a metallic plug was inserted at intervals into the strictured part of the larynx and allowed to remain there for a short time. The execution of the above processes was often attended with much distress, and their results were frequently most unsatisfactory. By the method of O'Dwyer a tube through which the patient can breathe is passed into the larynx and allowed to remain there as long as may seem desirable.

No great contribution made to surgery has ever been more modestly presented, nor has surgery often received a gift more indicative of important future results than the article published by Dr. O'Dwyer in the *New York Medical Record* for June 5, 1886, entitled "Chronic Stenosis of the Larynx Treated by a New Method, with Report of a Case." How thoroughly the author himself appreciated its value will appear from his own words: "Chronic stenosis of the larynx is one of the most unsatisfactory diseases which the physician is called upon to treat. Tracheotomy must be resorted to sooner or later to save the patient from a painful death, and, as a rule, in such cases the tracheal tube . . . must be worn through life. Various dilating instruments have been invented for this class of cases, notably by Morell Mackenzie, Navratil, Whistler, and Schrœtter,

[1] Read at a meeting of the New York Academy of Medicine, under the auspices of the Section on Laryngology and Rhinology, March 3, 1898.

Of these, the metallic plugs of Schrœtter are the best. In using them, however, it is necessary that the patient should be wearing a tracheal cannula, and the progress of the treatment is slow, tedious, and, in the end, often unsatisfactory. . . .

"Although I have treated only a single case of chronic stenosis with my laryngeal tubes, *I am fully convinced that they will prove infinitely superior to anything yet devised* for the relief of this unfortunate class of sufferers.

"In the use of these tubes tracheotomy is never indicated, and anesthesia rarely. They are inserted through the mouth, and rest solely in the larynx and trachea, the upper end being completely below the epiglottis. They facilitate rather than interfere with respiration, and permit the patient to swallow solids and semi-solids, and, to a certain extent, fluids."

Two years after the foregoing was published Dr. O'Dwyer, in the following remarkable statement, says:

"Had intubation of the larynx proved a complete failure in the treatment of croups, I would still feel amply repaid for the time and expense consumed in developing it, for *I believe that it offers the most rational and practical method yet devised* for the dilatation of chronic stricture of the glottis."—*N. Y. Medical Journal*, March 10, 1888.

In this same paper he reports five cases successfully treated by his method, and he also presents a new device for the permanent dilatation of stricture of the trachea.

From the date of the work recorded in the above articles up to the end of his life Dr. O'Dwyer was constantly laboring and writing in this field. The store of information which his large experience gave him was always digested to the best advantage, and the sound reasoning of his clear mind, aided by a judgment remarkably free from predjudice or conceit, caused his deductions to be of final value. Indeed, in the present connection I do not believe that it can be found that a single one of them of any real importance has ever been set aside. His work is on record, freely given to the profession, and so accurately and minutely explained that all may read and learn.

Meanwhile, the world has not been slow to profit by it. Although his invention was of evident value there were not wanting the inevitable carpers who objected to its features and actively opposed its adoption. It is interesting to observe how many of these have since become warm advocates of his method. Many of the ablest men both here and abroad at once recognized its great value and welcomed it accordingly.

While instances of chronic stenosis of the larynx are not very common, a considerable number of cases have already been reported by various operators, and several contributions to the literature have been made which not only confirm Dr. O'Dwyer's predictions, but prove that his method has been unanimously accorded a permanent place. Among the first to adopt it in this country was Dr. W. K. Simpson of New York, and, after him, Gerster (*N. Y. Med. Jour.*, April 20, 1890) and Dillon Brown. Lefferts, at the Tenth International Congress in 1890, presented a résumé of O'Dwyer's work, together with a report of five cases operated upon and a general statement of the indications for the use of the O'Dwyer method. Four successful cases were reported about this time by Simpson (*N. Y. Med. Jour.*, February 22, 1891).

Annandale of Edinburgh (*Brit. Med. Journal*, March 2, 1890) was the first foreign authority to recognize the application of the O'Dwyer method to these cases, and in his article recommends intubation "in certain cases of laryngeal stenosis from chronic inflammation, or from accidental or surgical conditions." Later, Ranke (*Münch. med. Woch.*, November 28, 1890) accepted it, and reported a successful case. In *Sajous' Annual* for 1892 the whole progress of intubation during that year is reviewed by Dr. O'Dwyer himself. In this he refers to two successful cases, and records a veritable triumph in the statement that "Professor Massei of Naples, after first strenuously opposing the introduction of intubation into Italy, is now an enthusiastic advocate of the operation, especially in the treatment of chronic stenosis, for which he has employed the method in twelve cases. F. E. Hopkins reports an interesting case of intubation for stenosis in tuberculous laryngitis (*N. Y. Med. Jour.*, February 27, 1892). In *Sajous' Annual* for 1893 O'Dwyer gives the records in fourteen cases. These occurred in the practice of Drs. C. H. Knight of New York, Nicolai of Rome, Schmiegelow of Copenhagen, and Sutherland, Pitts, and Brooks of London. The closing remark of his report is indicative of the progress of his ideas in the world at large. He says: "In this paper I have dwelt particularly upon intubation in chronic stenosis because the value of this procedure is beginning to be recognized, and serious mistakes are being made."

During the year 1894 no less than twenty-four cases were reported. Of these W. K. Simpson reported five, and added to their histories, in the words of Dr. O'Dwyer, "a practical and instructive thesis on the treatment of chronic stenosis of the larynx."

Rosenberg of Berlin, in by far the best report yet given from abroad, relates the histories of eleven cases treated by him at Professor Fränkel's clinic, while Baer of Zurich reports six, and Waxham of Chicago and Thrasher of Cincinnati each report a case. About this time O'Dwyer himself devised a very ingenious fenestrated tube for the removal of new growths of the larynx. In 1895 Baumgarten of Stuttgart reports two cases, Chiari of Vienna one, and Cheatham of Louisville two. Schmiegelow, in his paper on the subject, speaks especially of the difficulty of intubating in close strictures of the larynx. Up to 1896 about 100 cases had been reported. The results of these were in a large proportion of cases brilliantly successful. In the few that were unsatisfactory the evident explanation lay in faulty technic or bad judgment in the selection or management of the case. Since the beginning of 1896 the most important contribution to the subject of intubation for acute stenosis in the adult is by Dr. W. E. Casselberry of Chicago. (*Trans. Amer. Laryngological Ass'n*, 1896.) This paper contains many suggestions of practical value in chronic stenosis.

From the number and variety of cases operated upon by himself and reported by others it was easy for O'Dwyer to study the conditions in which intubation is applicable. Thus, it is effective in:

1. Cicatricial stenosis, due to the results of injury to the soft parts from (*a*) syphilis, (*b*) irritants, and (*c*) traumatisms.

2. In narrowing of the space both above and below the vocal bands from the products of chronic inflammation—simple, tuberculous, specific, malignant, or otherwise, and including such conditions as the so-called pachydermia laryngis, and chorditis vocalis inferior hypertrophica.

3. It is especially valuable in cases in which tracheotomy has been performed, and, when the tracheal cannula having been worn for a considerable length of time, the upper part of the trachea is filled with granulations and the laryngeal muscles have become weakened from disuse. In this condition intubation has effected many brilliant cures.

4. In papilloma of the larynx it has been found helpful in a fair proportion of cases, although its results in this disease are less satisfactory than in most others in which it has been employed.

5. In the rare condition known as a web of the larynx, hitherto very difficult of removal, but easily cured by the use of a tube for a few days.

6. Deformities of the larynx from injury or disease of its cartilaginous framework, which have resulted in constriction of the caliber of the organ, have been cured by it.

7. It has also been used, with excellent results, in anchylosis of the crico-arytenoid articulations, and in arthritis deformans of the same part.

8. It is useful in various affections of the nerves of the larynx; for instance, in (*a*) bilateral paralysis of abduction[1] and in (*b*) hysteric contraction of the abductors, "aphonia spastica."

The value of intubation is shown (1) in the relief of urgent dyspnea; (2) the promotion of absorption, by pressure, of inflammatory products; (3) the stretching of contracted tissues and of cicatricial bands and adhesions; (4) the forced motion of anchylosed or stiffened crico-arytenoid articulations, and in (5) the separation of the vocal bands in cases of paralysis for a sufficient length of time to overcome the difficulty or to admit of successful treatment by other means.

In the performance of intubation for chronic stenosis the method may be applied in one of several ways, as follows: (1) By progressive dilatation, a tube of smaller size being replaced from time to time by a larger one. (2) By forced introduction, the tube being worn continuously for a considerable period. (3) By preliminary division of cicatricial or other constricting or obstructing bands, followed by dilatation.

The last method is useful in a variety of conditions, including cicatrization from syphilis, irritants, and traumatism, injury of the laryngeal cartilages, and web of the larynx. The incisions may be made from above, by the aid of the laryngoscopic mirror, or may be effected through a tracheotomy wound, from below upward.

In an excellent article, Ernest Schmiegelow of Copenhagen, writes as follows: "If the stricture is so great as to prevent the introduction of tubes large enough to allow the patient to breathe, the treatment becomes complicated. This difficulty may be overcome (*a*) by dilating the stricture by endolaryngeal operations until sufficiently large tubes can be introduced; (*b*) by commencing with the introduction of Schrœtter's bougies, and continuing until the stenosis is so far dilated that the tubes can be introduced; (*c*) by the immediate performance of laryngofissure in order to remove the obstruction caused by the stenosis, and then proceeding to intubation. Complete obliteration of the larynx should be treated by laryngofissure, with excision of the diaphragm, and then by intubation, to prevent its recurrence.

This last suggestion should be taken with great reserve, as an ordinary web of the larynx can be perfectly cured by simple endolaryngeal incision and the use of a tube for a short time. In such a case laryngofissure is entirely out of place, because unnecessary. To Schmiegelow's first proposition, also, exception is taken, and Simpson very properly

[1] O'Dwyer, "Trans. Ninth Internat. Congress," vol. iv, p. 125; also, *N. Y. Med. Jour.*, December 25, 1895.

says that "while it may be necessary in a few cases to employ some form of dilatation prior to the attempt to pass the smallest tube, such instances, however, are rare, for if any instrument whatever can be passed, it is usually possible to insert an intubation-tube sufficiently large for breathing purposes" (*N. Y. Med. Jour.*, September 19, 1896).

With regard to the process by which the tube should be introduced into the larynx, several good descriptions have been given, though it is always O'Dwyer to whom we are indebted for the first and the best. Thus, writing in 1892, he says: "I believe that in chronic cases in which the throat has become more or less accustomed to the use of instruments intubation can be performed with greater facility and less discomfort to the patient by the aid of the laryngoscopic mirror than by the usual method." If the above manipulation should not prove successful, the tube may be inserted without the aid of the mirror, as in a child.

An excellent description of this method of introducing the tube by Dr. Simpson (*loc. cit.*) is as follows: "If possible, the tube should be introduced by the aid of a mirror, in the same way as in making a laryngeal application, the pharynx and larynx first having been anesthetized with cocain. After the point of the tube is seen to enter the stricture, the mirror should be dropped, and the forefinger of the mirror hand transferred to the head of the tube, making pressure upon it while the introducer is being removed. It may be necessary in a long-standing case, in a very tall patient, or when a tracheotomy-tube has been worn, for an assistant to elevate the larynx externally. During the passage of the tube the mouth should be opened as widely as possible and the tongue well protruded. The string should remain in for a few hours at least, especially if the tube be of small caliber, so that it may be easily withdrawn in the event of difficulty in breathing. Sometimes it may be necessary to etherize the patient, in which case the tube is inserted in the usual manner by the sense of touch. Instruments for tracheotomy should always be on hand during this procedure. The most difficult cases for intubation are those in which a tracheotomy-tube has been worn for a long while. First, because the larynx from long inactivity is prevented from rising, so that the tube must be passed to a deeper level in the throat; and, second, there is generally an added stricture or even complete closure at the superior part of the tracheotomy wound which may require dilatation from below before the intubation-tube can be successfully inserted. In the after-treatment of these cases the same care must be exercised as in children. The tube must be removed if it becomes occluded and replaced if expelled by coughing. The process of feeding may be carried on also, as with younger patients, by placing the patient in Casselberry's position, that is, lying upon the back with the head thrown backward until it is below the level of the body."

I have had several successful cases of intubation for chronic stenosis in my own practice. The last occurred two weeks ago, under circumstances so unusual as to make it worthy of note.

I was called to see a patient at the Sloane Maternity Hospital who was said to have something wrong with her throat. I found a German woman, aged about thirty years, with advanced pulmonary tuberculosis, pregnant, and well through the first stage of labor. As she was brought before me, I saw that she was suffering from urgent dyspnea. Her lips were blue, her expression haggard and anxious, and with each effort at inspiration the air was drawn through the larynx with a strident sound by severe muscular exertion of the chest-walls. Rapidly demonstrating the larynx with the throat mirror, I found its cavity filled, both above and below the vocal bands, with a dense, fibrous-looking mass of tissue, which had so encroached upon the glottic aperture as to leave a slit so narrow that it seemed impossible that enough oxygen could pass through it to sustain life. The distress for air was severe and was rapidly increasing and meanwhile the pains of the second stage of labor had begun. The situation was most critical for if mother and child were to be saved not a moment was to be lost. Leaving the patient in the hands of the House Surgeon, I sent an assistant for tracheotomy instruments, and went myself in greatest haste to the Vanderbilt Clinic, which adjoins the Sloane Maternity Hospital, for a set of adult intubation-tubes. By rare good fortune, I not only secured them, but also found my friend, Dr. Simpson, who accompanied me back to the patient with all speed. As quickly as possible we applied cocain to the patient's throat, made the arrangements preliminary to the introduction of the tube, and when all was ready, attempted its insertion. This proved a difficult matter, owing to the great density of the infiltrated tissue, the smallness of the glottic aperture, and the fact that the thickening filled the interior of the larynx to a level so high above the vocal bands that its cavity was practically obliterated. Still, it seemed possible to pass the tube, and under the circumstances we were anxious, for obvious reasons, to avoid tracheotomy. Following each attempt to introduce the tube, labor pains of so sharp a character would come on that a second intubation could not be undertaken until they had subsided. I succeeded in passing a small tube, but it was immediately coughed out. Meanwhile, the pains came faster and harder, the dyspnea became more and more severe. No situation could have been more perilous to the patient nor fraught with greater anxiety to those in charge. It was an exciting moment when, in an effort made with great skill and with the application of considerable force, Dr. Simpson carried the end of a tube, too large to be expelled, past the obstruction, and accurately downward into its proper place. After having been nearly strangled for a few seconds, the patient began to breathe easily, and the cyanosis disappeared. Hardly had she taken three good inspirations when she whispered, in great agitation, that the baby was coming. She was quickly lifted upon a stretcher and taken to the operating-room, while I stayed behind to gather up the throat instruments for use in case any accident should happen to the tube. Reaching the operating-room within three minutes after the others had arrived there, I was greeted with the announcement, "We are all through, the baby is born; he is sound and hearty, and the mother's condition is perfect."

As I stood by the side of the poor woman and witnessed the immeasurable relief which had come to her, as I saw that voiceless patient's gratitude beaming from her eyes, and felt it carried to to me in the eloquent grasp of her hand, the recollection of the brave, unselfish, noble soul, to whom she was so deeply and so doubly indebted, came over me with a mighty rush, and I could but echo the sentiment which we have all so often heard as it has arisen from the depths of many another thankful heart, "God bless Dr. O'Dwyer."

TREATMENT OF ARTERIOSCLEROSIS.

By HENRY B. FAVILL, M.D.,
OF CHICAGO, ILL.

IN a text-book discussion of arteriosclerosis there is usually expressed a certain hopelessness in regard to therapeutic measures, which, I am frank to say, is not shared by the author of this paper. This skeptical attitude is, however, not at all extraordinary in consideration of the character of the text-book discussion of the subject which has hitherto prevailed. When the consideration of arteriosclerosis is extended past the aorta, temporals, radials, and larger arterial trunks in general, there may be some hope of incorporating it in a logical relation to disease processes the therapeutics of which are tangible. As well might one dispose of the complications of a water system which tends to occlusion, by discussing the scale in the mains; very pertinent, it is true, as to accidental bursting, but utterly worthless in an analysis of the dynamic relations of the process.

The portrayal of the ravages of arteriosclerosis in the aorta is graphic. Is the description of what occurs in the finest arterioles equally impressed? And yet, not until the subject is approached from the side of the capillary and the fine arterial twig is the remarkable symptom-complex of this affection even vaguely comprehensible. Furthermore, not until one struggles to fathom the relation between cell perversion and its nourishment, or between vitiated pabulum and tissue degeneration, or between circulatory dynamics and innervation, can he hope to establish an etiology upon which to rear therapeutics. It is not my privilege to dwell upon etiology, nor do I desire to more than allude to classification. All treatment must find its reason in consideration of three general factors: (1) The cell and its natural endowment. (2) The character of the supply from which the tissue derives its support. (3) The controlling influence which determines its nutrition and functional activity.

Great was the day of cellular pathology. Greater is this day of investigation of morbid-cell physiology, the natural exponent of morbid anatomy. The endowment of the cell is the resultant of its inheritance and its adaptation to environment, cooperative, or antagonistic, as the case may be; the management of its difficulties must involve the just estimate of these factors. That the cell has a morbid physiology long before there is demonstrable organic change, admits of no question. To determine the elements of this malfeasance is the task of the future. Inseparable from this problem is the consideration of the vital experience of tissue as determined by the nutrient current to which it is exposed. Hence, we come to regard as a determining influence in morbid development the vitiated blood-supply which reaches the part. Thus, does cell pathology reach back into the darkness and lead forth for its own elucidation, a new and enlightened humoral pathology.

To deal with arteriocapillary fibrosis in respect to innervation is a most venturesome undertaking. Of the facts in question we know nearly nothing. Analogy, however, and clinical observation compel the conclusion that the relationship is pronounced; on the one hand trophic influence, and on the other, functional control, combine to furnish the activities which finally develop the defects resulting from the malnutrition above suggested.

The treatment of arteriosclerosis, or, as more suggestively called by Gull, arteriocapillary fibrosis, should be regarded from various standpoints. Unquestionably, the better knowledge of the process which the future has in store will admit of great advance in prophylaxis. The process once established demands relief for one or both of two reasons: either because of general disability, or because of special predominance in organs which demand specific consideration. It is not too trite to repeat that "a man is as old as his arteries." No relative estimate of age compares with this. It implies that arterial degeneration is the physiologic index of decadence. It becomes a pathologic condition when it anticipates years, or what is the same thing, exceeds the reasonable expectancy of a given period. Whatever conditions contribute to this maladjustment and the possibilities of modifying them, determine treatment. As a rule, before the arterial degeneration affords distinct symptoms there is evidence of the toxemia that is behind it. The character of the toxemia varies. It is the result of poisons ingested, or infection, or auto-intoxication. Of the first two, as of plumbism or syphilis, little may be said; their therapeutics are well defined. Of the third much must be said, inasmuch as it includes the greater number of all cases. The common factor in the various types appears to be defective food metabolism. The active agency inducing this defect varies. We find it in the overfed and in the underfed; in the inactive and in the over-active; in the young, middle-aged, and old. In its earlier stages it usually is associated with good digestion; rarely with dyspepsia. It is a post-digestive development. The most constant factor in a series of cases is evidence of incomplete disposal of nitrogenized materials.

Chemically, we determine this by the defective excretion of urea. This means lessened manufacture of urea, or faulty separation of urea, or both. Clinically, we detect the condition in symptoms of nitrogenous intoxication, the so-called uric-acid manifestations. It is by these that our attention is primarily attracted, and in this analysis we are enabled to early demonstrate arterial change. That the true toxin is uric acid is doubtful. That the poisonous agents generated in this way are several is highly probable, but philosophy must reach far ahead of our full knowledge and outline the probable. These facts are not asserted as ultimate. Unless lightly held as provisional data they are likely to mislead. They do, however, furnish the clinical characteristics, more or less demonstrable, which serve as a basis for the conclusion that the essential agency in this process is toxic, and for the most part autotoxic. The treatment at this stage of the disease is essentially hygienic. The initial proposition is how to adapt the individual to his environment. In general the elements of food and physical expenditure are at fault. The important requirement is that food should be adequately introduced and thoroughly eliminated when no longer useful. Decided failure in either direction is destructive. For any given individual, "Is his food adapted to his work?" should be asked. To meet this query what do you demand? That his eliminating organs yield the proper representation of his ingesta. You see at once that our diagnostic resources do not cover such elaborate investigation, and yet we are not without resources.

Clinically we have well-recognized evidences of toxemia by which to measure condition. Believing that the toxic agents are nitrogenous, we have approximate means in the estimation of urea and total nitrogens excreted with the urine. Marked departure of these from the standard average of health demands explanation and correction. So far as our present knowledge goes it points to defective combustion as the efficient cause of these conditions. At once this opens the most complicated questions of relative combustibility of foods. Into this we cannot enter. Sufficient to say, that quantity is quite as important as quality.

Given a good digestion, a mixed diet may be right or wrong according to the quantity. The "rendering" capacities of the body have definite limitations, and react accordingly. Clinically we encounter, as a rule, the necessity to diminish the nitrogenous food, or to change the form of its use. That the struggle against this gradual toxemia may be more successfully waged by attention to this line of procedure I have not the least doubt. Practically it amounts to the gradual adoption of a mixed milk and vegetable diet, and experience fully warrants the advocacy thereof. It is remarkable how broadly applicable this simple regulation may be. Alone it frequently is the efficient means of correcting the phenomena associated with this pathologic state. Of these may be mentioned, nervousness, sleeplessness, shortness of breath, faintness, and a number of allied conditions, dependent for their causation upon the interplay between a toxic blood and pathologically limited capillary distribution.

It is true that the arteriocapillary limitation may be complex; in fact, usually is; that in addition to structural encroachment upon the blood-vessels, there is usually muscular over-action spasm, if you like, in the arteriole wall; that the result is a raising of general blood-pressure by the participation of these elements in various degrees. Attention should be directed in this connection to the distinction between arterial pressure and arterial rigidity. Associated as a rule, they may be far apart. It is not rare to find a great arteriosclerosis with arterial rigidity widespread, together with a dangerously low blood-pressure. Of the complication so arising we shall say a word later. The important question is: To what extent may the mischief of heightened arterial pressure be avoided by attention to this nerve reaction? In response, I adduce as the next measure of treatment, and not second in importance, the adoption of an even, equable life. It ought not to require a demonstration into which we cannot now enter to show how vital is the principle involved in this question.

All of the life influences which tend to exhaustion, incoordination, and perverted nerve control range themsélves upon the one hand; all of the forces residing in deliberate, coherent, even though forceful activities, oppose themselves—to the end that it lies within reasonable demonstration that the poise of life is fully as determinative of its physical destiny as are the factors which we are superficially in the habit of regarding as crucial. When we come to consider more specific pathology, and search for indications for treatment less general, we find that the occasion arises in connection with organic change in many vital organs. Three distinct relations between special organic change and general sclerosis are possible, and frequently coexist. The special change in an organ may be a direct consequence of the general process; or it may be a part of the general process, that is to say, participating, or it may be in a measure causative of the general process. Without pausing to discuss these relationships it is possible to state that the clinical phenomena bear a constant relation to intra-arterial pressure.

Of these the most prominent are hypertrophy of the heart and polyuria. The heart hypertrophy occurring as a truly conservative process in response to enforced labor. The polyuria, occurring *pari passu* with the sclerosis in the kidneys, becomes an equally compensatory event. In so far as these conditions maintain a due relation, little can be done to alter them. It is at the point of failure upon one side or another that interference becomes necessary. If, for example, the heart hypertrophy begins to yield to its excess, and the *vis a tergo* is withdrawn, the effect upon circulatory conditions becomes enormously exaggerated. This exaggeration follows the fact that in the typical condition resistance in the capillary area has been met by increased force of the heart, with the result of creating an intra-arterial pressure sufficient to maintain the circulation. Withdraw even slightly the heart power, and you have left all the resistance resulting from altered caliber minus the blood-pressure; hence, ensues stagnation quite out of proportion to the amount of heart failure involved.

The result of these changes upon the function of the kidney is in all cases pronounced. The immediate effect is to reduce the bulk of the urine. At the same time, the solid excreta of the urine fall short and there supervenes a more or less intense uremia. Almost the same description will apply to circumstances in which the blood-pressure has been suddenly reduced from other causes. The chain of serious consequences is finally chargeable to undue disturbance of a blood-pressure which has become quasi normal.

It is important to estimate these phenomena at their true value. The therapeutics follow absolutely this analysis. The indications for treatment are two: To restore the balance between impelling power and resistance, and usually, to protect the interests of organs which have grown dependent upon an altered pressure. Therefore, it will not do, if it were possible, to bring down the peripheral resistance to the capacity of the heart; the pressure must be restored, and hence the invariable rule: When the subject with arteriosclerosis begins to fail in the maintenance of the new balance, as a primary move, conserve the energies to the utmost by reducing expenditure in every direction. Hence, put the patient in bed. Regarding the tendency to toxemic complications, as most threatening, it becomes imperative to reduce the problem of nourishment to its simplest terms; that is, to the point at which the system most nearly protects itself from toxic accumulations. Hence, reduce the diet, perhaps to consist simply of milk. Promote the interchange of fluids in the tissues, bringing fresh materials and carrying away effete, by means of baths and massage. Secure the highest possible functional perfection in the organs whose efforts control food and tissue metabolism, particularly the liver, by the small and long-continued administration of calomel; thereby contributing in the highest degree to the final and indispensable demand, *viz.*, that elimination be not allowed to flag.

In the kidney we encounter the most serious obstacles. An organ, primarily or secondarily cirrhotic, dependent upon a high blood-pressure, finds itself choked by these conditions. It must be relieved. To this end the following measures may be instituted: In the absence of great edema provide sufficent fluid ingesta. Restore the equilibrium of the circulation, to accomplish which administer strychnin for its benefit to the heart, and digitalis for its effect upon the peripheral arterioles. Recall the fact that digitalis may not be indefinitely used in these conditions without resulting damage; but remember also, that in an emergency like this, it is indispensable.

In thus touching here and there a salient point of this subject, I have striven to keep in mind the fact that the efficient treatment of the degeneration in question lies in prevention.

To know the signs of the predegenerative state, and forestall them, is the highest usefulness of the physician. Once the disease is well established, the treatment becomes a treatment of complications and emergencies. Thoroughly investigated in the beginning, the therapeutic possibilities are far more gratifying.

CLINICAL MEMORANDA.

A CASE OF TRIGGER FINGER.

BY J. B. NICHOLS, M.D.,
OF WASHINGTON, D. C.;
CLINICAL ASSISTANT, BARNES' HOSPITAL, UNITED STATES SOLDIERS' HOME.

As trigger finger is not a common condition, the case here reported seems worthy of record. In an examination of the hands of one thousand adult men to determine the frequency of the occurrence of certain lesions of the hand and fingers I did not find a single instance of trigger finger. The present case developed in a man, when he was forty years of age, as the result of traumatism, and exhibits an impediment in extension of the third finger of the right hand. The particular lesion which causes the locking of the finger in this case is not determinable from the appearances present.

N. P. N., male, was born in 1854 in Denmark. He was a soldier in the United States army from 1880 to 1895; was last discharged during January, 1895, and rejected for re-enlistment on account of defective vision. He has done but little work since. He had an attack of rheumatism in the shoulders during 1889, and his eyesight has been failing since 1890, though his general health has been good. During March, 1895, he stumbled in the dark and fell on his right hand dislocating the distal phalanx of the thumb, lacerating the little finger, and contusing the third finger. The hand remained in a dressing nearly two weeks, and on removal of the latter a trigger condition on extension of the third finger was found to exist, which has continued without material change to the present time. Previous to the accident the hand had not been affected in any way.

Examination revealed the following conditions: After firm flexion of the third finger of the right hand its middle phalanx frequently became locked and flexed on the proximal phalanx at slightly less than a right angle. Considerable force was required to free the finger, release occurring suddenly with a jerk and further extension being accomplished without hindrance. There was no impediment to flexion, the finger becoming locked only during extension and at only one point. The finger did not usually become locked when flexed with little force, but when it was firmly flexed, as when the fist was tightly closed, it usually became fixed. A jerk could be felt and a slight click could be distinctly heard both when the finger locked and when it was released. When the middle phalanx was locked the distal phalanx was slightly flexed, and the act of extending this phalanx with the other hand seemed to aid in unlocking the joint. When the finger locked a pain was felt in the affected joint. When it was released, either by passive or active force, there was pain in the extensor tendon of the finger, most marked opposite the proximal end of the metacarpal bone. There was frequently also, on release, pain in the upper half of the forearm just internal to the ulna and near the course of the ulnar nerve.

There were no cicatrices, thickenings, or other evideuces of any old injury or disease of the affected third finger. There was no nodule or swelling on its flexor tendons; no perceptible luxation or lesion of the joints, and no anatomic abnormality of any kind perceptible about the finger, either when locked or free, sufficient to account for the condition. There was an old unreduced dislocation of the last phalanx of the right thumb and a cicatrix from an old laceration on the middle phalanx of the little finger.

CHANCRE OF THE ESOPHAGUS, ACQUIRED THROUGH TOBACCO.

BY WESLEY G. BAILEY, M.D.,
OF PEKIN, ILL.

Not being able to find an example of the initial lesion of syphilis in the situation above mentioned, after a careful search through the literature, I venture to believe the case a rare one, and the method of conveying the infection also somewhat unique.

On December 26, 1895, I was called to see a young man, J. H., aged thirty years, who complained of a severe sore throat. On inspection, the right side of the pharynx showed considerable tumefaction very low down. The soft palate and tonsils were but little involved, and the voice was free and clear. Breathing was not interfered with. There was great dysphagia. The external cervical glands immediately contiguous to the site of the tumefaction in the throat were somewhat swollen. On the 30th I was again summoned to see the patient, and found the whole right cervical region, anterior to the sternocleidomastoid muscle and below the angle of the jaw, intensely swollen. The mouth could not be sufficiently opened to permit examination. The employment of a hot antiseptic spray and the application of hot fomentations externally enabled me, by January 2d, to make a fairly satisfactory examination. Below the epiglottis, on the upper margin of the gullet, I could see an intensely red ulcerated spot, at this time apparently nearly well. There was nothing distinctive about the ulceration, though it was sufficiently suspicious to justify the institution of antisyphilitic treatment. He denied having a sore penis or having kissed any one but a pure girl, whom I myself knew well, and in regard to whom there could be no suspicion. It was several months afterward that to me the real source of his infection became known; for as he had developed true secondary symptoms there could be no doubt of the nature of his disease. In replying to the query had he smoked any one else's pipe, he said, "No," but recollected having taken a "chew" from another "fellow's" plug, and on returning the tobacco he had noticed that its owner's neck was covered with blotches of an ugly appearance. As the sore throat commenced within a day or so of three weeks after the fatal "chew" was taken, and as the secondary symptoms also developed in regular order, it seems justifiable to think that the disease was inoculated into the gullet by the saliva containing the virus of syphilis from the unfortunate "chew" of tobacco.

CYST OF THE RECTUM.

BY JOSEPH M. MATHEWS, M.D.,
OF LOUISVILLE, KY.;
PROFESSOR OF SURGERY AND CLINICAL LECTURER ON DISEASES OF THE RECTUM IN THE KENTUCKY SCHOOL OF MEDICINE, ETC.

THE following case is, to me, unique in rectal surgery, and especially interesting because it was wrongly diagnosed.

A gentleman from a town in western Kentucky was recently referred to me. He presented a history of having had a fall several months before his first visit to my office. He fell a number of feet and struck upon his back. He had some pain in the rectum following the fall, also pain in the back, which was more or less aggravated according to the position he assumed, but his fecal evacuations appeared to be normal in every way.

Upon examination I found no special disease just inside the rectum. I examined the coccyx, which seemed to be normal. About 3½ inches up the rectum, situated a little to the left, but encroaching upon the center of the sacrum, I felt a tumor. Its base must have been two inches in diameter, and in surface it was as large as a small orange. The base was very hard, and on top it gave the impression of a rubber ball. It did not feel exactly like a cyst. I concluded that the patient had a sarcomatous growth of the rectum. I called Dr. W. O. Roberts in consultation, and upon examining the patient, without knowing my conclusion, he said that the condition was the most perfect demonstration of sarcoma of the rectum he had ever seen. The patient was removed to the hospital of the Kentucky School of Medicine, where he was prepared for operation and taken into the amphitheater. I expected to perform a Kraske operation, thinking I could remove the growth without any difficulty. While the patient was on the table he was examined by Dr. William L. Rodman, who also pronounced the growth a sarcoma. Dr. James M. Holloway, who was also present, concurred in this opinion.

Under chloroform I made a long incision down from the sacrum to the anus, and dissected out the coccyx, thinking that this procedure would be sufficient, and paying little attention to the tumor during the manipulations. I then, to provide space in which to work, cut off the side of the sacrum, as is done in the Kraske operation. This provided sufficient space, and I knew that I could bring down the entire rectum if it were thought desirable. Placing my hand in the space behind and inserting a finger into the rectum, I discovered that the growth was a cyst, and not a sarcoma. After this predicament I simply went into the cyst from behind (through the inflammatory deposit), tapped it and evacuated a cupful of clear fluid. The cyst at once completely collapsed, and the wound was closed.

This is the only cyst of the rectum which I have ever seen, nor do I remember to have read of one. The way we were deceived, I think, was that in pushing against the base of the tumor with the examining finger it was pushed against the sacrum; thus the inflammatory deposit was felt over the promontory of the sacrum. We were also deceived by the pain, and the idea was conveyed to at least three physicians that the growth was attached, that it was a true tumor, or at least that it was in all probability a sarcoma. The tumor was in the wall of the rectum, and was easily handled after I had cut down into the space. In my opinion the trouble was distinctly inflammatory in character, and in no sense malignant.

FOUR CASES OF EXTRAGENITAL CHANCRE.

BY I. N. BLOOM, M.D.,
OF LOUISVILLE, KY.;
CLINICAL PROFESSOR OF GENITO-URINARY DISEASES IN THE UNIVERSITY OF LOUISVILLE; DERMATOLOGIST TO THE LOUISVILLE CITY HOSPITAL, ETC.

CASE I.—Mr. B., thirty years of age. On November 23, 1896, the patient presented himself to me and exhibited a small ulcerated patch on the upper surface of the tongue, one-half inch from the tip and a little to the right of the median line. It was about half the size of the cross-section of a lead-pencil, slightly ulcerated, and presented no typical features. It had been first noticed two days before, on November 21st, and did not give pain or inconvenience. The patient was somewhat of a hypochondriac, having been afflicted since infancy with valvular heart trouble, and so was inclined to watch himself and any symptoms he might present extremely close. Within a few days the erosion disappeared, and in its place an elevated papule, twice the size of the previous patch, became evident. This slowly grew larger, and on about the tenth day a zone of induration formed around it which was about as large as a 25-cent piece, and never exceeded that size. In the meantime the elevated portion, roughly circular in form, began to assume a cartilaginous hardness. With the forefinger on the sore and the thumb against the lower surface of the tongue it felt almost as hard as gristle.

This condition of affairs persisted until the patient's departure to New York on January 24, 1897. He had early been made acquainted with the nature of the affection, and being quite hypochondriacal, greatly feared his trouble might be epithelioma, so that I had an opportunity of observing him every two or three days during this time. There was no glandular enlargement in the neck until the first week of January. At which time one moderately enlarged gland could be felt on the affected side just below the angle of the jaw, and another, more decidedly enlarged, beneath the belly of the sternocleidomastoid muscle. The eruption was delayed and only the faintest signs were visible on January 21st. These consisted of a few erythematous spots on the patient's bald head. They were very faint and undecided in character.

As the patient was to pass some three or four months in New York, I referred him to Dr. R. W. Taylor, to whom he presented himself three days after I saw him last. Dr. Taylor concurred in the diagnosis.

CASE II.—Miss D.—When the patient first presented herself, December 5, 1896, she had a chancre in the median line on the upper lip from which the induration was fast disappearing. It was about the size of a 10-cent piece, decidedly indurated above the mucous membrane of the lip, and was situated at the mucocutaneous juncture. The lesion had existed "about two months or more," just how long she could not say. The cervical glands showed some slight signs of enlargement; indeed, it is possible that they existed previous to the onset of the present affection. She had a papular syphilide on the trunk and arms, and a trace of roseola. Two weeks later tubercles were found within the greater labia, and mucous patches on the vestibule were also noticed. Only when these disappeared was there any inguinal glandular enlargement, and that but slight. Under appropriate treatment the chancre entirely disappeared, while the other symptoms were still present when the patient was last seen about one month ago.

CASE III.—Physician, twenty-five years of age, practising in a neighboring town. On October 1, 1896, he noticed a papule on the index-finger of his left hand, which grew slowly and without ulceration until it was about the size of a silver dime. It was only slightly indurated and was painless. He made a crucial incision through the lesion, and was surprised not to find pus. Without a suspicion as to the real nature of the lesion he applied a mercurial plaster, and two or three weeks later the sore had disappeared. When I saw him he had an erythematopapular syphilide covering the trunk and the arms, two or three small mucous patches in the mouth, and as many scabs on the scalp. There was general adenitis to a moderate extent. I have not seen the patient since.

CASE IV.—Mrs. G., aged forty years, widow, came to me on September 3, 1896, requesting a thorough examination. On the body, arms, and legs there was an extensive papulopustular eruption, the genitals were covered with mucous patches, and there were nodules in the labia. She had shaved her head and wore a wig, but scratched papules were visible all over the head when the wig was removed, as was also alopecia syphilitica. The mouth, especially around the tonsils and back of the last molar teeth, contained large mucous patches. Her right nipple hung by a shred, and around an eroded sore involving the areola was a thick, deep, infiltrated zone. There was no other evidence of the initial lesion. She had been bitten, she claimed, on the nipple by her lover several months before. She located the time of the first appearance of the nipple trouble as nine months before. The patient did not impress me as being a reliable person, and, as I have not seen her since, I am able to present but a brief account of the case.

I used every endeavor to discover the method and site of entrance of the syphilitic poison in the three cases first reported. In Case I. the patient was thoroughly reliable and afforded me every facility for discovering the mode of entrance of the infection. He had not been indiscriminate in his sexual congress during the previous six months, and, living as he did with his grandmother, he knew of no way in which he could have been exposed. His habits were very much those of a man in the better walks of life, and the origin of his trouble will remain forever unknown.

In Case II. the patient had had intercourse with but one man, and denied having kissed any other for many months. I was unable to secure an interview with this man, although I endeavored to do so.

Case III. has already been sufficiently discussed. The patient acknowledged to having had four lovers at the same time, any one of whom might have been the cause of the trouble.

A CASE OF CONGENITAL MALFORMATION.

BY S. J. MCNAMARA, M.D.,
OF BROOKLYN, N. Y.

THE infant whose case is here related was born October 22, 1897, of Irish parents. The father was twenty-four and the mother twenty-one years of age. The couple had been married four years. They had one child who was well-formed and healthy and at the time of writing twenty months old. The mother had a miscarriage when she had been married one year, during the fifth or sixth month of gestation, and the fetus, I was told by the father, was deformed, both lower limbs being fused together and the genitals being placed on one side.

The labor which resulted in the birth of the third child was short and easy. The breech presented in the left sacro-anterior position. The infant at birth weighed four and a half pounds and had a fairly developed trunk and head. The left arm was missing from the middle third, and the right, from the elbow, with the exception of a rudimentary finger on which was what could have been taken for a finger-nail. One lower limb was absent from the knee-joint, while on the other was a poorly developed leg with a foot which was twisted backward. The mother, a woman of a somewhat nervous, self-conscious, and secretive disposition, accounts for the deformity by the following incident:

About the middle of June, or when she was in mid-pregnancy, while standing at the door of her house, she was asked for money by a beggar with no legs who was seated on a tricycle playing an organ, and was being drawn by another man. She was about to give him some money when she found she had no small change. She regretted the fact very much, and felt very sorry afterward that she did not give him what she had, although it was more than she could really afford. She remembered the incident several days, when it slipped her mind, but she again saw this same man and the second meeting recalled to her mind all that she had gone through on first seeing him. Moreover, the night of her confinement she said she saw this man at the foot of her bed and stated that she was not very much surprised at the baby being deformed.

MEDICAL PROGRESS.

A Simple Method of Collecting the Urine from Either Kidney.—HARRIS (*Jour. Amer. Med. Assn.*, January 29, 1898) has devised a method of obtaining urine from either kidney alone or from both separately, which is both simple and reliable and applicable to patients of either sex. The advantages of separate urine are at times so great that all sorts of measures have been devised to obtain it. Various instruments have been made to compress one ureter, and surgeons have not hesitated in certain cases to expose one ureter, in order to compress it more accurately, or by opening it to obtain urine from its kidney. Pawlick was able by an unusually delicate touch to catheterize the ureters; with the help of the cystoscope this has been repeatedly done, though the procedure has ever remained a difficult one, even in the hands of an expert. Simon devised a urethral speculum for the female, through which the ureters may be seen by reflected light and catheterized as the bladder becomes distended with air. Kelly has popularized this method, but it is still one which requires special training, and sometimes the pain is so great as to require an anesthetic; sometimes it is impossible even for the most skilled surgeon to find the ureters in a reasonable length of time.

The instrument devised by Harris does away at once with all of these disadvantages, and, moreover, allows of the separation of the urine in the male as well as in the female. It consists of a septum which, when passed into the rectum or vagina, and pressed against the posterior bladder-wall, makes a watershed in the median line of the bladder; also, of two small silver catheters, the straight middle portions of which are enclosed in a thin sheath. They can be rotated in this sheath, and when so rotated the curved upper and lower ends are separated. The ends within the bladder slip into the two pouches formed by the rectal septum, and the ends outside the body are connected by rubber tubes with two bottles. By means of slight aspiration the urine is sucked out of the bladder-pouches, right and left, before enough collects there to make possible any overflow from one side to the other. In this manner as much urine as is desired can be collected separately from the two ureters without any discomfort to the patient. The catheters should be inserted and rotated before the septum is placed in the rectum. The inventor has tested the instrument upon one patient who had had one kidney removed, and the demonstration was perfect that there was no overflow of urine from one side to the other.

THERAPEUTIC NOTES.

Treatment of Obesity.—ROBIN (*Rev. de Therapeut.*, December, 1897) treats obesity as follows: At eight A.M. the patient receives a boiled egg and two-thirds of an ounce of lean meat or fish—the whole to be eaten cold and dry. A third of an ounce of bread and a cup of weak and very hot tea without sugar complete the repast. At ten o'clock a second meal is given, consisting of two boiled eggs, one-sixth of an ounce of bread, and five ounces of water, wine, or tea. At noon the meal consists of as much cold meat as is desired, without bread, but with salads served with salt and lemon-juice. If the patient craves bread very badly, an ounce may be permitted. He also receives from three to five ounces of green vegetables served with butter. Farinaceous articles, and those extremely sweet, are absolutely forbidden. Three to five ounces of raw fruit may be allowed as dessert. Two glasses of water may be drunk with this meal, and a quarter of an hour later a cup of weak tea without sugar. Another cup may be given at four o'clock. Finally, at seven o'clock, the same meal may be taken as at eight in the morning, with the fish or meat warmed, if preferred, the amount not to exceed three ounces. The patient should walk half or three-quarters of an hour after each repast; that is to say, five times daily. He should take vapor baths, followed by general massage; should never sleep in the daytime, and not more than seven hours at night. Of the various systems of medication proposed to reduce flesh, Robin has this to say: The thyroid preparations are unreliable and are not without danger. Iodid of potassium will diminish the amount of flesh, but produces accompanying ill effects, such as shrinking of the glands. Treatment by mineral waters is only efficacious as long as it is continued, and should be regarded as a mere adjunct of diatetic treatment.

Treatment of Vomiting of Pregnancy.—GEOFFROY (*Bull. Gen. de Therapeut.*, December 15, 1897) is convinced that the condition of nausea and vomiting of pregnant women is due to reflex contracture of the digestive tube; that such contracture is located either at the pylorus and the different portions of the small intestine, or more particularly in the iliopelvic angle of the colon, and that this painful contraction at this angle is a pathognomonic sign of reflex hyperesthesia of the intestinal canal, of which the morbid symptoms vary from slight pain about the heart to simple nausea or to uncontrollable vomiting. By the slow, light, progressive movements of massage, with the balls of the fingers, he is able to cause the passage of gas and liquid through this region with gurgling sounds distinguishable both to the physician and to the patient. Usually two or three séances of this light massage are sufficient to cause the vomiting to cease altogether, though the treatment may be repeated as often as necessary without fear of ill results. This procedure has been employed by the writer with complete success in a number of obstinate cases.

The Best Treatment for General Edema.—A writer, in *La Médecine Moderne*, says that the best treatment for general edema of the legs is the introduction of a fine cautery-point some seven or eight centimeters (three to three and a half inches) above the external malleolus, the skin first being carefully prepared with antiseptics. Two punctures are made on each leg, one above the other, passing clear through the skin. Hemorrhage is rare. The leg should be enveloped with compresses soaked in a weak antiseptic solution, after having been smeared with borated vaselin. The dressing should be changed several times daily. From the punctures a large amount of serous fluid escapes, and the improvement of the patient is manifest within a short time. When the openings close it is necessary to repeat the punctures in another place. This method yields better results than punctures with trocars, or with a lancet. It is, in fact, superior to any other method that has yet been suggested.

THE MEDICAL NEWS.

A WEEKLY JOURNAL

OF MEDICAL SCIENCE.

COMMUNICATIONS are invited from all parts of the world. Original articles contributed *exclusively* to THE MEDICAL NEWS will after publication be liberally paid for (accounts being rendered quarterly), or 250 reprints will be furnished in place of other remuneration. When necessary to elucidate the text, illustrations will be engraved from drawings or photographs furnished by the author. Manuscripts should be typewritten.

Address the Editor: J. RIDDLE GOFFE, M.D., No. 111 FIFTH AVENUE (corner of 18th St.), NEW YORK.

Subscription Price, including postage in U. S. and Canada.

PER ANNUM IN ADVANCE	$4.00
SINGLE COPIES	.10
WITH THE AMERICAN JOURNAL OF THE MEDICAL SCIENCES, PER ANNUM	7.50

Subscriptions may begin at any date. The safest mode of remittance is by bank check or postal money order, drawn to the order of the undersigned. When neither is accessible, remittances may be made, at the risk of the publishers, by forwarding in *registered* letters.

LEA BROTHERS & CO.,
No. 111 FIFTH AVENUE (corner of 18th St.), NEW YORK, AND Nos. 706, 708 & 710 SANSOM ST., PHILADELPHIA.

SATURDAY, MARCH 19, 1898.

WAR AND PESTILENCE.

IN these days of warlike preparation and patriotic commotion so much dust is kicked up that many public affairs of great vital importance demanding instant action are completely lost sight of. Millions of dollars are appropriated for national defense against a very problematic enemy, while at our very doors, perhaps within our borders, lurks a foe against which no adequate precautions have been taken. It is the opinion of our best sanitarians that with the coming of warm weather yellow fever is likely to again break out in our Southern States. If such fears are groundless, and if, as some hope, the epidemic of last summer has been stamped out, there still remain conditions which call for unusually strict sanitary precautions and rigid and uniform quarantine regulations.

Be there war or peace, our near neighbor Cuba has seldom, if ever, been in a state so potential for evil as at present. Impoverished by fire and sword, swarming with starving natives and unacclimated, non-immune soldiers, it must, during the coming summer, become a pestilential menace alike to friend and foe. Within a few hours' sail of Florida and many of our Gulf ports is Havana, where yellow fever is endemic and perennial. It is definitely known that this disease has been continuously endemic and frequently epidemic in Havana since 1761. It is impossible to estimate how many times our country has been infected from this source in all the years since 1761, but more recent data will show what a long-standing, constant, and present menace this hive of disease is. From 1807 to 1894 we have escaped yellow fever only during seven years. According to the report of the Marine Hospital Service for 1896, the source of the infection is known in only 41 of the 87 years; in 12 of these 41 years the origin of the disease is given as simply the West Indies, which may or may not mean the island of Cuba; but in 23 of the years the source is definitely given as Havana.

Between 1862 and 1894 yellow fever invaded the United States during twenty-six different years. The source of infection was known in 19 instances, and for 16 years could be traced to Havana. Oftentimes several of our ports have been simultaneously infected from this source, and to it our last two great epidemics were directly traced. The epidemic of 1878 invaded 132 towns, killed 15,934 persons, and entailed upon us a pecuniary loss of over $100,000,000, a sum that would support an efficient national quarantine for a century and a half. It is pretty well known that Havana was once free from yellow fever, but the reasons for the introduction and fostering of the disease are not difficult to determine. The only sanitary measure of importance ever, we may say, introduced into Havana, has been the rather recent acquisition of a fairly good and abundant water-supply; but this, without a commensurate increase of sewer capacity. As a result the soil and houses are damper than before, and the dangers attendant thereon are multiplied by the increased water-supply.

The condition of Havana is a sad commentary upon the general sanitary enlightenment of the age. The circumstances perpetuating the disease there are many; the "annual mean" temperature is high, ranging from 77 to 79° F., and frost is unknown. The soil upon which much of the city is built consists of mangrove swamps filled with refuge and garbage; the air is polluted, and the streets, most of them, are narrow and filthy. The houses, of the poor especially, are low, crowded, and damp, and many of them have in dangerous juxtaposition, stable, privy, cesspool, kitchen and sleeping-quarters. The harbor is small, almost land-locked, and shallow; it receives all the drainage and refuse from the city, and because of the small influx of river water and the low tides (only about two feet) stands a stagnant cesspool. The death-rate is over 40 per 1000. The city suffers not alone from the ravages of yellow fever, but also has a tremendous mortality from phthisis, diarrheal diseases, malignant malaria, and smallpox.

Cuba as a country and Havana as a city are commercially most closely linked with us. Dangerous in times of peace, what would happen in case of war with Spain, and that during the rainy, pestilential season? The Spanish forces would naturally seek to hold Cuba as a base of operations, and the initial movement on the part of our Government would be to dislodge them.

Our shores might be invaded by alien, infected troops; they certainly will be invaded in any event by Cuban refugees; our soldiers or sailors may be compelled to land upon and perhaps occupy Cuba, and the sure result, in any of these three exigencies, would be an infection of our tide-water towns, and the possibility of the worst epidemic of yellow fever that we have ever experienced. War is bad enough, and the ordinary diseases following in its wake kill more than combat, but what shall be said of the coexistence of war and pestilence?

Instead of helping the quarantine authorities, the Government has just crippled them by converting the Dry Tortugas into a military post. No locality equally good for a National quarantine station exists in that neighborhood, but the best available should be assigned to them at once.

Congress, by immediate and unanimous action, or the President, by proclamation, should grant the Marine Hospital Service power to increase its personnel and money to prepare tents and hospital supplies with such liberality that it would be able to locate hospitals and detention-camps whenever and wherever they may be needed. An epidemic of yellow fever would mean the loss of millions in money and thousands of lives, which could be prevented by the speedy endowment of the quarantine authorities with a little more power and a few thousands of dollars.

The results of rigid and enlightened sanitation elsewhere have shown that it is possible to stamp out infectious disease due to uncleanliness, a proof of which is the fact that Vera Cruz, once a hot-bed of disease in general, and yellow fever in particular, has purged itself, kept itself clean, and recently stood in the anomalous position of decreeing a quarantine against the United States, and had in lazaretto a steamer from one of our Gulf ports with three cases of yellow fever on board.

Local boards of health should see to it that their towns and cities are clean, so that if alien diseases evade a rigid quarantine, they will find a sterile nidus and not become epidemic.

THE GIFT OF THE NEW YORK HOSPITAL LIBRARY TO THE ACADEMY OF MEDICINE.

THE gratifying announcement of the gift of the books of The New York Hospital Library to the Academy of Medicine has recently been made. No more appropriate beneficiary could possibly be found. Although the library of the Academy of Medicine has had an astonishingly active growth during the past decade, no one who patronizes it to any considerable extent can fail to discover that it is lacking, particularly in rare and ancient books, possessions which enormously increase the worth of any library, and which make it invaluable to the real student. By the gift of the New York Hospital Association this hiatus in the shelves of the Academy library has been obliterated, and the library is at once lifted to rank, in point of number of volumes, second of the medical libraries of this country, and first of the private libraries.

Books are of far greater importance in contributing to the education and mental prosperity of a community than colleges and post-graduate schools. This is no less true of medicine than of other departments of learning, and New York greatly enhances her claim of being the medical center of the Western Hemisphere by the possession of the library of the Academy of Medicine.

This would seem to be an appropriate occasion to urge upon the trustees of the Academy the institution of needed reforms in the conduct of the library. There can be no doubt that its usefulness would be materially enhanced if it were open on holidays, and until at least 11 o'clock in the evening. Furthermore, we have never been able to see the wisdom of denying every one not a member of the Academy entrance to the library after 6 P.M. This unnecessary exclusiveness is surely of no advantage to members, as we feel quite safe in saying that there has always been ample elbow-room in the library after sunset, and it unquestionably prevents many non-resident physicians who come here for investigation and study from making complete use of the opportunities which the Metropolis affords. We say this despite the fact that strangers have access to the library in the evening if vouched for by a member. There should be no such senseless formality. On the contrary, every inducement should be offered to make the library of the Academy the pleasantest and most profitable place for the large number of physicians who visit this city every year to do post-graduate work to spend their evenings.

The trustees of the Academy have an emulable example in the library of Columbia University, the managers of which are successfully striving to make it the most important as well as the most accessible feature of that institution.

ANOTHER MEDICAL PARASITE.

CURRAN, in one of his memorable speeches, said that it "is the common fate of the indolent to see their rights become a prey to the active, and that eternal vigilance is the price of liberty." These must be the sentiments of every true physician who is brought in contact with the loathsome, nauseous literature which is incessantly put forth by the cormorants of the medical profession—the advertising quacks. We are approaching the time of year when these pestiferous creatures seem to double their sinister efforts, and the secular press and the mails alike are sorely burdened with their emanations. Of the entire class the sexual quack is by far the most malignant and irrepressible. His name is legion. He springs up like a toadstool in the night and is as fatal to those who mistake him for a genuine physician as the former article is to those who confound it with the salutary mushroom. He is, like the tubercle bacillus, widely distributed, and to be found in the most unexpected places, yet his favorite location seems to be in the Middle West of our country. It is with the hope of interesting the State and County Societies, which in the majority of cases have the power to deal deservedly with this species of depraved man, that we call attention to a very flagrant offender who burdens the town of Mechanicsville, Iowa, with his presence, and who poisons the youthful mind of many other States with his disgusting circulars and testimonials. His game is a diagnosis for any one who will send his name, age, sex, and a lock of hair, with four cents in postage stamps. On receipt of these, Dr. C. E. Batdorf, for it is thus he signs himself, will contribute a letter urging the beguiled and deluded sufferer to send one dollar in payment for a box of sexual pills or uterine regulators, whichever he thinks is most needed, and a warning that the unfortunate victim is on the verge of disaster. A sample of such letters, handed to us by a Philadelphia physician to whom it was given by one of the victims, reads as follows: "Your liver is inactive, the bile does not flow. Kidneys and sexual organs affected. Loss of vital fluid. Nervous at times, bilious and dull headache. Blood impure. The whole system is run down from dissipation, you will know what kind. We can cure you. Send $2 for magnetic powders and $1 for sexual pills. Do not delay. Please return this letter. Dr. C. E. Batdorf."

The last edition of "Polk's Medical Directory of the United States" gives no indication that such an individual as the one just named is practising medicine in Mechanicsville, Iowa, and we venture to think that in thus calling attention to him he will decide that the climate is not sufficienty salubrious for him to tarry there longer. We trust that the physicians of that community will assist in furthering our efforts.

ECHOES AND NEWS.

Drug-Clerks' Bill.—The bill restricting the working hours of drug clerks of New York City has passed the Senate by a vote of 27 to 3.

Dismissals in the Health Department.—President Murphy of the New York City Department of Health, on the 12th inst., discharged about forty of the employees of the old board, and appointed as milk inspector Richard V. Croker, a distant relative of the Tammany chief.

Salaries of Coroner's Physicians.—A bill increasing the salaries of coroner's physicians from $3000 to $5000 a year in the Boroughs of Manhattan and Brooklyn, and fixing them at $3000 for the Boroughs of the Bronx, Queens, and Richmond, was recently introduced in the New York Senate.

Obituary.—Sir Richard Quain, Bart., physician extraordinary to Queen Victoria, President of the General Medical Council, and editor of the "Dictionary of Medicine," recently died in London. He was born October 30, 1816, was a fellow of numerous medical societies, and the author of many scientific and medical works.

The Lewis Carroll Endowed Bed.—A fund to endow a bed in the Children's Hospital, Great Ormond Street, London, as a memorial to the author of "Alice in Wonderland," has been opened by the editor of the *St. James's Gazette.* The bed will be called the "Lewis Carroll Bed," the name under which Mr. Dodgson wrote his admirable books.

Ohio State Medical Society.—At the coming meeting of this Society, to be held at Columbus, May 4, 1898, the address on surgery will be delivered by Dr. Nicholas Senn. The local committee of arrangements is already actively engaged in preparations for the convention, and unusual efforts will be made to attain the fullest possible membership and attendance.

Board of Health and Hydrophobia.—The New York City Board of Health is now prepared to treat without charge cases of hydrophobia by the Pasteur method. During the past six months experiments with antirabitic serum have been conducted in the bacteriologic laboratory of the Health Department, and the results obtained have led the board to adopt the treatment.

Graduates of Local Medical Colleges Exempt from Examination.—A bill has recently been introduced into the Legislature of Iowa which exempts from the examination required by the "medical-practice" law all graduates of the the Medical Department of the University of Iowa. It is said that a similar bill will be drafted in Maryland, exempting graduates of the University of that State.

Fourth International Congress of Physiologists. — The Fourth International Congress of Physiologists will be held at Cambridge, England, August 23 to 27, 1898. There will be an exhibition of physiologic apparatus in connection with the Congress. Exhibits may be contributed by members of the Congress, by directors of physiologic laboratories, and by makers recommended by any member or director.

Entertainment in Aid of a Convalescent Home.—A musicale was recently given at the Astor Gallery, New York, in aid of the Rest for Convalescents, a charitable institution at White Plains, N. Y. This institution is open all the year, and receives Protestant women who have been discharged from hospitals or who are worn out with overwork. Its beneficiaries pay a nominal sum for their board, but are lodged without charge.

Liniment Exploded.—The explosion of a mixture of benzine and turpentine which was being used as a liniment recently resulted in the painful burning of a man and his wife in New York. The man was suffering from rheumatism, and his wife was rubbing him with the mixture. The application smarted so much that the woman lighted a match to see if there was an abrasion of the skin, and the explosion followed.

St. Mary's Hospital (Brooklyn) Loses a Bequest.—By a verdict recently rendered in the Surrogate's Court in Brooklyn, St. Mary's Hospital loses a bequest of $30,000 willed to it by Mrs. Jane Cunningham, widow of John Cunningham, who was at one time Charities Commissioner of Kings County. Mrs. Cunningham died in St. Mary's Hospital after a year's illness. Her relatives contested the will on the ground of undue influence with the result that it was declared void.

Bequests to Charities.—By the will of the late Amos R. Eno, the following charitable institutions of New York will each receive $5000: Colored Orphan Asylum, Demilt Dispensary, Protestant Half-Orphan Asylum, Association for the Relief of Respectable Aged and Indigent Females, Home for Old Men and Aged Couples, New York Cancer Hospital, Society for the Relief of Ruptured and Crippled, New York Training-School for Nurses, and the Institution for the Blind.

Plague Riots in Bombay. — Despatches from Bombay bring news of a riot which broke out among the low-caste Hindus and Mohammedans against the Europeans. It orginated in an attack upon a plague search-party. The mob attacked the hospital, burned the offices and stores, and savagely attacked the doctors, killing one of them. Detachments of police, of the Shropshire regiment, and of artillery were hurried to the scene, and a volley was fired into the mob, killing several persons.

The Practitioner and the Footpad.—Dr. A. A. Hallock of Massilon, Ohio, was recently the victim of a highway robber. While on the way to see a patient he was confronted with a revolver and a demand for money. The robber is said to have secured $20 in cash and $110 in checks, while the doctor received in return a bullet through his left foot. It is a poor sign of returning prosperity when the lonely country practitioner is called on by a highwayman to stand and deliver. It must have been an act of desperation.

Stolen Instruments and a Chicago Doctor.—Dr. C. A. Simmons, assistant demonstrator of anatomy in the Northwestern University and lecturer on anatomy and surgery at the Chicago Post-Graduate Medical School, has been charged with having in his possession $2000 worth of surgical instruments alleged to have been stolen from Chicago physicians. The stolen instruments were traced to Dr. Simmons' office by the arrest of a negro thief, who confessed that he had robbed the offices of several doctors and sold the stolen instruments to Dr. Simmons. The latter denies all guilt in the transaction.

Dr. William Gowers, Knighted.—Dr. Gowers of London has recently been knighted by his sovereign and dined by those of his fellow practitioners who are addicted to stenography. It has been said of Sir William that some of his works on nervous diseases have been translated into nearly every Continental language. At a dinner given last November, the honored guest related a reminiscence of his student life, going to show that his expertness as a shorthand writer was a matter of critical importance to him early in his career. Because of his ability to use phonography he became secretary to Sir William Jenner, which appointment prevented his acceptance of a partnership in a practice at Bournemouth. This proved to be the turning-point in his life.

Navy Needs Assistant Surgeons.—The Surgeon-General of the Navy has recommended that authority be immediately granted to enlist acting assistant surgeons for service on ships to be placed in commission and on auxiliary cruisers which may be impressed by the Government. He states that there are already eighteen vacancies in the lower grade of the medical corps, and, in the event of war, the medical department would be seriously crippled for lack of surgeons. The Surgeon-General recommends that additional inducements be offered for doctors to enter the navy, and that he be authorized to enlist any number of assistant surgeons deemed necessary. Secretary Long has the subject under consideration, and will probably recommend that the Surgeon-General's suggestion be approved.

Scarlet Fever from Blueberries.—One of the ways by which scarlet fever may be transmitted is illustrated by the following account which has been sent by a subscriber: A physician last summer attended two children in the same family having this disease. Since both were taken sick at the same time, and since there were no other cases known to exist anywhere in the community, not a little speculation as to its origin was occasioned. Finally, it was discovered that a few days previously both of these children had eaten of raw blueberries procured of a backwoodsman, whose family had doubtless picked them, and several of whom had been known to have scarlet fever the previous spring. The circumstances of this family were such that thorough disinfection was practically impossible except by fire.

New Competitors in the Medical Field.—In spite of the vigilance and persistence practised by the medical profession in suppressing irregularities in its domain, some unexpected dragon is constantly protruding his obnoxious head. The latest surprise comes in the form of spiritulistic mediums who are supplying prescriptions written by celebrated physicians, many of them long forgotten, who have left the terrestrial for the spirit world, but who, nevertheless, have not lost their interest in the practice of medicine. A specific instance of this has recently occurred in England, and the question has arisen whether such prescriptions can be recognized and compounded by a legitimate chemist, and also as to who is to assume the responsibility of the effect of such prescriptions on the individuals taking them.

The Troubles of a Practitioner.—A well-known physician of irreproachable character was recently arrested in New York on a criminal charge of manslaughter in the second degree, which was based on the allegation that in April, 1897, nearly a year ago, he had been guilty of culpable negligence in prescribing medicine for the infant child of the complainant, an actor, thereby causing its death. The physician was arraigned before a magistrate in the West Side Police Court, and was held for examination in $5000 bail, which was furnished later in the day, but not until the doctor had been locked up in a cell a number of hours awaiting the coming of his bondsman. In connection with this there seem to be two points calling for comment. One is the unseemly and barbarous manner in which a citizen and an honorable member of the medical profession was haled by the authorities and thrust into prison; and the second is the very surprising comments attributed to various members of the medical profession which were published in the daily papers in connection with the case. If the opinions attributed to them were expressed as reported, nothing that we can say would probably add to the humiliation which overwhelmed them when the specter of their words appeared before them. If they did not express the opinions attributed to them, no time or space should be too brief in which to set themselves right before the profession and the community. The facts of the case are not all in. There are two sides to every question, and no man should be condemned until he has been heard.

CORRESPONDENCE.

MIDWIVES IN NEW YORK.

To the Editor of the MEDICAL NEWS.

DEAR SIR: In regard to Dr. Cole's letter in the issue of the MEDICAL NEWS, March 5th, purporting to offer a correction of a statement in the beginning of my paper on "Midwives," published in the NEWS, February 19th, I have only to say that I do not know who had formulated the bill referred to, but I do know that Dr. Warden and I were sent to Albany at the expense of the County Medical Society to oppose its passage.

The acute stage of the recent agitation of the midwifery question is passed. The resolutions offered in societies have for the most part not been carried, and the committees appointed to report on the matter have been dismissed. No attempt will be made to obtain any legislation on the subject during this session of the legislature, but there is hardly any doubt that the question will come up again, and it would be desirable if, in the meantime, those who agree on the main points would come to an understanding about minor details.

Between the two extremes of those who want midwives officially recognized, examined and licensed, and those who want them "wiped out," the writer occupies a median position. Although fully aware that European methods are not applicable to the peculiar conditions of the United States, and especially the State of New York, and that a licensing bill would only lead to an increase in the number of midwives without any great improvement in their quality, he takes the fact into consideration that in cities with a large foreign element a considerable proportion of the population, ignorant of the dangers to which they expose themselves, are in the habit of employing midwives, and wish to continue to do so. Nor does he overlook that those who are engaged in this practice, and who by registering have complied with all that any authority has required of them, have obtained a certain right to be left alone. All lawyers consulted on the question declare that the law of 1895 regulating the practice of medicine does not prevent midwives from practising in normal cases for the reason that the courts and many members of the medical profession hold that childbirth is a physiologic act not appertaining to the domain of the practice of medicine.

The writer not only holds a position midway between two extremes, but a position which has the advantage of having been unanimously endorsed by the Section on Obstetrics and Gynecology of the Academy of Medicine at its meeting of January 27th (see MEDICAL NEWS, February 19, 1898).

Since then the writer has found a valuable ally in the Board of Midwifery of the City of Rochester, one of the two places in which examination, licensing, and supervision of midwives have been prescribed by a State law. In his paper read before the Section on Obstetrics the writer predicted that a licensing act would not prove satisfactory, a prediction which is fully supported by the following letter addressed to me by the Secretary of the Rochester Board which I herewith append.

H. J. GARRIGUES, M.D.

NEW YORK, March 10, 1898.

MY DEAR DOCTOR: Your recent paper on the subject of "Midwives" before the N. Y. Academy of Medicine was so timely and important, that at a recent meeting of the Rochester Board of Midwifery a resolution was passed which instructed the secretary of this board to communicate with you and say that it is the sense of this board that the present law enacted by the State Legislature for the purpose of regulating the practice of obstetrics in the City of Rochester is inadequate for the purpose designed.

To state also that this board is ready to cooperate with you in an endeavor to obtain some kind of general State remedial legislation.

Personally we agree entirely with your statement that there is no place for midwives. They are not only unnecessary, but are a menace to the public health. The final day of the midwife has come; she is obsolete, and must pass out of existence.

Any instruction you or your committee may have to offer will be gladly accepted.

(Signed) Respectfully yours,
N. W. NOBLE, Secretary.

ROCHESTER, N. Y., February 17, 1898.

OUR PHILADELPHIA LETTER.

[From our Special Correspondent.]

CECAL HERNIA—JURGENSEN'S SIGN—PARASITIC CHYLURIA—ALTERATIONS IN THE BUILDINGS OF THE MEDICO-CHIRURGICAL COLLEGE—STATE CARE OF CRIMINAL INSANE AND THE EASTERN PENITENTIARY OF PENNSYLVANIA.

PHILADELPHIA, March 12, 1898.

THE results of a careful study of sixty-three cases of cecal hernia were reported at the last meeting of the Philadelphia County Medical Society by Dr. J. H. Gibbon, tending to prove that the condition in question is rather more commonly met with than is generally supposed. Cecal hernia occurs more often in early childhood than at any other period of life, and is nearly always congenital; on the other hand, when it happens in adults, it is usually acquired and occurs after middle life. The speaker showed that in 642 herniotomies performed by Halstead and by Coley for femoral and inguinal herniæ, the cecum or appendix was found in the sac no less than 21 times. Of these 21 patients only 3 were over 15 years of age. Of the 63 cecal herniæ referred to by Gibbon, 36 were in patients under 15 years of age; in 5 the subjects were between 15 and 40 years of age; in 7 between 40 and 50 years, and in 15 past 50 years. The condition is rare in females owing to the anatomic differences. Of the series of 63 cases but 8 were in women. The right inguinal is the variety of hernia in which the cecum is most likely to be found, 44 cases of his series being of this nature, while 6 were right femoral, 6 left inguinal, and a single case left femoral. The congenital cecal hernia was thought to be more easily accounted for than the acquired variety; by the fact that in fetal life the cecum is not firmly fixed in the right iliac region and has been proven to possess some fibrous and muscular attachments to the testicle. Hence, in the descent of the testicle, the cecum or appendix is liable to be brought down with it. From a study of the present series of cases it would seem likely that a preexisting hernia of the ileum might act as a predisposing cause in the acquired cases. It was also added that other predisposing causes should be sought in the facts that some ceca are more movable than others, and that some are also of comparatively small size. That these conditions coexist is shown by Treves, who has demonstrated that when the cecum fails to become fixed in its normal situation it usually is of smaller size than normal. The idea that the sac of a cecal hernia is often deficient or absent is no longer tenable, and in very few of the reporter's cases was the sac incomplete. As to the condition of strangulation: of the 63 cases 28 were strangulated, and only 12 were reducible on account of adhesions, which were often so dense that reduction was impossible. Complicating disease of the appendix was comparatively rare, never being noted except when this part of the gut was the sole occupant of the hernial sac; in such cases the process was usually far advanced. The relative infrequency of appendical complications, noted by Gibbon, differs from the views of other observers with whom a much larger percentage of appendix inflammation is generally reported. In the speaker's series, foreign bodies were found in two instances, and perforation existed in five cases. As to the diagnosis of cecal hernia, it can be only positively made when the appendix can be felt by palpation; this may be readily done in young children and in the aged, in which the coverings of the hernia are thin. The hernia is usually of large size when the cecum is contained in the sac. Concerning the treatment of the condition, Gibbon is inclined to be governed by the same operative rules applicable to other herniæ, except when the appendix is known to be in the sac, and will, in all probability, give rise to strangulation and become itself diseased. In such instances the removal of the appendix will depend upon its condition, and the attitude of the operator will be governed by the general question of its removal.

Jürgensen's sign, a usually pathognomonic sign of miliary tuberculosis, was faithfully simulated in a recent case reported by Hamill before the College of Physicians, in which the condition was later proven not to have been miliary tuberculosis, although it was at first so considered. Hamill's patient, after a period of pyrexia and delirium, developed suspicious pulmonary signs, and later on a friction fremitus over the lungs which corresponded characteristically to the description given by Jürgensen to the sign produced by the rubbing together of fine subpleural tubercles and the costal pleura. Subsequent developments in the clinical history of Hamill's case, however, proved that the sign had been misleading.

A case of parasitic chyluria, due to infection by the filaria sanguinis hominis, was recently reported to the College of Physicians by T. H. Dunn. The case, so Dunn claimed, was indigenous to this locality, the patient having always lived in the immediate vicinity of Philadelphia. The chief symptoms noted were paroxysmal attacks of cephalalgia, gastro-intestinal disturbances, and periods of anuria. Following these periods of anuria, which occasionally continued as long as two days and a half, the patient's urine became chylous, albuminous, and fatty, and contained, in addition to granular leucocytes and red blood-cells, numbers of actively motile embryos of the filaria sanguinis hominis. A casual relation between the infection by mosquitoes, and the present case was deemed not improbable. It may be recalled that in 1896 F. P. Henry reported in the MEDICAL NEWS a case of filarial infection in this city in which the blood of the patient was rich in embryos of the filaria nocturna. Henry's patient was not, however, a native of Philadelphia, having come to this city from South Carolina, where instances of filariasis are not unknown. It may be interesting to note that in this case of Henry's the filarial infection is still active without deleterious effects on the health of the patient. Your correspondent recently had an opportunity to examine the blood of this patient several times, and found without difficulty the embryos of the parasite, though the number of filariæ was less than at first reported, two years ago.

Extensive alterations in the buildings of the Medico-Chirurgical College are to be made this spring for the purpose of erecting additions to be used as a college of pharmacy, soon to be established by this institution, and also for dispensary purposes. A number of buildings adjoining the present college have been purchased by the trustees, and will be torn down at the close of the present term, in May, to make room for the improvements. This move on the part of the "Medico-Chi" puts it in possession of the entire front of the block on Cherry Street from Seventeenth to Eighteenth Street.

The authorities of the Eastern Penitentiary in this city, one of the largest penal institutions in Pennsylvania, are urgently demanding State care of the criminal insane in a separate place of confinement especially devoted to this purpose. General insane hospitals will not answer for insane criminals, they argue, and their reasoning seems sound when one recalls the fact that of seven so-called insane criminals removed last year from the Eastern Penitentiary to the Norristown Hospital for the Insane, by order of the Court, three were sane enough to effect their escape, and one received fatal injuries, in attempting to escape, three days after his arrival. The Legislature is to be asked to at once remedy this defect by establishing a separate prison building at the Eastern Penitentiary for the use of the insane criminals confined in this prison. This class is the most dangerous element in prison life, and it is necessary that their segregation from the rest of the prisoners be effected without delay on account of the overcrowded condition of the penitentiary.

The number of deaths in this city for the week ending March 12th was 464, a decrease of 16 from those reported last week. Of the total number of deaths, 177 were of children under 5 years of age. There were 88 new cases of enteric fever, with 7 deaths; 76 cases of diphtheria, with 19 deaths, and 73 cases of scarlet fever, with 2 deaths.

OUR BERLIN LETTER.

[From our Special Correspondent.]

THE "LONDON TIMES" ON THE PRIVAT-DOCENTS AND PROFESSOR VIRCHOW—DISCUSSION AS TO THE VALUE OF KOCH'S NEW TUBERCULIN AT THE CHARITE—EASTER VACATIONS AND THE GERMAN MEDICAL AND SURGICAL CONGRESS—OESTREICK ON THE ANATOMIC BASIS OF SOME HEART CONDITIONS.

BERLIN, March 10, 1898.

THERE has been some little amusement in medical circles in Berlin lately over an almost unaccountable mistake in *The* (London) *Times*. One day last week an editorial in this paper discussed the question of the new law with regard to Privat-docents at the German univerities in a very masterly way. The obvious advantage of thorough freedom of teaching and the assurance it gave of unhampered evolution of new ideas in social and political science, sciences in which above all an untrammeled environment is a necessity to development, was pointed out. Some of the readers of the MEDICAL NEWS will remember somewhat similar views expressed in this column some weeks ago.

The editorial in the *Times* was opportune, and, as the representative of the best conservative English opinion, carried a good deal of weight here, and was very widely read. One of the salient facts pointed out was that the greatest German professors, the representatives of what is best in German educational life, were thoroughly opposed to any measure that would tend to make the younger men in the universities too dependent upon governmental or political influences. Among others, the great Virchow, and here was the joke of the matter, "the universally known professor of physiology at the University of Berlin," was outspoken in his opposition to the proposed law.

Thackeray defined glory somewhere as "being wounded severely in battle to-day and having one's name spelled incorrectly in the next day's gazette." A great medical reputation would seem to be no more sacred from the desecration of carelessness. One scarcely expects, however, to find the supposedly omniscient leader-writers of the great "Thunderer" making such egregious errors as this, and metamorphosing, without even by your leave, the father of modern pathology, into a professor of physiology.

The last two meetings of the hospital staff of the Charité (which constitutes a sort of medical society with bi-weekly meetings) have been occupied with a discussion of Koch's new tuberculin—tuberculin R. In April it will be a year since the authoritative publication of the new method and announcement of the remedy. Some definite conclusions, it would seem, might be reasonably expected. The drift of opinion was all against the tuberculin R and most of the clinicians did not hesitate to compare it to the old tuberculin in its effects, and some of them, in its possible dangers.

Dr. Huber, an assistant in Professor Leyden's clinic, has attempted to immunize animals in the way in which Koch immunized the animals which served as the basis for his conclusions in his last communication, but utterly failed. The experiments seem to have been carefully carried out, the dosage of tuberculin was exact and sufficent, and the observations numerous enough to do away with the idea that perhaps coincidence played a rôle in the results obtained. Yet he failed to get the desired immunity. The full details of the experiments are to appear in the next number of the *Zeitschrift für klinische Medizin* of which Professor Von Leyden is the principal editor. After supposed immunization all the animals died when inoculated with tuberculous material, and interestingly enough, most of them before the control animals inoculated with the same material at the same time.

In Professor Von Leyden's clinic there has been absolutely no success with the new tuberculin. Patients acquire an immunity to reaction from the tuberculin itself, but no curative effects on tuberculous deposits were noted. At times some improvement occurred, but there was never complete disappearance of any physical signs of the disease which had been previously noted. In patients with fever even Koch himself does not recommend it, and there is no doubt that it can, and often does, do harm in such cases.

Non-tuberculous patients may react to even small doses of tuberculin R, so that the employment of any such reaction as a sign of the presence of a tuberculous process in a given case is said here to be utterly delusive. The conclusion of the experience in the medical clinic is that it is not a specific. Therapeutically it is no better than other forms of treatment which are not near so costly, and not near so worrying to the doctor; for in no case can this treatment be employed except under a doctor's immediate supervision. These conclusions are shared by the workers in Professors Gerhardt and Senator's clinics.

Even Professor Fränkel, the throat and nose specialist, who on the strength of some lupus and laryngeal cases in which at first improvement seemed very rapid, was for some months an advocate of the new treatment, now admits that it is practically no better than many other forms of treatment for these affections, that it often fails to produce a change in the course of the disease, and never produces radical cure. Only Professor Briger, Professor Koch's assistant in the Institute for Infectious Diseases, makes any claims as to the value of the tuberculin treatment. The history of the second tuberculin forms an interesting commentary on the enthusiastic reception of the first. Here it has had practically the effect of destroying faith in all so-called specific remedies for tuberculosis. Constitutional treatment, especially such as can be given in favorably situated, specially arranged consumption hospitals, is now the only method receiving any attention.

With the first of March the University closed for the Easter vacations. The semester is supposed to begin October 15th and end March 15th, but fifteen days of grace, corresponding to the academic fifteen-minutes' grace always taken before a lecture, is allowed the lecturers at the beginning and the end of each semester. The summer semester is supposed to begin April 15th, and will really get under way May 1st, so that after about three and one third months of work (not counting the twenty days vacation at Christmas) there comes a solid break of two months in the regular work of the year. This is taken advantage of by many to do special work, but for most it must be just vacation in the ordinary sense of the word. The summer semester is supposed to end July 15th and really closes July 1st, while there is fully a week free at Penticost, so that a German medical year is absolutely only five months of required attendance at lectures. Our American course with four years, each of almost eight solid months of work, is not so far behind in requirements as is usually and at times a little sneeringly remarked over here.

German doctors take advantage of the freedom of the University men to hold the annual congresses in medicine and surgery. The German is essentially an animal *sociale* and is rather ready to attend meetings of almost any kind. Meetings of medical societies, notwithstanding their frequency, are magnificently attended. The Berlin Medical society has five hundred to eight hundred members at its meetings every Wednesday night and the society for Internal Medicine, two hundred to three hundred every Monday night. Needless to say that the congresses are well attended.

The medical meeting to be held this year from April 13th to 16th at Wiesbaden promises to be of universal interest. Professor Von Ziemssen of Munich and Professor Von Jaksch of Prague, who may be taken to fairly represent the old and the young among the great German professors, are to open the discussion of the methods to be employed in the clinical teaching of medicine. Professor Müller of Marburg, a colleague of Professor Behring's, and Professor Brieger of Berlin, whose work in bacteriologic chemistry is well known, are to read papers on auto-intoxication and intestinal antisepsis. Professor Schott of Nauheim, whose method of treating chronic heart disease has of late years attracted so much attention, is to talk on the treatment of muscular affections of the heart.

The Annual German Surgical Congress is to meet at Berlin at the same time as the Medical Congress in Wiesbaden, and while its program has not yet been defiitely announced, some hints of what are to be interesting features are known. The question of the use of gloves at operations will be discussed, and probably favorably; operative interference in heart wounds will be advocated, while performance of radical ear operations for chronic purulent otitis media will be discouraged except when these are urgent symptoms.

An interesting article on "Some Mechanical Factors Which Influence Pathologic Conditions in the Heart Muscle and Valves" occurs in the last number of *Virchow's Archivs*, from the pen of his assistant, Dr. Oestreick. Some two years ago this author's article on fragmentation of the myocardium attracted a good deal of attention, and its conclusions were very generally accepted in Germany. French clinicians still insist that it is in their realm and may be diagnosticated and yet recovery follow. Unfortunately the diagnosis has not been confirmed by autopsy often enough to make the interesting symptom-complex sketched for it of much practical importance.

Dr. Oestreick's present article, besides interesting descriptions of the pathologic appearances of pure mitral stenosis and mitral insufficiency in actual specimens (some clinicians and pathologists deny their existence), discusses the question of dilatation from a new standpoint. The muscle of the whole ventricle or auricle does not dilate equally under the strain put upon it, but certain parts are more protected because of papillary and trabecular origins in them, and so suffer less. Then to, when the blood stream, owing to the contraction of the mitral orifice, for example, and the hypertrophy of the auricle, is forced in a narrow-pointed stream seventy times a minute against a particular part of the wall of the ventrical, a mechanical factor to which not much attention has been paid heretofore, is brought into play in the production of atrophic patches of muscular tissue. These atrophic spots under these circumstances become the so-called aneurisms of the heart. Dr. Oestreick thinks these impossible to diagnose clinically, since even post-mortem they easily escape notice. Young clinicians will, however, I suppose, still presume on the diagnosis. The whole article is extremely suggestive, and shows that there is still room for new work in so old a field as the heart.

TRANSACTIONS OF FOREIGN SOCIETIES.

London.

OBLITERATIVE ARTERITIS — PERIPHERAL NEURITIS FROM ARSENIC—AN OPERATION FOR CHRONIC ULCER OF THE LEG—IMMUNITY AND LATENCY AFTER OPERATIONS FOR REPUTED CANCER OF THE BREAST—SOME REMARKS ON RECTAL SURGERY—EMERGENCIES OF ANESTHESIA.

AT a meeting of the Clinical Society, January 14th, SPENCER exhibited a man, twenty-seven years of age, suffering from *obliterative arteritis*. The first symptoms appeared during August, 1897, in the left leg, and amputation for gangrene was soon required. The femoral artery was found to be obliterated. After this the disease remained stationary. This case was similar to that reported by Gould during 1884, in which the disease came to a standstill after progressing for about three years.

COLMAN exhibited a case of *peripheral neuritis caused by arsenic*, occurring in a girl aged twelve years, who had been given arsenic for chorea. She had received 15 minims of liquor arsenicalis (Brit. Ph.) three times daily during several weeks. At the close of the treatment the chorea was apparently perfectly cured. Two weeks after the use of arsenic had been discontinued the patient complained of weakness and tingling of the leg, soon followed by ankle-drop, and later, by paralysis of all muscles below the knees, with well-marked reaction of degeneration. There was also some weakness and diminished faradic reaction of the extensor muscles of the forearm. The patient was placed in bed and treated by massage and galvanism, and is now rapidly recovering. The case is interesting as showing that heroic doses of arsenic, so often used in chorea, are not without risk.

WALLIS showed a man upon whom he had *operated for ulcer of the leg* by making incisions at some distance from the edges of the ulcer, raising the strips of skin, dissecting out the ulcer with its base, and bringing the two lateral skin-flaps together in the middle, thus leaving for granulation two distinct wounds in healthy tissue. These were later covered with Thiersch grafts. Both the ulcer and the lateral incisions completely healed.

At the meeting of January 28th, HERRINGHAM read a paper on *sudden death in acute rheumatism*. A girl, aged sixteen years, suffering with a first attack of rheumatic fever, many joints being involved, grew gradually worse, and then suddenly died. An autopsy revealed edema of both lungs and fatty degeneration of the walls of the left ventricle, with much increase of the cells in the interstitial connective tissue—that is to say, acute myocarditis. This acute change in the heart is probably the usual cause of the few cases of sudden death from acute rheumatism. Suspicion should be aroused if with cyanosis, for which there appears no sufficient cause in the lunes, there is considerable pain in the epigastric or precordial regions.

MACLAGAN said that he never gave salicylate of soda in cases of rheumatism in which he suspected involvement of the heart, but preferred to give salicin, as it has been stated that the bad effects which sometimes follow the administration of salicylate of soda are due to the presence of impurities in the form of creosotic acid. He said that the symptoms, delirium, pain, dyspnea, and tendency to cyanosis, were not in themselves proof of a genuine inflammatory condition of the cardiac substance, but were more probably due to some toxic product of rheumatism.

DUCKWORTH said that he had learned to recognize such cases clinically, and sometimes to avert the attacks by proper treatment. He thought that enough attention is not usually given to the existence of myocarditis, and to the fact that it is the result of the influence of the rheumatic poison. He had seen pericarditis spread into the myocardium, but he had also observed its development from endocarditis. He thought that if the myocardium became affected salicylate of soda should be either withheld or combined with brandy, but under such circumstances he preferred to omit it altogether, and to administer in its place iodid of potassium and quinin.

At a meeting of the Royal Medical and Chirurgical Society of January 25th, SHIELD read a paper on *immunity and latency after operations for reputed cancer of the breast.* Every surgeon of experience, he said, is able to quote notable exceptions to the generally received rule that rapid recurrence is invariable after operations for cancer of the breast. An investigation into the subject led him to believe that even the old or incomplete operation does not give as universally bad results as is generally stated. In some of the cases in which life had been longest preserved it was remarkable that local recurrences had been removed one or more times. Some of the best results obtained must be due to a peculiarity of the growth or of the individual, rather than to the character of the operation. Shield mentioned eighteen cases occurring in private practice, the post-operative histories of which he had been able to follow, in which there had been no recurrence after ten years. In none of them was the so-called complete operation performed.

The analysis of seventy-two cases by Bryant showed that in eighteen per cent. the patients lived from five to ten years or longer after operation. It was noticeable that recurrence rarely took place in the axilla, but usually below it, or in the scar. Hence, he always explored the axilla, but did not clear it out unless there was positive evidence of the presence of malignant disease. In eight cases of recurrent carcinoma he had known cutaneous tubercles to persist for six months and then disappear without treatment. Formerly he considered such tubercles disseminated new growths, but, in the light of his experience, a surgeon need not hesitate to remove a distinct recurrence of the cancer, even though cutaneous nodules are present.

BARWELL spoke of late recurrence of cancer. In one case the disease recurred seven years after operation, and in another sixteen years after. In his opinion, granular infection is less apt to occur when the disease is on the sternal side of the breast. He also said that recurrence is less likely to follow in the scar if healing is prompt.

At a meeting of the Medical Society, January 24th, BRYANT made *some remarks on rectal surgery.* He lamented the fact that practitioners so readily accept, without examination, a patient's diagnosis of piles. By such carelessness many trivial cases pass into a serious chronic condition. During examination the patient should lie in the Sim's position on the edge of a bed or couch. Bryant advocated an early incision of abscesses in the anal region in order to relieve pain and prevent deep burrowing. Before opening the abscess the surgeon's finger should be passed well into the rectum so as to press the abscess cavity out toward the skin of the perineum. After being freely opened the cavity should be irrigated with iodin water. It should not be packed with gauze, as it is desirable that its walls should at once adhere. A small slip of gauze should be placed in the incision in the skin. The same principle of dressing applies to fistulæ, which should be thoroughly opened and well scraped. The bowels should be kept open, but the stools should not be liquid, for liquid stools are apt to excoriate, and are more painful than pultaceous ones.

GOODSALL said that in ninety per cent. of all cases of disease of the rectum and anus the affection is situated in the first two inches of the bowel, and may be missed if the finger is introduced too far. A T-shaped incision into an ischiorectal abscess gives the patient the best chance of avoiding a fistula. EDWARDS said that fifty per cent. of the cases of pruritus ani were unassociated with rectal disease. Forcible dilatation continued long enough to cause temporary paralysis of the sphincter, with scraping of the eczematous part, will usually effect a cure. In some cases of uncomplicated piles he preferred the injection of a 1-to-5 solution of carbolic acid in glycerin to any other mode of treatment.

The methods of treatment of the *emergencies of anesthesia* were discussed at the Society of Anesthetists, January 20th. The various measures usually employed fall under one of six heads: (1) Those which excite respiration by external irritation, *e. g.*: cold to the epigastrium or ammonia to the nostrils. (2) Those which excite respiration by mechanical means, *e. g.*: rhythmic traction of the tongue (Laborde) or dilatation of the sphincter ani; (3) stimulation of the heart by mechanical and electrical means, including acupuncture; (4) artificial respiration; (5) measures counteracting circulatory failure; by *e. g.*, amyl nitrite, strychnin, atropin, etc. Hot and cold applications to the skin and precordial percussion were adversely criticised. The influence of posture on the circulation was said to be not clear at present, probably a good deal depending upon the degree of arterial tone and the influence exerted by gravity. In circulatory failure inversion and pressure over the abdomen were recommended. BOWLES said that in cases of pus or blood in the pleura, for instance, empyemia—patients should be placed with the affected side down and the Silvester method employed with one arm only, the supine posture being carefully avoided.

SOCIETY PROCEEDINGS.

THE NEW YORK ACADEMY OF MEDICINE.—SECTION ON LARYNGOLOGY AND RHINOLOGY, BEFORE THE ACADEMY.

Stated Meeting, Held Thursday, March 3, 1898.

THE President, E. G. JANEWAY, M.D., in the Chair.

A MEMORIAL ADDRESS ON THE LATE JOSEPH O'DWYER, M.D.,

was read by DR. WILLIAM P. NORTHRUP.

Joseph O'Dwyer, M.D., the inventor of intubation, died at his home on Lexington Avenue, New York City, January 7, 1898, in the fifty-seventh year of his age. He was born October 12, 1841, in Cleveland, Ohio; spent his boyhood near London, Ontario, in which city he received his early education, and took his first studies in medicine with Dr. Anderson. He attended lectures at the New York College of Physicians and Surgeons in

1864, and was graduated from this institution in 1866. Just at this time the staff of the Charity Hospital on Blackwell's Island was made a separate body, and, after a competitive examination in which Dr. O'Dwyer stood first, he was appointed sanitary superintendent of the institution. Shortly after his assumption of duties there an epidemic of cholera broke out in the workhouse, and Dr. O'Dwyer contracted the disease in the performance of his duty. His recovery was complete, without complication or sequelæ.

1868–9 Dr. O'Dwyer was appointed examiner of patients applying for admission to hospitals under the control of the Board of Charities and Correction, and about this time he opened an office with Dr. Warren Schoonover on Second Avenue, between Fifty-seventh and Fifty-eighth Streets, where he began an extensive obstetric practice, ultimately reaching the number of 3000 cases.

In 1872 Dr. O'Dwyer moved to Lexington Avenue near Sixty-fifth Street, in close proximity to the New York Foundling Asylum, which had likewise moved uptown, and was about to open its new building, with which he became connected, together with Drs. Reynolds and J. Lewis Smith. From 1873 to 1880 tracheotomy was on trial in this institution, but met with no success. In 1880 Dr. O'Dwyer "began thinking" on croup and some method for providing a channel for the passage of air and secretions through the larynx without the complication of an open wound. How to hold apart the swollen false and true vocal cords until the disease should run its course and the stenosis be relieved was his first thought. The most natural resource was a skeleton wire spring. This, however, soon gave way to a small bivalve speculum formed on the model of a bivalve vaginal speculum, and fitted with a spring to force the two valves apart when placed in position. This laryngeal spring or speculum served to keep the air-passages open, but had important faults. The space between the open valves allowed the swollen mucous membrane to crowd in, and ultimately cause a recurrence of the stenosis. If the spring was too weak, it would not separate the blades; if too strong, it caused ulceration from pressure. The mouth-gag had not been devised at this time, but a shield, consisting of two metal discs about the size of a silver quarter of a dollar, bent to fit the proximal phalanx, and held together with rubber elastic bands, was worn on the index-finger of the left hand.

The first intubation recorded at the New York Foundling Asylum is as follows:

"October 21, 1882. Dr. G. M. Swift, House Physician. Female, aged four years; severe croup, pseudomembrane in pharynx; dyspnea urgent; temporary asphyxia relieved at 1:40 A. M., by introduction into the larynx by Dr. O'Dwyer of one of his "springs." Eight hours later the spring was removed, and the child again became asphyxiated. Tracheotomy and death. *Autopsy:* Pseudomembrane in pharynx, larynx, and bronchi down to the finest bronchioles, continuous, tenacious, and the thickness of wet blotting-paper."

In this and two other cases two points had been demonstrated: First, that the larynx would tolerate a tube; and, second, that air could gain entrance and the secretions find exit. Dr. O'Dwyer's only idea at this time was to temporarily keep a channel open for the short distance between the false vocal cords and the beginning of the trachea. The bivalve laryngeal speculum or spring, with all its faults, had one recovery to its credit—the first case of membranous croup which had recovered after operation during the thirteen years of the existence of the Foundling Asylum.

After three years of experiment the idea of accomplishing the desired result with a bivalve laryngeal speculum was abandoned, and, after some time spent in studying the healthy larynx and the larynx swollen and lined with pseudomembrane, Dr. O'Dwyer appeared one day in the dead-house with a tube—a tube longer than the speculum, narrow, oval or flattened laterally, and having a collar at its upper end. The first mention of a "tube" occurs in a recorded history in the dead-book, April 25, 1894, "Dr. O'Dwyer put in a 'tube' at night; dyspnea relieved, breathing fairly good until death occurred sixteen hours later." A foot-note in connection with this case states that the question whether the lungs were collapsed or pneumonic was of much interest to Dr. O'Dwyer. He and Dr. J. H. Ripley discussed this question at great length, Dr. Ripley contending that the lungs in such cases did not show pneumonia, but rather were collapsed. Dr. O'Dwyer was much pleased with the relief afforded by this tube for sixteen hours, and with the fact that it was not coughed up.

The second case in which the tube was employed resulted in recovery. The patient was a girl four years of age, who shut her teeth tightly upon the metallic shield upon the finger and imprisoned the Doctor until chloroform relaxed her jaws. A new need was presented by this case, and this led to the invention of the mouth-gag, but new difficulties were still to be met. The tube contained a little slit into which the extractor hooked when the tube was removed, and into this slit the mucous membrane likewise booked and held fast, thus causing damage to the soft tissues when the tube was withdrawn, so the slit had to be dispensed with. The tubes were also made longer to reach to the bifurcation so that they would not be coughed up, as had happened up in this time in some instances. Then a second shoulder was made below the point of contact of the vocal cords, with an abrupt shoulder above and a vanishing wedge below, the cords resting in the space between the shoulders. The head of the tube was blunt, rounded, and of odd shape. This tube remained in position too well, and it was almost impossible to get it out, so it was abandoned. Then came a long period of thinking, of measuring larynges, of modeling putty on the middle of tubes and putting them into specimen larynges, and of taking plaster casts. The result at last came in the form of the retaining swell—a fusiform enlargement of the middle portion of the tube lying within the trachea. To avoid pressure and ulceration at the base of the epiglottis, within the cricoid ring, and where the lower end of the tube rested, a backward curve was given to the upper portion of the tube, and its lower end was thickened and rounded off. Finally, the tubes were made of much smaller caliber. To-day the perfect intubation-tube is made of hard rubber. Lime salts do not form upon it; it does not corrode or require replating; it can be easily boiled and disinfected, and can be indefinitely worn without the necessity of frequent removal.

Two years after intubation was given to the public, and half a year after the first ovation to its inventor at the International Medical Congress in Washington, Mrs. O'Dwyer died. It is not difficult for those who knew the man to understand how much he needed all which is comprehended in the word "home." He was a retiring man, of few words, sensitive, conscientious, diffident, always thinking. A congenial home atmosphere was the one thing necessary to a man of his disposition, and his wife was of the kind to produce that congeniality, for she was hopeful, sympathetic, encouraging, and absolutely devoted to him. He felt her death keenly.

If I were asked what most contributed to Dr. O'Dwyer's medical excellence, I would say his habit of thinking and his good logic. He had a good medical mind, good medical judgment—that quality which allows a man to grow after the age of forty. To the New York Foundling Asylum, with which Dr. O'Dwyer was connected for twenty-five years, he was everything; to the maternity service he was the expert obstetrician; in intubation he was the teacher; in general service his was the constant consulting mind; to the Sisters of Charity he was the physician, the friend, the general regulator of the household. All adored him.

What the world knows of Dr. O'Dwyer is his genius as an inventor, his achievement in adding a great operation to the equipment of the profession and thus making the most conspicuous real contribution to medical progress within the last fifty years. This the world knows and has acknowledged. To us there is another and a pleasant duty—to testify that with this genius there was all that goes to make a man. His home life, his religious life, his civic life, his professional relations with both colleague and patient, his hospital relations were such as befit a high-principled man. As highly as we esteem him as an inventor and genius and practitioner of wide knowledge, as much as we valued his superior medical judgment, we would write upon the monument of his achievements, "O'Dwyer, the Man."

DR. WILLIAM K. SIMPSON then read a paper, entitled

INTUBATION IN DIPHTHERIA (see page 353).

DR. CHARLES H. KNIGHT followed with a paper on

INTUBATION IN ACUTE NON-DIPHTHERITIC STENOSIS OF THE LARYNX (see page 357).

DR. D. BRYSON DELAVAN closed with a paper on

INTUBATION IN CHRONIC STENOSIS OF THE LARYNX (see page 360).

DISCUSSION.

DR. H. W. BERG: I have seen a number of cases in which intubation was employed, and in some instances, in which the tube was withdrawn after it had been worn four, five, or six days, it has been necessary to reintroduce it. A second and third removal of the tube was followed by such severe dyspnea that reinsertion was necessary, and in this way the patient has gone on wearing the tube weeks and months, and, in one case which I recall, the months became years. Two of these cases were seen by Dr. O'Dwyer, who thought this due to cicatricial contraction or to adhesions produced by ulceration at the upper border of the cricoid cartilage. It seemed to me that the trouble was due to paralysis of the vocal cords caused by pressure upon them, but Dr. O'Dwyer did not agree with me. Some authorities attribute this condition to the general paralysis which often follows diphtheria, but it is hardly probable that a post-diphtheritic paralysis would affect only the muscles of the throat. The cause and treatment of this inability to breathe without the tube is still an unsettled question. Dr. O'Dwyer himself tried removing the tube for a few minutes at a time in these cases, but with little success. Then the insertion of a smaller tube was tried, but this was generally coughed up by the patient. The condition is still but little understood, and forms an interesting problem which as yet awaits solution.

DR. SIMPSON: Dr. O'Dwyer, I think, attributed the inability to do without the intubation-tube after its prolonged use to loss of the cricoid cartilage. He quotes a case in which autopsy showed entire loss of this cartilage. I think all the points mentioned by Dr. Berg are thoroughly discussed in Dr. O'Dwyer's book. I agree with the speaker that this Section might well make this subject a matter of study.

A very handsome collection of gold- and silver-plated and wire tubes, showing the evolution of the tube from a one-inch "spring" to the present perfect rubber tubes, together with the mouth-gag, extractor, and other instruments employed in intubation, was exhibited. These and the case containing them were presented to the Academy of Medicine by Mr. George Ermold, the instrument-maker, who for years made the tubes for Dr. O'Dwyer.

REVIEWS.

MANUAL OF PATHOLOGY, INCLUDING BACTERIOLOGY, THE TECHNIC OF POST-MORTEMS, AND METHODS OF PATHOLOGIC RESEARCH. By W. M. LATE COPLIN, M.D., Professor of Pathology and Bacteriology, Jefferson Medical College, etc.; being a second edition of the author's "Lectures on Pathology." Rewritten and enlarged. Philadelphia: P. Blakiston, Son & Co., 1897.

THE author has revised and enlarged his "Lectures on Pathology" written three years ago, and in the volume before us has attempted to give to the student in pathology all the more important facts pertaining to laboratory technic. Most of the essential data which a student should know are touched upon, to some is given considerable attention, while others receive but a passing mention, and as a result the work is not as complete and satisfactory as some others which have recently appeared.

The book is divided into three parts. Part I. includes post-mortem examinations, histologic methods, and the technic of urine, sputum, and blood examinations. Parts

II. and III. are devoted to general and special pathology, respectively.

The directions for making a post-mortem examination of the brain occupy but half of one page, and are by far too superficial for the beginner. Under histologic methods only two stains are mentioned, *viz.*, Grenacher's borax-carmin and Delafield's hematoxylin. These are all very well for ordinary routine work, but in a book of more than 600 pages one has a right to expect more than this.

The chapters on special and general pathology are more satisfactory, but we are amazed to discover that diseases of the entire central nervous system have been omitted. If this be an oversight it is a serious one indeed.

The book is fully illustrated, many of the reproductions from drawings being especially well executed. At the end of each chapter is a list of questions directed to the student on the preceding text. An alphabetic index of illustrations has been introduced. We trust that in a future edition the few omissions noted will be supplied, for as the books stands we cannot unhesitatingly recommend it as a complete manual for students' use.

PATHOLOGICAL TECHNIQUE. A PRACTICAL MANUAL FOR THE PATHOLOGICAL LABORATORY. By FRANK BURR MALLORY, A.M., M.D., Assistant Professor of Pathology, Harvard University Medical School; Assistant Pathologist to the Boston City Hospital, etc.; and JAMES HOMER WRIGHT, A.M., M.D., Director of the Laboratory of the Massachusetts General Hospital; Instructor in Pathology, Harvard University Medical School. With 105 illustrations. Philadelphia: W. B. Saunders, 1897.

IT would be difficult to find a better example of the progress made in laboratory technic during the last decade, than to note the rapidity with which new books on this subject have appeared. We have had great satisfaction in reading this latest addition to the subject, and we feel convinced that a book written on such a high scientific plane and at the same time in so practical a manner will be welcomed as a helpful guide to all laboratory workers.

The book is one of 397 pages, including the index. It is well printed on heavy paper, and is supplied with many excellent illustrations, some of which are in colors. We cannot review all the sections in detail and must confine ourselves to the general plan of the book.

Part I. is devoted to post-mortem examinations, and most of the drawings are borrowed from Nauwerck's admirable work, but are poorly reproduced and much diminished in size. The customary directions for performing autopsies are clearly stated, and many valuable hints to beginners are given. Part II. is taken up with bacteriologic examinations, and includes a description of bacteriologic apparatus, culture media, methods of obtaining pure cultures, the inoculation of animals, staining methods, and a short description of the commoner forms of micro-organisms. At the end of this section is a chapter on clinical bacteriology which contains many useful hints for advanced workers as well as students. The authors claim that Löffler's blood-serum is the best medium for the routine examination of all bacteria, and a simplified method for its preparation, by which the tedious fractional sterilization is dispensed with, is given. In staining for flagellæ by the Löffler's method, we are pleased to note that the authors do not consider it necessary to add an acid or an alkali to the stain as recommended by Löffler, depending on the different species of bacteria. In this section of the book, however, there are too many repetitions in the preparation of culture media and in the inoculation experiments.

Part III., which deals with histologic methods, is the most valuable section of the book, and contains chapters on examination of fresh material, injections, fixing reagents, decalcification, embedding, section cutting, staining, and examination of the blood, as well as a few hints on examination of the gastric content, feces, and urine which come within the provinces of the pathologist. Weigert's new neuroglia stain is described for the first in any American laboratory manual, we believe. The albumin method for fixing paraffin sections to the slide is given, but the far better method by distilled water is not mentioned. Among the staining methods we are surprised to find Heidenhain's iron-hematoxylin missing. This is far too valuable a stain to be entirely neglected.

Only a few defects have been mentioned, for, all in all, the work is a good one and the authors have produced a book which is bound to receive recognition and take a high place among all workers in the laboratory. The one chief objection is in the title, and we are more than astonished at the substitution of the French "technique" for the English "technic." This is a blunder which will no doubt be corrected in a subsequent edition.

VADE MECUM OF OPHTHALMOLOGICAL THERAPEUTICS. By DR. LANDOLT and DR. GYGAX. Philadelphia: J. B. Lippincott Company, 1898.

IN their introduction to this little work the authors state, as their aim, to put into the hands of the profession in a concise form the indispensable facts of special therapeutics, and "to give a constant companion, a true friend to the busy practitioner and to the student preparing for examination." As far as comprehensiveness is concerned, there is little to criticize, as we find no less than 326 headings between accommodation paralysis, and zona ophthalmica. The therapeutic hints are in general, up to the mark of modern ophthalmology, as, indeed, we are entitled to expect from the reputation of the authors. The enumeration of all the varied ocular affections with the corresponding treatment does not preserve the general level of excellence.

In the consideration of accommodative spasm, as in that of blepharitis and conjunctivitis, no mention is made of the importance of correcting errors of refraction. The directions are often exceedingly vague. Thus, "36. Cataract. Surgical treatment"; "132. Hemiapia. Etiologic treatment"; while, in other instances, they are decidedly at variance with the best teaching: as, "104. Embolism of Central Artery. Repeated paracentesis of the anterior chamber"; "129A. Goiter. Exophthalmic. Preparations of thyroidin. In severe cases extirpation of the cervical sympathetic"; "138. Hyphema. Paracentesis made at the lower margin of the cornea"; "293. Staphyloma, total corneal. Tattooing or *ablation* with strict antiseptic precautions."

In general it may be said that the suggestions are so condensed and abbreviated as to the practically presuppose familiarity with all the methods. The entire subject of refraction error, for instance, is disposed of in less than three diminutive pages. Although the little volume contains many valuable suggestions, as in the chapter on specific treatment and ophthalmia neonatorum, most of the therapeutic procedures would require much additional elucidation before we could put them into practice. If they are to be "crammed" by the student solely for the purpose of enabling him to pass an examination, the volume may serve fairly well as a quiz-compendium. For any practical purpose it is entirely inadequate.

As to the "busy practitioner" he had better send his eye-cases to a specialist, or prepare himself for their treatment by work in an ophthalmic hospital. Therapeutics cannot be learned by cook-book recipes.

THE FAT OF THE LAND AND HOW TO LIVE ON IT. By ELLEN GOODELL SMITH, M.D. Amherst: Carpenter & Morehouse, 1896.

ADORNED by a portrait of the authoress inserted as a frontispiece, this work deals with the virtues of vegetarian diet in its first part, emphasizing the frightful sequels of the eating of meat. Part I. abounds in much of the usual specious argument against the food of fish, fowl, and cattle, interspersed here and there with digressions on religion, morality, intemperance, and kindred favorite topics. Part II. contains directions for preparing vegetarian food, and, as far as the reviewer is able to judge, is good. Part III. is a pseudo-scientific harangue embodying a denunciation of most of what is pleasant and good in life, and contains a lament from the author that physicians are able to earn a living from the practice of their profession. Books of this character are necessary, we suppose, in a cosmopolitan civilization, but the necessity of reading them is a mournful task.

A TREATISE ON GYNECOLOGY, MEDICAL AND SURGICAL. By DR. S. POZZI of Paris. Third revised edition, Translated by DR. BROOKS H. WELLS of New York. One volume, of 950 pages, royal octavo, illustrated by over 600 wood engravings. New York: William Wood & Company, 1897.

THE appearance of the first edition of Pozzi's work on gynecology, seven years ago, marked a distinct advance in gynecologic literature. The cosmopolitan character of the work signalized the author as a man of exhaustive research and of judicious appreciation of the work of his collaborators throughout the world. The broad spirit in which the work was written led the author into rather exhaustive discussions of the opinions held by different writers and operators with the desire to allow each reader the opportunity of forming a personal conviction upon the points discussed. Elaborate accounts of the evolution of various surgical procedures were also inserted, which gave the book a completeness most acceptable to advanced specialists. An elaborate bibliography was appended to each chapter, which afforded the reader the opportunity to consult the original sources of the author's information. This completeness necessitated the division of the work into two large volumes. The present edition is in one large octavo volume. The bibliography of each chapter has been omitted, but the other features are retained. Some of the chapters have been rewritten, and in many instances additions have been made. The work still stands as an excellent reference book, but is too elaborate for the average medical student or the general practitioner.

THERAPEUTIC HINTS.

For Influenza in Children salipyrin is said to be an efficient remedy. For a child of five years the dose is 4 grains, and for one of ten years 8 grains, to be administered three times daily.

For Spasmodic Croup.—STIMPSON advises the following treatment, which, in his hands, has proved successful even in very severe cases: The child is first given an emetic in warm water in teaspoonful doses. It is then put in a hot bath, and after this, flannels wrung out of hot mustard water (four teaspoonfuls of mustard to the quart) are applied to the neck and chest. A two-per-cent. cocain spray is of great service in overcoming the laryngeal spasm. After the immediate danger is past, the following mixture should be given until the catarrhal symptoms have disappeared:

℞		
	Syr. scillæ	ʒ iss
	Tr. opii camphorat.	ʒ ii
	Tr. tolutan. } aa Glycerini }	℥ i
	Aq. dest. q. s. ad.	℥ iii.

M. Sig. One-half teaspoonful every three hours during the day, and every four hours at night.

Tonic for the Scalp.—

℞		
	Quin. hydrochlor.	gr. xv
	Ac. tannici.	gr. xl
	Tr. cantharidis	♏. xxxvi
	Glycerini	ʒ iv
	Eau de Cologne	ʒ liss
	Vanillæ	gr. 1/3
	Pulv. santali	gr. 1/6
	Alcoholis	℥ vii.

M. Allow the mixture to stand five days, and then filter it. S. Apply to the scalp, with friction, every other day.—*Deitrich.*

To Allay Vomiting Following Anesthesia.—

℞		
	Cerii oxalat.	gr. xii
	Codeinæ sulphat.	gr. i
	Hydrarg. chlor. mit.	gr. 3/5.

M. Ft. pulv. No. VI. Sig. One powder every half hour for four or five doses.

For Spermatorrhea.—

℞		
	Cornutine citrat.	gr. iiss
	Boli alb.	ʒ i gr. xlv
	Mucilag. tragacanth.	q. s.

M. Ft. pil. No. L. Sig. Two pills daily.

THE MEDICAL NEWS.

A WEEKLY JOURNAL OF MEDICAL SCIENCE.

VOL. LXXII. NEW YORK, SATURDAY, MARCH 26, 1898. NO. 13.

ORIGINAL ARTICLES.

MIGRAINOUS VERTIGO AND THE SUBSTITUTION OF VERTIGINOUS SEIZURES FOR ATTACKS OF SICK HEADACHE.[1]

BY CHARLES L. DANA, M.D.,
OF NEW YORK;
VISITING PHYSICIAN TO BELLEVUE HOSPITAL, ETC.

To better elucidate the subject it may be expedient to ask attention for a moment to a matter of physiology. It will be remembered that the eighth cranial nerve is usually described as the acoustic, though this conveys but half the truth, as it is the nerve of space as well as of hearing. In reality then, the eighth pair of cranial nerves constitute four nerves, two for the sense of hearing and two for that of space. The latter are distributed to the semicircular canals and have their origin in the cerebellum. When they are diseased the patient loses his spatial relations; his bodily equilibrium is disturbed; he feels as though he were being whirled about; when walking he tumbles from side to side, or is forced violently backward or forward. The feeling and power of adjustment to the external world are gone.

The symptoms above enumerated are often associated with disturbances of the nerve of hearing, so that the patient is found to be more or less deaf; he hears buzzing sounds in the head, or, by diffusion of the irritation to the medulla, suffers from nausea, vomiting, and a condition of speechlessness or even syncope may supervene. The purely space-sense symptoms, without any auditory complications, are observed in seasickness.

When the peripheral ends of the space-sense and acoustic nerves are the seat of a progressive organic process, as in disease of the labyrinth, there occurs the mixture of vertiginous and aural symptoms clinically known as Ménière's disease. Often there are slight changes in the middle or external ear, which cause somewhat similar symptoms. This condition is called functional or irritative labyrinthine vertigo. In such a case the middle-ear disease directly leads to a neurosis of the eighth nerve; or this nerve, by reason of its irritated condition, becomes the starting-point in the production of a general neurosis, the special symptoms of which originate in, and are dictated by, the local affection.

[1] Read at a meeting of the Northwestern Medical and Surgical Society of New York, February 16, 1898.

As illustrative of the foregoing I wish to submit the history of a case. It is purely a clinical report, having no terminal adornment in the shape of an autopsy—nor, indeed, is the dead-house needed to unravel its mysteries. Sometimes cases occur in which the study of the symptoms throws a light upon the cause and pathology of disease which is much more luminous and satisfactory than that obtained from the most ample enlargements of the microscope or most virulent cultures of bacilli. Cases may be reported, also, because they are rare or unique, or have about them a certain piquancy of incident or sensuous fulness of detail which makes them beautiful to medical minds, well attuned to the harmonies of vagrant tissue life. However, my case, I think, furnishes more than a purely interesting recital. It shows the evolution of one affection into another, and proves a kinship between two diseases, which taken together might seem entirely independent one of the other.

We all know that migraine in its various forms is one of the most common of neuroses—indeed, one of the most familiar diseases to the practitioner of every branch of our art. Beginning, usually, in the early part of the second decade of life, it increases in the activity and severity of its manifestations for a number of years, and then is gradually dissipated by the maturing of the organism, leaving the patient, generally, at middle life. In a good many cases, however, this nervous instability, instead of disappearing, changes its manifestation from the sensory centers, in which it first started, and shows itself in another form; it may be, in some neuralgia or recurrent paralysis, or in some convulsive affection. In the following case it will be seen that the migrainons diathesis took a peculiar and unusual turn:

CASE I.—Mr. A. P., aged twenty-four years, a native of the United States, draughtsman by profession, was referred to me by Dr. D. B. St. John Roosa, during June, 1894. His father had been subject to migraine. His mother was healthy, and there were no severe neuroses or psychoses, no consumption or inebriety in the family. The patient had been well as a boy, except from an attack of measles when he was eleven years old, and but for the fact that he had had from his sixth year attacks of ordinary sick-headache, which recurred with considerable frequency up to his twentieth year, that is, four years before I saw him. From early childhood he had been very sensitive to the effects of swinging, and was easily made giddy. On the other hand, he was not subject to seasickness, he was not affected by climbing to great heights, or by being in positions requiring skill and presence of mind in the adjustment of equilibrium.

His attacks of migraine came on with nausea and vomiting and at times with a slight temporary deafness and ringing in the ears. When he was twenty years old the migrainous seizures began to change their character. They began to come upon him during the day, and were first manifested by sensations of nausea, with pain in the head, similar to his ordinary sick-headaches. These symptoms were soon followed by an intense vertigo, so severe that he would be obliged to lie down. After an hour or two he would become drowsy and go off to sleep, sleeping profoundly, like a person who had had an epileptic attack. He never, however, at any time lost consciousness or had any convulsive movements. For four years he suffered once or twice a month from attacks of this nature. During this period he had at times some tinnitus and a little deafness, especially in the left ear, for which he consulted a local ear specialist, who treated him in the usual way for middle-ear catarrh. The ears were syringed, Politzerized, the throat treated, and counter-irritation was applied back of the ear. This did him no good whatever, and as the attacks continued, he finally consulted Dr. Roosa, who, after examination, decided that there were no indications for local treatment, and referred him to me. Dr. Roosa wrote: "He has some chronic catarrh of the middle ears, as it seems to me, but in connection with this he has seizures which do not appear to me to be aural."

When first seen by me, during June, 1894, the patient presented the appearance of a healthy young man, of good color, with no objective evidence of nervous or other disease. His heart, lungs, abdominal viscera, and kidneys were all normal. His eyes also, which had been examined by Dr. Roosa, were also found to be normal. He had none of the stigmata of a neurotic degenerate. Examination of his hearing showed at this time a very considerable degree of deafness in the left ear, especially by bone conduction, and a less degree to aerial conduction. The right ear was normal. His description of his symptoms was unusually clear and explicit.

He stated that he was then suffering from the seizures at the rate of five or six a month. They would occasionally come on with no premonitory symptoms of any kind, but usually he had some headache and nausea. While standing or sitting he would suddenly feel as if he were being toppled over backward, and he had to cling to some object near by to support himself. He felt at the same time an intense desire to go to stool, a variety of aura, which is sometimes experienced in epilepsy. If he was able to go to the closet he had two or three watery evacuations. As soon as possible, in any event, he would lie down, and in a little while would pass into a condition in which he could neither speak nor cry out. As soon as he lay down the sense of rotation which he felt while standing changed its character. Instead of feeling as though he were being thrown back and revolved vertically, it seemed as if objects were whirled around him, sometimes from left to right, and in other attacks, from right to left. This whirling of the objects was not continuous but of a pulsating character, and at first these pulsating objects going past him, went slowly, then more rapidly, until finally, on account of their rapidity, the pulsations could hardly be distinguished at all. After a time they slowed down again. If he closed his eyes while lying down, this objective whirl disappeared, and in place of it, he felt as though he himself were being whirled vertically backward on a horizontal axis, just as he did when standing erect. He lay there, therefore, between the devil of an objective and the deep sea of a subjective vertigo; for while standing, or while keeping the eyes closed in the lying posture, he felt himself in a terrific cart-wheel progression, but while lying down, with open eyes, the world dashed past him like an express train.

The nausea and vomiting from which he sometimes suffered, disappeared after he lay down and he had no headache after the attack set in and usually none at any time. After a period of fifteen minutes to half an hour the vertigo would lessen, and he would go oft into a profound sleep. He woke in a few hours, with the symptoms nearly or quite gone. The attacks would usually come on during the daytime, and under the most varied conditions; for instance, they would sometimes occur while he was sitting quietly at his work, and sometimes while engaged in active exercise, such as playing tennis. The attacks occurred also in different degrees of severity, and this was especially the case after treatment at my hands. In the light seizures, he simply had nausea followed by moderate vertigo, and he was sometimes even able to go on with his work until, in the course of half an hour or an hour, he would feel all right again. He occasionally had two or three mild attacks in one day, but never more than one severe one. He was always better in summer, but the conditions were not particularly improved by any change in his diet or mode of living, except that, when he got very tired or lost sleep, he would be more likely to have them.

My diagnosis, at the time, was that he was suffering from a migrainous neurosis of the eighth nerve, and that it was perhaps allied to, or indicative of, a developing epilepsy, and it was on this basis that treatment was begun. During the succeeding years he has been under my care at more or less regular intervals, and the attacks have gradually diminished. Between 1890 and 1894 he had over twenty attacks; during 1894 only fifteen, and none during 1895; during 1896 he had eight, and the attacks, though lighter, would sometimes occur suddenly without any premonitions. During the past year, 1897, he had but two, and his general condition has been very good.

The patient presented himself to me again during January, 1898. I had not, at that time, seen him for nearly a year, and during that interval he had been practically well, having had only two mild attacks during the summer. He complained ot suffering at times from a loud buzzing in the right ear, and he stated that any loud noise would make him stagger or sway toward the right side, but only when the ear was buzzing, this tinnitus not being constant. The examination in January last, nearly four years from his first visit, showed that he heard the voice normally with each ear. The watch was heard three inches from the right ear, and one inch from the left. A tuning-fork on the mastoid was heard imperfectly, but more so in the left ear, and was not heard as a musical note, but as a buzzing, both by bone and by aerial conduction. He could not hear a loud tuning-fork on the forehead at all; on the whole, bone conduction was much more imperfect than aerial. This condition of bone-deafness, however, he stated only existed when the buzzing was present. At other times he heard perfectly well. He was having no attacks of vertigo, headache, or nausea.

I sent him again to Dr. Roosa, who examined him and wrote me that "the voice and tuning-fork tests show that the lesion, of whatever nature, is in the labyrinth or the trunk of the nerve. His hearing is better than when I saw him first, in 1894, but the left ear is the one which exhibits an increase of hearing. He requires no local aural treatment."

We have, therefore, the case of a man who, during fourteen years, had typical attacks of migraine, and had also a migrainous hereditary history. At the age of twenty the typical migrainous attacks became modified, and instead of having the headache he had objective and subjective vertigo associated with forced movements, often preceded by an aura of desire to go to stool and followed by a lethargic sleep. As the condition progressed the nausea and vomiting also ceased, and he had for a time only attacks of severe vertigo with forced movements, and a subsequent tendency to sleep. This condition was associated with some bone-deafness and a very little local disease of the left ear. While he probably had at some time a slight degree of chronic middle-ear catarrh, this has been very insignificant, and any organic disease of the middle ear can be almost excluded from the fact that his hearing, when he feels well, as he does most of the time, is perfect in both ears to both bone and aerial conduction.

The case seems to me to show that the migrainous tendency, which is so often manifested in various forms, located itself upon the eighth nerve and produced disturbances of its function.

In my personal experience I have had other cases which suggest this same transformation of pathologic energy.

CASE II.—I was called to see a lady, sixty-four years of age, who all her early life had suffered from attacks of migraine, and also from pains along the spine and in the back of the neck, which we associate with the name "spinal irritation." She still had occasional (not very severe) attacks of migraine and at times severe pains in the back of the neck and along the spine. When I saw her, however, she was suffering from an attack of most intense vertigo, with extreme nausea and sense of weakness, lasting in all eight to ten hours. The symptoms were, as she described them, almost precisely like those which she had experienced during an attack of seasickness. In this case there were no objective disturbances of the eighth nerve, her hearing being normal, and, furthermore, there was no tinnitus or evidences of middle-ear catarrh. The attack could not be attributed to any disturbance of digestion or abnormal condition of the eyes, and, in fact, she was apparently physically sound. These attacks she had five or six times during the course of two years, and they were brought on by overwork and fatigue, just as occurs with migrainous attacks. At that time I made the diagnosis of a neurosis affecting the eighth nerve and similar in character to the crises which affect the spinal and cranial nerves in spinal irritation. I believe now that it was a migrainous neurosis of the eighth nerve.

Other cases of this kind, though less marked, have occurred in my experience, and doubtless have been observed by others.

The interesting and practical points connected with such cases, of course, are those of therapeusis. In the case which I have related at so much length the treatment consisted largely in the use of hydrobromic acid and the bromids, careful attention to condition of the stomach and bowels, regular life and abundance of sleep, so necessary to young neurotics, and avoidance of work which would lead to excessive fatigue. The salicylate of soda was also occasionally given, and at times cannabis indica. This line of therapy is much the same as we pursue in the treatment of migraine itself, and is usually helpful or curative with these cases when they are seen early and proper conditions of life can be brought about.

For a good many years the association of migraine with eye trouble has been very strictly insisted upon, and I always make it a point to have the eyes carefully examined and errors of refraction corrected. I hear from my ophthalmologic friends of many cases in which migraine has been cured by treatment of the eyes, but in my personal experience I have never known of a single case of this kind. I have known migrainous attacks to be lessened in frequency, and the conditions generally ameliorated, but for some reason the eye-treatment of migraine has been of little assistance in the cases which have come under my observation. I should, of course, add that I do not often see migraine in its early and easy stages, whereas, no doubt, the oculist meets many such, owing to the prevalent view that chronic headaches are so often associated with disorder of the eyes.

The conclusion of the whole matter is that periodic vertiginous seizures, not due to organic ear disease, occurring in young or even in old persons, if there is a migrainous history, are really only forms of migraine. Local treatment accomplishes nothing, and therapy must be applied on the general principles directed to the care of the constitutional neurosis.

NOTES ON THE WIDAL SERUM-REACTION AND ON THE METHOD OF HISS.[1]

By JEROME B. THOMAS, JR., M.D.,
OF BROOKLYN, N.Y.

About one year ago I had the pleasure of presenting to this Society a paper which briefly described the history and the principles of the Widal serum-reaction and contained a report of fifty-seven cases in which I employed the method at the Hoagland Laboratory. The specimens examined were all of dried blood. At that time the necessity of using cultures of moderate susceptibility and serum in high dilution was not generally appreciated, and in consequence the method presented many sources of error which more careful methods have since eliminated. In a circular published early last year Wyatt Johnston emphasized the importance of diluting the dried blood with water till the solution became a light pink, and one of the conclusions deduced from a study of my cases was that high dilution of the suspected blood was necessary to exclude the rare cases in which normal blood or blood from patients suffering from disease other than typhoid gives the serum reaction. This reaction, as you will perhaps remember, consists in the paralysis and agglutination of typhoid bacilli when mixed with the blood of a patient having typhoid fever or of an animal immunized against typhoid.

During the past year a vast amount of careful work has been done on this subject and literally thousands of cases have been reported, with the general result that the procedure has been purged of most of its imperfections, and is held by those who are best acquainted with it to be of the very highest value as an aid to the diagnosis of typhoid fever; in fact, the presence of the reaction falls very little short of being pathognomonic of the disease.

To exclude all possibility of error the serum to be tested should be diluted fifty times with water, in regard to which point Professor Welch says: "Hitherto it has not been shown that the reaction ever occurs with non-typhoid serum in dilutions exceeding 1 to 50." He also requires that a reaction consist of both agglutination and paralysis, and not one of these phenomena alone. This excludes many so-called positive reactions reported from time to time. Some cases have been recorded in which the diagnosis of typhoid was made on the basis of a serum-reaction, and the authors, judging from later developments, considered them free from typhoid infection. Professor Welch in his paper before the American Medical Association last June mentioned two or three cases in this connection which are extremely suggestive, and prove that the presence of the reaction may reveal a typhoid infection which clinical symptoms and the autopsy-knife fail to demonstrate.

A patient with obscure symptoms, the blood giving a positive reaction, died at Johns Hopkins Hospital, and the autopsy showed no intestinal lesions. The patient did not present a history of having previously had typhoid fever. Dr. Flexner isolated typhoid bacilli in large numbers from the gall-bladder of this patient.

Pick has reported a case with marked positive serum-reaction in which no typhoid intestinal lesions and no enlargement of the spleen were found at the autopsy, though bacteriologic examination demonstrated the presence of typhoid bacilli.

Guinon and Meunier have reported an interesting and suggestive case in which, during life, there had been symptoms of typhoid fever and acute miliary tuberculosis combined. The serum-reaction was positive. At the autopsy the lesions appeared to be simply those of miliary tuberculosis. There were also small intestinal ulcers typically tuberculous in appearance. Typhoid bacilli, however, were cultivated from the spleen and other organs. As the symptoms of typhoid indicated that this disease was disappearing, the case, if examined somewhat later, might readily have been placed to the discredit of the positive value of the serum-test.

Such cases as these very strongly point to the probability that the typhoid bacillus sometimes develops a set of symptoms resembling but slightly those commonly attributed to it, and further they suggest that the few cases in which the serum-test has been discredited as disagreeing with the clinical phenomena may have been more correctly interpreted by the bacteriologic phenomena. In illustration of this point, Dr. N. E. Brill of Mt. Sinai Hospital has quite recently published a report of "seventeen cases of a disease clinically resembling typhoid fever," but failing to give the Widal reaction. These patients had many symptoms resembling typhoid, and yet the disease was mild, all cases recovering with no sequelæ, and in none was there intestinal hemorrhage. The bowels were, as a rule, constipated, and in nearly all the cases the fever suddenly fell to normal on about the tenth or

[1] Read at a meeting of the Kings County Medical Association, February 8, 1898.

twelfth day, and remained there, the patient at once recovering from all symptoms except weakness. Of the undoubted typhoid cases treated during the year in the same hospital (80 in all), 78 gave a positive serum-reaction, or 97¾ per cent. The blood of 212 non-typhoid patients was examined, of which 211 gave no reaction, and the one case which gave a reaction was that of an ignorant woman who was not sure of her previous history.

Dr. R. C. Cabot of Boston recently published statistics of the Widal test in the *Journal of the American Medical Association*. His collection numbered 3475 cases, of which 3434 (98.8 per cent.) gave a positive reaction. More recent statistics presented by Brill bring the total of reported cases up to 4879, of which 4781 (97.9 per cent.) gave a positive reaction—a remarkable result considering the great number of cases and the various examiners with many varieties of technic.

Still more remarkable are the results of the following skilled bacteriologists:

Widal and Sicard, 163 cases of typhoid; 162 positive reactions.
Courmont, 116 cases of typhoid; 116 positive reactions.
Chantemesse, 70 cases of typhoid; 70 positive reactions.
Johnston and McTaggart, 129 cases of typhoid; 128 positive reactions.

A more accurate conclusion may be reached by considering these last results in which the examinations were conducted by men of unquestioned skill and ability.

It seems to me that the present status of the Widal test may be summarized as follows: (1) It is in the doubtful and mixed cases that the test may be said to find its greatest usefulness; for not more than sixty per cent. of all cases give a positive reaction before the twelfth day, a period at which the clinical symptoms are ordinarily sufficient to determine the diagnosis. (2) If made with proper dilution and culture, a positive reaction is practically pathognomonic of typhoid infection. In this connection the history as to previous attacks should receive consideration. (3) If repeated daily examinations of the serum in a suspected case fail to give the reaction, the presumption is very strong that the case is not one of typhoid. The fact that the reaction may in rare cases not occur until late in the disease prevents the positive exclusion of typhoid.

At the meeting of the American Medical Association at Philadelphia, June 4, 1897, the following was given as a summary of the views expressed by those discussing the serum diagnosis of typhoid fever: "Without being absolutely infallible the typhoid reaction appears to afford as accurate diagnostic results as can be obtained by any of the bacteriologic methods at our disposal for the diagnosis of other diseases. It must certainly be regarded as the most constant and reliable sign of typhoid fever, if not an absolute test."

The cultivation of the bacillus of typhoid, when obtained unmixed with other organisms, as in puncture of the spleen, is an easy matter, but the procedure becomes complicated and fraught with difficulties when the bacillus is mixed with other germs, as in the fecal discharges. Elsner's method of differentiation, by using a medium containing a small quantity of potassium iodid, has failed to be of practical value. The method of isolation devised by Dr. Hiss of the New York City Health Department offers more promise, though its value has not yet been fixed by general experimentation. My personal experience with the method has been limited and unsatisfactory.

I have examined samples of feces in seven cases of undoubted typhoid fever from the wards of St. Peter's and the Long Island College Hospital, and have been unable to isolate the specific bacillus in any case, though control-plates made from stock cultures of typhoid and colon bacilli have presented a characteristic appearance in all cases. My culture-media were prepared by a skilled chemist, my colleague, Mr. Randolph, and I have discussed the technicalities of the work with Dr. Hiss himself.

Whether my failure to isolate the germs in the cases mentioned was due to faulty technic or to the possibility that the series may have been an unfortunate one, I am unable to say, but I would certainly not presume to base an opinion on the examination of such a small number of cases or cast any discredit on the results of Dr. Hiss. In four of my cases the patients were constipated, a fact which lessens the likelihood of finding the specific germs in large numbers. Orders were given to the nurses to take that portion of the stool which was passed last, and they may or may not have carried out the instructions. I mention these facts to demonstrate the possible sources of error.

In view of my results my main excuse for bringing the matter before you to-night is the fact that the method has been added to the routine diagnostic work of the Bacteriologic Bureau of the Health Department, and is, therefore, a matter of some interest to the practitioners of the Borough of Brooklyn.

The method depends upon the behavior of the micro-organisms of the feces, in certain culture-media which Dr. Hiss has worked out by experimenting with many combinations of nutrient material of varying degrees of acidity and alkalinity. The media he has found to best differentiate the typhoid bacilli from other fecal organisms are two: a tube and a plate medium. Both consist of certain proportions of agar, gelatin, beef-extract, glucose, and salt, acidulated with a definite amount of hydrochloric acid. If the tube medium be inoculated with typhoid bacilli and incubated at 37° C. (98° F.) for sixteen to eighteen hours, it will be found to be quite uniformly cloudy, the medium becoming semifluid at that temperature, and permitting the motile bacilli to spread rapidly through it. The less motile colon bacillus grows along the puncture and the paths of gas-bubbles formed by it. Very motile colon bacilli may cloud the medium in a manner similar to typhoid germs, but will differ in forming gas-bubbles which find difficulty in escaping from the semisolid medium and remain entrapped therein if the medium be allowed to cool. This forms a striking picture, and is a very convenient method of testing the gas-forming properties of any organism.

The plate medium contains a larger percentage of agar, and thus, by its greater solidity prevents rapid permeation by the germs. Increased acidity also aids in checking their multiplication. After incubation at 37° C. (98° F.), for sixteen to twenty-four hours, the deep typhoid colonies are, under low power, seen to be very small with shaggy edges composed of tiny threads. Some of the smallest colonies are entirely composed of threads without a thickened center. The colon colonies are much larger, more opaque, and have more clearly defined edges.

In testing a suspected sample of fecal matter the specimen is shaken up with five cubic centimeters of beef-tea, from which plate-cultures are made and incubated as described. After incubation they are examined with a low-power lens, and typical or suspicious colonies are isolated and planted in the tube medium for verification. The whole procedure does not occupy more than thirty-six to forty-eight hours.

In regard to other fecal organisms besides the colon bacilli which simulate typhoid, Hiss says: "These organisms must be rare, for in all the samples of feces and water subjected to test (about 200 on December 20, 1897) none have been found giving an appearance not readily distinguishable from that of the typhoid bacillus cultivated at 37° C. (98° F.)."

According to Hiss' preliminary report to the Academy of Medicine, he has succeeded in detecting the bacillus in about fifty per cent. of cases examined once, and in 89.5 per cent. of a series of twenty-six cases repeatedly examined in the New York Hospital. Bacilli were isolated as early as the sixth and late as the thirtieth day, and in a case of relapse, on the forty-seventh day. As a rule, they rapidly disappeared after the fall in temperature, and when they persisted there was special liability to relapse. They were most plentiful from the tenth to the twelfth day of the disease. Thus, it will be recognized that we have in this method simply an additional aid in diagnosing typhoid fever, and, even if experience and experiment prove it to be as useful as its author claims, it presents such a large working error that it will probably be used only in doubtful and atypical cases, in conjunction with the Elsner method and the Widal serum-test. Comparing Hiss' method with the Widal test I believe the latter to be more useful because the working error is not so great, the method is more simple in its application, and the result of an examination may be obtained much more rapidly.

The New York City Health Department is doing most interesting and valuable work in determining the true value of the Hiss method, and to this end offers to examine specimens of feces and urine from any suspected case of typhoid fever in the greater city, reporting the result to the physician within thirty-six to forty-eight hours. Outfits and blanks will soon be obtainable at all the Brooklyn stations for diphtheria cultures.

PUERPERAL MYELITIS.[1]

BY ARTHUR CONKLIN BRUSH, M.D.,
OF BROOKLYN, N. Y.;
ASSISTANT NEUROLOGIST TO THE KINGS COUNTY AND BROOKLYN EYE AND EAR HOSPITALS; NEUROLOGIST TO THE BROOKLYN CENTRAL DISPENSARY; CONSULTING NEUROLOGIST TO THE BEDFORD DISPENSARY.

PARALYTIC conditions due to organic disease of the central nervous system are unfortunately not a very rare complication of the puerperal state. In the majority of the cases, however, they are due to some pathologic condition of the cerebral blood-vessels which causes rupture or obstruction by an embolus or thrombus, and less commonly they are the result of multiple neuritis. Paralysis, due to inflammatory changes in the spinal cord, are rare as puerperal complications. The obstetric text-books which I have consulted make no mention of this complication, and works on neurology are, as a rule, equally silent. The only reference to this condition which I have been able to find is that of Gower's, who describes acute myelitis as sometimes due to puerperal septicemia. Dr. J. C. Shaw informs me that even in his large experience he has observed but one case.

During the past two years it has been my good fortune to see in the wards of the Kings County Hospital no less than five cases of myelitis occurring as a complication of the puerpery. These cases, brief histories of which are appended, were all of the subacute or chronic type, and in them various portions of the cord were involved.

[1] Read at a meeting of the Kings County Medical Association, February 8, 1898.

CASE I.—A. S., aged twenty-nine years; German; presented a history of always having enjoyed good health. Four years ago she was delivered by means of forceps, following which there was slight fever lasting a few days. Upon recovery she found that she was gradually losing power in the lower limbs, and two years ago she became unable to walk. This condition was at first associated with sensations of numbness and formication in the lower extremities, as well as retention of urine, but at the present time these symptoms are much less marked.

Examination, November 19, 1896, revealed the following condition: The patient is unable to walk or stand. Only very slight voluntary movements are possible in the lower extremities, but marked involuntary movements occur at times. All the muscles of the lower limbs are in a spastic condition, with increased reflexes and ankle clonus. There is a diminution of all forms of sensation in the feet and legs. There is slight ataxia of the arms. The act of urination is feeble and incomplete.

CASE II.—C. M., aged twenty-two years; American; unmarried. The patient had always enjoyed good health until her confinement one month previously. During the labor both cervix and perineum were lacerated. Ten days later she rapidly developed the following condition, which continued up to the time when I first saw her.

Examination, September 22, 1896. Patient is unable to walk or stand. There is complete paralysis of the lower extremities, with absence of reflexes and all forms of sensation. She complains of pain referred to the hips and pelvis. There is incontinence of urine.

During the next four months the patient improved so much as to be able to walk a few steps with the aid of a cane, the gait being shuffling, and the lower limbs in a state of spastic paraplegia. Sensation finally returned, the reflexes were exaggerated, and the incontinence of urine was much improved.

CASE III.—N. S., aged thirty-five years; American. The patient's previous history was good. One year ago she was delivered of a dead child. The labor was followed by fever and pelvic pain, lasting about ten days. One week after delivery she suddenly developed marked weakness in the lower extremities, associated with numbness extending upward over the lower part of the abdomen, and girdle sensations at the level of the umbilicus. At the end of twenty-four hours the loss of motion and sensation was complete and there was incontinence of both urine and feces.

Examination, September 10, 1896, revealed the following condition: There is complete paraplegia, associated with partial loss of all forms of sensation and absence of reflexes, though there was no incontinence of urine. There was no improvement in the patient's condition, which ultimately resulted in atrophy of the paralyzed limbs.

CASE IV.—M. S., aged thirty-five years; American. Two months previously the patient had been delivered by means of forceps, and five days afterward she developed within a few hours a complete paraplegia, associated with feeling of weight and numbness in the lower limbs, girdle sensation at the level of the umbilicus, and vesicle incontinence.

Examination, March 31, 1897, showed that there was almost complete loss of power in the lower limbs. Slight motion in the toes being the only voluntary movements possible. The knee-jerks were increased, and there was partial loss of sensation in the feet and legs, associated with both vesicle and rectal incontinence. This patient improved so much that at the end of six months she was able to walk, though with a spastic gait, and at this time sensation had fully returned, and the control over the bladder and rectum were much improved.

CASE V.—S. G., aged twenty-seven years; Belgian; unmarried. The patient's previous history was good. One year previously she had been confined, and during the labor both the cervix and perineum were lacerated. Ten days later she began to notice difficulty in moving her lower limbs, and at the same time experienced sensations of numbness in her feet and legs.

Examination, May 13, 1896, showed the following condition: The patient can stand, but is unable to walk. There is partial loss of power in the lower extremities, associated with increased reflexes and partial loss of sensation. The bladder occasionally empties itself involuntarily, while at other times there is retention of urine. The condition gradually improved so that at the end of four months she was able to walk, though with a spastic gait; sensation had returned, but the vesical symptoms did not improve.

From the brief histories presented it will be seen that in all five cases the myelitis occurred as a complication of the puerpery. In no instance was there any evidence of previous disease of like nature, all of the patients having been in good health up to the time the disease in question made it appearance. The cause, therefore, of this complication must be sought in the labor itself or in the puerperal period, or in some recognized cause of myelitis which happened to operate at this time, the last being most probable, for the reason that it is not likely, in such a rare complication of the puerpery, that there would be any special etiologic relation between the two conditions.

The recognized causes of myelitis are exposure to cold, severe muscular exertion, blows or falls injuring the spine, fractures and sprains of the spine, extension of inflammation from the vertebræ, syphilis, infective fevers, and septicemia. From the histories presented we are warranted in excluding as causes of the myelitis all but the last, and in regard to this, septicemia, there is sufficient evidence to warrant consideration of the possibility, at least, that it was the etiologic factor in the production of the spinal affection.

In Case I. there was a history of instrumental delivery and a febrile movement lasting several days; in Case II., of laceration of the cervix and perineum; in Case III., of stillbirth, followed by fever and pelvic pain; in Case IV., of a forceps delivery, and in Case V., of lacerations of both perineum and cervix. In all of the cases, therefore, there was either a history of a febrile movement, not due to any other assigned cause, or of injuries through which septic infection might readily have entered.

One fact, however, in regard to these cases is peculiar: In all but Case III. the evidence of septic infection was slight or wanting, and though myelitis is a well-authenticated sequela of severe septicemia, both in puerperal and non-puerperal states, I can find no evidence of its occurrence as a complication of such mild cases as those mentioned. It is possible, therefore, that there may have been some other etiologic factor which has escaped detection.

A CASE OF INTESTINAL OBSTRUCTION DUE TO MECKEL'S DIVERTICULUM.[1]

BY C. P. GILDERSLEEVE, M.D.,
OF BROOKLYN, N. Y.

ON December 11, 1897, I observed the following case in consultation with Dr. Thayer of this city: The patient, a young man, twenty-one years of age, of slight build, presented the following history: The preceding Thursday, three days previously, about 11 A.M., he complained of pain in the bowels, as he expressed it, and for which he took several doses of Jamaica ginger. He remained at his business all that day and came home at 9 P.M. He remarked to his room-mate that he had been troubled with cramps all day. He went to bed, and hot flannels were applied to his abdomen. He soon became restless, and suffered so much pain that at 4 A.M. Dr. Thayer was sent for. The doctor found him with pulse about normal, and temperature 99.5° F. There was considerable pain and tenderness, most marked about two inches below the umbilicus and to the right of the median line, for which ¼-grain of morphin was administered hypodermically. An enema was also given, but without result. A few hours afterward another enema was given and was followed by a fair movement. During the day he did not vomit except after taking something into the stomach. I saw the patient the next morning about 9 o'clock, at which time his pulse was 90, and his temperature 100.5° F. There was considerable tenderness and pain, the tenderness being most marked about two inches below the umbilicus and slightly to the right of the median line. Dr. Thayer had diagnosed the case appendicitis, and I concurred in his opinion, although the location of the tenderness was not at the point most commom in appendicitis.[2]

[1] Read at a meeting of the Kings County Medical Association, February 8, 1898.

[2] I have observed cases of appendicitis (one in particular in which I operated two months ago) in which the point of most pronounced tenderness upon pressure was about in the same place as in this case.

I advised removal of the patient to St. Peter's Hospital, and he was taken there about noon, but the family had such a strong objection to an operation that I did not at once urge it, his condition at that time being by no means alarming. At 7 o'clock that evening the patient was apparently better; there had been little vomiting, though the bowels refused to act, notwithstanding that he had received six doses of magnesium sulphate (1 dram in hot water every hour). In addition to this several enemata had been given. I now realized that I was dealing with a case of intestinal obstruction, caused, I believed, by a fecal impaction. I ordered the administration of high enemata during the night.

I was called to the hospital the next morning and found my patient in a condition bordering collapse. His pulse was 150 per minute, and extremely weak, respirations rapid, skin cold and moist, and vomiting had become excessive and stercoraceous. There was increased tenderness, marked tympanitic distention, and complete obstruction of the bowels. He was in such a desperate condition that I did not believe that he would live through an operation, and, although I realized that delay was dangerous, I considered it better for the time being to attempt to combat the impending collapse. With this object in view he was surrounded with hot-water bags and given ¼-grain of spartein, $\frac{1}{30}$-grain of strychnin, and 10 drops of digitalis every three hours, and whisky each hour; but in spite of this, the condition did not improve. About 5 o'clock the family consented to an operation, although I had explained to them that it was easily possible that the patient might die upon the table. I then prepared to open the abdomen, but, after examining patient once more, concluded that he had absolutely no chance and refrained from operating. He died within an hour.

At the autopsy the following morning, Dr. Baldwin assisting, I found complete obstruction of the ileum caused by a Meckel's diverticulum, which had become so thoroughly twisted upon itself that it was mechanically impossible for its contents to return to the ileum. The diverticulum terminated in a fibrous cord which formed a complete ring, through which the ileum passed. I believe that the condition was congenital, and that the fatal constriction was due to the twisting of the sac upon itself, thus causing the fibrous ring to tighten its grip upon the ileum so firmly that nothing could pass through the intestine. Even had the constriction not been sufficient to cause complete obstruction the patient was bound to die from the condition of the diverticulum itself, as it contained considerable material which had entered it from the ileum, and, as communication with the intestine had been rendered impossible by the twisting to which it had been subjected, the occurrence of perforation and septic peritonitis would have been but a question of time.

Meckel's diverticulum is said to exist in about two per cent. of all subjects, and is due to a defective closure of the vitelline duct. I have not had time to look up the literature of the subject, but cases of obstruction from this cause have been reported from time to time. Dennis speaks of two cases which occurred in the Massachusetts General Hospital, in both of which a diagnosis of acute appendicitis was made. In one of these cases operation was successfully performed, and the patient recovered. In the second case the diverticulum was found distended and gangrenous, and the patient died.

In my case, judging from the ease with which the condition was located at the autopsy, I belive that the patient's life would have been saved had I operated shortly after the symptoms referable to obstruction developed. The determination of the point of obstruction was rendered comparatively easy by the fact that beyond the constriction the intestine was nearly collapsed, while above it, the distention was very great. The mere division of the fibrous ring would have released the ileum, and at the same time would have resulted in untwisting the diverticulum itself, after which its contents would have found their way back to the ileum, and the danger of gangrene and perforation would have been averted. But we all known that these acts are much more easily performed at an autopsy than upon the operating-table. It is our duty to appreciate the fact that acute intestinal obstruction which is not relieved by medical measures and is not due to a paralysis of peristaltic action, such as is observed in general peritonitis, constitutes a condition which means one of two things: Death of the patient, or relief by means of an operation, and, while I know that the average surgeon enters the peritoneal cavity with a feeling of perfect composure for the purpose of removing a diseased appendix or some other lesion the location of which can be definitely determined before the incision is made, I believe that in cases of intestinal obstruction, a condition which, with the exception of hemorrhage, is second to no other surgical emergency from a standpoint of gravity, and further, that the element of uncertainty and the fear of failure to locate the obstruction, knowing as we do that it may be at any part of the entire intestinal tract, causes us to be too apt to defer operation until too late.

NOTES ON THE PREVALENCE OF FRAMBESIA AMONG THE FIJIANS.

BY A. O. TREBECK, M.D.,
OF CHARLOTTESVILLE, VA.

FRAMBESIA is almost extinct in England, but is found in some parts of Scotland, in France, and in the South Sea Islands. It is supposed to have been carried from Africa to Southern America and the West Indies by the importation of slaves, and was introduced into Ceylon by Portugese traders, where, on account of its origin, it is called *Parangi lede* (foreigner's evil). Captain Cook and other explorers of the South Seas also make some mention of the disease *tona*, as it is called, in their records.

The premonitory symptoms of frambesia, or *yaws*, are difficult of detection, consequently the disease is insidious in its inception, and it is only by the physical signs that one is aware of its existence.

FIG. 1.

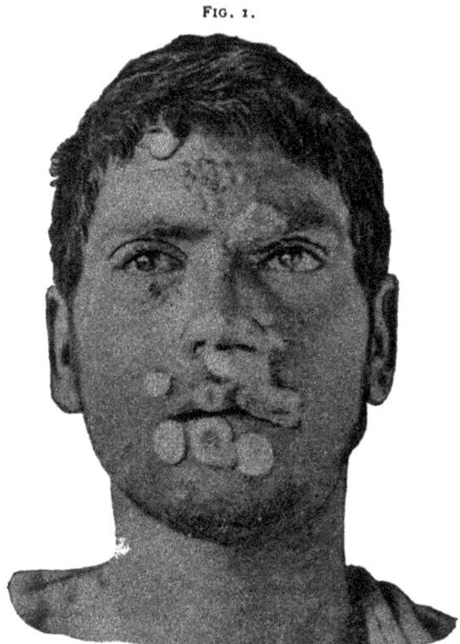

Showing lesions of frambesia.

The appearance of the sores is accompanied by a certain amount of pain in the limbs, rise of temperature and restlessness, and these are the first indications that the patient is infected. The first sore varies in size from one to two inches in diameter, and is soon surrounded by other smaller ones. It is called by the natives *tina-ni-coko*, or "mother yaw," and appears on the site of a wound or scratch, and not infrequently on the lips. Other sores soon develop on the neck, groin, or axilla, and at mucocutaneous junctures. In some cases crops of papules appear in an irregularly distributed eruption; the case is then called *coko-se-ni-nin*, on account of the resemblance to the budding flowers of the cocoanut palm.

In the next stage a soft warty excrescence works its way through the true skin without destroying its substance, and when these appear on the soles of the feet of people unaccustomed to wearing boots their extrusion is extremely painful, on account of the outside horny growth. When the warts reach the surface of the skin they exude a stinking, viscid fluid, which is highly contagious. As it dries the raised scab with the granulated and mulberry-like sore beneath is characteristic of the disease; hence its name.

In some cases the crusts form a curved outline, not unlike syphilitic rupia, and are consequently called *coko-balewa*, or "lempet-yaws." When healing they form circular or horseshoe patterns, and the center heals before the edge. Not only do the excrescences force their way through the plantar skin, but the whole surface becomes cracked and ex-

FIG. 2.

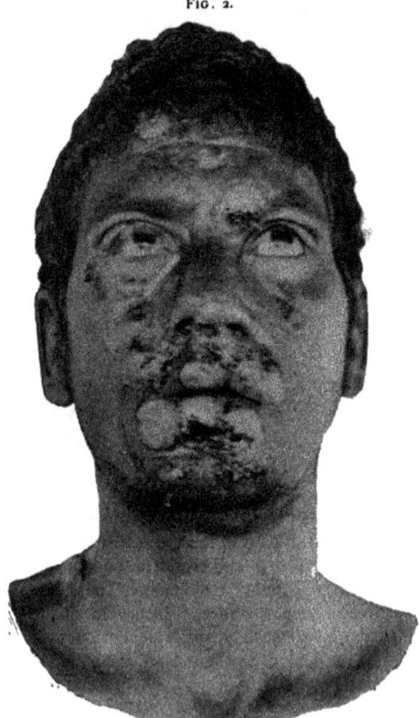

Showing lesions of frambesia.

coriated; this is said to be nearly as painful as the sore itself. The Fijians regard the communication of the disease as due to mysterious influences, and consequently they do not take any means to treat the malady, and look on the interference of a medical man with anything but favor.

It is well known by those who have had communications with the natives that Fijian mothers think that if their children do not contract *yaws* they will not be able to withstand attacks of future diseases. They, therefore, hail its appearance with delight, make no attempt to treat the ulcers, and allow the disease to uninterruptedly run its course. It is only when the eruptions prematurely disappear that they think there is any danger. This state they call *maca-vaka-ca* (dry in the manner bad). The majority of children contract yaws between the ages of two and six years, but the children of chiefs in many instances are kept from associating with other children of the village till they are older and more physically fit to endure its effects on the constitution.

In mild cases the sores disappear within three or four weeks. They may remain, however, for as many years. Weak children are more severely affected, and become susceptible to diarrhea, marasmus, and even paralysis. In many instances the health of those attacked has been completely shattered, and tertiary effects strongly resembling those of neglected syphilis have proved no less severe than irremediable. The results are impairment of the nutritive and digestive functions, inflammation of the joints, ulcerations, and constitutional weakness, rendering the patient liable to attacks of dysentery, pneumonia, etc.

Cases in which Europeans have been attacked with yaws have come under observation in Fiji, inspiring, on account of its repulsive appearance, fear and disgust. When an adult Fijian gets yaws a favorite form of treatment is to rub a red-hot knife over a cut lemon and apply it to the sores as a caustic. The experience of European medical men has shown that the free use of the iodid of potassium internally, with an ointment of nitrate of mercury and lactic acid, have been beneficial, especially with a plentiful nitrogenous diet, and iron tonics.

The East Indians imported into the country for work on the sugar plantations frequently contract yaws. The accompanying illustrations show two patients thus affected.

THE USE OF GLOVES AT OPERATIONS.[1]

BY EDWARD MILTON FOOTE, M.D.,
OF NEW YORK;
SURGEON TO RANDALL'S ISLAND HOSPITALS.

I DESIRE to call attention to some gloves which have been recently recommended by a German surgeon, and which are a very decided aid in the prevention of infection by the fingers in operating.

It is unnecessary in so brief a sketch to go into the details of sterilization of the hands. It has been proved that this can usually be accomplished by a series of washings and brushings with soap and water,

[1] Read at a meeting of the Section on Surgery of the New York Academy of Medicine, March 14, 1898.

and various disinfectant solutions; but it has been equally well proved that this result can be reached only by a sacrifice of time and epidermis, and by a painstaking attention to detail, of which, unfortunately some of the best surgeons are incapable.

To stop this bacterial leak into the wound some surgeons long ago tried to remove the hands from the operative field altogether, by covering them with gloves of rubber or wash-leather. Thick gloves of whatever material naturally diminish the sensitiveness and dexterity of the fingers, and to avoid this very thin rubber gloves were tried, and are still employed by some surgeons. Zweifel has used rubber gloves for years, covering the arms with linen sleeves, which fit close to the gloves at the wrist. His gloves have no finger-tips, but separate finger-cots of thin rubber are used instead. This is a considerable saving in expense, as a very thin rubber glove is easily pricked or torn in tying ligatures and in suturing. Rubber gloves of an extra fine quality, though not very thin, were shown at the last meeting of the Surgical Society by Brewer, who expressed himself as well satisfied with their use.

Within the past few months Mikulicz has recommended the employment of fine silk or Lisle-thread gloves, which may be sterilized without damage in a steam sterilizer and which may be changed during an operation as often as they become soiled. As they readily absorb blood, it is necessary to disinfect the hands before putting them on, but they are superior to rubber gloves in several respects. They are far less clumsy. To tie a knot of fine silk with the hands encased in rubber gloves is a difficult procedure. They are more durable. They are pervious to air, and, therefore, far more comfortable. The increased perspiration of the hands when rubber gloves are worn, may become a positive danger if removal of the gloves is necessary during an operation. They do not compress the fingers. They will adhere slightly to a slippery tissue, so that dissection of fascial planes with the fingers, as in done in inguinal hernia, is made surprisingly easy.

Attempts have been made to render such gloves impervious to moisture, by saturating them with oil, turpentine, and other substances. This has been most successfully accomplished by Menge, an assistant in the Frauenklinik at Leipzig. The gloves are first dried in an oven and then soaked in absolute alcohol, then in xylol, again in fresh xylol, and then during fifteen minutes in a ten-per-cent. solution in xylol of paraffin of a low melting-point. This is exactly the series of steps used to impregnate microscopic specimens with paraffin, before embedding them. The process sounds complicated, but is really not at all so. It is only necessary to have four wide-mouthed bottles containing these solutions, and to pass the gloves through the different solutions one after another. In fact, all that is actually necessary is to have one bottle containing a ten-per-cent. solution of paraffin in xylol, and to soak the thoroughly dry gloves in this solution. When taken out and dried they are ready for sterilization. When soiled they may be washed with soap and water, dried, re-paraffined, and sterilized, and are then again ready for use.

These gloves are not absolutely impervious to moisture, but are sufficiently so for practical purposes. If water is poured slowly upon them, it flows off as from any oily surface. If rubbed into them, a certain amount will be absorbed. In this respect the cotton gloves here shown are inferior to those made of silk, but even they are so good that it is a pleasure to use them; and if an operator has cleansed his hands even superficially, and operates by the dry method, and has consideration enough for his patient to keep his fingers on the handles of his instruments and not in the wound, he ought never to see pus. I cannot refrain from emphasizing this last point. Most of the minor surgical operations and some of the major ones can be performed without direct contact between the fingers and the patient. After a little practice, ligatures and sutures may be tied with forceps or clamps; and when a man finishes an operation without a stain of blood on his fingers he is sure that he has not introduced germs from his hand into the wound. Quite recently I had the pleasure of assisting the secretary of this Section, Dr. Walker, in suturing a badly fractured patella. The joint had been widely opened and contained clots of blood, though the skin was not torn. The blood-clots were wiped away, the patella was sutured, and the incision was closed, neither of us having touched the wound nor any part of any instrument or suture which came into contact with it. It is scarcely necessary to add, that the knee never presented a symptom of inflammation.

To summarize briefly, the best means to avoid infection by the hands are as follows: (1) Keep them out of the wound. (2) Wash them, dry them, and cover them with sterilized gloves. (3) For operations within the serous cavities, and for difficult dissections, thoroughly disinfect the hands according to the well-known methods before drawing on the sterilized gloves.

Floating Naval Hospital.—Surgeon-General W. K. Van Reypen, U. S. N., has been inspecting the steamship "Grand Duchesse" with a view to recommending that the vessel be purchased by the Government for use as a hospital ship in the event of hostilities between this country and Spain.

CLINICAL MEMORANDUM.

TWO CASES OF TUMOR OF THE CEREBELLUM.

BY HOWELL T. PERSHING, M.D.,
OF DENVER, COL.;
PROFESSOR OF NERVOUS AND MENTAL DISEASES IN THE UNIVERSITY OF DENVER.

CASE I.—J. D., aged thirty-five years, was first seen October 16, 1893, in consultation with Drs. A. K. Worthington and W. P. Munn. His mother was subject to headaches, one sister was insane, and one brother died of consumption. The patient was well until September, 1892, when he was kicked by a horse in the right frontal region, and fell, striking on the occiput. After the injury he was unconscious about three hours and vomited. Within a few days he had apparently recovered and went to work. About two weeks after the accident he began to have spells of dizziness in which he was forcibly turned to the left, sometimes being whirled quite rapidly. His own expression was that he "went around like a chicken with its head off." Any change of position caused dizziness. For three weeks the patient was unable to work, but then gradually improved and was apparently as well as ever until August, 1893, when dizziness on motion gradually returned and grew worse, being often accompanied by stiffness of the neck, especially in the morning. Nevertheless, he continued to work until the end of September, when he was obliged to desist on account of dizziness, vomiting, and severe headache. Syphilis was positively denied.

Examination, October 16, 1893, revealed the following condition: The gait is reeling and is about the same whether the eyes are closed or open. Staggering is toward the left, and the left leg is weaker than the right. Motions of the arms, face, and tongue are normal. The knee and heel reflexes are lively and greater on the left side. The pupils are equal and react to light. There are about five degrees of insufficiency of the external recti muscles, causing diplopia when one eye is covered with a red glass. Vision is very slightly below normal in each eye. Both eyes show beginning optic neuritis. Taste and smell are intact. Hearing is slightly impaired by bilateral otitis media. Sensibility to touch and pain is normal in face, hands, and legs. The skin reflexes are lively. The patient's talk is often silly. The examination is somewhat difficult on account of severe headache which is much aggravated by any movement.

During the following month the patient was kept under close observation in St. Anthony's Hospital and treated with inunctions of mercury and large doses of potassium iodid. Nevertheless, he grew steadily worse; the intellect became more and more dulled, vomiting continued, the optic neuritis became more intense, especially on the right side, the right pupil became larger than the left, and the right external rectus was distinctly paralyzed. The knee-jerks disappeared and finally the right side of the face was paralyzed. There was no hemianopsia. During this time the temperature was generally slightly below normal, never above; the pulse varied from 52 to 70 per minute.

The diagnosis of tumor of the right side of the cerebellum being clear and the condition being otherwise hopeless, an operation was decided upon and performed by Dr. Munn, assisted by Dr. Worthington, November 16, 1893. The patient's condition was bad at the beginning of the operation. The occipital bone was rapidly trephined just below the superior curved line. The dura bulged strongly into the opening but did not pulsate. Beneath it was found a mass of very dark, somewhat softened tissue, evidently a glioma, which was scooped away until apparently normal cerebellar tissue appeared in place of the tumor and there was no longer any bulging. The whole amount removed was about one hundred and eighty grains. After the operation the patient was nearly moribund, but under the influence of stimulants revived and spoke rationally. The evening temperature was 101° F. and the pulse 135. The next day the mind was perfectly clear, the facial paralysis had disappeared, and swallowing was much better than it had been for some time before the operation, but the pulse was very weak and vomiting frequently occurred throughout the day. In spite of the administration of stimulants and hot salt solution, both subcutaneously and by rectum, he grew weaker and died thirty-six hours after the operation. An autopsy showed that the brain was elsewhere normal, and that the glioma had been completely removed except for some insignificant ramifications. The tumor had been entirely within the right cerebellar hemisphere.

As this case is reported at this rather late day only for the purpose of placing its symptoms and the result of operation on record, I shall not discuss any of the interesting features it presents. It should be said, however, that judging from the general result of operations for the removal of cerebellar tumors it would have been better to trephine for the relief of pressure without attempting removal or even opening the dura.

CASE II.—H. C., aged six years, was examined in consultation with Drs. Clough and Seebass, November 29, 1895. The parents and a younger brother were perfectly well, and the most careful investigation failed to reveal any hereditary taint or possibility of syphilitic infection. A year before the examination the patient had complained of occipital pain, but it had passed away. During the summer of 1895 he had a mild attack of whooping-cough, the paroxysms of which seemed to cause a return of the occipital pain, which had afterward persisted, and had been decidedly worse, being also occasionally accompanied by vomiting, during the month preceding examination.

Examination, November 29, 1895, showed the following condition: The gait is staggering, with feet wide apart. There is no other motor defect. Exertion causes pain in the occiput, and the nuchal region is somewhat tender. The skin and tendon reflexes are lively and equal on both sides. Sensibility to touch, pain, smell, taste, hearing, and vision is normal, but there is intense optic neuritis on both sides and the left pupil is greater than the right. The head is proportionately considerably larger than that of the brother, who is eighteen months younger, its circumference being 17.9 inches. The urine contains an excess of urates, but is otherwise normal. The temperature is normal, and there is no sign of suppuration in any part of the body.

The diagnosis of tumor in this case scarcely admitted of doubt. In the absence of alcoholism, plumbism, and uremia, the association of intense optic neuritis with headache and vomiting made the existence of organic disease within the cranium quite certain. Chronic meningitis could hardly be suspected except in the presence of syphilis, of which there was not the slightest indication, and the intensity of the optic neuritis militated against a diagnosis of meningitis. On the other hand, the combination of symptoms and their gradual onset were strongly indicative of brain-tumor. In the absence of other localizing symptoms the staggering gait and nuchal tenderness pointed to the cerebellum as the probable seat of the growth. There was no positive indication of the nature of the tumor. Gumma, however, was excluded, not only by the history and condition of the child and of his parents, but also by the extreme rarity of intracranial gummata in children and of cerebellar gummata at any age. Tubercle seemed more probable than any other form of growth simply because in children it is far more common than any other. The favorable result of treatment strengthens this probability, for, excepting gummata, tuberculous tumors are the kind most likely to be favorably influenced by internal medication. The prognosis given the parents was necessarily very grave, but not altogether hopeless.

The child was vigorously treated with inunctions of mercury and with iodid of potassium internally, alternating with iodid of iron. At the end of two months the ataxia was somewhat worse and the other symptoms remained about the same. Within four months, notwithstanding occasional attacks of headache and vomiting, and the persistence of optic neuritis with distinct impairment of vision, a general improvement was manifest. From that time the optic neuritis began to slowly improve and it finally disappeared altogether without resulting in atrophy. The attacks of headache and vomiting ceased, and the gait steadily improved, so that for nearly two years the parents have regarded the boy as quite well.

It should not be thought, however, that treatment has actually removed the tumor. What may be inferred is that its growth has been arrested and that an excess of fluid in the ventricles has been absorbed.

The main value of this case is that it illustrates the advantage, in a case of tumor, even though it be non-syphilitic, of a patient trial of mercury and iodids before resorting to more radical measures, and, also, of refraining from an absolutely unfavorable prognosis even though the diagnosis of an incurable disease be practically certain.

Kings County Inebriate Home.—A bill has been introduced in the New York Senate dissolving the corporation known as the Inebriate's Home of Kings County. The institution is situated at Fort Hamilton, Brooklyn Borough.

MEDICAL PROGRESS.

Immunity of the Negro to Certain Diseases and the Causes Thereof.—CLARK (*Maryland Med. Jour.*, January 8, 1898) calls attention to the fact that negroes present a certain degree of immunity to yellow fever, malaria, chorea, and other diseases. In the case of yellow fever, one attack renders an individual less likely to contract another, and, therefore, it is easily understood why the survivors of a race always subjected to the disease should be to some extent immune to it. In the case of malaria, one attack predisposes to others, so that those individuals prone to have malaria will long ago have succumbed. Hence, those who remain, are less likely to contract the disease than the members of other races. In this writer's experience the susceptibility of a negro to malaria is not more than one-fourth that of a white person. The immunity of the negro from chorea is well-known. This is apparently due to his more stable nervous organization. Clark also cites the fact that an enlarged prostate in a negro is a very rare affection, and that this is the more remarkable when one considers that it is a fibroid condition, and that the female negro is especially prone to fibroid disease of the uterus. He gives as a reason for this immunity from enlarged prostate the fact that but few negroes reach the age at which this gland usually begins to cause trouble, say about fifty-five years.

Use of the Gigli Wire Saw to Open the Skull.—KEEN (*Philadelphia Med. Jour.*, January 1, 1898) describes his experience with the Gigli wire saw, a new instrument consisting of a twisted steel wire with sharp edges and two handles attached. The wire is passed from one trephine opening to another, and the action of the instrument is similar to that of the old-fashioned chain saw. In this way an osteoplastic flap of any desired size may be removed. The advantages of the saw are first, that one is able to bevel the edge of the bone-flap in such a way that it will not sink into the cavity of the skull when replaced. There is practically no loss of bony tissue, as the saw is so thin. The second advantage is that when a bone-flap has been sawed on three sides it is possible with the saw to cut from the inside outward through the fourth side of the flap, thus avoiding the ragged, broken edge which is invariably present when the flap is pried out by main force. The third advantage is that the saw avoids the jarring produced by a mallet and chisel. This advantage is a purely theoretic one in Keen's opinion, as he has never seen unpleasant effects follow the use of a mallet and chisel which could be attributed to jarring. The wires of the saw can be used only once, as being so very fine they quickly wear out and curl up. A number of them of various sizes should be prepared for each operation.

The Significance of Mucus in Stools.—SCHMIDT (*Fortschr. der Med.*, January 1, 1898) says that the characteristics of mucus in the stools are not sufficiently exact to enable one to diagnose therefrom a special form of membranous enteritis, as Nothnagel has attempted to do. The mucous origin of the so-called yellow mucous grains, "gelben Schleimkörner," is, moreover not proved. The basic substance of the membranes is mucus or mucin, and they contain considerable amounts of fat and soap. Fibrin has not been definitely proved to exist in their composition. Unless there is a very rapid passage of the intestinal contents through the large bowel, particles of mucus from the small intestine can scarcely reach the anus without being dissolved.

Resection of the Saphenous Vein for Ulcers of the Leg.—HEINTZE (*Deut. Zeit. für Chir.*, vol. xlvii, p. 107) lauds resection of the saphenous vein in the treatment of chronic ulcers of the leg. He advocates the removal of from two to five inches of the upper end of the vein in order to resect it below some of its largest branches. Patients are kept in bed three weeks or longer, and the ulcers are dressed with any suitable salve. He cites a list of seventy-nine cases in which this operation has been performed, thirty-five times upon women and twenty-eight times upon men. Only nine of these patients (it is worth remarking) were more than fifty years old. The results were excellent. At the time of discharge from the hospital all of the ulcers excepting four were completely healed.

Heintze explains the good effects of this operation upon the supposition that the valves which ought to shut off the saphenous vein from the femoral often act imperfectly. In consequence blood passes from the vena cava backward into the saphenous vein, and from there into the deep veins of the leg, where the current, assisted by muscular action and valves, is again upward into the vena cava. Even if an actual back-flow does not take place in the manner indicated, there is a stagnation in the current which interferes with the nourishment in the skin of the leg, and thus the least scratch causes ulceration. That the improvement noticed in his patients was not simply due to rest in bed, was shown by the fact that a number of them were kept in bed for some days before operation, without any marked change in the condition of the ulcers. The time is yet too short to form an opinion as to the permanence of the cure in these cases.

How Bacteria Are Influenced by Prolonged Exposure to Roentgen-rays.—BONOMO and GROS (*Centralbl. für inn. Med.*, December 31, 1897) have established the interesting fact that long exposure of bacteria to Röntgen-rays lessens their power of growth and their virulence. If two or three successive generations are exposed to the rays these alterations become evident, and are associated with diminution of the power of motion and changes in chromogenous power in such bacteria as possess this function. Spore formation is also destroyed, especially in the case of the anthrax bacillus. Unfortunately, as far as any practical application goes, even prolonged exposure to the rays for two or three generations, did not entirely destroy virulence.

The Influence of Morphin and Ether upon the Pains of Child-birth.—HENSEN (*Archiv. für Gynek.*, vol. 51, p. 129) says that morphin in doses of ¼-grain or less is without any influence upon the contractions of the uterus or the abdominal pressure during child-birth. Ether, on the other hand, when administered one or two minutes reduces the force of the pains and lengthens the intervals between them. In five to twenty minutes after suspension of the ether the contractions are again normal. In ether narcosis the abdominal pressure is lessened. These results show the advantage of ether over chloroform, for the latter exerts an unfavorable influence upon the pains, sometimes lasting for two hours after its administration has been discontinued. For example, when version is necessary, or it is wished to apply the forceps, in complete narcosis, and to allow Nature to finish the labor in partial narcosis, ether is far preferable to chloroform. It is for the same reason less likely to produce atony of the uterus which so often follows the administration of chloroform.

THERAPEUTIC NOTES.

Instantaneous Cure of a Long-Standing Case of Borborygmus.—VEIRE (*Bull. Gen. de Therapeut.*, January 8, 1898) reports the case of a girl, aged fifteen, who for more than two years had been troubled with borborygmus. The noises were so loud that they could be heard in the next room. After an attack of borborygmus had continued several hours a great quantity of gas would be brought up, and for a short time the noises would cease. Veire made a diagnosis of ectasia and ptosis of the stomach. He prescribed a close-fitting bandage. A month afterward the patient stated that from the time when the bandage was first applied the noises and formation of gas had entirely ceased.

How to Administer Creosote.—In order to obtain the best results from the use of creosote more attention should be paid to the method of administration. According to a writer in *La Méd. Moderne*, December 29, 1897, the best of all the numerous methods suggested is to give the drug by mouth in capsules, each one of which contains $^{1}/_{16}$-grain of pure creosote, emulsified with 1 grain each of cod-liver oil and balsam of tolu. In this manner the disagreeable taste and odor are avoided, while this emulsion is one of which all the ingredients exercise a favorable influence upon the respiratory tract and do not irritate the mucous membrane of the stomach. Many writers have at different times reported great satisfaction with the administration of this drug by inhalation, friction, introduction into the rectum, and by subcutaneous injection, but none of these methods have stood the test of experience.

Puerperal Sepsis and Antistreptococcic Serum.—CLARK (*Boston Med. and Surg. Jour.*, January 13, 1898) gives the history of two cases of puerperal sepsis in which Marmorek's antistreptococcic serum was employed, 20 cubic centimeters being injected at one time into the gluteal region. In one case, particularly, the improvement was so prompt after the serum had been injected, and the patient was before in such a bad condition, that Clark felt sure that recovery was due to the serum alone.

THE MEDICAL NEWS.

A WEEKLY JOURNAL

OF MEDICAL SCIENCE.

COMMUNICATIONS are invited from all parts of the world. Original articles contributed *exclusively* to THE MEDICAL NEWS will after publication be liberally paid for (accounts being rendered quarterly), or 250 reprints will be furnished in place of other remuneration. When necessary to elucidate the text, illustrations will be engraved from drawings or photographs furnished by the author. Manuscripts should be typewritten.

Address the Editor: J. RIDDLE GOFFE, M.D.,
No. 111 FIFTH AVENUE (corner of 18th St.), NEW YORK.

Subscription Price, including postage in U. S. and Canada.

PER ANNUM IN ADVANCE	$4.00
SINGLE COPIES	.10
WITH THE AMERICAN JOURNAL OF THE MEDICAL SCIENCES, PER ANNUM	7.50

Subscriptions may begin at any date. The safest mode of remittance is by bank check or postal money order, drawn to the order of the undersigned. When neither is accessible, remittances may be made, at the risk of the publishers, by forwarding in *registered* letters.

LEA BROTHERS & CO.,
No. 111 FIFTH AVENUE (corner of 18th St.), NEW YORK,
AND NOS. 706, 708 & 710 SANSOM ST., PHILADELPHIA.

SATURDAY, MARCH 26, 1898.

THE EFFECT OF THE MODERN BULLET.

THE credit, if credit there be, for the development of the most deadly fire-arms the world has ever known belongs to Germany. The Germans have also been most painstaking in figuring out the exact effect upon a person who stands in the range of a high-velocity bullet. In these days of rumored war, a review of a book recently published upon this subject by Köhler, will doubtless be of interest to army surgeons as well as to many a possible target for rifle practice.

When a bullet of very high velocity strikes a receptacle containing a fluid or semi-fluid, there is a destruction of the receptacle entirely out of proportion to the size and direction of the missile, so that the force under these conditions has been spoken of as an explosive one. This is manifest if the head or stomach or intestine is encountered, provided, of course, that the viscus be full. Scientists have been at a loss to explain this manifestation of great force, and it has been loosely spoken of as "hydraulic," some men claiming that the hydraulic power shown in such cases was equivalent to the force of the bullet distributed over the whole surface of the skull, and others stating that every portion of the skull, equivalent in area to the cross-section of the bullet, was by reason of this hydraulic power, impinged upon with a force equal to the impact of the projectile, *i.e.*, a true hydraulic pressure.

Köhler says that these hydraulic theories are unsupported by facts. The true explanation of the great destructive force of high-velocity missiles, is that they do not give the fluid time to move out of the way. It has, therefore, the resistance of a solid body. Now a blow on a solid body is distributed in ever-widening circles, as can readily be seen in the chipping of an arrow-head, or from a large scale which a bullet breaks off from the reverse side of a plate of sandstone, if its power is not sufficient to penetrate it. The following experiment also shows the slowness with which fluids recede before a very swift projectile. A board is placed a few inches below the surface of the water, and a bullet at low velocity fired into it. The bullet passes through the water and penetrates the board. Let the speed of the projectile be great enough, however, and it is shattered into pieces on the surface of the water, and the board is unharmed.

If this lack of mobility of a fluid is difficult to understand, one has only to think of the difference in the feeling when the hand strikes the surface of the water, slowly, and when it strikes with great speed, and then to consider that a modern bullet moves at such a rate that it takes only the 2000th part of a second to traverse the skull. This amount of time is far too brief, according to Köhler, for any hydraulic power to manifest itself, for before it could begin to act, there would be two holes in the skull, one of entrance and one of exit, out of which the fluid could escape and so relieve pressure.

"Suspended lability" is the name suggested for this new theory, which at least bears the semblance of truth.

DR. CLEAVELAND AND HIS ACCUSERS.

THE arrest and indictment for manslaughter of a well-known physician of this city a few days ago, charged with having prescribed salol and resorcin for a child six weeks old, which caused its death nearly a year ago, was referred to in last week's issue of the MEDICAL NEWS. The matter is of such importance that it seems to call for more than passing notice, and that for several reasons. Aside from the fact that both salol and resorcin are not ordinarily looked upon as lethal drugs, the description of the child's illness contained in the public press corresponds so completely with the symptom-complex of an attack of cholera infantum that at first sight it is difficult to conceive the grounds taken by the District Attorney in the conduct of the prosecution. There was no necroscopic examination, and the physician who saw the patient in consultation after the collapse symptoms developed, a man of great skill and an authority on the action of drugs, is quoted as supporting in every way the physician under indictment.

The prosecution apparently rests on the affidavit of a physician of this city who avers that, in his opinion, the child was poisoned to death by the drugs used. This opinion is said to be concurred in by a number of physicians, most, if not all, members of the profession in good standing, who have reached this conclusion after listening to the mother's story. In brief, it would seem to the unimpassioned observer that the prosecution of the defendant is in reality a persecution by his professional brethren. If this be true it is a most deplorable state of affairs, and one of serious consequence to the medical body politic. A number of physicians in this and in other cities have been interviewed by the mother of the dead child, and by her agents, with the object of getting an expression of opinion as to the lethality of the drugs given. Naturally, the majority of these physicians refused to discuss the merits or demerits of the case without other knowledge of it than the mother's *ipse dixit*. Others were not deterred from making known their views and of embodying them in letters or in verbal communications which have been available to the public press. Some of these expressions were couched in such extravagant language that they bear unmistakable marks of exaggeration by the reporter, and lead to the conclusion that the speaker was either tricked into some unguarded admission or induced by mutual friends to innocently state his hypothetic opinion. Nevertheless, the lesson is a most pertinent one that absolute silence under such circumstances is the only just attitude.

No one will question the right of an individual to personal opinion, but it is a universally admitted fact that an opinion based on hearsay evidence is well-nigh valueless as testimony. We have no doubt that the courts will deal justly with the defendant in question, and that justice meted out to him will be an honorable acquittal. There is a question of duty to one's fellow man—and of ethics—involved in this matter that should not be allowed to pass unremarked. If the *esprit* of the medical profession has come to such a pass that it will tolerate the gratuitous persecution of one of its members by others who are in no way concerned, then we should cease discussing canons of conduct, and forget with all possible haste the maxim: "Do unto others as you would have them do unto you."

We feel sure that when Dr. Cleaveland is placed on trial he will not be lacking the volunteered service of the medical men of this city, and of this country if needs be, whose opinion is worth having. We have abundant faith in their willingness and desire to maintain that the character of a man, who in the eyes of the law is innocent, shall not be snatched from him by the inflammable misquoted words of a few professional brethren.

THE BLOOD-SUPPLY OF THE HEART-MUSCLE AND THE INFLUENCE OF DIGITALIS UPON IT.

ONE of the great difficulties which stands in the way of rational therapeutics is our lack of knowledge as to the actual living functions of certain vital parts of the human body. Researches in morbid anatomy reveal to us the results of disease, and the study of pathology, or morbid physiology, is often rewarded by valuable discoveries, while investigations in the realm of physiology proper give us clear ideas of healthy functional activity. Far too little is really known as to minute but important facts concerning the blood-supply of vital organs, and this is particularly true of the heart, an organ whose living functions in man cannot be minutely studied. Interference with its blood-supply, of a severe and suddenly developed form, may speedily produce death, as, for example, in disease of the coronary arteries, and changes in the myocardium, secondary or primary, may so result. These facts we know chiefly from post-mortem findings. Of the action of drugs upon the cardiac functions we know only facts demonstrable by an examination of the thorax and the pulse, the effect on the general condition of the patient, and from studies of a more direct character made upon the circulatory apparatus of animals.

For many years it has been known that digitalis does good in most cases of failing compensation following cardiac valvular lesions, and basing our views upon animal experimentation, fairly satisfactory statements of how it does good in the various diseases have been offered. Almost all of these have dealt with its mechanical influence upon the blood-current, and only imaginative reasoning has been utilized in explaining how the final good effects are produced; for it certainly is a fact that in some cases at least the beneficial influence of digitalis does not cease as soon as the use of the drug is discontinued, but persists for a long time after all its direct and immediate effects have passed away. In other words, digitalis not only has a direct stimulant effect upon the heart-muscle, but under its influence this tissue obtains a better tone, its nutrition is improved, and it is in every way more fit for the proper performance of its duties.

Aside from the well-known regulation of the cardiac beat produced by digitalis through its effect upon the pneumogastric nerve, how does it improve cardiac nutrition and power? This is the question which is important, and the answer to which has not been forthcoming until recently, except in a hypothetic manner. It has been hinted that the stimulation of the vagi not only slows the heart-beat, but that these nerves, being the trophic fibers, their stimulation results in an improved nutritional process. Again, it has been thought that the mere slowing of the heart-beat and prolongation of diastole produced by digitalis allowed of a better blood-supply to the heart-muscle, with improved nutrition as an indirect result of vagal stimulation, but these views have been rather theories than statements based upon facts, as we have already pointed out.

Wood teaches that the supply of blood to the heart is driven into the coronary arteries during diastole, and that the force which propels it is derived from the arterial system; or, in other words, that while all the other arteries in the body are filled by systole, the coronary arteries are filled by diastole. This is, however, only partly, if at all true; for Rabatel (Paris, 1872) has proved that the blood wave under systole is synchronous in both the general arteries and those of the heart itself; that is, the coronary arteries are filled during systole. This fact has recently been confirmed by W. T. Porter (*American Journal of Physiology*, March 1, 1898), who has proved, as has Pratt, that the systole of the heart which fills the coronary arteries also results in such a pressure upon the terminal intramural arteries that they are emptied, and thus allows the free entrance of fresh blood as soon as diastole begins. In other words, an increased systolic contraction of a ventricle not only fills the coronary arteries with blood, but at the same time urges on the blood already in the intramural vessels, and so a greater blood-supply is brought to the heart-muscle in a minute if its systole is complete and forcible than if it is incomplete and feeble. These results, obtained in the laboratory, are in direct confirmation of the hypothetic explanation given by the writer of this article in his work on "Practical Therapeutics" (p. 567) as to the manner in which the heart-muscle is nourished under digitalis.

The next question of interest is whether improvement in the heart-muscle is simply one of tone or due to an actual increase in its muscular growth and power. The answer to this question is that both effects are produced. That the tone is improved is self-evident to the clinician who uses the drug properly in suitable cases. That the muscle-fibers are strengthened and hypertrophied is indicated by a research recently published by the writer of this article in the *Therapeutic Gazette* for December, 1897. In this investigation two sets of young pigs belonging to the same litter were carefully weighed and prepared for the experiment. One set of five received ascending doses of normal liquid digitalis for a period of four and a half months, and the other set were reserved as a control experiment. After the lapse of time named both sets were killed and the hearts of all carefully examined macroscopically and microscopically. Both these methods of study revealed an increase in the size of the hearts under digitalis, and the muscular tissue when cut was firmer in these hearts.

Finally, it is interesting to note the results reached by Dr. Ida H. Hyde in a study of the effect of distention of the ventricle upon the flow of blood through the heart walls (*American Journal of Physiology*, March, 1898) in which she shows that this condition, even in moderate degree, may diminish the flow of blood through the heart-muscle. Distention of the heart is well recognized as a resült of violent muscular exercise, and is frequently seen in persons who habitually lift heavy weights and in mountain-climbers, athletes, and hod-carriers. In this connection Hyde's study would seem to indicate that digitalis by stimulating the heart-muscle may overcome the distention and improve cardiac action by improving the cardiac circulation.

H. A. HARE, M.D.

ECHOES AND NEWS.

Yellow Fever in Rio de Janeiro.—Yellow fever is prevalent in Rio de Janeiro, and for a week past twelve deaths from the disease have occurred daily.

Appropriation for Care of Epileptics.—The bill appropriating $161,000 for the Craig Colony of Epileptics has been passed by the New York Senate.

Bacterial Treatment of Sewage.—The British Government has decided to appoint a Royal commission to inquire into the bacterial treatment of sewage.

Bequest to Jefferson Medical College.—By the will of the late S. C. Shain, Jefferson Medical College, Philadelphia, has received $7000 for scholarships and prizes.

Donation to Pomona College.—Dr. E. D. Pearson of Chicago has donated $25,000 to Pomona College, Pomona, Cal., to be used by the trustees to defray the expense of erecting a new science building.

Commission to Study the Propagation of Tuberculosis.—The Paris Academy of Sciences, upon the motion of M. Brouardel, has appointed a commission to study the question of the propagation of tuberculosis.

St. Vincent's Hospital Asks for Appropriation.—A bill recently introduced in the New York Senate authorizes the payment by New York City of $30,000 a year to St. Vincent's Hospital for the maintenance of indigent patients cared for in that institution.

The Sheppard and Enoch Pratt Hospital.—In order that it may receive the $1,500,000 bequeathed to it by the late Enoch Pratt, the Maryland Legislature has passed a bill allowing the trustees of the Sheppard Asylum to change the name of that institution to the Sheppard and Enoch Pratt Hospital.

Bellevue Hospital and the State Board of Health.—President William R. Stewart of the New York State Board of Charities, calls attention in his report to the unsanitary condition of the cellars of Bellevue Hospital, New York City, and also refers to the overcrowding of the alcoholic wards.

Investigation of Zymotic Diseases.—A gift of $5000, to be used in promoting the study of the diseases of the Congo, has been received by the Society of Colonial Studies of Brussels, and the Society offers two prizes of $500 for some notable addition to the knowledge of the evolution of the hematozoon of Leveran and for the discovery of the origin of hemoglobinuric fever.

St. Mary's Hospital (Hoboken).—An addition to St. Mary's Hospital, Hoboken, N. J., has just been completed. The new wing is 228 x 175 feet, affords accommodation for an additional two hundred patients, and cost $225,000. There has also been added a dissecting-room and a chapel, the latter capable of holding six hundred people. The hospital is non-sectarian and is under the care of the Little Sisters of the Poor of St. Francis.

Inspection of Lodging-houses.—The New York houses for lodgers are said to number 113, at least that is the number on record in the Department of Health as being operated under an official permit. In consequence of the disastrous fire which recently occurred at one of the Bowery houses a simultaneous inspection was made of the entire number on a given night. The result was quite satisfactory, as only five of the houses were discovered to be conducted in violation of the terms of their permits or of the requirements of the lodging-house law.

Absence of the Diaphragm.—An unusual case of diaphragmatic hernia occurring in a new-born infant is referred to in a recent number of the *British Medical Journal*. At birth the child was very livid and the heart could be felt beating on the right side of the chest. Various methods of artificial respiration proved unavailing, and the child soon died. Autopsy showed that the left half of the diaphragm was absent and that the abdominal viscera had entered the thoracic cavity, pushing the heart to the right, and compressing the left lung into a very small solid mass.

Quarantined Patients without Food.—At Middlesboro, Ky., forty cases of variola and twenty-nine suspects are quarantined in the pest-house and there are no funds to pay for their care. Dr. McCormack, chief inspector of the State Board of Health, says the State has no funds to be used for this purpose, the county refuses to make an appropriation, and the city is bankrupt. Surgeon Wertenbaker of the Marine Hospital Service, who was sent to investigate the situation, is anxious and willing to render Federal assistance, but can only do so on invitation of the State Board of Health. Dr. McCormack vigorously opposes Federal intervention and states that if the county does not render the necessary aid, he will withdraw and release the patients. Meanwhile the latter have been without food for two days and threaten to make their escape.

Unsanitary Bombay.—According to the correspondent of the *Lancet* (London), the conditions in which the native poor of Bombay live are terrible in the extreme. The present epidemic has given opportunities for inspecting the over-crowded houses, and the dark, unventilated rooms, filled with the fumes of cooking and burning wood—there are no chimneys. A large number of houses were found in which the rooms, especially on the ground and first floors, were without windows and absolutely pitch dark. In many of the houses an imperfectly covered drain runs through the hallway on the ground floor, and privies are often placed in dark and totally unventilated corners. The night-soil is collected in baskets placed beneath the native form of closet, and the habits of the natives are so filthy that the condition of these places is beyond description. To make matters worse, the floors and passages are smeared with cow-dung, which is put to such a variety of purposes in India that it is considered heresy to complain of it. It is collected in the streets by the women, and messed about the house with utter indifference as to the danger of its polluting the food and drink. The first step toward reform should be the abolishment of the use of this material. As might be expected, the over-crowding is excessive. In one large room thirteen families, with their separate cooking-stoves and domestic conveniences, were counted. The people work hard, especially the women, and their fare is a meager diet of rice and flour, with butter of some sort, and perhaps vegetables and fruit.

Diphtheria Statistics in New York City.—The following statistics relative to the occurrence of diphtheria in this city (Boroughs of Manhattan and the Bronx) well illustrate the reduction in mortality attendant upon the use of antitoxic serum:

DEATHS FOR JANUARY AND FEBRUARY, 1894-1898.

	1894	1895	1896	1897	1898
January	350	210	208	162	91
February	260	175	187	133	109[1]
Total	610	385	395	295	200

DEATH-RATE FROM DIPHTHERIA AND CROUP FOR THE MONTHS OF JANUARY AND FEBRUARY, 1894-1898.

1894	1895	1896	1897	1898
2.03	1.23	1.23	0.89	0.59

Diphtheria antitoxin came into use in New York City in the autumn of 1894. The Department of Health placed its serum in use January 1, 1895.

Liquid Air Readily and Cheaply Produced.—Professor Peckham of the Adelphi College of Brooklyn, has made the first public demonstration of the new discovery of Mr. T. C. Tripler of Manhattan, comprising the liquefaction of air. For many years chemists have been searching for the absolute zero. Scientists had been on this hunt with as much eagerness as explorers had been searching for the North Pole. The announcement had been made that at 273° C. below zero, 460° F., all heat would cease. About 330 degrees in liquid oxygen had been reached. The first scientists to liquefy oxygen did so at a cost of $2500 a quart. Mr. Tripler has recently discovered a method to produce it at a nominal cost with a forty-horse-power engine. He could make from two to three gallons every hour of a liquid air, which can in this form be drawn out in pipes and can be handled as easily as water. As soon as it comes out it begins to boil violently until the air about it is frozen and cooled, then it ceases to boil. Those present witnessed the novel sight of a mercury hammer. The professor took a handful of fluid mercury and placed it in a kind of mold. This was placed in a pot of liquid air, and before it became hard a rod of iron was inserted in the mercury. In a moment the professor drew out what appeared to be a hammer with a silver head. The mercury had become frozen so hard that a nail could be driven with it. Several other curious experiments were made. This discovery is regarded by Professor Peckham as second only in importance to that of the Röntgen-ray.

[1] To February 26th, inclusive. Monthly returns not as yet made up.

Obituary.—Dr. Alexander Russell Strachan died March 1st at his rooms in the St. Cloud Hotel, New York, from bronchopneumonia following la grippe. He was born in Canada about seventy years ago, and named after his uncle Lord Alexander Russell. His preceptor was the great Dr. Rolph, founder of the Rolph School of Medicine. He was graduated from Victoria College, Toronto, in 1861, and in 1862 and 1863 served as resident physician in St. Luke's Hospital, New York, then in its youth. He was a member of the Academy of Medicine, County Society, and Society of Alumni of St. Luke's Hospital, but had not of late years attended many medical meetings because of marked deafness. However, his love of books provided him plenty of entertainment at home. He was a gentleman of the old-school type, and much beloved by all who knew him. Almost the last time he was seen on the street was the day he sprang to rescue a woman and child from a cable-car. He saved them but was himself knocked down. Dr. Strachan left no family.—Dr. John T. Conkling recently died at his home in Brooklyn, New York City. He was born in 1825 in Smithtown, L. I. He studied medicine in the College of Physicians and Surgeons of New York, and was graduated from this institution in 1855. He settled in Brooklyn and established a practice there. In 1866 and 1867 he was sanitary superintendent of the Brooklyn Board of Health and was in charge of the Board of Health during the cholera epidemic. In 1874 he was appointed Health Commissioner of Brooklyn, and served in that capacity during the following three years. Dr. Conkling was a member of the Practitioner's Club of Brooklyn, of the Hamilton Club, and of the Medical Society of the County of Kings.

An Ointment to Abort Furuncles.—

℞		
Europhen	. . . . . .	gr. lxxx
Ol. olivæ	. . . . . .	ʒ iiss
Vaselini } aa	. . . . .	ʒ vi.
Lanolini }		

M. ungt. Sig. Apply to affected area, covering with sterilized gauze.

CORRESPONDENCE.

THE CLEAVELAND CASE—A PERSONAL STATEMENT BY DR. NORTHRUP.

To the Editor of the MEDICAL NEWS.

DEAR SIR: Allow me to avail myself of your columns to state my connection with this unfortunate indictment of Dr. Cleaveland. First, as to my connection with the affair at all. A personal friend called at my office, bringing an Assistant District Attorney and Mrs. Carhart. After the attorney had stated his wishes, my first words were: "Am I wanted as an expert witness?" His answer was: "Yes." I then said: "An expert witness has the right to decline, has he not?" He said: "Yes; but in the interest of humanity I hope that you will not." I replied: "I do decline, and on no account will I have anything to do with it." To everything he had to urge, I reiterated my refusal with absolute positiveness. After this, the mother narrated the case at the suggestion of my personal friend, without giving either names of persons or localities, and asked my opinion upon it. Let it be remembered that until I saw the account in the newspaper I did not know the name of the Doctor or whether he lived in New York or New England.

Having declined to serve and supposing that what I now said was merely of a private nature, I expressed myself as nearly as I can remember as follows: "As the facts are represented to me my first impressions are that there is some causal relation between the size of the dose and some of the symptoms." I have no remembrance of using any such flamboyant expression as has been attributed to me in the press. To my surprise and annoyance, a few days later, I was summoned before the Grand Jury. The substance of my testimony there was that I had no experience that would unable me to give any answer to the question whether the dose mentioned was dangerous.

W. P. NORTHUP, M.D.

NEW YORK, March 21, 1898.

SMALLPOX IN ALABAMA.

To the Editor of the MEDICAL NEWS.

DEAR SIR: Apropos of your editorial on the smallpox epidemic in Alabama, which appeared in your issue of March 12th, I offer for your consideration the following: The Board of Health of Jefferson County, Alabama, declared smallpox epidemic in Birmingham in July, 1897. The local papers all made the announcement.

Every county in Alabama has a Board of Health which has well-defined powers and a legal status. Every county health-officer in the State is required by law to furnish vaccine free of cost at all times. There is, however, no compulsory-vaccination law in the State code. There is a large proportion of our populution who will not submit to vaccination when it is voluntary.

Under the charter of the City of Birmingham the Council has power to pass a compulsory-vaccination law, and upon request of the Board of Health proceeded to pass it as soon as smallpox was declared epidemic. A corps of vaccinators, house-disinfectors, and inspectors was appointed without delay, and during the next three months the vaccinating-corps went over the city four times.

Every day reports were published in the papers—every day a report was made by our local health-officer, by request, to the Surgeon-General of the Marine Hospital Service. These reports were published regularly by the Surgeon-General, and must have been sent to your journal. After some three months the epidemic was so much under control that most of the inspectors and vaccinators were discharged, and later, when no new cases were reported during four weeks, the epidemic was declared to be at an end. Cases soon, however, began to appear, being imported into the city and county, and the health machinery, consisting of pest-house, detention-camp, inspectors, ambulances, etc., was continued in operation until Dr. McGruder took charge.

Good and efficient work has been done by the Marine Hospital Service, but perfect results have not been attained—for smallpox has not been eradicated. More than $20,000 has been expended by our county and city authorities, besides the money spent by the Marine Hospital Service in its eight-weeks' work. The reasons for this failure are plain: absence of State compulsory-vaccination law, a predjudice against vaccination, and lastly, the mildness of the disease during the present epidemic. Had the disease been of the ordinary type, as regards severity, it is safe to assume that the systematic concealment of cases would not have been practised by our colored population. The truth has been that many of them seemed to dread the sore arm incident to vaccination more than they did the mild smallpox, which, in not a few instances, did not even confine them to bed. This mildness was especially observed in children, contrary to the usual rule. Regular detective work was required of the inspectors in their efforts to find the cases —such were the expedients employed to conceal them.

When smallpox will be eradicated from Alabama and adjoining States is problematic; certainly not until compulsory-vaccination laws are passed, accompanied by large appropriations for their enforcement. The disease has been in lower Alabama for nearly a year and a half, having been introduced from an adjoining State.

From a medical standpoint the interesting feature has been the extreme mildness of so many of the cases.

Very truly,

THOS. D. PARKE, M.D.

BIRMINGHAM, ALA., March 17, 1898.

PROTARGOL: A NEW REMEDY FOR GONORRHEA.

To the Editor of the MEDICAL NEWS.

DEAR SIR: Through your valuable journal I wish to make the medical profession acquainted with the results attending the use of protargol in gonorrhea in the polyclinic of Drs. E. Frank and A. Lewin at Berlin.

Since the discovery of the bacterial cause of gonorrhea by Professor Neisser of Breslau, not only has the diagnosis of specific urethritis been rendered more easy and certain, but new impetus has been given to the attempts to discover a specific treatment for the disease. So long as no such specific existed, the more conservative men have always warned against active interference, *i. e.*: injections, during the first ten days or two weeks of the disease at least, because they have too often seen a gonorrhea posterior acuta follow such treatment. The reason thereof is clear: none of the remedies thus used were able to destroy the gonorrheal virus, and, therefore, they often only transplanted it into new areas.

Of late years Janet has claimed splendid results by the frequent irrigation of the urethra and bladder with a solution of permanganate of potash. He does not claim that the gonococci are directly destroyed, but that the soil is rendered so unfavorable to their development that they cannot thrive or even live thereon. Not only is this treatment tedious and expensive, since the patient must be seen twice daily, but the results, in other equally skilful hands, have been far from satisfactory. This is likewise easily explained. In the first place, the remedy is not a specific; and, secondly, it occasions, very often, extremely severe irritation.

Professor Neisser and his followers have, therefore, endeavored to discover some substance which would directly destroy the gonococci, and, at the same time, produce no marked irritation of the urinary tract. Nitrate of silver has long been used in the so-called abortive treatment of gonorrhea, and occasionally with the most brilliant results, but, as a rule, it produces an intense irritation of the urethra and often epididymitis and other complications. Nevertheless, bacteriologic experiment has demonstrated that silver is the most active poison for the gonococcus. The unsatisfactory results attending its use are due partly to the above-mentioned irritation and partly to the fact that nitrate-of-silver solutions are precipitated by albumen and by solutions of sodium chlorid.

Urine or pus, adhering to the walls of the urethra, thus reduces the silver to an inactive compound before its destructive effects upon the gonococci can be exerted. The coating so formed prevents the contact of the silver which remains unprecipitated with the diseased areas. The same holds true of the recently recommended silver compound, argentamin.

Persistent efforts in this direction have, however, been finally rewarded by the production of two efficient and almost non-irritating silver preparations, argonin and, very recently, protargol. Argonin is non-irritating, and certainly exercises a destructive influence upon the gonococci, but the length of time until their final disappearance (eight to twelve days) is so great that they are able to migrate deep into the mucous and submucous tissues, as well as into the posterior urethra, the prostate gland, and the epididymis.

Professor Neisser published the first report concerning protargol in the Berlin *Dermatologische Centralblatt* (edited by Dr. Max Joseph) for October, 1897. This substance is a chemic combination of silver (manufactured by Friedr. Bayer & Co., Ebberfeld) with a proteid body in the form of a fine yellow powder; it is easily soluble in ordinary water, and is not precipitated by albumen, salt solution, dilute muriatic acid, or caustic soda. It is fully as non-irritating as argonin, and its retention in the urethra, even for half an hour, produces no disagreeable symptoms whatever.

On the other hand, its effect upon the gonorrheal process, as shown by microscopic examination of the secretion, is immediate and decided. In several cases the gonococci, which were abundant on the first day of treatment, totally disappeared from the secretion within twenty-four hours, never to reappear, and the pus-cells themselves began to look swollen and disintegrated, and the nuclei to lose their characteristic form. This rapid action is due to two causes: first, the large percentage (eighty-three per cent.) of silver; second, the fact that no possible condition of the urethra is able to precipitate it from its solution. The protargal solution (1 part to 200 of water) was used according to the method of Professor Neisser in the cases to be related. A syringe containing 2½ fluid drams (a smaller quantity of liquid does not smooth out the urethral folds, and thus fails to reach every part of the surface) is injected three times daily and retained thirty minutes. Where this is impossible the injection is retained half an hour morning and evening, or evening only, and finally for ten minutes three or four times during the day.

Fifteen cases of specific urethritis have been treated with protargol in this polyclinic during the past four weeks, in all of which gonococci were microscopically ascertained to be present, and their subsequent appearance in the secretion noted. In 6 cases the gonococci disappeared from the urethral discharge within 24 hours; in 5 cases they vanished within 2 days, in 2 cases within 3 days, and in the remaining 2 cases within 4 days.

In one case in which the gonococci disappeared within one day a urethritis posterior developed six days later, and the prostatic secretion, obtained by expression, was found to contain gonococci. This case had been treated seven weeks, according to the Janet method. During this period the gonococci had abundant opportunity to migrate to the posterior urethra and prostate gland. In another case in which they disappeared within two days, they were again found in the discharge eighteen days later in consequence of the introduction of a sound. In this case the gonorrhea had existed a long time (several months) before treatment was begun, and a small colony of gonococci had without doubt established itself in the prostate; hence, the irritation of the sound caused migration into the urethra again.

These cases were treated by massage of the prostate gland and expression of its suppurating secretion, followed by irrigation of the urethra and bladder by a solution of nitrate of silver (1-5000 up to 1-1000).

In two other cases, one of ten-months', the other of two-weeks' standing when they came for treatment, a secondary inflammation developed later, characterized by the presence of diplococci and streptococci, but no gonococci. These cases have been treated by the injection of corrosive sublimate (1 to 15,000) which acts as a stimulant to any remaining gonococci, but the latter have not reappeared in either case. The remaining cases have run a smooth course. One patient returned eight days after his first treatment, after drinking beer, for examination. He had no secretion whatever, and both the first and second portions of his urine were clear (Thompson's test). Another came sixteen days after the first treatment to announce that in spite of liberal use of beer and alcoholic liquors, as well as indulgence in sexual intercourse, the discharge had completely vanished. In another case there was no discharge whatever after four-days' treatment. Several others of those first treated have not recently appeared, and it is to be supposed that they no longer have any symptoms.

The catarrhal (aseptic) discharge which often persists some time after the disappearance of the gonococci is treated by injections of zinc sulphate (1 part to about 150 of water).

If subsequent results prove as favorable as those hitherto noted no argument is necessary to show the superiority of this over any previous treatment.

In closing, attention should be called to the need of more careful treatment of acute gonorrhea by the general practitioner. As a rule, the case is either left to itself during the first two weeks or longer, with the possible exception of internal treatment, or any one of a long series of astringent remedies is injected, the only possible effect of which is to extend the inflammation to adjacent parts. Only in case the profession at large adopts and carries out the principles of Professor Neisser, both as to diagnosis and treatment, can it be hoped that the ravages caused by this disease will be less frequently observed by specialists than is the case at present. What one observes in the after course of so-called healed cases of gonorrhea passes belief. A few only need be mentioned here, for example: chronic anterior and posterior gonorrhea, prostatitis, strictures, chronic cystitis, and, worst of all, the infection of the wife with its dread sequence—bartholinitis, metritis, salpingitis, ovaritis, ovarian cysts and tumors, often ovariotomy, and not infrequently death, not to dwell upon the mental and moral suffering of an unhappy marriage. Respectfully,

E. WOOD RUGGLES, M.D.

BERLIN, February 16, 1898.

OUR PHILADELPHIA LETTER.

[From our Special Correspondent.]

THE INCREASE IN THE PAUPER INSANE—INFLUENZA MILDLY EPIDEMIC—EXPERT EVIDENCE FROM THE STANDPOINT OF A WITNESS—CHESTER COUNTY HOSPITAL FOR THE INSANE—A SYMPOSIUM ON ANEURYSM—THE SCHOTT TREATMENT OF CARDIAC DISEASES.

PHILADELPHIA, March 19, 1898.

STARTLING as the statement may appear, it is, nevertheless, a fact that during the past ten years there has been an increase of eighty-five per cent. in the number of cases of mental diseases treated at the Insane Department of the Philadelphia Hospital, the population of this branch of the hospital having increased from 394 inmates in 1888, to 1323 inmates at the present time. On the other hand, the number of paupers cared for by this institution during this period has materially decreased, not only in point of actual numbers, but in direct proportion to the population of the city. As your correspondent has had occasion to note before, the accommodations of Blockley for this additional number of patients has not kept pace with the increased demand, but the long-contemplated additions to the insane quarters of this hospital are now almost finished, and in the near future the inmates who at the present moment must be content to occupy cots in the passageway and in the aisles of the hospital, will be moved to suitable dormitories. About 300 patients will be benefited by the opening of the new buildings, and the congestion will also be lessened to some extent by the consolidation of the outlying poor-districts of Germantown, Frankford, and Roxborough, each provided with its separate insane hospital.

Influenza, which has been more or less in abeyance for two or three years past, has, according to the experiences of a large majority of general practitioners, again become of widespread prevalence in this city. The large clinics and hospitals do not, however, show a material increase of influenza cases over the number usually met with at this season of the year, but this is due, most probably, to the mild nature of the epidemic, if it may be dignified as such, and to the fact that the sufferers are among that class of people who do not patronize dispensaries—if there be such a class! Even if the present malady is not as severe as the disease which played pandemic havoc among all sorts and conditions of men nine years ago, it possesses sufficiently active characteristics to cause no little discomfort among a large portion of the citizens, and gives rise to very evident objective signs of its presence wherever people are congregated, whether it be on the street, in the theater, or in a place of public worship.

Among the causes of the evils attending the employment of expert evidence of a medical nature are, according to Dr. F. X. Dercum, himself an alienist and experienced expert witness, the manner of calling the expert, the bias of the expert himself, and the mistaken idea on his part as to the nature of his functions, and the manner in which the expert, because of his lack of knowledge of evidence, presents his testimony. The absurd and unfortunate propounding of hypothetic questions, and the lack of recognition of the fact that very properly legal truths and scientific truths do not always correspond, are other minor causes of confusion. These views were among those expressed by Dr. Dercum in a paper on "Expert Evidence from the Standpoint of a Witness," read before the New York Society of Medical Jurisprudence on March 14th. Dr. Dercum went on to say that it should be the imperative duty of the court to determine for itself the qualifications of the expert and to communicate to the jury in the trial in question the opinion thus gained, and that, further, the court should be empowered, in all instances in which the precaution is deemed necessary, to call independently an expert to advise the court as to the scientific facts presented by the expert witnesses engaged by the various lawyers. The court should absolutely rule out all hypothetic questions, which, as a whole, or in part, are misleading, and are often intentionally so construed that it is impossible to base a scientific judgment upon them; hypothetic questions are always needless, and they never, at best, accurately represent, nor are they the equivalents of, the case under trial. The duty of the expert on cross-examination is to answer questions freely, regardless of the benefit or injury to the side by which he is engaged, to confine his answers as far as possible to the simple "yes" or "no," and to exhibit at all times a coolness and an entire self-possession which will prevent the expert lapsing into an address of explanation to the jury of the facts in the case.

The new Chester County Asylum for the Insane, plans for the erection of which have just been adopted by the county authorities, will be situated on the well-known County Home Farm, a few miles from this city. The new building will be of a colonial style of architecture, three stories in height, and in addition to the facilities which it will possess for the modern methods of treating the insane, it will contain apartments for the physicians and for the nurses of the institution, as well as an amusement-hall, with a stage, provided for the entertainment of the inmates. The new hospital will be erected at an expense of $85,000, and by its operation the Poor Directors of Chester County estimate that they will save at least $10,000 annually in the care of the county's insane.

The last meeting of the Section on General Medicine of the College of Physicians of Philadelphia, held March 14th, was conspicuous because of the fact that it partook of the nature of a symposium on aneurysm. In addition to a number of papers read on other subjects, no less than twenty-three cases of aneurysm were reported by several of the Fellows of the College. Dr. F. A. Packard presented two cases of aneurysm of the aorta, and reported two cases of pulsating tumor, most probably aneurysmal in character, one of the abdominal aorta, and the other of the carotid artery; he also showed a specimen of aneurysm involving the entire arch of the aorta and the superior portion of the descending part of the thoracic aorta. Dr. S. Mc C. Hamill showed a case of aneurysm of the descending portion of the arch of the aorta, of eleven-years' duration, in a woman of middle age, who had passed through a number of severe illnesses from other causes during this period. The physical signs of bruit, thrill, pulsation, and thoracic prominence, which were marked when she first came under observation, are at the present time either entirely absent or greatly modified in intensity. This patient received the usual internal medication. Dr. A. O. J. Kelly exhibited nine specimens of aneurysmal tumors of the abdominal and of the thoracic aorta, of the arch of the aorta, and ofthe subclavian artery. Almost every variety of aneurysm was comprised in this collection. Dr. Judson Daland showed four specimens of aneurysm of the aorta, one of which had dissected downward and ruptured into the pericardial sac, and two of which had perforated into the bronchi. Dr. D. D. Stewart spoke of three cases of aneurysm in which he had introduced into the aneurysmal sac a gold wire for the purpose of producing thrombus formation by electrolysis. A patient with aneurysm, recently operated upon by Dr. H. A. Hare, and whose case he will report in ful at a later date, was said to be at the present time, a week after the introduction of the wire and the electrolysis of the contents of the sac, in an improved condition, both as to objective and subjective symptoms.

The Schott method of treatment of cardiac diseases by baths and resistance-movements was explained with great detail in a lecture at Professor Hare's medical clinic at the Jefferson Medical College, March 14th, by Dr. H. N. Heineman of Nauheim, Germany. Dr. Heineman divided the cases for the Schott treatment into three classes: those receiving the baths alone, those receiving the exercise alone, and those receiving both the baths and exercise. The waters of the Nauheim springs are of value chiefly because of the saline, alkaline, and chalybeate constituents which are found in them, to which is to be added a large percentage of carbonic acid gas. The duration of a bath should not be longer than ten minutes, and a safe rule governing its use is that it should never be continued so as to cause any discomfort to the patient. If, for any reason, such, for instance, as marked intermission of the pulse, the resistance-movements are contraindicated, walking is the form of exercise to be employed; these walks should be taken over a level stretch of ground, or over a slightly inclined plane constructed for the purpose, but should not consist of mountain-climbing, as some recommend, a form of exercise far too severe, in Dr. Heineman's opinion, for the average case of organic cardiac lesion. The treatment outlined above was greatly augmented, in suitable cases, by the practice of pulmonary gymnastics. In order to produce a lengthening of the diastole of the heart, the speaker described a sort of cardiac massage, consisting in making forcible and gradually more and more prolonged pressure over the precordium during systole, and suddenly relaxing the pressure during diastole. thus educating, as it were, the heart to prolong the ventricular contraction. The effect of the Schott treatment, as practised at Nauheim, was attributed to various reflex actions, and the *régime* was highly recommended as a rational method of therapeusis, particularly in cardiac lesions with signs of lost compensation.

The typhoid epidemic seems to have at last quite run its course, and the diminution in the weekly number of cases of this disease reported during the past three or four weeks confirms the hope that finally the infection has dwindled to what we, here in Philadelphia, are pleased to consider a normal proportion of cases. For the week ending March 19th, the report of the Bureau of Health shows 57 new cases of enteric fever, with 12 deaths from this cause, a decidedly comforting contrast with the reports of a month to six weeks ago, when double to quadruple this number were returned each week to the health authorities. During the week there were also reported 81 new cases of diphtheria, with 24 deaths; and 53 new cases of scarlet fever, with 4 deaths. Diseases of the lungs, including tuberculosis, pneumonia, and congestion were responsible for 151 deaths. No deaths from influenza were recorded, although, as noted before, the disease widely prevails at present.

OUR BERLIN LETTER.

[From our Special Correspondent.]

MULTIPLE SCLEROSIS AND A HITHERTO UNDESCRIBED MICROSPORIDION PATHOGENIC FOR MAN—PROFESSOR BAGINSKY ON THE DISEASES OF SCHOOL-CHILDREN AND ON SERUM IMMUNIZATION FOR DIPHTHERIA—FORMALDEHYD FOR DOMESTIC DISINFECTION—FURTHER REGULATION OF THE SALE OF PATENT MEDICINES IN GERMANY.

BERLIN, March 17, 1898.

AT the conclusion of Dr. Jürgen's paper at the Berliner Medicinische Gesellschaft (Medical Society) meeting on Wednesday evening last, there were some hearty cries of bravo, and then a murmur of interested remarks on the contents of the paper. Such a demonstration was unusual, and meant that something which was considered distinctly new had been reported. It was a series of sclerotic patches in heart and brain, in which there was found a parasite hitherto unknown to occur in man.

The case was that of a child who died shortly after admission to the hospital, but whose history contained the account of a number of epileptiform attacks. The sclerosed areas involved only the brain, but affected both white and gray matter, seemingly without distinction. They did not have the usual grayish-yellow color of the ordinary lesions of multiple sclerosis, or the translucent appearance so characteristic of that disease. They were normal in color, rather paler than usual perhaps, and were distinctly more resistent to the touch than the neighboring tissues. Microscopic examination showed that despite their hardness the sclerosed areas did not contain much connective tissue. There was a zone of round-celled inflammatory exudation surrounding them, but their increased consistency seemed to be due to the presence of a large number of the parasites.

If the condition thus described has a relation to ordinary multiple sclerosis it is as an acute preliminary stage of that disease as it is known to us—when the acute inflammatory reaction has given way to the chronic sclerosis consequent upon the death of the parasite and the overgrowth of connective tissue in the resulting scar.

The parasite would seem to be closely related to, if not a member of, the family of the Glugea, a microsporidion described by Professor Pfeiffer of Weimer as occurring in Cyclops, a species of Diatom, and in Daphnia. Inoculation experiments in animals were successful in this case, and the lesions produced were similar to the original lesions in the child. One of the animals not yet dead has had certain larval epileptiform attacks, followed by paralytic symptoms, seemingly indicating that metastases to the central nervous system have occurred.

The parasite itself is as ordinarily seen an oval-shaped cell with a nucleus. It takes the usual stains somewhat as do the nuclei of cells, but may be easily distinguished from them by its larger size, its more regular outline, and its greater affinity for the stains, which give it a deeper color. In the heart it occupies the interior of muscle fibers, whose substance usually has more or less disappeared, as if eaten away. In the brain they occur in the midst of degenerated nerve-cells and fibers.

Professor Baginsky concluded a course of lectures on the diseases of school-children last week, in which some thoroughly conservative opinions were expressed. It is consoling to hear from so distinguished an authority on children's diseases, that he does not think attendance at school responsible for so many of the ills of childhood as it has of late become the fashion to claim. For him there are three dangers to which special attention should be given, *viz.*, scoliosis, myopia, and overwork in delicate ambitious children, and in girls about the time of puberty. For these teachers must be ever on the watch.

As to the serotherapy of diphtheria (he was talking mainly to school-teachers and non-medical listeners) he could not say enough in praise. He begged them never to be misled by the carping articles which sometimes appear in the secular press (here as well as in America!) in opposition to the new method of treatment. It was undoubtedly one of the greatest, probably the greatest therapeutic discovery ever made.

As to the occurrence of diphtheria in schools, he believed that the appearance of a case ought to be the signal for the immunization with antitoxic serum of all the children in attendance at the school, certainly all of the children who occupy the same classroom as the sick child. He thought further, that the teachers should be ready to consider such a procedure as the proper one, and impress it as such upon the minds of parents. An unfortunate accident, not due to the serum itself, but to a mishap during the injection, had been followed by the death of the child in one of the first cases in which immunization was tried in Berlin (the Langerhaus case). He looked to the teachers to dispel the groundless prejudice occasioned by this. He, himself, would willingly take all responsibility in the matter of serum immunization.

When a case of diphtheria occurred in the surgical wards of the Kaiser and Kaiserin Friedrich Spital, of which Professor Baginsky is the Director, he immediately had all the other children immunized. In private families, when a case of diphtheria occurs, he does not consider immunization so necessary. Prompt segregation often prevents the disease from spreading to other members of the household, and, as the Doctor in such cases is in daily attendance, the serum-treatment may be begun as soon as the first suspicious symptom is noticed in another child. Antitoxin, when given thus early in the disease, he considers an unfailing remedy. In patients injected during the first forty-eight hours of the disease there is absolutely no mortality.

As Professor Heubner has for some time made it a practice to immunize all the children in his wards at the Charité every three weeks, it may be seen what a prominent place immunization has taken here during this last year. For awhile Professor Heubner had to give up his immunizing injections, because the hospital directorate thought it savored too much of experimental investigation on the children, and might arouse popular indignation. They were resumed after an interval of only two months, however, as it had become clear that they were wonderfully efficient in preventing the development of diphtheria in the wards of the hospital. Absolutely no inconveniences have resulted from the practice.

The results of some very interesting work on the disinfection of rooms with formaldehyd gas have just been published by Dr. Fairbanks of Boston, from the laboratory of Professor Grawitz in the Charlottenburg Hospital here. The conclusions are confirmatory of other work in this line, as regards the thorough disinfecting power of the vapor of formaldehyd. Practically all pathogenic micro-organisms, with the exception of anthrax spores, are killed by it, even when they are enclosed in several layers of cloth, provided the covering is not so thick as to be impervious to the gas. Especially interesting are the personal experiments and those on animals, showing that the gas is almost entirely non-destructive, even when present in quantities sufficient to accomplish disinfection, ordinary upholstery or clothing material not being affected by it. The finest silk in the most delicate shades remains absolutely uninjured, and leather, after exposure for hours to the fumes of the gas, remains as smooth, polished, and flexible, as before the experiment.

Here in Germany the formalin and formaldehyd disinfectant methods are rapidly replacing all the other methods which were previously in vogue, which besides their distinct limitations, had a number of serious disadvantages.

It is forbidden to sell "secret remedies" in Germany, and the Ministry of Commerce and Industry has just announced for the guidance of the courts what is meant by a secret remedy. This will remove the last loophole of the patent-medicine people, for, taking advantage of discordant legal decisions, they had been able to keep certain preparations on the market. All remedies not sold under a prescription from a doctor must have the formula of its contents printed on the label. This formula (and here is where the new instructions define the law) must be written not in Latin, but, when possible, in the vernacular. It must be intelligible not only for a doctor or pharmacist, but for any one who wishes to buy, and it must be sufficient to enable a buyer to decide whether the ingredients contained therein are such as may be reasonably expected to give relief, and whether he is paying a not unreasonable price for the amounts of the different drugs which are being bought.

As the merit of the invention (if there is any) is the method of composition of the remedy, this need not be given if there is a real discovery in it, so that the inventor does not lose the benefit of his idea. This decision would strike one as a thoroughly common-sense way of dealing with a difficult question, and one calculated to eradicate the immense swindle patent medicines usually involve. *Quousque tandem?* How long, then, before Americans will be able to point to some such sensible law.

TRANSACTIONS OF FOREIGN SOCIETIES.

Berlin.

EPIDEMIC OF ALOPECIA AREATA—THE TREATMENT OF GONORRHEA AMONG PROSTITUTES—TIC GENERAL CURED BY A SUGGESTION—ECHINOCOCCUS CYSTS OF THE KIDNEY—TRAUMATIC MYOCARDITIS—TREATMENT OF OCCIPITAL NEURALGIA.

AT a meeting of the Medical Society, January 12th, BLASCHKO described a small *epidemic of alopecia areata*, occurring among boys who were playmates, eight being effected. This disease has been held by most of the German physicians to be a nervous affection, while the French have for a long time said that it is contagious, and one of their number, Sabouret, claims to have isolated the microbe and to have caused alopecia by the injection of a pure culture thereof, as well as by the injection of its filtrate. It has sometimes been suggested that the lesions of so-called contagious alopecia areata are in reality patches of eczema seborrhoicum; but in these boys the characteristic appearances left no doubt of the nature of the trouble.

BEHREND read a paper upon the *treatment of gonorrhea among prostitutes*. He took the position (1) that in cases of acute gonorrhea in men treated by rest in bed and the application of ice, with frequent injections of ice-water and light astringents, the clinical evidences of disease, together with the gonococci, soon permanently disappear; (2) that in women this is not always the case. The clinical symptoms may disappear while the gonococci persist, or the reverse may be true. It is, therefore, extremely difficult to say when a woman is incapable of communicating the disease.

Acute gonorrhea in the female presents two kinds of lesions: (1) Those which are really gonorrheal in character and are located in the vestibulum vaginæ, and possibly in the cervix, and (2) lesions which are simply erosions and which occur upon the outer genitals and in the vagina.

Behrend has little faith in the great number of new remedies proposed, and relies chiefly upon astringents, especially alum and chlorid of zinc. Swabs of cotton saturated with a solution of alum, and frequently changed, are kept upon the vulva and in the vestibule, while twice a day a five-per-cent. solution of zinc chlorid is brought into contact with the cervix through a speculum. No applications of any sort are made to the urethra. In general he expressed the opinion that the clinical appearances of gonorrhea are a far more reliable guide to treatment than the microscopic examination of the pus.

At the session of February 16th, STEIN presented a little girl aged twelve years, who had suffered four years with *tic general*, with the usual symptoms of twitching of the muscles of the face, movement of the extremities, inarticulate sounds, etc., all to a marked degree. Treatment at the hands of various neurologists, including attempts at hypnotism, had failed to give the slightest relief. During five weeks she was treated by application of magnets, the treatments lasting one-half hour each, three times in a week. Stein treated the child by suggestion, her hypnotic state being one more of waking than of sleep. Attention was first directed to the use of the hands and arms, and in five days the little girl was able to write her name. After two-months' treatment control of the muscles was perfectly restored. As the patient had continued well for six months there was good reason to regard the cure as permanent, especially in view of the fact that for four years preceding treatment there had been no remission of the symptoms. The improvement in the girl's general health was most striking.

POSNER showed a patient, aged sixty-two years, who sought treatment because he had noticed that at urination he frequently passed little round, elastic bladders. These were found to be *echinococcus cysts*, and a large tumor was felt in the right hypochondriac region. Upon cystoscopic examination the left ureter appeared normal. The right ureter was greatly enlarged. As the condition of the patient did not improve an incision was made in the right loin, which allowed the escape of a quantity of pus and a great number of echinococcus cysts. The patient rapidly recovered, the tumor disappeared in great part, and four months later the right ureter, when examined through the cystoscope, appeared normal. In view of these facts it was thought that the echinococcus had developed in the right kidney.

MENDELSOHN read a paper upon *traumatic myocarditis* before the Union for Internal Medicine, January 17th. A patient, who at the time of accident enjoyed good health, was crushed by a horse against the side of a stall and held in this position a considerable time. He was not compelled to go to bed, but was troubled with weakness, pain in the chest, and shortness of breath. Three weeks later there was well-marked dilatation of the heart, with frequent and arhythmic pulse. A short time previously the man had been examined for military duty, and his heart was pronounced normal. There can, therefore, be no doubt that the cardiac affection was the result of the severe and prolonged strain to which the patient had been subjected.

JASTROWITZ spoke of the *treatment of occipital neuralgia*. In one patient who had been frequently exposed to severe weather the auricularis magnus, the occipitalis minor, and at times the occipitalis major, were the nerves affected. The affection was confined to the left side. There was a burning pain in the skin of the ear and back of the head, the affected areas being reddened and slightly thickened. At times paroxysms of most intense pain came on, and the ear would become scarlet or violet, and more swollen than usual, and the head would be jerked violently backward. After this had continued nearly five years, and all other remedies had proved of no avail, neurectomy and stretching of the nerves was performed. This resulted in the diminution of the swelling and pain, and relief from the jerkings of the head. Jastrowitz urged his hearers not to postpone operation too long in similar cases.

SOCIETY PROCEEDINGS.

NORTHWESTERN MEDICAL AND SURGICAL SOCIETY OF NEW YORK.

Stated Meeting, Held February 16, 1898.

THE President, L. DUNCAN BULKLEY, M.D., in the Chair.

ECTOPIC GESTATION.

DR. JOHN F. ERDMANN showed a specimen removed from a case of ectopic gestation. The patient was twenty-eight years of age, married ten years, and the mother of two children, the youngest being eight years of age. During November, ten days after her last menstruation, she had a yellowish vaginal discharge and some abdominal pain, and was admitted to the hospital as a case of pyosalpinx. When first seen by the speaker, February 1st, she had a pulse of 128, a temperature ranging between 99.5° and 101° F., and abdominal tenderness. A tumor in the left side was found, reaching to the lumbar region, and to within three-finger's breath of the umbilicus, and the uterus was fixed in the general pelvic mass. There was no especial history pointing to ectopic gestation. An aspirating-needle was passed into the posterior fornix and blood and serum withdrawn. Abdominal section was then performed. The mass was found to consist of a partially decomposed blood-clot. The fetus, which was three-fourths of an inch long, was found among the blood-clots on a towel just before the wound was closed. The patient made a good recovery.

DISCUSSION.

DR. J. RIDDLE COFFE: The diminutive fetus shown by Dr. Erdmann suggests an explanation of the frequency with which the product of conception fails to be discovered in cases giving many evidences of ectopic gestation. That his microscopic eye should have picked it out from the mass of clots and débris was evidently a happy accident. One week ago to-day I had the good fortune to rescue a woman from the impending dangers attending ruptured ectopic. The stage of advancement of pregnancy at which rupture occurred was much later than in the case presented by Dr. Erdmann. The fetus was completely formed, measured 3½ inches in length, and the sex was clearly revealed. The patient presented a history of more or less irregular menstruation for three months—as the apparent result of interference for the purpose of inducing menstruation. For five days preceding the date of my first visit she had had severe pains in the pelvis which had been controlled by rest in bed and hypodermics of morphin. The patient resided in Yonkers and I was called in consultation with the intimation that there were products of conception in the uterus, and that I was to come prepared to empty the uterus if necessary. Upon obtaining the history and making a thorough examination I diagnosed ectopic gestation with rupture, and advised operation. The uterus was slightly enlarged and was crowded forward against the symphysis pubis, the posterior half of the pelvis being filled with a large irregular and somewhat boggy tumor reaching up to the abdominal wall.

The patient was placed in St. John's Hospital, Yonkers, where I operated, with the assistance of Dr. Sherman of that city, on February 9th. The abdominal incision was employed and the patient placed in Trendelenburg's position. Upon incising the peritoneum its inner surface was found adherent to a large, firm blood-clot, which had to be peeled off. This clot was adherent not only to the abdominal peritoneum, but also to the coils of intestine, the omentum, and to the entire posterior surface of the uterus and broad ligaments. By passing my hand down the posterior wall of the uterus, dissecting off the clot, and then sweeping the hand all aroung the circumference of the pelvis, the main part of the clot was set free and lifted out *en masse*. It was found to be thoroughly organized, being held in compact form by threads of plasma. The fetus was found at the bottom of the cul-de-sac underneath the clot and—a fact which I neglected to mention in connection with the diagnosis—was quite plainly outlined by the finger in the vagina. The appendages upon the left side were quickly seized, brought up into the wound, and removed after a ligature had been thrown around them. The tube was greatly enlarged, and a rent was found along its free border over two inches in length through which the fetus had evidently escaped. This rent extended through the fimbriated end of the tube. The fimbriated end was patulous and it was apparent that an effort at abortion had been made by Nature through the end of the tube, which, however, resulted in rupture on account of the large size of the fetus.

The vermiform appendix was found firmly embedded in the blood-clot to which it was adherent. On account of its large size and congested condition it was removed. Branches of blood-clot reached from the main mass up into the abdominal cavity among the coils of intestine and omentum, and had to be torn away from their attachments. The pelvis was thoroughly flushed with hot-salt solution, and an iodoform-gauze drain placed in Douglas' pouch and brought out through the lower angle of the wound. Convalescence has been steadily progressive with the exception that the patient's stomach has been very irritable and her bowels constipated. On the fourth day some peculiar mental symptoms developed; the patient was at times irrational and incapable of recognizing her friends. This condition rapidly disappeared after the removal of the gauze and flushing of the pelvic cavity. I am inclined to think that the irritable stomach and the mental symptoms were due to iodoform poisoning. There were no symptoms of infection, the drainage from the abdominal cavity being sweet and free from any sign of sepsis.

DR. CHARLES L. DANA: I would like to ask Dr. Goffe what would have been the probable result in his case had no operation been performed.

DR. GOFFE: There are cases of ectopic gestation on record in which the condition was not recognized at the time of rupture, and in which the fetus has become encysted, or has sloughed into the rectum or vagina, I can understand how Nature might throw out an exudate which would surround the fetus and shut off the pelvic cavity and no bad result follow, provided, of course, that there had not been much hemorrhage.

DR. S. H. DESSAU: I have been struck by the number of cases of ectopic gestation which have been reported of late. At the December meeting of this Society I was called away to see such a case. At the Harlem Medical Association meeting on Monday last a case was reported, and two cases have been reported here to-night—four cases in all within a few months. The case reported at the Harlem Medical Society was very interesting, the fetal sac being attached to an accessory tube.

DR. CHARLAS L. DANA then read the paper of the evening, entitled

MIGRAINOUS VERTIGO.

(See page 385.)

DISCUSSION.

DR. S. N. LEO: The paper is one of peculiar interest. The general practitioner very frequently meets with cases in which there is vertigo associated with migraine. I recall the case of a boy who had had his ears boxed by a playmate, in which pain and inflammation of the superorbital foramen supervened. After this subsided he complained of vertigo. Treatment did not relieve him and the condition continued three years, when it spontaneously disappeared.

I recently saw a little boy who suffered from quite severe convulsions resembling those of epilepsy. He complained of vertigo and pain in the ears, first on one side and then on the other. He was given bromid and the symptoms disappeared. Not long ago I attended a woman who suffered from migraine of the worst variety, and also from hysteria. She informed me that a physician had told her she had a "fracture of the cauda equina." There were evidences of fracture of the last dorsal vertebra.

The pathologic facts stated by the author are very interesting. Such changes in the cranial nerves in old people are associated with the most diverse symptoms. What these changes are it is difficult to say, but it is strange that the special senses are not more often impaired. In the first case I referred to there was marked deafness on the right side. The boy also complained of an occasional flash of light before his eyes, and which was invariably followed by a desire to pass water.

DR. E. S. PECK: I fear I can add little to the subject, but I wish to express my pleasure at hearing so graphic aud clear an elucidation of it by Dr. Dana. I know of no one who is better able to differentiate these abstruse conditions. Auditory vertigo is undoubtedly due to congestion about the sixth pair of nerves in the labyrinth, either just beyond the ampulla, in the cochlea, or in the semicircular canal. Ménière's disease of the text-books is not what was originally described by that observer as deduced from the well-known experiments of Flourens. Every exhibition of aural vertigo is not Ménière's disease. I think we ought to designate vertigo as aural, laryngeal, nasal, and gastric, although it is sometimes difficult to tell where aural vertigo ends and gastric vertigo begins. I once had a case in the City Hospital which puzzled me. The man was hemiopic on the nasal side of the field of vision; he had migraine; he had laryngitis; he had vertigo, but he did not have Ménière's disease. He was seen by my colleagues of the hospital staff and by neurologists. The symptoms continued a number of years, and the man became blind just before he died. He was supposed to have a gumma in the optic tract. Many of these cases are diagnosed as syphilis. This man was given iodid of potassium in very large doses with no apparent benefit. Attention to nutrition and the administration of nerve tonics are, perhaps, the measures upon which we should rely in cases of this kind.

DR. JOSEPH COLLINS: The paper is of such a unique

character that discussion seems unnecessary. I have kept in mind the fact that one of the objects of the communication was to show the possibility or the reality of the transformation of one degenerative neurosis into another in the same subject. This Dr. Dana has done in such a convincing manner that there is nothing to be added, except to say that one has, or has not, had similar personal experiences. I am prompted to say a word concerning the necessity of closely differentiating migraine from other forms of headache and of distinguishing Ménière's disease from diseases having some clinical resemblance to it.

The case related by Dr. Leo was not, I venture to say, one of migraine, which is always a degenerative disease. It seems to me rather to have been a traumatic or hysteric headache and neither Ménière's disease nor true hemicrania. Ménière's disease is a symptom-complex due to organic disease of the labyrinth, the prominent symptoms being vertigo, and it always entails deafness. It is an accidental disease, not a degenerative disease. Vertigo which alternates with or is replaced by a hemicrania, on the other hand, in most likely, it seems to me, to be of a degenerative nature; a condition depending upon prenatal influences, possibly antedating several generations. In diseases of this latter kind there is nothing like the departure from the normal which attends the ordinary pathologic condition, nothing inflammatory, and nothing of a gross or microscopic nature. I think they are the natural conditions incident to a man or woman who is in a certain stage of biologic evolution. The histories of such cases as Dr. Dana's, and, moreover, the transformation of one symptom-complex into another, will, I think, bear me out in this view.

Migraine is a degenerative neurosis. One symptom does not make the disease—it is the entire symptom-complex. I recently had a case of hemicrania which has impressed upon me the clinical transformation of one disease to another. A young girl of sixteen, who had many somatic stigmata of degeneration, was brought to the clinic suffering from severe attacks of migraine. The attacks were typical, ushered in by nausea, vomiting, a feeling that she wanted to be left alone, and prostration. Then came the lethargic state, from which she finally awoke, feeling that the world was an agreeable place to live in. When I came to examine her, I found that she was like one without a mind. She was incapable of the simplest mental association; memory was very defective, and she was quite lacking in the capacity to indulge in introspection or retrospection; in short, she was in a mental condition very similar to that found in some epileptic patients and in those suffering from other diseases of a degenerative nature. It does not seem to me that we should look for symptomatic transformations in accidental diseases; such transformations are inimical to our conception of them.

In regard to Dr. Peck's case, I do not think I saw the patient. If I had, I do not know that I would have advised large doses of iodid of potassium. The possession of three such symptoms as aural vertigo, hemianopsia, and profound asthenia would not lead me to look for syphilitic disease unless there were some more pointed indications of that affection.

DR. ROBERT MILBANK: I have only a word to say, and that is in regard to the effect of air or absence of air upon that branch of the eighth nerve which presides over the sense of equilibrium—the nerve of space. I think the action of the air upon it is often seen in patients who complain that when diving in deep water and even when bathing in shallow water the equilibrium is lost when the ears become filled with water, and there is an inability to stand until this runs out. I have a patient who has no ear disease, and yet he has twice fallen and often staggers if he allows water to enter his ears, even when bathing them.

DR. FRUITNIGHT: The paper of Dr. Dana in regard to the transformation of one degenerative neurosis into another is on a very interesting and suggestive subject and offers much food for thought. This transformation doubtless occurs much oftener than is suspected and may explain many obscure phenomena occurring in the course and development of neurotic affections. Personally, I have had no experience with cases of vertigo depending upon the aural neuroses, those which I have had under observation having been due rather to digestive disturbances, which, as we all know, cause the most frequent variety of vertigo.

THE PRESIDENT: All of us must have noticed that there is a free passage of urine in these cases before and after an attack. No mention has been made of this in the paper. I have seen a number of cases of vertigo which we have always looked upon as due to stomach or liver disorder, and in which relief has always followed administration of the proper remedies. I would like to make a line of definite therapeusis in such cases. I would like to recommend the administration of the alkalies half an hour to an hour before meals in cases of migraine, together with nux vomica and cascara. The alkalies should be given before eating, as their effect is then very different. Dr. Dana has not mentioned the effect of diet in these cases. I would like to know if he has been able to trace any of the attacks to the period of secondary digestion—two, three, or four hours after meals.

DR. DANA, in closing: The attacks in the case mentioned bore no relation either to diet or to meal-time so far I was able to discover. They all bore a relation to nervous exhaustion. Overwork and loss of sleep brought on an attack. There are two kinds of aural vertigo; one is a progressive disorder due to disease of the labyrinth, always advancing and ending finally in deafness. This is Ménière's disease. In the other the vertigo is functional or nearly so, and there may be no progress. This includes all cases not of the Ménière group. It is to these latter cases that I refer. I do not see any such thing as the gastric vertigo of Trousseau. Such is probably an autotoxemia. I have been very much interested in Dr. Collins' remarks about the mental deterioration which occurs in migraine patients, similar to that which is seen in epileptics. I know that this deterioration does occur, especially in individuals with not very strong brains.

KINGS COUNTY MEDICAL ASSOCIATION.

Stated Meeting, Held February 8, 1898.

THE President, J. S. BIERWIRTH, M.D., in the Chair.

A paper, entitled

REPORT OF A CASE OF INTESTINAL OBSTRUCTION,

was read by C. P. GILDERSLEEVE, M.D. (See page 392.)

DISCUSSION.

THE PRESIDENT: I am sure the Association must be very much indebted to Dr. Gildersleeve for reporting this case; in the first place, because of the rarity of the occurrence, and, in the second place, as he very correctly points out, because of the reluctance of opening the abdomen in cases of intestinal obstruction; more especially in this instance on account of the location of the pain to the right of the median line and in the vicinity of the point at which is usually found the greatest tenderness in cases of appendicitis. The difficulty of making a diagnosis in cases of appendicitis is sometimes extremely great. During the past two weeks I have had two cases in which in my opinion a diagnosis of appendicitis would have been impossible, aud yet I think that in both cases the appendix was involved, though in neither did the inflammation progress to suppuration, and in neither was operation performed. In both cases there was pelvic inflammation; in one due to abortion caused by drugs, and in the other due to severe uterine and ovarian cramps, the cause of which was not determined. However, in both cases the pain was located in the pelvis and chiefly on the right side; the tenderness was strictly on the right side. In one case I saw the patient at short intervals, expecting hourly to be obliged to decide upon operation, and in the other case there was considerable inflammatory action about the uterus and ovaries—the case of abortion—and the patient was seen by Dr. Baldwin, and he fully agreed that it was impossible to distinguish between the right ovary and the appendix. So that cases of supposed appendicitis, like the one mentioned in the paper and the two just related, are not so very infrequent. We hear of the easy diagnosis to be made in all cases of appendicitis. I must confess that I have seen a good many cases in which the diagnosis was far from easy, especially if there were any complications.

DR. J. D. SULLIVAN: I have a case in mind that I saw last Saturday morning. The patient came into the hospital with no symptoms except intestinal obstruction and vomiting. He had been taken sick the preceding Monday with vomiting and symptoms of appendicitis, so far as could be made out, but he was not sent into the hospital until Friday evening. I saw him Saturday morning; his temperature was about normal, pulse 70, very little pain, and he appeared to be in good condition. My diagnosis was appendicitis, although the grounds for such a diagnosis were very few and obscure; but he was operated upon and the appendix found gangrenous, as was also the ascending colon. There was sufficient vitality in the base of the appendix to permit removal of the gangrenous portion, and then I packed the operating field because I felt quite sure from the gangrenous condition of the ascending colon that it would give way. The operation was performed about noon on Saturday. Sunday morning the patient seemed remarkably well. I was surprised to find him in such a good condition, but yesterday —Monday—he suddenly died. An autopsy revealed perforation of the intestine and a great many gangrenous spots in the ileum as well as in the ascending colon.

THE PRESIDENT: I would like to relate the history of a very curious, perhaps a unique, case. The specimen should have been taken out and the case reported. The patient was an old gentleman eighty years of age, who presented a history of repeated fecal accumulation, which I washed out a number of times, enormous quantities of fecal matter being removed by means of the high injection. I cautioned him to be very careful in regard to his bowels and keep them open, but my caution was of no avail. I was sent for and found him in collapse. He died within twenty-four hours after my first visit, and at the autopsy a condition was found which was very curious. During life the patient appeared stout, having had quite a large abdomen. He looked like a fat man, as far as his abdomen was concerned, and I had been very much astonished when I washed out his colon and saw his abdomen exposed at that time, to find how very thin the abdominal walls were. There was a curious feeling of the contents of the abdomen, and at the autopsy, on making the incision through the skin, instead of finding the omentum, we saw two columns—as if I took my two arms and laid them on my abdomen in the shape of a U —and we were at first puzzled by the condition; but, passing a bougie into the rectum, it was found that the instrument entered this U-shaped tube, which was about eight inches in diameter. It was determined that the rectum had become dislocated in front of the omentum, and was enormously enlarged. It was certainly four or five times the normal size in every direction—in length as well as in circumference. Notwithstanding the fact that shortly previous to his collapse he had been thoroughly washed out, enormous quantities of feces were removed, and we estimated that the contents of this dislocated and enlarged gut weighed from fifteen to twenty pounds.

REPORT OF FIVE CASES OF PUERPERAL MYELITIS

was the title of a paper by Dr. A. C. Brush. (See page 390.)

DISCUSSION.

DR. SULLIVAN: I would like to ask if there is any prospect of recovery in any of the cases mentioned in the paper.

DR. BRUSH: The prognosis will be the prognosis of myelitis in general. As a rule, the paralysis is most extensive at first. The disease originates in a hemorrhage or septic inflammation and shock. At first the disturbance is exaggerated by the shock. As the lesion gradually improves the cord recovers some of its lost power. If the lesion is in the lumbodorsal region and the bladder and rectum are not affected, the prognosis is better than when it is lower down. When it is higher there is spastic paraplegia, due to the fact that the influence of the brain is removed, but under such circumstances the lower centers still act, nutrition is maintained, and the patient can walk with a peculiar shuffling gait. It is impossible without a careful examination to state whether the case is one of true lateral sclerosis or myelitis and hemorrhage into the cord. Of course, if the lesion is low down, absolute paralysis of the bladder and rectum and atrophy of the muscles and death is the only outcome, and, as a rule, bed-sores rapidly develop, the patient lives a few months on a water-bed, and dies with cystitis, bed-sores, and pneumonia. When the lesion is higher up the prognosis is better, and the patient may walk a little with the aid of a cane or sit up in a chair. Under these circumstances patients may live a number of years. Life, although not directly in danger, is probably shortened, as it is very rare to find an old person with any one of these affections.

DR. SULLIVAN: Does Dr. Brush think that all the elements of the cord are involved; that is, the sensory as well as the motor tracts?

DR. BRUSH: In myelitis there is not inflammation of the column so much as of the spinal centers. In these cases the sensory portion of the cord recovers more rapidly than the motor; just as in neuritis, the motor is not involved as soon and recovers more slowly, while in the sensory tracts recovery is more rapid. In all the cases mentioned in the paper except one there was more or less recovery of sensation, while the motor paralysis improved more slowly, or not at all. In one of two, I think, recovery of sensation was fairly complete.

NOTES ON THE WIDAL SERUM-REACTION AND ON THE METHOD OF HISS

was the title of a paper by DR. JEROME B. THOMAS, JR. (See page 388.)

THE PRESIDENT: It was especially interesting to listen to the paper for the reason that Dr. Thomas a year ago presented to us what was then a comparatively new method, and he has now given us in concise form the results of a year's experience with the Widal test, in addition to the new method of Dr. Hiss.

DR. J. D. RUSHMORE: There is one statement the Doctor made—and I have heard it before from bacteriologists—in regard to which I would like to inquire, and it is: What are the difficulties in isolation of the typhoid bacillus in fecal matter?

DR. THOMAS: The special difficulty is that other organisms contained in the feces rapidly overgrow the typhoid bacillus, and the object of this particular medium is to keep other organisms from growing, and at the same time not interfere with the growth of the typhoid bacillus. The colon bacillus is an exceedingly hardy organism, and is inclined to overgrow the typhoid bacillus, its colonies spreading over and contaminating colonies of other germs. I should have said, perhaps, that one of the main points in the matter has been to accomplish isolation rapidly, so as to make the test of practical value.

DR. SULLIVAN: I would like to ask if this peculiar element which paralyzes the typhoid bacillus is a toxin or antitoxin?

DR. THOMAS: It is supposed to be a product of infection rather than an antitoxic product. This point has been carefully worked out by some of the Germans who have studied the subject. I think it pretty well settled that it is a product of intoxication rather than an antitoxic product. It has been called "paralyzin" and "agglutinin," naming it from its peculiar action on the typhoid bacillus, but the substance in question has never been definitely isolated.

REVIEWS.

A CLINICAL TEXT-BOOK OF SURGICAL DIAGNOSIS AND TREATMENT. By J. W. MACDONALD, M.D., Professor of the Practice of Surgery and of Clinical Surgery in Hamline University, Minneapolis. Illustrated. Philadelphia: W. B. Saunders, 1898.

THE medical public is well supplied with books on medical diagnosis, but this is the first attempt, so far as the reviewer is aware, to gather into a single work the data essential to surgical diagnosis supplemented by the appropriate treatment of each condition. The wisdom of writing a practical work on surgery at the present time without any reference to surgical pathology or bacteriology, or even to surgical principles,—the wisdom of such a course may be questioned. The author finds himself at a disadvantage, for example, when he discusses puerperal septicemia; for no reference is found to the serum treatment of this condition. That it was not omitted because it is not invariably infallible cannot be the case, for the ancient and discarded methods of the treatment of hemorrhoids, for instance, are all given a place (p. 327). Aside from this objection, which is raised on grounds purely scientific and by no means utilitarian, the author has undoubtedly fulfilled his purposes well. He has covered, as will be seen, an enormous field, and has taken evident infinite pains to be complete. A quite careful perusal of the volume has shown that little in the way of surgical diagnosis is omitted and that the greater part of the treatment recommended is in accord with modern surgical notions.

Chapter I. deals with the general examination of the patient, including age, sex, heredity, and individual peculiarities. Chapter II. takes up the vascular system; Chapter III. the osseous system, its diseases and injuries. Chapters IV. and V. treat of the diseases of the muscles, tendons, and bursæ, and the injuries and diseases of the joints, including a short but excellent treatise on orthopedic surgery. The next chapter includes the surgical ailments of the digestive system, beginning with the lips and ending with the anus, and embracing the surgery of all the abdominal organs. The recent methods of intestinal surgery and the surgery of the gall-bladder are all found mentioned and discussed. The author is in favor of the removal of any appendix which has once been inflamed. His discussion of appendicitis is particularly good.

The genito-urinary system is next considered in its surgical light, and is followed by a very complete chapter on cranial surgery. The spine and nervous system are next taken up. Under the heading of the respiratory system we find no mention of the subphrenic abscess. The diagnosis and treatment of syphilis and of tumors occupy the two succeeding chapters. Chapter XIV. takes up the diseases and injuries of the neck, Chapter XV. those of the breast. Following the next chapter, on the surgery of the female generative organs, is the concluding chapter on the use of Röntgen-rays in surgical diagnosis.

It will be seen that the work covers quite completely the surgery of the day. Throughout the book particular stress is laid upon diagnosis and differential diagnosis, the usefulness of the latter being enhanced by several tables. The practical nature of the work is further increased by the consideration of appropriate treatment under the discussion of each disease or injury. The few remarks on the preparation and after-treatment of operative cases might be extended with benefit. In the main the views expressed are those sanctioned by highest surgical usage and endorsement, and one can come to no conclusion but that the book is a safe and valuable guide, as it is a novel one, for both practitioner and student. It takes up a method not before presented in the English language and will undoubtedly receive the endorsement it deserves.

We should like to see the next edition contain articles on the ear, eye, and skin, omitted from the present one because the diseases of these organs are usually left to the care of specialists. The same argument holds true in respect of the diseases of the female generative organs; and certainly most communities which possess specialists in the domain of the eye, the ear, and the skin have gynecologists as well. The chapter dealing with gynecology is, we feel in duty bound to add, rather behind the others in point of modern thought, and would benefit by considerable revision and improved proof-reading.

The impression left by the reading of the book is that of a thorough and complete work on surgical diagnosis and treatment, free from verbiage and padding, full of valuable material, and in accord with the surgical teaching of the day.

The publisher's work is well done. The printing and paper are good, and the illustrations, many of them from original photographs, are well executed. Several radiographs enhance the value of the book.

THE PRACTICE OF SURGERY. By HENRY R. WHARTON, M.D., and B. FARQUHAR CURTIS, M.D. Philadelphia: J. B. Lippincott Co, 1898.

THIS latest contribution to the numerous text-books on surgery is a synopsis of the subject in a single volume of 1214 pages, with 925 excellent illustrations and a very elaborate index of 25 pages.

The commonplace affections receive full consideration, and there is a brief rendering of the unusual ones, among which, we note the omission of coxa vara, painless whitlow, and trigger-finger.

The first 261 pages are devoted to the principles of surgery, wherein bacteriology and surgical pathology are duly emphasized, and the technic of asepsis and antisepsis is briefly expounded; then follow the chapters on minor surgery and anesthesia. In the latter it is stated that chloroform may be administered by pouring one-half to one dram on a cloth. This is decidedly wrong. The "drop method" is the only correct one. In regard to cocain we should have preferred to teach a one-per-cent. solution as adequate for all purposes.

The remainder of the work deals with a regional description of the surgical affections, and passing to a review of these, a few instances, to dissent from, have been singled out.

In presenting the theories of shock, Goltz's classic experiment should have been introduced. For tamponing the posterior nares in epistaxis, Belocq's canula ought never to be employed, but the catheter always. Under tracheotomy the description of Rose's method of dividing the fascia transversely at its attachment to the lower margin of the cricoid cartilage, thus rapidly reaching the trachea, is wanting. Referring to the diagnostic value of the examination of fluids accumulated in the abdomen, so important a disease as tuberculous peritonitis has been overlooked.

After all, these are but errors of omission and, in so extensive a treatise, are pardonable. The epitomized style, the rather too frequent omission of author's names in connection with diseases and methods, and the entire absence of reference to literature, may detract from its usefulness to the general practitioner, yet we heartily commend the perusal of this book to the student, as embodying methods and teachings well tried and tested at the hands of two surgeons engaged in very active practice.

TRANSACTIONS OF THE CONGRESS OF AMERICAN PHYSICIANS AND SURGEONS. Fourth Triennial Session held at Washington, D. C., May 4, 5, and 6, 1897. New Haven: Published by the Congress, 1897.

THE complete transactions of the Fourth Congress of American Physicians and Surgeons are here presented in a handsome bound volume. The proceedings of the Congress were duly chronicled in the MEDICAL NEWS at the time of the meeting, so a review of the details of the meeting is unnecessary now. The volume is edited by Dr. William H. Carmalt of New Haven, is finely printed on heavy paper, and is profusely illustrated.

A MANUAL OF LEGAL MEDICINE FOR THE USE OF PRACTITIONERS AND STUDENTS OF MEDICINE AND LAW. By JUSTIN HEROLD, A.M., M.D., Formerly Coroner's Physician of New York City and County; Late House Physician and Surgeon of St. Vincent's Hospital, New York, etc. Philadelphia: J. B. Lippincott Co., 1898.

THE author of this admirable book draws attention to the fact, so well known to us all, that the teaching of legal medicine in the medical colleges of this country is very defective: "The well-educated physician, even though he be acquainted with all the other branches of medicine, is utterly incapable of solving important questions of medical jurisprudence. He is completely baffled when confronted by such intricate questions as those embracing infanticide, strangulation, drowning, or others," and this for the reason that "none of the conditions of forensic importance are subject to solution by theoretic principles, but are comprehensible only when studied alone as facts."

With these truths ever in mind, the author has given us a work which is in every way complete and satisfactory, and it is a pleasure to follow to a conclusion the practical and oftentimes simple hypotheses which he has drawn. The first portion of the book (142 pages) is devoted to toxicology, and embraces the methods of administration and the effects of poisons, the diseases simulating poisoning, and the rules to observe in poison cases. The entire range of poisons, from mineral agents to ptomains, is exhaustively treated, and the section ends with remarks on embalming from a medico-legal standpoint.

Part II., on forensic medicine, is very complete. Beginning with the powers and duties of coroners, the subjects relating to legal medicine, with the exception of insanity, are treated *in extenso.* Many famous cases bearing upon the respective points are cited, and the author clearly and concisely elucidates the lessons which are to be learned therefrom. Altogether this book is an exceedingly valuable addition to those of like nature already published.

HOW TO LIVE LONGER AND WHY WE DO NOT LIVE LONGER. By J. R. HAYES, M.D., Medical Examiner, Bureau of Pensions. Philadelphia: J. B. Lippincott Co, 1897.

THERE is much in this little work of 180 pages to commend itself to thoughtful people, especially to those who desire longevity. It is hard to believe that an ascetic life induces length of life, and it is difficult after reading this work to think that it does not. Although we do not like the religious tone of the book, devoted as it is to purely physical considerations, it is written honestly, we have no doubt, even to the tacit acceptance of Christian Science. There is much that could be combated on scientific grounds, but since the book is intended for lay readers, there is no need of further consideration at our hands.

LIPPINCOTT'S POCKET MEDICAL DICTIONARY, Including the Pronunciation and Definition of Twenty Thousand of the Principal Terms Used in Medicine and the Allied Sciences, together with Many Elaborate Tables. Edited by RYLAND W. GREENE, A.B. Philadelphia and London: J. B. Lippincott Company, 1897.

THIS little book aims to supply the requirements of a pocket medical lexicon, handy in size, clear, reliable, and up to modern requirements. An effort has been made in its compilation to eliminate obsolete terms and to insert only those which are necessary in modern medical literature. It has a flexible cover, but on account of its thickness, would probably be found rather cumbersome to carry about.

LECTURES ON PHYSIOLOGY. FIRST SERIES. ON ANIMAL ELECTRICITY. By AUGUSTUS D. WALLER, M.D., F.R.S. London, New York, and Bombay: Longmans, Green & Co., 1897.

THIS book contains part of the material of a course of lectures on animal electricity delivered by the author before the Royal Institution of Great Britain, in which he is the Fullerian Professor of Physiology. The matter is presented so clearly and precisely that any one who reads this little book cannot help retaining the facts of animal electricity. The lectures are a model of conciseness, yet are complete in every respect. Teachers of physiology are reminded that there is much in this book which will be of value to them in class demonstrations.

HANDBOOK OF MATERIA MEDICA, PHARMACY, AND THERAPEUTICS. By SAMUEL O. L. POTTER, A.M., M.D. Sixth edition. Philadelphia: P. Blakiston, Son & Co., 1897.

ANY book which has passed to its sixth edition within a little more than ten years has reasonably answered all doubt as to its usefulness, and there is usually little left to be said by the reviewer. To its former acquaintances it may be of interest to remark that the sixth edition presents an increase of nearly one hundred pages, with a consideration of forty-six new subjects. The work appears to be quite accurate in its vast details, and highly convenient as a volume for quick and easy reference. If any adverse criticism is merited, one might be pardoned for suggesting that the scientific correlation of subjects has been too often sacrificed to convenience in classification, and the broad principles of therapeutics are less prominently taught than is desirable in a text-book. The mechanical preparation and general appearance of the book compare favorably with the previous editions.

THERAPEUTIC HINTS.

For Syphilides of the Scalp the following ointment is highly recommended, especially for the impetiginous variety:

℞ Hydrarg. ox. rubr. } aa . . . ʒ ss
Zinci ox. }
Resorcini . . . . . . gr. xv
Vaselini . . . . ℥ ii.

M. Sig. For external use.

For Painful Parotiditis Complicating Influenza.—The following ointment should be rubbed into the skin over the affected gland three times daily, and then a cotton-wool dressing should be applied:

℞ Ichthyol } aa . . . . gr. xlv
Plumbi iodid. }
Ammonii chloridi . . . . ʒ ss
Adipis . . . . . . ℥ i.

M. Sig. For external use.

For Bronchopneumonia in Infants.—

℞ Lactophenini . . . . . gr. xv
Ac. benzoici . . . . . . gr. v.

M. Ft. pulv. No. VI. Sig. One powder every four hours.

For Epilepsy.—

℞ Zinci oxidi } aa . . . gr. xviii
Pulv. rad. valerianæ }
Pulv. rad. belladonnæ . . . . gr. ii
Saponis . . . . q. s.

M. Ft. pil. No. XII. Sig. Four pills daily.—*Voisin.*

THE MEDICAL NEWS.

A WEEKLY JOURNAL OF MEDICAL SCIENCE.

VOL. LXXII. NEW YORK, SATURDAY, APRIL 2, 1898. NO. 14.

ORIGINAL ARTICLES.

SPLENECTOMY.[1]

BY FRANK HARTLEY, M.D.,
OF NEW YORK.

KOLLIKER, Bizzozero, Salvioli, Rindfleisch, and others considered the spleen both a hematolytic and hematogenetic organ; that is, one containing the materials out of which hemoglobin is formed, as well as one in which food products are appropriated and further elaborated. Metchnikopf also believes that the spleen takes part in the war with microbes; since animals without spleens are less resisting to the action of germs. It is the opinion of Sykoff that after splenectomy the medulla of bones acquires an augmented activity which partly compensates for the loss of the spleen's function. This belief is supported by the fact that such increased functionation on the part of bone-marrow occurs in all acute infectious diseases, and also in many chronic affections, but not to a degree fully compensatory for the loss of the spleen. The differences in the condition of the blood in patients in whom enlargement of the spleen is either primary or secondary to general infection led Vulpins to assume that the function of the spleen may be vicariously assumed by other organs. When a portion of the spleen has been extirpated there is but little hypertrophy. of what remains, this being the opinion of Peyran, who has given especial attention to this point.

Accessory spleens are common in young people, having been found to exist in a ratio of from 1 to 400 to 1 to 16. After splenectomy, nodules have appeared in the omentum of animals, but microscopic examination (Mosher) has shown them to be hemorrhagic telangiectatic lymphomata. Many writers, including Bardeleben and Zesas, think the thyroid gland competent to assume the function of the spleen, but Tauber, Ughetti, and Mattei were able to save animals in which both organs had been removed. In man, hyperplasia of the thyroid following splenectomy has been observed three times, but in these cases the enlargement was so transitory that when combined with its rarity and the results of experiments on animals we can hardly say that it was more than accidental, and, of course, not functionally compensatory. General enlargement of the lymphatics has not infrequently been observed after removal of the spleen, yet there remains a large number of cases in which such enlargement has not been observed. Tritons, which have no lymph-nodules, have had their spleens removed without causing death (Pouchet), and fish, which have no bone-marrow, do not suffer from splenectomy (Pouchet).

In splenectomized dogs, Mosher and others found the bone-marrow red and congested, which condition they believed to be a functional hyperemia. Observations substantiating this theory have not been made in man.

It is the opinion of Vulpius, provided the spleen is a blood-making organ, that its function may be assumed by other structures; but since, after splenectomy, enlarged organs are not constantly found, he considers doubtful the supposition that the spleen is a hematogenetic organ. His conclusions, however, are as follows: (1) Red blood-cells undergo disintegration in the spleen. (2) The spleen is increased in size in acute general anemia. (3) The removal of this organ causes a transient decrease in the number of the red, and an increase in the white cells of the blood. (4) The thyroid gland as regards function has no relation to the spleen. (5) Lymph-glands and bone-marrow are more active after splenectomy has been performed. (6) Regeneration of the blood is retarded in persons who have undergone splenectomy.

The early history of splenectomy is practically comprised in the operations of Zaccarello (1549), Ferrarius (1569), Küchler (1855), Quittobaum (1826), and Sir Spencer Wells (1865), in which all patients, except that of Ferrarius, died. Pean, 1867, had the second successful case. Since that time, 1867 to 1894, over 100 splenectomies have been performed, with a mortality of fifty per cent. (Vulpius). In all I have been able to find recorded 126 splenectomies. Of these, excluding the operations performed for leucocythemia, the mortality was 20.5 per cent. Arranging the cases of splenectomy according to the conditions existing at the time of the operation, it is found that in leucocythemia there are 29 cases, in which 25 patients died from the immediate effects of the operation (20 of hemorrhage, 2 of septic peritonitis, 1 of shock, and 2 in which no cause was mentioned, though, as Vulpins suggests, probably from hemorrhage, since death occurred within five hours). Three patients

[1] Read at a meeting of the New York Clinical Society, January 28, 1898.

survived the operation, 1 of whom died of the disease thirteen days after the operation; 1 lived eight months, and finally died of the disease. One patient, in whom the disease was of a mild type, lived, and in this case the blood-count was normal within three months. The mortality from splenectomy in leucocythemia is, therefore, 89.3 per cent.; recoveries from operation, 10.7 per cent.; permanent recoveries, 3.9 per cent. From these results it naturally follows that the operation is not justifiable when leucocythemia exists, and only when the spleen, by its enlargement, causes dangerous symptoms, would one entertain the thought of extirpation.

Malarial Enlargement of the Spleen.—Vulpius collected the records of 26 splenectomies for malarial enlargement performed up to 1894, in 11 of which there was a fatal result, giving a mortality of nearly fifty per cent. Jonnesco collected 36 cases up to 1897, with a mortality of fifty per cent. From 1887 to 1896, there were 25 cases, with a mortality of 31.7 per cent. Since 1896 the last-mentioned writer collected 15 cases, with a mortality of 15.4 per cent. I know of two cases in which the operation was performed during 1897, and which are not included in Jonnesco's statistics, one of Olgiati, and one of my own, in both of which recovery occurred, so that the mortality for these seventeen cases last recorded is about 13.5 per cent.

Idiopathic Hypertrophy.—Vulpius collected 21 splenectomies for idiopathic hypertrophy up to 1894, with 2 deaths, and a mortality of 22.5 per cent. Since that time I have collected 9, with 2 deaths. (In 1894, 2; in 1895, 6; in 1896, 1.) This makes in all 30 cases, with a mortality of about 22.1 per. cent.

Wandering Spleen.—Vulpins collected 19 cases, with 2 deaths, giving a mortality of 10.5 per cent. I have added to these 4 cases (4 in 1895), with 2 recoveries, and a mortality of 8.7 per cent.

Axial Rotation (with or without an infarction).—I have collected 4 such cases (2 each in 1894 and 1895), with 1 death—a mortality of twenty-five per cent.

Echinococcus Cysts.—Vulpius, up to 1894, reports 5 cases of this affection, with a mortality of forty per cent. Since then Snegirjopf, Hahn, Jonnesco, and Douval have each had a case in which splenectomy was successfully performed. There are, therefore, altogether 9 such cases, with 2 deaths, making a mortality of 22.2 per cent. There may be added here 2 splenectomies for blood cysts; 1 performed by Mijerowitsch and 1 by Schalita, both resulting in recovery.

Sarcoma of the Spleen.—Six cases have been recorded. In 3 there was recovery from the operation, but subsequent death from recurrence. In 1 case death occurred immediately after the operation, and in 2 cases (Herzcel's and d'Antona's), in which the sarcoma was small, the patients are still alive. To summarize: 1 patient lived two years after the operation, and 1 for one year—33.33 per cent.; 3 patients died from recurrence—50 per cent., and 1 patient, 16.66 per cent., died immediately after the operation.

Chronic Congestion of the Spleen and Amyloid Kidney.—Up to 1894 Vulpius reports 3 cases with 3 deaths.

Syphilis.—One case of splenectomy for syphilis of the spleen has been reported. In this case the patient recovered.

Rupture of the Healthy Spleen.—Up to 1894 the statistics of splenectomy for rupture of the spleen gave a mortality of nearly 100 per cent. In my case (1894), in Czerny's, and in Riegner's there was recovery. In a case of Trendelenburg's there was a fatal result, and Lane had 2 fatal cases. There are recorded, therefore, 6 cases, with a mortality of 50 per cent.

The Blood in Laparosplenectomy.—In leukemia the blood has been examined in only 3 cases; in each both before and after the operation. The blood-count ratio was from 1–74 to 1–105 before operation; whereas after operation, in 1 case, it was normal within three months; in another, 1–50 within five months, and in a third 1–7 to 1–3 thirteen days after the operation. In leukemia splenectomy is contra-indicated, since the general disease advances after the spleen is removed, and in my opinion in this disease the operation should never be undertaken under any circumstances. A blood-count ratio of 1–50 is certainly to be considered, however severe the pressure symptoms and local pains may be, the limit outside of which operation is not justifiable.

In wandering spleen the blood has been examined in 7 cases, both before and after operation (Vulpius). The blood-count ratio ranged from 1–65 to normal before operation to 1–30 and 1–160 three weeks after operation, and, finally, to normal within two or three months after removal of the organ in question.

In hypertrophy the blood has been examined in 4 cases. It ranged from 1–200 and 1–430 before to 1–62 two days after operation, and normal within five months.

In splenectomy for malarial enlargement the blood has been examined in 10 cases, including 4 of Vulpius, 1 of my own, and 5 of Jonnesco's. In these the blood-count ratio ranged from 1–100 and normal before operation, to 1–150 one month afterward (a slight diminution in red cells), and a normal condition within two to three months after operation. The diminution in red cells and the leucocytosis after operation are transitory.

In echinococcus cysts the blood has been examined in one case. The ratio was normal both before and after the operation.

In sarcoma the blood-count ratio varied in two cases from 1–500 to normal before operation to 1–100 to normal at the end of six weeks.

In rupture of the spleen no blood-count has been made either before or after splenectomy; this is true of both Czerny's and Riegner's case, as well as of my own. The condition of the blood previous to the injury is, therefore, unknown, and the same is true of the period following operation—a time when there was a condition of traumatic anemia. In my case the blood was not examined until the fourth day after operation. At this time the blood showed a deficiency of red cells, and an increase to 75,000 of the white cells (1–28), which on the tenth day showed 125,000 to 1,900,000, *i.e.*, 1–15. On the twenty-third day after operation the ratio was reduced, and continued to diminish until 107 days after operation, when the red blood-cells were nearly normal in appearance, but slightly deficient in hemoglobin. Five months afterward the blood was normal.

The *contraindications* to the operation of splenectomy are exemplified in leukemia and amyloid degeneration of the spleen, in both of which the mortality is very high, and removal of the spleen does not avoid the continued advance of the general disease. Leukemia, with its mortality of 25 out of 28 cases, and with only 1 permanent cure, as well as amyloid spleen with its mortality of 100 per cent., render the operation quite unjustifiable under these circumstances.

Splenectomy for sarcoma of the spleen may also be regarded as probably of no particular benefit. Primary tumors of the spleen are very rare, while metastatic sarcoma and carcinoma, especially lymphosarcoma are more frequently found in this organ. Hence, except in benign tumors or primary sarcoma, operative interference is contraindicated. Could an early diagnosis be made in benign tumors or in primary sarcoma, the mortality, reasoning from the combined statistics of wandering spleen and sarcoma, would be between 8.5 and 20 per cent., and would justify operative interference, provided the symptoms, in a benign process, indicated removal on account of their severity.

In certain instances the size of the spleen has been thought to be a contraindication to operation. Valpius and Pean consider interference unjustifiable when the spleen weighs more than 3000 grains. Jonnesco does not believe that the size of the spleen is a contraindication to removal, and has operated successfully upon three malarial hypertrophic spleens, weighing respectively 3350, 4620, and 5750 grains, and one echinococcus cyst of the spleen weighing 4000 grains. Vulpins maintains that from the study of the cases of hypertrophy and wandering spleen it is shown that the limit of safety is 3000 grains; whereas, in malarial spleens no relation seems to exist between the size of the tumor and the mortality. It is difficult to say just what extent and degree of adhesion to surrounding structures will contraindicate operative procedures. If the general condition of the patient is such that a prolonged operation cannot be borne, if ascites is present, and these two conditions are combined with extensive adhesions, operation is certainly contraindicated. If, on the other hand, the adhesions are extensive, but not very vascular, they may be removed by working upon the abdominal wall and not upon the spleen; so that extensive adhesions, under other favorable conditions, may be effectually dealt with without prolonging the operation. If adhesions are vascular, especially in the neighborhood of the phrenico-splenic ligament, great care is necessary to prevent injury to the diaphragm and solar plexus. The time expended in this and in the ligation of the adhesions will necessarily prolong the operation. So much depends upon the surgeon (the ability to work quickly and carefully) that, as said before, it is difficult to state just what extent of adhesions render an operation inadvisable. Undoubtedly, a severe malarial cachexia contraindicates an operation, yet it is here difficult to judge, except by the anemia present, whether or not a successful termination may be reasonably expected. In reference to the anemia, it can only be said that a hemoglobin per cent. of .30 here, as elsewhere, contraindicates operative procedure (Mikulicz).

Indications for Splenectomy. — In the malarial spleen the inefficiency of internal medication and suitable climate, with a beginning cachexia, will, when the pain and pressure symptoms from the enlarged spleen are severe, indicate splenectomy. In the echinococcic wandering, or hypertrophic spleen, in benign tumors, and in large cysts from bematomata, the pain and pressure effects alone will indicate operation. In abscess of the spleen, whether caused by injury, primary infarction, or echinococcus disease, the indications for splenectomy are present. In some cases the operation becomes necessary on account of the danger of sepsis or invasion of neighboring structures. In axial rotation of a wandering and enlarged spleen, with or without sepsis, the indication is for operation, either splenectomy, or, in some instances, splenopexis. In primary sarcoma, provided the diagnosis is made, the indication is for removal of the affected organ. If the growth is secondary, or cachexia is present, an operation is contraindicated. In trauma of the spleen, the indication is for a splenectomy when a traumatic anemia follows the injury, or, in some cases, splenotomy and suture (Tiffany and Lamarchia).

The prognosis will depend upon the particular disease affecting the spleen and its mortality. The degree of mobility of the organ will also influence the prognosis; since, if the spleen be immobile, the adhesions to the abdominal wall, the short pedicle, and the difficulty of working upon the phrenicosplenic ligament without producing injury to the neighboring structures or causing severe hemorrhage are elements which may make the operation exceedingly difficult. If the spleen is movable and situated in the left hypochrondrium, the necessary procedures are not difficult and tearing and bleeding are avoided. In the case of a wandering spleen the operation becomes very easy of execution. In twenty-seven such cases only two deaths occurred.

CASE I.—*Malarial Hypertrophy of the Spleen—Splenectomy.*—A. G., twenty-four years of age, born in Boston, but of recent years a resident of Georgia. During the four previous years he had repeatedly suffered from malaria. During the spring and winter of 1897 he had the tertian form of malarial fever. He had been treated with antimalarial remedies during these years, and especially during the last two or three months. He became easily exhausted, and was unable to endure his usual work (accountant) any longer. He suffered daily from headache, dizziness, and irregular pain in the lower limbs. On examination he showed a well-marked anemia and some edema of the lower extremities; pulse, 120; respirations, 22; temperature, 99.5° F.

In the left hypochrondrium and iliac fossa could be seen a large mass which was found to extend to the median line and into the hypogastric region. The enlarged spleen was slightly movable, though for practical purposes it could be called fixed. The patient was very desirous of being relieved of the tumor, and after considering the danger, decided to have the operation performed.

Operation, March 20, 1891. A median abdominal incision was made, extending from the xiphoid cartilage to below the umbilicus. On entering the abdomen the adhesions were not so extensive as was supposed from the apparent immobility of the organ. The adhesions upon the abdominal wall were first separated and ligated, but few of them being vascular. Adhesions to the omentum were slight and were easily ligated, and were absent in the neighborhood of the phrenicosplenic ligament, so that the ligation of this structure was easily accomplished, the spleen being pushed down and held to the left side of the abdomen. It was much more difficult to separate the gastrosplenic ligament and to ligate the pedicle. This latter was accomplished by means of three ligatures encircling both branches of the splenic artery and the branches forming the splenic vein. After this ligation, *en masse,* and a careful avoidance of the pancreas, the pedicle was divided and the spleen removed. The branches of the splenic artery were then separately tied. The bleeding during the operation was slight. The space left after removal of the spleen presented in many places an absence of peritoneum. A small sterile gauze handkerchief was placed at the former site of the spleen, and was brought out through a counter incision in the lumbar region. The intra-abdominal pressure soon closed the space, and brought the wounded surfaces in contact with the gauze. The gauze was used because of the fear of oozing—a fear which, however, I now think was without foundation. The abdominal wound was closed with silk sutures. Catgut was used within the abdominal cavity. There was but little shock, and after the operation the pulse was 140, respiration, 25, and temperature, 99° F.

March 21st to 23d.—Patient gradually improving; pulse, 120; respirations, 20; temperature, 99° to 100° F. The gauze was removed through the lumbar incision.

March 29th.—Patient continues to improve, the pulse being 110, respirations, 18, and temperature, 99° F. The wound healed by first intention.

April 15th.—The anemia is less marked, and the patient's appetite is good, and the pulse, respiration, and temperature practically normal.

April 30th.—Patient has left the bed and intends to return home within a few days. The weight of the spleen removed was 2565 grains.

The blood examination before the operation showed 1,000,000 red and 4000 white blood-corpuscles (1–250) to the c.mm., and the hemoglobin, forty per cent. Three days after the operation examination showed 2,300,000 red and 10,000 white cells, that is, 1–220; hemoglobin thirty per cent. On the ninth day the ratio was increased, inasmuch as the ratio of red to white-corpuscles was 1–300; hemoglobin forty per cent. The blood condition gradually improved until, on April 30th, the ratio was 1–350 and the hemoglobin fifty-five per cent. After the patient returned home he continued to steadily improve.

CASE II.—*Traumatic Rupture of the Spleen—Splenectomy.*—Fred. H.W., admitted to Roosevelt Hospital May 27, 1896, age nine years, American. He was a delicate child and had been subject to malaria. May 6th, three weeks before entering the hospital, he had a chill, which was followed by slight vomiting and cramps in the abdomen. He remained in bed one day. Three days later, May 9th, he had completely recovered, and was apparently well. On May 23d (four days before coming to the hospital and fourteen days after the former illness) he fell and struck his abdomen upon a coal-scuttle, following which a small, bruised spot made its appearance to the left of the umbilicus. He did not seem to be inconvienced by the accident. May 25th (two days later), while still attending school, he complained of a loss of appetite, but nothing else. On returning from school on the same day he was seen staggering and doubled up with intense pain over the abdomen. The pain was slightly more intense upon the right side. He was put to bed, and was apparently suffering from shock, having cold extremities, pinched face, and a pulse and temperature which were about normal. At 1 A.M. the next day (May 26th) he began to vomit, and the pulse increased to 120. The abdomen became tympanitic and tender. Both internal medication and enemata were unsuccessfully employed in an effort to move the bowels. He was slightly delirious. He did not pass any blood, either from the rectum or bladder.

Examination, shortly after entrance to the hospital, showed him to be slightly jaundiced and only partly conscious. The breathing was largely thoracic. The abdomen was tense and distended, chiefly over the hypogastrium and the right iliac fossa. No mass could be detected in the abdominal cavity. Rectal examination proved negative. A small bruised spot, the size of a 1-cent piece, could be seen just to the left and above the umbilicus. The pulse was compressible and about 146 per minute. The temperature was 102° F. The history, according to the opinion of the family physician, pointed to a commencing peritonitis from rupture of the appendix, it being supposed that the rupture occurred May 25th (two days before admission).

As the condition of the patient seemed to contraindicate operation, he was stimulated, and, after a quick response to restorative measures, operation was performed under ether anesthesia. From the history, symptoms, and the location of the pain and tenderness in the hypogastrium and right iliac fossa, I could not but think that I had to deal with a morbid process in the pelvis and right iliac fossa, and probably, since the bruise near the umbilicus apparently had no significance, an appendicitis and peritonitis. I made an exploratory incision to the right of the rectus muscle, in order to obtain a good view of the iliac fossa and interior of the pelvis. The tissues were divided down to the peritoneum, through which could be seen a mass of blood in the iliac fossa. In separating the delicate adhesions and endeavoring to determine the source of the blood the cecum was found ecchymotic, but not torn. The appendix was normal. The pelvis was found to contain about three-quarters of a pint of blood. The incision was increased in length, and the left iliac fossa was found to be perfectly free from blood. The blood in the pelvis was removed, and the intestines and mesentery were then carefully examined in the hope of discovering the source of the hemorrhage, but with none but negative results. Some clots of blood were seen among the coils of the small intestines, in the space occupied by the ascending colon, mesentery of the small intestines, and transverse colon. No blood was seen in the neighborhood of the pancreas, in front of or behind the peritoneum, nor in the neighborhood of the right kidney. The omentum contained a single blood-clot. The blood apparently flowed down to the left of the mesentery of the small intestines, then into the pelvis and right iliac fossa. The splenic flexure of the colon and ligamentum colico-lienale, were found to be covered in places with a few clots of blood.

Finally, a rupture of the spleen was discovered, the wound in this organ being filled with a large and adherent clot. A part of the latter was removed by the hand during the examination of the abdominal contents. The tear was found upon the outer or convex surface of the spleen. The injured organ was firmly grasped by the hand at its pedicle, and, with the other hand, an oblique incision was made below the eleventh rib and running downward and forward a distance of six inches. The tissues were rapidly divided down to the peritoneum, which was opened. The blood-clot was seen in the spleen, lying within a rupture upon the antero-external surface. The pedicle, with the vessels, was tied with catgut. The blood-clot in the omentum was loosened and removed, and the bleeding vessels tied. The spleen was then removed. The abdominal cavity was irrigated with salt solution until all clots were washed away. The two wounds in the abdominal walls were rapidly closed with catgut, layer for layer. The skin was sutured with silk. In the midst of the operation the child's pulse became very weak, and it was necessary to administer stimulants; strychnin, in divided doses, and 1½ pints of salt solution by the intravenous method. The patient left the operating-room in good condition. A temperature of 105° F. and a pulse of 140, were recorded soon after he was placed in bed, but both gradually improved until, within twelve hours, the temperature was 101° F. and the pulse 112.

May 29th.—Patient in fair condition; no vomiting or pain in the abdomen. Stimulants not so frequently required.

May 30th.—At 1 P.M. the temperature rose to 104° F.; pulse, 120. The wound was dressed; it looked well. No evidences of infection present. The abdomen was soft and not tender. An enema resulted in a movement of the bowels.

May 31st.—The patient had a chill. Temperature rose to 104° F., pulse to 120.

June 1st.—The temperature and pulse were normal.

June 2d.—Quinin and ginger were administered every two hours, beginning eight hours before the expected fever. Only a slight rise in temperature was recorded. The wound was dressed and all packing removed.

June 6th.—Wound dressed. Slight serous discharge from the sinus left by the removal of the packing. No rise of temperature.

June 11th.—Wound dressed. Temperature and pulse normal.

June 14th.—Temperature 105° F., pulse 126, but both were down again within two hours.

June 26th.—Wound solidly healed. Patient well.

In attempting to explain the occurrence of a laceration of the spleen in this case, it seems probable that on the fourth day before I saw him the patient he received, from his fall upon the coal-scuttle, a subvisceral tear[1] in the spleen, and possibly through its capsule, but without injury to the peritoneum. The rupture into the peritoneal cavity evidently occurred on the second day after the injury.

In forty-two cases of rupture of the spleen Mayer found two subvisceral tears, in both of which the laceration subsequently broke through the peritoneum following more or less violent contraction of the abdominal muscles and diaphragm. Vincent, who has carefully examined after death 100 cases of rupture of the spleen, believes that many of the cases in which the tear is slight result in recovery. Some lacerations give rise to secondary bleeding, more or less severe, but the majority are the cause of a rapid and severe hemorrhage at the time of the injury, or, at a later period, of abscess, peritonitis, or exhaustion. In the case reported it is very probable that the tear in the spleen and its capsule, had the patient remained quiet, would have healed with a cicatrix, or subsequently caused an abscess, tumor, or a cyst.

In addition to the studies of Meyer and Vincent, we have the statistics collected by Edler and Trapp, in which they analyzed 78 of these cases with reference to operation and complications. In 57 of the 78 cases the spleen was the only or the principal organ involved, and in 33 of the 57 the spleen was found to be healthy; 24 times it was found to be diseased. In the cases in which the spleen was normal recovery ensued in 4; in those in which it was abnormal, 6 cases resulted in recovery. In the remaining 47 cases death was in 42 instances ascribed to bleeding, and in 5 to peritonitis. In 13 cases death occurred within an hour; in 9 cases within a few hours; in 1 case after a day; in five cases after 3 days; in 2 after 8 days; in 3 after 14 days; in 2 after 3 weeks; in 12 the time was not stated.

In Vincent's 100 cases death occurred from hemorrhage alone in 75. The mortality, then, probably ranges between the autopsic record of Vincent (seventy-five per cent.), and the statistic record of Elder and Trapp (89.3 per cent.).

The spleen is the subject of subcutaneous laceration in about twenty-eight per cent. of all cases of injury to the organ, and when diseased, may be ruptured from muscular contraction alone. The diagnosis is difficult unless there is a history of splenic disease or evidence of the occurrence of an injury sufficient to cause a rupture; since the symptoms of rupture are completely masked by the bleeding into the peritoneal cavity.

In the case reported evidence of hemorrhage might have been obtained before the operation had less credence been placed in the history and had a blood-count been made. In my opinion, the blood-count, quite as much as urinary analysis, should be made in every case of severe injury in which shock is present, and is possibly complicated with hemorrhage, as well as in slow and less severe hemorrhages, such as may be observed in ruptured extra-uterine pregnancy, or following injury to the kidney, liver, or spleen, when no history is obtainable. As a differential point between shock and hemorrhage, a blood examination is of inestimable value in furnishing a clue to the immediate use of the salt solution, and as an indication for or against operative procedure.

The examination of the blood of the patient whose case has just been reported was made by Dr. Ewing, pathologist to the hospital. The first examination was made June 2d, four days after the operation. His report reads as follows:

The blood is extremely pale. The red corpuscles are much diminished, and show very little tendency to form rouleaux. About forty per cent. of them are very large-sized megalocytes, and many are very fine and deformed microcytes and poikilocytes. The hemoglobin is extremely deficient. There is present a small number of normal nucleated red cells. The leucocytes are very much increased in number, and are estimated at 75,000, of which twenty-three per cent. are monocular and seventy-seven per cent. polynuclear. The so-called splenocytes are abundant. A moderate number of myelocytes are present, indicating some similarity to the blood of leukemia. The neutrophile granules appear to be deficient. The plasma is distinctly stained, indicating some solution of the hemoglobin. Many red cells stain a dark brown with eosin, indicating a change of hemoglobin to met-hemoglobin.

June 12th.—Red cells 1,900,000 to the c.mm. They show very little change from that previously noted. The hemoglobin has slightly increased in quantity; the leucocytes are 12,500 to the c.mm.

June 25th.—The red cells are much increased in number and in their hemoglobin contents. Rouleaux are abundant, and there are only moderate differences in size and form of the corpuscles. The leucocytes appear normal in number and proportion, but there still appears to be a deficiency in the number of granules. This is the twenty-third day after operation.

September 17th.—The red cells are nearly normal in appearance, showing only a slight deficiency in hemoglobin. Some megalocytes are still present.

[1] It may be that malaria, by causing congestion of the spleen, will render this organ more friable than usual, but it cannot be positively said that malaria was present in this case, there being no evidence of malarial infection other than the chills and fever following the operation, and the physician's statement that the patient had been subject to malaria. An examination of the blood following the operation did not reveal the presence of the plasmodium of malaria, nor did the treatment given him indicate the existence of this affection.

Leucocytes are present in normal numbers, and in the following proportions:

Lymphocytes....................15 per cent.
Large monocular cells............20 per cent.
Polynuclear cells.................62 per cent.
Eosinophile cells................ 3 per cent.

The neutrophile granules are distinctly deficient. This is the 107th day after the operation. The only abnormality in the blood appears to be a slight general deficiency in the amount of hemoglobin.

Unfortunately, no records of blood analyses are accessible in those cases of rupture of the spleen in which the organ was not diseased. In those cases in which such a record exists, either the general system or the spleen was involved, and the records cannot be compared in value with experiments on animals in which a healthy spleen was removed. Both Czerny's, Regnier's, and my own case were complicated with a traumatic anemia, and cannot be strictly compared with the animal experiments in splenectomy, in which such anemia does not complicate the case. Yet I do not think it amiss to state here the similarity in such comparison when it exists. The experiments on rabbits and goats by Vulpius and Zesas show that the leucocytes increase more than 100 per cent. within nineteen days after splenectomy, and then gradually sink to the normal on about the sixty-fifth day. In my case, though there existed a traumatic anemia, and certainly malaria was not present, the examination of the blood showed a deficiency of the red blood-cells with an increase of the leucocytes to 75,000 on the fourth day after the operation, and on the tenth day the ratio of white to red cells was 12,500 to 1,900,000, or, 1 to 15. On the twenty-third day after operation this ratio was reduced to normal, and so continued until the 107th day, at which time the red blood-cells were nearly normal in appearance, but slightly deficient in hemoglobin. Some megalocytes were still present, but the leucocytes were normal in number.

After five months from the time of operation no abnormality in the blood existed except a slight general deficiency in the hemoglobin. In a case examined by Tschistowitsch, with reference to the condition of the blood during the first and second years after operation, the red blood-cells and the hemoglobin were found to be at least equal to the normal. During the first year there was an increase of leucocytes. After this period the leucocytes diminished and the eosinophile cells increased.

The conclusion, then, to be drawn from my case is, simply that after splenectomy the red blood-cells and hemoglobin are greatly diminished, and the leucocytes increased, and that shortly after operation (ten to twenty-three days) the red blood-cells and leucocytes are again normal in ratio. There is, however, a deficiency in the amount of hemoglobin which persists, in slight degree, for some months.

MATERNAL IMPRESSIONS AND THEIR INFLUENCE UPON THE FETUS IN UTERO.

BY CLAUDIUS HENRY MASTIN, M.D.,
OF MOBILE, ALA.

IT is a well-established conclusion that all animal monstrosities do not arise in the original organization of the embryo, but from subsequent accidents occurring after conception, during the term of uterogestation. An evidence of this fact is illustrated by those preternatural appearances of, or rather upon, the fetus, which now and then result from frights, or the so-called "longings" of pregnant females, constituting what are known as "nævi materni," or "mothers' marks," the sequences of maternal impressions.

I am well aware that diverse and opposite opinions are entertained upon this subject and that a large amount of scientific and well-digested literature, based upon correct physiologic grounds and bearing upon the subject of conception and gestation, has been produced to controvert such ideas; while, on the other hand, much has been written which sustains the popular belief of the laity on this subject, a belief also held by not a few of the best informed in our own profession. Many well-recorded cases have fallen under the observation of scientific men who are not given to hasty or immature conclusions, but who, after careful analysis of the cases which have come under their immediate notice, have been compelled to give their unqualified endorsement to the belief in maternal impressions.

The simple fact that these "mothers' marks" are not seen upon *every* child, although we know that during the nine months of uterogestation almost every expectant mother, at one time or another during her pregnancy, passes through stages of mental excitement or undergoes cravings and longings which are common to her condition, without the means or power of gratifying her appetites or pleasing her fancies, and still there may be no stain or blemish upon the face or the form of the infant after birth. Even though this be true, it is no argument against the fact that maternal impressions, under certain conditions and at certain stages of pregnancy, may and do occur as the direct result of powerful or prolonged disturbance of the nervous system.

We know from our personal observations that every child which is born into the world is not stamped with the trade-mark of its mother's fancy, or the evidence of her alarm and terror. But because this is true in many instances we cannot accept it as an invariable rule, and thus deny the truth of the aphorism of Chelius: "The probable is not always, the improbable is occasionally true."

We are aware that many pregnant women are alarmed without consequences, and the most varied fantasies may cross their idle brains without any ill results. It is an axiom, as true as it is forcible, that "when a circumstance may proceed from many causes we do not universally reject any one, because it is frequently alleged without reason;" and so it is, there are too many well-authenticated cases before us to justify doubt of the powerful effects of the maternal impressions. Just here I must acknowledge that for years past I have been a pronounced skeptic on this subject, so much so, that I was unwilling to accept even the evidence of the sacred writer who recorded in the Book of Genesis the following:

> And Jacob took him rods of green poplar, and of the hazel and chestnut tree; an piled white *stakes* in them, and made the white appear which was in the rods. And he set the rods which he had piled before the flocks in the gutter in the watering-troughs when the flocks came to drink, that they should conceive when they came to drink. And the flocks conceived before the rods, and brought forth cattle ring-straked, speckled, and spotted.

This description from the Mosaic writings shows the antiquity of the belief in the impressions made by external objects upon the impregnated ovum. So prevalent was this idea among the ancients, and especially so with the Spartans, that it was an established custom among them to place beautiful pictures and other agreeable objects before their pregnant women, so that they might be constantly in their sight, and thus have an effect upon the unborn child. So common was this that, by a law of Lycurgus, it was ordered that the pregnant women of the empire should have constantly in view the images of Castor and Pollux, thus to insure the beauty and strength of the expected infant.

It is a widespread and popular belief that pregnant women are impressed by external objects, and, as a rule, the majority of popular ideas have foundation in fact; yet very many absurd notions and ridiculous stories arise from ignorance and superstition, and hence become general among the uneducated. This is evidenced by many superstitious people who attribute a great deal to the supernatural and very much more to the sympathy of people. Butler, in Hudibrastic lines, gives an amusing description of this sort of sympathy, and absurdly illustrates it in his description of the Taliacotian operation: "So learned Taliacotius, from the brawny part of porter's bum, cut supplemental noses, which would last as long as parent breech,

> "'But when the date of Nock was out,
> Off dropped the sympathetic snout.'"

The idea of sympathy has a powerful hold upon the popular mind; and a widespread notion prevails among horticulturists, which they assert is true, that "a graft will dry up and drop off, if perchance the tree from which the graft was taken is cut down, or otherwise should perish." Although this idea is not sustained by actual results, it is, nevertheless, believed to be true. Another rather curious and strange fact, or, we might more correctly say, coincidence, is that wine which has been kept in wooden vessels will, at certain seasons of the year, almost always set up a feeble fermentation, and, as a rule, about the same time of the year when the vine commences to blossom. A rational solution would be, the vine begins to blossom when the warm weather sets in, and the fermentation in the wine-cask is doubtless due to change of temperature, and the setting free of gas which had been fixed by the cold weather of winter.

If, however, there be a sympathy exerting an influence upon organic bodies, whether animal or vegetable, a something intangible, which we denominate *a sympathy*, then how or why should we question the possible, nay, the probable result of impressions made upon the most sensitive of all structures—the nervous system?

When I speak of coincidences I simply dodge the question, and I dodge it because I have no other more rational explanation to offer; and I am free to admit that it is as irrational as to pronounce a manifestation of a natural law "a miracle," because the finite mind has not been taught to comprehend the workings of the infinite.

When we see a child upon whose person there is a nævus bearing some resemblance to a fruit or to a flower, which the mother tells us she had "longed for" during her pregnancy, we may doubt and be skeptical, yet we cannot deny that the phenomenon shows that there does exist a wonderful sympathy between external objects and the uterine system of nerves—a sympathy born of a powerful impression made upon the mind of the woman at a time when of all others she is most impressionable.

The strangest part of the so-called superstition or popular belief is that the sympathetic impression remains even after the birth of the child, and is subsequently observed between the marks and the objects they are said to represent. This is illustrated by the coincidence which seems to have a shade of authenticity, that when these marks bear a certain resemblance to fruits they assume a tinge of maturity when said fruits are ripening, and become gradually more pale when the fruits are going out of season. I have had my attention directed to this point, and have seen persons whose marks evidently were more colored at one season of the year than they were at others. But I solaced myself with the belief that this change was most probably due to a systemic condition of the individual at that particular season of the year.

It is not at all strange that with the existing belief in the popular mind we should see marks of almost every conceivable description depicted upon the skin of children. I myself have seen what the mothers have told me were "dried peaches," "strawberries," "raspberries," "port-wine stains," and a variety of other objects. The most notable of these was in a little negro boy, about eight years of age, whom I saw a year ago. This little fellow was the subject of a most horrible deformity of the face, which gave him more the appearance of a wild beast than a human being—his countenance was distorted by a roll of rough skin which increased his facial angle, making him prognathous in the extreme; it was covered with coarse, rough hair, and he was unlike anything else than a lower animal. As I examined him and wondered at the mysterious ways of Providence, I was forcibly reminded of the lines written by an old poet of the long ago, one not much read nowadays, namely, Peter Pindar, who described a person whom he had seen: "A pair of leathern cheeks composed his face, from which there sprang many a hairy sprig — resembling much the bristles on a pig." This similarity was sustained by the mother of the boy to whose case I just referred. She assured me that it was a birthmark, and had been produced by her intense desire, when pregnant, for roast pig. I was skeptical on this point, and doubted the possibility of one of the freedmen of the present day, longing for pig-meat, and not gratifying the desire!

Fright or sudden alarm has a powerful impression upon the pregnant female, and there are many instances in which premature delivery has taken place as the consequence of such shocks, showing the influence upon the general nervous system; while shock of less intensity may produce less serious effects upon the gravid uterus and its contents. In evidence, I may mention a case in which a lady in the early stage of her pregnancy was very much shocked at the sight of some leeches upon the foot of a relative; her child was born at term with the mark of a leech, coiled in the act of suction, upon an identically similar spot upon the foot of the child. Another lady gave birth to an infant whose mouth was filled with globular tumors growing from the tongue, tumors which bore a strong resemblance in shape to a bunch of grapes, both in form and color. It was established that the mother had craved grapes during her pregnancy, which was at a season of the year when that fruit could not be obtained. During the same pregnancy she had also been very much alarmed by a turkey-cock, and when the child was born, in addition to the globular tumors in the mouth, it had upon its breast a red excrescence exactly resembling, in figure and color, a turkey's wattles. This double mark may have been a coincidence, and, if these growths had been carefully examined, it is not at all improbable that the microscope would have revealed a case of multiple fibroma.

There are so many curious stories related of these mother's marks that it would consume too much time to go further into a detail of them, but it may serve a purpose if I, in conclusion, mention one or more which have been related by men of such known reputation for veracity that we cannot, with propriety, question their truth, even though we may doubt the causes. A French writer of eminence, whose name at this moment, without some reseach to find it, has escaped my memory (but I think it was Colmbat. del'Isere), mentions a case which was brought before a commission appointed to investigate and report upon it, and which was to the effect that a lady was delivered of a child, upon the iris of whose eyes was clearly depicted the dial of a watch—not an imaginary or simple representation, but the figures clearly outlined. This is rather a difficult story to credit, but since the case has the authentic indorsement of reliable professional men, we may content ourselves with placing it among other remarkable medical curiosities.

In the classic work of Professor W. F. Montgomery, and there is no other more authentic and reliable treatise on pregnancy, are found some most curious and remarkable cases taken from his own practice; one or two of which I will quote in his own words, as substantiating the truth of maternal impressions. Dr. Montgomery says:

> A lady, pregnant for the first time, to whom I recommended frequent exercise in the open air, declined going out as often as was thought necessary, assigning as a reason that she was afraid of seeing a man whose appearance had greatly shocked and disgusted her. He used to crawl along the flagway on his hands and knees, with his feet turned up behind him, which latter were malformed and imperfect, appearing as if they had been cut off at the instep, and he exhibited them thus and uncovered, in order to excite commiseration. I afterward attended this lady in her confinement, and her child, which was born a month before its time and lived, although perfect in every other respect, had the feet malformed and defective, precisely in the same way as those of the cripple who had alarmed her, and whom I had often seen.

Another more remarkable case than this is given by Professor Montgomery, as having occurred in his own practice, and, therefore, not to be questioned. He says:

> Mrs. N., the wife of a clergyman, came to Dublin for her confinement, and a lady who was with her told me

that she had been very uneasy in her mind from an impression that her child would be born with a deformed hand. Her anxiety had been induced from the following occurrence: The mistress of a school which she frequently visited had been delivered of a child with a deformed hand; and as Mrs. N. was known to be at all times very nervous and easily alarmed, and was then a short time pregnant, great pains were taken to prevent her seeing the child's hand. It one day so happened, however, that she walked unexpectedly into the room where the child lay asleep, and sat down by the cradle to look at the child, which at that moment happened to have the deformed hand fully exposed to view. She felt greatly shocked, and afterward alluded to what she had seen, and expressed her conviction that her child would be born with a similar deformity. I delivered her, and very soon after she was attended to she expressed an anxious wish to see the infant, which was brought to her wrapped up in a flannel in the usual way; she instantly drew out the child's arm and exclaimed, "Oh, the dreadful hand!" and there it certainly was, with exactly the same deformity as that which had excited her disgust and terror several months before. The deformity (in each) consisted in the absence of one finger, and the complete union of the middle and third fingers, the united extremities of which were covered by one nail, and presented a very disagreeable appearance.

Can we doubt these statements at the hands of such a man as Professor W. F. Montgomery? Notwithstanding such evidences, we are constrained to feel that it is altogether inaccurate to attribute such consequences entirely to the influence of the mother's imagination, while they are in reality truly effects of physical causes of a very obvious kind, and in no way fairly ascribable to the power of imagination alone. To whatever conclusions we may come as to the precise agency of such causes, it will be always safe and prudent to act upon the presumption that such consequences may follow certain causes, from exposure to which it should be our endeavor to save the pregnant woman; for, although we do not credit all the idle stories which we hear, there certainly are cases wherein it seems to me to be very hard to depart totally and altogether from the opinion which is common to some of the greatest men. So, then, the question whether mental emotions do influence the development of the embryo must be answered in the affirmative, because instances undoubtedly have occurred in which maternal impressions, such as violent shocks or fright, have given rise to malformations; and, since many malformations originate in an arrest of development, it is frequently the case that they do bear a certain resemblance to various animals, so also it is conceivable that the development of the embryo may be so arrested by maternal emotions and so accidentally occasion a likeness between the object which produced the impression and the resulting malformation. The question is yet a moot one as to the kind or degree of impression required to modify the condition of the embryo, so as to develop a malformation; as it is to decide whether it be produced simply through the agency of the mind of the woman, or is the result of a direct shock to the nervous system itself.

These prefatory remarks will enable me to present a brief history of a case of very great interest, and, since it has occurred under my own immediate observation, I can vouch for its truth:

Wm. Y., aged twenty-two years, was shot on the morning of September 24, 1894. The ball, a 38-caliber, was fired from a Winchester rifle, and entered the rear of the chest on the left side, just below and to the outer side of the angle of the scapula; at this point it penetrated the chest between the seventh and eighth ribs and, passing through the entire chest, emerged from the intercostal space between the fourth and fifth ribs, 2¼ inches from the left nipple on the inner side. The exact measurement of the man's chest shows that the distance from the midsternal line in a transverse direction to the center of the left nipple is 4¼ inches—a line drawn from the wound of entrance to that of exit passes directly through the location of the right ventricle, and it is upon this anatomic fact that I diagnosed the case to be one of direct heart penetration.

I shall not consume time with a detail of the case, which has been the subject of a paper upon "Gunshot Wounds of the Heart," which was read before the American Surgical Association at its New York meeting in 1895, and published in Volume 13 of its transactions. At the time when this man was shot his wife was near by, and reached him very soon afterward. In attempting to render what assistance was in her power her hands were stained with blood, and she also had her face covered with blood. When I saw the patient late that afternoon I found her very much agitated, and seemingly as much exercised on account of her condition as she was for her husband's safety. She then informed me that she was pregnant, and felt certain that her child would be born with a "bloody face." I asked her why a "bloody face," and she said, "Because I put my bloody hands to my face and covered it with blood, and I know my child will be born with a bloody face." She was an ignorant countrywoman, and filled with superstitious notions. I calmed her fears as much as I possibly could, and dismissed the subject from my mind. After a long and tedious convalescence her husband was able to be taken home in the country, and I thought no more of the case, beyond the remarkable recovery from so severe a wound.

During the succeeding spring (1895) the man and his wife came to the city and called at my office, bringing with them a new-born infant. She said to me, "Doctor, my baby has not got a bloody face, but it has got the holes where the ball went through Bill's breast." Upon examination of the child I did not find "the holes" which she said were there, but in place of them I discovered bright red marks, clearly shown upon the chest of the child; they were not simply discolored spots, but elevated nævi, and bright carmine-colored spots, easily to be seen at a a distance of a hundred feet. There they were, on the left side of its chest, and although not in the exact anatomic location of the wound on the father's chest, still so near the spot that they are easily recognized as resulting therefrom. The mother had seen the wounds in her husband's chest, and had told me during his illness that they made her sick every time she looked at them.

Interested now in the condition of the case, I made accurate inquires as to her pregnancy and the date of her delivery. She informed me that her pregnancy had passed as was usual in former ones, with the exception that she had been very nervous, and that the motions of the child had been more violent and were brought on by any noise or excitement. Her labor took place on May 10, 1895, was about as previous deliveries. Assuming the term of gestation to be 280 days, and this child having been born on May 10, 1895, it is fair to calculate that her conception took place about August 3, 1894, and from that date to September 24th, the date on which the father was shot, gives us fifty-two days. The question is, Was the maternal excitement at the sight of the wound in her husband's chest the cause of the marks upon the child with which she was then pregnant? I present the facts and leave the reader to answer.

THE WOULD-BE RIVALS OF THE PHYSICIAN IN PRACTICE.[1]

BY REYNOLD W. WILCOX, M.D.,
OF NEW YORK;
PROFESSOR OF MEDICINE AND THERAPEUTICS IN THE NEW YORK POST-GRADUATE MEDICAL SCHOOL AND HOSPITAL; PHYSICIAN TO ST. MARK'S HOSPITAL.

WHEN the metropolitan profession is being agitated over the dispensary and hospital abuse and our country brethren are disturbed by the descent of the city physician upon the various summer-resorts, and the latter generally becomes more eminent the farther he gets from his hearthstone, it may seem trifling to take up the time of the reader with a brief consideration of our would-be rivals in practice. Yet, it has been brought each year more forcibly to mind that the proper field of the physician is being gradually usurped to a greater and greater extent by those whose pretensions are only equaled by their audacity. I have no intention of discussing the evils within the profession, the pauperization of the masses, for which we are in a large measure responsible, the specialism, pseudospecialism, and the fadism, which we often unwittingly encourage, or the tendencies toward trade methods which we, as a class, ignore, but rather the illegitimate rivals or preferably the parasites which fatten upon us, and are sources of irritation to every thoughtful physician. Nor shall I consider the Christian Scientists whom the theologians declare are not Christian and whom we know are not scientists, nor the Faith-Curists who are usually successful in curing their dupes of faith, nor the Mind-Curists who are named *lux a non lucendo*, because neither operator nor victim possesses any mind.

The laws of our State prevent those grossly incompetent from openly exercising the functions of the physician. On their execution there is much upon which we may congratulate ourselves. Thanks to the energetic work of the Medical Society of the State of New York the portals of medical practice are properly guarded. We could wish that the requirements were more rigid, the medical course longer and more thorough, and the preparatory education upon a higher plane, and the entrance examinations more rigorous, but in comparison with the past the outlook is hopeful.

It seems to be a national weakness of ours that we desire a title, and, failing in its attainment, some are content with an epithet: such as the "Doc.," which apparently satisfies the druggist. "Prescribing-druggists" have been the theme of countless diatribes, and their number never seems to diminish. The popular opinion appears to be that the man who sells drugs is perfectly competent to direct their use. The public are of the opinion that he knows the "what," little realizing that the "how much" and "when," which are entirely beyond his knowledge, are of quite as much importance. So long as this opinion prevails the corner dispenser of morning pick-me-ups, purveyor of cigars and proprietary medicines, with prescription annex, will have his liver-persuader, pectoral-balsam, female-regulator, and dyspepsia knockouts. We ourselves are partly responsible; for when the druggist knows that physicians prescribe the various hypophosphite preparations, tonic compounds, and trade-marked, shot-gun concatenations, of which they know little and can guess less, he sees no harm in joining in. This evil will probably never be checked, but it is time to call a halt on barefaced counter-prescribing such as selling two ounces of creosote to an ignorant woman who wanted something to rub on a painful shoulder. A severe burn of large dimensions followed, and the druggist, when called to account, could not be made to see anything wrong in his conduct. I have not discovered any method of checking the indiscriminate repetition of prescriptions. One druggist told me that he thought that the *nonrepetatur* at the bottom of my prescription was some medical motto, and the injunction, "This prescription must not be repeated without my written order" stamped in red ink across the face of the prescription was observed by less than a dozen druggists in the City of New York.

[1] Read at a meeting of the Harvard Medical Society of New York, February 26, 1898.

My own practice now is to supply all prescriptions containing opiates, chloral derivatives, and powerful drugs from my private stock, and so disguised that no apothecary is likely to ascertain what they are. Probably the cleverest trick, and one that has been very disagreeably brought to my notice, is the compounding of a prescription which has been regularly prescribed for a patient by a physician and vending the same at an exorbitant price to any chance comer, the vendor confidently stating that "this is Professor Blank's remedy for malaria, in regard to which his patients all speak well"; then the affair is complete! If the victim is not relieved and visits the writer denouncing the remedy, the surprise of the physician in having attributed to him something of which he himself is guiltless, is only equaled by the audacity with which his brains are borrowed.

It is a hopeless task to educate a public that is fully satisfied with the ecbolic department of the religious press, the seductive advertisements in the street-cars, and the "tommy-rot" of the Doctor's Column of the *Daily Yellow Liar*. It would be equally unsatisfactory if, as is quite generally recommended, the physician should dispense his medicines. He would quite likely degenerate into a tablet-triturate fiend and give N. 631 X & R., forgetting of what it is composed. Notwithstanding that some manufacturers have tried to think for the practitioner, by naming their products as disease or symptom remedies, these are not so constructed that their attempts at thinking can result in other than confusion to the physician and dissatisfaction to the patient. When the retail druggist thinks, the results are likely to be peculiar; for instance, the substitution of oleum rusci for oleum betulæ volatile in a mixture intended for internal use, and the very latest powdered althæ for taka-diastase, "but he knew althæ was harmless and he had never heard of taka-diastase." On writing a prescription containing a small amount of apomorphin in the treatment of certain forms of bronchitis I always add tincture of sanguinaria to prevent the druggist from assuring the patient that "It is an excellent emetic."

The remedy for all this lies with the physician; when his encouragement is sufficient to maintain a pharmacy for the compounding of prescriptions, for their original owner only, without repetitions, and when each druggist shall possess a pharmacopeia, which most of them do not, and when there is no vending of notions, patent-medicines, and no counter-prescribing, then, and not before, will pharmacy take its proper place and become an efficient aid to the science and art of healing. Druggists and the "Docs." of the corner will then be as extinct as the dodo. As matters now are the physician of six prescriptions is the one popular with the druggist, for he knows that as number six is reached number one is shortly due.

The druggist complains that we oblige him to carry an unnecessarily large stock. This is undoubtedly true, and our time is wasted in argument whether malt in a short fat bottle is better or worse than in a tall slim bottle; for probably both are equally useless excepting as bad beers. At present the average druggist is a stumbling-block of no mean dimensions to therapeutic progress. This would be reduced if he would keep in stock even the official drugs many of which are obtained with great difficulty. Whether a properly conducted pharmacy would be profitable or not I cannot say, for I have never known of the experiment being tried.

The surgeons complain that the same state of affairs obtains with the instrument- and appliance-makers; the making of an instrument or appliance confers a knowledge of its use. It is probably that the abuse is not so widespread as with druggists and is chiefly limited to the truss-makers. These have frequently found to their sorrow that trusses fail to give relief when the pad is applied over a bubo or an undescended testicle. Yet, many physicians and occasionally the surgeons deem the maker or even a druggist a proper person to apply the instrument, as a few instances, which have come under my personal observation, prove. That this habit is fairly widespread among physicians has been shown by the circulars which have been received on several occasions offering a commission upon all apparatus supplied by the manufacturer.

The contest with the refracting opticians is too recent to admit of additional statement. The success of the battle in the legislature shows that the public generally are not inclined to give to the glass-grinder the privilege of treating diseases of the eye, nor to others of similar trades which claim equal qualifications, the microscopic- and photographic-lens manufacturer.

The audacity of these people may be inferred from the statement of one of that class of artisans who recently assured me that he could "find the correct glass for any case of mixed astigmatism in five minutes." Here the remedy is the same as for druggists: patronize no optician who prescribes glasses or sells them without a prescription from an oculist. Incidentally, it should be observed that the financial arrangements between opticians and oculists should be discontinued to the benefit of both parties.

The Pedic Society claims the right, I believe, to perform all operations and apply treatment to the feet. Just how far their powers, as defined by legislative enactment, go I know not, but their claims tread upon the rights of the general orthopedic surgeon so far as concerns diseases and injuries of bones, cartilages, and muscles, which precludes their giving attention to bunions, while the skin and nails are within the province of the dermatologists, and this restrains their activity as regards corns and ingrowing nails. Whether they will be content with the application of plasters, or wish to cover the whole field, is not apparent; if the latter, edema of the feet will attract their attention, and by an early step they will advance to the treatment of diseases of the heart, liver, and kidneys, thus directly competing with the physician. The remedy appears simple. The unoccupied would-be surgeon can erect a new specialty and pedic surgeons will doubtless find plenty of employment, if only in demonstrating to the public that pedic differs from orthopedic—straight pedic surgery.

The barbers occasionally afford instances of the abuse of their occupations, aside from the vending of their depilatories, dyes, and hair-restorers. An instance recently came under my observation of a young girl who consulted me for an ailment of the digestive system. She called my attention to a small patch of inflammation on the forehead at the edge of her hair. Presumably there had existed a seborrhea which had been regularly treated by a barber for several months by application, so far as I could judge from her description, of a solution of iodin and silver nitrate. On assuring her that if it was let alone it would get well she departed. On her return two weeks later the inflammation had disappeared.

An amusing instance of the shoemaker not sticking to his last was found in the person of a man who complained of strangury, bloody urine, and painful erection, for which no physical cause could be found. Investigation, however, showed that a bald area upon his head had been treated by a barber with vigorous inunctions of his "capillary embrocation" with the result that the said area was well blistered. A cessation of the barber's treatment was followed by a relief of the symptoms. The supposition is that the "embrocation" contained cantharides.

For years it has apparently been the custom for bath attendants to prescribe for all sorts and conditions of ill-health. Many establishments advertise the removal of superfluous hair by electrolysis, and of late, since the Schott-Nauheim treatment for heart disease has been vulgarized, we find rubbers of high and low degree alike recounting the wonderful results accruing from the giving of saline carbonated baths and the application of resistive gymnastics. How far they carry out these upon their own responsibility it is not easy to say, but since most of them profess acquaintance with an English pot-boiler it is likely that some patients are not treated under a physician's direction. One instance has come under my observation: The book in question deserves severe condemnation for its general inaccuracy and positive untruthfulness. The author claims that some of the alleged illustrations were printed upside down; it is charitable to suppose that the text met the same fate. Sooner or later some one will die under treatment and an indictment for manslaughter will determine how far the physician's rights are encroached upon.

Trained and untrained nurses are frequent offenders in the way of prescribing, not for the person whom they are waiting upon, but generally for other members of the family. It is by no means uncommon to find that several members of a family are taking medicines upon the recommendations of the nurse. Some of these are patent, some are simple—generally remarkably simple and, therefore, adapted to those who take the wisdom of nurses for gospel—and occasionally some prescription "which has cured me of the trouble you have." The best way to deal with these offenders is to admonish them, and, in case of failure, to procure their discharge. One point deserves attention: never allow a nurse to talk of "his or her patient." Warn nurses at once that physicians only have patients and that nurses are only to obey the orders which they receive from them.

Bartenders have some reason but no excuse for practising medicine. Since they dispense poisons I presume they feel obliged to administer antidotes. The various bitters, malaria cures, and dyspepsia mixtures to be found in barrooms are not so objectionable if chloral and various coal-tar products could be kept out.

The worst offenders against decency and law are the midwives. If a Coroner in the city of New York is to be believed, the majority of them are midwives only in name, and infanticide, feticide, and murder can be justly charged against them. Under the existing laws there is no pretense of ascertaining the qualifications of these persons. Their legitimate work should be limited. When we take into consideration the large number of junior physicians who are willing to work for the same fees as do the midwives, and who would value the experience gained, there seems to be no reason for the perpetuation of what has become a crying evil. Besides this, many labors among the very poor could be utilized for the instruction of undergraduate medical students, under proper supervision, thus benefiting both student and patient. If the plea is made that this would throw out of employment a worthy class of women, the reply could be made that a superfluous vocation is abolished and that those engaged in it could become scrub-women, for which there is always a demand. The few midwives whom I have met, and that was during my residence in hospitals, were apparently only fitted for that somewhat laborious but certainly honest employment.

It is a curious fact, but I have never known of a veterinary surgeon prescribing for human beings, yet they are far better qualified than any of those previously mentioned.

I have not touched upon the illegal and brazen-faced encroachment of local boards of health upon the province of the physician, for this subject demands far more time than can be spared in this paper.[1] Their carrying out gratuitous vaccination, compulsory inspection of school children, segregation of patients afflicted with diseases assumed to be contagious, engaging in the manufacture and sale of vaccine and antitoxins, call for something more than a protest. The height of their impudence is their receiving an appropriation of public money for the printing and distribution of their defence. Pseudo-science is no less harmful when disseminated by the boards of health than by an individual, and much that has emanated from them would have received speedy and severe condemnation had it not been labeled as official.

The evils of which we may justly complain are of long standing and deeply seated. They undoubtedly arise partly from the desire of unqualified persons to assume knowledge which they do not possess, and, therefore, are willing to take risks which physicians would not, and partly from the ignorance of the public. It is useless to attempt to punish interlopers by process of law, for that is too tedious and altogether uncertain. Besides, any effort in that direction always excites the sympathy of the public, who are content with inferior products and who always take the side of those whom they deem to be persecuted. The public are beyond the possibility of education in medical matters. As Dr. Samuel Johnson said more than one hundred years ago: "The uncivilized, in all countries, have patience proportionate to their unskilfulness, and are content to attain their ends by very tedious methods."

To-day it is evident that the general public is, so far as medical matters are concerned, entirely uncivilized, in that they prefer those who pretend to those who possess scientific knowledge. The advancement of medical science comes only from the self-denial and devotion of the profession. On the part of the public there is no demand for the educated physician, for it is quite content with the pretense of the ignorant. The crowning honor of our profession lies in the fact that it is the only one which has raised its standard far above that demanded by the people and has maintained this position unaided by those who profit from its high place.

[1] Greanelle, *New York Medical Record*, December 25, 1897.

A FEW REMARKS ON THE DIET AND GENERAL CARE OF CONSUMPTIVES COMING TO SOUTHERN CALIFORNIA.

BY GEORGE L. COLE, M.D.,
OF LOS ANGELES, CAL.

ONLY a few days ago a patient consulted me who recently had been sent to this section by his physician from one of the middle Eastern States. He said that he had been told to go to Southern California, find a place suitable to live in, and to derive as much benefit as possible from the climate, and not waste his money on either physicians or drugs. He was expected to use his own judgment, and when he thought best, return to the East. Many similar cases met with here have impressed me with the fact that a few words on the subject may result in benefit to some who may seek such a change in the future.

Please imagine the responsibility thus laid upon the patient. How shall he find the place suitable for him? How shall he know where to find suitable lodgings and board? How shall he learn the proper clothing to wear in a climate wholly different from that which he has left? Most of all, how is he to judge competently of the improvement made at the end of three, six, or twelve months, in order that he may know whether it will be best to remain longer or to return to his home? He comes here during the winter months, and because he finds himself transported from snow and ice to a country in which sunshine and flowers abound he immediately dons his summer clothing and succeeds in contracting a cold, if nothing worse. He takes his first day's outing to an orange grove and proceeds to demoralize his digestive apparatus by picking and partaking of the golden fruit which at that time is unripe and unfit to eat. He returns to his temporary quarters at a hotel and awakens the next morning in anything but an amiable mood in which to set out in search of a permanent location—his stomach upset, and suffering from the effects of the cold he has contracted. He finds some pleasant rooms situated on the north side of a building where he does not notice the absence of the sun's rays from morning till night, but rather has his attention called to the "beautiful mountain view" by his would-be landlord, who is quietly reserving his sunny rooms for others more experienced in the requirements of the invalid. The patient does not notice that his room has no contrivance for providing proper artificial heat, or if he does notice the fact, he is promptly informed that one of those abominations with which the country abounds—a kerosene heater—will answer all purposes. In such quarters he takes up his abode, and succeeds in prolonging his cold until he has a genuine attack of bronchitis, and, augmenting his diet with green fruit, continues the disorder of his digestive organs, until, at the end of three or six months, he concludes that his own Eastern climate with home comforts is about as good for him as California and constant dyspepsia and bronchitis. And really he has now arrived at the proper conclusion. He begins to wonder if his lungs are in any better condition than when he came to such an abominable climate. He seeks a physician who has no data of his condition at the time he arrived in California, but who tries to put him aright in matters pertaining to location, clothing, diet, suitably heated, sunny apartments, and other matters connected with his general welfare and comfort, possibly suggesting some remedies which may tend to relieve the bronchitis and dyspepsia which he has contracted. The patient stays a month longer and returns to his Eastern home in a worse condition than when he left.

What a different picture is that presented by the patient who, on first going to a new section in which the conditions present such a contrast to those of his former home, seeks medical advice and is started out correctly at the beginning of his new experience. A careful physical examination is made and recorded, so that at some later time he may be intelligently informed as to the progress he has made, and some definite reason given why he should, on the one hand, remain longer, or, on the other, return to his home. By knowing his history and physical condition, the physician can direct him to a suitable location; and some location well suited to nearly every individul can be found within a radius of one hundred miles from Los Angeles. Any altitude from sea-level to six thousand feet can easily be secured, with comfortable quarters, and the patient may at the same time be guided to sections varying greatly in relative humidity.

Do not misunderstand me as pleading in behalf ot our local physicians for remunerative fees. It is not this; but the manifest injustice done by many Eastern medical gentlemen to their clients in this respect when sent to California has caused so much needless suffering among this class that I cannot forbear a word of criticism. At the same time I commend the host of Eastern physicians who provide their patients with suitable letters to physicians, who, while not infallible, nevertheless, do better in guiding the patient than he can do himself.

Successor to Tarnier.—Dr. Pierre Budin has been chosen to succeed Dr. Tarnier as clinical professor of obstetrics in the University of Paris.

THE CULTIVATION OF THE GONOCOCCUS.[1]

BY F. C. BUSCH, M.D.,
OF BUFFALO, N. Y.

THE gonococcus, which was discovered by Neisser in 1879, was first cultivated and thoroughly studied by Bumm in 1885. He succeeded, by inoculating with a culture of the twentieth generation, in producing a gonorrhea in the male urethra. The culture-medium employed by him was human blood-serum obtained by expression from a recently delivered placenta. Upon this medium but a scanty growth was obtained, and that with difficulty. The germ soon died out and had to be reinoculated every eighteen to twenty-four hours.

Since Bumm's monograph the gonococcus has been studied by a number of observers, using a variety of culture-media with more or less success. Schröter and Winkler in 1890 reported success in the use of albumen from the egg of the pewit. Anfuso, in 1891, cultivated the germ in knee-joint effusion from gonorrheal arthritis. Finger, Ghon, and Schlagenhaufer, in June, 1894, reported that sterile urine-agar made a favorable medium, and Turro, in the following month, reported success with acid-gelatin and gelatin-gelose.

Recent observers have been unable to repeat Turro's results, who neglected to state whether or not his diplococcus was stained by Gram's method. Bockart used a mixture of blood-serum and gelatin. Wertheim successfully employed a mixture of blood-serum and nutrient agar-agar. He was able to isolate the gonococcus by plating cultures while this mixture was in a liquid condition. Wright of Boston has recently used, with good results, a mixture of sterile urine (one part), serum (one part), and agar-agar (two parts). Heiman of New York, in 1895, and also in December, 1896, reported excellent results with a mixture of chest-serum and agar-agar. Upon this medium the gonococcus grows more readily than the pyogenic cocci, with the exception of the streptococcus. Hence, it can be used to separate the gonococcus from other organisms occurring in gonorrheal pus.

In endeavoring to obtain cultures of the gonococcus I have used the medium advised by Heiman. It was prepared in the following manner: Chest-serum was obtained from a patient with pleurisy and collected in a sterile flask. Agar-agar, which had been previously sterilized on three successive days, was melted and cooled to 40° C. (104 °F.). The chest-serum was heated to the same temperature. Equal parts of chest-serum and agar were thoroughly mixed and poured into tubes which were allowed to cool on the slant. These were sterilized in the steam steril-

[1] First Prize Essay, MEDICAL NEWS Prize Contest.

izer, at a temperature not exceeding 65° C. (149° F.), for one hour, on seven consecutive days. They were then placed in the incubator, at a temperature of 35° C. (95° F.) for forty-eight hours. The tubes which were without growth at the end of this time were stored in a cool place to prevent evaporation of their moisture. Tubes were also prepared with ascitic fluid in place of chest-serum. It is advisable, according to Heiman, to have the medium neutral in reaction. This can be accomplished by allowing the agar to remain slightly acid, trusting the serum to neutralize it. The neglect of this in my medium may account for several unfavorable results.

In most of the cases in which I was able to obtain the discharge the disease was of more than two-weeks' standing. There was present in all a small diplococcus which occupied the pus and epithelial cells and decolorized by Gram's method. Other micrococci were also present in most of them, and some showed a small diplococcus outside of the pus-cells which stained by Gram's method. This may have been the diplococcus urethræ of Heiman. The pus was obtained for examination and inoculation in the following manner: After the parts had been cleansed externally, the patient was instructed to squeeze several drops of pus from the urethra. A sterilized looped needle was then inserted well into the fossa navicularis and the adherent pus smeared on a slide or the surface of the culture-medium. Another method recommended, particularly when the discharge is slight, is to have the patient urinate into sterilized tubes of a size to fit the centrifugal-machine. These are then centrifuged and the sediment employed for examination and inoculation.

As a check on my results, tubes of plain agar-agar, as well as of chest-serum tubes, were inoculated in each case. The gonococcus practically does not grow on agar: that is to say, a scanty growth may very rarely be obtained upon this medium. Preparations made from the pus and from cultures were stained in all cases both by Löffler's solution of methylin-blue and by Gram's method. The gonococcus decolorizes by Gram's method and may be thus distinguished from other similar diplococci occurring in the male urethra which stain by this method. It is therefore evident that the use of the method mentioned is of primary importance in the identification of the gonococcus. Gram's method was employed in the following manner: The preparation, whether of pus or from culture, was stained one and one-half minutes in anilin violet water. Without washing, Gram's solution of iodin was then added and kept in contact with the specimen one and one-half to two minutes. The preparation was then washed in absolute alcohol ten seconds and in ninety-five per cent. alcohol from three to five minutes. I found that in all cases in which the gonococcus was present it would be decolorized within this time.

In several cases of my series cultures of the staphylococcus pyogenes aureus and albus were obtained upon agar agar without any growth upon chest-serum agar. In one case, large, white, glistening colonies of a diplococcus were obtained both upon agar-agar and chest-serum agar. This diplococcus was somewhat larger than the gonococcus and stained by Gram's method. In the following cases I succeeded in obtaining pure cultures of the gonococcus:

CASE I.—Male, aged twenty-one years, who had not been treated before the examination of his discharge and inoculation from it. He had been exposed to infection eight days before and had had a discharge three days. The discharge was copious and creamy. Specimen stained with methylin-blue showed pus-cells filled with small biscuit-shaped diplococci. Slides stained by Gram's method showed cells filled with diplococci which decolorized. There were also present a few larger diplococci, some micrococci, and a few short bacilli which took the stain by Gram's method. Two tubes of chest-serum agar and one of agar-agar were inoculated and placed in the incubator at a temperature of 35° C. (95° F.). At the end of forty-eight hours there was no growth visible upon the agar-agar. The chest-serum agar showed a light gray film along the line of smear with here and there a small, round, glistening, grayish-white colony. This growth, within the next forty-eight hours, increased until it covered a space 2 mm. wide along the line of streak.

Preparations made from the culture showed a small diplococcus which stained by methylin-blue and decolorized by Gram's method. Reinoculation from the original culture into chest-serum agar, showed, within the thirty-six hours, numerous colonies along the line of smear. These were small, round, and glistening, with opaque centers and translucent peripheries. Stained preparations showed the characteristic biscuit-shaped diplococci which decolorized by Gram's method. Reinoculations were made from culture to culture up to the tenth generation. A successful reinoculation was made from the original culture after being in the incubator twelve days.

CASE II.—A young negro, who had a slight discharge from the urethra four days after exposure. Stained preparations showed a diplococcus in the pus and epithelial cells, which decolorized by Gram's method. Inoculation on agar-agar was negative at the end of forty-eight hours. Inoculation on chest-serum agar showed isolated colonies similar in appearance to those obtained in Case I. Stained preparations showed a biscuit-shaped diplococcus which decolorized by Gram's method.

CASE III.—In this case the discharge had existed a week. Slides showed the diplococcus in the pus-cells, decolorizing by Gram's method. On the chest-serum agar colonies of the gonococcus were obtained within thirty-six hours. In several cases the ascitic fluid agar was employed, but without success.

Turro's method has also been tried in our laboratory, but without success. Concerning the diagnostic value of culture-methods in gonorrhea, I am at present not in a position to make any statement. Recent investigators report positive results in a large majority of cases, both acute and chronic, using chest-serum agar and urine-serum agar. It has been reported to me verbally that at Johns Hopkins University the gonococcus is being cultivated in albuminuric urine and agar.

Welch has been able to demonstrate the gonococcus, by stained preparation, in the blood of a patient with malignant endocarditis. By placing a drop of the patient's blood upon agar-agar a pure culture of the gonococcus was obtained, and the results were subsequently confirmed post-mortem.

Heiman states that he has been able to obtain the gonococcus in culture from tripperfäden when he couuld not demonstrate it by staining methods. If this can be done it will be of the utmost importance in determining whether or not the gonococcus is still present in individuals who have had the disease and have been apparently cured. The detection of gonococci in old tripperfäden might prevent much of the infection and misery of innocent women who become infected through their husbands.

MEDICAL PROGRESS.

Glycosuria in Primary Cancer of the Pancreas.—BARD and PIC, who have made a study of glycosuria in connection with cancer of the pancreas, have come to the following conclusions in regard to this affection: (1) Glycosuria, in these cases, presents itself under two conditions. Sometimes there is an abundant glycosuria accompanied by the symptoms of diabetes; sometimes there is a slight glycosuria with or without symptoms of diabetes. (2) Diabetes is independent of cancer of the pancreas, but it may in some measure assist in producing the former disease, and, conversely, the development of cancer may reduce or even cause diabetic phenomena to disappear. (3) Slight glycosuria is due to sclerosis of the pancreas, produced by cancerous obstruction of the canal of Wirsung. It is only found in a few cases. (4) Secondary sclerosis of the pancreas increases step by step with that of the liver. This parallelism may be clinically useful in the diagnosis of primary cancer of the pancreas.

Improved Method for Detecting Casts in Urine.—HAINES and SKINNER have described a combined subsidence and centrifuge method of detecting casts in the urine, which for ease and certainty leaves little to be desired. It is especially useful in those doubtful cases in which, if casts are present at all, they can be detected only after repeated examinations.

The method practised is as follows: About 250 c.c. or more of urine, as freshly voided as possible, are poured into a cylindric glass percolator, such as is used by druggists in making tinctures and fluid extracts. The opening at the bottom of the percolator is closed with a perforated rubber or cork stopper through which passes a piece of glass tubing about 4 cm. long, and this is connected with a short piece of rubber tubing provided with a pinch-cock. The entire apparatus, before the urine is poured in, should be washed thoroughly clean and sterilized. After pouring in the urine a gram or two of chloral hydrate, dissolved in a few cubic centimeters of warm distilled water, are added to retard decomposition. The percolator is now covered with a glass plate and set aside in a cool place for eighteen or twenty-four hours. By opening the pinch-cock on the rubber tubing the sediment is drawn off and collected in one or two centrifuging tubes. In all cases the first cubic centimeter or two may be rejected, as it contains little or none of the sediment. The centrifuge-tubes, which now contain 20 or 25 c.c. of urine, and practically all the sediment from the specimen, are placed in the centrifuge and submitted for a few minutes to about 3000 revolutions per minute. By this treatment the sediment is condensed to a small deposit at the apex of one or two tubes, from which it is removed by a pipette and examined under the microscope. With suitable care essentially the entire sediment from 250 c.c., or even 500 c.c. of urine from the average patient with suspected cirrhosis of the kidney, may by this procedure be reduced to from one to four small drops, in which, it is evident, are practically all the casts originally contained in the large volume of urine employed.

Singular as it may seem, the chief defect for clinical purposes in this method is possibly its too great delicacy. By its use the writers have found that if sufficient time and care be given to the microscopic examination, casts may be found in the majority of samples of urine even from persons in perfect health.

Scarlet Fever a Local Disease.—FLEMING (*Med. Record*, January 15, 1898) describes scarlet fever as a self-limited, acute, infectious, local disease of the throat, presenting marked general symptoms. It is the twin-sister of diphtheria. The idea that the desquamated skin is the source of the germ, and in consequence that the desquamatory period is most dangerous, is incorrect. Both diseases attack the mucous membranes of the throat, especially in children. Both have a tendency to invade the nares and trachea, and both likewise produce false membrane, the membrane being extensive in diphtheria, and slight in scarlet fever. Both diseases produce poisons similar in their destructive action upon the blood-corpuscles, as is exemplified in purpuric cases. In scarlet fever, however, the poison exercises a most marked irritative power on the organs by which it is eliminated; if by the bowels, it produces diarrhea; by the kidneys, nephritis; and by the skin, dermatitis. In several cases of scarlet fever recently observed, there was disease of the throat in all, varying in intensity from violent inflammation to severe involvement of all the cervical tissues. In one case there was a nasal discharge, as though the seat of the infection was in the nose. As a general rule the severity of the general symptoms in scarlet fever is in direct proportion to the severity of the local lesion in the throat. The rash is of more importance in a prognostic than in a diagnostic sense. Severe scarlet fever may exist without a rash. The rash indicates that the poison is being eliminated by the skin; whereas, an absence of rash indicates that it is being eliminated by other organs, usually the kidneys.

There are two cardinal rules for the treatment of scarlet fever. One is to practise disinfection at the seat of the disease, namely, in the throat, and the second, is to protect the kidneys at the expense of the skin. To accomplish the first, mild antiseptic mixtures should be given either in the form of throat douches or in teaspoonful doses to be swallowed. If scarlet fever and diphtheria are specific infected wounds of the throat, he who treats them locally on antiseptic principles is surely carrying out the idea and teachings of Lister.

How to Prevent Typhoid Fever in Rural Districts. — BASHORE (*Med. Record.*, January 15, 1898) says that the introduction of cisterns in rural districts will almost entirely eradicate typhoid fever. As an example he cites the experience in a town in Pennsylvania in which cistern water is used almost exclusively for drinking purposes because the limestone underlying the soil makes it impossible to obtain good well water. In this town, within the last five years, there have been only three cases of fever which were plainly typhoid, but even calling them so and reckoning one death for every twenty-six cases, would make the death-rate in this community from typhoid fever something like one per ten thousand. The unpleasant taste of cistern water is due to decomposing vegetable matter. This can be in a great measure avoided by having a "cut-off" by which the first water of the rainfall is turned into the street and not into the cistern. Further improvement in the water can be readily obtained by dividing the cistern by a brick partition, filling one-half of this to a depth of three feet with a filter of coarse sand and broken stone. The water is allowed to run into the side which contains the filter. It then passes through the filter and through holes at the bottom of the partition into the other side of the cistern from which it is pumped out for use. In this manner pure water may be obtained at small expense, and the family using it will absolutely avoid the possibility of having typhoid fever.

Gloves for Operative Purposes.—WOLFLER (*Fortschr. der Medicin*, November 15, 1897) says that he tried to find gloves suitable for operative purposes in England, America, and France, but without success, though as long ago as 1892 he obtained from Berlin a silk tricot glove covered with rubber which fulfils his purposes admirably. He employs it in case the rectum or vagina requires an investigation during operation, and also in septic operations. In ordinary aseptic operations he uses the usual leather army glove, which remains in a three-per-cent. solution of carbolic acid and glycerin when not in use. Before being used it is well washed with sterile salt solution, and afterward it is boiled and again placed in the carbolic-glycerin solution. Wölfler uses these gloves regularly, but while convinced of their value, he has not as yet prepared any figures showing the better results which he obtains by their use.

Protection of a Baby's Eyes.—BALDWIN (*Jour. Am. Med. Assoc.*, December 18, 1897) calls attention to the unfavorable conditions in which babies are usually placed while getting their daily outing in a baby-carriage. A glaring white blanket close to its eyes, and a white or mottled parasol with a deep fringe or ruffle waving or flapping in the sunshine, produce a needless strain upon the eyes, sufficient to explain the squinting which we so often see under these circumstances. This description applies to things at their best, and to those annoying conditions must usually be added the jolting of the carriage, and a careless arrangement of the parasol by a nurse whose attention is often fixed upon anything but the baby.

THERAPEUTIC NOTES.

Internal Use of Ichthyol in Respiratory Diseases.—LE TANNEUR (*Wien. med. Blätter*, December 2, 1897) has employed ichthyol internally in doses of 4 grains, eight times daily, with success for more than two years past in diseases of the respiratory tract. This success has followed not only in cases of a chronic character, such as tuberculosis, dry and purulent catarrh, and bronchiectasis with offensive expectoration, but more recently he has used the same remedy with equally good results in the acute attacks of bronchitis, which often arise in phthisical patients; as well as during attacks of acute bronchitis in otherwise healthy individuals. In some instances, within three days after the remedy was first given, the cough entirely ceased.

It is important to give the ichthyol in capsules of gluten, so that the capsules will reach the intestinal tract before being destroyed. Ichthyol is best taken immediately after eating, half of the daily dose after one meal, and half after another.

Treatment of Chronic Constipation by Creosote.—Creosote, according to HOLSTEIN (*Bull. Gen. de Therapeut.*, January 8, 1898), is an excellent remedy for chronic constipation if given in doses of 7 or 8 drops immediately after lunch and dinner, in a glass of milk, beer, wine, or water. As the dose which is necessary to relieve constipation is different for different persons it is well to commence with a single drop and to increase the amount by one drop daily, until the required dose is ascertained. Creosote, when administered in this way for several months, will not only relieve chronic constipation but will bring back the appetite, improve the general condition, and clear up the skin. Under its influence the stools become regular, soft and abundant, and are not accompanied by any pain or any sign of intestinal irritation. The drug is supposed to act by neutralizing an intestinal toxin which in chronic constipation paralyzes the intestine.

THE MEDICAL NEWS.

A WEEKLY JOURNAL

OF MEDICAL SCIENCE.

COMMUNICATIONS are invited from all parts of the world. Original articles contributed *exclusively* to THE MEDICAL NEWS will after publication be liberally paid for (accounts being rendered quarterly), or 250 reprints will be furnished in place of other remuneration. When necessary to elucidate the text, illustrations will be engraved from drawings or photographs furnished by the author. Manuscripts should be typewritten.

Address the Editor: J. RIDDLE GOFFE, M.D., No. 111 FIFTH AVENUE (corner of 18th St.), NEW YORK.

Subscription Price, including postage in U. S. and Canada.

PER ANNUM IN ADVANCE	$4.00
SINGLE COPIES	.10
WITH THE AMERICAN JOURNAL OF THE MEDICAL SCIENCES, PER ANNUM	7.50

Subscriptions may begin at any date. The safest mode of remittance is by bank check or postal money order, drawn to the order of the undersigned. When neither is accessible, remittances may be made, at the risk of the publishers, by forwarding in *registered* letters.

LEA BROTHERS & CO.,
No. 111 FIFTH AVENUE (corner of 18th St.), NEW YORK, AND NOS. 706, 708 & 710 SANSOM ST., PHILADELPHIA.

SATURDAY, APRIL 2, 1898.

A LIVING SUTURE.

THE man who is "hoist with his own petard" is an old acquaintance, but we must bid him good-by. Times are changing, and he must move on to make room for the man who is stitched with his own thews. The kangaroo, too, may sit undisturbed on his third hind leg. No longer will he be hunted for his tendon. Let the word go forth to the operating-rooms of two hemispheres that a better suture has been found,already sterile and fastened at one end—hidden in each patient like the lion in a block of marble, waiting for the artist who can see it and bring it into being.

The discoverer of this secret is a Parisian surgeon named Faure, who thus describes the operation for ventral hernia as performed by him with success:

An elliptic piece of skin is removed from the hernia, which is in the median line, and the edges of the separated recti muscles are freed by delicate dissection. This is done without opening the peritoneal cavity. From the anterior portion of the sheath of the rectus muscle, on either side, there is then cut a strip about six inches long, and a half an inch wide. Upon the left side this strip remains attached to its upper end, upon the right side at its lower end. These strips are then used as continuous sutures, the upper half of the wound being closed with the left strip and the lower half with the right strip, the suture passing through the recti muscles. These autosutures are knotted in the middle, and the knot, to make it more secure, is bound about with catgut. The wound in the skin is sutured with silk. In the case narrated primary union resulted, and three months later the abdominal wall was perfectly solid. Faure claims for this suture that it is a living one and will, therefore, unite with the portions of the body which are sewed by it. Though some skeptical surgeons may dispute the propriety of speaking of a strip of aponeurosis six inches long and half an inch wide as "living," yet surely none will be so mean-spirited as to deny to Monsieur Faure a corner position in the main aisle in the International Exhibition of Surgical Inventions.

THE SUPERIOR RESISTING POWER OF THE FEMALE PERITONEUM.

SOME months ago Haberkant published a series of statistics of operations of various sorts, from which it appears that the results obtained in abdominal perations are markedly better in women than in men. Thus, in his tables, pylorectomy in men was performed 70 times with a mortality of 64.3 per cent., and in women 140 times, with a mortality of only 52.8 per cent.—not a large difference, but still large enough to be noticeable. The difference in gastro-enterostomy was much greater. There were 117 operations in men, with a mortality of 54 per cent., and 96 in women, with a mortality of 35 per cent.

This difference is far too great to be set down to chance, and several scientific explanations have been offered. Perhaps the best of these is that of Terrier, who says that the lower mortality is due, not to a greater power of resistance in the woman, but to the fact that she comes earlier to operation. This results from several causes. If a woman has borne children her abdomen is flaccid, and so permits of an easier diagnosis. Women are more prone than men to seek medical advice, and to their credit be it said, more ready to follow it when given. For these three reasons Terrier believes that the affection at the time of operation is usually less severe in women than in men, and hence the lower mortality.

This explanation will appeal to many, but the simple statement that the power of resistance is greater in women than in man, will doubtless be given the preference by those women at least, who look forward to a happy day when the world will be run by women for women, and man, like the male spider, will be tolerated for a time, for breeding purposes, and then put out of the way as being too weak to live.

THE TRUE MEANING OF THE WINGATE-SPOONER BILL.

THE bill for a Commission of Public Health—variously called the Wingate Bill, from its putative parent, the Spooner Bill, from the Senator who introduced it by request, and falsely named by its friends as the Bill of the American Medical Association—means one of two things, a measure to obliterate the Marine Hospital Service, or a measure to provide forty-five gentlemen with public positions. That it certainly does the latter cannot be denied, for one of the chief sources of support which it has attained thus far has been the representatives of the State Boards of Health, who have provided for themselves these forty-five places of chief advisers in the great deliberative commission created by this measure. Until lately, it has been the policy of the framers of the Wingate Bill to protest that it meant no harm to their professional brothers who are officers in the Marine Hospital Service. It became necessary to do this in order to explain away satisfactorily to the friends of the Service the suspicion that the wholesale looting of its plant, as provided for in the bill, was simply technical language to provide for the ultilization of the Marine Hospital Service in its fullest and widest extent; that no humiliation was meant or intended, and that the promoters of the Wingate Bill had only sentiments of the highest consideration for the work and record of the Marine Hospital Service. All this masquerade has been carried on with the hollowness of theatric love-making. It was meant simply to amuse and deceive the public by a show of amity.

In such plays as this some member of the troupe can be relied upon to expose the true character of the performance. It now appears in a circular issued by the President of the American Public Health Association, which has been sedulously distributed to members of Congress, officers of medical colleges, health boards, and other kindred bodies, that the real purpose of the Wingate Bill is to wipe out the Marine Hospital Service.

In a circular addressed to members of Congress, dated Boston, March 1st, 1898, this official says: "The American Public Health Association, the largest sanitary body in the world at the present time, at its Twenty-fifth Annual Meeting, held in Philadelphia, during October last, voted to approve this bill, and the Committee of the American Medical Association is urging upon the Fifty-fifth Congress the necessity of establishing this Commission of Public Health, *which will take the place of what is now known as the Marine Hospital Service.*" This author, however, neglects to state that the vote by which this bill was approved, consisted of nineteen for, and seven against the bill, notwithstanding the fact that it was stated by its proposer that it had received the endorsement of the American Medical Association. A vote of twenty-six members out of nearly 1000 is not a conclusive expression of opinion.

In another circular, dated March 3, 1898, which is being sent to medical bodies, the same expression appears, that the American Medical Association (which has never approved this bill of Dr. Wingate) is urging upon Congress "the necessity of establishing a National Commission of Public Health, *which will take the place of what is now known as the Marine Hospital Service.*" No reason is given for the intended abolishment of the Marine Hospital Service, except the statement that the proposed commission is "broader in scope." This attack upon professional brothers engaged in a public-health service, as are the officers of the Marine Hospital Service, then, has no better basis than that it is "broader in scope." Reduced to its final terms this problem becomes a case of substitution. The support which it has is of two kinds—natural and artificial. It has the natural adhesion of officers of health boards of nearly every State, who see in it an office in the commission. It has the artificial support of one or two mercantile associations, whose knowledge of these conditions is based largely upon misunderstanding of the true character of the bill.

International Sanitary Convention.—The annual conference of State and Provincial Boards of Health of North America will take place at Detroit, Mich., August 9, 10, and 11, 1898. Benjamin Lee, M.D., of Philadelphia, is president of the Sanitary Conference.

ECHOES AND NEWS.

Dr. Biglow Appointed Examining Physician.—The Commissioner of Charities has appointed Dr. Horace Biglow examining physician at Bellevue Hospital, New York City.

A Hydrotherapeutic Clinic.—The Baden Legislature has voted the sum of 10,000 marks toward the establishment of a hydrotherapeutic clinic in the University of Heidelberg.

Crozer-Griffith Lectures at Bellevue.—Professor J. P. Crozer-Griffith of the University of Pennsylvania, Department of Diseases of Children, lectured by invitation of the Faculty before the Bellevue Hospital Medical College on March 22d. The subject of the lecture was "Typhoid Fever in Infants and Children."

Dr. LaPorte Acquitted.—The Court of Appeals has acquitted Dr. LaPorte who was recently convicted in Paris by the Court of First Instance of having caused the death of a patient by performing craniotomy. In addition, the Advocate-General has withdrawn all accusations against him. Dr. LaPorte is earning his living as a shorthand reporter.

New Hospital for New York.—The New York State Board of Charities has been requested to approve the incorporation of "The Storrs Memorial Hospital" of New York City. The hospital is intended as a memorial to the late Richard A. Storrs, Deputy Comptroller of the City of New York, and for nearly forty years connected with the comptroller's office.

Diphtheria in Brooklyn School.—The prevalence of diphtheria among the children of the kindergarten department of Public School No. 9, Borough of Brooklyn, has led to the closure of the school by the sanitary inspector of Brooklyn. The school is attended by nearly 1000 children, and twenty-six teachers are employed there. Fifteen cases of diphtheria have occurred.

Pasteur Institute at Florence.—A Pasteur Institute is to be established at Florence, Italy, for the treatment of rabies, its prophylaxis and cure, and snake-bite, the latter being of common occurrence in Tuscany, where most of the population is engaged in agriculture. Milan, Rome, and Naples are already provided with institutes in which the Pasteur treatment is employed.

Vital Statistics of Chicago.—The February bulletin of the Chicago Department of Health shows that during that month the total number of deaths from all causes was 2023, or 1.26 per thousand. In 105 instances death was due to violence. Of the 2758 births reported during the month, 1429 were males and 1329 females. There were also 162 premature and still-births.

A Specialist Wanted to Fill a Professional Chair.—The Chair of Diseases of the Eye, Ear, and Throat at the Medical College of Virginia, made vacant by the death of Professor Charles M. Shields, will be filled at the annual meeting of the board of visitors of the college, April 21st. All applications, accompanied by credentials, should be forwarded to Christopher Tompkins, M.D., Dean, Richmond, Va.

A Blow at "Face Specialists."—A bill has been introduced in the New York Assembly to put a stop to the work of unprincipled persons who make a business of removing facial blemishes and making dimples. The bill provides that such work may not be done by any but practising physicians. A fine of $250 and imprisonment for six months will be the penalty for the first offense, a fine of $500, and a year's imprisonment for a subsequent conviction.

Congress of Gynecology and Obstetrics.—The second periodic French Congress of Gynecology, Obstetrics, and Pediatrics will be held at Marseilles, France, from October 8th to 15th, under the presidency of Professor Pinnard (Section on Obstetrics), Professor Pozzi (Section on Gynecology), and Professor Broca (Section on Pediatrics). All communications should be addressed to Dr. Queirel, General Secretary of the Congress, 20 Rue Grignan, Marseilles.

Changes in the New York Sanitary Department.—Dr. Charles S. Benedict, who has been the Chief of the Bureau of Contagious Diseases in the New York City Health Department for a number of years, was recently removed by the commissioners and assigned to the minor post of diagnostician. Dr. Alonzo Blauvelt, the chief of the medical school inspectors, was appointed to Dr. Benedict's old place. The position made vacant by the transfer of Dr. Blauvelt was filled by Dr. E. J. Aspell, Dr. Benedict's former deputy.

Pension for Medical Officers.—A bill was recently introduced in the New York Senate providing that "any medical officer who has been in the service of the State in any of its institutions for the care of the insane for the term of fifteen years or longer shall, in case of being physically disabled, receive annually for life a sum equal to one-third the annual salary received at the time the pension is granted. If the officer shall have been in the service continuously for twenty years, his pension shall be one-half his annual salary."

Astoria Hospital to Close.—The Astoria (L. I.) Hospital, which was established by the women of the Astoria section of Long Island City, is to close its doors as soon as the patients now in the institution are well enough to be removed. Under the new charter the city authorities state that they cannot send public patients to the institution, and it cannot be successfully conducted without the income derived from them. The hospital was built three years ago through the generosity of Mrs. Hagameyer, who contributed $6000 to the building fund with the understanding that the managers should raise a like amount.

The Coroner's Jury.—One of the city's watchful representatives in the State Senate is worried over the pending bill to abolish that ancient implement of investigation, the coroner's jury. It is no rash plunge into the unknown, no reckless experiment beyond the field of experience, that the advocates of this bill are urging. Other States made this change years and years ago, and they not only survive, but prosper. In Massachusetts, for instance, no coroner's jury has exercised its owlish wisdom on a mysterious death since 1877. Before that, Suffolk County, which is Boston's, had forty-seven coroner's all to itself. The entire forty-seven, and their almost innumerable jurymen, were then supplanted by just two officials, who have continued to do, in an entirely satisfactory manner, all the probing of mysteries to which the police and other regular courts did not attend. Here are some figures as to the relative expense of the Massachusetts and the New York system: For this coming year it is estimated that the coroners of the five city boroughs will use up $239,050; that is what they ask for, and it means a tax of 7 cents per capita on the city's population. The cost for Massachusetts will be $30,600, a tax of 1⅓ cents per capita for the whole State. Still our able representative says we are not prepared to risk a change!—*New York Times.*

Secret, Proprietary, and Trade-marked Medicinal Preparations.—*The Philadelphia Polyclinic*, March 19th, makes the following editorial comments: "We are very sorry to be obliged to differ from our highly respected contemporary, the *Philadelphia Medical Journal*, on so important a question as the legitimacy of certain medicinal preparations; nor can we altogether admire the tone of its reply to the criticisms of the *Pennsylvania Medical Journal* on this subject. Surely the 'holler-than-thou' epithet is not argument, and its use should be left to the nostrum-defenders. The confusion which these latter gentlemen like to throw about the main question, especially when advertisements are under consideration, seems, very strangely, to have affected in some degree our usually clear-sighted contemporary of Philadelphia. Undoubtedly the true line of cleavage between the permissible and the non-permissible, *cæteris paribus*, is the line of secrecy. Our contemporary rightly insists on this, but it fails to apply the principle correctly. Secrecy takes many different forms, and some of these are the more objectionable that they are sought to be cunningly concealed so that the secret nostrum may masquerade as a preparation devoid of taint. Hidden secrecy is not a paradox or a hyperbole, but a fact well known in the drug trade. Or, most perverse of perversions, there may be a claim or hint of secrecy when no secret exists. But in such a case, fraud is intended. Our contemporary has admitted to its advertising columns preparations that the *Polyclinic* has consistently refused to advertise. Herein there may be only differences of judgment; one editor or publisher may be as easily mistaken as the other. Neither should call names. Our contemporary is right in saying that everything is proprietary; but at the same time it knows, or ought to know, that by a 'proprietary medicine' is meant one that is made by a proprietor and cannot be made by others, because of the trade-mark, patent, or secrecy. With our contemporary we prefer to drop the word altogether, and thus be able to fight secrecy in all its forms, cunning or foolish, without confusion or false issues."

Preliminary Program of the Thirteenth Annual Meeting of the Association of American Physicians, to Be Held in the Arlington Hotel, Washington, D. C., May 3, 4, and 5, 1898.—1. President's Address, F. C. Shattuck, Boston. 2. Discussion—"Is a Uric-Acid Diathesis an Important Factor in Pathology?"; referee representing physiological chemistry, V. C. Vaughan, Ann Arbor; referee representing clinical medicine, Wm. H. Draper, New York; co-referee representing clinical medicine, James Tyson, Philadelphia. 3. "Bacillus Icteroides (Sanarelli) and Bacillus X" (Sternberg), George M. Sternberg, Washington. 4. "Comparative Studies of Bovine Tubercle Bacilli and of Human" (sputum), Theobald Smith, Boston. 5. "Actinomycotic Forms of the Bacillus Tuberculosis; an Experimental Study," Simon Flexner, Baltimore. 6. "Gastric Syphilis, with the Report of a Case of Perforating Syphilitic Ulcer of the Stomach," Simon Flexner, Baltimore. 7. "Some Observations on Cardiac Syphilis," I. Adler, New York. 8. "Danger of Error in Diagnosis between Chronic Syphilitic Fever and Tuberculosis," E. G. Janeway, New York. 9. "Two Attacks of Temporary Hemiplegia Occurring in the Same Individual as the Result of the Use of Peroxid of Hydrogen in a Sacculated Empyema" (pleural), E. G. Janeway, New York. 10. "Acute Interstitial Nephritis," Wm. T. Councilman, Boston. 11. "Chronic Interstitial Nephritis" (by title), I. N. Danforth, Chicago. 12. "Acute Leucemia," M. H. Fussell and A. E. Taylor, Philadelphia. 13. "Bacteriology of Cheese," V. C. Vaughan and Julian T. McClymonds, Ann Arbor. 14. "A Chapter in Peripheral Pathology; the Circulation in the Feet," Morris Longstretch, Philadelphia. 15. "A Case of Chronic Infective Endocarditis, with Streptococci Found in the Blood before Death Treated by Antistreptococcus Serum, and Experimental Researches upon the Effects of Injections of Antitoxins upon the Kidneys," W. H. Thomson, New York. 16. "Nephritis of Malarial Origin," W. S. Thayer, Baltimore. 17. "Experiments upon the Localization of Micro-organisms in the Spleen and the Importance of a Lesion of an Organ for the Localization of Bacteria within It," S. J. Meltzer and T. M. Cheesman, New York. 18. "Congenital Stenosis of Pylorus in Infants," S. J. Meltzer, New York. 19. "Paralysis of the Left Recurrent Laryngeal Nerve in Mitral Stenosis," Wm. Osler, Baltimore. 20. "Combined Symptoms of Myxedema and Exophthalmic Goiter," Wm. Osler, Baltimore. 21. "The Renal Form of Enteric Fever," J. C. Wilson, Philadelphia. 22. "Gastric Carcinoma Associated with Hyperchlorhydria," D. D. Stewart, Philadelphia. 23. "The Diffuse Infiltrating Form of Secondary Melanosarcoma of the Liver" (by title), L. Hektoen, Chicago. 24. "A Case of Myxedema and Albumosuria; Treatment with Thyroid Extract; Death," R. H. Fitz, Boston. 25. "Some Usually Overlooked Physical Signs in Chest Diseases," Norman Bridge, Los Angeles. 26. "Studies of Antitoxins for Tuberculosis," E. L. Trudeau and E. R. Baldwin, Saranac Lake. 27. "Report of a Case of Madura Foot," J. H. Wright, Boston. 28. "Antitoxin Treatment of Pneumonia," A. H. Smith, New York.

ANNOUNCEMENT.

ANNUAL MEETING OF THE AMERICAN MEDICAL ASSOCIATION.

THE forty-ninth annual session of this Association will be held in Denver, Col., Tuesday, Wednesday, Thursday, and Friday, June 7, 8, 9, and 10, 1898. By a circular letter recently issued by the officers of the Society, attention is called to the fact that in future each delegate or permanent member when he registers shall also record the name of the section, if any, which he will attend, and in which he will cast his vote for section officers. An amendment to the constitution and by-laws of the Association will be presented whose sentiment favors greater liberality in the matter of membership. It reads thus: "Any State or local medical society or other organized institution whose rules, regulations, and code of ethics agree in principle with those of this Association, may be entitled to representation on the advice or agreement of the Judicial Council." The general addresses will be as follows: Presidential Address, George M. Sternberg, Washington, D. C.: Address in Surgery, J. B. Murphy, Chicago; Address in Medicine, J. H. Musser; Address in State Medicine, not yet determined. The officers of the various sections are as follows

Practice of Medicine.—S. A. Fisk, Denver, Col., chairman; A. A. Jones, Buffalo, N. Y., secretary.

Surgery and Anatomy.—W. L. Rodman, Louisville, Ky., chairman; Clayton Parkhill, Denver, Col., secretary.

Obstetrics and Diseases of Women.—Joseph Price, Philadelphia, Pa., chairman; C. Lester Hall, Kansas City, Mo., secretary.

Ophthalmology. — Harold Gifford, Omaha, Neb., chairman; Robert L. Randolph, Baltimore, Md., secretary.

Laryngology and Otology.—B. Alexander Randall, Philadelphia, Pa., chairman; S. E. Solly, Colorado Springs, Col., secretary.

Diseases of Children.—J. P. Crozer Griffith, Philadelphia, Pa., chairman; Edwin Rosenthal, Philadelphia, Pa., secretary.

Materia Medica, Pharmacy, and Therapeutics.—John V. Shoemaker, Philadelphia, Pa., chairman; C. C. Fite, New York, N. Y., secretary.

Physiology and Dietetics.—Randall Hunt, Shreveport, La., chairman; A. H. Tuttle, Cambridge, Mass., secretary.

Neurology and Medical Jurisprudence.—Charles H. Hughes, St. Louis, Mo., chairman; Hugh T. Patrick, Chicago, Ill., secretary.

Cutaneous Medicine and Surgery.—A. W. Brayton, Indianapolis, Ind., chairman; T. C. Gilchrist, Baltimore, Md., secretary.

State Medicine.—I. N. Quimby, Jersey City, N. J., chairman; Arthur R. Reynolds, Chicago, Ill., secretary.

Stomatology.—G. V. I. Brown, Duluth, Minn., chairman; Eugene S. Talbot, Chicago, Ill., secretary.

Permanent Secretary.—Wm. B. Atkinson.

These officers are already active in securing interesting programs, and those which have been issued give promise of a most instructive and delightful session. Moreover, the medical profession of Denver and of the State of Colorado give every assurance that a good time will be in waiting for all their visitors upon this occasion. The generous hospitality of that magnificent city of the Rocky Mountains is neglecting nothing which will add to the comfort and pleasure of her guests. Excursions are being planned to reveal the rugged grandeur of the mountains and the interesting products of the deepest mines, and opportunities will be given to experience the qualities of Colorado's rarefied, health-giving atmosphere, and to investigate those features of climate and soil which make Colorado a boon to all those who require the most healthful environment.

CORRESPONDENCE.

THE GERMAN UNIVERSITY WORKING YEAR.

To the Editor of the MEDICAL NEWS.

DEAR SIR: Your Berlin letter in the issue of the MEDICAL NEWS for March 19th, contains some errors which might be said to offset the mistake of *The Times* mentioned. The summer semester in German universities closes officially August 15th, really in the last week of July, and not July 1st. The course, therefore, equals seven months, including the Christmas and Whitsuntide vacations. About the end of every semester there is usually some talk in university and other circles of adhering to the official dates, but for many reasons, some of them obvious, this is not done.

Several things might be said in favor of the German arrangement, but even if agreed upon it would be difficult to apply in American schools.

Sincerely yours,
GEORGE DOCK.

ANN ARBOR, MICH., March 21, 1898.

A LONG APPENDIX.

To the Editor of the MEDICAL NEWS.

DEAR SIR: In an article by Dr. Bryant (Notes on Appendicitis, with Report of Interesting Cases), in the last issue of the MEDICAL NEWS, he mentions a case in which operation was performed at St. Vincent's Hospital and in which he removed an appendix measuring four and one-half inches in length. In his verbal illustration of the "interesting and somewhat unusual features" of this particular case he uses the words "marked length." This recalls to my mind the unique case of Grant Price, a colored male convict, aged twenty-six, suffering from chronic relapsing catarrhal appendicitis, upon whom I operated during April, 1892, at the State Prison Hospital, Frankfort, Ky., removing an appendix nine and one-half inches in length. The specimen is now in the possession of Dr. William A. Bolling of Frankfort, Ky.

I have often thought of reporting this case, but as its only interesting feature was the extreme length of the appendix I failed to do so until now. I hope it may prove of worth, since one four and three-quarter inches shorter is considered by so good an anatomist as Dr. Bryant as worthy of special comment.

I am not familiar with the extremes in the length of this organ. Anatomists and operators give it as varying between three and six inches. The latter figure seems to be the exception, this being the only case that I have ever known to go beyond or even reach it.

Respectfully,

WALLER H. DADE, M.D.

CHICAGO, March 7, 1898.

OUR PHILADELPHIA LETTER.

[From our Special Correspondent.]

ANOTHER "DIVINE HEALER"—DIETETIC VALUE OF EDIBLE MUSHROOMS—MEETING OF THE ASSOCIATED HEALTH AUTHORITIES OF PENNSYLVANIA—NATHAN LEWIS HATFIELD PRIZE ESSAY—CHANGE IN THE PLANS OF THE PAY HOSPITAL FOR CONTAGIOUS DISEASES—ANOTHER BEQUEST TO THE PENNSYLVANIA HOSPITAL—DR. ALFRED STENGEL—WILLIAM PEPPER MEDICAL ASSOCIATION.

PHILADELPHIA, March 26, 1898.

THE presence in this city of another "divine healer" of the Schlatter type again proves the truth of the sage oxiom of the late Mr. Barnum concerning the gullibility of the great mass of the public. This new medical impostor, who styles himself Father Girand, has during several weeks been industriously "healing" large numbers of the hyponchrondriac lame, halt, and blind, and the crowd of medical-bargain seekers which applies to him for relief from real and fancied ills is at times so great that one must possess both patience and a knack of insinuating one's self through a throng in order to reach the presence of the "healer." Girand, who claims to be a regularly ordained priest of the Roman Catholic Church, has been denounced as "a capital fraud" by the Archbishop of Philadelphia, and has been ordered by this prelate to immediately leave the city. But despite the Archbishop's denunciation and his mandate, this pseudo-healer refuses to give up his occupation—in fact, the added notoriety which the Archbishop's notice has given him has served rather to increase than to decrease his clientele, and he is at present daily consulted by hundreds of persons. It is a curious fact that a large number of his patients are Catholics, who continue to express their belief in this object of the head of their church's disapproval. Aside from the general consideration of the lamentable effects which must be produced upon the credulous and the ignorant of the community by the unchecked progress of the gigantic burlesque, the incident serves to demonstrate once more the absolute impotence of our laws to prevent the perpetration of such swindles as this. What, with faith-curists, homeopaths, antivaccinationists, and antivivisectionists, the already too much befooled public have enough to stagger under, without this last swindle, instances of which, since Schlatter's advent here, have become of too frequent occurrence. We have laws to prevent the adulteration of the food intended for our stomachs, but no laws to prevent the dissemination of food like this for our minds.

The report of the recently concluded investigations of the physiologic properties of edible mushrooms and other fungi, made by the American Physiological Society, at the instigation of Dr. S. Wier Mitchell, has shown the fallacy of the popular belief in the great nutritive properties possessed by these articles of food. According to these investigations, the total amount of available proteid present in these fungi is never more than two or three per cent., and their nitrogenous elements chiefly consist of non-proteid bodies. The amount of fat, cholesterin, soluble carbohydrates, fibers, and organic substances found in mushrooms corresponds very nearly to that found in such common articles of vegetable diet as potatoes, corn, and peas. The commission in charge of this study consisted of Professors Mendel and Chittenden of Yale University, Professors Bowdich and Pfaff of Harvard University, and Professor Abel of Johns Hopkins University. The report of these gentlemen seems to prove that, while mushrooms may be of service as dietetic accessories, they far from deserve the term "vegetable beefsteaks," with which the popular mind is prone to associate them.

The fifth annual meeting of the Associated Health Authorities of Pennsylvania will take place in Lancaster, May 18th and 19th, next. Inasmuch as funds are lacking for the purpose of making this meeting a representative State sanitary convention, the aim will be to broaden the scope of the convention in other ways and to embrace subjects not usually treated at a meeting of health authorities. Educational hygeine, for instance, is to be a special feature of the meeting, in view of the large State educational institutions situated in the immediate vicinity of the place of meeting, these institutions serving a very practical purpose for the elaboration of this particular topic. Part of the proceedings will be held in conjunction with those of the Pennsylvania State Medical Society, which convenes in Lancaster at the same time. The annual address will be delivered by that authority on forestry, Professor J. T. Rothrock, Forestry Commissioner of Pennsylvania, his subject being "The Highlands of Pennsylvania in Relation to Sanitation and Public Health." By invitation of the State Board of Health the attending members will inspect the celebrated Lancaster County Vaccine Farms at Marietta, a few miles from the city of Lancaster. The meeting will be presided over by the First Vice-President, Crosby Gray, Esq., Superintendent of the Bureau of Health of Pittsburg.

The subject for the initial competition of the newly founded "Nathan Lewis Hatfield Prize" will be announced this fall by the committee of the College of Physicians of Philadelphia. The scope of the competitive essays will be limited to some subject in general medicine, medical pathology, or therapeutics. The value of the prize is never to be under $500, to be awarded triennially, under the usual rules governing such competitions, to members of the medical profession of the United States. The successful essay will be published in book form by the college, whose property it will become according to the terms of the deed. The deed of trust conveying the sum of $6000, the principal of the award, to Drs. J. M. Da Costa, Herbert Norris, and R. G. Le Conte, has just been executed by Walter and Henry Hatfield of this city, the donors of this memorial to their father, the late Dr. Nathan Lewis Hatfield.

The officers of the proposed Pay Hospital for Contagious Diseases now announce that they have resolved to abandon their first plan of beginning the new hospital in a small way, and that they require for their more extensive efforts a sum of not less than $100,000 for the purchase of grounds and for the erection of buildings. The establishment of this new hospital, which will certainly fill an urgent need, seems an assured fact, and it is hoped that no delay will ensue in the erection of this institution, in which persons suffering from contagious diseases may be treated by their own physicians at a cost proportionate to their means. The charter has already been granted for the hospital, and a full board of officers has been elected.

The Pennsylvania Hospital of this city has long borne the reputation of being one of the most richly endowed hospitals of its kind in America. To its already ample funds has just been added another legacy, estimated to be worth between $50,000 and $75,000, by the will of the late William J. Headlam, who died in this city this week. The entire estate of the donor is bequeathed to the Pennsylvania Hospital. This last gift recalls the huge sums of which this institution has been recipient in the very near past, and it is found that within the past six weeks no less than $500,000 has been left outright to it, not to mention a contingent bequest of $2,000,000, which in every probability will revert to the hospital in the course of time. It is of interest to note that the Pennsylvania Hospital does not receive a penny of State aid, being supported entirely by the gifts of individuals.

Dr. Alfred Stengel o the University of Pennsylvania, has left for Cleveland, Ohio, where he is to deliver a course of lectures on topics of internal medicine by invitation of the Cleveland Medical Society.

Dr. William Pepper, according to his annual custom, gave a large reception on March 25th, in remembrance of the thirty-fourth anniversary of the William Pepper Medical Association. The reception was attended by a large number of prominent Philadelphia medical men, and by many physicians from the vicinity of the city.

OUR BERLIN LETTER.

[From our Special Correspondent.]

SECONDARY INFECTION WITH TUBERCLE BACILLI—A RETURN TO SOME OLD OPINIONS—FRESH AIR AND OXYGEN IN PNEUMONIA—INTEREST IN DIABETES.

BERLIN, March 24, 1898.

THE discussion of the question of secondary infection with tuberculosis, raised by Professor Hansemann's paper at a recent meeting of the Berlin Medical Society, is interesting as an example of the way the pendulum of medical opinion swings now this way and now that, let us hope with each swing remaining a little nearer the dead center, where truth lies, than before. With the discovery of the tubercle bacillus came an era when at least the younger pathologists explained all the pathologic anatomic lesions in which the presence of the tubercle bacillus could be demonstrated as due to the activity of this germ and the toxins to which it gave rise.

Then came a second era, not so long ago, here we are yet in the midst of it, when it began to be realized that many of the worst pathologic lesions of so-called tuberculous processes were really due to the presence of a secondary infection with the ordinary pus cocci, the staphylococci, and certain forms of streptococci. The significance of this secondary infection has been so overvalued (the over-swing of the pendulum once more) that most of the symptoms ordinarily considered to be characteristic of tuberculosis have been attributed to it. The chill and fever, the sweating, the hectic temperature, the breaking down of pulmonary tissue, much even of the cachexia, has been accredited to the presence of pus cocci and the absorption of their toxins into the system.

Professor Fränkel, from whom the Fränkel-Weichselbaum diplococcus pneumoniæ derives its name, said decidedly, at the meeting referred to, that an infection with tubercle bacilli alone may cause the remittent fever and the hectic temperature, exclusive of secondary infection.

Now comes the other phase of secondary infection: How often does the tubercle bacillus gain its foothold because there is already a lowering of vital resistance from prior infection? Professor Heubner reported some cases not long since in which patients with bronchiectasis had become infected with tubercle bacilli, and in many more cases than has been so far suspected this would seem to have been the case. Professor Hansemann added a number of other conditions in which the tuberculous infection might be considered secondary, in which in fact, the most careful bacteriologic examination seemed to demonstrate this.

Certain enlarged glands, not alone from the cervical region, but also from the mesentery, were shown to contain tubercle bacilli, though in other glands from the same individual even the delicate test of inoculating guinea-pigs with the suspected material failed to disclose their presence. Ordinary microscopic examination is of no value for negative results, but these negative inoculations Professor Hansemann considers sufficient to justify the conclusion that some of the enlarged glands did not owe their enlargement to tubercle bacilli; for the glands taken for inoculation were not the cheesy masses in which the process of degeneration had, as has often been noted, led to the disappearance of the bacilli, but the ordinary enlarged glands of comparatively recent infection.

In these cases the enlarged glands would seem to be secondarily infected with tubercle bacilli, and Professor Hansemann considers that many scrofulous cases are of this character. The cervical glands in an especially unresistant subject, readily enlarge as the result of infection through carious teeth, through the tonsils, through small wounds, or the lesions of eczema, or by means of parasitic diseases of the hairy scalp. These enlarged glands, with sluggish lymphatic circulation, incomplete metabolic processes, and defective oxygenation, form an excellent nidus for the development of the tubercle bacillus.

It is the complete justification of the old medical saying, formulated by Niemeyer in the dualistic tubercle days: "The greatest danger a scrofulous person is in, is the danger of becoming tuberculous." Many of the older pathologists, Professor Virchow among the number, have never admitted that all the pathologic lesions noted in tuberculous cases are due to the tubercle bacilli. To them, this atavistic reversion to an older opinion under a new name must be a little amusing. During the discussion it was evident that many of the prominent medical men were believers in this secondary infection with tubercle bacilli.

Professor Senator, especially, was frankly outspoken in his opinion that injured or diseased tissue was much more unresistant to tuberculous infection. I have mentioned secondary infection in glands alone, because in these the question is at its simplest. Other striking examples were given: Tuberculous intestinal ulcer after and on the remains of a typhoid ulcer; tuberculous infection of fibrinous and syphilitic pneumonia; tuberculous invasion after injury to, or venereal disease of, the testicle, prostate, seminal vesicles, and Fallopian tubes.

Something of the importance placed on the therapeutic value of fresh air in pneumonia, may be judged from the fact that when pneumonia patients are brought before a clinic, at the Charité for instance, they are never kept in the clinic-room more than the few minutes necessary to demonstrate the physical signs of the disease. Professor Gerhardt says that he has seen patients have a sudden change for the worse after having been kept in the clinic-room some time and that under circumstances such that he could not but attribute it to their confinement in a room with vitiated air; for it does not seem to be so much the mere fact of the diminution of oxygen in the air, as the presence of morbid, organic, respiratory products, which breathed into a partially consolidated lung are more easily retained there.

With regard to oxygen in pneumonia, experience with it here has not been favorable. After a thorough trial, its use has been completely abandoned, despite the fact that at first there seemed to be some excellent results in severe cases.

The special invitation to Professor Leo of Bonn to talk on the therapeutics of diabetes at the coming German Congress for Internal Medicine, to be held at Wiesbaden during the middle of April, is an index of the present lively interest in diabetes in Germany. All the clinicians and neurologists, for of late years its connection with the nervous system symptomatically and etiologically has been its specially interesting feature, are agreed that the disease is on the increase. This is not a relative increase due to more careful or to more accurate methods of diagnosis, but an actual increase of the number of people whose metabolic faculty for sugar consumption has become defective.

Toward the end of the semester I heard Professors Senator, Gerhardt, and Mendel each express this opinion in clinical lectures. Each of them at the same time called attention to the feature of the disease which is at present attracting so much attention, *viz.:* its proneness to occur in a notable percentage of cases in husband and wife. There seems to be no doubt that this is the case too often for it to be merely a coincidence, and that the theory that it is due to the family abuse of certain articles of diet, especially the carbohydrates, is not sufficient explanation. There is some closer etiologic connection.

Here, in all cases of diabetes, syphilis is looked for in the history, and often a course of mercury and iodids is tried as the first thing in treatment. The characteristic lesions of syphilis in the liver, the kidney, the base of the tongue, and the testicle are looked for at autopsies, and it is not very infrequently that at least some of them are found. This is a time of syphilophobia, and since the connection between tabes and many of the chronic nervous diseases has been demonstrated, the etiology of most obscure pathologic processes is looked for in syphilis. In pernicious anemia, for instance, the pathologic anatomists and the clinicians are agreed that it plays an important etiologic rôle.

With regard to the therapeutics of diabetes, Professor Gerhardt, in talking of diabetic coma in his last lecture of the semester, said that he had never seen the slightest good result from the subcutaneous injection of alkalies. It was considered theoretically possible to thus neutralize the toxic acids (oxybutyric and diacetic), whose presence in the blood is thought to cause the coma. Naunyn, from Strassburg, has reported some excellent results from the practical application of the theory by the injection of bicarbonate of soda. The improvement did not last long, but there was a distinct remission in all the symptoms, sometimes to the extent of complete restoration of the patient to consciousness for some hours. Professor Gerhardt, to whom medicine owes the iron-chlorid test for the presence of the acid toxins in the urine, as a warning of the approach of diabetic coma, and for whom the subject has always been a favorite study, does not think that by this means he has ever lengthened life by an hour, or given a moment's consciousness that would not have come of itself. In his hands, too, the injections of large amounts of saline solution—the so-called washing of the blood—and so removing toxins, has had no effect.

TRANSACTIONS OF FOREIGN SOCIETIES

Paris.

SURGERY OF THE STOMACH—TREATMENT OF NIGHT-SWEATS OF PHTHISIS WITH ACETATE OF THALLIUM—SUPRASPINOUS LUXATION OF THE EXTREMITY OF THE CLAVICLE—OPERATIVE TREATMENT OF BADLY UNITED POTT'S FRACTURES—ARTHROTOMY FOR OLD DISLOCATIONS AT THE SHOULDER-JOINT—HEMORRHAGE CONTROLLED BY GELATIN—AN UNUSUAL FOREIGN BODY IN THE STOMACH—THE FUNCTION OF THE LARGE OMENTUM.

AT the session of the Academy of Medicine of February 8th, DOYEN announced that he had performed 146 operations for different diseases of the stomach with 30 deaths, 20 being in malignant cases. Of the last 55 operations in benign cases, 50 were successful. It appears, therefore, that surgical intervention in non-malignant affections of the stomach is not so very serious.

Doyen advocated gastro-enterostomy not only for pyloric disease but also for those patients afflicted with gastric hyperesthesia, dilatation, and ulcer, either with or without hematemesis. The mortality of gastro-enterostomy has been greatly reduced by improved methods and instruments.

At the session of February 22d, COMBEMALE read a paper upon "The Treatment of Night-sweats of Phthisis with Acetate of Thallium." He has had only one failure in the treatment of thirty patients. The remedy also exercises a beneficial effect upon chronic catarrh due to bronchial dilation, emphysema, etc. The daily dose is from 1 to 2 grains, given in pills about one hour before bed-time. It should never be given during more than four successive days.

At the Surgical Society, February 2d, REYNIER spoke of supraspinous luxation of the extremity of the clavicle. This luxation is sometimes called post-acromial. Reynier was called to see a patient who had been run over by a carriage. A supraspinus luxation of the clavicle was easily demonstrated. It was, however, impossible to bring the bone into its normal position, and when partially reduced, the deformity had a tendency to recur. An incision was therefore made, and muscle-fibers of the trapezius were found to intervene between the clavicle and scapula. The conoid and trapezoid ligaments were ruptured. Recovery after operation was perfect.

At the session of February 16th, KIRMISSON discussed the operative treatment of badly united Pott's fractures. The subject of the paper was a man aged forty-six years, upon whom a double osteotomy had been performed, that of the fibula being linear and that of the tibia cuneiform. A month later the deformity of flat-foot was reproduced; the peroneal tendons were then cut and the normal condition of the foot was restored. Still, the patient had very little use of it. The difficulty lay, according to Kirmisson, in the fact that the operative effort was not expended upon the tibiotarsal articulation. By resection of a portion of the tibia, coupled, if necessary, with division of the fibula, he had in eight cases restored the function of the joint. Reynier said he had usually found supramalleolar osteotomy sufficient in simple cases. At times the irregularities of the articular surface of the tibia may require excision.

At the session of February 23d, NELATON read a paper upon "Arthrotomy for Old Dislocations at the Shoulder-joint." He made a distinction between (1) cases primarily irreducible on account of the position between the bones of the capsule of the joint or some tendon; (2) those cases in which it is still the capsule which prevents reduction, but in which a considerable interval of time has elapsed, though less than six weeks, and (3) those cases in which more than six weeks have elapsed and in which the joint is therefore already destroyed. The treatment recommended in the first class is immediate operation, and in the second, operation is also indicated, with a sufficient division of the capsule to permit the reduction of the head of the bone. In the third class, it is useless to attempt to put the head of the bone back into the joint cavity which no longer exists.

At the Medical Society of the Hospitals, February 11th, SIREDEY said that he had treated with success nine cases of metrorrhagia, and one of severe epistaxis, using tampons containing gelatinized serum. This is made by dissolving gelatin in normal salt solution to the extent of five to ten per cent. It should then be sterilized fifteen minutes on two succeeding days, and, when wanted for use, it can be melted by placing the vessel containing it in boiling water.

HAYEN gave an illustration of the retention in the stomach of a curious foreign body which examination showed to be composed chiefly of butter. The patient had been sometime upon a milk diet.

At the session of the Biological Society of January 19th, ROGER said that the large omentum acted as a sort of lymphatic ganglion to protect the system against invasion by germs introduced into the peritoneal cavity. To establish this hypothesis he excised the omentum in rabbits and guinea-pigs. Such animals were proved to have diminished resistance to infection. One may therefore conclude that the great omentum plays an important part in the protection of the peritoneum.

Vienna.

SIGNIFICANCE OF CONGESTION—TRICHINA DISSEMINATED THROUGH LYMPH-CHANNELS — TABETIC PATIENTS IMPROVED BY FRAENKEL'S MOVEMENT TREATMENT.

At a meeting of the Imperio-Royal Society of Physicians, February 11th, FREUND spoke of the significance of congestion of mucous surfaces. This it is which prevents the stomach from being digested by its own secretions, and recent investigations have led to the belief that a congested condition of the mucous membranes prevents the passage through them of bacterial invaders. The mere stretching of the membrane seems to aid in this direction. Thus, if capsules of parchment be filled with agar-agar and glue in solution and suspended in water, the parchment will be tightly stretched. These little bags and others similarly treated, except that the latter were only partially filled with agar-agar, were placed in cultures of bacteria. The tightly stretched bags resisted the entrance of the bacteria from eight to fourteen days, while the others did so only one day. It is reasonable to suppose that a living membrane will have even more power than a dead one to prevent the passage of bacteria.

At the session of February 18th, KRETZ showed the lesions of healed trichinosis in the organs of a patient who had died of carcinoma of the stomach. There was no history to indicate the age of the embedded trichinæ. It is well known that they may exist ten or twenty years in the muscles. In this patient they were scattered throughout the muscle of the extremities, as well as in the diaphragm and larynx. There were also several calcified nodules in the lungs, but as here not only the fibrous envelop was calcified, but also the trichinæ themselves, it is certain that their life had become extinct. This general distribution of the trichinæ is of great importance as showing that the view, still so widely held, that the parasites penetrate the intestinal wall and find lodgment in the diaphragm, is not the correct explanation of the phenomenon. There is now no doubt that the dissemination occurs through the lymph-channels, and this has been proved by experimental feeding of rabbits with trichinous meat. In the light of this discovery it is easy to understand why living trichinæ are sometimes found in the blood, at the height of an acute attack, and why pneumonic patches develop in the second or third week, as the invasion evidently proceeds from the thoracic duct into the systemic and pulmonary circulations.

At the Medical Club, February 9th, BUM showed a patient suffering from tabes dorsalis whom he had treated by the Fränkel method (MEDICAL NEWS, February 12, p. 219, 1898) of voluntary movements, and who had improved so that from going about with two sticks he had regained the power to walk alone, either forward or backward, or with the eyes shut. Bum has used the treatment in nineteen cases, and is, on the whole, well pleased with the results. Sometimes the treatment had to be suspended on account of lancinating pains. There were also cases in which improvement and relapse rapidly alternated, and in these it was considered wise not to push the treatment. Complicated apparatus is by no means necessary.

SOCIETY PROCEEDINGS.

THE NEW YORK CLINICAL SOCIETY.

Stated Meeting, Held January 28, 1898.

THE President, FRANK W. JACKSON, M.D., in the Chair.

SPLENECTOMY.

DR. FRANK HARTLEY read a paper on this subject. (See page 417.)

DISCUSSION.

DR. A. J. MCCOSH said that his experience with splenectomy had been limited to one case of leucocythemia. The patient lived a few months after the operation. Some years age he had seen eight or ten splenectomies performed by other surgeons, and, if he remembered correctly, in about seventy or eighty per cent. the patients had died, usually from shock and hemorrhage. Most of the spleens had been enlarged as a result of malarial infection. The hemorrhage was enormous at the time of the operation, and the veins were so friable that the ligature cut through at once. In several of the cases the patient almost died on the table from this great loss of blood. There seemed to be an excellent field for the histologist in the study of enlargements of the spleen and their relations to the general blood condition. At the present time our knowledge of the subject is extremely meager and unsatisfactory.

DR. FRANK W. JACKSON said that from a medical standpoint he had been deeply interested in the fact that apparently the ultimate effect on the blood of removal of the spleen had been practically nil.

DR. G. M. SWIFT said that in connection with this subject it might be of interest to refer to a case seen at St. Mary's Hospital two years ago. A child had a large spleen, appeared very anemic, and the blood examination showed only forty per cent. of hemoglobin. The patient eventually died, and at the autopsy, in addition to the enlarged, amyloid spleen, there was a very extensive hydronephrosis which no one had suspected, as there had been no symptoms or urinary signs pointing to such a condition.

PUSTULAR ACNE FOLLOWING PROFUSE HEMORRHAGE.

DR. J. H. EMERSON said that he had recently seen in the Out-Patient Department of the New York Hospital a woman who had been operated upon for a laceration of the cervix at one of the large private hospitals. The operation had been a failure. According to the history, on the third day after operation there had been a very profuse hemorrhage, sufficient to necessitate the use of saline enemata, and a second hemorrhage had occurred some days afterward. The face and side of the neck were covered with an eruption, which, she stated, had immediately followed the saline injection. The eruption was an ordinary pustular acne, which was diminishing at the time the patient was first seen. There was no other history bearing upon the case, and he reported it to learn, if possible, if such a result is common after the occurrence of severe hemorrhage.

DR. HARTLEY thought the case could be explained by diminished resistance of the organism following upon great loss of blood.

PERICARDITIS AND ITS PHYSICAL SIGNS.

DR. G. M. SWIFT said that last summer a child had entered St. Mary's Hospital with rheumatism and pericarditis. On one occasion the temperature suddenly rose higher than it had been before, and the physical signs showed dulness, bronchophony, and bronchial breathing over one lung. Death occurred within three or four days. It had been stated by a well-known English observer that a reliable sign of pericarditis was a quadrilateral area of dulness on the left side. In this case he had been led astray by the transmission of the sounds in an unusual manner. The autopsy showed that there had been little effusion into the pericardial sac.

DR. JACKSON remarked that the physical sign referred to was applicable to surgical pericarditis, *i.e.*, when there is distention of the pericardium. He did not think it is very uncommon to find transitory bronchial breathing around the edges of the lung.

SIMULTANEOUS SCARLATINA AND CHICKEN-POX.

DR. WALTER MENDELSON reported an interesting example of the simultaneous occurrence of two infectious diseases in the same person. The case, also, throws some light on the period of incubation of chicken-pox. The patient was a boy, who, exactly eight days after the appearance of chicken-pox, developed a well-marked rash of scarlet fever. Twelve days after the beginning of the chicken-pox a younger brother became sick with it, so that the latter had a chicken-pox eruption, while the scarlet-fever eruption was beginning to fade. The case was interesting as showing that although an active inflammatory process like that of scarlet fever was going on in the body it did not interfere with the germ or poison of chicken-pox. This is the only instance of the kind which had come under his observation.

DR. L. EMMETT HOLT said that several years ago there had been at the same time an epidemic of scarlet fever and one of chicken-pox at the New York Infant Asylum. Quite a number of children had both diseases at the same time, usually one subsiding as the other developed. Regarding the incubation of measles, he said that it is ordinarily stated to be from nine to fourteen days, and that after two weeks there is but little danger of infection. Recently he had had under observation two cases in which the incubation period had been definitely fixed at eighteen and nineteen days respectively. A year and a half ago he had kept a child, suspected to have been infected with measles, in quarantine for twenty days. It was released on the twenty-first day, and immediately came down with the disease. This was the second time that he had observed an incubation period of twenty-one days in measles. This prolonged period of incubation is a matter of importance to those who are responsible for the health of a large number of children in an institution.

DR. HARTLEY said that at one time he had operated upon a boy suffering with pseudoleucemia in the hope of relieving distressing dyspnea by the removal of the enlarged glands which were causing pressure on the trachea. The second day after the operation the boy developed an attack of measles. His brother had had measles two weeks before. Notwithstanding the measles the extensive wound of the neck healed by primary union. He had always understood that when there is an attack of scarlet fever or measles, any existing wound is likely to break down, but in this instance the union had been unusually good.

AN INCOMPLETE URETHROTOMY AND ITS CONSEQUENCES.

DR. WOOLSEY reported the case of a man who had been subjected to urethrotomy at a hospital in this city, the operation being performed under cocain anesthesia. Six weeks later he had come to Bellevue Hospital with the perineal wound still unhealed. No sounds had been passed for three weeks. The house surgeon introduced a sound to a depth which seemed to indicate that the instrument must have entered the bladder, but it did not feel free, as though in the bladder, and its withdrawal was followed by copious hemorrhage. Dr. Woolsey said that when he operated, he could not find the proximal end of the urethra, but discovered two large pockets. He then opened the bladder from above, passed his finger down into the urethra and distended the prostatic portion. Only a small sound—No. 10 or 12 French—would pass through. There was a stricture in the membranous portion which had not been divided, showing that at the first operation the operator had not passed the instrument into the bladder.

A TUBERCULOUS APPENDIX AND LOCALIZED TUBERCULOUS PERITONITIS.

DR. WOOLSEY also reported the following case: On January 24th last he had operated for appendicitis upon a patient who appeared fairly healthy, but who gave a history of having had a slight pulmonary hemorrhage about two years before and of having lost some flesh during the past year. The history also indicated that the appendicitis had come on gradually. There was an ill-defined and not very sensitive tumor in the right iliac fossa. The incision opened into a cavity containing a few drops of purulent fluid. This cavity was located between the peritoneum and a much-dilated appendix. To this appendix the omentum was adherent, and over the surface of the omentum and in the neighborhood of the appendix were numerous tubercles. The appendix seemed to be the primary focus of the tuberculous peritonitis. There was no effusion into the peritoneum, and the tuberculous peritonitis did not seem to be general. The pathologist had not yet reported upon the case, but the gross appearance had been very characteristic.

ENLARGED GLANDS AND OPERATIONS FOR APPENDICITIS.

DR. SWIFT referred to the case of a small boy who had been operated upon last summer for appendicitis. A large number of mesenteric glands appeared in the wound, and these the operator considered tuberculous.

DR. HARTLEY remarked that it was not at all uncommon to find these enlarged glands in appendicitis, and he did not consider any operation for appendicitis complete which does not include their removal. Neglect to do this is often responsible for those secondary infections which have been so frequent and annoying after operations for appendicitis.

NEW YORK NEUROLOGICAL SOCIETY.

Stated Meeting, Held February 1, 1898.

THE president, B. SACHS, M.D., in the Chair.

DR. MARY PUTNAM-JACOBI presented a boy of three years who had talked well when he was two years old. About September 2, 1897, the mother noticed that the left arm trembled. About a week later the child fell down in the street, and a wagon ran near, but not over him. A policeman insisted that the child had been injured, and he was taken to a hospital, where the doctors stated that he had a hemichorea due to fright. As the trembling of the arm had preceded the fall, it was hardly possible to attribute it to this fright. A little later, the child had quite a severe attack of measles, with pneumonia, during which the tremor ceased. In November he was taken to the Presbyterian Hospital, and there was seen by a number of physicians. It was noted shortly afterward that his leg also trembled. Iron and arsenic were freely given, but with no benefit. He was taken home on November 25th. There was then weakness in both the leg and arm, which since that time has steadily increased. On January 3, 1898, Dr. Putnam-Jacobi first saw the child. There was then a condition present which the mother had not noticed, *i. e.*, a deviation of the right eye outward and also a marked dilatation of the pupil as well as very slight reaction to light. Vision was good. At present, there is a noticeable drooping of the left angle of the mouth. Another new symptom is an inclination of the head to the left side, with slight resistance on attempting to straighten it. The disposition of the child is good. His speech is indistinct, but this may be because he is so young. The spontaneous tremor in the leg has disappeared, but an attempt to walk causes incoordinate movements in the leg. Sensation and electric reactions are normal. The knee-jerk on the affected side is decidedly increased. The diagnosis seems to rest between hemichorea, with consecutive paralysis, post-hemiplegic chorea, and multiple sclerosis. Two or three physicians who had seen the case made a diagnosis of tumor, but this seemed to be excluded by the absence of vomiting, convulsions, headache, or alteration of character. The existence of ocular symptoms on the opposite side would seem to militate against a diagnosis of chorea. A lesion in the inner part of the right thalamus, or under the aqueduct of Sylvius, would explain the symptoms. The extreme youth of the child would not exclude such a diagnosis, for several such cases are on record.

DR. L. STIEGLITZ said that two years ago he had exhibited to this society the brain of a child of two and a half years, with a tubercle in the right crus. In this case a very similar symptom-complex had been observed; *i. e.*, left hemiplegia with a characteristic crossed third nerve paralysis. There was also a very similar tremor which persisted a long time and which was present both during rest and movement. Finally total paralysis occurred. Gowers states, in his book, that "stationary tubercle not infrequently produces an intentional tremor." The speaker had found recorded as many as thirty-five cases of disseminated sclerosis in young children. One should be careful not to base the diagnosis upon the presence of intention-tremor alone. It would be interesting to know if there had been choked disk in the case just presented. He would venture to predict that the case would progress to a fatal termination, and that tubercle would be found post-mortem. In his own case the choked disk had developed only very shortly before death.

DR. C. A. HERTER said that this little patient had been referred to him about one month ago. After careful examination he had leaned toward the diagnosis just made by the last speaker, as he did not regard the presence of a tumor as in any way antagonistic to this view. Two years ago he had a case of crossed paralysis of the same general character, and Dr. Starr had coincided in the diagnosis of tubercle of the crus, and within a few months the child died. In view of the fact that tubercle of the brain is a much more common condition than multiple sclerosis in children, such a diagnosis is the more probable one. He thought that the child's eyes had been examined with a negative result.

DR. SACHS said that he had seen this child about three months ago, when the condition had been quite different. On examination he had found slight rigidity in the lower extremities and increased reflexes in the upper extremity and in both lower extremities. The statement had been made at that time that the examination of the fundus of the eye was entirely negative. At the time he had made a tentative diagnosis of post-hemiplegic tremor or a post-hemiplegic ataxic tremor. He now thought it exceedingly probable that there is a neoplasm in the brain. In a case published by him some time ago there had been very marked ataxic movements, and the autopsy had shown a lesion in the crus. In all the cases of this kind which he had seen the movements had been observed only on attempting to move the arm, whereas in this case the movements are continuous.

DR. PUTNAM-JACOBI said that the occurrence of measles and pneumonia after the beginning of the nervous symptoms, without the development of pulmonary tuberculosis, seemed to be against a diagnosis of tubercle. If a tumor were present, as had been suggested, there should be a total paralysis of the third nerve, whereas there is only an associated paralysis. Another point is that there was no hemiplegia until some time after the development of the tremor.

LOCALIZED SYRINGOMYELIA.

DR. L. STIEGLITZ presented a woman, thirty-eight years of age, who two years ago began to complain of pains in the left shoulder, arm, and forearm. Shortly after this, she noticed some weakness in her left hand, and subsequently wasting of the muscles of the hand. The fingers then became contracted. Examination during August, 1897, showed complete atrophy of the thenar, hypothenar, interossei and other intrinsic muscles of the left hand, and contractures of the long flexors of the fingers, especially of the three ulnar fingers. Along a narrow strip of the inner surface of the left arm sensation was disturbed. The left eye is markedly sunken, and the left pupil is small and remains so in a dark room. It does not dilate under cocain, but is at once dilated by atropin. The speaker said that it is known that the fibers to the sympathetic leave the spinal cord with the first dorsal anterior root, and also that the muscles of the hand are represented in the cord at the level of the first dorsal root—in other words, this is a case of very marked localized spinal lesion in the anterior part of the left side of the spinal cord. He thought an inflammatory condition, such as myelitis, could be excluded. There is no history or evidence of syphilis, and the condition was not changed by specific treatment. This clinical picture might be produced by a neoplasm at the level of the anterior horn, or by a gliomatosis. The patient had been under observation six months, and practically had developed no new symptoms. He was inclined to regard the condition as one of syringomyelia localized for the present at the level of the first dorsal root.

In connection with this case he exhibited a classic example of syringomyelia, in which there were the same conditions of the eye. This patient, twenty-one years of age, is a porter by occupation. Two or three years ago he first noticed a stiffness of the left hand, and this became steadily worse, and the hand always felt cold. Examination showed the left shoulder to be considerably higher than the right, and a marked scoliosis to the left in the middle and upper dorsal regions. There was almost complete atrophy of the small muscles of the left hand, and marked atrophy of the muscles of the left forearm,

arm, and shoulder. When the skin of the left hand is injured, the wound heals very slowly. There is analgesia of the entire left arm, and of a large part of the left chest and scapular region. Tke temperature sense is less affected on the left than on the right side. The left palpebral fissure, the left eyeball, and the left pupil are smaller than on the opposite side. The left pupil is not dilated by cocain, but readily reacts to homatropin. The speaker said that this condition of the eye is not uncommon, but is sometimes overlooked when both eyes are alike affected. A very excellent point in the differential diagnosis in the test with cocain.

Dr. C. L. Dana said that some years ago he had a patient with a very typical variety of progressive muscular atrophy. It ran the usual course and terminated fatally. In the early stage there were precisely the same conditions of the eye, so that he always considers this part of the usual symptomatology of the disease. For that reason, it seemed to him that the diagnosis of progressive muscular atrophy is admissible in the case just presented. The eye symptoms could hardly be of any particular value except in localizing.

Dr. Leszynsky said that when he had first seen the patient some time ago he had been inclined to think that the case was one in which the dorsal root of the brachial plexus had become involved. Not having had an opportunity to further examine the case he had not been able to confirm his opinion.

Dr. Stieglitz said that he could not positively exclude progressive muscular atrophy. Before the clinical picture of syringomyelia had been well known quite a number of cases were diagnosed as progressive muscular atrophy; moreover, syringomyelia often begins without sensory symptoms, because the gliomatosis commences in the anterior part of the cord.

UNILATERAL REFLEX IRIDOPLEGIA.

Dr. W. M. Leszynsky read a paper with this title, and presented a patient illustrative of the condition. He said that the term "unilateral iridoplegia" was applied to an ocular condition in which one pupil does not react directly to light, while its reaction in convergence is preserved. The other pupil reacts normally. The pupil may be either dilated or contracted, or both pupils may be dilated. It is not usually accompanied by any interference with vision, or changes in the fundus. It might also be called a unilateral Argyll-Robertson pupil. Absolute iridoplegia of recent origin had been known in a few instances to disappear under the administration of mercury and iodid of potassium. It had been erroneously inferred that this unilateral form of iridoplegia is associated with tabes. The patient presented, a woman of thirty-eight years, was first seen by him in December, 1896. Her second husband had had syphilis some years before marriage, and had since then given abundant evidence of the disease. The patient had never been pregnant after this marriage. The patient herself had been somewhat intemperate. Her left pupil is larger than the right, and she says that this has been so during at least three years. All of the external eye muscles act normally. There is none of the usual evidence of syphilitic infection, but the other signs and symptoms seem to warrant the diagnosis of cerebrospinal syphilis. She improved somewhat under antisyphilitic treatment. At the second examination it was found that both patellar reflexes were lost. In January, 1898, the pupils were found to be the same. This case could be considered an atypical case of tabes, or of cerebrospinal syphilis.

He had found that only seventeen other cases had been reported. From a study of these it would be seen that in nine there was a definite history of previous syphilitic infection, and in four the nervous manifestations justified a suspicion of antecedent syphilis. In thirteen cases the left pupil was affected; in eleven the iridoplegic pupil was dilated. The condition of vision or refraction seemed to have no bearing on the condition of the pupil. Apparently, unilateral iridoplegia is a very rare condition, though systematic examinations would probably show that it is more frequent than is supposed. In three unrecorded cases of tabes he had observed unilateral iridoplegia at the first examination, but this had disappeared within a few weeks. He was inclined to think that in his patient, when the pupil became affected, there was a sudden ophthalmoplegia interna, and that the muscle-fibers had only partially recovered, thus leaving the pupil in its present permanent condition.

After an extensive review of the literature, particularly as to the various theories which have been propounded regarding the nervous control of the pupil, Dr. Leszynsky expressed his preference for the view that the ciliary and sphincter nuclei are separate and have independent muscular fibers. His conclusions were: (1) That unilateral reflex iridoplegia is a condition which may arise in tabes or paretic dementia, being confined to one side for an indefinite time before the other pupil becomes affected; (2) that it often occurs in cerebrospinal syphilis and as a remote result of disease or injury of the third nerve; (3) that it is always indicative of degeneration of the oculomotor nerve; and (4) that the lesion is situated in the centrifugal portion of the reflex mechanism, as shown by its occurrence with, or as a consequence of, oculomotor paralysis.

Dr. Carl Koller was invited to take part in the discussion. He said that unilateral loss of light-reflex is not such a rare condition as might perhaps appear from neurologic literature. Of course, the loss of reflex to light is brought to our attention in two ways—one during neurologic examination, and the other when the patient comes to the ophthalmologist because of eye symptoms. The latter is more frequent. He called to mind three cases, observed in private practice during a number of years. Two of them had been followed eight years, and when first observed these patients had dilated pupils and loss of accommodation. In the beginning, with the loss of reflex there had been also a loss of the power of accommodation. This had, in part, returned after a time. In two cases the loss of reflex appeared in the other eye, and also without loss of accommodation. From his own experience he would be inclined to believe that it is a nuclear affection (1) because the accommodation is but slightly interfered with, and (2) because in most of the cases the nucleus on the other side becomes subsequently affected. In the majority of cases he believed syphilis to be the cause.

DR. HERTER thought the conclusions reached by the reader of the paper were justified by the facts. In one or two instances he had noted this one-sided iridoplegia and had been puzzled by it. He had looked upon the lesion as a simple one of syphilitic origin.

DR. SACHS thought the condition extremely common, and that for this reason it had not been oftener recorded. It seemed to him that unilateral reflex iridoplegia is invariably specific, and indeed a very important diagnostic symptom. Its mere presence had caused him to suspect specific disease. Unilateral immobility, and especially double complete immobility, is an extremely characteristic sign of syphilis. He did not see how it could be anything else than nuclear in its nature.

DR. LESZYNSKY, in closing, said that the experience of Dr. Sachs was opposed to that of a number of observers who had studied a large number of cases of pupillary phenomena without finding more than a few examples of the affection under consideration.

REVIEWS.

TEXT-BOOK OF NERVOUS DISEASES.—Being a Compendium for the Use of Students and Practitioners of Medicine. By CHARLES L. DANA, A.M., M.D. Fourth edition, revised and enlarged. New York: Wm. Wood and Company, 1897.

THE fact that this book has gone through three editions within five years demonstrates its popularity with the students and with the profession. The changes in this edition are confined to the chapters on the histology and general anatomy of the brain and spinal cord, which are practically rewritten, and to the revision of the articles on sclerosis and encephalitis. A new chapter has been added on alcoholic meningitis, a bad term of the author's for a condition which positively is not an inflammation of the meninges.

PRAXIS DER HARNALYSE. Von DR. LASSAR-COHN, Universitäts Professor zu Königsberg. Hamburg und Leipzig: Leopold Voss, 1897.

PRACTICAL URINALYSIS. By DR. LASSAR-COHN, Professor in the University at Königsberg. Hamburg and Leipsic: Leopold Voss, 1897.

THIS little manual gives in rather extended form and with scientific accuracy the data for quantitative and qualitative examination of the urine. Microscopic examination is not considered. As an appendix, the author has given the chemic methods of examination of the gastric contents, and in a table shows the reagents necessary for the determination of the various elements.

REFERENCE-BOOK OF PRACTICAL THERAPEUTICS. By various authors. Edited by FRANK P. FOSTER, M.D. Vol. II. New York: D. Appleton & Co., 1897.

THE second volume of this extremely practical work has just come to hand. The various articles contained in it show the same careful and painstaking work which characterized those of the first volume. This, however, was to be expected in view of the ability of the men who are associated in the preparation of this work on therapeutics.

The articles on opium, quinin, serum-therapy, thyroid treatment, transfusion and infusion are especially noteworthy for their thoroughness.

The entire work deserves, by reason of its intrinsic merit, a place in the library of every physician.

THERAPEUTIC HINTS.

Intestinal Antiseptic Mixture in Typhoid Fever.—

℞ Salol . . . . . . ʒ i
Thymol . . . . . gr. xxxvi
Bismuthi subnit. . . . . ʒ ii–iv
Mucilag. acaciæ . . . . ℥ ii
Syr. tolutan. . . . . . ℥ iv.

M. Sig. One teaspoonful three times daily.

For Tinea Tonsurans.—

℞ Ac. carbolici . . . . . . ʒ i
Tinct. iodi } aa . . . . ʒ ii
Ol. terebinth. }
Glycerini . . . . ʒ iii.

M. Sig. Apply twice daily to affected spots with camel's-hair brush.

For the same affection SOLARES recommends the following treatment by which he has effected rapid cures. The diseased areas are first shaved, then brushed for ten minutes with formalin, and finally sprayed with the same, so that no part escapes disinfection. This treatment is applied daily or on alternate days, according to the degree of reaction shown.

For Vaginismus.—

℞ Zinci valerianat. . . . . . gr. x
Quinin. valerianat. . . . . gr. xviii
Ext. opii } aa . . . . gr. ii.
Ext. belladonnæ }

M. Ft. pil. No. XII. Sig. Three to six pills daily.

In conjunction with the above the following should be applied locally:

℞ Cocain. hydrochlor. . . . . gr. xii
Ext. belladonnæ . . . . gr. vi
Strontii brom. . . . . . gr. xvi
Ol. theobrom. . . . . . ʒ v.

M. Ft. suppos. vaginal. No. IV. Sig. Use one suppository daily.

For Chronic Follicular Pharyngitis.—

℞ Iodi pur. . . . . . . gr. iii
Potass. iodid. . . . . . gr. v
Ac. trichloracetici . . . . gr. vi
Glycerini } aa . . . . . ℥ ss.
Aq. dest. }

M. Sig. Apply by means of cotton applicator in full strength, or diluted as may be indicated.

THE MEDICAL NEWS.

A WEEKLY JOURNAL OF MEDICAL SCIENCE.

VOL. LXXII. NEW YORK, SATURDAY, APRIL 9, 1898. NO. 15.

ORIGINAL ARTICLES.

GRADUAL DILATION VERSUS CUTTING IN THE TREATMENT OF URETHRAL STRICTURES.

BY GEORGE T. HOWLAND, M.D.,
OF WASHINGTON, D. C.;
SURGEON, GENITO-URINARY DEPARTMENT, TO THE SOUTH WASHINGTON FREE DISPENSARY AND HOSPITAL.

PERHAPS there is no branch of genito-urinary surgery in regard to which so many good surgeons vary on the question of treatment as in strictures of the urethra. Ten years ago this difference of opinion was more marked than it is to-day. Then it was the practice to cut and dilate the urethra to a large caliber, very little attention being paid to what was cut or how it was cut as long as the urethra could be made to admit a large-sized sound. The best genito-urinary surgeons throughout the world are now decrying the practice of using the knife at the first sign of a stricture of the urethra.

This is good surgery and should be even more generally practised. The writer is frequently asked if dilation of a urethral stricture is advisable and if the results attending its application justify the surgeon in using it. To this there is but one answer: This method of treatment is always advisable and more often successful than is generally believed among surgeons. On this subject Dr. R. W. Taylor, in his recent work on "Sexual Disorders of the Male and Female," makes the following appropriate remarks: "The trend of thought as regards the treatment of urethral stricture of late years has been so unswervingly toward cutting operations that many surgeons are wholly unaware of the benefit and lasting effects of gradual dilation. I am to-day more than ever convinced that cutting operations should be a last resort, and that intemperate incisions and over stretching are very frequently the cause of never-ending suffering and inconveniences." A very careful and prominent genito-urinary surgeon of Boston, in conversation with the writer on this subject, stated that he was obtaining excellent results from the gradual dilation of urethral strictures.

The more I observe stricture of the urethra, the more firmly I am convinced that the hard stricture may be successfully treated by gradual dilation. Stricture of the membranous portion of the posterior urethra is now successfully treated by this method. At the present time the writer has under observation a number of patients with stricture in this part of the urethra who are doing exceptionally well under this method of treatment. Other surgeons have informed me that they are having equally good results in treating stricture of the posterior urethra by this method. The greatest drawback in its application is to get patients to continue the treatment long enough; for in the majority of cases it requires some time before the surgeon is justified in saying that a cure has been attained. To state just how long a period is necessary to effect a cure is difficult; it depends to a great extent both upon the patient and the stricture. The time will be shortened if the patient presents himself for treatment at stated intervals. The quickness of cure also depends both upon the length of time the stricture has existed and its location in the urethra. The time required for a cure may be stated as being from three to twelve months. The longer the period of treatment, the more lasting and permanent the results.

When the time necessary is explained to the patient he occasionally hesitates, and in some instances, rare as far as my experience goes, prefers the cutting operation; but if it is explained to him that even after the stricture has been cut he will still have to submit to the passage of sounds at regular intervals, that the cure is not as permanent as when obtained by means of gradual dilation, and that by patience and perseverance there is every reason to believe that success will follow non-operative treatment, then, as a rule, objections are no longer raised; as the patient perceives the improvement he will gain confidence and seek, rather than shun, the treatment. In the past we have been advised to dilate the urethra up to 40 French, and even to a greater caliber. Such a degree of dilation is no inconsiderable factor in producing the train of symptoms so common after excessive stretching of the urethra. I have observed the best results from gradual dilation up to and not exceeding 32 French, and if a urethra thus treated can be maintained at a caliber of 28 or 26 French, it is all that will be required.

The gradual dilation of a stricture, as the name implies, should be conducted slowly and with great care, and an advancement of more than two sizes should not be attempted at one sitting, and the sitting can be at intervals of one week or less, providing the urethra does not rebel. It is just here that the knowledge of the surgeon stands him in hand, and he can tell when to give the urethra a rest before the patient feels any inconvenience from inflammatory reaction. At the slightest sign of blood-oozing the treatment must cease, and the irritated membrane of the urethra should be treated by the instillation or irrigation of some of the different astringent preparations. The writer has of late resorted to irrigations of plain water at a temperature of 105° to 110 F., one quart being used at a sitting. The results have been very encouraging.

It is claimed by some that complications may arise from treating stricture by this method, such, for instance, as urethritis, urethrocystitis, fever and chills, pyemic abscess, hemorrhage, temporary retention, and rheumatism. All of these, and many more ills to which flesh is heir, may arise from the injudicious use of the sound; but by care and cleanliness the likelihood of the occurrence of any of these distressing complications may be reduced to the minimum.

It is a common practice on the part of some physicians, following the cutting operation, to instruct the patient in the use of the sound, and advise its use once or twice a month or oftener, thus preventing a more rapid return of the trouble. The patient may reason, and perhaps justly, from his imperfect knowledge, that if he will be benefited by passing a sound once or twice a month, why will he not be cured quicker if he uses the sound at shorter intervals, say two or three times a week? The writer recalls an instance when the patient was cut seven times for as many different strictures in the anterior urethra (?), and then his urethra was dilated by steel sounds up to 40 French. He drifted into the habit of passing a 36 French sound once a day and continued to do so for several months. Under appropriate treatment he was relieved of the distressing symptoms caused by such a pernicious habit. It is now over a year since a sound was passed, and there is marked improvement in his health. This patient informed me that he never could correctly pass the sound, and that it would always catch just as it was about to go under the arch. I have under observation a patient who passed a 38 French sound anterior, twice a day, morning and evening. The condition of his urethra can be imagined far better than it can be described. Yet, on stopping the use of sounds and with the instillation of nitrate of silver, he is making rapid progress toward health.

These two incidents represent cases which are observed more frequently than is necessary, and which are the result of carelessness on the part of the surgeon and a too great desire on the part of the patient to take the treatment in his own hands.

To avoid this never allow a patient to pass sounds upon himself. It is far better that he should be untreated than to practise this method of self-treatment.

CASE I.—On August 26, 1888, J. W., aged twenty-five years, consulted me on account of a urethral stricture. He had gonorrhea two years before. There had been more or less discharge since, which was more pronounced if he indulged to excess in alcoholic liquors. The stream of urine was small and there was dripping after the act was apparently finished. This had troubled him during the previous six months, and was gradually growing worse. Bougie *à boule* No. 8 passed freely into the bladder; No. 9 would not pass. The stricture was two inches from the meatus. Gradual dilation was advised, and the treatment accepted. Anterior sounds were passed until 30 French was reached. Up to this time the treatment was at weekly sittings. When size 30 French was attained the sittings were at intervals of two weeks. The entire treatment occupied eight months. At no time was there hemorrhage from the urethra. Up to the present time he has had no trouble from his stricture. The stream is voided with vigor, and has not decreased in size. There are no symptoms pointing to a return of his trouble.

CASE II.—On October 15, 1888, W. K., aged forty years, consulted me on account of urethral stricture, which he said he knew he had had at least eight years. He would occasionally have sounds passed, but never regularly. He had contracted gonorrhea several times. The last attack occurred, as near as he could remember, about ten years before. During the previous year he had suffered much annoyance from the stricture, especially with dripping of the urine. The stricture was four inches from the meatus, and would admit a bougie *à boule* No. 9 French. Gradual dilation was commenced and carried up to 30 French. The treatment occupied a period of ten months. I saw him about six months ago, and he told me that he had never had any trouble from his stricture since treatment was stopped, about nine and one-half years before.

CASE III.—On January 2, 1889, I was consulted by G. C., aged thirty-five years. He had had gonorrhea three years before, and during the previous year had had more or less trouble in voiding his urine. The stream was small, and about two or three minutes were required in which to empty the bladder. Bougie *à boule* No. 7 French was passed; stricture three inches from the meatus. Straight sounds were passed up to 32 French. Time required for treatment was eight months. Reports no trouble from the stricture up to the present time.

In all of these cases the strictures were hard, yet with patience on the part of both patient and physician they responded to treatment by the method advised in this paper. The writer does not believe that all strictures can be cured by gradual dilation, but he does believe that a great number can thus be successfully treated. In those cases in which gradual dilation has no effect on the stricture, and they are few, then we must resort to the knife, but it is fair to your patient as well as to yourself to give him the benefit of the doubt and first try gradual dilation.

TUBERCULOUS LARYNGITIS.

BY ELLET ORRIN SISSON, M.D.,
OF KEOKUK, IOWA;
PROFESSOR OF ANATOMY AND DIRECTOR OF THE MICROSCOPIC AND BACTERIOLOGIC LABORATORIES IN THE COLLEGE OF PHYSICIANS AND SURGEONS, KEOKUK, IOWA.

TUBERCULOUS LARYNGITIS was first described by Petit in a treatise which appeared in 1790, and this was followed two years later by a more important work by Portal. Suavee in 1802 collected these writings in a monograph which fully established the main features of the malady, but it was not until 1819 that Laennec insisted upon the tuberculous nature of the disease. Louis disputed this view a few years later, and attributed the ulceration to the corroding effects of the sputa in pulmonary phthisis. Hasse was the first to describe the deposit of tubercles in the mucous membrane of the larynx with anything like detail. Heinze, in an exhaustive monograph, placed the pathology of the affection on a thoroughly scientific basis.

The etiology of tuberculous laryngitis resolves itself into the question: Does it occur as a primary affection or is it always secondary to pulmonary phthisis? The majority of authors and investigators are inclined to the view that in every case it is secondary. Heinze, pathologist to the Leipzig Pathological Institute, in 1876 made most minute pathologic investigations upon the bodies of fifty persons who had died of pulmonary phthisis. In forty-seven of these there was tuberculous ulceration of the larynx or trachea, and in no instance did it appear that the deposit in the larynx or trachea had preceded the pulmonary involvement.

During life it is difficult to determine the existence of primary tuberculosis of the larynx, as the most careful physical examination may fail to detect cheesy deposits or indurated spots in the lungs, especially when they are of long standing and deeply situated; it is also impossible, by means of the laryngoscope, to be absolutely sure that any deposit in the larynx is actually tuberculous. A few cases have been recorded in which, at the autopsy, tuberculous disease of the larynx has been found without any deposit in the lungs. Dr. Gottlieb Küer reports three cases of primary pharyngeal tuberculosis substantiated by post-mortems, and Hans Ruge reports what he believes to have been a case of primary tonsillar tuberculosis.

The predisposing cause may be a severe catarrh. A chronic weakness of the vocal organ may also be developed by persistent overexertion of the voice, as in the case of public speakers, singers, etc. Under such circumstances some special laryngeal affection is ultimately produced, which, if tuberculosis be present in the system, is very likely to culminate in the local phenomena of laryngeal phthisis. Dr. Marcet did not, however, find the excessive use of the voice a frequent cause of the disease in the seventy cases reported by him, but attributed its occurrence rather to sedentary indoor occupations. Men are more frequently affected than women, and the greatest number of cases occur between the ages of twenty and thirty years.

In 500 cases of marked laryngeal phthisis examined by Mackenzie there were 365 males and 135 females, or 2.70 males to 1 female, and in 100 autopsies he found the same ratio.

In primary tuberculosis of the larynx there are found on the mucous membrane, singly or in groups, small, roundish nodules, sometimes attaining the size of a pin-head. In secondary tuberculosis of the larynx, two stages are recognized: (1) that of infiltration; and (2) that of ulceration. The first stage is characterized by a swelling of the mucous membrane from infiltration of the mucosa and submucosa, the overlying epithelium appearing normal. Microscopically, there is a general thickening of the mucous membrane affecting both the mucosa and submucosa so that these structures become three or four times their ordinary thickness. Tubercles are more numerous in the upper layers of the mucous membrane. These tubercles sometimes undergo fatty degeneration or such complete caseation that only their walls remain. They occasionally appear to be placed laterally in relation to arteries, but this may be accidental, the irregular course of the vessels in the laryngeal mucous membrane not being favorable to the exact determination of any such relationship. Sometimes they are close to the dilated ducts of the mucous glands. In parts both acini and ducts are dilated, and, while containing small, round-cells, they are surrounded by a considerable amount of cellular infiltration. Perichondritis is characterized by an abundance of pus-cells between the cells of the perichrondrium. The suppuration is sometimes so active that the whole structure may disappear, and the cartilage lie loose in an abscess.

The stage of ulceration is characterized by softening and breaking down of the tubercles, forming superficial ulcers, which, by extending to the deeper tissues, causes extensive destruction of the parts.

The symptoms of tuberculosis of the larynx, because of the important functions of the parts involved, are necessarily of a distressing nature. The ones commonly present are hoarseness, dysphagia, cough, and dyspnea of greater or less severity. Hoarseness, which may be considered essentially a laryngeal symptom, may be caused by an implication of one of the recurrent laryngeal nerves (more commonly the right), in a lesion of the lung or of the bronchial glands. Cough is almost invariably present, and is accompanied in nearly every case by expectoration. Dyspnea of sufficient moment to necessitate tracheotomy is rare, but shortness of breath on slight exertion is almost a constant symptom. Of the most painful and characteristic of the symptoms of laryngeal phthisis is dysphagia due to the swollen and ulcerated condition of the larynx, and especially of the arytenoids. If the epiglottis is ulcerated there is acute pain on swallowing. Laryngoscopically, one of the earliest signs to suggest the onset of tuberculous disease is pallor of the laryngeal mucous membrane. Simon says: "That a partial anemia, that is, pallor limited to the epiglottis, ventricular bands, and the mucous membrane covering the arytenoids, is more suggestive than a general anemia.

Cohen describes an acute form of tuberculous laryngitis in which congestion of the mucous membrane is a marked feature. This condition, which resembles an acute catarrhal laryngitis, passes, in the course of two or three weeks, into a chronic laryngeal catarrh, and it is only later that the tuberculous nature of the affection becomes manifest. The latest stages of laryngeal tuberculosis are very characteristic. There is generally a pyriform swelling of the arytenoids which prevents the approximation of the vocal cords, and the epiglottis becomes involved in a like manner, presenting a turban-like appearance. The aryepiglottic folds may become infiltrated so that the glottis may be almost occluded by a pale, puffy swelling extending around it. The swollen mucous membrane has a tendency to ulcerate, and the ulcerated surface is bathed in a milky white secretion that is very characteristic.

The vocal cords may to a great extent escape this destructive process, though they usually lose their shining appearance. There are, however, cases in which the brunt of the disease falls upon the cords, which then become injected and thickened, and after a time ulcerated, or there may be loss of mobility in one or both cords without any gross alteration in structure. In some cases the cords become fixed, almost in the phonatory position, giving rise to symptoms of laryngeal stenosis and simulating a bilateral abductor paralysis.

Tuberculous laryngitis being secondary to phthisis pulmonalis in the majority of cases, it is easily recognized, and in the stage of ulceration, when it might be confounded with syphilis or cancer, the discovery of tubercle bacilli in the secretions will settle the question of diagnosis.

The prognosis of this affection is grave. The statistics of Morrell Mackenzie show that in 100 cases (submitted to post-mortem examination) 26 of the patients died within the first twelve months, 56 within eighteen months, and 75 within two years; and only 12 lived upwards of two and one-half years.

As Sajous aptly says: "Although the number of well-authenticated successful results reported is not large, a possibility of recovery under appropriate treatment has been sufficiently demonstrated to place the practitioner under the stress of considerable responsibility." The constitutional treatment of laryngeal tuberculosis differs in no respect from that which has been found useful in pulmonary tuberculosis. Sommerbrodt, from an experience of over 5000 cases, maintains that creosote is not merely a useful drug for the systematic treatment of tuberculosis, but that it exerts a specific influence upon the disease by the resistance it offers to the cultivation of tubercle bacilli. As regards the climatic treatment of laryngeal tuberculosis, Hall says: "The cold, dry, rarefied air of high altitudes has been found to act unfavorably." In the way of local treatment, Schmidt highly recommends the inhalation of balsam of Peru. Hall claims to have had excellent results from the insufflation of iodoform, and Semon says: "Regular applications of iodoform in powder to the ulcerations of laryngeal phthisis produce cleansing, and in many cases diminution in size of the ulcers, often diminution of the surrounding edematous infiltration, decrease of pain and soreness, and frequently considerable improvement of the dysphagia, which had previously formed one of the most distressing and serious features of the disease. Fronstein speaks very highly of the action of resorcin applied in a ten- to twenty-per-cent. solution by means of a brush, or a two-per-cent. solution used as a spray, he claims it acts more satisfactorily in allaying the pain and distress caused by laryngeal ulceration of tuberculous origin than does cocain.

The plan of treatment suggested by Heryng and Krause, *viz.*, the application of lactic acid to the ulcerations with or without previous curetting, has met with much favor at the hands of a great number of laryngologists at the present time. It is advisable to begin with a weak solution, say twenty per cent.

If there is very little local reaction as a result of the application, the strength of the solution may be increased at the next sitting. A fifty-per-cent. solution is said to usually suffice to effect cicatrization, but sixty-per-cent. and eighty-per-cent. solutions, even the pure acid, have been employed. It is rubbed into the ulceration by means of cotton wool firmly wrapped around a rectangular laryngeal forceps, but when there is simply an infiltration or tuberculous out-growth, a still more radical plan of treatment is necessary to bring the lactic acid into contact with the submucosa. In simple infiltration, Heryng advises that the acid should be injected beneath the mucous membrane by means of a sharp-pointed syringe he devised for the purpose, or the surface can be scraped with the curette and the acid rubbed into the raw surface. In all cases, before applying the lactic acid or curetting, the affected surface should be freely swabbed with a twenty-per-cent. solution of cocain. Hedderich made a trial of paramonochlorphenol in the treatment of thirty cases of laryngeal phthisis in the clinic of Professor Jurasz at Heidelberg, and reports that after the second application all patients were relieved of pain, the breathing became easier, the ulcers healed, and infiltration diminished. In severe progressive cases no improvement was perceptible. Dr. Hajek recommends insufflations of iodol, because of two advantages which it possesses: (1) It is insoluble and capable of forming a true protective antiseptic covering upon the surface of the ulcer with which it comes in contact, and (2) it is an admirable disinfectant. After two or three applications the ulcer loses its dirty appearance and becomes covered with healthy granulations. Dr. W. Scheppegrell of New Orleans, in a recent article on the treatment of laryngeal tuberculosis read before the Southern Section of the American Laryngological, Rhinological, and Otological Society, described the principles of cataphoresis and his method of applying it to the larynx in the treatment of tuberculosis of this organ. He has experimented with a number of substances, such as creasote, guaiacol, iodin, chlorid of zinc, and oxychlorid of copper. Guaiacol was found useful when alleviation of pain was the principal object; the oxychlorid of copper possesses marked bactericidal properties and stimulates the tissues to a healthy reaction. In applying cupric cataphoresis, he uses spheric bulbs of pure copper, one-eighth to one-fourth inch in diameter, attached to an insulated handle. These bulbs are connected with the positive pole and are applied directly to the tissues, a current of two to five milliamperes being used from three to ten minutes, and the sitting being repeated every two or three days. A dispersing electrode connected with the negative pole is applied to the back of the neck. The copper in contact with the tissues is electrolyzed, and the oxychlorid of copper which is produced passes into the tissues. Cocain anesthesia (five-per-cent. solution) is necessary in the majority of cases.

He gives the clinical history of three cases in which the method was used with satisfaction. In the first two the ulcerations were cured and the infiltration diminished when the treatment had to be discontinued on account of the aggravation of the pulmonary disease. In the third case, in which no pulmonary disease could be detected, but in which the bacilli of tuberculosis were found on repeated examination of the sputum, and in which the clinical signs of tuberculous laryngitis were very marked, the patient had lost twenty-five pounds, and was so weak that he could walk only when supported. Deglutition was so painful that he could swallow only with the greatest difficulty. There was no history of any specific affection. Antiphthisin had been used without effect. The arytenoid region was much infiltrated, with extensive ulceration of the interarytenoid fold extending to the left, over the ventricular band. The epiglottis was tumefied with ulceration of the left anterior portion. The cataphoric treatment was at once commenced; at first every three days and afterward twice weekly. Improvement was noted after the third application, and after the ninth the ulcerations had healed so far that the patient could swallow semi-solid food with but little pain. The patient continued to improve, and eight weeks later was entirely cured, with the exception of a slight huskiness due to injury of the vocal cords. Six months later the larynx showed no return of laryngeal disease.

Tracheotomy is only to be advised in cases in which life is threatened by laryngeal stenosis. Percy Kidd has ably summarized the advantages and disadvantages of tracheotomy in laryngeal phthisis, and points out that the weight of evidence is against the performance of this operation, except in cases of stenosis. By this brief *résumé* of some of the existing literature on this subject, we have forced upon us the following conclusions:

First. That to the microscopic investigations and to them alone is due the present thorough knowledge of its pathology.

Second. That no one line of treatment can be laid down at the present time.

Third. That there is too great a tendency on the part of the medical profession at large to place this disease in the list of incurable affections, and to use only palliative treatment, and not take the interest that they should in the reports from the few untiring investigators, who, in the face of apparently insurmountable obstacles are endeavoring to find some cure for this dread malady. When we stop and think of the progress that has been and is being made in the treatment of other diseases as destructive in their nature as this, and which were less than ten years ago classed with it as incurable, we are justified in predicting that the time will come, and that it is not far distant, when laryngeal tuberculosis will take its place among them, and be classed as a curable disease.

SOME PRACTICAL CONSIDERATIONS OF GASTRIC STAGNATION.

By A. L. BENEDICT, M.D.,
OF BUFFALO, N. Y.;
PROFESSOR OF PHYSIOLOGY AND DIGESTIVE DISEASES, DENTAL DEPARTMENT, UNIVERSITY OF BUFFALO.

CASE I.—During the spring of 1895, a young woman, a teacher in a public school, consulted me on account of a troublesome dyspepsia which had persisted some months, notwithstanding the application of the usual treatment, including regulation of the diet. The patient had gradually abandoned one kind of food after another until she was taking little but toast and milk. As the diet was reduced the power of digestion had steadily declined, so that she felt herself no freer from disagreeable symptoms than at first, while a logical pursuit of the plan of treatment seemed to promise nothing better than starvation. There was the customary history of a sensation of fulness in the epigastrium, of gas formation in the stomach, and, to a less degree, in the bowels, and of occasional nausea without vomiting. Food was said to "lie heavy in the stomach" for several hours after a meal. It is surprising how frequently the last symptom is found to be reliable, and, in this instance, there was no reason to doubt it. Under treatment with strychnin to improve the motor power of the stomach, gastro-intestinal antiseptics, etc., she improved, but relapsed during examination week, recovering during the summer vacation. During the following year she had a return of the trouble, and her stomach was found to be dilated, reaching to the level of the umbilicus.[1] The same line of treatment was carried out, and, on August 28th, nearly three months from the first visit of this year, the stomach was in practically normal position and the patient was discharged. Since then she has practically remained well.

In a simple case of atonic dyspepsia, the prognosis depends almost entirely upon the general physical and nervous state of the individual, present and potential. Appropriate treatment of the motor and chemic disorders will usually cause marked relief, but in a certain proportion of cases patients lack the necessary stamina to dispense with medicines. Strychnin represents in a temporary and superficial manner the much-needed influence upon the general vital capacity. Rest, amusement, out-door exercise of an exhilarating but not too severe character, often an entire change of life, are demanded, and the ultimate prognosis depends upon the possibility of fulfilling this demand. The season has some influence upon the prognosis, many patients simply holding their own during the winter and making a rapid recovery as soon as pleasant weather sets in. It may be said that the sagging of the lower border of the stomach indicates something more than a dyspepsia of atonic form, that we have to deal with an organic lesion. To a certain extent this is true, but practically it is impossible to distinguish between the symptomatology and the course of stagnation of purely functional cause and that due to mild grades of dilation; and from the standpoint of the pathologist, dealing with a non-fatal condition which does not permit the study of morbid anatomy, it is questionable whether the sagging of the greater curvature is a genuine dilation or a functional stretching.

[1] Unfortunately, the notes of the position of the stomach at the first visit of the patient have been lost.

CASE II.—A young man, now aged twenty-eight years, overworked since boyhood, and with vitality impaired by a severe attack of typhoid fever, which resulted in the necrosis of most of one side of the lower alveolar arch, has been under observation several times within the last three years. He is employed in the stock-yards, partly as bookkeeper, partly as superintendent. His worst seasons are those when the weather is best, and when he is most actively engaged in out-door work. This paradox is explained when we remember that out-doors, for him, means a filthy yard crowded with sheep or pigs, with the air always foul and usually dusty with pulverized excrement. His stomach was prolapsed, though not markedly enlarged, and several examinations established the existence of a-chlorhydria, with some fermentation but no lack of pepsin. From June to August, 1895, the fundus of the stomach rose an inch, though he kept at work, and by September the stomach was practically normal. During August, 1896, he returned, complaining of the same symptoms as before, and with the same chemic condition, but differing from the previous condition in that his stomach had remained in normal position. Yet, the course of the trouble was more obstinate than during the first series of observations and, in September, he was compelled to take a vacation. The opinion was frankly expressed that he could not hope for complete and permanent recovery in his present circumstances and that he must seek out-door life—in other words, must leave this climate for a semitropical one—before he became much older, or his chances for improvement would be gone.

Yet, in July, 1897, an examination of the stomach by the writer's method of obtaining a fluoroscopic shadow of a capsule containing bismuth, showed that the stomach had retained its normal contour. The subjective findings were also satisfactory.

CASE III.—By one of the curious coincidences of practice, the writing of this article was interrupted by the arrival of the patient whose case it was intended to report next, and the latest examination somewhat modifies the original conception of the condition. This patient first called two years ago, complaining of the general symptoms of gastric stagnation, his stomach being at the umbilical level. There was diminished secretion of hydrochloric acid. The main etiologic factor seemed to be irregular and hurried meals, due to his vocation, which was that of a trainman. Although hygienic measures could not be fully carried out, treatment was quite successful, and the patient remained well until the following fall. During the winter of 1896–7, only temporary relief could be obtained, and the stomach could not be restored to its normal level. The patient has since been occasionally seen, but no careful examination has been possible until the date of writing, when inspection revealed a significant feature to which too little attention has been called. Along the lower part of the chest, in a wavy line corresponding quite closely to the attachment of the diaphragm, was seen a series of vertical venous twigs, disappearing quite abruptly by diving deep beneath the skin to seek internal anastomoses. Each one of these parallel venous lines is about an inch in length. The writer hesitates to claim originality in regard to this sign, but would urge its importance as a diagnostic feature of sclerosis of the liver. On auscultatory percussion, the stomach was found as before, but the liver, previously normal in area, extended only from the fifth rib to the ninth, a vertical distance in the mammillary line of only ten centimeters. Of course, those clinicians who are accustomed to rely upon ordinary percussion and to reckon the absolute flatness of the liver, must discount this figure very materially. It represents a contraction amounting to at least a rib both above and below. The presence of ascites or jaundice could not be demonstrated.

The connection between hepatic sclerosis and gastric catarrh has been long known, and atony and moderate dilation of the stomach is also a frequent accompaniment of the hepatic affection. Whether the motor change depends upon the catarrh or directly upon the influence of increased back-pressure is not decided. Hemmeter calls attention to a point which most of us overlook, namely: that hepatic sclerosis obstructs the arterial flow through the celiac axis, thus throwing more blood into the arterial supply of the stomach at the most dilatable part of the organ. The obstacle to the venous current from stomach to liver has long been emphasized.

Almost nothing has been said as to the chemic examination of the stomach contents in these cases. As a rule, hydrochloric acid is deficient, as determined by the usual tests or by the writer's effervescence test which obviates the use of the tube, although it is of crucial value only in distinctly acid or non-acid cases. The ferments rarely fail, so rarely, indeed, that it is rather a matter of physiologic study than of practical importance to perform the digestive tests. Constipation is the rule, atony of the whole alimentary tract existing. Even the deglutition murmur is often heard after a very appreciable delay, indicating slow esophageal peristalsis. However, the deglutition murmurs have only slight practical value. The writer has elsewhere protested against the tendency to make fine discriminations in gastric disorders, perhaps he has gone too far and has left certain conceptions confused in the mind of his readers. To some degree, confusion is necessary, as it is an analogue of the pathologic condition. While classing atony and mild dilation as motor failures of the stomach, it must be remembered that mere delay of the passage of food through the stomach cannot produce serious harm, unless secretory failure or secondary fermentation or putrefaction occurs. On the other hand, if the secretory power of the stomach alone fails, the chyme is swept on to the intestine before serious fermentative changes can occur and gastric digestion is so unimportant when compared with that of the intestine and its tributary glands that the former function is scarcely missed by the organism. In other words, however valuable for purposes of theoretic study may be the classification of the various functions and diseased conditions of the stomach, in the study and care of the particular case all of the existing conditions must be made out and treatment directed accordingly. If there is subacidity, as is usually the case, the fact that we conceive of such cases as essentially motor does not lessen the indication for hydrochloric acid. If excessive fermentation is in progress, we must not neglect such active internal antiseptics as salacetol, menthol, gaultheria, etc. The word active is used with due apologies to the surgeon and the bacteriologist who deal with more virulent micro-organisms and who are not so easily satisfied with the mere subduing of germ activity. The slurs which have been so often thrown at gastro-enteric antisepsis are based upon a total misconception of the problem which confronts the practitioner and upon the unwarrantable assumption that the principle *Porcus totus aut nullus* applies to him as well as to the surgeon or the sanitarian.

The three cases reported might be accompanied by dozens of others. They represent the commonest form of stomach trouble and comprise probably half of a practice limited to digestive affections, *i.e.*, one including gastric, hepatic, intestinal, and occasionally esophageal and pancreatic cases. These cases are fairly typical and stand between mere gastric atony on the one hand and true gastric dilation on the other. Just where we must cease to consider the gastric muscle as functionally stretched and regard it as pathologically dilated, it is not profitable to discuss. It often happens that patients with a stomach absolutely normal in area will suffer more from motor and secondary or concomitant secretory weakness than will those who show a moderate sagging of the greater curvature. Such patients rarely die unless from intercurrent disease, and the forbidding of autopsies, almost universally demanded by sentiment, prevents a study of the morbid anatomy. The attempt to solve the pathologic problem by microscopic examination of epithelium from the stomach is useless, judging from the writer's somewhat limited experience. Even if the particular specimen shows well-marked degeneration, we must still ask whether it is not an exfoliated bit of tissue which has ceased to be part of the organism. The impossibility of forming positive conceptions of pathology and of making sharp differential lines has led the writer to hesitate to use technical terms, especially the more or less correct but very imposing Greek terms which are now somewhat in vogue. Even the simple term gastritis is often applied with difficulty. Cases have been so diagnosed simply because the patient has swallowed pharyngeal or respiratory mucus or because the stomach tube has collected a hyalin mass from the esophagus. Excluding these sources, it is quite impossible to mark the boundary between normal mucus production and catarrh. The difficulty of diagnosing the state of the epithelium has already been referred to. Many writers consider deficiency of hydrochloric acid as indicating the presence of gastritis. This is as simple and comforting a rule as can be found, but who will guarantee its accuracy in a particular case?

The prognosis in these cases depends very largely upon underlying conditions, and it is well to watch a case some weeks before committing oneself to a positive statement. In one case in which the stomach sagged only slightly below its normal level, in a young woman in whom the diagnosis of cancer could be almost certainly excluded, matters went from bad to worse. Hydrochloric acid was deficient, intestinal digestion failed, digestion and curdling tests with the stomach contents were exceedingly weak and a diagnosis of anadenia with correspondingly grave prognosis was given. Two or three months after the writer's last visit, the patient died under the care of a thoroughly competent clinician who made the diagnosis of Addison's disease from clinical manifestations of late development, but who could not secure an autopsy. This diagnosis had been considered and set aside for lack of evidence during the writer's attendance. The question in this case, whether actual degeneration of the gastric glands existed or whether the abeyance of function was due to nerve weakness, is still undecided.

In a young girl with gastric atony without dilation, no progress could be made by treatment supposed to be appropriate. After a time a pleurisy coming on without apparent cause gave the first hint of the underlying dyscrasia and she was transferred to another physician for the treatment of tuberculosis. In a highly respectable middle-aged widow, a dyspepsia of the form here considered baffled first her family physician, and was no more than temporarily relieved by the writer. Meningeal symptoms developed, along with a swelling of the knee. Tuberculosis was considered, but neither the writer nor the surgical attendants were satisfied as to the validity of the diagnosis. A physician, called on account of the nervous manifestations, suggested syphilis and although there was no further basis for this diagnosis than the admission that the patient's husband had not been a model of virtue, specific treatment cured the remains of the lesion of the knee and also the meningitis, and the patient has remained well ever since so far as the atonic dyspepsia is concerned. The rôle of the liver in such cases has been alluded to in one of the three cases detailed above, and the production of a mild gastric catarrh and dilation, with symptoms similar to those of essentially functional atony, is to be expected in circulatory lesions which have passed the stage of compensation.

Aside from serious underlying causes which are comparatively rare, the prognosis is almost always good so far as immediate relief is concerned, while ultimate recovery, so that the patient can be free from medical care, depends largely upon the patient's vitality. Occupation and surroundings are important secondary factors, as has been noted in the three cases at the beginning of the paper.

It is a great mistake to lay too much stress upon purely hygienic treatment in such cases. In mild cases of atony, without change in the size of the stomach and without serious disturbance of secretion, recovery undoubtedly occurs, usually without medical care, and in too many instances, in spite of misdirected efforts with pepsin and bismuth. But cases of the degree referred to are very apt to develop in persons leading fairly hygienic lives. They are particularly common in the country, so that we must be cautious about sending patients away from the city with the idea that farm life is distinctly curative. Some patients who have taken this course on their own responsibility have returned in the fall sadly disappointed. Gymnastic courses are also of questionable utility, unless very closely supervised, and the off-hand recommendation to go to a gymnasium is likely to result in an exacerbation of the trouble. Curious enough, medical treatment must be the foundation of hygienic treatment. The physician can almost certainly cure the patient, but only physical vigor and avoidance of depressing causes will keep him well. Medical treatment has been sufficiently alluded to, with the exception of local measures. Lavage is sometimes necessary, sometimes not. Seldom is it advisable to disturb the stomach oftener than once a week and usually a very few local séances suffice. With lavage, the writer uses his method of gastric inflation and medication with menthol vapor.

THE RELATIVE VALUE OF EXPERT TESTIMONY, AS ILLUSTRATED BY THE RECENT INVESTIGATION AT THE EASTERN PENITENTIARY, PHILADELPHIA.

BY HERBERT R. GOODRICH, M.D.,
OF PHILADELPHIA.

THE following bit of history has come to me incident to my duties as resident physician in one of the largest penal institutions in our country—an institution which is unique for its system of separate confinement, and which for years has been the study and admiration of those experienced in the care of the criminal classes.

A few months since this prison became an object of investigation by one of the judges of Philadelphia's Court of Common Pleas, and His Honor pursued the investigation with great vigor and with a manifest purpose of discovering, at any hazard, a large percentage of insane and abused prisoners.

Acting upon his prerogative, the judge finally appointed a commission of two laymen and four physicians whom he was pleased to designate as alienists; they repeatedly visited the prison, threw open the door of every cell, explained their charitable mission to the convicts, and asked for complaints of any and all kinds.

Of course, the distribution of cigars and tobacco to the prisoners, an act distinctly prohibited by law of the Commonwealth, could have no effect upon the general character of the complaints elicited, and is perhaps too trifling to deserve mention.

Given the moral tone of the men who compose the criminal class, and the fact that these men appreciated the power of their champion, it is hardly strange that the judge soon found his grist to be a fine one. The normal element of malcontents grew apace in numbers and audacity, while malingerers appeared on all sides, and what was of custom considered to be an excellent disciplinary effect was seemingly threatened with disintegration.

The press accounts of flagrant abuses in the prison so aroused the surrounding community that a State Senatorial Committee was appointed to investigate the methods of the prison and, specifically, the charges of abuse alleged by the judge and his commission of experts.

Space will permit but a brief review of the many interesting details brought out in the course of this investigation, but the following condensed history of a particular case under question, with extracts from the sworn testimony of several experts, including those of the judge's commission and others of equal and greater experience, is pertinent.

To this will be added references to a few of the "star" cases which were made the cause of diagnostic fancy-flights on the part of the judicial commission of experts.

The history of the first case is as follows:

Convict 7897. Male, large, muscular; shrewd, criminal face; regarded as a dangerous man; of little schooling, but broad experience in crime. He served one term in Sing Sing, from which prison he was sent to the asylum at Matteawan, N. Y., because of suspected insanity, and from this asylum he ultimately escaped. While at the last-named institution he had evidently improved his chances for observation, for he could speak very glibly about delusions, hallucinations, and other phases of insanity.

After admission to the Eastern Penitentiary his conduct for several months was exemplary, and the work assigned to him was well and cheerfully done. Then he began to be restless, asked his cell-mate concerning the treatment of convicts who became insane in this prison, said he had successfully feigned insanity in other prisons, and that at Matteawan, where he was sent from Sing Sing because of insanity, he had recovered too soon and was sent back to Sing Sing. He was thus compelled to go through the malingering process the second time, to be again sent to Matteawan, from which asylum he finally escaped.

He boasted to his cell-mates of a very successful robbery perpetrated in New York City, where he and his pals had planned to break into a jewelry store. A few days before the robbery he was seized with a violent maniacal attack upon the streets of New York and was taken by the patrol-wagon to the station-house. The next morning, being perfectly rational, he told of occasionally being afflicted with such attacks, and he was thereupon released. Later the jewelry store was robbed and he was caught red-handed, but with no plunder, and in a fit of mania. Upon ascertaining his former record he was sent to an asylum from which he escaped shortly after to "divide the swag," which he said was a "rich one," with his confederate. In his words "playing crazy was the easiest snap going."

After being confined in the Eastern Penitentiary for several months, he announced to his cell-mate that he "always made it a point to get crazy" if he thought he could gain anything by it, and he would have played crazy here if he could have gained his point. A few days after this statement he began to show signs of extraordinary devotion to religious subjects, praying frequently, and exhorting his cell-mate to do so. The cell-mate stated that he took little stock in that sort of religion, for when 7897 was not praying, he was cursing or planning some bit of deviltry. In the cell-mate's words, "I thought it was a poor way to be good—to be religious one minute and then telling all kinds of rascalities." He began to be uneasy, said he had never been used to being penned up for so long; that he had been used to getting into some insane asylum and then escaping from it.

With these prodromes, which are somewhat indefinitely diagnostic in value, 7897 was one night seized with a violent maniacal attack, in which he beat his cell-mate, attacked the officers of the prison, threw and held himself upon the hot steam pipes used for heating the cell, thereby inflicting upon himself deep and painful burns, and otherwise behaved in a most impetuous manner. He shouted aloud and prayed to God, saying that he must purge away his sins through this burning inflicted upon himself; he was destructive and filthy in his personal habits, fought his attendants, and tore the bandages off his burns, slept little, and refused to eat. Within a month and a half he had completely recovered, and was shortly afterward put to work in the yard, where he had more companionship and liberty. Fourteen months afterward, during which time he had been entirely tractable and rational, he was able to recite with remarkable accuracy every detail of the attack just described, recounting minutely the extreme keenness of the pain he felt at the time of his injuries, and announcing that he had at that time suffered from an attack of "religious mania." At the end of this period, which would seem to be one of voluntary sanity, and after having several interviews with the afore-mentioned judge and his experts, he was one day removed to the court that he might give testimony concerning the treatment of convicts who become insane while confined in this prison.

The incidents of this inquiry were sensational in extreme—a most humane and sympathetic judge, an outraged and denunciatory commission of experts giving clinical demonstrations to the jury, and incidentally to the representatives of the press. As a result, the convict was subjected to a rather more than ordinary period of mental excitation. Immediately upon his return to prison, during two days, there followed a period of what seemed to be nervousness and depression, when another outbreak of violence occurred; this time of a milder character than the first, and he was filthy in his habits and refused to wear his clothes, but he offered no injury to his person. On the sixth day of this attack, after he had destroyed several suits of clothes, he was again dressed and threatened with the strait-jacket if he further refused to be clad. He gave no trouble after this, and on the tenth day of the attack had completely recovered and remained entirely rational in talk and behavior until his discharge a few weeks later. This man was observed during this latter attack by two alienists, not included in the judge's commission, and they declared themselves unwilling to state that he was insane. This history is written from an almost daily personal observation and from the correlative testimony of those associated with the prisoner.

The following is abstracted from the testimony of several experts summoned before the Senatorial Investigating Committee and examined by that body. To avoid personalities each expert will be designated by the letters of the alphabet, the three members of the judge's commission taking precedence and being considered, as it were, for the prosecution, while the gentlemen whose testimony follows may represent the defense.

Dr. A. (Judge's Commission):

7897 had religious mania. He gave a very connected account of himself. He was very emotional and cried a great deal in the description of his condition. This man had a wonderful memory — a memory for the minutest details. He was not insane when I examined him. I think he was a man easily excited into a maniacal condition.

Dr. B. (Judge's Commission):

At the time I examined 7897 he did not give evidence of being insane, but in the history of the case I should say he undoubtedly had an attack of insanity. I was told his prior history. I think he will have recurrent attacks of mania. My examination I regarded as careful. That man should be removed instantly to some asylum. I think it better that a violent criminal should escape than that the reason of one man be overthrown by his detention here.

Dr. C. (Judge's Commission):

We examined 7897. This occupied several hours and he was heard on two separate occasions. We received a history from 7897; he had been confined at various asylums previously. We had that and the authoritative fact that cases of mania are very prone to recur. The tendency of modern writers is to place mania among the recurrent insanities. I have a great deal of credence in the statement made by 7897. I have been familiar with the detailed accounts which patients in mania give of their experience. Those of us who have examined such cases of insanity know how good an account they can give of their experiences—especially in cases of simple mania. There was no conclusion open to the commission save that the man had a bona-fide attack of acute mania. I say that detailed accounts of this mania are very striking; and that the patients give an almost stenographic account of what occurred; that the existence of memory (in these cases) is a well-known fact and that it has received a technical name—being known as hypermnesia. It looks as if the attack of mania originated in a few hours. Sometimes we have attacks of mania which are termed explosive—in the epileptic form; but I do not believe that the attack in this case was of that kind. Let me tell you that malingerers, unless they are educated persons or have some medical knowledge, are not capable of playing their rôle and doing it well. This case was a clear A-B-C case to an alienist.

Dr. D. (alienist of wide experience, not of Judge's Commission):

Persons feigning insanity would injure themselves to any extent at all. They will burn themselves as that man did.

Dr. E. (not of Judge's Commission):

At the time I saw 7897 he impressed me as being a man in full possession of his faculties and having a rather acute intellect. I found him with his mind fully intent upon his own future interests, and particularly so as to how individuals acquainted with his testimony would be disposed to look out for him when he got outside. He obtained the addresses of some of them from me and seemed to think he ought to be taken care of in a very proper manner.

Q. For doing what?

A. For testifying. He did not specify except to say that it might be of interest to know that the burns he received, in one respect, were unfortunate: he said he was a pickpocket by occupation, and his future usefulness was limited by the scar on his right hand. He seemed to be rather grieved in that respect. He told me, with remarkable elaboration, how the burns occurred. He dwelt especially on his own feelings, and he rather made an analysis of his own mental condition that led him to inflict the burns, and said he inflicted them because he felt it diverted himself from the contemplation of his misfortunes. I have seen people mutilate themselves; it is not unusual; but it has never been my experience to see an insane man who was able to analyze the sentiments under which he did mutilate himself. The impression that I gathered was that he had done this for a purpose. I would certainly think it possible for this man to be a malingerer.

Dr. F. (not of Judge's Commission):

From his subsequent history I would look upon him with suspicion. He admitted to me that he had feigned insanity at other times, but said that he was really insane at this time. He had been in an asylum for some time, and could talk very learnedly about delusions, showing that he had used his wits while in the asylum. He said he was at Auburn. and added: "I wasn't there for nothing." He had chances to observe cases of insanity, and if he did want to simulate he was thereby enabled to be that much more expert at it.

Dr. ——'s diagnosis of the case was acute mania. Now, as he had a constant delusion that he was burning himself to do penance for his sins, and thought he deserved that burning, he could not possibly have had acute mania.

If this prisoner was insane, he had melancholia agitata. Acute-mania patients are exalted, and whatever they do is done because they are exalted. A case of acute mania would not maintain a delusion for days and weeks as 7897 did; the patient would have occasional delusions that would come and go. Moreover, it is impossible for a patient in acute mania to remember everything that happens. He may or may not have a hazy recollection of what has happened to a certain extent; he does not have clear-cut recollections of everything that has happened.

Another patient, diagnosed by the entire commission as primary spastic paraplegia, had none of the symptoms characteristic of this disorder, with the single exception of increased tendon reflexes. He positively lacked the spastic muscular condition and the characteristic gait, while his apparent loss of power in the lower limbs was simply the expression of faulty coordination. Some curiously reckless higher power had given these experts the ability to diagnose this disease (as was expressed by one of their number) "not by any particular line of symptoms, but by the general appearance of the patient."

A third man, declared by the commission to be afflicted with chronic mania, was, during the time of their visits to the prison, violent in the extreme. A strong, muscular negro, a degenerate, criminal type; he would by day be comparatively quiet, but at night the silent corridors would resound with his almost continuous shouting and singing. He was destructive and filthy to an extreme degree. During all this time his appetite was good and the bowels normal in action. He maintained a constant body weight, could be bribed and thus induced to behave himself, and had a good memory for recent and past events, with an ability for reasoning. After the cessation of the apparently disturbing visits of the commission he was placed at work in the yard, where aside from occasional exhibitions of deviltry, evidently given for the purpose of creating laughter among his companions, he behaved rationally.

At the expiration of his sentence he was discharged from the prison, and shortly after his case came to the notice of Professor Horatio C. Wood, who exhibited the negro at his clinic, where was shown some of the possibilities to which the malingerer, if he wishes, may attain. At the time, being asked if he thought he could again deceive the prison officials, he replied: "I don't know. A burnt child is scared of the fire."

It is a well-known fact that, however much a bad man may have menaced and terrorized society while in possession of his liberty, as soon as prison gates shut him out from the inquisitive gaze he becomes the object of sympathy and pity of a strangely unreasonable community, which is ever ready to believe him of necessity abused and maltreated by those who have him in keeping; and the individuals who, before his incarceration, demanded little short of his immediate extermination, now say: "Poor fellow; how great must have been his temptations."

Granting that such a condition is to be expected from our untutored masses, who may read but do not reason, is it too presumptuous to ask that the minds of our leaders in thought—our professional men—be disabused of such idiocy?

Prisons hold within their walls the most desperate and depraved of our kind—men who are wont to take infinite pains that they may abstain from honest toil, and for precisely this reason the discipline of a prison is strict; and, since it protects the honest man in the enjoyment of his property and rights, this discipline should be respected.

The conditions and circumstances incident to prison life are so impossible to the community at large as to be absolutely incomprehensible to the average person in possession of his liberty, and often to those versed in the management of penal institutions.

To the prisoner who has a desire to make himself amenable to the rules the life is necessarily irksome —from the deprivation of his liberty—though it is by no means intolerable; but it is to the professional malcontent—the man who constantly schemes to wrong his fellow-man, in prison or out, that prison enormities occur. To such a man, who has perhaps been checked in the perpetration of some trifling infraction of the rules, any and all rules are obnoxious; and thereafter he will take any risk and go to all lengths to attain an end which to the average person would seem almost too trivial to act as a factor. Considering the machine methods of our American politics, it does not create so much wonderment to discover now and then instances of the perversion of public services to private ends, even in our judiciary. But to whom shall we turn if our men of science give us as their profound and deliberate opinions results which are derived from cursory examinations and incomplete knowledge of conditions? Formerly the sworn testimony of a man versed in medicine or one of its allied sciences had great weight and was accepted as high authority, in the minds of the jury, as bearing upon this or that phase of a case in question; but to-day there is found within call of the court-room the parasitic expert, who, after a casual glance at the details of a case, and for a consideration, coupled with the gratification of a few press notices, will eructate ponderous opinions, favoring either defense or prosecution, according to orders. Such facultative philanthropists, while seeking to pose as benefactors of the oppressed, are actually, to the extent of their limitations, prodigies in wrong-doing.

A glance at the press comments upon expert testimony in many of our murder trials will indicate the derision in which such evidence is coming to be held by people who are in the habit of thinking.

DOES THE THEORY THAT TYPHOID FEVER CAN BE ABORTED CONFLICT WITH ANY ESTABLISHED LAW OF PATHOLOGY OR WITH ANY KNOWN SCIENTIFIC FACT?[1]

BY JOHN ELIOT WOODBRIDGE, M.D.,
OF CLEVELAND, OHIO.

THROUGHOUT the ages medical writers have deplored their helplessness in the presence of the grave fevers and have admitted their inability to cure them. Hippocrates alludes to epidemics in which the fever ran forty, sometimes eighty, and in one reported case, one hundred and twenty days. An important adjunct, if not an essential part, of his treatment of "many diseases" was the bath, for which he gives minute directions. According to Pliny, Asclepiades of Bithynia was also a distinguished advocate of the use of the bath. Francis Adams said, "However much the advocates for a bold system of treating disease may be disposed to deride the 'expectant method' of Hippocrates, which Asclepiades contemptously denominated 'the contemplation of death,' it does not want the sanction of a name which is second only to Hippocrates in the literature of epidemic fevers, *viz.*, Sydenham. Avicenna, 'the most illustrious of Arabian physicians,' whose 'canon was for five centuries regarded as the highest authority in the schools of Europe,' said of semitertian fever, 'It is apt to be protracted and pass into the hectic. It is said to be generally protracted to the fortieth day.'"

John Huxham in 1750 said, "In many cases only time itself seems to wear it off."

Watson in 1858 said, "The treatment of continued fevers has been at all times a stumbling-block to young practitioners, and a subject of dispute even among physicians who have built it upon their own experience. . . . It was once a favorite practice with physicians to attempt to cut short the fever at its outset, and the two expedients which were chiefly relied upon for that purpose were emetics and cold affusions. They have both of them, in this country, gone very much out of fashion." Sir William Jenner says: "I have never known a case of typhoid fever to be cut short by any remedial agent—that is, cured. The poison which causes any of the acute specific diseases (to which typhoid fever as much as smallpox belongs) having entered the system, all the stages of the disease must, as far as we now know, be passed through before the patient can be well. The ordinary duration of a fully-developed attack of typhoid fever is from twenty-eight to thirty days."

Moore of Dublin says: "There is no specific for enteric fever, any more than for typhus." And he adds: "Although we cannot cure the disease we must treat it."

Flint says: "It must be admitted that the known resources of therapeutics do not afford reliable means for the arrest of these fevers or even for shortening the duration of the febrile career." Allbutt says: "We have as yet no specific treatment of enteric fever. We do not know of any drug which destroys the typhoid bacillus or checks its growth in the intestinal glands or other organs, nor of any agent to counteract or neutralize the action of the toxins of the bacillus circulating in the blood."

Hare says: "Before going farther, however, the

[1] Read at a meeting of the Medico-Surgical Society of New York, February 7, 1898.

writer desires to insist very strongly upon one fact, namely: that a case of typhoid fever is not curable in any degree. No remedy yet found, except it act through the prevention of complications, can shorten its course." Wilson says: "No drug or method of treatment is at present known by which enteric fever can be aborted. . . . Enteric fever, like the other acute specific febrile infections, runs a course uninfluenced by medicines. . . . In the words of Osler, 'no known drug shortens by a day the course of the fever. No method of specific treatment or of antisepsis of the bowel has yet passed beyond the stage of primary laudation.'"

Osler says: "We are still without an agent which can counteract the gradual influence of the poisons which develop in the course of acute febrile diseases, such as typhoid fever, pneumonia, and diphtheria."

The text-books and medical journals from which the above quotations are taken, bear testimony to how firmly intrenched in the minds of the greatest teachers of medicine is the theory that typhoid fever cannot be cured, and how fondly ancient tradition, modern science, and even the most recent discoveries, have been evoked to sustain these erroneous theories of a bygone age.

If, in discussing this subject some of my utterrances seem too forcible, please bear in mind that my denunciations are not directed against the distinguished gentlemen who have criticised my theories, but against their false deductions and their erroneous interpretations of facts, and against these because the sacred name of science has been invoked to sustain false dogmas—stumbling blocks in the pathway of progress—which are responsible for the sacrifice of enormous numbers of human lives and which militate against the highest interests of the human race and of the medical profession. If the theories or arguments advanced savor of want of reverence for the authority of the great teachers, you will hear me more patiently if you realize that while I have not imitated the ancient physicians of whom Sir William Roberts says: "The writings of Hippocrates, Aristotle, Ptolemy, Galen, and other masters were studied and searched, not for inspiration to new inquiry and higher development, but these great names were erected into sacrosanct authorities, beyond whose teachings it was vain, and even impious to penetrate," I have, on the contrary, studied to profit to the utmost from these writings; I have accepted their teachings with a too confiding faith, and have rejected such of them only as have been, by absolutely apodictic evidence, proven erroneous. I have fully realized the responsibility of making such rejections, and I have given all of the best years of my life to the verification of a principle—before promulgating it.

The theory that typhoid fever can be aborted and the abortive treatment of typhoid fever have been so often and so persistently denounced as unscientific and irrational that my duty to humanity, no less than my obligation to the physicians who have volunteered in my defense, demands the refutation of these charges (notwithstanding the fact that they are mere bald assertions entirely unsupported by scientific data or sound arguments) because to those who are fully informed as to what is and what is not science, these denunciations—unreasonable, illogical, and unscientific as they are—are equivalent to a sentence of outlawry pronounced against every physician who cures typhoid fever.

Therefore, without awaiting the more specific arraignment which should have accompanied the charges, without waiting to learn from the devotees of science what especial law or edict forbids the jugulation of typhoid fever or condemns the abortive treatment for this disease, I shall endeavor to show that there is no warrant either of science or reason for the denunciations so wantonly hurled at the theory under consideration. All allusions to the scientific aspects of this subject have been purposely thus far deferred, because it was known that the simple enunciation of the fact that typhoid fever can be aborted, an idea so at variance with all teaching, would elicit a sufficiently exciting discussion, and that the declaration that erroneous interpretations of science were being invoked to sustain fallacious arguments would have unmasked an adversary in every scientist, and the result would have been that rational medicine would have been buried in oblivion under an avalanche of reprehension. But the weakling theory of 1880 is an established principle to-day, and, although there is still a majority of the physicians of the country who do not believe in the abortive treatment, which with its wide range of usefulness and application to the cure of a large class of microbic diseases, has, by its results, endeared itself to the hearts of thousands of the best clinicians in the United States, Canada, and Mexico, it has become so firmly established that no power can uproot it. When a very respectable minority of the physicians of the country have become enthusiastic enough to report their results and have highly commended a method of treatment which has been so sharply criticized as the one under consideration, its future status is assured, because the most learned and intelligent class of the most enlightened people on the earth does not court martyrdom for the sake of opinions or theories of the correctness or validity of which they entertain the slightest doubt.

The science of to-day is built upon the correction of the errors of yesterday, and much of that which a hundred years ago was treasured and defended as science is to us a conglomerate of stupid blunders, and some of the errors which we are now teaching will a century hence be laughed to scorn. Revolutions in science are sometimes rapid, and it is not always necessary to scrutinize long periods of time to observe the changes which are taking place. He who a few months ago would have spoken of looking through those substances that were then regarded as opaque would have been an unscientific dreamer, and he who, before Laveran announced to the world his great discovery, exhibited a specimen of paludal blood under the microscope and said that it could be disinfected by a single dose of quinin, would have been promptly consigned to the scientists' Hades. In fact, there is now lying on my desk a copy of a medical journal, in which the associate editor, ——, A.M., M.D., a professor of clinical medicine, who occupies a place in the scientific world, has published under his signature a leading article to prove the absurdity of the theory under consideration by showing that in an individual of average development *there will be* from sixteen to eighteen pounds of blood, and he adds that "he knows of no remedy but turpentin which can be administered in large enough doses to 'effect' (?) the blood;" but quinin aborts ague and ague is a specific infection. The author adds that, "the upper portion of the (alimentary) canal being acid and the lower portion alkaline, a drug which would be absorbed in one place would be slow of action in another, and as a result, of little avail." These are scientific deductions which the veriest tyro would laugh at, but they do not seem more ridiculous to those who know better than are many of the lessons in science that are gravely inculcated in this the closing decade of the Nineteenth Century.

I give—without endorsement—a few citations of various authorities to show that among scientists, who have devoted their lives to investigations in the departments of knowledge which they discuss, there is so much divergence of opinion upon questions of vital importance, there are so many admissions of want of "final" proof of the validity of some of the fundamental principles of modern science upon which depends not only the value of all the deductions which are drawn from them, but also the permanence and stability of some of the accepted interpretations of the sciences themselves, and that even among these learned savants there is such a limitation of positive and exact knowledge of essential facts as would militate against the value of any opinion which even they might entertain upon this important subject.

You, no doubt, all believe that the bacillus of Eberth sustains to typhoid fever the relationship of cause and effect, but you have no positive knowledge of this fact, if it is a fact. Sternberg says: "Recent researches support the view that the bacillus described by Eberth in 1880 bears an etiologic relation to typhoid fever, and pathologists are disposed to accept this bacillus as the veritable 'germ' of typhoid fever, notwithstanding the fact that the final proof that such is the case is still wanting." Thoma says: "Klebs, Eberth, Koch, and Gaffky have identified what is in all probability the cause of this disease." Dr. Frangulea of Roumania read a paper at the recent International Medical Congress, entitled "The Pathogenesis of Typhoid Fever, and the Errors of the Current Microbian Theory," in which he said: "Typhoid fever may, under certain conditions, arise spontaneously—that is, without the presence of the bacillus of Eberth. The bacillus coli communis may, under favorable conditions, acquire pathogenic properties and produce typhoid fever. It can preserve and transmit these new qualities to future generations. These new generations may adapt themselves to new conditions, and, obeying the law of atavism, return to their primitive state. It is incorrect to say that a germ must always and everywhere preserve its form and specificity, especially an absolute specificity."

Dr. Peckham has, by a carefully conducted series of experiments, shown that nearly, if not quite all the characteristics which serve to distinguish the bacillus of Eberth from the bacillus coli may be obliterated or transposed, and, giving a table of seventy cultures, lays stress upon the anomalous results obtained, and says: "We conclude, as others also have done, that there is a series of closely related forms which may be regarded as intermediate or transitional, and which serve to establish a biologic relationship either near or remote, between these two typical members" (the typhoid and colon bacillus).

Professor Behring thinks that "in the light of serum-treatment all our older views must vanish." "Cellular pathology," he says, "has become unfruitful for therapeutics. It is vain to treat the organs that are affected." Serum-treatment, if we may judge from the summary of his paper, is alone efficient.

Professor Liebreich, in the Fifteenth German Congress for Internal Medicine, spoke "at length of the modern medicinal therapy. He was strongly opposed to Behring's school and its methods. . . . He was opposed to the recognition of a bacterium as the cause of an infectious disease. Especially did he oppose serotherapy."

Dr. Saundby is of the opinion, "not only that the

recent discoveries with regard to pathogenic organisms and their products open up an altogether new prospect in therapeutics, upon the threshhold of which we are now standing," but that "the system of pharmacology is about to pass into the limbo of the forgotten."

Wilson says: "It has been demonstrated that the pathogenic bacilli do not appear in the stools earlier than the tenth day, very often not before the sixteenth or seventeenth day. . . . The toxins which result from their growth are evolved within the tissues of the organism itself, not in the intestinal canal. Intestinal antisepsis, in so far as the pathogenic organisms of enteric fever are concerned, is, therefore, directed against germs not present in the bowel prior to the breaking down of the intestinal lymph-elements and must, for that reason, be largely inoperative. . . . From clinical and pathologic considerations alike, the whole subject of the antiseptic treatment of enteric fever falls to the ground."

F. Wallis Stoddard says: "The isolation of the typhoid bacilli from sewage and polluted waters is a problem which in spite of the large amount of attention bestowed upon it may be said to remain unsolved. Of the now numerous instances in which this separation has been announced, few, if any, have been supported by convincing evidence. . . . I have been exceptionally favored as regards opportunities of carrying out this research. . . . I have never been able to demonstrate the presence of any organism (in water or milk) which I could conscientiously accept as the typhoid bacillus, and in one instance only—the Poultney epidemic—did I find a bacillus so closely resembling typhoid as to make it a matter of some difficulty to decide upon its non-specific character. These failures, however, fade into insignificance, when compared with the experiences of Lawe and Andrews in London, and Dr. Nicolli in Constantinople. The report of the former to the London County Council is too recent to require further comment. The latter investigator not only failed to find the typhoid bacillus in sewage or even in stools, but roundly declared that the presence of the colon bacillus presented an insuperable obstacle to the separation of the typhoid bacillus from such material."

The Chairman of the Section on Pharmacology, at the recent meeting of the British Medical Association, said: "At one time it seemed that with the increase of knowledge of the nature of disease and the action of drugs and of the constitution of remedies, pharmacology would march straight to victory, and we had only to accumulate information relating to antiseptics and to determine more accurately the influence exercised on tissues and organs, by groups and compounds, to acquire the power of successfully opposing all forms of evil, but we found no drugs which act as mercury does in syphilis, and the action of this and also of some of the best known of our remedies remained undetermined."

Hare says: "We cannot explain how salicylic acid does good in rheumatism, or how mercury does good in syphilis, because we have no knowledge of the essential nature of rheumatism or of syphilis." This distinguished author might have added—or of the action of either of these or of hundreds of other common remedies.

Behring has said, "antitoxins are not chemic substances, but natural forces."

Wilson says: "The toxins are poisonous chemic compounds." Liebreich says: "The theory that antitoxins are not chemic substances but natural forces is a daring hypothesis." Virchow says: "Life is in the cell. He who speaks of serum as a vital force apart from cells is wrong. The grand truth of cellular succession may be assailed in the future as it has been in the past, but it will never be thrown to the earth. It will shine through all the long years of the Twentieth Century." In an editorial which recently appeared in the *British Medical Journal*, it was said: "Standing as we do on the verge of a new era in treatment, it would be rash indeed to attempt to predict the future of therapeutics."

We have not yet solved the great problem of life. We have not yet solved the mystery of the life of a single cell. We do not know how cell-life is influenced or how it influences the organism of which, minute as it is, it is a vital part. We do not know how medicines affect or influence the metabolism of cells, and yet it is probably here that we must come to study the action of medicines and to formulate the science of therapeutics, for it is just as true to-day as when Pareira wrote it in 1836: "The exact way in which medicines influence tissues is involved in impenetrable mystery." There is, therefore, but one way in which their action or their value can be established, *viz.*, by the clinical experience of a large number of observers extending over a long period of time and in an enormous number of cases scattered over a large area. Discussing this point Sir William Jenner says: "I do not in the least degree underestimate the immense importance of numeric analysis for arriving at truth on medical subjects; and if it were possible to find the value of the several remedies proposed for the treatment of typhoid fever or of its symptoms by numeric analysis, the results of such an analysis would be real steps in our knowledge; for facts would replace opinions, and doubts in regard to the influence of remedies would be impossible. Each special act of treatment would then be based upon firm grounds instead of being as it now is—an experiment performed by the medical attendant."

Unfortunately, the abortive treatment of typhoid fever must be discussed as a curative rather than an abortive treatment, because the efficient application of antiseptic (?) medicines in the inchoative stage of the disease will generally prevent the development of its pathognomonic symptoms, and thus all ideally aborted cases are lost to science. Therefore, while the 179 deaths no doubt include all of the fatalities which have occurred under this treatment in the hands of physicians who have reported their cases, the 9487 cases reported certainly do not include all of the cases treated. But a death-rate of 1.88 per cent. in so large a number of cases in the hands of so many physicians, a very large number of whom applied the method in an emergency or as a *dernier ressort*, with little faith in its value, and no previous experience in its application, is a phenomenal result, quite as surprising to me as to any one, because, knowing the difficulties which had so often interfered with my own success, I fully appreciated the dangers which would always lie in the pathway of the inexperienced. In one of my earlier papers I anticipated and strove to discount the adverse reports which I confidently expected. It has, therefore, been a most gratifying surprise that so many physicians have given expression to their highest approval of the method, and that, so far as I know, there are but fourteen dissentients among those who speak from experience.

Presenting these statistics, I ask the devotees of science to name one of her laws which they violate, or with which the theory *that typhoid fever can be aborted* is not in perfect harmony. As every possible effort has been made to invalidate the statistics on the ground that they are vitiated by "errors of diagnosis," I may be excused for reverting to the subject, although this puerile and untenable contention was conclusively refuted in a recent issue of the *Medical Record.*

In the words of Sir Francis Palgrave, "I have never shunned repetition of any sort or kind when I have found repetitions necessary. Repetitions are not superfluities, or is it surplussage to reiterate the same thought or factor under diverse combinations." As this is the most important contention in the most important subject before the medical profession, repetition and reiteration are justifiable. I, therefore, present the history of a case which has already been published:

James K., aged twenty-four years, on March 30th, was very ill. He sent for a physician on April 1st, who (according to the statements of the family) made a diagnosis of influenza. On April 6th Dr. Cunningham was called to see the patient, and diagnosed typhoid fever. On April 7th I was called in consultation. When the abortive treatment was instituted the patient had a morning temperature of 104° F., and an evening temperature of 105° F. His abdomen was excessively tender and tympanitic; his nervous symptoms exceedingly bad; his tongue tremulous, very dry and brown; he had persistent hiccough, and also was delirious. The next morning he was so wildly delirious that he could with difficulty be held in bed or forced to swallow medicines. At the end of five days of treatment his temperature had dropped to 99° F.; all of the grave symptoms had disappeared; his tongue was moist; his head clear; his abdomen quite flat and entirely free from tenderness; tympanites was very slight, and he was sleeping naturally and had a good appetite. At this time intussusception developed and ultimately caused his death. There can be no doubt as to the correctness of the diagnosis in this case, and the extensive ulcerations of Peyer's glands found post-mortem exclude it from the category of the so-called "abortive" cases.

It is, therefore, an unquestionable fact that the abortive treatment did, in this instance, reduce the temperature practically to normal; dissipate the wild delirium and the tympanites; relieve the abdominal pain and tenderness; steady the nerves; restore the appetite, and cause natural sleep. It moistened and cleared up the dry, brown tongue. It rendered the urine normal in quantity and appearance; it deodorized the alvine dejections, asepticized the alimentary canal, and placed the ulcerated Peyer's patches in a healthy condition, and had it not been for the unfortunate accident (intussusception) which caused his death, they would have healed within four or five days, and the patient would have been well.

Case 9178 illustrates the effect of the abortive treatment when properly applied early in the course of the disease, and it emphasizes the importance of verifying the clinical diagnosis by the diazo reaction of Ehrlich and by the serum-test of Widal; because, although the patient was treated two days by an able and skilful physician, and was then sent to the writer with a diagnosis of typhoid fever, and, although the symptoms indicated a remarkably severe attack of the disease in the seventh or eighth day of its course, it would have been difficult to establish a diagnosis of typhoid because the malady yielded so promptly to treatment that no rose spots appeared.

It would, perhaps, be improper to say that undue attention has been given to the morbid anatomy of this disease; but that undue importance has been attached to certain anatomic lesions of typhoid is susceptible of most positive proof; *e.g.*, the swelling and ulceration of intestinal glands have been regarded as the essential feature of the disease, and this lesion has given it a name—an error which it is to be regretted is being perpetuated by an important department of the government of the United States. The very constant and characteristic lesion has not only been studied, described, and regarded as *the disease*, but the time required for the healing of the ulcers has given a measure to its duration, and their presence has been declared an insurmountable obstacle to the shortening of the course of the fever. Another double delusion, embodying two errors: First, an abrasion of like size and depth on the surface of a healthy body, in an aseptic condition, would be completely cicatrized within three or four days. Second, aside from the danger from hemorrhage or perforation, the intestinal ulcers, in a properly asepticized alimentary canal, are ordinarily of no more consequence than would be like abrasions on the surface of the body. They will not, under the circumstances named, cause an elevation of temperature of one-fifth of a degree. They will not give rise to tympanites or pain, they will not cause perceptible acceleration of the pulse or respiration, and they will not cause headache or delirium. These are the manifestations of the toxemia, and the toxemia is the disease. It follows, therefore, that a rapid decline of temperature from 105° F. to nearly or quite normal in a severe attack of typhoid, with a like diminution of the frequency of the pulse and respiration, the entire dissipation of enormous tympanities, and of profound delirium, complete restoration of the appetite and of ability to sleep naturally throughout the night, and of an appearance and feeling of almost perfect health, do not prove that the ulcerations of Peyer's glands have healed; nor does the presence of these ulcers prove that the real disease—the toxemia—was not aborted.

The case of James K., which illustrates all these and many other important points, if accepted and interpreted correctly, will negative many of the arguments deduced from erroneous interpretations of facts, the mere mention of which is prohibited by the limitation of time. For instance, clinicians have taught us that diarrhea and intestinal hemorrhage should be guarded against by the administration of opium and astringents; whereas, a proper and judicious use of antiseptics, not only obviates all danger from diarrhea, but makes the administration of laxatives necessary to secure even normal activity of the bowels. Moreover, the free exhibition ot laxative which are capable of emptying the intestinal canal and increasing peristaltic action, minimizes the danger of both hemorrhage and perforation. Another grave error which has been repeated and emphasized in almost every society in which the subject has been discussed is: "nourish and sustain the patient and avoid the use of laxatives as too depressing and weak." Hippocrates said: "Impure bodies, the more you nourish and cherish the more you hurt them," and experience sustains the wisdom of the aphorism, as any physician who has tried to "nourish and cherish" a typhoid patient and has seen the flesh melt away and the strength fail week after week may satisfy himself by first making the body pure and watching the patient's strength and symptoms improve while the toxins are being neutralized and eliminated, even though the bowels are moving six or eight times daily.

I know of no other disease which may be accompanied by so many concurrent affections, followed by so many dangerous sequelæ, and in the course of which so many grave complications may develop. It is highly important, therefore, to apply scientific treatment as early and as efficiently as possible. Your distinguished townsman, Dr. Jacobi, in discussing another subject spoke so aptly that I cannot refrain from quoting his words. He said: "What cannot be cured need not be endured—it ought to be prevented. We were on the wrong track when we spoke of the necessity of a so-called 'expectant' treatment. This waiting, Macawber-like, for something to turn up, is fraught with great danger, and has caused the sacrifice of many lives."

These are words of living truth, and especially applicable to the subject under discussion, and it is equally true that he who awaits the development of such symptoms as will make a positive diagnosis of typhoid fever possible, will often lose the golden opportunity of aborting the disease and will consequently expose his patients to the dangers of numerous complications and sequelæ.

In view of the unequivocal evidence here presented of the limitations of our positive knowledge of the bacteriology, etiology, pathology, and therapeutics of typhoid fever, it is puerile to contend that these sciences or any or all of them can furnish any reliable data upon which to ground the theory that typhoid fever cannot be aborted or that any method of treatment that has produced satisfactory results is unscientific. The subject is entirely beyond the realm of *a priori* reasoning, and it is as futile to argue that because the scientist in his laboratory has not pointed the way to abort the disease that it cannot be aborted. The same argument might be applied to malaria.

The German formula and the laboratory are, in their proper sphere, excellent servants and assistants to medicine. I avail myself of their aid on every possible occasion, but they are unsafe guides, intolerable masters, and dangerous leaders; they may point the way, but the true clinician will pursue it warily. They may verify results, and the proudest discoverer will bow his head in gratitude for their encouragement. But when scientists demand that the strong evidence of clinical experience shall be measured by their imperfect standards and shall conform to their *ipse dixits*, and when they assert that the thousands of observers who have cured typhoid fever have been mistaken in their diagnoses, they demand more than the present state of their knowledge will justify and they assert what is not true.

It is an insult to the intelligence of this enlightened age to argue that—because no one ever has cured typhoid fever—ergo—no one ever can cure typhoid fever. Equally insolent is it to ask the medical profession to accept as an immutable law a senseless tradition born of the ignorance of an almost prehistoric time and handed down from age to age—growing more dogmatic as one pseudo-scientist after another stamps his egotism upon it, until from a simple admission that the fever generally runs to the fortieth day, it becomes an affirmation that typhoid fever cannot be cured and a shibboleth by which to condemn those who do not accept it.

Justified and sustained by the clinical evidence here and heretofore presented, I demand that they correct their interpretations of science in accordance with established facts. The abortive treatment of typhoid fever is rational and scientific. The physicians who apply it to the cure of disease are the true scientists. The knowledge which accords with their observations and experience is science, and that which does not is scientolism, and will fall to earth.

Addendum.—After this paper was read, and during the discussion, the following histories of cases of typhoid fever were reported by the President of the Society, Dr. John Blake White, who said that "they were the last of a series of cases in which he had used this method of treatment, and in which the clinical diagnosis was positively verified by the Widal-test, which was made by the Bacteriologist of the Board of Health of the City of New York."

Mrs. F. J. B., married, native born, consulted me for some special complaint requiring slight operation, which was performed Saturday, December 11, 1897. Convalescence satisfactory until last week in December, when she had headache, backache, nausea, prostration, tongue coated, with red edges; abdomen tympanitic, with pain in right iliac fossa, and gurgling on pressure; no diarrhea, but discharges when induced by enema or laxative medicines were offensive, ocher-colored, with mucus and fibrinous shreds; some pieces of mucus appeared like an organized exudate several inches in length. Stool always accompanied by pain. Rise in temperature, with exacerbations night and morning. Woodbridge treatment begun January 1, 1898. A characteristic and extensive rose-colored eruption appeared upon abdomen and chest, January 5th. Widal reaction confirmed diagnosis, January 6th. Temperature normal, January 11th, and, with slight fluctuations, continued so. Diet increased on January 12th, and solid food allowed after January 22nd. Patient sitting up and walking about the room by January 28th. Some mucus expelled per rectum about this time, for which 5 minims of spirits of turpentine in soft capsule, were prescribed every night for a week, after which no mucus was observed.

Miss A. O., native born, single, aged thirty years. About November 20, 1897, she experienced pain in back, frontal headache, sense of chilliness, constant lassitude and languor, with feverishness increasing every afternoon. This condition continuing until November 28th, I was summoned in the afternoon, and found her with tongue furred, edges red. Temperature, 103° F.; pulse rapid; bowels loose; abdomen resonant, and soreness and gurgling in right iliac fossa. Rose spots appeared at the end of the second week. On the fourteenth day there was pulmonary edema, with cough. Woodbridge treatment was begun January 30th, without calomel addition. Seventh day of treatment morning temperature declined to 99.2° F.; temperature went up to 101.5° F. in the evening; was normal next day, and thereafter convalescence was uninterrupted and satisfactory. The patient took solid food on the twentieth day. Diarrhea was controlled by the antiseptic treatment alone. This case was characteristic in every respect, except the usual lengthy convalescence, the prolonged fever, and the great debility, which is always a part of the typhoid condition.

MEDICAL PROGRESS.

Death from Urethral Sound.—ZUCKERKANDL (*Monatsh. für Prakt. Dermatol.*, vol. xxv, No. 10) was consulted by a patient whom he had treated two years before for stricture of the urethra. In the intervening time sounds had been frequently passed by different physicians. After the passage of a small sound, No. 12 French, the patient was seized with vomiting, chills, and profuse diarrhea. He then went into collapse, and died within six hours. The autopsy showed that there was a narrow stricture in the membranous portion of the urethra, near which were numerous false passages, one leading into the prostate. The man's heart was also badly degenerated.

Vesico-Umbilical Fistulæ.—According to VON TROGNEUX (*Monatsh. für Prakt. Dermat.*, vol. xxv, No. 10), such fistulæ are by no means so rare as one might suppose. They may be congenital or develop after birth. They are often complicated by umbilical hernia, hypospadias, imperforate prepuce, absence of urethra, etc. In the cases which develop in later life the history usually shows that a fluctuating tumor in the region of the umbilicus followed some slight blow or accident.

After a certain time this opens, either spontaneously, or is opened by the surgeon. Both the acquired and congenital varieties are the result of patency of the urachus.

Different Forms of the Meatus Urinarius.—PASTEAU (*Centralb. für Chir.*, November 6, 1897), who has examined 500 patients with reference to this point, finds that the situation and the breadth of meatus urinarius varies greatly in different individuals, so that it is impossible to speak of a normal type. In one-third of the cases the narrowest portion of the canal is situated from four to five millimeters behind the orifice of the urethra. In the majority of instances a No. 22 French sound is the largest which will pass the meatus. If there are several openings in the end of the penis the lowest one of all is invariably the real urethral opening.

Lipoma of the Spermatic Cord.—GABRYSZEWSKI (*Centralb. für Chir.*, November 6, 1897) describes an unusual tumor occurring in a man of advanced years and connected with the right spermatic cord. It grew until it reached the size of a child's head. The organs in the vicinity were very little affected, either in condition or in their relations to each other. Examination of the tumor showed it to be of a lipomatous nature. It weighed five pounds, and was removed without great difficulty.

The Management of Children with an Inherited Tuberculous Diathesis.—STICKLER (*Jour. Am. Med. Assoc.*, January 1, 1898) gives some practical advice concerning the management of children whose parents are tuberculous. The opinion that a tuberculous diathesis is inherited has been held by many recognized authorities. Thus, Squire of London, from a study of 1000 cases, concludes that heredity accounts for nine per cent. of all cases of tuberculosis among children born of phthisical parents, in excess of cases among children born of non-phthisical parents. It is at least safe to say that children born of tuberculous parents are apt to develop tuberculosis; but furthermore, with proper care and management, the inherited diathesis may remain latent or be entirely overcome.

The first thing to be done for an infant whose mother s tuberculous is to secure a healthy wet-nurse. Should artificial feeding be necessary, unusual care should be observed in the selection and preparation of the food, and digestion should be watched from day to day, and assisted if necessary. It is important to maintain an even temperature of the child's room by day and night. The child should never sleep in the same room with a tuberculous mother; if this rule cannot be observed, the cradle should not be placed near the mother's bed.

As the child grows older continuous city life is most undesirable. If such children can spend all day out of doors and when indoors can still live in a pure atmosphere, they will do well. Older children may practise gymnastics with great benefit, such movements, for example, as those advocated by Butler in the *New York Medical Journal*, October 20, 1894. The physician does not do his duty by such children unless he keeps them away from school. As a rule they are precocious, and prefer books to sports. Under such circumstances it is all the more necessary that the medical adviser should insist upon an outdoor life, though in many instances, of course, a few simple lessons may be taught each day without danger.

By attention to these common-sense principles the most satisfactory results may be obtained. It is, moreover, worth remembering that about one-half of the cases of tuberculosis in children make their appearance between the first and fourth year, so that the prognosis improves very much as age increases.

Differential Diagnosis between Gastritis and Cancer of the Stomach.—CHAUFFARD (*La Méd. Moderne*, December 29, 1897), recognizing the difficulty in differentiating hypopeptic gastritis from cancer of the stomach, says that variation in weight of the patient is a sign of great value. As a general rule, if a cancerous patient is put upon suitable diet and is given a great deal of rest, his weight will slightly increase, perhaps to the extent of three or four pounds. Such increase in weight is invariably followed by a progressive loss which continues without interruption until the patient is emaciated. A dyspeptic patient, on the other hand, will continue, under suitable treatment, to gain weight until a maximum point is reached, at which the weight is constantly maintained—a point which may be fifteen or twenty, or even thirty pounds in excess of the weight at the beginning of the treatment.

Comparison of Cigarette- and Cigar-Smoking.—In the *Virginia Medical Semi-Monthly*, January 28th, SOHON discusses the injury received from smoking cigars as compared with that from smoking cigarettes. He emphasizes the harm of smoking before the body is fully developed. Locally, the effect of cigar- or pipe-smoking is far worse than that of cigarettes. The cigarette-smoker rarely has a chronically inflamed throat, as is invariably the case with cigar-smokers. Cigarettes, unless used inordinarily, do not produce a cough. Few singers can smoke cigars, while many of them smoke cigarettes. The difference seems to be in the choice of a profound intoxication at longer intervals or a transient impression which can be repeated oftener. He thinks that one can better judge of the dose of nicotin by the cigarette. He admits, however, that one is more likely to over-indulge in cigarettes on account of the greater satisfaction derived from inhaling.

Massage as an Occupation for the Blind.—BENNETT, in a paper read before the New York Medical Association, October, 1897, suggested massage as an occupation for the blind. According to statistics, not more than eight per cent. of the entire blind population of the United States are able to support themselves. Probably the actual figures would show even a smaller proportion than this. The idea that blind persons are especially musical and can earn their living by such a talent he showed to be an erroneous one.

The proposition to make massage the profession of the blind seems rational. Their touch is more delicate than that of a seeing person, presumably from practice only. However that may be, few seeing people possess such sensitive fingers as blind persons. A second respect in which a blind masseur would be superior to one not blind is in the blindness itself. Many persons object to expose themselves and their little imperfections to such a stranger as a massage operator usually is. With a blind person this difficulty would be at once removed. In the third place, if the custom became general the fees charged would be so small that massage could be taken advantage of by people in moderate circumstances, especially as a blind person would be satisfied with such fees as would insure him a comfortable living. A fourth advantage would be the development physically of the blind themselves, as they would require strength and health in order to carry on this occupation. The tremendous therapeutic value of massage will be recognized more and more, and the time seems ripe for a such a plan as Bennett proposes. He advocates for it a fair trial in institutions which can afford to support a massage operator.

Formaldehyd as a Disinfectant.—HARRINGTON (*Amer. Jour. of the Med. Sciences*, January, 1898), who has made careful experiments to determine the disinfectant power of formaldehyd, finds that this gas, if produced in the atmosphere in sufficient quantities, has extraordinary power as a surface disinfectant. An atmosphere produced by about 10 ounces of formalin to each 1000 cubic feet will kill ordinary pathologic bacteria within half an hour. Less quantities are not of much practical value. Unfortunately, the experiments demonstrated the fact that while the gas will penetrate dry substances to a certain extent, such as cotton cloth, hair, absorbent cotton, etc., in the presence of moisture its penetrating power is practically nil. It must, therefore, be employed and regarded as a surface disinfectant, and can never be anything else. This conclusion is in accord with that of numerous other investigators.

DOTY, who published in the *New York Medical Journal*, October 16, 1897, the results of experiments made with formalin pastils burned in Schering's apparatus, reached substantially the same conclusions, *viz.*: that formaldehyd is valuable as a surface disinfectant, and as it does not injure the most delicate fabrics or papers, it can be used in any apartment with safety. It failed, however, to kill germs wrapped in newspapers, although forty pastiles were used in a room containing 1000 cubic feet of space, the time of exposure being twelve hours. Forty of these pastills contained about 1½ ounces of formalin—only one-seventh the quantity recommended by Harrington. The apparatus manufactured by Schering overcomes the difficulties which at first greatly interfered with the production of large quantities of formalin vapor within a short time.

Significance of a Green Color in Strangulated Gut.—BEGOIN (*Gaz. Heb. de Méd. et de Chir.*, January 27, 1898), in discussing the different colors of strangulated bowel and their significance, says that he has been able to artificially produce shades of yellow, yellowish green, and olive in loops of human intestine by means of human bile obtained at autopsies, as well as by the bile of dogs; but that he has never been able to reproduce the Florentine bronze which he has seen in some fatal cases of obstruction. The practical outcome of his investigations he thus sums up: (*a*) A clear green tint may exist without alteration of the intestinal wall. (*b*) Yellow green, dark green, bottle green, and black green have a more sinister significance. They do not necessarily indicate the death of the tissues of the bowel, but the latter may occur with these colorations. At any rate, it is desirable to use other methods to determine this point, such as irrigation with hot water or pricking of the intestine. (*c*) The same precautions should be employed in the presence of that beautiful green color known as Florentine bronze. In the two cases under the observation of the author in which this color existed, there was gangrene of the gut; but the evidence is too limited to say that such is of necessity the case.

A New Situation for an Artificial Anus.—MAYER (*Rev. Med. de la Suisse Rom.*, January 20, 1898) advocates a novel situation for an artificial anus in those cases in which it is necessary to make a permanent opening into the large intestine. The site is none other than the symphysis pubis. A medium incision is made, and in the lower angle of the wound the symphysis is exposed, and a U-shaped depression is chiseled out of it to the depth of an inch or more. The abdominal cavity is then opened, and the sigmoid flexure is secured and brought out through this notch and fastened in position. Two days later it is opened. The advantages of an anus in this novel situation are those of greater convenience. The patient is able to empty the bowel by leaning well forward in a sitting posture, and is thereby enabled not only to care the better for the opening, but to conceal from others his deformity more readily than is the case with iliac and lumbar openings. The bandage is also more easily kept in position, and the artificial anus is protected from friction by a shallow hard rubber cup. The inconvenience is very slight indeed. This operation has been performed twelve times at Lausanne.

Significance of Arrhythmia of the Pulse.—CLAYTOR (*Univ. Med. Mag.*, January, 1898), having made a special study of arrhythmia of the pulse, concludes that although this symptom in the majority of instances may not be of serious import, still it is often a result of grave nervous or cardiac changes, so that when recognized a careful investigation of its origin should be made. He says: (1) That the prognosis in arrhythmia of purely neurotic origin is more favorable, so long as the patient is unaware of the disordered heart-beat, since anxiety and worry have a marked tendency to increase the trouble. (2) That an arrhythmia which is present only occasionally is of less importance than one which is persistent. (3) That the disappearance of arrhythmia upon exertion is, of course, favorable, while one which becomes more marked is correspondingly unfavorable, as indicative of myocardial incompetency. (4) That, generally speaking, an allorrhythmia (rhythmic arrhythmia) is of graver prognosis than an irregular arrhythmia, since this form is so often associated with myocardial degeneration.

THE MEDICAL NEWS.

A WEEKLY JOURNAL

OF MEDICAL SCIENCE.

COMMUNICATIONS are invited from all parts of the world. Original articles contributed *exclusively* to THE MEDICAL NEWS will after publication be liberally paid for (accounts being rendered quarterly), or 250 reprints will be furnished in place of other remuneration. When necessary to elucidate the text, illustrations will be engraved from drawings or photographs furnished by the author. Manuscripts should be typewritten.

Address the Editor: J. RIDDLE GOFFE, M.D.,
No. 111 FIFTH AVENUE (corner of 18th St.), NEW YORK.

Subscription Price, including postage in U. S. and Canada.

PER ANNUM IN ADVANCE	$4.00
SINGLE COPIES	.10
WITH THE AMERICAN JOURNAL OF THE MEDICAL SCIENCES, PER ANNUM	7.50

Subscriptions may begin at any date. The safest mode of remittance is by bank check or postal money order, drawn to the order of the undersigned. When neither is accessible, remittances may be made, at the risk of the publishers, by forwarding in *registered* letters.

LEA BROTHERS & CO.,
No. 111 FIFTH AVENUE (corner of 18th St.), NEW YORK, AND NOS. 706, 708 & 710 SANSOM ST., PHILADELPHIA.

SATURDAY, APRIL 9, 1898.

INTERSTATE QUARANTINE AND THE MARINE HOSPITAL SERVICE.

THE organization and administration of external or coast quarantine is a comparatively simple problem. Disease is introduced through well-known and easily watched commercial channels, and severe penalties follow infraction of well-understood regulations which are enforced by ample State or national authority.

In the administration of internal quarantine, on the contrary, the conditions are entirely different. In the last and recent epidemic of yellow fever nowhere was mismanagement so flagrant as in this department. Under the laws which then existed, and which exist to-day, such must inevitably be the case. Many places, even towns of considerable size, have no health organization, and when boards of health do exist a lack of uniformity in their regulations causes turmoil among the inhabitants and lax enforcement of what laws they have.

Few cities, and, indeed, few State Boards of Health, are ready and able to confine and strangle an epidemic in its early inception, for the reason that their organizations are not sufficiently compact and trained to enable the enforcement of regulations with military-like speed and thoroughness. This was illustrated in the recent epidemic, and many communities and municipalities lost confidence in their local health authorities, and promptly appealed to the Marine Hospital Service.

Until national uniformity in sanitary laws is secured interstate quarantine will be impossible. Past experience has shown, and the last epidemic confirmed the fact, that when a disease like yellow fever is pronounced epidemic within our borders, panic seizes upon the inhabitants of the infected locality, and to avoid contagion an effort is made to fly in all directions. They are unwelcome guests wherever they go. All feelings of humanity are thrown to the winds, and harsh measures of quarantine, even personal violence, result. Town is pitted against town, city against city, and State against State. Almost as much animosity is manifested against innocent and probably uninfected fugitives as though they were plague-ridden aliens instead of fellow-citizens deserving of all pity, protection, and help.

The General Government, seeing this weakness in local administration, has provided for just such emergencies, and some local authorities have not been slow to avail themselves of the aid of the Marine Hospital Service, which, by an act approved February 15, 1893, was granted additional quarantine powers, and had imposed upon it additional duties.

Section 3 of this Act provides, first, that the Supervising Surgeon-General of the Marine Hospital Service shall examine the quarantine regulations of all municipal and State Boards of Health, and, under the direction of the Secretary of the Treasury, shall cooperate with such boards in the enforcement of their rules. Second. That, where existing quarantine regulations are considered inadequate, or where cities or States have no such regulations, the Secretary of the Treasury shall make such rules and regulations as seem necessary for the protection of public health, expecting the State or municipal authorities to enforce them. Third. If State or municipal authorities shall fail or refuse to enforce such rules and regulation, "the President shall execute and enforce the same, and adopt such measures as in his judgment shall be necessary to prevent the introduction or spread of such diseases, and may detail or appoint officers for that purpose."

This section not only provides for warding off disease from our shores but is also intended to prevent the spread of infectious disease from State to State, from State to Territory, or from either to the District of Columbia, or vice versa.

In the recent epidemic the Marine Hospital Service did good work wherever it could (*i.e.*, wherever its aid was asked or allowed). When summoned, its officers confirmed or disproved diagnoses, aided in works of relief, helped enforce quarantine, superintended the establishment of detention-camps and rendered other services for which their training and discipline specially fitted them. In this body of workers was found ample material for the prompt and efficient establishment of intermunicipal or interstate quarantine.

The insufficiency of the present law consists in permitting valuable time to be lost while waiting to see whether local authorities fail or refuse to put into operation proper and efficient quarantine regulations. This, the Caffery bill which is now before Congress efficiently overcomes; all coast quarantine is vested in the Marine Hospital Service and so becomes a National institution with uniform laws adapted to uniform conditions; the authority of the Marine Hospital Service in local sanitation and in local and interstate quarantine whenever an epidemic arises is also greatly extended, so that it is not necessary to wait until the local authorities have tried and failed to control the disease, but upon order of the President the Marine Hospital Service can at once assume control.

To an unbiased mind nothing seems more reasonable than that an organization which has proved itself efficient not only in the management of coast quarantine but also in the control of epidemics whenever its services have been requested (even when such request has been delayed to the stage of general demoralization of the community) should have its powers extended and its authority enlarged to enable it to fulfil the duties of Health-Officer of the Nation.

The danger of a renewed outbreak of yellow fever in the South with the advent of warm weather is most imminent. Already emphatic expressions of belief in and fear of such a calamity come from New Orleans and other Southern cities. This is no time for untried experiments with complicated commissions and official bureaus. The conditions demand the services of a well-trained and well-equipped organization whose especial duty is quarantine and sanitation, and which through previous experience will command the immediate confidence of the people.

THE PENNSYLVANIA EASTERN STATE PENITENTIARY.

JUDGING from recent newspaper reports there is less brotherly love among Philadelphians, lay and medical, at the present time than there has been since the immortal Penn forsook the Arcadian simplicity of the town on the banks of the Schuylkill. The citizens of Philadelphia seem to be divided into two hostile camps; those who are convinced that the Eastern State Penitentiary is, or has been grossly mismanaged, and those who believe that it is a model of its kind.

The facts of the matter seem to be that a year or so ago, after much discussion and deliberation, a commission made up of laymen and medical experts was appointed by the courts to inquire into alleged abuses, particularly the retention of insane criminals and the cruel, inhuman treatment of them. One of the results of the commission's labors was to show that there were insane convicts within the institution walls, and there was much evidence pointing to negligence and improper treatment. The verdict of the commission was not cordially received by many individuals, and at the time of the report the atmosphere seemed to be so full of personal feeling that, so it was charged, scientific deliberation and accuracy of judgment seemed to be quite impossible.

The whole matter roused a great deal of personal ill-feeling which has since continued. One of the prisoners, who was held up as a particular example of the inhuman treatment to which many were subjected, and who was afterward released, was recently made the subject of a clinical lecture on feigned insanity before the medical class of the University of Pennsylvania by Dr. H. C. Wood. In commenting in the public press on this clinic, Judge Gordon, who appointed the commission and who had deputized, unawares to the professor, a court stenographer to report the lecture, says: "This erotic paranoiac was only restrained by the deprecating outcries of the students and the interdiction of the professor from transforming a medical clinic into a Phallic symposium." Judging from the reported interviews with other neurologists of Philadelphia there is considerable doubt that the patient exhibited as an example of feigned insanity is not a striking example of paranoia, who, like most paranoiacs, exhibits a degree of cunning and mentality greater than many of his sane fellows. Moreover, it has been insinuated that the professor in question went far out of his way to attempt to discredit the work of his professional brethern on the committee by delivering a lecture on insanity when he is not the professor of mental diseases in the institution. Be that as it may, the publicity which the matter has received from the daily press is to be deprecated, as no possible good can come from the publication of such matter, or from the vilification of one citizen by another such as the calling of the learned professor by the learned judge a mountebank and circus manager.

This investigation by the commission has been the subject of careful analysis by Dr. Goodrich, the result of which appears in this issue of the MEDICAL NEWS. The value of expert medico-legal testimony is evidently as problematic as ever.

ECHOES AND NEWS.

Johns Hopkins Relief Bill.—The House of Delegates of Maryland has passed by a vote of 56 to 22 the bill appropriating $50,000 per annum for the support of Johns Hopkins University.

Craig Colony for Epileptics. — Governor Black has appointed Dr. Frederick Peterson of New York County one of the managers of the State Colony for Epileptics at Sonyea for the ensuing term.

Ginger-beer and the Teetotallers.—Ginger-beer is a favorite drink of teetotallers because it is cooling and refreshing. It is a matter of fact, however, that it contains about two per cent. of alcohol.

Responsibility for Typhoid Fever.—The heirs of a man who died of typhoid fever, contracted, as they assert, while he was imprisoned in the jail at Wayne, W. Va., on a charge of highway robbery, are about to bring suit against the county for $10,000 damages.

Typhoid Sufferers Sue Water Company.—Several hundred of the sufferers in the recent typhoid epidemic at Maidstone, Eng., have decided to bring a combined action against the water company to obtain compensation for the losses which they have sustained.

Proprietary Medicines. — Of 217,000 prescriptions written in Chicago, New York, Boston, Washington, Baltimore, Denver, San Francisco, New Orleans, and St. Louis, 11.25 per cent. called for proprietary articles, says the *International Medical Magazine.*

Surgeon Banks a Delegate to the International Congress of Hygiene.—Surgeon C. E. Banks of the Marine Hospital Service, has been detailed to represent the Service at the Ninth International Congress of Hygiene and Demography, Madrid, Spain, April 10–17, 1898.

The La Caze Prize.—The La Caze prize of 10,000 francs has been awarded to Röntgen by the Paris Academie des Sciences, which also awarded a like sum to Professor Lenard of Heidelberg. It was the latter's work on the cathode-ray which led to Röntgen's great discovery.

Railroad Rates to the American Medical Association Meeting.—The Committee on Arrangements announce that the Western Passenger Association will issue round-trip tickets, with a thirty-day limit, at the rate of one fare, plus $2, and are hopeful of procuring the same rates throughout the United States.

Deaths under Anesthesia.—According to Dr. Robert Bell of Glasgow, "the jubilee year of chloroform, after fifty-years' experience of its use, has gone out with a record of ninety-six inquests held in England alone on cases of death in persons of both sexes and of all ages. This is the largest number of deaths from anesthetics reported for any one year."

A Fellowship in Medicine.—The authorities of Magdalen College, Oxford, have announced that they will shortly offer to Oxford graduates a Fellowship for proficiency in medical science. This is the second time that the claims of medicine have been recently recognized by Oxford colleges, Pembroke being the first to offer a fellowship in medicine.

The Value of Commas.—A newspaper proprietor was recently sued for damages by a patent-medicine man for an error which was made in printing a testimonial. By the omission of a comma the testimonial was made to read thus: "I now find myself cured, after being brought to the very gates of death by having taken only five bottles of your medicine."

Preparing for War's Ravages.—The Surgeon-General of the Army has placed with certain instrument-makers of New York City large orders for capital and minor operating-cases and other apparatus. One firm received an order for 950 probes and 500 field tourniquets. Adhesive plaster has been ordered up to nearly 4000 yards, and 2000 spools of antiseptic ligatures.

A Faithful Nurse Decorated.—The Cross of the Legion of Honor has been conferred upon Mlle. Marguerite Bottard, who, for more than fifty-six years, has served faithfully as nurse and superintendent in the Salpêtrière Hospital in Paris. Charcot had the highest opinion of this faithful woman, and frequently remarked that she richly deserved the distinction which has now been accorded to her.

Scientists Honored.—The Emperor of Germany has conferred decorations upon the members of the German deputation for research into the plague in India. Professor Gaffky of Giessen has received the second class of the Red Eagle Order, and Professor Pfeiffer of Berlin, Dr. Sticker of Giessen, and the Bavarian army surgeon Dr. Dieudonne, have received the fourth class of the same order.

Alcoholic Milk.—According to the *Lancet* (London), a

German chemist has discovered that it is possible to get "straight from the cow" milk which contains alcohol. Upon examining some milk which had an irritating taste it was found to contain 0.96 per cent. of alcohol. The cow from which it was obtained was one of a herd belonging to a distillery, and had been fed on waste which contained alcohol.

London's Epidemic of Measles and the Circus.—It is said that the Barnum and Bailey Circus, by bringing together a large number of children, has done much toward spreading the epidemic of measles which has prevailed in London for some months. The death-rate of this disease in that city for the week ending January 1, 1898, was ninety-one. This figure has not been reached since, although as yet there is no evidence of any very material decline in the epidemic.

Bellevue House-Staff Offer Their Services to the Government.—At the suggestion of Dr. G. Boling Lee, a nephew of Consul-General Fitzhugh Lee and senior house-physician of the Fourth Medical Division of Bellevue Hospital, twenty-one of the thirty-two members of the house-staff of that institution recently signed their names to a document in which they offer their services to the Government in the event of war between this country and Spain.

Contamination of Rivers To Be Investigated.—A bill was recently introduced into the United States Senate by Mr. Cockrell providing for an appropriation of $3000 for an investigation to be made by the Marine Hospital Service of the source of contamination of rivers and other natural sources of water-supply where the sanitary condition of the people of more than one State or Territory is affected, or threatened to be affected, by such pollution. The bill provides that the first investigation shall relate to the Potomac River.

A Motor Tricycle.—A correspondent writes to the *British Medical Journal* recommending the use of motor tricycles by medical men in country practice. Petrol or doubly distilled benzoline is the oil used, and it costs about twenty-four cents per 100 miles to operate the tricycle. The speed can be regulated anywhere between four and twenty miles an hour by means of a small lever immediately in front of the rider. Any ordinary hill can be climbed by it, but a little pedaling is necessary to ascend a very steep incline.

Rush Medical College.—Liabilities amounting to $71,000 have been wiped from the ledgers of Rush Medical College, and its complete affiliation with the University of Chicago is now practically assured. This was one of the conditions set forth when the scheme of annexing the medical school to the University was first mentioned. The principal donors were Drs. Ephraim Ingals, Nicholas Senn, and E. Fletcher Ingals. Hereafter the Board of Trustees will be chosen from representative business men instead of from the Faculty, in accordance with another condition.

Cerebrospinal Meningitis in Massachusetts.—In the ten weeks ending March 12, 1898, there have been in Boston twenty deaths from cerebrospinal meningitis, ten in Holyoke, nine in Worcester, and fourteen in Malden, Chelsea, and nine other towns; sixty-three deaths in all from this disease in that period having been registered with the State Board of Health. The largest number of fatal cases in any one week was nine, in the week ending March 5th. There were eight deaths the week ending January 8th. These returns show the widespread distribution of the disease and its very uniform prevalence during the cold weather.

Divine Healers in Kansas.—According to the New York *Times*, Attorney-General Boyle of Topeka, Kas., has recently rendered an opinion to the effect that "divine healers" cannot be prosecuted by the State Board of Health under the anti-quack law. He holds that the State Board may proceed against magnetic healers and hypnotists as "quacks" because they pretend to possess personal healing powers, but that divine healers are exempt from prosecution because they declare their power to come from Jehovah, and Jehovah, he explains, is not amenable to the laws of the State.

Professor McLane Resigns His Professorship.—Dr. James W. McLane after thirty years of service as a teacher has resigned the Chair of Professor of Obstetrics in the College of Physicians and Surgeons of New York. In accordance with the wishes of the Medical Faculty Dr. McLane was made Emeritus Professor of Obstetrics, and retains his position as Dean of the College. The vacancy in the Chair of Obstetrics was filled by the appointment, with the title of Lecturer in Obstetrics, of Edwin B. Cragin, M.D. Dr. Cragin is a graduate of Yale College in the class of 1882, and of the College of Physicians and Surgeons, 1886. He will have professional charge of the Sloane Maternity Hospital.

Red Tape in Hospital Administration.—The following instance of hospital red-tape is related by the Paris correspondent of the *British Medical Journal*. A workingman with confluent smallpox, sent to a hospital near his commune, was refused admittance because there was no isolation ward; he was, therefore, sent to Charix, his birthplace. The Mayor of Charix ordered that he be sent to the Bourg Hospital, and the man traveled to the latter place in an ordinary railway carriage. When he arrived there no conveyance would transfer him to the hospital. Finally, a tender-hearted porter wheeled him there in his wheelbarrow. Admission was refused because the papers were not *en règle*. After being sent to the Mairie, and then to the Prefecture, the patient was admitted as an urgent case, and death occurred the following morning.

Philadelphia Personals. — Dr. W. A. N. Dorland was elected assistant surgeon of the Second Troop of Philadelphia City Cavalry at the last meeting of the troop, held on April 2d.—Dr. John H. Packard expects to sail for Europe the latter part of this month. He will spend some time in London during the first part of his vacation, and later intends to go to the west coast of France, where he will spend the remainder of the summer.—Dr. Abner F. Chase, one of the best-known practitioners in West Philadelphia, died on April 2d, in his fifty-sixth year. Dr. Chase had been a member of the medical staff of the Charity Hospital for more than twenty years, and had been physician to the out-patient department of the Presbyterian Hospital, and to St. John's Orphan Asylum. He was a graduate of the Jefferson Medical College in the class of 1874.

The Author of "Hugh Wynne."—One of the prominent London medical journals has discovered that "this stirring and exquisitely written historic romance is from the pen of no less a person than the *late* Dr. Weir Mitchell, and we learn for the first time that this author *was* an accomplished writer as well as a sagacious physician." It is not surprising, perhaps, to discover that our plodding friends across the water are now learning, for the first time, of the literary accomplishments of Dr. Weir Mitchell. It is sad, however, to find them speaking of him so completely in the past tense. We are pleased, therefore, to inform our contemporary that Dr. Weir Mitchell is still giving suffering humanity the benefit of his sagacity, and at the same time is writing another romance, his third or fourth by the way, which is appearing in current numbers of a monthly magazine.

Salutary Reduction in Poisoning by Phosphorus. — It appears that the use of white phosphorus in match-making is not interdicted in England, as it is in France and elsewhere. An inquiry in the House of Commons on this subject led the Home Secretary to make a statement that speaks most favorably for the results which have followed sanitation in respect to the match industry. He stated that the use of white phosphorus had been found less open to objection than has been asserted; on the contrary the information in his possession is that in some important countries—such as Germany, Austria, and Belgium—its use is not prohibited. In England the use of white phosphorus is regulated by special rules, which have been so far successful that last year only two cases of phosphorus-poisoning occurred, neither of which was fatal. In these circumstances he did not think there is sufficient cause for further legislative action.

Hospital Ventilation in Hot Countries.—A novel feature of the new General Hospital for Europeans in Calcutta, India, the corner-stone of which was recently laid, will be a system of ventilation during the hot and rainy seasons by cold and dried air. The idea originated with Brigade-Surgeon Lieutenant-Colonel Crombie, the superintendent of the hospital, and like most new ideas met with a great deal of opposition, although the advantages of the system are obvious. During the hot and rainy seasons Calcutta has a temperature ranging from 85° to 95° F., and a humidity which frequently reaches ninety per cent. Dr. Crombie proposes to establish a uniform temperature in the wards of from 75° to 80° F., and a humidity reduced to about sixty per cent., as a necessary part of the process of cooling the air. As the cool, dry air is to be passed through screens of cotton wool, there will be no mosquitoes, and accordingly no necessity for punkahs and mosquito curtains.

Artificial Fecundation.—The recent death in Paris of Dr. J. Gérard recalls a little incident showing the disfavor with which artificial fecundation is looked upon in France. In 1885 he presented as his graduation thesis an essay, entitled "A Contribution to the History of Artificial Fecundation." The subject had been approved by the president of the Faculty, but while it was being printed the Faculty became alarmed and ordered that the printing should be stopped and all finished copies destroyed. The thesis was of little scientific value, but an attempt was made to represent Gérard as a martyr to the foolish prudery of the Faculty. Two years prior to this incident, a French law court had shown itself much opposed to this method, the Bordeaux tribunal having declared, in giving judgment in a case, that the practice of artificial fecundation was a veritable danger to society, and could not be recognized as a legitimate form of medical practice. The question has also been referred to the highest ecclesiastic tribunal in the Roman Church, which decided that the practice is contrary to the teaching of the church.

Professor Grimaux and the Zola Trial.—According to the *British Medical Journal*, M. Grimaux, formerly professor of the Faculty of Medicine of Paris, and still a member of the Academy of Science and professor at the Ecole Polytechnique, was subpoened as a witness for M. Zola in the recent trial of the latter. When upon the stand he gave it as his opinion that the famous writer had done right in publishing his letter of accusation against the *Etat Major*, adding that both M. Zola and Captain Dreyfus were completely unknown to him. M. Grimaux' testimony caused great excitement among various officers, many of whom had been pupils of his at the Polytechnique, and much ill feeling was displayed toward him. In consequence of this, the Minister of War, in whose hands are the direction of the Ecole Polytechnique and the nominations of the professors, suspended M. Grimaux from office upon the ground that his position would be intolerable with regard to his pupils. Soon after, at a meeting of the Society of Biologie, Professor Richet made a little speech when Professor Grimaux made his appearance. He reminded the members that it was the custom in that society to congratulate any member who had recently attained any distinction or decoration or had been nominated to any important post. He, therefore, thought they ought to congratulate Professor Grimaux on account of his suspension, for it was an honor to him as showing the independence and dignity of his character. Professor Grimaux was much affected and expressed his thanks. The Society then voted that its congratulations be entered on the minutes.

Hypodermic Treatment of Malaria.—

℞ Cinchonidin. sulph. . . . . . gr. xvi
Ac. tartarici . . . . . . gr. xii
Aq. dest. . . . . . q. s. ad ℥ i.
M. Sig. Fifteen minims for one injection.

CORRESPONDENCE.

OUR PHILADELPHIA LETTER.

[From our Special Correspondent.]

A MEETING OF HOSPITAL PHYSICIANS AND MANAGERS TO CONSIDER THE QUESTION OF MEDICAL CHARITIES—THE WAR FEVER AND THE MEDICAL STUDENTS—DEATH OF DR. OLIVER A. JUDSON—DR. BENJAMIN LEE'S DUAL POSITIONS—LATE BEQUESTS TO PHILADELPHIA HOSPITALS—MEDICO-CHIRURGICAL COLLEGE—AN ENDOWED BED FOR TRAINED NURSES—POST-TRAUMATIC NEUROSES—THE CASE OF WILLIAM HENDERSON.

PHILADELPHIA, April 2, 1898.

A DEFINITE step in the proper consideration of the question of hospital abuse has been taken by the officers of the Philadelphia Polyclinic, by the issuance of a circular letter to hospital physicians and hospital managers inviting their representation at a meeting to be held at the College of Physicians, May 4th, for the discussion of this topic. The action of the Polyclinic at once removes that element of personal antagonism which unfortunately existed in other quarters at the time the agitation of the question first began, and the solution of the difficulty is now in the hands of competent, representative men. These communications have been sent to members of the boards of managers and of the medical staffs of every hospital and dispensary in the city, and it is hoped that this general and unlimited representation will result, by the cooperation of all concerned, in checking the demoralization of public charities, and in the proper regulation of the whole question, by dispassionate and fair methods of procedure. The call is signed by Dr. Howard F. Hansell, President of the Faculty, and by Dr. John B. Roberts, President of the Board of Trustees of the Polyclinic. It should be recalled that during more than a year past this hospital has required of all who apply for gratuitous treatment a signed statement as to their inability to pay a physician's fee, and that this system has been adopted by several other institutions to a certain extent, without, however, having as yet become a conspicuous element in dispensary services.

The probability at this moment of a war with Spain has caused no little excitement among the student bodies of the various medical schools of the city, and the majority of the undergraduates have expressed an eagerness to enlist as hospital stewards or as assistants in this department of the navy. At an informal canvass of one of the classes at the University, taken yesterday, more than two-thirds of the members signified their willingness to serve in these subordinate army positions. There is also a rumor, which your correspondent is unable to verify, that the senior classes of the Medical Department of the University of Pennsylvania and of the Jefferson Medical College will be given their final examinations earlier this year, so that the members of the class may be qualified without delay to compete for army and navy medical commissions. Although, with the exception of the Philadelphia Medical Emergency Corps, a local organization cooperating with the police and the fire departments, and whose members formally tendered their services to the Government two weeks ago, no organized union of Philadelphia medical men has yet been effected for the purpose of volunteer army duty. Such a union is generally talked of, and should the need arise, the project will be realized under the sponsorship of many experienced veterans of the late war, whose past experiences will stand in good stead at the present moment. In the event of hostilities there will be a surfeit of volunteers for the medical corps of the army and navy, both for field and for hospital service.

Dr. Oliver A. Judson died at his home in this city March 30th, in the sixty-eighth year of his age. Dr. Judson was graduated from the Jefferson Medical College in 1851, and was engaged in a lucrative practice in this city until the outbreak of the Civil War, when he at once entered the Medical Department of the United States Army. After serving throughout the war in responsible executive positions connected with the medical corps, as well as in the field as brigade-surgeon, Dr. Judson resigned from the service with the rank of lieutenant-colonel, and was obliged, a little while later, to retire from active practice because of his breakdown in health from the effects of his long and arduous services in the army. During his professional life he was one of the visiting physicians to the Philadelphia Dispensary and to the Howard Hospital, consulting physician to the Philadelphia Hospital, a manager of the Children's Hospital, and vice-president of the Pennsylvania Institution for the Instruction of the Blind. At the time of his death he was a Fellow of the College of Physicians of Philadelphia, a member of the Academy of the Natural Sciences, and of many other scientific, military, and social organizations.

Active political influences are being enlisted by interested individuals in an effort to compel Dr. Benjamin Lee of this city to relinquish one or the other of his two official positions, as secretary of the State Board of Health and as Health-Officer of the Port of Philadelphia. For the former position Dr. Lee receives a salary of $2500 a year, while to the latter position an annual salary of $7000 is attached. A number of applicants for one or the other of these positions—with a distinct leaning, naturally, toward the $7000 job—are importuning the Governor to compel Dr. Lee to confine his efforts to one position, and local ward-politics have been dragged in by the opposition. The City Solicitor is quoted as giving an informal opinion to the effect that the dual-positions held by Dr. Lee are not illegal, inasmuch as there is not the slightest interference in the duties of the two offices, and that, so far, it is not apparent that any legal incompatibility exists to require his resignation. Meanwhile, Dr. Lee performs his two-fold duties, and will probably continue to do so until requested to alter his course by Governor Hastings.

The trustee's account of the estate of the late George S. Pepper, who died in Philadelphia during 1890, shows that the following hospitals, among a long list of other beneficiaries, have been bequeathed the following sums: University Hospital, $19,750; Presbyterian, Episcopal, Pennsylvania, and Jefferson Hospitals, $18,500 each; Orthopedic, Charity, St. Joseph's, St. Christopher's,

Children's, and Maternity Hospitals, $9250 each. The total amount of bequests left to other charitable institutions and to scientific societies is approximately $500,000. The Pennsylvania Hospital, by the will of the late Mordecai D. Evans, receives a bequest of $10,000, to be applied to the general endowment fund; and also, as a contingent bequest, this hospital further receives one-ninth of the residuary estate of the donor, amounting, it is said, to considerably over $100,000.

An amendment to the charter of the Medico-Chirurgical College was granted this week by the courts, empowering this institution to establish a college of dental surgery and pharmacy and to grant degrees in these branches. The two new schools will, it is understood, be inaugurated this fall, a number of the members of the faculties attached to them having been already engaged.

The class of 1897 of the Nurse's Training School of the Woman's Hospital is endeavoring to secure funds sufficient to endow a permanent bed in this hospital for graduate nurses. This training school is the oldest in America, and the efforts it is putting forth should be realized without difficulty, on account of the excellent standing of the graduates, and of their widespread acquaintance.

Putnam of Boston, in an address delivered by invitation before the Philadelphia Neurological Society, March 28th, gave an interesting account of his personal experiences with "The Nature and Symptoms of Post-Traumatic Neuroses." Post-traumatic neuroses should be considered, in many instances, said the speaker, as entirely preventable affections; for, it was argued, the proper exhibition of therapeutics at the proper time, during both the prodromal and active stages of the disorder, not infrequently prevents in some cases, and modifies in others, the development of symptoms. Functional disturbances were held accountable for more traumatic neuroses than are caused by organic lesions; and such causal factors of a social nature as straightened circumstances, whereby the patient's confinement to bed means to him financial loss and consequent mental unrest, the fear of the word "accident," as applied to his individual case, and a general personal neurotic temperament, all influence the production of the condition. The point was also emphasized that while it is true that serious non-legal cases sometimes occur, cases involving legal questions are, as a rule, by far the more serious, and the course of such cases is usually very favorably influenced by a verdict sustaining the interests of the patient. The influence of the mode of production of the trauma was deemed important as bearing upon the patient's mental state at the time the accident was received. Bicycle and foot-ball injuries which may produce trauma just as severe as those received by accidents of a more unusual nature, rarely, if ever, produce neuroses. While the indirect influence of violence undoubtedly is a cause of the condition in many instances, it was considered very probable that the actual injury played a more important rôle in the etiology of the neuroses in question.

The trial of fourteen-year-old Samuel Henderson, who murdered his five-year-old playmate under peculiarly atrocious circumstances last January, has resulted in the unsatisfactory verdict of murder in the second degree. This trial attracted interest because of the large amount of expert medical testimony submitted by both sides, and of the prominent alienists who figured in the case. Dr. Martin W. Barr, the physician-in-chief of the Pennsylvania Training School for Feeble-Minded Children at Elwyn, was the principal witness for the defense, and although he maintained that the prisoner was an incurable imbecile, and that he plainly bore such stigmata of degeneration as marked asymmetry of the skull, face, and ears, together with many other marks of degeneracy described by Lombroso and others, the Commonwealth's experts, Drs. Chapin, Morton, Dercum, and Butcher proved conclusively that the defendant's mental condition was not abnormal, and that the so-called signs of degeneracy upon which the expert for the defense laid such stress, were in reality but gross artefacts. The trial was a good illustration of the present status of expert medical testimony, and the complete failure of the defense in relying upon stigmata of degeneration to prove the insanity of the prisoner has attracted no little attention in medico-legal circles.

During the week ending April 2d, the total number of deaths reported to the Bureau of Health was 448, a decrease of 56 as compared with those of last week, and an increase of 16 over those of the corresponding period of 1897. Of the total deaths, there were 140 of children under five years of age. There were 84 new cases of diphtheria, with 18 deaths; 64 new cases of enteric fever, with 12 deaths; and 42 new cases of scarlet fever, with 3 deaths.

OUR BERLIN LETTER.

[From our Special Correspondent.]

THE PRUSSIAN GOVERNMENT AND LEPROSY—NEUROLOGISTS AND THE DIFFERENTIAL DIAGNOSIS OF SYRINGOMYELIA AND LEPROSY—PROFESSOR VIRCHOW'S HABILITATION ESSAY AS PRIVAT-DOCENT FOR THE UNIVERSITY OF BERLIN—A MODIFICATION OF THE THOMA-ZEISS CELL-COUNTER—A MINISTER OF PUBLIC HEALTH FOR GERMANY, RUSSIA, AND THE UNITED STATES.

BERLIN, March 31, 1898.

THE Prussian government is the first to take official action upon the recommendations of the Lepra Conference, held here last October. A careful census of all the lepers living in the country, their present condition, their abode, and the circumstances in which they are living, has just been completed. The majority of the lepers are in the Memel district, where leprosy has become insidiously endemic. In all of the cases except those in the Memel district, the lepers had lived some time in other countries where leprosy is known to be endemic, notably India and Venezuela. Measures are to be at once instituted to prevent any further spread of the disease, and by careful segregation of the affected it is hoped to eradicate it completely. A home for the lepers of the Memel district has just been begun which will ensure segregation there, and lepers living with their relatives are to be subjected to certain stringent regulations. A note of warning is sounded as to lepers in hospitals kept for purposes of study. The absolute immunity of nurses and attendants which has often been put forward as a proof of the non-contagiousness of leprosy is no longer accepted. Lepers kept in hospitals will be subjected to more thorough segregation than has been the custom in the past.

The attitude of the German neurologists with regard to syringomyelia, since the Lepra Conference, is very interesting. No one presents a case of syringomyelia at a medical society, or even at a clinic, without stating that he has taken all diagnostic precautions to demonstrate that it is not leprosy. The nasal and conjunctival secretion are always examined for the lepra bacillus (they are said to occur in these secretions in more than eighty per cent. of all cases of leprosy), the nerve-trunks are carefully examined for the characteristic lepra nodes, and in cases in which there are no severe trophic symptoms to contraindicate it, a blister is applied to affected parts and the serum examined for bacilli. Characteristic signs of syringomyelia which could not be due to leprosy, such as hemiatrophy of the tongue or pupillary differences, are carefully searched for and their significance pointed out.

Some of the German medical men who have been in India studying the plague assert that they have not the slightest doubt that among the lepers of the East there are a number of cases of pure syringomyelia. Some of the mutilations which are considered most characteristic of leprosy, and that in the East would assure without further ado the sending of the patient to a leprosery, have been noted in cases in which no evidence of leprosy in the history or bacterial examination could be found.

The gradual dwarfing of the fingers, a general atrophic process affecting all the tissues and yet unaccompanied by ulceration, has been considered especially pathognomonic of leprosy, yet it has been found here in a man in whom the first symptoms of the disease were noted over thirty-nine years ago, and there is still no ulcerative process, no unsightly mutilation of the fingers; in a word, none of the characteristic symptoms to which leprosy would give rise during so long a time.

At the late conference this case was pronounced leprosy by several distinguished experts in leprology, yet there seems no reason to think that the case is leprosy. The result of the Lepra Conference is then to be two-fold in practice: While it makes the neurologists and dermatologists much more circumspect in their diagnoses of cutaneous trophic diseases, it is going to react on the leprologists, too, and make them less final in their diagnosis in doubtful cases. This will save many a poor creature whose malady is but a nervous one, though absolutely incurable, from the living death of having to eke out his life among lepers without any good reason for it.

The last number of *Virchow's Archives* contains the essay written by him on the occasion of his habilitation as a privat-docent at the University of Berlin. It was packed away at that time unpublished, and it was only when the question of the celebration of the fiftieth anniversary of his privat-docentship was broached and the committee from the faculty came to offer their congratulations that it was found among some other old papers relating to the time.

It is written in Latin, a Latin for which the distinguished Latinist of maturer years apologizes, but of which, I think, he need not be ashamed. It was written when he was twenty-six years old, and yet contains the ear-marks of genius in a way that few of the earlier works of great men do. The subject is "The Pathology of Bone," and some of the opinions advanced are those which years later Virchow himself, after exhaustive study of this difficult subject, gave as his final views in the matter.

It is written with the intuitiveness of genius, which, after reviewing the state of the question as it then was, picks out of the elements thus brought before it those whose effectual development is to constitute the real explanation of a most difficult pathologic question, in which, up to that time, the most confusing obscurity had reigned. It is an example of the method of genius in being able to skip from the first premise to a sure conclusion while ordinary mortals must plod on wearily from premise to premise, often going back to assure themselves they have not wandered from the way.

Though published in this modest apologetic way, the habilitation essay is an important document as mirroring the mental processes of the young Virchow in the midst of the unsatisfactory pathology of his day, at an age when most young men are not quite able to grasp a master's teaching and do not think of branching out into the fields of thought for themselves.

A modification of the Thoma-Zeiss blood-counter, which allows air to enter the chamber in which the blood-corpuscles are counted, has just been placed on the market. This will, it is said, do away with the error introduced by variations in barometric pressure, an error which has only been discovered as the result of the further investigation of the supposed increase of red blood-cells at high altitudes. It is thought that this new modification will obviate a number of objections to the counting apparatus, errors introduced by incomplete coaptation of the ruled space and its cover glass, more or less pressure within the space, etc.

For some time prominent German medical men have been endeavoring to have the governmental care of medical matters transferred from the Ministry of Public Worship and Education, the *Cultus ministerium* as it is known, to the Ministry of the Interior. It was hoped that this would obviate a number of difficulties in the management of public-health affairs and physicians' privileges and duties which the profession has been endeavoring to remedy, a phase, you see, of the same medical question which is occupying medical attention in the United States—public health and the question of its consistent regulation by the general government.

Here, as the medical journals all claim, the ideal would be attained in a Ministry for Public Health and medical matters alone. It is announced that in Russia a separate ministry for Public Health is to be established. Those who attended the Congress there will not be surprised, for it is not in that alone that our some time Tatar friends are leading the world in matters medical.

TRANSACTIONS OF FOREIGN SOCIETIES.

London.

RECURRENCE AFTER OPERATION FOR CANCER OF THE BREAST—SURGICAL TREATMENT OF MICROCEPHALY—REMOVAL OF ENTIRE UPPER EXTREMITY FOR RECURRENT CARCINOMA OF THE BREAST—VALUE OF LAPAROTOMY PER SE—A TUMOR OF THE PULMONARY VALVE—RELIEF OF PRESSURE PARAPLEGIA IN SPINAL CURVATURE.

AT a meeting of the Royal Medical and Chirurgical Society, February 22d, the discussion upon recurrence after operation for cancer of the breast was resumed. GOULD said we were hampered by ignorance of the processes and conditions under which the disease develops. Cancer of the breast is particularly variable as it may remain confined many years to one spot or it may within a few months spread all over the body. The average duration of the disease in twenty-six patients who died without operation from cancer of the breast was forty-five months. The extremes were four months and twelve years. Forty-eight patients who died alter operation for cancer of the breast had an average duration of life of forty-six months. Here the extremes were four months and twenty-five years. Subsequent attacks of cancer are to be regarded not as a fresh attack but as metastases. The influence of operation is merely the removal of affected tissue. Hence, cancer can no more be said to be cured by operation than gangrene of the leg can be said to be cured by amputation.

CHEYNE said that of twenty-two patients operated upon by the new method thirteen were alive and free from recurrence more than three years after the operation. Under the old methods from ten to eighteen per cent. remained free three years or more. He objected to calling the modern operation by the name of Halsted. Investigations were made and the rules for operation laid down by Heidenhain and Stiles, and patients had been operated upon and their cases published both in England and Germany before Halsted published his cases.

TREVES said that our knowledge of the nature of cancer has advanced little from its position at the beginning of the century. The geographic distribution of cancer, the variations in the course of the disease, and in the rapidity of recurrence, the disappearance of cutaneous nodules, and the effect of the removal of the ovaries, are at present quite unintelligible. He doubted whether we are even justified in assuming that excision is the right and proper treatment, although it is the best available at the present time. He thought that when the pathology of cancer is properly understood many of the present methods of treatment will be discredited. Deformity, disability, and pain in patients in whom recurrence takes place after operation by the new method is often very great.

SHEILD said that he could not accept the view of some surgeons who regard secondary growths as fresh attacks. They are common in glands and in bones, situations in which primary scirrhus rarely occurs. Recurrence is most common in the lungs and liver, organs which are in direct lymphatic connection with the breast. In operating, the axilla should always be opened. He does not remove the pectoral muscle, as a rule, but when he wishes to clear out the axilla very thoroughly he removes the sternal part of the pectoral muscle, which gives him plenty of space. Removal of the breast has been referred to as an easy operation, but he wished to insist that it requires the greatest care and skill. He thought that some cases had fallen into the hands of surgeons in whom a due sense of proportion is lacking. He considered the operation of sawing through the clavicle and removing the arm in order to clear out the axilla quite unjustifiable. The term "cure" can never be used in connection with cancer in the sense that it is used in speaking of the removal of a lipoma, and he thought it important that in dealing with malignant diseases the terms used should be accurate and unequivocal. He thought that the cases he had collected justify the surgeon in encouraging patients, although a definite prognosis of cure cannot be given.

At the meeting of March 8th, GRIFFITHS read a paper on microcephaly and its surgical treatment. He detailed a case in which he had performed linear craniectomy upon a megacephalic idiot, aged sixteen years, who also presented muscular rigidity, especially of the lower limbs. Recovery was complete, and there was marked diminution of the muscular rigidity, while the boy for the first time in his life showed a desire to play with toys. Two weeks later an artificial lambdoid suture was made on the left side, and the patient died from infection and septic meningitis. Autopsy showed the skull was deformed on account of lack of brain-pressure rather than from any disease of its component parts. A prematurely synostosed skull over a normal brain is a purely hypothetic condition. It is conceivable that a craniectomy may be of benefit in such a case. Otherwise, in megacephalic cases, unless symptoms of cortical irritation are present, the operation is contraindicated.

DENT read a paper upon "The Removal of the Entire Upper Extremity for Recurrent Carcinoma of the Breast." This seemingly daring operation was performed without difficulty and with the loss of only two or three ounces of blood. The wound healed readily and the patient was relieved from the distressing neuralgic pain caused by the extension of the growth around the axillary vessels and nerve-trunks. When last seen the patient had recurrences in the thorax and liver, but was in a fairly comfortable condition.

At the Medical Society, February 28th, TREVES read a paper upon "The Value of Laparotomy *per se*." In tuberculous peritonitis seventy per cent. of 308 patients were reported as cured after an exploratory incision. The reader mentioned a number of cases of chronic inflammation in different parts of the abdomen which showed marked improvement after simple incision. In some of them the appearance was such at the time of operation that the patients were considered to be in a hopeless condition. It is less surprising that hysteric and other nervous patients have been benefited by a cut through the abdominal wall. Treves warned against a hasty resort to exploratory operation.

At the Pathological Society, March 1st, CRAWFURD

showed a heart with a tumor of the pulmonary valve. The case was remarkable clinically for the reason that the patient suffered no inconvenience from its presence until his sudden death at the age of seventy-two years. It was two inches in length and more than one inch in its transverse diameter, and it almost filled the pulmonary artery, temporary occlusion of which had caused the death of the patient. The tumor was made up of granulation tissue of different ages, replacing an initial thrombus.

At the Clinical Society, February 25th, three patients were shown who had suffered from spinal curvature resulting from pressure paraplegia. In all three the symptoms had much improved; twice as a result of laminectomy, once after forcible reduction. The last patient, a child aged five years, was chloroformed and the spine straightened during September, 1897. Power of movement in the legs began to return within a week, and improvement steadily progressed. The jacket was removed within five months and the patient was to all appearances completely cured.

SOCIETY PROCEEDINGS.

NEW YORK ACADEMY OF MEDICINE.

Stated Meeting, Held January 6, 1898.

THE President, EDWARD G. JANEWAY, M.D., in the Chair.

DR. BEVERLEY ROBINSON read a paper on

CLINICAL OBSERVATIONS ON MALARIA AND ITS TREATMENT.

He said that although microscopic examinations are often valuable in establishing a diagnosis of malaria, still he could not regard Laveran's great discovery as final in all cases. There certainly are cases of malaria in which even experts cannot find the specific parasite. It is a wide conviction in the profession that quinin must and will cure malarial fever; yet time and again he had given quinin in large doses, both by mouth and by rectum, without benefit, and then improvement had promptly followed the administration of Huxham's tincture of bark, in teaspoonful doses, every two or three hours. This statement is particularly true of cases in which there is a certain degree of anemia present. It is an old observation, but none the less a valuable one, that Virginia snake-root combined with Peruvian bark often gives quicker and more permanent results than quinin; that is, relapses are fewer than when quinin alone has been used. Good bark contains two active substances, *viz.*: (1) the alkaloids, or febrifuge principles, and (2) tannin, the tonic element. Tannin has been recognized as a valuable ingredient in preparations of bark, and quite recently F. Alix claimed that the administration of tannin in solution is very efficacious in cases in which quinin itself had failed. Of course, many persons cannot possibly take quinin, on account of the eruptions, annoying tinnitus, etc., produced by it.

It is not uncommon for children suffering from malaria to suddenly become languid and desist from their usual amusements. After an hour or two of such prostration the child will often resume playing. It has become quite a general opinion that malaria is less common in children than in adults, but Dr. Robinson said that, according to his experience, just the opposite is true. The explanation is probably to be found in Dr. Holt's statement that malaria in children is often overlooked because of the irregular types presented. In his summer practice by the sea, the speaker said, he had seen many cases of malaria, and in these the specific organism had been more easily found. In localities having a rocky soil and a substratum of clay, malaria of a most pronounced type often develops. The physician should be on the alert for unusual sources of malarial infection, for example, in houses in which the cold-air flue of the furnace communicates with the damp and unwholesome air of courts or uncemented cellars. Sewer-gas poisoning and malarial infection are often confounded, and experience has demonstrated that the same preparation of quinin or of bark will be of benefit in both disorders. Patients with severe and obstinate malaria are often very strikingly benefited by a change to a high inland region. Much has been said about enlargement of the spleen as a diagnostic sign in malaria, but the speaker was positive that the spleen often remains of normal size in cases in which the existence of malarial poisoning cannot be questioned.

In considering the question of treatment, it is perhaps well to bear in mind that the way in which quinin is administered probably has much to do with the production of tinnitus; it is better when an aural affection complicates the case to administer the drug by the rectum. In the treatment of the mild forms of malaria, while the preparations of bark may not act so rapidly as quinin, they will be found more efficacious, and after their use the paroxysms are not so prone to recur. Moreover, the anemia will be less marked, the appetite keener, and the strength less impaired than when quinin is used. As a substitute for the compound tincture of cinchona, one may employ with advantage the compound fluid extract of bark, as the latter does not contain as much alcohol as the compound mixture, and has five times its alkaloidal strength. The fluid extract may be given in glycerin, simple elixir, or in some palatable syrup, in doses of ½ to 1 dram. Some years ago the late Dr. Gaspar Griswold published an article advocating the hypodermic administration of 1/5 of a grain of the muriate of pilocarpin, claiming to have succeeded by this treatment in aborting malaria. Dr. Robinson said that he had tried the method, using, however, only doses of 1/12 to 1/10 of a grain, being fearful that larger doses might induce pulmonary edema. He had not been able to substantiate the claims made for pilocarpin in the treatment of malaria. For treatment during the chill he knew of nothing better than a large dose of chloric ether, though he occasionally employs the hot-air bath.

In closing, Dr. Robinson made some remarks on the diagnosis of malaria and the significance of the malarial plasmodium. He insisted that clinicians should not allow themselves to be swayed too much by laboratory investigation, albeit the latter is often of much value.

DR. A. H. SMITH: I think we cannot enter very profitably on a discussion of this subject until we are agreed as to what is meant by the term "malaria." My own opinion is that if we cannot find the specific organism we should at least insist upon a certain degree of periodicity as a test of the existence of malaria. The physician should be careful not to make a diagnosis of malaria simply because chills are present. I well remember a case which I saw last summer after a number of physicians had already been called in. The patient had chills and more or less fever, and although the blood did not contain the plasmodium, free pigment granules were found in it. The patient insisted, when questioned, that he had no tender or painful area anywhere, yet the diagnosis was not determined until an ischiorectal abscess made its appearance. On opening this abscess and evacuating the pus, the whole clinical picture of malaria vanished. I have time and again observed the development of malaria at the seashore, although this disease was not indigenous to the locality. I have also noted a recurrence of this malarial infection during several successive seasons. It is a popular belief, for which there is a certain foundation of fact, that a person who has once been severely ill with malaria is liable to have a recurrence of the disease for many years afterward. Persons who exhibit an idiosyncrasy toward quinin should be treated by a combination of quinin and hydrobromic acid or the bromids. I prefer the muriate to the sulphate of quinin, as it is more soluble and has a greater alkaloidal strength. If it be true that quinin acts directly upon the malarial organisms in the blood, it is certainly not necessary to give large doses of this drug, for in doses of 5 grains it has been estimated that it would form with the blood a solution of the strength of 1–16,000, and experiment has shown this to be amply sufficient. In the ill-defined cases of malaria in which quinin proves unsatisfactory, arsenic, although slower in its action, will prove efficacious and its good effect more lasting.

DR. LOUIS F. BISHOP: When the Home for Consumptives was transferred from Fordham to St. Luke's Hospital many of the patients were having chills. These were at first thought to be due to a septic process associated with the tuberculosis, but more careful study of the temperature charts seemed to reveal a malarial element, and this part of the temperature curve was quickly eliminated by the administration of quinin. I recently observed a case in which the action of quinin was slow and uncertain until this drug was combined with the bromids.

DR. ALBERT W. WARDEN: It has been my experience that if the secretions are much altered arsenic will not be well tolerated. I have found capsicum and taraxacum useful adjuvants to quinin, and the favorable action of this drug has seemed to be augmented by encouraging the patient to drink freely of lemonade. The syrup of iodid of iron is, in my estimation, a very valuable remedy in the cases of chronic malaria.

DR. HENRY DWIGHT CHAPIN presented a paper, entitled

CLINICAL OBSERVATIONS UPON THE HEART AND CIRCULATION IN DIPHTHERIA.

Owing to the lateness of the hour, only portions of the paper were read. It was based upon observations made last summer in the Willard Parker Hospital. Dr. Chapin said that in septic cases of diphtheria death nearly always results from a steady and rapid failure of the heart—a condition very slightly influenced by cardiac stimulants. The occurrence of vomiting in connection with a very weak pulse should be regarded as an exceedingly bad omen; it is as uncontrollable as the weak heart action. He had noted that a distinctly marked slowing of the pulse-rate is not infrequent in these grave cases. This slowing may take place either before or after a marked quickening in the action of the heart. If the slowing is extreme it is almost invariably followed by death. In one case, cited in the paper, the pulse dropped on the fourth day from 128 to 66 per minute, but its strength continued good. By the next day, however, it was rapid and feeble, beating 120 to 138 per minute; then stupor and vomiting supervened, and death occurred three days later. In another case, a boy of five years had a rapid heart action for a few days; then the pulse-rate was reduced to 28 per minute. At this time auscultation showed the heart sounds to be fairly distinct. Repeated hypodermic injections of whisky, nitroglycerin, and other heart stimulants were given, but death occurred within two days. A slow pulse alone does not necessarily constitute a fatal indication. In still another case the pulse went down to 40 per minute, but there were no other symptoms, and recovery took place.

The author said that it is very important in these severe septic cases to insist that the patient should be kept a long time in the recumbent posture, as the tendency to heart failure often persisted through many weeks. In some of the mild cases, however, improvement seemed more rapid when the children were allowed to be out of bed, although previously the pulse had been week and intermittent. The heart tonics which he had employed had been chiefly whisky, strychnin, nitroglycerin, and, in some cases, digitalis, the latter being administered hypodermically when the stomach was irritable. In children who are very restless and in whom the pulse is weak and irregular, small doses of morphia ($\frac{1}{32}$ to $\frac{1}{16}$-grain according to age, (given hypodermically) are often very effective.

DR. A. JACOBI: What is meant by this very common expression, "heart failure"? When the muscles are anemic, there is muscular failure, and if this condition is present in the voluntary muscles, it will also obtain in the heart-muscle. It is evident then that it is possible to have the heart dangerously weakened without having associated with it any marked anatomic changes. The result of such an enfeeblement of the circulation may be the formation, first of small and afterward of large thrombi in the heart, and as these cannot be removed, they constitute one cause of death. In the course of infectious diseases the heart may undergo interstitial change, with the usual results—hyperplasia and subsequent cicatrization. In most of the cases of parenchymatous inflammation the muscular tissue becomes degenerated and quite friable. The extremely slow action of the heart, referred to in the paper, is a result of the incompetency of this organ. It should be remembered that when the second sound of the heart is feeble, or the intervals between the sounds equal, that danger is imminent. Many lives are sacrificed to the so-called expectant plan of treatment. The heart failure should be anticipated by early and judicious administration of heart stimulants.

DR. JOSEPH E. WINTERS: I do not think we possess much knowledge in regard to the important subject of the heart failure so commonly observed in diphtheria. Why is it that the toxins of diphtheria at one time affect the inhibitory fibers of the pneumogastric, and at other times the vaso-excitor fibers? The text-books hardly mention the very slow pulse of diphtheria, and I have personally observed it only during the past two years. Although I cannot say that there is any connection between the two, I have noticed that these cases of slow pulse have been more common since large doses of antitoxin have been freely employed. It is far more dangerous than the very rapid pulse—I can only recall two recoveries in cases in which this symptom has been marked. In the case reported in the paper, in which the pulse fell to 28 per minute, 6000 units of antitoxin were given. I cannot agree with those who believe that in many of these cases the heart failure can be prevented by the timely use of stimulants; in some cases it occurs in spite of every precaution. It is probably to be explained by varying individual susceptibility to the toxins of diphtheria. I cannot say that I have seen any benefit from the present generally accepted practice of giving strychnin. and in this belief I am supported by Dr. W. M. Welch of Philadelphia, who has made a constant study of diphtheria during the past thirty years, nor do I see anything in the physiologic action of strychnin which should lead us to expect that it would be efficacious in cases of heart failure. I would place alcohol first on the list, and would give it in very large doses, preferably without other remedies, as as when given in this way it is less likely to provoke vomiting.

DR. H. W. BERG: Fully eighty per cent. of all cases of diphtheria exhibit nothing characteristic in the pulse. The specific effect on the circulation sometimes observed—the slow pulse noted by the reader of the paper—is a not infrequent phenomenon in very severe cases. I recall a case, seen with Dr. Jacobi fourteen years ago, in which this slow pulse was present, so it is evident that this is not a peculiarity of the cases treated with antitoxin. Moreover, although antitoxin was used in large doses in the hospital during my time of service, I did not see any cases exhibiting this peculiarity of the pulse.

REVIEWS.

OUTLINES OF ANATOMY. A Guide to the Methodical Study of the Human Body in the Dissecting-room. By EDMUND W. HOLMES, M.D., Demonstrator of Anatomy, University of Pennsylvania. Avil Printing Co., 1897.

DR. HOLMES has succeeded in his effort to produce a good outline or working manual for use in the dissecting-room. It is a valuable little book, which we commend to medical students. We feel sure that it will aid many in acquiring systematic habits of work, and, if faithfully followed, will "contribute to orderliness and discipline in the dissecting-room," thus accomplishing the object of the author.

THE ROLLER BANDAGE, with a Chapter on Surgical Dressing. By WILLIAM BARTON HOPKINS, M.D., Surgeon to Pennsylvania Hospital. Fourth edition. Philadelphia: J. B. Lippincott Co., 1897.

THIS little volume gives a short description of the methods of application of the most common bandages, together with a series of definitions and general rules for bandaging. The short chapter on the dressing of wounds which has been added to this fourth edition had best have been omitted. The illustrations constitute the most valuable portion of the book—if such a term can be applied to any part of the little volume. Altogether, we think, that the multiplication of books of this kind is of little use to the medical student.

THERAPEUTIC HINTS.

For Rheumatic Phlebitis.—HIRTZ recommends the external application of salicylic acid as follows:

℞		
	Ac. salicyl.	ʒ iv
	Morphin. hydrochlorat.	gr. v
	Lanolini	℥ i.

M. Sig. Use as an inunction twice daily.

For Congestion of the Liver.—

℞		
	Bryonin	gr. ii
	Sacchari lact.	ʒ i
	Acaciæ	gr. xv
	Syrupus	q. s.

M. Ft. pil. No. C. Sig. One pill every two hours until the bowels are thoroughly evacuated.

For the Vomiting of Appendicitis.—

℞		
	Menthol	gr. iv
	Cognac	ʒ v
	Tinct. opii	♏. lxxv.

M. Sig. Ten to twenty drops several times daily.—*Pigk.*

Protargol in Affections of the Eye.—DARIER employs protargol in preference to nitrate of silver, because, while its action is non-irritating and painless, it is a powerful germicide, remains stable in solution, combines well with cocain, and is not precipitated by alkalis, albumen, etc. He prescribes it as follows:

1. For acute catarrhal conjunctivitis.

℞		
	Protargol	gr. xxiv
	Aq. dest.	℥ ss.

M. Sig. For cauterization, at first daily, later every other day.

2. For blepharitis and blepharoconjunctivitis.

℞		
	Protargol	gr. xxiv
	Zinci oxidi / Amyli } aa	gr. xvi
	Vaselini	℥ ss.

M. Sig. Salve for eyelids.

THE MEDICAL NEWS.
A WEEKLY JOURNAL OF MEDICAL SCIENCE.

VOL. LXXII. NEW YORK, SATURDAY, APRIL 16, 1898. NO. 16.

ORIGINAL ARTICLES.

REPORT OF A CASE OF PROSTATIC HYPERTROPHY IN A VERY OLD MAN; OPERATION BY BOTTINI'S METHOD.

BY LEONARD WEBER, M.D.,
OF NEW YORK;
PROFESSOR OF MEDICINE IN THE POST-GRADUATE MEDICAL SCHOOL; VISITING PHYSICIAN TO THE POST-GRADUATE HOSPITAL; CONSULTING PHYSICIAN TO ST. MARK'S HOSPITAL.

IT is about ten years since I first learned of Dr. Bottini's operation for the relief of prostatic hypertrophy. He said that by burning three or four superficial grooves into the prostate with a galvanocautery loop, moving like a Maisonneuve urethrotome, in an instrument similar to that for crushing a calculus in the bladder, the sore distress of the sufferer would be relieved and the use of the catheter might be dispensed with.

Bottini's proposition did not receive the attention it deserved, mainly I believe, because surgeons are as a rule not much inclined to operate with the galvanocautery in the dark, and partly also, I take it, because the author failed to state in his early communications on the subject what he expected to take place after the operation. Was it to be simply new and permanent channels made and maintained by the cutting of the cautery, or the restoration of the natural prostatic urethra by a certain degree of atrophy following the superficial morcellation of the gland, or both? Possibly also a strong suspicion of the very uncertain work of the incisor may have induced us to stand aloof and assume an expectant attitude. Meantime, various operations, some of them mutilating, have been tried for the relief of this distressing condition—from the recent division of the spermatic cord to castration and excision of the prostate. So it was not until quite recently, when Bottini's instrument had been modified and improved by Freudenberg of Berlin, and a few successful operations at that city had been performed with it, that the profession in general began to be interested in the cautery operation.

After reading Dr. Willy Meyer's report of his case and demonstration of the Bottini incisor, I laid the matter before my patient, a man aged ninety-three years, comparatively hale and hearty in spite of his great age, who had been a prostatic sufferer during the previous five years and showed, besides the vesical catarrh, symptoms of pyelitis during the last twelve months, though the muscular force of his bladder continued to be fairly good. His consent to the operation having been obtained, my associate Dr. F. Torck, obtained one of Freudenberg's instruments, and an instrument-maker furnished us a portable storage-battery supplying a steady current of four volts, which is sufficiently strong to heat the platinum loop to a red heat and keep it at the same temperature as long a time as is required for performing the operation. The day before the operation Dr. Torck and myself had made ourselves thoroughly familiar with the working of the instrument and battery.

Having repeatedly examined the patient *per rectum*, I knew the right prostatic lobe to be much more enlarged than the left, and it was therefore agreed that an upper, a lower, and a right lateral cut should be made. Everything being ready, the patient was anesthetized with a mixture of chloroform and ether, equal parts. I felt quite certain that the patient would bear the chloroform-ether mixture, and we were not disappointed.

No difficulty was experienced in introducing the instrument far enough to have its short beak within the neck of the bladder. Having turned on the full current, and having counted slowly from one to five, Dr. Torck proceeded. A cut was made about 1½ centimeters in length without difficulty, and another, and then a third, but there was neither any sizzling nor odor of burnt flesh. There was, however, considerable oozing of blood from the meatus. What was the matter? We had forgotten to close the short circuit in the instrument, and it was the cold steel only, which, plowing along the prostatic urethra, had produced a superficial laceration. Our chagrin was great, but there was only one thing to do, *i. e.*, do the operation over again. After the first cut now there was a very decided odor of burnt flesh, and the subsequent cuts were readily made. The cooling apparatus attached to the instrument along its entire length worked admirably, and gave us no trouble.

When I first examined the instrument used in this operation, it struck me that the arrangement for closing and opening the circuit in the instrument itself was unnecessary and would tend to complicate matters in the handling of a tool, which is not a simple apparatus by any means, but requires much care in its use. By means of the switch of

Vetter's storage-battery, the current is under complete control and one is able to instantly turn it on or off.

The operation was performed on Wednesday, January 5th, at noon. At 1 P.M. the patient was in bed, and at 2 P.M. he was fully conscious. He had as good a pulse as before and during the operation. There was no nausea or other unpleasant symptoms. A hypodermic injection of morphia, ¼-grain, was given. At 4 P.M. he took some food, at 6 he passed urine, the half of which was blood, and continued to do so every half hour until 6 A.M. of January 6th, when the hemorrhage ceased and did not recur. In all, he lost about half a pint of blood, his pulse remaining good, and his temperature normal. Ice-bags applied to the perineum and about the symphysis pubis appeared to be effective in controlling hemorrhage.

January 6th: Temperature, 99.5° F.; pulse, 86; frequent micturition of rather clear urine, one to two ounces at a time; general condition good; appetite excellent; Vichy water was freely given.

January 7th: Temperature, 99°F.; pulse, 84. The patient was made more comfortable as to tenesmus by suppositories containing morphin and extract of belladonna, ¼-grain each, two being inserted during the twenty-four hours.

January 8th: Temperature and pulse practically normal. A gentle attempt to introduce a flexible catheter into the bladder was successful, and during the two weeks following the operation the bladder was irrigated twice daily with a weak solution of boric acid.

The patient continued to do well. While there was generally between three and four ounces of residual urine before the operation, but one and a half to two ounces are now drawn before washing the bladder. Micturition, to be sure, is still very frequent, about every twenty minutes, and since January 9th there has been some fine detritus in the urine, but no shreds of mucous membrane, nor has the microscope shown anything worth noting.

From January 10th to January 24th the patient still suffered considerably from acute exacerbation of his chronic cystitis, undoubtedly in consequence of the operation. After the latter date he rapidly improved, and February 3d was able to be about again.

February 15th: There is about two ounces of residual urine; he can hold his water sometimes from two to four hours, but more often passes it hourly, and has to get up five or six times during the night to micturate.

From about February 5th to March 1st the patient's bladder was irrigated twice daily with a 1–8000 solution of nitrate of silver, but vesical catarrh is still present with discharge of slightly turbid urine. Now and again there will be a gush of muco-purulent urine. The acute symptoms have all passed away, and the patient goes about, drives, and enjoys life in the way he was used to, and can void his urine without using a catheter. There has been practically no change in the amount of residual urine. True, there is more often one ounce than two or three. March 1st, I examined the prostate *per rectum;* the size and configuration of the gland are the same as before the operation, in fact, I did not expect any appreciable atrophy to follow the cauterization.

It is but two months since the operation was performed, and too early to say more than a single thing in regard to success in this case: The patient is able to micturate voluntarily and to empty his bladder down to line of residual urine, while before the operation he could not do more than press out from a few drops to an ounce without using a catheter. For just so much the prostatic portion of the urinary tract has been improved by the galvanocautery operation, and it is reasonable to hope and believe that this improved condition may be maintained. As to reduction of the size of the hypertrophied prostate, nothing has been gained as yet, nor is such reduction likely to occur.

The cuts might be made deeper than they probably were made in this case by holding the handle of the instrument more firmly up and toward the abdomen, while an assistant endeavors to hook the prostate, with finger in the rectum, and press it against the incisor as it is burning into the gland. But even so, nothing more than cuts one-half centimeter in depth can be made, which, when healed, will have led to the formation of grooves, one to three millimeters in depth, and the patient is not likely to be benefited more than our patient has been. Cutting into the gland with the knife or cautery-loop is not equal to resection and cannot induce an appreciable reduction in the size of the hypertrophied organ.

It is not my province to say anything about the management of prostatic hypertrophy; the less so, as everything that can be said and advised has quite recently been stated by Dr. Bolton Bangs in both a concise and comprehensive manner in a paper published in the MEDICAL NEWS for February 12, 1898. So long as we succeed in keeping the bladder aseptic and the patient is contented to lead a catheter life, there is no indication for an operation; but when a patient objects to the further use of the catheter or the bladder has become infected, I would be inclined to advise the performance of a Bottini operation first of all, as it appears to be a good and safe method to rescue the patient from catheter slavery. In the presence of pyelonephritis to any extent or chronic nephritis, I would not do this or any other cutting operation within the bladder nor allow any to be done upon a patient of mine, unless some vital indication were presented. I have performed a few operations for stone—not more than fifteen altogether. I have cut for stricture of the urethra many times. In my earlier experience I operated on some patients in that way who had chronic kidney disease complicating vesical calculus; they all died of acute exacerbation of the nephritis soon after the operation. With all patients whose kidneys were relatively sound, I had no trouble. And judging by what I have learned in my intercourse with surgeons of large practice in diseases of the urinary organs, their experience coincides with my own.

THE QUARANTINE LAWS AND NATIONAL CONTROL OF QUARANTINE.[1]

BY JAMES H. McCALL, M.D.,
OF HUNTINGDON, TENN.

THE recent researches of Sanarelli and Sternberg show, to all practical purposes, that yellow fever is caused by a specific virus which when inoculated into the body of a human being will produce the characteristic symptoms of this disease. It is not the scope of this paper to determine which of these distinguished bacteriologists has priority in this discovery, but suffice it to say, that the germ has been isolated in a sufficient number of cases of typical yellow fever to conclude that it is the cause of the disease.

The natural habitat of this germ is in the tropical regions and not in the United States; however, if it is transplanted from its native soil to our Gulf Coast, experience has shown that it thrives wonderfully, and is even more virulent here than in the tropical regions, and it is even more fatal in our Middle Southern States than on the Gulf Coast, as the records of the epidemics which have invaded Memphis and New Orleans will show.

So far, all quarantine regulations to prevent the introduction of yellow fever into the United States have utterly failed. In the recent epidemic it seems that the first case developed at Ocean Springs, Miss., a summer-resort. The disease soon became epidemic at Ocean Springs, and immediately spread to Biloxi, New Orleans, Mobile, and a number of other southern cities and towns, reaching as far north as Cairo, Ill., and Memphis, Tenn., and had it not been for the lateness of the season we no doubt would have had a repetition of the disastrous epidemic of 1878. In this as in other diseases prevention is of more importance than treatment, and since it is agreed that yellow fever is caused by a specific microbe, the only rational prophylaxis is the prevention of the ingress of the specific germ into our country.

Our present quarantine laws are not by any means what they should be. They cause the people to feel a sense of security until they are confronted with the fact that the disease is in their midst.

There are at present 68 quarantine stations on our seaboard, 44 of which are simple inspection stations and 24 quarantine stations proper. Of the former, 6 are National and 38 are State or local. Of the quarantine-stations proper 11 are National and 13 are State or local; *viz.*, 17 stations are under National control and 51 under State or municipal control. The National stations are, of course, operated under but one law, but the 51 State or municipal stations are operated under fifty-one separate and distinct laws. With this difference in laws and regulations it is impossible to institute an effective and uniform quarantine. An infected vessel would naturally seek to enter a port at which the quarantine laws were most lenient. We have about 12,000 miles of seacoast, and this vast territory is under the control of 68 quarantine stations, an average of 176 miles of seaboard under the jurisdiction of each station. It can be readily seen that the number of stations is altogether too small, compared with the territory involved, if satisfactory work is to be accomplished.

Legislation in the direction of improvement in quarantine laws has indeed been retrogressive, as is shown by the fact that the laws, with but few amendments, under which our quarantine regulations are enforced were enacted one hundred years ago. Following the great yellow-fever epidemic of 1796, Congress passed an act directing the use of the Revenue Service in carrying out the quarantine and health laws of the several States. This law was repealed in 1799, and an act was passed in which the possession and exercise of quarantine powers by the States was fully and distinctly recognized, and certain Federal officers, such as the custom's officials, masters of revenue cutters, and military officers commanding posts or stations on the seacoast being required to aid in the execution of the health laws of the States according to their respective powers and within their respective precincts, and subject to the direction of the Secretary of the Treasury. This law, passed in 1799, is the one under which our quarantine regulations are enforced. Indeed, a few acts have been passed by Congress since that time, with a view of experimenting with the subject, these, however, were all repealed after a few years' trial. In 1878, Congress passed an act empowering the Surgeon-General of the Marine Hospital Service to frame rules and regulations for the purpose of preventing the introduction of contagious diseases into the United States,

[1] Read at a meeting of the Medical Society of the State of Tennessee, held at Jackson, Tenn., April 14, 1898.

which rules and regulations should be subject to the approval of the President, but should not conflict with or impair any sanitary laws or regulations of any State or municipal authority which then existed or might thereafter be enacted. One of the orders published under the authority of this act prohibited all vessels from the Black Sea, conveying rags, furs, clothing, etc., and all vessels from the Mediterranean and Red Seas, carrying such articles from Russia, from entering any port of the United States. This bill was greatly opposed by New England commercial bodies, and in subsequent legislation was modified. In March, 1879, an act was passed authorizing a National Board of Health, consisting of seven members to be appointed by the President, not more than one of whom was to be from any one State, and four National representatives detailed from the Attorney-General's Department, the Medical Departments of the Army and Navy, and from the Marine Hospital Service. The most important duties of this board were: "To obtain information upon all matters affecting public health, to advise the several different departments of the Government, the executives of the several States, and the commissioners of the District of Columbia on all questions submitted by them, whenever in the opinion of the board such advice may tend to the preservation and improvement of public health."

In June, 1879, Congress authorized the National Board of Health "to cooperate with, and so far as it lawfully could, aid State and municipal boards of health in the execution and enforcement of the rules and regulations of such boards." The National Board of Health was also authorized to make rules and regulations to be observed by vessels sailing from any foreign port at which were contagious or infectious diseases to any port of the United States, and to obtain information of the sanitary condition of foreign ports from which contagious or infectious diseases might be brought into the United States. The last section of this act states: "That this act shall not continue in force for a longer period than four years from the date of its approval." This law expired at the end of four years, a reenactment was prevented, and Congress placed an epidemic fund in the hands of the President to be used at his discretion in preventing and suppressing epidemics and maintaining quarantines at exposed points. This fund has been transferred to the Treasury Department, and the expenses of the refuge stations established by the National Board of Health are now paid from it by the Marine Hospital Service. With the exception of the action of Congress in creating this fund there has been no National legislation within the past hundred years—which protects the country from invasion by exotic diseases—and our facilities for preventing the introduction of contagious diseases are but little better now than they were in the epidemic of 1798, which devastated Philadelphia, New York, Boston, and other northeastern cities.

In 1888 an act was passed authorizing the establishment of seven additional quarantine stations, which were placed under the control and management of the Marine Hospital Service. In 1893 an act granting additional powers and imposing additional duties upon the Marine Hospital Service was passed, and at the same time the act of March 3, 1879, establishing a National Board of Health, was repealed, and the Secretary of the Treasury was directed to obtain possession of any property, records, etc., which were formerly the property of the National Board of Health. The Marine Hospital Service was given practically the same power as was given the National Board of Health in the act of March 3, 1879, and has accomplished a great amount of good for humanity, notwithstanding the difficulty of operating under the different laws of the various States.

Dr. H. E. Brown, U. S. A., by joint resolution in Congress in 1872, was authorized to make a thorough inspection of southern ports exposed to yellow fever, and in his report says: "These quarantines, being established by State or municipal authority, lack that uniformity which is absolutely necessary to their efficiency, are not founded on rational views of the pathology of the disease, and are generally defective in their administration." The same condition found by Dr. Brown in 1872 exists to-day.

The entire system of quarantine should be in the hands of the National Government, and instead of the Government assisting the States in epidemics, the States should assist the Government. A system of sanitary inspection should be inaugurated, under the control of the Federal Government. The sanitary inspectors should have the cooperation of the State and local health boards and railroad officials.

In the recent outbreak of yellow fever in the South the execution of the quarantine laws in the different localities worked a greater hardship on the commercial interests of the country than the disease itself. Each municipal and county board was supreme authority within itself, and recklessly quarantined against any and all points upon the slightest rumor, without any investigation to ascertain the facts in the case. One county in Western Tennessee went so far as to station a shotgun brigade on the county line for the purpose for preventing any trains from passing through the county. These trains carried United States mail, and it took the Federal authorities but a short time to show the county officials the ridiculousness of their order. Such a condition of affairs is not only a great inconvenience to the traveling public, but is also the cause of great financial loss to the transportation companies.

There are at present before Congress three bills, the object of each being to place the National Government in control of all quarantine laws. One bill provides for the establishment of a Bureau of Public Health, under the control of the Treasury Department. Another bill provides for an executive department to be known as the Department of Public Health. The other bill is an amendment to an act granting additional quarantine powers and imposing additional duties upon the Marine Hospital Service, and transfers the execution of the quarantine laws from the States to the National Government. Each of these bills is a step in the right direction, and it is to be hoped that Congress will act favorably upon one of them at an early date.

Immediate steps should be taken by the Marine Hospital Service to thoroughly disinfect every house in which there was a case of yellow fever during the past season; then, if Congress will place the quarantine laws absolutely under Federal control, there will be no danger of a recurrence ot yellow fever in the United States.

TROPHIC KERATITIS, WITH THE REPORT OF A CASE OCCURRING IN CAISSON DISEASE.

BY GEORGE C. HARLAN, M.D.,
OF PHILADELPHIA.

J. B., aged twenty-nine years, came to the Eye Clinic of the Pennsylvania Hospital, October 22, 1895. He had been employed on the construction of the bridge built across the Delaware by the Pennsylvania Railroad Company, and had worked in a caisson under an atmospheric pressure of from eighteen to thirty pounds per square inch. He had commenced in June, and had worked in the caisson eight hours a day continuously until sixty feet below the surface, and then six hours a day, three hours at a time, with an intermission of three hours. Several of his fellow workmen had been taken from the caisson unconscious, one had died, and one was paralyzed. We made a search for the latter, but were not successful. In the latter part of July the patient suffered much from giddiness, debility, loss of appetite and nausea, and finally from frequent vomiting. After the first of August there was occasional numbness of the whole right side. Early in September, when he was obliged to stop work, the right eye commenced to be irritable and painful.

There was a superficial ulcer of the cornea about three millimeters in diameter, near the outer border, with irregular, ill-defined margins and a grayish, infiltrated surface, and the whole cornea was steamy. There was a dense pericorneal zone, but no corneal vessels. Some slender post-synechiæ showed a moderate iritis. The fundus could not be seen. There was anesthesia, almost complete, of the cornea, conjunctiva, and of all parts of the face supplied by the ophthalmic and superior maxillary branches of the fifth nerve. There was also loss of taste on the right side of the tongue. There was no other sensory paralysis and no motor, unless for a slight weakness of the masseter muscle, which was not positively determined. The temperature on the right side of the mouth was three-fifths of a degree higher than on the left.

Four days later the area of the ulcer had increased and a small hypopyon appeared, which, however, lasted only a few days, and by the middle of November there was a decided improvement in the condition of the cornea. The ulcer was filling up, and there was a raised line of demarcation about its margins, and several small, deep, corneal vessels were noticed. On December 10th a well-defined opacity occupied the position of the ulcer, and the whole cornea had become vascular. There was little or no improvement in sensation.

The only general treatment adopted was at first mercury and iodid, administered about a month with a view to the possibility of specific complication, though there was no evidence of such, and afterward the internal use of quinin and strychnia, with good diet and hospital care. Locally, atropia and boric acid, hot stupes, and an occlusive bandage were used. About the last of January the patient's general condition had improved so much that he felt well enough to go to work, and was allowed to leave the hospital, an ankyloblepharon having been first performed to insure protection to the insensitive cornea. He soon afterward went to a distant city, and his new address could not be obtained.

It can hardly be claimed that exposure to irritants was a prime cause here, as the keratitis persisted months after the cornea was carefully protected, though it is possible that if this had not been done the disease might have proved more destructive. Then, too, the iris was involved in the early stages, before the corneal affection had reached its height. Several subjects of interest are suggested by this case; for example, the unusual cause of the disease, the influence, or the existence, of trophic nerves, and the pathology of so-called neuroparalytic ophthalmia.

Anesthesia has been much less frequently recorded as a symptom of caisson disease than has motor paralysis, and both usually occur in the extremities; but the more important symptoms can always be referred to the brain and spinal cord. According to Dr. Bauer of St. Louis, "in grave cases there is paralysis of different degrees, from slight paresis to complete loss of sensation and motion," and "cerebral and spinal congestion, edema of the arachnoid, and softening of the brain and spinal cord" are found post-mortem. Some or all of these lesions, with, in some cases, the addition of more or less extensive extravasations of blood, were found in the nine post-mortems on the bodies of workmen who died during the building of the St. Louis and Brooklyn bridges. The cerebral and spinal lesions are explained by Dr. Andrew H. Smith and others on the theory that the brain and spinal cord, being contained in bony cavities, are less exposed to the effects of increased atmospheric pressure, and that consequently blood is driven into them from the periphery and the soft tissues. However this may be, there is no doubt that intracranial lesions do occur, and they might readily involve the Gasserian ganglion, or the fifth nerve, or its central nuclei.

The question of trophic nerves may be considered still unsettled. Of two recent prominent writers Berger says, that "experimental and clinical researches seem to prove the existence of trophic fibers in the trigeminus"; while Knies states that in neuroparalytic keratitis "we evidently have to deal with a traumatic loss of substance which is infected from the conjunctival sac. The assumption of special trophic nerves is superfluous." The subject is by no means so easily disposed of as the latter author seems to imply, as any one who attempts to explore the mass of literature which has gathered about it will be ready to admit.

Charcot says: "Defective action of the nervous system has no direct immediate influence upon the nutrition of peripheral parts; on the other hand, it is at least very probable that morbid excitation, irritation of nerves, or nerve centers will, under certain conditions, provoke the most various trophic troubles at a distance. Do these trophic lesions depend upon irritation of these hypothetic nerves, which anatomy does not recognize, and which are sometimes designated *trophic nerves?* — the theory of special trophic nerves of which Samuel has been one of the chief advocates." Charcot, while he does not admit the theory, considers it worthy of consideration because it explains better than any which preceded the pathologic phenomena observed in practice. He is inclined to attribute these phenomena to an irritation conveyed by sensitive fibers, but admits that the question still awaits solution.

According to Gowers, "Nutrition of tissue elements is largely under the influence of the nervous system. Whether this influence is exerted through special 'trophic nerves,' or through the motor, the sensory, and especially through the vasomotor nerves, is a question that has been much discussed and is still undecided. The balance of evidence is against the existence of special tropic nerves. In the case of the fifth nerve, acute trophic changes occur in the eyeball chiefly when the disease involves the Gasserian ganglion or the nerve in front of it." The author likens these changes to the acute trophic changes which occur in the skin.

The corneal lesions which follow section of the fifth nerve, or its paralysis from other causes, were formerly attributed to the loss of the trophic influence of this nerve, but since Snellen and Büttner reported that in their experiments upon rabbits these lesions did not occur if the eye were protected, they have been quite generally attributed, at least in the text-books, to loss of sensation of the cornea and its consequent injury by external irritants. Numberless cases have been recorded, and we have all met with such, which would prove this contention most satisfactorily if there were not others which, if less numerous, are equally positive on the other side of the question and can be better explained by recourse to the older theory. They are too numerous also to be set aside as exceptions, and I have seen a sufficient number of them myself to make me quite sure, while still in doubt as to the true pathology of the disease, that the mechanical theory is insufficient. I merely wish to comment on some of these cases without attempting to review the extensive literature of the subject, which would lead far beyond the limits of this paper and is, besides, familiar or accessible to all. The results of physiologic experiments have been too various and even contradictory to be conclusive. What some experimentalists have claimed to establish others have almost invariably failed to confirm, even if they have not reached opposite conclusions. Some have thought it proved that the keratitis is due to mechanical injury depending upon loss of sensation; others that it is the result of depriving the cornea of the influence of trophic nerves; and still others that it is a phenomenon, not of paralysis, but of irritation, while some authorities attribute it to a paralysis or an irritation of vasomotor fibers as distinct from trophic, and in some experiments the removal of the superior cervical ganglion alone has caused the phenomenon in question, but in others has prevented its occurrence, even when the fifth nerve has been divided.

The cornea will sometimes slough, if exposed, though perfectly sensitive, but it will by no means always do so when insensitive. An example of the former fact is found in the case of a farmer who came to me a few years ago with a corneal fistula due to complete peripheral paralysis of the facial nerve, following exposure to cold while filling his ice-house. The fifth nerve was quite healthy. The actual cautery and a protective compress promptly restored the anterior chamber, and a subsequent ankyloblepharon prevented any recurrence of the trouble. The lid margins were united a little to the nasal side of the middle, and the patient could see well enough for all his purposes through a partial opening of the outer half of the commissure.

Among many examples of the resistance of a sensitive cornea to exposure may be mentioned the case of a patient whose eye had been completely exposed during six years by the entire destruction of the lid by a burn, but the cornea remained perfectly clear. As for the insensitive cornea, in a case which I reported some years ago a haziness of about a fourth of the cornea, which occurred during the acute stage of an infection of the fifth nerve, probably gouty, was permanent, but the rest of the cornea remained clear and bright many years, though the sensation never returned.

In absolute glaucoma, the insensitive cornea never sloughs or presents anything like the picture of neuroparalytic keratitis. It may even remain clear. Proofs are not wanting that the sensibility of the cornea and the state of its nutrition are not necessarily associated. Instances of loss of corneal sensation without inflammation are not very infrequent; and so-called neuroparalytic keratitis without loss of sensation has been observed. So, also, we may have typical neuroparalytic sloughing of the cornea without exposure.

In a case which I reported in the *Philadelphia Medical Times*, vol. iv, p. 166, the cornea, which had remained clear under prolonged exposure, commenced to suffer at the very time when it was protected by paralysis of the levator palpebræ muscles. The cranial nerves were involved one after another in the progress of an extensive sarcomatous disease of the temporal bone. The patient, a child three years of age, was brought to the Children's Hospital, August 4th, with a purulent discharge from the ear, a large polypus in the meatus, and a fluctuating swelling over the mastoid. There was complete paralysis of the facial nerves, and the left eye could not be closed. The cornea was clear and bright, and, as the eye showed no symptoms of irritation, no means were adopted to protect it. More than three weeks later, August 29th, the disease involved the third pair of nerves and produced ptosis, and it was noticed at this time that the cornea was dim. On September 1st, three days afterward, the whole cornea was hazy and its lower fourth infiltrated. At the end of three more weeks, September 17th, there was a sloughing penetrating ulcer; as the child's mother said, "the eyes seemed to be melting away." The little patient died a few days afterward, but no post-mortem was allowed beyond a partial removal of the growth which had appeared externally.

Dr. Norris has reported a case of neuroparalytic ophthalmia from intracranial disease in which the insensitive cornea sloughed, though it had been carefully protected.

Such cases are comparatively rare, but the positive proof which they offer that the cornea may suffer in connection with lesions of the fifth nerve, under conditions which exclude the mere loss of sensation as a cause, cannot be ignored. No doubt in some cases simply exposure, either with or without loss of sensation, particularly when combined with pressure, as in the case reported to the Society last year by Dr. Green and as frequently occurs in exophthalmic goiter, is competent to induce destructive keratitis; but it is equally certain that in other cases inflammation of the cornea, and even of the deeper structures of the eye, occurs as an evident result of lesions of the fifth nerve, though exposure to external irritants can be positively excluded as a cause. It is well known that the cornea is not always alone involved, but even in the earlier stages of the disease the iris is often found to be affected; and in some experimental cases hypopyon has occurred while the cornea remained sound and clear.

Instead of the sloughing or ulcerative keratitis usually met with in this form of ophthalmia, an increase of nutritive action, resulting in vascular turgescence and hypertrophy, may occur, as is illustrated by the case of a farmer's wife, forty-four years of age, who applied at the Wills Hospital with a painful affection of the left eye from which she had suffered a year. The sight was gone, and the patient complained of intense and constant pain in the eyeball, brow, and side of head. There was complete loss of sensation in the cornea and in all the other parts supplied by the fifth nerve, except a just perceptible sensitiveness of the ocular conjunctiva. There was no other paralysis and no indication of herpes. The palpebral conjunctiva was enormously thickened and the bulbar conjunctive engorged, while the cornea presented the densest pannus crassus that I have ever seen. The other eye was sound and the patient's general health was good.

The literature of this disease includes comparatively few post-mortem examinations, but Serres, Romberg, Alison, Genkin, and Haase found lesions of the Gasserian ganglion; De Schweinitz found the ciliary nerves normal, which points to a central cause though it does not exclude disease of the ganglion, and Duval and Laborde claim to have proved by extensive experimentation that there is a bulbar central nucleus a lesion of which produces the same sensitive and nutritive alterations in the eye as follow intracranial section of the fifth nerve. Panas thinks that, "we are authorized to conclude that neuroparalytic keratitis has its point of departure in an alteration of the Gasserian ganglion, or of the nuclei of the fifth pair of nerves," which is perhaps about as far as we can confidently go in the present state of our knowledge, leaving it still undecided whether this alteration is of a paralytic or an irritative character, and whether its effects are produced through the medium of sensitive, vasomotor, or special trophic fibers.

TREATMENT OF POST-PARTUM HEMORRHAGE.[1]

BY FRANK E. LOCK, M.D.,
OF BUFFALO, N. Y.

UNDER the term post-partum hemorrhage may be included any bleeding which occurs after the delivery of a child from any part of the parturient canal. By general consent however, the term is commonly applied only to hemorrhage from the site of the placenta.

In a considerable number of instances this is a preventable accident, oftentimes depending upon causes within the power of the physician to overcome. It follows, therefore, that there must be three lines or periods of treatment: (1) prophylaxis, (2) control of the hemorrhage when it occurs, and (3) the after-treatment of the patient.

Hemorrhage from the uterus after child-birth is normally prevented by the contraction and retraction of the muscular fibers of this organ, which compress the vessels in the uterine wall, and also by thrombus formation, pressure of the fetus, if present, and by the contraction of the arteries themselves. Any condition in the mother or in the uterus which tends to prevent these factors from operating may be an exciting cause of this alarming accident. The contractile power of the uterus may be lessened by an exhausting labor, rapid artificial delivery, excessive distension due to multiple pregnancy or hydramnios, or by general or nervous disturbances on the part of the mother.

Contraction and retraction are also rendered more or less ineffectual by foreign matter in the uterine cavity, such as clots, pieces of membranes or placenta, and also from tumors, adhesion from old pelvic inflammatory disturbances, or by an over-distention of the rectum or bladder. Thrombosis may be prevented by defective contractions, or by restlessness, coughing, vomiting, or excessive movements of the patient.

Prophylaxis consists of the treatment of the patient during pregnancy, especially during the latter months, and in the proper management of labor. Any abnormality or departure from health which is amenable to treatment should be corrected. Examinations of the urine, for albumin, urea, and total solids should be frequently made. If the patient be run down, weak, or anemic, general tonic and hygienic measures must be instituted. Good results follow the administration of quinin in tonic doses during the last three or four weeks of pregnancy, especially when given in connection with the compound syrup of hypophosphites. Care should be taken to have the diet nutritious, and directions should be given in regard to proper clothing, exercise, rest, and other matters which tend to promote the general health and tone of the body.

There is much depending upon the proper management of the labor itself. It should not be allowed to continue too long, as the patient or the uterus may become exhausted: neither should it be too rapid, as thereby contractions may be delayed and the time may be insufficient to allow of thrombus formation. When necessary labor must be artificially terminated and the uterus made to contract by gentle kneading through the abdominal wall. As soon as the child is delivered it is good practice, although thought inadvisable by many, to administer ʒ i of the fluid extract of ergot by mouth or hypodermically, in order to inhibit any tendency to relaxation of the uterus should such be present. The third stage must not be hurried, and manipulation and pressure should be maintained until the placenta is delivered.

During the third stage of labor the patient should lie upon her back so that fluids may escape from the vagina without clotting. In manipulating the uterus to expel the placenta, by Credé's method, care must be taken to make pressure in the proper direction, and all traction upon the cord must be avoided. The placenta and membranes should be inspected for assurance that everything has been expelled, and intermittent pressure made over the fundus to insure firm contraction. The attendant should remain within call for at least an hour after the placenta is delivered, and should make occasional examinations of the uterus, by abdominal palpation, in order to note any tendency to unusual relaxation.

During the second stage of labor the physician should see that the following articles are accessibly placed: Davidson's syringe, in working order; ice in small pieces, brandy or whisky, ergot, morphin or laudanum, a hypodermic syringe, vinegar, iodin, hot and cold sterilized water, a large pitcher, and a Kelly's pad or substitute for it.

Unfortunately the physician often has no previous knowledge of his patient and sees her for the first time when called to attend her in labor; thus, he has no opportunity for previous preparation or treatment of the case. The occurrence of severe hemorrhage after an apparently normal delivery comes as a

[1] Second Prize Essay, MEDICAL NEWS Prize Contest.

great surprise and calls for prompt action, a steady hand, and the coolest judgment.

The physician should endeavor to call to mind Nature's methods of controlling hemorrhage and imitate her by securing contractions, thrombus formation, or, these failing, by the employment of pressure.

The pillows should be removed from beneath the patient's head to prevent syncope and the hand placed over the uterus to stimulate contractions. A hypodermic injection of a standard preparation of ergot, such as Squibb's fluid extract, or the normal liquid ergot should be administered, preferably in the anterior or outer aspect of the thigh as approximating the part against which its action is directed. If necessary cold may now be applied over the lower abdomen by means of cloths wrung out of ice-water; this should be done at short intervals, two or three seconds at a time only, in order that the shock may act as a factor in stimulating contractions. Ice may be used for the same purpose by gently rubbing with it, or cold water may be dashed over the abdomen.

In case the uterus cannot be palpated through the abdominal wall, the hand must be introduced into the vagina and any clots removed as quickly as possible. The hand may be placed within the uterus itself and its walls scratched with the fingers, being kept in until forced out by the uterine contractions. A small piece of ice may be carried in with the hand, but if so it must be quickly removed.

Having rapidly tried the foregoing methods without result we must endeavor to secure effectual contractions by the introduction of substances which act upon the uterus locally, as irritants. The substances are forcibly thrown in by means of a Davidson syringe, which it is well to have provided with a return-flow tube in order that the cavity of the uterus may not be distended.

Water, as hot as can be borne by the hand (about 120° F.), should first be tried, as this, in addition to being an excellent styptic, causes contraction of the uterine walls and blood-vessels, and also prevents abstraction of heat from the patient, who is already more or less cold and exhausted. This may be followed in case of failure by vinegar or iodin.

The iodin to be used should be the compound tincture made in accordance with the formula of Dr. Churchill, as this is the best preparation for use in an emergency. A sufficient quantity is added to water to produce a dark amber color, and the injection made as before. It rarely fails to control the most frightful hemorrhage. In favorable cases when proper agents are not at hand a temporary cessation of the flow may be secured by compression of the abdominal aorta.

A faradic battery, if at hand, may be employed to stimulate contractions, by placing one electrode in the uterus and the other over the fundus upon the abdomen.

When necessary to resort to packing of the uterus, strips of iodoform gauze should be used, sufficient to tightly fill the cavity of the organ up to the fundus, the walls of the uterus being squeezed down upon it. This is removed after twenty-four hours and a hot antiseptic douche given.

Monsel's solution should rarely be employed as a styptic, as the clot produced is removed with difficulty, and, being a foreign body in the uterus, may be a cause of secondary hemorrhage or a nidus for septic processes. It can usually be relied upon to stop the flow but should be reserved until all other methods have failed.

Having succeeded by means of some of the foregoing measures in securing a stoppage of the flow, a firm binder should be applied and the patient's condition carefully considered. The depression following an excessive loss of blood will be considerable and its effects upon the circulatory and nervous systems will be immediately manifested. The skin is cold and clammy, and there is distress, restlessness, small, frequent pulse, rapid respirations, and possibly fainting or convulsions due to the effects of the anemia upon the brain-centers.

The treatment of this stage is most important. The patient's head should be lowered and the foot of the bed raised; hot applications should be made to the extremities and warm compresses to the head. The circulation must be stimulated by the hypodermic use of cardiac stimulants, of which ether is probably the most rapid in its action, which may be followed by alcohol in some form or strychnin. If syncope threatens the limbs should be elevated and a tourniquet applied over the femoral artery, or a Martin's rubber bandage, including the entire lower extremity, may be employed in order that the blood may be confined as much as possible in the upper part of the body. The hypodermic use of morphin or laudanum, as a cerebral congestant, is also advisable.

If these measures fail to improve the pulse, warm coffee may be thrown into the rectum in small quantities frequently repeated, with brandy or whisky, if desired, as small quantities of fluids are rapidly absorbed from the rectum under these circumstances. Transfusion may be employed, or, what is usually more practicable, the intravenous or intracellular injection of salt solution, which, by increasing its bulk, tends to improve the condition of the circulation. The solution must be sterile, at about the temperature of the body, and should contain ʒ i of sodium chlorid to Oi of water. About half an hour is necessarily consumed in introducing the solution by means of a small trocar, rubber tube, and funnel, all of which have been previously sterilized. An ordinary large-size hypodermic syringe may be used, but necessitates a great many pnnctures.

When the circulation has been restored the patient must be nourished by the administration of small quantities of hot fluids by mouth, repeated at frequent intervals. Brandy and water may be first used, and gradually milk and broth may be added, and the quantities gradually increased. Great care is necessary in order to avoid nausea.

Headache, restlessness, and pain, when present, must be controlled by the administration of opiates, and the thirst, which is usually piesent, relieved by giving the patient ice and water in the intervals of feeding.

TENDENCIES IN MEDICINE.

BY J. S. TRIPLETT, M.D.,
OF HARRISONVILLE, MO.

IN discussing the tendencies of medicine of to-day, it seems that the question which stands out most prominently and the one which is receiving the most consideration from investigators is the etiologic factor in the production of disease; and since an overwhelming majority of diseases are due either directly or indirectly to micro-organisms, the subject resolves into a study of these minute bodies; or, in other words, a study of bacteriology. I do not wish to convey the idea that progress has been delayed in other departments of medicine, but I do wish to emphasize the fact that researches in other departments of medicine have been, for the most part, greatly facilitated by the application of the principles of bacteriology.

It has been remarked that "no other man of our time has been such an epoch-maker in the history of surgery as Lister." This is certainly true, but it was only through the application of those principles which have for their object the perfect cleanliness of wounds, that the approbrium of surgery has, in a large measure, been removed. A careful reading of Lister's masterly address before the London Congress of Medicine one year ago, will impress one with the fact that aside from the remarks on anesthesia and the Röntgen-ray, the subject matter relates almost entirely to questions which belong to the domain of bacteriology. He tells in a plain and characteristic style of the process by which he was enabled to place surgery upon the scientific basis it now occupies; and, now, the entire medical profession stands debtor to the painstaking labors of this great man.

However skilful the surgeon may be, or perfect his technic, the entrance of pathogenic bacteria into the wound often frustates the object of the operation and menaces the life of the patient. Concerning this point Lister says: "Nothing was formerly more striking in surgical experience than the difference in the behavior of injuries according to whether the skin was implicated or not. Thus, if the bones of the leg were broken and the skin remained intact, the surgeon applied the necessary apparatus without any other anxiety than that of maintaining a good position of the fragments, although the internal injury to the bones and soft parts might be very severe. If, on the other hand, a wound was present communicating with the broken bones, although the danger might be in other respects comparatively slight, the compound fracture, as it was termed, was one of the most dangerous accidents that could happen. What was the cause of this astonishing difference? It was clearly in some way due to the exposure of the injured parts to the external world. One obvious effect of such exposure was indicated by the odor of the discharge, which showed that the blood in the wound had undergone putrefactive change by which the bland nutrient liquid had been converted into highly irritating and poisonous substances. I have seen a man with a compound fracture of the leg die within two days of the accident, as plainly poisoned by the products of putrefaction as if he had taken a fatal dose of some potent toxic drug. These and many other considerations had long impressed me with the greatness of the evil of putrefaction in surgery. I had done my best to mitigate it by scrupulous ordinary cleanliness and the use of various deodorant lotions. But to prevent it altogether appeared hopeless while we believed with Liebig that its primary cause was the atmospheric oxygen. But when Pasteur had shown that putrefaction was a fermentation caused by the growth of microbes, and that these could not arise *de novo* in the decomposable substance, the problem assumed a more hopeful aspect. If the wound could be treated with some substance which without doing too serious mischief to the human tissue would kill the microbes already contained in it, and prevent the access of others in the living state, putrefaction might be prevented however freely the air with its oxygen might enter."

Thus, was put into operation a method which has so revolutionized the practice of surgery that every region of the body is now explored with impunity; and the dread of former unsatisfactory results and fatal terminations has been reduced to an insignificant minimum.

So universal is the prevalence of bacteria in nature, so absolutely indispensible are they to our well-being (saprophytic), so inseparable are they from disease (pathogenic), that the study and recognition of the science of bacteriology becomes our imperative duty. DaCosta sounds the keynote of modern tendencies when he says:[1] "Now, the recognition of minute organisms, their study, their artificial culture and modes of growth, their secretions, their chemic character, their likes, their antagonisms, have let us into the secrets of another world, and are showing us the way in which infective maladies originate, and the laws they obey. We are looking for infection in every disease; we are often keenly pursuing it where it probably does not exist, at all events, not in the shape of bacteria, which in our day we accept as a term almost synonymous with infection."

Inasmuch as the subject of bacteriology is only in its developmental stage (its systematic study does not exceed a decade and a half) the data cannot be obtained whereby we are enabled to state the proportion of deaths or the number of cases of disease of parasitic origin, as compared to the whole number of deaths and the whole number of cases of sickness. Moreover, we must take into consideration the fact that diseases the etiology of which has hitherto been obscure and unsettled are constantly being added to the infective list.

In illustration of the first part of the above paragraph a brief consideration of cancer is apropos. As yet its specific cause is not established; still many eminent men believe it to be of parasitic origin, and have observed an organism upon which they base their belief. On the other hand it has *not* been proven to be of non-parasitic origin. When an organ becomes the seat of carcinoma, distant organs and parts will in time become similarly involved (inoculated?), and again, quite a number of inoperable cases have been successfully treated with antistreptococcic and other serums, both of which facts argue for a parasitic origin. And, in regard to the latter part of the paragraph referred to, we do not have to search far to prove its correctness. Perhaps the disease the specific cause of which has been most recently discovered is yellow fever. Thus, as research continues and our knowledge of disease widens, the percentage of infectious maladies is ever higher and higher.

I might state here, as a matter of statistic importance, that Robert Koch in 1881 at the London Congress of Medicine, showed the bacterium which is responsible for more deaths among mankind than any other known disease. The tubercle bacillus causes one-seventh of all deaths, and Vaughan states after a careful investigation, that one-third of all men are affected with tuberculosis at some period of their existence.

[1] MEDICAL NEWS, vol. lxx.

Let us now inquire what relation bacteria bear to animal and vegetable life and what rôle they play in Nature.

Unlike the higher order of vegetable plants, bacteria are devoid of chlorophyl and are forced to obtain their nutritive materials from organic matters as such, and, therefore, lead either a saprophytic or parasitic existence. Their life processes are so rapid and energetic that they result in the most profound alterations in the structure and composition of the materials in and upon which they are developing. Decomposition, putrefaction, and fermentation result from the activities of the saprophytic bacteria, while the changes brought about in the tissues of their host by the parasitic forms find expression in disease processes and not infrequently in death.

The rôle played in Nature by the saprophytic bacteria is a very important one. Through their presence the highly complicated tissues of dead animals and vegetables are resolved into simpler compounds, carbonic acid, water, and ammonia, in which form they may be taken up and appropriated as nutrition by the more highly organized members of the vegetable kingdom.

The chlorophyl plants do not possess the power of obtaining their carbon and nitrogen from such highly organized and complicated substances as serve for the nutrition of bacteria, and as the production of these simpler compounds by the animal world is not sufficient to meet the demands of the chlorophyl plants, the importance of the part played by the bacteria in making up this deficit cannot be overestimated. Were it not for the activity of these microscopic living particles, all life upon the surface of the earth would undoubted cease. Deprive higher vegetation of the carbon and nitrogen supplied to it as a result of bacterial activity and its development comes rapidly to an end; rob the animal kingdom of the food-stuffs supplied to it by the vegetable world, and life is no longer possible. It is plain, therefore, that the saprophytes which represent the large majority of all bacteria, must be looked upon by us in the light of benefactors, without which existence would be impossible. With the parasites, on the other hand, the conditions are far from analogous. Through their activities there is constantly a loss, rather than a gain, to both the animal and vegetable kingdoms.

Their host must always be a living body in which exist conditions favorable to their development and from which they appropriate substances which are necessary to the health and life of the organisms to which they may have found access; at the same time, they eliminate substances as products of their nutrition which are directly poisonous to the tissues in which they are growing.

When the pathogenic bacteria gain admittance to the body and there find conditions favorable to their growth, they produce alterations which we call disease and which we further specify by saying it is an infectious disease. Quite often, however, persons are exposed to contagion and escape infection; *i.e.*, they are not susceptible to that particular form of infection. How shall we explain this? After the bacteria have gained admittance one or two results follows: The invading organisms will multiply and by their poisonous products—toxins—produce death, or the protecting substances of the tissues—the alexins—will inhibit or neutralize the action of the toxins, and health will be resumed. In the latter mode of termination, when there is a failure to establish a condition of disease, the tissues are victorious and are said to be resistant or to possess immunity.

Immunity may be natural or acquired. Natural immunity may be peculiar to the individual, species, or race. Acquired immunity is observed in individuals (for some time at least) who have recovered from certain forms of infection, and have thereby acquired protection against subsequent similar attacks.

The most generally accepted explanation of acquired immunity, and the one worthy of the greatest confidence, assumes immunity to be due to reactive changes on the part of the tissues, which result in the formation in the tissues of antitoxic substances capable of neutralizing the poisons produced by the bacteria against which the animal has been immunized; and not as Metchnikoff would have us believe, due to phagocytosis, the principle of which is that the wandering cells of the animal organism, the leucocytes, possess the property of taking up, rendering inert, and digesting micro-organisms with which they may come in contact in the tissues.

A vast amount of research and experimentation has been required to place acquired immunity upon a working basis, but it has lead to the greatest triumph that has ever been witnessed in the history of medicine, *viz.*, the establishment of a therapeutic system founded upon Nature's own process of protecting the living organism against disease.

Let us notice a few of the diseases which are being treated by this process: Of these we are perhaps more familiar with *diphtheria* than with any other. The use of the serum treatment has been so general in this affection and its results so convincing that we are forced to accept it as the best known method of to-day. The serum treatment of diphtheria has reduced the mortality more than one-half as compared with other modes of treatment.

Tetanus.—Not being of such frequent occurrence as diphtheria, the treatment of tetanus by its antitoxin has not had the extended trial which has favored the antitoxin of the former affection, but we are safe in saying that better results have been obtained with this treatment than with other methods.

Bubonic Plague (Malignant Polyadenitis).—Yersin has so conclusively demonstrated the efficacy of the serum treatment of this infectious disease in India that he has begun the manfacture of the serum on a large scale. He is developing the antitoxin as rapidly as possible, for use not only as a specific against the disease, but also as a prophylactic. (Item, MEDICAL NEWS, January 30, 1897.)

Yellow Fever.—There seems to be no doubt that Sanarelli has discovered the bacillus of yellow fever. He prepared a serum-antitoxin and the results of his treatment are pronounced definitely convincing. (Item, MEDICAL NEWS, March 13, 1897.)

Tuberculosis.—When Koch's tuberculin treatment became known, the news was heralded through the world that a cure had at last been found for consumption; enthusiasm ran high, and an impatient populace was led to believe that in a short period of time the greatest enemy of mankind would be forever subdued. In justice to Koch we must say that rumor was far in advance of his most sanguine expectations. Koch's tuberculin has been, and is now of incalculable value in the diagnosis of bovine tuberculosis, thereby furnishing the means of stopping one important source of infection. The reaction following injections of tuberculin into tuberculous cows is so marked that it is our best means of diagnosis; and were this its only use, it must be accorded a high place.

However, our investigators are not yet through with the tubercle bacillus, and a successful method of combating tuberculosis is only one of the unsolved problems.

Pyogenic Infection.—In phlegmonous inflammations, spreading suppuration, puerperal infection, and septicemias in general of streptococcic origin, the antistreptococcic serum has been used with such satisfactory results as to merit its continued employment.

Other Miscellaneous Diseases.—Among other diseases which have been treated by antitoxic serums with varied success may be mentioned typhoid fever, leprosy, syphilis, Asiatic cholera, hydrophobia, pneumonia, erysipelas, anthrax, and many others.

From a review of the facts which have been set forth, are we not justified in claiming that more has been accomplished through the study of bacteriology, concerning the cause, nature, prevention, and cure of disease, than through the study of any other department of medicine, and are we not looking for the solution of most of the important questions in the study of bacteriology? Clearly the present tendency in medicine is in this direction.

WATER IN THE TREATMENT OF GASTRO-INTESTINAL DISORDERS.

BY JOHN A. LICHTY, M.D.,
OF CLIFTON SPRINGS, N. Y.

IN recent years the advocates of hydrotherapy have been receiving more attention and respect than formerly. Men acquainted with physiologic principles and able to judge as to the therapeutic value of a remedy have succeeded in establishing it upon a more rational basis. The Brand treatment in typhoid fever is no longer an experiment, and the pack in pneumonia is admitted to be a great aid to any internal medication which it may seem wise to employ. The principles which the empiric Priessnitz blindly followed in the early part of this century, have thus, through the experiences of physicians, been revealed in the various treatments of diseased processes. To-day, the text-book upon therapeutics which does not recognize water as a remedial agent and specify the mode of its application is not considered complete.

The famous Hoffman, a contemporary of Boerhaave, in writing upon the subject of water said: "If there exists anything in the world that can be called a panacea, a universal remedy, it is pure water; first, because it will disagree with no one; secondly, because it is the best preservative against disease; thirdly, because it will cure agues and chronic complaints; fourthly, because it responds to all indications."

But water is not a panacea, and those who have not kept this in mind when speaking of its efficacy in the treatment of disease are in the main responsible for the general disfavor into which hydrotherapy has so often fallen. Therefore, in writing upon the subject of water in the treatment of gastro-intestinal disorders, I approach it with care and candor, very ready to admit that it is not a cure-all, and to recognize the many other valuable remedies which are usually employed in the treatment of such affections, but with a growing consciousness that water is not as generally employed as it should be, and when employed, it is often in the most careless and haphazard way.

When a glass of water is ingested it probably has no other effect upon the mouth and esophagus than that of cooling, moistening, and cleansing them. From the interesting investigations of Von Mehring we learn that water is absorbed only in very small quantities from the stomach. At least nine-tenths of all the water taken into the stomach is passed into the duodenum. A glass of water will probably reach the duodenum within thirty minutes after being swallowed. If it is taken later than half an hour before a meal, a quantity will remain in the stomach to dilute the food and the gastric juice. This does not interfere with gastric digestion, since a glass of cold water taken during a meal does not disturb healthy digestion.[1] A greater amount than this, and especially if taken soon after a meal when the stomach is in the height of digestive activity, interferes with digestion. It is therefore best not to drink more than one glass of water half an hour before meals, one glass of cool water during meals, and to leave digestion undisturbed by water from one to two hours after meals, depending upon the known digestibility of the food taken.

After the water has passed into the small intestine it is absorbed. It has been found by experiments upon dogs that when a quantity of water is injected into the bowel the stream of chyle in the thoracic duct is but slightly if at all increased, thus showing that the water is absorbed by the blood capillaries of the intestinal villus, and not by the lacteal. It is therefore beyond dispute that water in the bowel is taken up directly by the rootlets of the portal vein, and must traverse the liver before it can reach the general circulation.

Not all the water, however, passes into the circulation, for some is held by the feces, which usually contain at least seventy-five per cent. of water. According to Landois and Sterling, the quantity of water taken has no direct effect upon the amount of water in the feces. Indirectly, however, it without doubt has some effect upon the feces; namely, that in a person who for some time takes a restricted amount of water, the feces will be dryer and harder than when water is freely ingested. I base my assertion upon the following facts, physiologic and clinical:

I have already shown that the water absorbed from the bowel must pass through the liver before it can reach the circulation. It is a well-known fact that this increase in portal circulation greatly augments the secretion of bile. (Reichert, unpublished lecture.) One of the main functions of the bile is to increase peristalsis; thus, it is called a "peristaltic persuader." Landois and Sterling admit that the more energetic the peristalsis the more watery are the feces. There can be no doubt then that increased ingestion of water will cause an increase of the water in the feces. I have always found in patients suffering from constipation that increased ingestion of water is followed by softer stools. This

[1] "Landois and Sterling's Physiology," p. 305.

principle, as I shall show later, in uncomplicated cases of constipation has frequently directed my treatment.

Pure water, when applied to an irritated mucous membrane, has a very soothing and quieting effect; in fact, it affects all tissue in this way. When an injury is sustained, usually the first impulse is to bathe the injured surface with water. It was this instinct which first led to the recognition of the therapeutic value of water.

The following facts, referring to the elimination of water, I base upon experiments upon myself and observations upon patients: When pure water is taken in large quantities (ten or twelve tumblerfuls, or eighty ounces a day) it produces a decided and constant effect upon the activity of the eliminating organs of the body. During the first few days the kidneys become very active, a large amount of urine is passed, which is pale and of low specific gravity, and the relation between urea and uric acid is very much disturbed, considering their usual relation to be one part uric acid to thirty-three of urea (Haig); during this disturbance I frequently find the proportion to be one to fifty-five—the uric acid being diminished about one-half, and the urea only slightly lessened. If the ingestion of this amount of water is continued a week or two, the excessive activity of the kidneys seems to diminish; the amount of urine passed in twenty-four hours is perhaps sixty instead of eighty ounces; it has a specific gravity of 1012, instead of 1006 or 1008; the uric acid remains diminished, while the urea is much increased, the proportion being, perhaps, one to seventy. For the first few days the specific gravity of the blood, if in the beginning it is above normal, remains the same, but it soon gradually diminishes to the normal. As the amount of urine lessens the feces seem to be more moist, and the bowels, if constipated, are inclined to become regular.

I have not followed out any clinical investigation showing the action of water upon the skin and respiratory tract.

In the treatment of diseases of the gastro-intestinal tract, I have learned that water must be employed according to the condition which is found, and that as much care must be exercised in prescribing it as in advising the employment of any other remedy. In acute gastritis small pieces of cracked ice are often all the stomach will endure. As the irritation subsides, frequently repeated drafts of water are tolerated, and finally liquid foods. The use of drugs is indicated in probably but one-fourth of the cases.

There is a peculiar idea among the laity, and I believe it is also cherished by some physicians, that as soon as any portion of the alimentary canal is affected by an abnormal condition attention must be turned, first and principally, toward dietetics, and that a successful issue of the case will largely depend upon how much the patient can be made to eat. This course is pursued unmindful of the fact that a human being can comfortably live several days without food, and that rest of function is of prime importance in treating any organ.

In chronic gastritis one of the chief difficulties to overcome is the accumulation of mucus in the stomach, as well as the chemic and mechanical irritation due to the presence of undigested food. Water, either in the form of lavage or in copious drafts, is the best remedy to overcome this difficulty. Lavage is the treatment, *par excellence*, but it is not always practicable, nor is it always necessary. I have found that drafts of water at the proper time and in proper quantity will wash out the stomach quite as satisfactorily as lavage, unless there be decided atony of the stomach or pyloric stenosis. In chronic gastritis there is usually a symptom-complex plainly showing that the patient has unconsciously or deliberately denied himself the proper daily amount of water. There is a urine of high specific gravity; blood not sufficiently diluted; a coated tongue, constipation, etc. These condition must be met, and the copious drafts of water which are taken to cleanse the stomach can be further used to flush the body.

Writers almost unanimously agree that in dilation of the stomach water should be sparingly used. Hemmeter says: "Not more than one and one-half quarts a day, including all drinks, coffee, soups, etc.[1] In these conditions water can be given in small quantities frequently repeated.

There are patients with dilated stomachs who are very much below the normal in weight. The loss of weight seems to be mostly due to the absence of the normal amount of fat about the abdomen. The condition is frequently associated with floating kidney and its sequelæ. Analysis of the stomach contents shows the gastric juice inert and not able to dispose of solid food to advantage. These patients do not gain in weight when placed upon a dry diet, and yet a decided gain in weight is essential to recovery. It is therefore frequently necessary to disregard the idea that fluids in large quantity will relax the stomach, and to prescribe a milk and raw egg diet. As the patient approaches the normal weight (and sometimes not until he is far above it) the diet can be gradually changed to solid food. I have found that a liquid diet taken while the patient is in bed will not have the same tendency to increase the dilation of the stomach as when the patient is up and about,

[1] Hemmeter, "Diseases of the Stomach," p. 593.

and that the stomach, especially in atonic dilation, will frequently contract as the patient accumulates fat about the abdomen.

In hyperchlorhydria, there is frequently a disturbance of the motor action of the stomach. A large quantity of water taken at any one time will usually aggravate this condition, and yet, water is very necessary in these cases as it keeps the highly acid contents of the stomach diluted and thus less irritating to the gastric mucous membrane Under these circumstances it is best to prescribe it in small quantities, frequently repeated.

There is no condition of the bowels which yields more happily to the use of water than chronic constipation. The causes of constipation are numerous and no treatment will permanently succeed which does not meet the cause. I have no doubt that in many instances the only cause of constipation lies in the ingestion of an insufficient quantity of water, and that in many more cases, whatever other cause may be found, it is secondary to, and induced by, a lack of water in the system.

I have already referred to the fact that the amount of water in the feces and the peristaltic action of the bowels depend, if not primarily, at least secondarily, upon the amount of water ingested. Clinically, my experience certainly accords with this. Patients suffering with constipation seem to have a sort of "hydrophobia." They will avoid water, and take all sorts of medicinal laxatives instead. These drugs, which act in the main by attracting water to the bowels, draw from the system some of the fluid necessary to the proper performance of the functions of the various organs and tissues. Under these circumstances the patient loses in weight, and the tissues become dry and more susceptible to disease. I could give clinical histories of numerous patients who have shown such unfavorable developments, and who have been permanently relieved by inducing them to drink sufficient water. I will, however, refer to only one:

Mr. E. L., aged fifty-three years, a manufacturer, consulted me first, January 9, 1897. He presented a history of constipation of twenty-years' standing. He had always taken medicine to make the bowels move; recently had taken aloin, strychnin, and belladonna tablets in ascending doses. He had a good appetite, and sometimes had distress in the abdomen about three hours after eating. One year previously he had had an anal fistula. He always ate rapidly.

Examination showed his weight to be 136 pounds, which was below the normal; conjunctivæ yellow; tongue coated; teeth poor, and breath fetid. This man was in the habit of drinking very little water.

I prescribed a diet of coarse food, such as cereals, green vegetables, and meat in small quantity. I also prescribed ten or twelve glasses of water to be taken daily at regular intervals. Within a few days the patient's bowels moved regularly, and have continued to do so ever since.

Not all cases will yield as easily as did this one, and other means must be employed, but in all cases, whatever system of treatment is adopted, the use of large quantities of water will be a great aid to the remedies and diets prescribed. Water is frequently used in constipation in the form of an enema. The "Hall treatment" some years ago became almost a household word. Too much cannot be said against the indiscriminate use of enemas. When an acute condition is to be met the enema may be employed, but in chronic constipation, while it may give the patient a feeling of immediate relief, it rarely if ever cures. On the other hand, it sometimes does great harm. The warm water produces a dilation and consequent inactivity of the lower bowel, and in women, a relaxed condition of the pelvic tissue as well as displacement of the pelvic organs.

Water used in this way cannot produce the same results as when taken by the mouth. It acts simply mechanically, and does not have the same physiologic effect as when ingested. It is sometimes a very difficult matter to persuade the habitué of the syringe to discontinue its use, but in all cases of chronic constipatiou it must be discarded if permanent relief is desired.

Water is a valuable aid in the treatment of the various forms of diarrhea and dysentery. When these conditions arise, the bowel makes an effort to free itself of an irritating material. After this has been thrown off peristaltic action continues because of the irritated and congested mucous membrane. Water in the form of an enema will frequently at once relieve the bowels, and should always be employed before a sedative or astringent medicine is administered. If the patient is strong and robust, cold water should be employed; if, on the other hand, he is weak or in a state of collapse, warm water is more desirable. The amount to be injected must somewhat depend upon the endurance of the patient; if the bowel is not too sensitive, from one and a half to two quarts should be slowly injected. If the distention of the bowels causes pain, it is well to insert a rectal tube, and inject small quantities of water at short intervals.

In dysentery nothing can be used which will give more general satisfaction then enemas of plain, cold water. They are grateful to the patient, do not produce nausea, and very largely relieve the tenesmus from the first. A noted physician has said of this treatment: "It changes a huge internal, into an external abscess, and enables us to cleanse the bowels of their putrid contents."

gation of the bowels with pure water is of such importance that, aside from proper dietetics, all other methods of treatment fall into insignificance. It is the most rational, and, I think, the most successful treatment which can be employed. It is very easily instituted. The nurse should be instructed to put on a rubber apron, and to take the child in her lap, laying it upon its abdomen. The lower end of the apron should be placed in a suitable receptacle to receive the wash water and excrement. The nozzle of a fountain syringe is then inserted in the child's anus, and the water allowed to flow continuously under slight pressure. Experiment has shown that there is no danger of rupturing the bowel, since the rectum in a child will expel the water after a certain pressure is attained. The child after two or three treatments of this kind will, in nearly every instance, be relieved.

Much has been written concerning auto-intoxication and its symptoms. Some conditions, such as epilepsy, melancholia, and neurasthenia, which have heretofore been obscure as to their etiology, are now referred rather to the absorption of toxic agents due to imperfectly digested foods: to the retention, or accumulation of normally produced materials that should be further elaborated and changed, and to the production of abnormal substances in the body. Physiologic and chemic research in this direction has been greatly stimulated, but not all which at first was hoped for has been demonstrated. The terms neurasthenia, melancholia, and not infrequently hysteria, have been made to include conditions which were entirely and only intestinal auto-intoxication. So eagerly has this idea been taken up by clinicians that there is now danger of referring all the functional neuroses, etiologically, to intestinal auto-intoxication.

In the treatment of intestinal auto-intoxication, water, taken in large quantities, is of great service. It especially accomplishes good results by aiding elimination. In this condition, the necessity of drinking a large amount of water to act freely upon the eliminating organs can well be compared to the necessity of using water for flushing out a general sewer system in a large city.

Such, in brief, are the indications for the employment of water in the treatment of gastro-intestinal disorders. Its use does not exclude the employment of any other rational therapeusis, on the other hand, it is a great aid to other remedial agents which may be indicated.

Gray's Anatomy in Chinese.—The president of the Medical Missionary Association of China, Dr. H. T. Witney, is translating "Gray's Anatomy" into Chinese.

A CONTRIBUTION TO THE STUDY OF THE FLAGELLATE FORMS OF THE TERTIAN MALARIAL PARASITE.[1]

By FRED P. SOLLEY, M.D.,
OF NEW YORK.

DURING the six months from May to November, 1897, a systematic study was made at the Presbyterian Hospital of the organisms occurring in the blood of eighty-seven patients suffering from malarial fever. The results of these observations, with an analysis of the cases, have been embodied in an article to appear shortly in the annual report of the hospital.

The interest attaching to certain of these observations, in view of very recent additions to our knowledge of the much-discussed flagellate bodies, prompted the publication of this excerpt.

The following are descriptions of three examples of flagellated forms of the parasite occurring in a case of tertian malarial fever:

1. The first form of the parasite to be observed was a pigmented extracellular body, ovoid in shape, at either pole of which was attached a rapidly vibrating flagellum. The movements of these appendages were so active that the pigment granules in the body were apparently shaken into a single crowded mass which lay almost motionless near one end of the ovoid. Later on, when the vibration of the flagella became slower so that their wavy outline could be seen, the pigment became more scattered and resumed the usual lively dancing motion. The flagella were finally withdrawn into the substance of the body, the latter expanding appreciably as it absorbed them. The pigment, still collected at one end of the body, continued its active vibratory motion as long as the organism was watched.

2. In the second form no flagellum was at first seen, but attention was attracted by a markedly rapid vibration exhibited by a group of the pigment granules at one side of the body, as if they were being violently shaken to and fro. The pigment in other parts of the body merely showed the ordinary dancing motion. This extremely rapid vibration was seen to become all at once much slower, then to almost cease, while a number of the pigment granules flowed out of the body into a single rather broad flagellum, revealing for the first time its presence and outline. After a few seconds the rapid vibration of the flagellum, and with it the violent to and fro movement of the pigment at that side of the body, again began. Except for one or two granules which remained caught here and there, the pigment which had entered the flagellum was now shaken back into the body. The flagellum itself, grown long and narrow, vibrated so rapidly that its outline could no longer be made out, and the pigment lodged in it showed only as one or two dark blurs. These intermittent vibrations continued some time, finally becoming slower and less frequent, the flagellum at the same time growing shorter, until ulti-

[1] An extract from the forthcoming Annual Report of the Presbyterian Hospital for 1897–8.

mately it was absorbed into the body. The pigment granules at the spot where the flagellum was absorbed continued to exhibit intermittent vibratory spasms some time longer. Finally, these ceased also, and the organism then appeared as an ordinary extracellular form with slowly dancing pigment. A clear nuclear space persisted near the center of this body through all these changes.

3. In the third flagellate form the presence of a flagellum was suspected on account of a peculiar intermittent oscillation among all the pigment granules at once. A disturbance among the surrounding red-cells was next noticed, and a long, slender flagellum was seen in active motion at that situation. A small bulbous projection was now observed protruding from the body near this flagellum. This protuberance gradually elongated, being at first straight, but beginning to bend as it still grew longer, then waving from side to side more and more rapidly.

It still slowly lengthened until it was about twice as long as the diameter of the body. Here it remained stationary a few moments, both flagella being now in extremely active continuous motion. A red-cell floating between them was actually whipped until it rotated like a top.

The vibratory motion of both flagella then became slower, allowing their snake-like undulations to be plainly seen. At this time both flagella began to grow longer, finally reaching a length of about four times the diameter of a red-cell. As they increased in length the body appreciably diminished in size, their growth being evidently at the expense of the protoplasm in the organism. Both flagella now became detached from the body, and during some seconds were seen actively wriggling about among the red-cells. They finally slid over the boundary of the field and were lost to view. The attenuated body remained as a small extracellular form with its slowly moving pigment granules crowded closely together. The nuclear clear space, which had been present at first, disappeared when the flagella broke away.

Since these observations were recorded an important advance has been made in our knowledge of the nature of the flagellate bodies. MacCullum of Baltimore published in the *Lancet* for November 13, 1897, and in the *Johns Hopkins Hospital Bulletin* for November, 1897, an account of the flagellate forms of a hematozoan occurring in crows, the Halteridium of Labbe.

The following is a brief summary of his description:

In the blood of these birds, full-grown forms of the parasite which have been extruded from the corpuscles are found in two distinct varieties. The protoplasm in one of these forms is granular, and readily stains with methylene-blue; in the other it is hyaline, and does not take this stain. The latter bodies frequently develop flagella; the former never do. The flagella when developed break away from the hyaline bodies and swarm about the nearest granular form, beating against its sides in an evident attempt to enter it. A single one of these flagella succeeds in inserting its rounded extremity or "head" into the body, and finally wriggles its way inside, churning up the contained pigment for a while after being absorbed. After fifteen to twenty-five minutes the granular form thus entered assumes an ovoid shape, the pigment being collected at one end in a small spheric appendage, while the opposite end is hyaline, and presents a conical process. This fusiform body is provided with a refractive nuclear area, and possesses remarkable power of locomotion. This is the body described by Danilewsky as a "vermiculus" ("Parasitologie Comparée du Sang," 1889). It moves about in the blood with great activity, puncturing the red-cells with its conical end, and sometimes dashing through a leucocyte, tearing it open and scattering its granules in the plasma.

The above changes, therefore, represent "a sexual process with a resulting motile form, occurring under unfavorable circumstances, analogous to similar processes in plants and lower animals. The vermiculus has power of penetration by means of its pointed anterior end, and may thus escape through the intestinal wall."

In the blood from a case of estivo-autumnal fever, MacCullum has seen this same sexual process, the flagella breaking away from the parent body and beating against a quiet extracellular organism in which the pigment was arranged in a ring. One flagellum finally plunged its head into this body, and was soon afterward absorbed, stirring up the pigment for some time after its entrance. No motile "vermiculus," however, resulted from this conjugation.

In the light of this discovery the three flagellate forms of the tertian parasite described above take on a new meaning. Let us briefly reconsider their salient features with the idea of the "vermiculus" in view.

1. The first was a fusiform body, into which, after a period of intense vibratory activity, *two* flagella entered instead of the single one observed to gain admission in the case of the Halteridium and the estivo-autumnal parasite. The final appearance presented by this body suggests the "vermiculus," the pigment, although more scattered than at first, being still collected at one end. The fact that the pigment was crowded into an almost motionless mass at the time when the flagella were vibrating most actively, would seem to indicate that the origin of the motion exhibited by this form was not in the body itself, but in the flagella.

2. In the second flagellate body it is still more strikingly suggested that the flagellum had become affixed to the body from without. Here the pigment showed violent commotion only at the point of attachment of the flagellum, the granules in the rest of the body being comparatively quiet. This single flagellum finally entered the body after a series of rhythmic vibratory movements which might well be purposeful. The pigment, at the spot where the flagellum was absorbed, was churned up for some time after the entrance of the flagellum. This body, moreover, presented throughout these changes the nuclear space found in the "vermiculus."

It is believed, therefore, that these two forms represent the first stage in the development of "vermiculi" after the attachment of the free flagella.

3. In the third flagellate body we are evidently dealing with a wholly different phenomenon. Here the rapid vi-

bratory motion simultaneously occurred in all the pigment granules and in the flagellum, indicating that the source of this motion was in the body itself. Moreover, a second flagellum was actually seen to develop from the substance of the body. Both flagella visibly grew in length at the expense of the body's protoplasm, and finally broke away, moving actively about as free forms in the field. The nuclear space present up to this time was obliterated in the shrunken remnant by invading pigment. This form, then, produced the free flagella designed to fertilize certain receptive extracellular bodies by the process observed in the first two forms.

In these forms, therefore, is represented an attempt on the part of the parasite to create a resistant body, the motile "vermiculus" apparently designed to escape from an unfavorable environment and perpetuate the existence of the organism elsewhere than in the blood. In this connection it is interesting to note the conditions obtaining in the patient whose blood furnished these specimens. In this case was presented a history of quotidian paroxysms, but after admission to the hospital showed only a tertian intermittent fever. In the blood two distinct generations of organisms were found, maturing at different times, corresponding to the quotidian paroxysms before entrance. One of these groups of organisms, however, was evidently dying out, very few of its representatives being found in the blood. This generation of the parasite was therefore present in too small numbers to cause a febrile reaction, and it was at the time of maturity of this group that the second and third flagellate forms described were found. Moreover, the patient had had a single moderate dose of quinin on the day before these blood-examinations were made. Add to these conditions the fact that the blood had been some time out of the body when these forms were observed, and we have a sum total of "unfavorable circumstances" which might well lead the parasite to assume a more resistant form.

The same sexual process, then, resulting in the fully developed "vermiculus" in the case of the Halteridium in crows, and demonstrated by MacCullum as occurring in estivo-autumnal infections in human blood, is here indicated for the parasite of tertian malarial fever.

MEDICAL PROGRESS.

First Care of a Baby.—HANSON (*Cleveland Med. Gaz.*, February, 1898) is one of those who believe that the baby who is started right stands a much better chance to grow up well and strong than if allowed to catch cold or get indigestion within the first few hours of life. He insists upon the following simple rules as being all important: (1) Do not expose the baby after birth to a greater change of temperature than is absolutely necessary. (2) Do not allow attendants to subject him to prolonged exposure while washing, but rub him over with lard (this usually being convenient), and quickly wipe him off and wrap him up warmly. (3) Do not use too fine a thread in tying the cord, and dress the same with dry, sterile dressings. (4) Give nothing but tepid water or some very weak aromatic tea until there is sufficient milk in the mother's breast for the child's requirements. (5) Notice the clothing and see that the abdomen and chest are not constricted thereby.

A New Vaginal Tampon.—BEUTNER (*La Méd. Moderne*, January 19, 1898) calls the attention of physicians to a new tampon especially recommended for patients while traveling. In the center of a little sac of cotton, to which is attached a string, is placed a ball of cocoa-butter, etc., in which have been incorporated the desired remedies. The tampon is introduced by the patient in the morning and taken out at night. The heat of the body melts the cocoa-butter and the therapeutic agent saturates the cotton and comes in contact with the mucous membrane. The inventor proposes a variety of soothing, astringent, antiseptic, and resolving remedies which shall be put up in this manner for the use of travelers.

THERAPEUTIC NOTES.

Rheumatoid Arthritis Treated by Lycetol.—NORWOOD (*Med. Times and Register*, November 6, 1897) says that the most that can be hoped for in rheumatoid arthritis is an arrest of its progress for a longer or shorter time and relief of the pains in the affected articulations. Galvanism, massage, baths, and an invigorating diet have been found of more or less value, as well as the administration of cod-liver oil, ferruginous preparations, and the iodids. A comparatively new remedy which seems to have a promising future before it in the treatment of this disease is lycetol. One of its distinct advantages is that, owing to its pleasant taste and freedom from irritating effects, its administration can be continued a long time. In two cases recently treated by Norwood the results were encouraging.

Lactophosphate of Lime for Acne and Furunculosis.—PURDON (*Dublin Jour. of Med. Sci.*, February, 1898) has been most successful with the treatment of acne and furunculosis with the syrup of the lactophosphate of lime. He regards it as "an agent of nutrition, and thinks it is appropriately given in the conditions above referred to, as they are "evidences of depraved nutrition." Be that as it may, the administration of this drug, coupled with the advice to the patient to wear Balbriggan linen undershirts, will prevent outbreaks of acne which occur from time to time on the shoulders and chest. If it is thought best to add cod-liver oil, the following prescription will be found palatable:

℞		
	Acaciæ	ʒ x
	Aquæ	℥ i
	Syr. calcis lacto-phosphat.	℥ iii
	Ol. morrhuæ	℥ iv
	Ol. amygd. amar.	*m.* iii.

M. Rub the gum, water, and syrup together until a smooth mucilage is made, then gradually add the cod-liver oil, with constant stirring, and lastly, the essential oil of bitter almonds. Thus made, each tablespoonful of the cod-liver oil and syrup of the lactophosphate of lime contains 4 grains of lactophosphate of lime and fifty per cent. of cod-liver oil.

THE MEDICAL NEWS.

A WEEKLY JOURNAL

OF MEDICAL SCIENCE.

COMMUNICATIONS are invited from all parts of the world. Original articles contributed *exclusively* to THE MEDICAL NEWS will after publication be liberally paid for (accounts being rendered quarterly), or 250 reprints will be furnished in place of other remuneration. When necessary to elucidate the text, illustrations will be engraved from drawings or photographs furnished by the author. Manuscripts should be typewritten.

Address the Editor: J. RIDDLE GOFFE, M.D.,
No. 111 FIFTH AVENUE (corner of 18th St.), NEW YORK.

Subscription Price, including postage in U. S. and Canada.

PER ANNUM IN ADVANCE	$4.00
SINGLE COPIES	.10
WITH THE AMERICAN JOURNAL OF THE MEDICAL SCIENCES, PER ANNUM	7.50

Subscriptions may begin at any date. The safest mode of remittance is by bank check or postal money order, drawn to the order of the undersigned. When neither is accessible, remittances may be made, at the risk of the publishers, by forwarding in *registered* letters.

LEA BROTHERS & CO.,
No. 111 FIFTH AVENUE (corner of 18th St.), NEW YORK,
AND NOS. 706, 708 & 710 SANSOM ST., PHILADELPHIA.

SATURDAY, APRIL 16, 1898.

ANOTHER DEAL AMONG THE MEDICAL SCHOOLS OF NEW YORK CITY.

JUST one year ago to-day the medical circles and medical journals of New York were rejoicing in the gratifying spectacle of the abolition of the last remaining proprietary feature from the medical schools of New York and the consolidation of Bellevue and the University Medical School under the fostering care of the University of the City of New York. This was welcomed as marking the inauguration of a new and progressive epoch in the history of medical education in the Metropolis. The circumstances of the withdrawal of Bellevue from this combination, which occurred a month later, brought disappointment to the friends of medical education, but the latent financial resources which that institution promptly exhibited and the elimination of proprietorship from at least one of the two institutions under consideration, were consoling circumstances. On the whole it was believed that the agitation had at least accomplished good. Both institutions settled down to their individual work and dropped out of special public attention.

But the Faculty of the University Medical School is resourceful, to say the least, in the field of surprises, and rumors are rife that it has severed, or is about to sever, its connection with the University, and active negotiations are under way for its affiliation with Cornell University as the medical department of that institution.

The history of the circumstances which have led to this final break between the Medical School and the University is interesting as tending to determine where the responsibility lies for this overthrow of an enterprise which gave to the profession such promise of worthy achievement in medical education. To understand all the circumstances it is necessary to review somewhat the history of the medical school and its relation to the university prior to the recent negotiations.

In the Medical Department of the University of the City of New York there were originally two distinct corporations, *viz.:* the Medical College Laboratory Association, which was the original foundation of the institution, and, second, the Loomis Laboratory Association. The property of the former institution had an estimated value of $230,000, and that of the latter, $225,000. These two corporations were legally distinct, each having its own board of trustees. Both of these boards were composed of members of the medical faculty and laymen in about an equal proportion of each. The University, previous to the agreement for consolidation, which was entered into during the spring of 1897, had no equity in either corporation, nor did it contribute any money to the support or running expenses of either, with the exception of a trifling sum of $2000 or $3000, which was raised for the benefit of the medical department about fifty years ago. The relation of the medical school to the university proper was, therefore, only a nominal one; that is, the chancellor of the institution signed the diplomas and the commencements were held under the auspices of the university, but the practical affairs were managed entirely by the faculty. Appointments to professorships and minor positions in the faculty were made by that body itself, although it was customary to go through the formality of submitting such appointments to the approval of the council of the university.

An effort was being constantly made, however, by the university to absorb more and more into itself the medical institution, and to this end about six years ago it seemed wise to the faculty to eliminate the feature of proprietorship from the school. The salaries of the various positions were fixed at a stated sum, and the university guaranteed the amount. With the intent of putting the medical department on a more substantial basis, and consolidating more firmly its relation to the larger institution so that it might become in fact as well as in name the medical department of the university, in the spring of 1897 an agreement was entered into by the Medical College Laboratory Association to transfer all of its property to the university and place the entire responsibility and management in the hands of the university council. As a part of the machinery for conducting the institution and as a guarantee to the faculty that its traditions, methods of instruction, and changes in its membership might be in the hands of those who were in immediate touch with it, it was agreed by both parties to the contract that a special medical committee of the council should be appointed to have these matters in charge. The inducement to the faculty to encourage its board of trustees to surrender the property was the expectation and assurance that under the fostering care of the university large sums of money could be procured to steadily advance the facilities for medical instruction and secure to the members of the faculty a degree of independence in the thoroughness of their instruction which would promote in every way the advancement of medical education. On these conditions, the property of the corporation known as the Medical College Laboratory Association, amounting to $230,000, was legally transferred to the university. Nothing was said about the property of the Loomis Laboratory Association, although it was expected by both parties to the contract that it sooner or later would follow in the wake of the older institution, and amalgamate with the university. Matters had reached this stage, and the success of the university council in accomplishing its aspirations of becoming a great university were steadily growing, when overtures were made to Bellevue Hospital Medical College to join with it, and together with the University Medical School establish a grand medical department.

To this proposition Bellevue acceded, and the execution of the agreement had proceeded to such an extent that the faculty composed of men from both of the schools was arranged and appointed. Here the misunderstanding began. The original faculty of the university, from the fact that it was the first of the two to form the alliance, inferred that its ideas should prevail and the power of directing the policy of the school should rest in its hands. When it was discovered that the chairs were equally divided between the two schools and the influence of Bellevue in voting power was equal to its own, an objection was promptly made. The council standing upon its decision that Bellevue should have equal influence and rights with the other school, the faculty of the latter institution had no recourse except to withdraw or ask the Bellevue faculty to withdraw. The latter was decided upon, and Bellevue, in response to a written petition, withdrew in a body from the university.

In the meantime the university had procured additional property adjoining the former medical school, and to meet the taxes and assessments upon this the resources of the medical school were drawn upon by the council. This necessarily diminished the amount of money available for professorial salaries, and the latter, therefore, have been reduced. Moreover, the medical committee, by failure of reelection of its members to the council and by resignation, has been disrupted. Friction has thus been generated and steadily increased as closer intercourse in the management of details became necessary, until finally the faculty was convinced that a further continuance of its relations with the university was unendurable. The petition was, therefore, submitted by the University Faculty, praying for release from their relations because of the failure of the council to carry out its part of the contract, and demanding a restoration of the property to its original holders.

In reply to this the council of the university affirms that it has carried out all the provisions of the agreement, and insists, moreover, that as the funds transferred to it are trust funds, it has no legal right to relinquish its trust by reconveying the property to the original holders. Moreover, the council, evidently fearing that the apparent estrangement of the faculty might lead them to be indifferent to the harmonious working of the university, sent to each professor a letter conditioning his reappointment for another year upon a promise that he accept the statute and rule of the university regarding the medical college, and that he use his influence to consummate the transfer of the Loomis Laboratory and its endowment to the university council. An answer was requested not later than March 31st. To this letter no reply was made by any one of the six professors, and the inference is that as the time for the reply has passed the appointments will expire with the college year, May 18, 1898. In this condition the matter now rests.

From certain aspects this whole matter may be regarded as a family affair, and therefore not coming properly within the domain of public comment; but any action of a medical school is legitimately the subject of review, comment, and criticism whenever it affects the standard and the quality of medical education. Where the responsibility lies for the disagreement under discussion the facts now at hand will not justify a decision.

THE FAILURE OF THE NEW YORK DISPENSARY BILL.

After a session of three months, replete with as disgraceful political jobbery as has ever been recorded in the annals of the State of New York, the Legislature has finally adjourned, and the nauseating odor of its misdeeds is strong in the nostrils of the rank and file of the two great political parties as a reminder of the misplaced faith reposed in their representatives. A majority of the honest bills introduced were allowed to die peacefully in committee, or, if favorably reported and passed, were so littered with amendments as to entirely defeat their original object; while those in connection with which there was a palpable "rake-off" for somebody, were railroaded through without conscience and with disgraceful haste.

Now that the curtain has been rung down on the final act, the calciums turned off, and the actors dispersed, it is not amiss to glance at the results for the benefit of that portion of the audience represented by the medical profession and determine wherein it has been the gainer or loser in its efforts to obtain just legislation. Undoubtedly the most important measure up for consideration was the so-called "Dispensary Bill," designed to correct the prevailing crying abuses of medical charity by placing all dispensaries under the supervision of the State Board of Charities. As is well known, this bill emanated from a joint-committee composed of representatives from committees appointed by twelve of the largest medical societies of the State, having their headquarters within the limits of Greater New York. It embodied the result of much painstaking investigation on the part of the committee, and was indorsed by the societies referred to, not once only, but in several instances a second time; not by a faction, as has been claimed, but unanimously. It was so framed as to provide for the welfare of the sick poor, and to facilitate the means by which they might receive medical aid. It was just in its provisions, equally to the laity and to the profession, and its enactment would have resulted in untold benefit to all concerned, whether viewed from a humanitarian, economic, or medical standpoint. Yet, after passing the Senate unanimously, thanks to the untiring efforts of Senator George W. Brush, to whom the entire profession of the State owes a hearty vote of thanks, the bill was allowed to die in the Committee on Public Health of the Assembly in spite of every effort on the part of its sponsors to have it reported.

The Assembly Committee on Public Health was composed of Miles W. Raplee of Dundee, Yates Co., chairman; Edger L. Vincent, Maine, Broome Co.; George A. Stoneman, Machias, Cattaraugus Co.; Dennis W. Evarts, Manning, Orleans Co.; Hyatt C. Hatch, Atlanta, Steuben Co.; Joseph Schulum, Dominick Mullany, and John F. Brennen, New York City; Otto Wicke (druggist), Brooklyn, and Cyrus B. Gale, Jamaica, L. I.

In exactly what way influence brought to bear upon the presiding officer of a legislative body percolates through devious channels and effectually gags a committee, is one of the secrets of the trade. Perhaps the contents of a loving-cup at times has something to do with it. The efforts of certain physicians of the regular school, and of a handful of dispensary managers, whose opposition to the bill was based wholly upon selfish personal motives, might have been successfully combated so long as the fight remained in the open, but some insidious and malign influence was too powerful, and so the plainly expressed demand of upward of 5000 reputable medical men for reform was refused and ignored.

The homeopathic opposition to the measure, previous to the date of the annual meeting of the State Homeopathic Medical Society at Albany, was wholly unexpected, as it was rightfully supposed that the provisions of the bill were equally favorable to both schools. It is to be regretted that the homeopathic practitioners of the State, and especially those residing in the City of New York, have seen fit to array themselves on the opposite side to those of the regular school in connection with efforts to obtain legislation, for it is natural to suppose that although they work in independent channels, their methods of organizing and managing dispensaries and hospitals must be much the same, the abuses the same, and their correction the same.

The adequate control of dispensary abuse is bound to come, and next year's session of the Legislature will find the same earnest workers on hand to further a bill having this object in view. More than this, another bill, of vital interest to every medical practitioner in the State, will be introduced and, it is hoped, will become a law. This bill, according to information just at hand, will contain three separate provisions: first, making a husband and wife jointly liable for a bill for medical services; second, making such a charge a first lien on a deceased patient's estate; and, third, in the event of judgment being obtained against a debtor whose income is derived from a salary, authorizing the creditor to obtain, and the proper court to grant, an order requiring the debtor's employer to set aside a percentage of his salary each month until the judgment has been satisfied. Such a law as the last-named is already in force in at least two States, and its working has produced excellent results. At the present time there is no law on the statute books of this State offering protection to the medical profession in this connection, and it is high time that combined and persistent effort should be made to obtain favorable legislation. Elections will occur in many of the Assembly districts of the State before the next meeting of the Legislature. Many of the present legislators will go before their constituents for reelection, and many new candidates for legislative togas will urge their claims. Much of the obliquity pertaining to the session that is past will be forgotten, and loving-cups for the time being will be relegated to the top shelf of an up-stairs closet. Unity of action and purpose on the part of the medical profession is imperative if success is to be achieved in legislative matters concerning the welfare of its members. Every physician should regard it as a personal affair; every prospective legislator should be interviewed and a pledge obtained in support of these bills. Personal support of a candidacy should be forthcoming only in the event of such a pledge being given. And the time to organize is *now*. It should not be deferred until a few days before election. We have all heard the cry "*Manana, Manana!*" too frequently repeated during the last few exciting weeks, and its sound is not a pleasant one.

THE EXPOSITION OF HYGIENE AT NEW YORK CITY IN MAY.

FROM April 25th to May 31st an International Health Exposition will be held at New York in the Grand Central Palace, Lexington avenue. The New York Household Economic Association and kindred organizations will cooperate with the management of the Exposition, which will embrace everything relating to health, both indoors and outdoors, and illustrate the sanitary and hygienic progress of the century. Mr. Charles F. Wingate is the supervising director. All exhibitions of this description should be encouraged, for they are of distinct benefit: first, in bringing together for comparison the latest sanitary appliances and methods, and, second, in educating the public in their use and benefits. The second point is perhaps the most important, because whatever sanitarians may do with regard to the improvement of their science, the resulting benefits to the health of the community must be tardy unless the public are ready to aid in the application of the improved processes. In our own country we have far too few of these exhibitions, and sanitary science would be much benefited if the public were better educated in this matter.

ECHOES AND NEWS.

A Medical Municipal Officer.—M. Navarre, the new President of the Municipal Council of Paris, is a member of the medical profession.

The Emperor of Abyssinia's Physician.—The physician to the family of the Emperor of Abyssina is a young Swiss woman, a graduate of the University of Zurich.

The Hospitals of Paris.—It is estimated that no less than $15,000,000 would be required to satisfactorily increase the bed accommodation and improve the sanitary arrangements of the Paris hospitals.

Quarantine against Jeddah.—Plague regulations have been ordered at Cairo against arrivals from Jeddah, where three deaths from the plague have occurred among pilgrims on their way to Mecca.

Medical Congress at the Paris Exposition.—Section No. 6 of the Congress to be held in Paris in 1900 will be devoted to medical science. A special building within the grounds of the Exposition will be reserved for the Congress.

A Doctor Dies from the Plague.—Dr. P. N. Davda, assistant medical officer of the Arthur Road Hospital, Bombay, died from the plague although he had been inoculated three weeks before with 10 cubic centimeters of Dr. Yersin's serum.

Feeding of Infants.—According to *Pediatrics* there is in France a law forbidding the giving of solid food of any kind to infants under one year of age without the written authority of a physician. The use of feeding bottles with long rubber tubes is also forbidden by law.

The Proposed Academy of Medicine. — Steps are being taken to form an Academy of Medicine in Toronto. The societies interested in the movement are the Toronto Medical Society, the Clinical Society, the Pathological Society, and the Toronto Medical Library Association.

Sanitary Mission.—A special sanitary mission, composed of five medical men, has been appointed by the Turkish Government and will soon leave Constantinople for Mecca. The object of the mission is to examine into the sanitary conditions of the pilgrims who will be gathering there.

The Plague in India.—The plague continues unabated in Bombay. Pneumonic symptoms are now a marked feature of the epidemic. It is also stated that influenza is prevalent. The mortality from all causes during the week ending March 26th is given as 2080—a rate of mortality of 130 per 1000 per annum, the average being 44 per 1000.

Long Island College Hospital.—The ex-internes of this hospital have associated themselves together in an alumni society, and during March last gave themselves a dinner. They are officered as follows: Dr. Frank E. West, president; Drs. Henry N. Read, J. A. McCorkle, and S. J. McNamara, executive committee, and Dr. B. O'Connor, secretary.

Contagious Disease Hospital for Orange, N. J.—It has been decided to erect by means of public subscription a hospital for the isolation of cases of diphtheria and scarlet fever, to be supported by the Board of Health and by fees paid by patients. The hospital will be in charge of a superintendent, and each patient will be attended by his own physician.

Red Cross Relief in Cuba.—The Cuban Red Cross bulletins have announced that the relief work in Havana hereafter will be under the supervision of Dr. Guzman, a Cuban, and Dr. Egan of the Red Cross Society. In case of a disagreement between them the American Consul-General is to act as arbitrator. The schedules show 171,000 persons in the island entitled to receive relief.

Additional Army Surgeons.—A bill was recently introduced into the House of Representatives providing for the appointment of fifteen additional surgeons for the army, with the rank of first lieutenant. The bill also authorizes the Surgeon-General to appoint as many assistants as he deems necessary in case of war with Spain, the salary of each to be limited to $150 per month.

The Free Home for the Dying.—There is in London an institution known by this name. It is absolutely free and the only passport to admission is a medical certificate to the effect that the applicant is believed to be dying. No distinction as to nationality, sex, age, or creed, is made. During the year 1897 forty-eight patients were admitted; of these thirty died, nine were discharged, and nine remain.

"Divine Healer" in New Jersey.—Considerable indignation has been aroused among the residents of Mount Holly, N. J., by the death of a young man who had been under the care of a "divine healer." Although he had been ill three months no physician was called to attend him. The attention of the Burlington County Medical Society has been called to the matter, and the Grand Jury will be asked to take action.

Woman's Medical College.—The formal opening of the new building of the Woman's Medical College of the New York Infirmary for Women and Children was held on the 21st ult., it having been rebuilt since its partial destruction by fire about a year ago. The building is now six stories high, has an amphitheater of large size, spacious recitation-rooms, and chemic and pathologic laboratories fitted with modern appliances and apparatus.

Resolutions on the Death of Dr. Sparkman.—At a recent meeting of the Georgetown Medical Society of Georgetown County, South Carolina, the following resolutions were read and unanimously adopted: "Resolved, That in the death of Dr. James R. Sparkman the medical profession of Georgetown, as well as the profession of the State, has lost one of its most accomplished and useful members; That our warmest sympathy be tendered to the family in their bereavement in the loss of this good and faithful servant, and that a page in our minute book be inscribed to his memory."

Rush Medical College.—Liabilities amounting to $71,000 have been erased from the ledger of the Rush Medical College, Chicago, and its complete affiliation with the University of Chicago is now practically assured. This was one of the conditions set forth by President Harper when the scheme of annexing the medical school to the University was first mentioned. The principal donors were Drs. Ephrain Ingals, Nicholas Senn, and E. Fletcher Ingals. Hereafter, in accordance with another condition, the Board of Trustees will be chosen from representative business men instead of from the Faculty.

An Important Decision by the Commissioner of Charities.—The first break in the present system of appointments to the visiting-staff of the public hospitals of New York has been made by the recent decision of the Commissioner of Charities, in which he has decreed that no member of the visiting-staff of any of the hospitals in the Department of Charities loses that position by resigning from the medical school in whose division he is serving. The effect of this must naturally be that men resigning from medical schools carry with them their hospital appointments and so gradually deprive the schools of the power to control hospital positions.

A Drinking-Fountain. — An ingenious drinking-fountain has been devised by a citizen of Rochester, N. Y., to supplant the use of cups and other drinking-vessels in public places. It consists of a marble pedestal about 3½ feet high, capped with a funnel-shaped basin twelve inches in diameter connected with the water-supply. Upon pressure of a lever at the base of the basin a jet of water shoots up from the center of the basin and into the mouth when the head is bent over, and in this way thirst is abundantly satisfied without the intervention of a drinking-vessel of any kind. A movement is on foot to have these fountains placed in the public schools of Rochester.—*Sanitarian.*

A Gift to the New York Academy of Medicine.—At a meeting of the New York Academy of Medicine held April 7, 1898, ex-President Grover Cleveland, in response to an urgent request, presented to the academy an autograph copy of the address delivered by him at the celebration of its semi-centennial anniversary. The manuscript consists of nine closely written pages of letter-paper, which have been artistically framed by Tiffany & Co., each page occupying a panel by itself. This gift from the ex-President supplies another invaluable feature to the rapidly accumulating collection of portraits, relics, and mementoes which decorate the walls of the Academy.

The American Hospital at Teheran. — The hospital conducted by the Presbyterian missionaries from this country to Persia has received a gift of more than $1000 from Persian officials, and the European colony, including Russians and Turks. The American Minister, Hon. Arthur Sherburne Hardy, organized an entertainment or concert with the help of the Persian Prime Minister, and a number of the diplomatic corps, by which so marked a success was achieved that the Shah requested a repetition of it at his palace. The Shah himself attended the second concert, and his distinguished guests were entertained, at its close, on his behalf, and further donations to the hospital were received from several Persian magnates.

Hydrotherapy and Foreign Spas.—It has always been a question as to how much of the benefit derived from treatment at foreign spas is due to the enforced regimen and how much to the waters themselves. From a recent discussion in the British Balneological and Climatological Society, it would seem that the waters have very little to do with it. One member declared that it is a matter of indifference whether the bath water be supplied at a German spa or by an English water-works company—the result is the same. A French physician from Aix-les-Bains admitted that he did not claim any special virtue for the water at that resort, and said that the good results abtained there are due to the method employed.

Medical Society of Kings County.—This society, through its organ, the *Brooklyn Medical Journal*, announces the receipt of a gift of $2000 as a library sustentation fund. The donor, Mrs. John L. Zabriskie, has chosen this as a means of commemorating her late husband's interest in this society, and its literary deeds and needs. Her design is that her gift shall *in perpetuo* be known as the Dr. John Lloyd Zabriskie Memorial Endowment Fund for the Library, and this library is already of such size and is in such good hands that there can be no doubt that she has in fact erected a living monument to her eminent husband. The name of the Zabriskie family has been identified with this society since 1829, in the person of Dr. John B. Zabriskie, father of the physician above mentioned.

Hygienic Laboratory in Costa Rica.—The National Institute of Hygiene of Costa Rica is situated at San José, the capital. The work of this department during 1897 included a considerable number of chemic analyses as well as many histologic and bacteriologic examinations of urine, feces, sputa, tumors, etc. Larvæ and ova of the ankylostomum duodenalæ were discovered in five out of sixteen samples of feces. The institute is amply provided with apparatus for the production of the Röntgen-rays and for microphotography. Dr. Emilio Echeverria, the director, incidentally mentions in his report that at the ordinary pressure at San José water boils at 95° C. (203° F.), a circumstance which, of course, shows that the town is situated at a great elevation. In connection with the institute there is a department, presided over by Dr. Bojas, for the preparation and inoculation of antileprous serum.

Obituary.—Dr. William H. Johnston, one of the founders and the Dean of the Birmingham Medical College at Birmingham, Ala., died of apoplexy on April 3d, in his eightieth year. He was born in Lincoln County, N. C., educated in the State University, and served gallantly in the Twenty-third North Carolina Regiment, Confederate Army. After the war he was graduated in medicine at the University of the City of New York, and served eighteen months at Bellevue Hospital, New York. For a short time he practised medicine in the latter city, moved to Selma, Ala., in 1872, and to Birmingham in 1886. A widow and four children survive him.—Dr. George S. Little of Brooklyn, died on the 30th ult., aged seventy-two years. He had been several years an inspector of the Board of Health of that city. He was a veteran officer of the late war, having served with two militia regiments. About forty years of his professional life was spent in Brooklyn.

Ants and the Plague.—A Bombay correspondent of the *Times of India* describes some remarkable observations which he made upon a nest of ordinary red ants, which infest the storerooms in India. The house in which the ants had their nest was infected with plague virus as shown by the number of rats and bandicoots which were daily found dead. One day it was noticed that the ants were moving and taking all their belongings to a new home about nineteen feet from the old nest. Further observation revealed that many hundreds of the insects were dead and dying, that the dead had been carried away by their companions about a foot distant from the new home until a little reddish heap was formed, and that much of the stores of rice had been cast away as if unfit for food. Two days later, the mortality still continuing, a further move was made, the dead ants and the discarded rice being left behind. This performance was repeated several times until an accident destroyed the nest and prevented further observations.

The Prescribing Druggist.—The evil of counter-prescribing was recently well illustrated at an inquest held in Derby, England, upon the body of a woman, seventy-five years of age, who died of pneumonia and in whom there also existed chronic Bright's disease and arteriosclerosis. A physician who was called in just before the patient's death found her under the influence of some narcotic, and it was ascertained that she had taken sixpennyworth of cough mixture which had been prescribed for her at a neighboring drug-store. At the inquest the druggist said that the cough mixture was his own and that he did not want to make the formula public, but he was directed to write it out for the benefit of the jury. In this way it was learned that two ounces of the mixture contained forty minims of morphia (presumably liquor morphia acetatis or hydrochloratis) besides compound tincture of camphor. The dose for an adult was one teaspoonful. This would contain about two and a half minims of morphia solution—not an excessive dose if not repeated, but there were no directions upon the bottle as to how often the mixture was to be taken. As it was clearly shown that the woman died of pneumonia, although the morphia may have hastened her death, the druggist was not held, but was strongly censured by the jury.

CORRESPONDENCE.

OUR PHILADELPHIA LETTER.

[From our Special Correspondent.]

TREATMENT OF ENTERIC FEVER BY SYSTEMATIC COLD BATHING AT THE GERMAN HOSPITAL—MUNICIPAL HOSPITAL—STATE BOARD OF MEDICAL EXAMINERS—MORE "FRESH-AIR PAVILIONS"—SUCCESSORS TO DR. PARVIN AT THE JEFFERSON MEDICAL COLLEGE—DR. W. M. L. COPLIN—DR. EDITH BAKER—$5000 FOR THE JEWISH HOSPITAL.

PHILADELPHIA, April 9, 1898.

ANOTHER valuable contribution to the treatment of enteric fever by the Brand method was made by Dr. J. C. Wilson in a paper, entitled "Observations upon the Treatment of Enteric Fever by Systematic Cold Bathing as Practised in the German Hospital, Philadelphia," read before the College of Physicians of Philadelphia, April 6th. This communication included the cases treated in this institution during the years 1896-97, since Dr. Wilson's last report was made. The total number of patients treated during these two years was 217, of which number 64 were treated in 1896, and 153 in 1897. The combined mortality, was 7.8 per cent., the mortality for 1896 being 10.9, and for 1897, 6.5 per cent. The average mortality of 403 cases of enteric fever treated in the Pennsylvania, Presbyterian, and Episcopal Hospitals of this city, by the more or less systematic application of the cold bath during 1896 (the latest statistics given by these institutions) was 9.92 per cent. The average mortality of 5484 cases in Philadelphia, treated by various methods, during the period covered by Dr. Wilson's report, was 14.76. The following statistics of the German Hospital cases were given: Combined per cent. of hemorrhage: 1896, 6.2 per cent.; 1897, 8.5 per cent. Hemorrhage in fatal cases: 1896, 2 cases, or 28.6 per cent.; 1897, 3 cases, or 30 per cent. Average day of disease on admission to the hospital: 1896, 9.3; 1897, 8.2. Average length of patients' stay in the hospital: 1896, 36.3 days; 1897, 35.2 days. Relapses occurred during 1896 in 12 cases, or 18.8 per cent.; during 1897 in 29 cases, or 18.9 per cent. Multiple relapses occurred in 2 cases, or 1.2 per cent. in 1897; none occurred in 1896. The average number of baths given in each case was 48.6 in 1896, and 51.3 in 1897. Albuminuria was noted in 30 cases or 46.9 per cent. in 1896; in 1897 in 59 cases, or 37.9 per cent. The following complications were noted: Nephritis, 1896, 12 cases, or 18.7 per cent.; 1897, in 44 cases, or 28.7 per cent. Phlebitis: 1896, in 1 case, or 1.6 per cent.; 1897, in 3 cases, or 1.8 per cent. Suppurative otitis media: 1896, in 1 case, or 1.6 per cent.; 1897, in 2 cases, or 1.2 per cent. Sciatica and rheumatic fever were noted each in 1 case, 0.6 per cent. in 1897. Pleurisy: 1896, 1 case.

With the exceptions of acute abdominal inflammation, hemorrhage, and perforation, the baths, repeated when the axillary temperature reached 101.4° F. three hours after a preceding bath, constituted the regular treatment. It is of interest to observe that during defervescence two baths daily were given irrespective of the temperature. Calomel, in doses of 7½ grains, was given at the beginning of the attack, but never after the tenth day of the disease. Cold compresses and ice-bags to the abdomen was recommended for pain and hemorrhage; and stupes and external cold were applied to the abdomen for tympanites. When specially indicated, aromatic spirits of ammonia, ammonium carbonate, strychnin, caffein citrate, the bromids, chloral, opium and its derivatives, and hyoscin were administered. For the anemia, iron, preferably in the form of Basham's mixture, proved beneficial. The results of these last two-years' work of Dr. Wilson in the German Hospital brings the total number of cases treated by him in this hospital from February 1, 1890, to January 1, 1898, to 741, of which number 55 were fatal, or a death-rate of 7.42 per cent.

As a result of a personal inspection of the Municipal Hospital for Contagious Diseases, Mayor Warwick, in his annual message to Councils, has drawn attention to the disgraceful neglect which has been shown by the authorities in providing the proper means for the improvement and maintenance of the institution. In the words of the Mayor, "the main building in its present dilapidated condition is a disgrace to our civilization and a reflection upon our humanity. The heating apparatus is most primitive, and the system of ventilation most incomplete. On the upper floors, where the sick are confined, the food is received in and distributed from bath-rooms which are in close proximity to a double row of water-closets." In spite of the handicaps to their work, the physicians and nurses of the hospital are commended in the highest terms for the cleanly condition of the institution and for their faithful performance of duty under such trying circumstances. The Mayor has requested the immediate appropriation by Councils of the sum of $136,900 for the erection of isolation pavilions, and for other improvements and extensions.

At the annual meeting of the State Board of Medical Examiners (regular profession) held in Harrisburg, April 5th, the following members were elected for the ensuing year: Dr. H. G. McCormick of Williamsport, president; Dr. W. S. Forster of Pittsburg, secretary and treasurer; Drs. S. W. Latta, A. H. Hulshizer, and Henry Beates of Philadelphia; Dr. W. D. Hamaker of Meadville, and Dr. J. K. Weaver of Norristown. The next examinations by the board will be held in Philadelphia and in Pittsburg on June 14th.

Encouraged by the success of last year's experiment in providing a "fresh-air pier" for the use of the public during the heated term, the city authorities have decided to erect several more of these pavilions along the Delaware water-front, to be completed before the commencement of the present summer. The plans, which have now been completed by the Bureau of Surveys, call for pavilions to be erected on several piers owned by the city. The lower decks of these pavilions are to be of granolithic pavement or of asphalt, and will be converted into a sort of public park, with flowers, seats, and electric lights. The upper decks will be used especially as childrens' playgrounds. The pier on which the first new pavilion is to be built is 554 feet in length and 80 feet in width.

The vacancy in the faculty of the Jefferson Medical College created by the death of Dr. Theophilus Parvin has been filled by the board of trustees by the election of Drs. Edward P. Davis and E. E. Montgomery to the chair of Obstetrics and Diseases of Women and Children. In this manner the work will be divided between Dr. Parvin's successors, Dr. Davis assuming the obstetric teaching and Dr. Montgomery having charge of the work relating particularly to gynecology.

At the annual meeting of the Lycoming County Medical Society, held at Williamsport, April 5th, the address on pathology was delivered by Dr. W. M. L. Coplin of this city.

Dr. Edith Baker, at present a physician in the Norristown State Insane Hospital, has been elected pathologist to the Delaware State Hospital at Barnhurst. Dr. Baker's term of service at Norristown will expire January 1, 1899.

The sum of nearly $5000 has been received by the Jewish Hospital Association as its share of the proceeds of the Hebrew Charity Ball, held in this city a few weeks ago.

OUR BERLIN LETTER.

[From our Special Correspondent.]

A SERIES OF TESTS FOR ORGANOTHERAPEUTIC REMEDIES — ACKNOWLEDGMENT OF THE WORK OF AMERICAN PEDIATRISTS—SMALLPOX AND VACCINATION IN PARIS AND BERLIN—CHILDREN'S SUICIDES, HYSTERIA, AND OVERWORK IN SCHOOL.

BERLIN, April 7, 1898.

SOME time ago at the Hufeland Medical Society (an organization founded in honor of the distinguished old German physician Hufeland), Professor Posner made a preliminary report, with demonstrations, of a series of tests for organotherapeutic remedies. Taking advantage of Ehrlich's observations as to the specific reactions produced in certain tissues and cells by various acid, neutral, and basic anilin dyes, he used these substances for the detection of the presence of specific tissues in the remedies as they are dispensed.

This preliminary report would seem to be substantiated by further observation, and it is hoped that this will enable the practitioner to decide, not alone whether a certain preparation said to contain an extract of a particular organ really does contain it, but also approximately how much of the extract is present. This will be a distinct step in advance, and will make these remedies comparable with the ordinary chemic compounds, which, in case of doubt, may be subjected to known tests. Meantime, the physician will not be obliged to depend so absolutely upon the manufacturer of the remedies for their authenticity and proportionate contents.

Professor Posner found that all the different organotherapeutic preparations offered for sale here in Berlin gave, within certain limits, the same reaction as all the others prepared from the same organ, except one series of prostatic preparations, which were distinctly different from those of other makers. This is all the more interesting, as it is not so long ago that medical Berlin was afforded a good deal of amusement by the story of the first prostatic preparations which were placed on the market here. Some one got the idea that extract of prostate might be good for prostatic hypertrophy; on just what grounds is not so clear.

A purveyor of remedies was found to furnish the preparation, and the experiments with it were begun. As is usually the case, in the hands of the man who thought out the line of treatment, it gave good results. Old men who had been persistently catheterized, and who had not been able to urinate voluntarily for years, regained their power of urination. There was residual urine of course, but improvement seemed to continue in some cases.

Reports of cases were published, and many physicians adopted the treatment. Other purveyors of drugs also placed prostatic preparations upon the market. The butchers at the general slaughter-house had been directed by the first firm to furnish them with a certain number of the glands lying at the neck of the bladder, and other firms were at once furnished with the same. The chemist of one of the drug houses was anxious to do some work on perfectly fresh prostatic glands in order to find, if possible, what the specific substance might be that was characteristic of the glandular secretion and played the supposed rôle in the therapeutic results. He went to the abattoir himself for the purpose of obtaining them, and found, to his surprise, that the butchers wanted to give him seminal vesicles, and not prostates, and that it was this that they had been furnishing the different firms about town who had prostatic preparations on the market. Thereafter the real prostate was substituted for the pseudo-prostate; the results continued to be at least as good as before, and there are a number of physicians in Berlin who use extract of prostate for prostatic hypertrophy and still cure their patients.

This was not the first time such a *mistake* has occurred in organotherapy. Some years ago, Owens of Manchester reported a series of cases of Grave's disease in which cure followed the use of thyroid extract; it turned out later that the butchers had furnished extract of thymus. Under such circumstances it is seen that a series of reliable tests, such as are likely to come from further study of the anilin color-reactions will be extremely welcome.

There is one specialty in medicine in which the work of Americans seems to be thoroughly appreciated over here, and that is in children's diseases. One often hears men like Heubner or Baginsky express the indebtedness of pediatrics to American workers, and Americans are more quoted in this department than in any other. Not long ago Professor Heubner, in a clinic on that special form of chronic nephritis, which he has recently described as occurring in children, and in which there are but very few casts, very slight albuminuria, though the affection is obstinately persistent despite all treatment, took occasion to mention Jackson's work in the same line, and to say a few very commendatory words of Emmet Holt's excellent work on nephritis in nurslings. One is tempted to hope that American pediatrists are prophets in their own country too—Scripture to the contrary notwithstanding.

Apropos of the history of smallpox in Paris since 1870, there has just appeared a comparison of the conditions which obtain in the two cities, Berlin and Paris. Vaccination is not compulsory in France, and since 1870 more than 20,000 people have died in Paris from smallpox. There have been two or three noteworthy epidemics, the epidemic of 1871 and 1872 being especially severe and fatal. Berlin has had no epidemic since the one that occurred among the French prisoners in the city in 1871. Vaccination is compulsory in Prussia, and school and military regulations are so framed that care is taken to provide for revaccination later in life, as well as the original vaccination in early childhood. Paris' lowest death-rate from smallpox for any year since 1870 was in 1895, when only seventeen deaths were reported. Of this state of affairs the health authorities were very proud, and not without reason, since the inability to require vaccination makes it extremely difficult to guard against the spread of the disease when once it has invaded a district. The next year, 1896, a few scattered cases of smallpox occurred in Berlin and two deaths were reported. The excitement over this was very great and a whole series of investigations were undertaken to discover, if possible, where the blame lay.

The comparisons are food for reflection for anti- or only half-hearted vaccinationists (it is hard to say which is the worst) and make a valuable lesson in public hygiene, scientifically and non-politically conducted.

The suicide of three school children within the last few months here in Berlin has called public attention once more to the question of overwork at school, especially to the ill-effects of prize competition and competitive examination. The question of overwork at school has been the subject of a good deal of discussion, and more than one voice has been raised in favor of abolishing competitions and examinations and limiting school work to the morning hours.

It is interesting to note in this connection that neurologists generally seem to be admitting the possibility of the occurrence of hysteria in children much more frequently than was the custom some few years ago.

Charcot thought hysteria in children extremely rare, while Krafft-Ebing and Henoch scarcely admitted that this neurosis occurred in a frank form in children. Emminghaus and Oppenheim have both pointed out that the disease is by no means so rare as has been taught.

Frankly outspoken, they have been able to demonstrate stigmata of the disease in a large number of cases in adults. The drain upon nervous force incident to the strain of school work, when the organism is using all the surplus energy at its command for developmental purposes, is considered to be at the root of the neurosis, and the older observers are not thought to have been mistaken in their judgment, but the new conditions are considered to have created a before unknown tendency to neurotic manifestations at tender ages.

SOCIETY PROCEEDINGS.

NORTHWESTERN MEDICAL AND SURGICAL SOCIETY OF NEW YORK.

Stated Meeting, Held March 16, 1898.

THE President, L. DUNCAN BULKLEY, M.D., in the Chair.

INTUSSUSCEPTION.

DR. SIMON BARUCH: I would like to report the case of an apparently healthy child, five years of age, who was suddenly seized with convulsions. These occurred every five minutes, the child being unconscious during the intervals, and continued all day and the following night, chloroform being administered to control them. Dr. Jacobi was called in consultation, but it was impossible to make a diagnosis at that time, 12 A.M. It was impossible to administer medicine by the mouth, and at 6 P.M. a No. 12 soft rubber catheter was introduced into the stomach through the nares, giving exit to a large quantity of bile and mucus. The stomach was then thoroughly irrigated, and an ounce of castor oil administered through the tube. At 12:15 A.M. the catheter was again introduced, and the castor oil, mixed with about six ounces of bile, escaped. I then felt convinced that the case was one of intussusception. Dr. Kinch, who also saw the child, was of the same opinion. The stomach was again irrigated, and eight grains of calomel was administered by means of the tube. The convulsions still continued. At five o'clock in the morning the child was inverted, and a quart and half of salt solution was injected into the bowel. At six o'clock there was an attack of rigidity with staring eyes, after which the convulsions ceased. At 6:30 A.M. the bowels moved. Shortly after this Dr. Jacobi made his second visit, and agreed with me that there must have been a partial intussusception. Before the bowels moved a tumor could be felt to the right of the median line. The child has since had attacks which resemble those of *petit mal*, and the temperature remains elevated. When she became conscious she displayed an enormous appetite, and constantly cried for food. She has taken large quantities of liquid food and seems to digest it all. The attacks of rigidity have occasionally recurred, and she has developed some strabismus. I suspected cerebrospinal meningitis, Dr. Jacobi agreeing with me, and bromids were given four or five days. The attacks, however, increased in frequency, and the child screamed a good deal. Dr. C. L. Dana was then called in and expressed the opinion that the child was not suffering from meningitis, and thought that the symptoms were more those of encephalitis, or a blood-clot irritating the brain substance. She was then given iodid of potassium, and is now improving, but the diagnosis is still obscure. The temperature has been high, reaching 104° F., at which time two baths at 95° F. were given. There are no signs of typhoid fever, and Widal's-test gave no reaction. She has not had nervous symptoms, except irritability, during the past few days. I mention the case in order to emphasize the value of introducing a catheter through the nose for medication and feeding in patients who are unconscious.

DISCUSSION.

DR. S. H. DESSAU: I recently saw an infant, two-months old, in convulsions. The child had undergone a surgical operation a few hours before—gastro-enterostomy, I infer, although its exact nature could not be ascertained, but it was said to have been performed for stenosis of the pylorus. I was at a loss to know what to do, as I did not know what had been done at the operation, but it occurred to me to give a hot rectal injection. I knew this could do no harm, for the nurse told me that she had been ordered to give two enemas of salt solution after the operation, and had done so. The child could not be put in a bath, for its body was all swathed in bandages. I, therefore, injected into the rectum about a pint of water at a temperature of 110° F., and the convulsions immediately ceased.

DR. ROBERT MILBANK: I have remarked that it is common at autopsies on children to find intussusception which seems to have taken place shortly before death, and to have had no pathologic significance.

DR. FRANK GRAUER: We often find this condition present at autopsies at the Children's Hospital. It probably occurs during the death struggle. I did not hear the paper, nor all of Dr. Baruch's remarks, but I infer that something has been said about rectal irrigation. I do not see how it can be expected that the irrigation fluid will reach high enough to do any good in cases of intestinal indigestion. In making a large number of autopsies on children I have noticed the peculiar shape of the sigmoid flexure of the colon, and how it occasionally dips deep down into the pelvis, and it hardly seems possible for any fluid to reach the iliocecal valve.

About seven weeks ago I saw a child six years of age who was suffering from severe gastro-intestinal disturbance. The child had had measles, and the mother had treated it herself with ordinary household remedies until it developed a severe cough. A physician living in the neighborhood was called, and he made a diagnosis of pneumonia, and prescribed a mixture composed of antipyrin and sweet spirits of niter. He was very much surprised on his next visit to find that it made a peculiar greenish-looking mixture, and thought the druggist must have made a mistake. The child meanwhile developed a high temperature, with vomiting and purging. For a week the patient had fifteen to twenty movements daily, bluish in color, and there can be no doubt that the gastro-intestinal inflammation was caused by this mixture of drugs, producing what is known as oso-nitroso-antipyrin. Professor Fischer of Breslau has called attention to the fact that sweet spirits of niter and any of the coal-tar preparations are incompatible, and should never be prescribed together. Although it is claimed by many chemists that oso-nitroso-antipyrin is non-poisonous, it certainly did produce symptoms resembling those caused by a mineral poison in this case, and for this reason I call attention to it.

DR. BARUCH: I fear there is too great a tendency to combine drugs, and it would be wiser if this were not done, for better effects are obtained when they are given separately.

DR. MURRAY: The following case is interesting because of the obscurity of the diagnosis. A young woman who had had recurrent attacks of pain in the left side was seized with severe pain in the right side in the ovarian region. As it was during her menstrual period she was supposed to be suffering from dysmenorrhea. I examined her *per rectum*, and found an enlarged ovary with an enlarged appendix attached to it. Signs of fluctuation were present. I am watching the case, and intend to operate as soon as the patient has a sufficiently high temperature to impress the parents with the fact that it is necessary to do something for her. I wish also to emphasize the value of a rectal examination in unmarried women. A diagnosis of appendicitis is easily made by this method of examination, more readily indeed, than by abdominal palpation alone.

DR. DESSAU: It is important to impress patients with the necessity of operating during an attack of recurrent appendicitis, but it is sometimes difficult to get the patient to consent. I recently had a case, the patient being a single woman in her second attack. There was a large exudation, and I was very much afraid there wa going to be suppuration. The patient expressed her willingness to submit to operation for removal of the appendix, but as soon as she recovered from the acute attack she went back to her business, and seems to have given up all idea of having an operation performed.

DR. S. HENRY DESSAU then read the paper of the evening, entitled

CHRONIC INTESTINAL INDIGESTION IN CHILDREN.

As chronic intestinal indigestion is one of the most common disturbances of health to which children are subject, the author considered it surprising that the condition has not been more widely recognized as a distinct disease. In children the occurrence of chronic indigestion is explained both by anatomic and physiologic data. The contents of the infant stomach are quickly propelled into the intestines, and the greater part of digestion takes place in the latter viscus. Over-feeding, even when the food is of good quality, is given by the author as the chief cause of intestinal indigestion, although the character of the food and its mode of preparation (when starchy) are important etiologic factors. Children who inherit a neurotic constitution are predisposed to derangements of digestion. A mixed diet, the main portion of which is best adapted to restore waste force and energy, best fulfils physiologic requirements. The carbohydrates and hydrocarbons in proper proportions have been proved by experiment to be the most appropriate. An excess of nitrogenous food should be avoided; for in children there is no great waste of muscular force which calls for large quantities of food of this character.

Infants, during the first four months of life, whether wet-nursed or artificially fed, should not be given more than four ounces at a feeding, and should not be fed oftener than every two hours during the day and every four hours during the night; from the fourth to the eighth month six ounces of food should be given every three hours during the day and once during the night; after eight months, eight ounces of food should be allowed every four hours during the day and once during the night. When the mixed diet is begun the starchy foods, such as oat-meal, barley, wheaten grits, etc., should be cooked not less than one hour, and never more than four ounces should be allowed as a portion.

In older children, milk and not tea or coffee should form the usual beverage until the age of seven, and, instead of fresh bread, stale bread toasted or a crusty roll should be allowed. Meat, not fried or overdone, should be given at the mid-day meal only, and it is best not to give it every day. Cheese, sweets, pastry, and any form of boiled dough should not be allowed. The child should be instructed to eat slowly and thoroughly masticate its food. Between meals the drinking of pure water should be encouraged.

The general appearance of a child suffering from chronic intestinal indigestion is one of disturbed nutrition. It is languid and pale or has a dingy complexion. The circulation is poor, and the hands and feet are cold and blue. There is often some discoloration under the eyes. The skin becomes harsh and rough over the arms and trunk, and in advanced cases there is loss of flesh. There is an irritation about the nostrils and anus. Sleep is restless and disturbed, and the child talks in its sleep or has attacks of night-terror. A curious irritability of temper is a characteristic feature. The appetite may be fairly good, but is appeased by the first few mouthfuls. Thirst is often marked, and occasionally a craving for acids is noted. Abdominal pain is often a prominent symptom, the attacks of which are sometimes very severe. The tongue is moist, glossy, and covered with a thin gray fur. There is often a denudation of epithelium in sharply defined patches, a condition described by Batlin as "wandering rash of the tongue." The urine is clouded with phosphates or contains large quantities of uric acid and oxalate of lime crystals. As a rule, there is constipation, although sometimes the movements are loose and contain thick mucus. The stools are pasty, light yellow in color, and more or less coated with mucus. Prolapse of the rectum is a frequent complication, but, unless of long standing, it disappears without any treatment other than that directed toward improving the condition of the entire intestinal tract.

In the treatment of chronic intestinal indigestion more depends upon the faithful execution of precise instructions in the management of diet and other hygienic requirements than upon any remedies which the physician may prescribe, although such will always prove useful. The diet, therefore, should first be regulated. These children should not be allowed, except in the most limited quantity, any of the starchy foods, such as potatoes, corn, rice, and the breakfast cereals, unless one of the amylolytic ferments, such as diastase, taka-diastase, or peptenzyme, has previously been added. Coffee and tea, also fats and sugar, except in the smallest amount, should be forbidden. Meat will be found to agree with the child better than anything else for a time, until the digestive function is restored. Soups and extracts should not be be given.

Hydrotherapy in the form of warm wet packs followed by a cold sponge douch at 60° F. to the spinal column and abdomen, with brisk friction, as recommended by Baruch, are indicated to promote oxidation of tissue and elimination of waste matter. In the constipation of infants, cold wet compresses to the abdomen followed by massage along the line of the colon will be found beneficial. Rectal irrigation with water at a temperature of 110° F., by means of Kemp's tube, is an excellent way to relieve the attacks of abdominal pain.

In infants, the principal indication is to relieve the constipation and flatulence by means of drugs. For this purpose calomel and bismuth are the only drugs which are recommended. The former should be given in doses of from 1/20 to 1/10 of a grain, in the form of tablet triturates, every two or three hours, from three to five days at a time, and again administered after an interval of a week or ten days. When there is excessive flatulence or an eruption of urticaria, bismuth, either in the form of the subnitrate or subgallate, should be given in doses of 5 grains three times daily.

After the period of dentition is passed, a tonic-laxative,

consisting of cinchona and nux vomica with senna or cascara sagrada, is indicated. To this may be added spigelia on account of its effect in preventing the development of intestinal worms:

℞ Ext. spigeliæ fl. }
Ext. sennæ } aa . . . ʒ ii
(or ext. cascaræ fl.) . . . ʒ j
Tr. nucis vom. . . . . ʒ i
Tr. cinchonæ comp. . . . ʒ iv
Syr. sarsaparillæ comp. . . . ʒ ii.
M. Sig. One teaspoonful three times daily.

If an intercurrent infectious disease has aggravated the symptoms, 2 grains of iodid of potassium may be added to each of the above doses; or, if sleep is disturbed or enuresis troublesome, 3 to 5 grains of bromid may be added in the same manner. If prolapse of the lower bowel occurs, 3 to 5 drops of the fluid extract of hydrastis may similarly be added.

If the child is anemic, the use of iron is indicated, and the administration of the spigelia mixture may be alternated a month at a time with the elixir of the manganate of iron.

When the round worms or their ova are found, santonin in ½-grain doses should be given three times daily, either with or without calomel, or the combination of fluid extract of spigelia and senna in dram doses may be given night and morning during one or two days.

The remedies mentioned should be administered three months, in alternating courses of three weeks each. After an interval of three or four weeks, the same medication may be again employed with advantage.

DISCUSSION.

DR. BARUCH: At the conclusion of the paper the author said that his purpose was not to propose anything new, and that he had simply gathered together the manifestations common to this disease and considered them under the head of chronic intestinal indigestion. I should go further and abolish the term "chronic intestinal indigestion," for it is only a symptom. I think it would be beneficial to do so, for we would them cease to treat the various manifestations, such as constipation, etc., and would treat the disease itself which, in my opinion, is subacute enteritis of the upper part of the intestinal canal, in other words subacute duodenal catarrh. It is as such that I treat all these cases. Dr. Eustace Smith has shown wisdom in calling this condition "mucus disease," for that is really what it is, and in its treatment calomel is a most valuable agent for cleansing and antisepticizing the upper intestinal tract. Hot water by the mouth is also of great value, because it is not absorbed by the stomach but is immediately poured into the intestine. More valuable than anything else is the rectal irrigation which I very frequently employ. I have seen cases in which it at once reduced the temperature and caused the symptoms to disappear. I employ irrigation daily, injecting from a pint and a half to a quart of warm water; it acts by increasing the peristaltic action of the intestine. It certainly does not reach the duodenum, but I am sure it does reach the iliocecal valve. Whenever peristalsis is thus mechanically increased, important changes in the condition of the patient will follow. In addition to the irrigation, I apply a wet compress at 60° to 65° F. to the trunk. When the temperature is above 101° F. I order a full bath at 95° reduced to 85° or 80° F., according to the amount of fever, and followed by friction. I have not found any necessity for treating such cases medicinally as recommended by the author.

DR. MURRAY: In these cases I generally give broth made of mutton and barley, instead of meat. I find that this seldom disagrees with the child in either acute or chronic intestinal indigestion. These intestinal disturbances are usually preceded by clay-colored, hard, and offensive stools. Calomel and bichlorid of mercury act in two ways, *viz.*, as antiseptics and by promoting the flow of bile. The bichlorid is a more powerful antiseptic than calomel. Another good remedy is eudoxin, a preparation of bismuth which prevents the formation of gas. The dose for a child is 3 grains. I have employed the injections of cool water and know that they increase peristaltic action, diminish tenesmus, reduce the temperature, and cause a free flow of bile.

DR. WILLIAM STEVENS: I can add nothing to what has been said. I think that if the general plan of treatment laid down by the author is carried out, it will be followed by good results and will prevent many serious complications, such as intussusception and convulsions.

DR. L. D. BULKLEY: Since the discussion has wandered somewhat I will relate an experience I had with my own children. One summer while in the mountains they developed intestinal indigestion with diarrhea which could not be checked. I read in an old book that such disturbances sometimes result from cold, contracted by throwing off the bedclothing at night, and that this is especially liable to happen in mountainous regions, where the nights are cool. I acted upon this suggestion, and had the children wear their winter flannels, with the result that the diarrhea ceased without further medication. I have frequently followed this plan in private practice with good results.

DR. DESSAU: The main point which I wished to emphasize is that over-feeding, as a rule, is the great source and origin of chronic intestinal indigestion in children. It begins early and increases as the child grows older. Should the infant escape, it is apt to develop later on.

In regard to distension of the abdomen, in rachitic cases there is always abdominal distension, but we do not usually observe it in other conditions, except in infants. As to nitrogenous food, too much of this is not desirable in a certain class of children—those of neurotic parentage. After the trouble has begun the child is unable to digest starches, and then a nitrogenous diet must be employed. So far as irrigation is concerned, I recommend it for the relief of pain in older children but have never used it in infants except in cases of summer diarrhea. Dr. Baruch speaks of the term subacute enteritis being more suitable to this condition. Possibly this may be so, particularly because there is seldom any lesion. Both Holt and Rotch have made a point of the fact that there is no pathologic lesion in this condition, and for this reason they consider it a functional affection. In regard to the treatment employed by Dr. Baruch, I shall take advantage of his experience and shall employ it in the future, especially in infants. I doubt if it would have a good effect in older children, and it is in the latter that we see the disease well developed. In this class I believe drugs are required as well as regulation of diet. Chronic intestinal indigestion is frequently mistaken for other conditions, such as malaria, intestinal worms, etc.

MULTIPLE FIBROID TUMOR OF THE UTERUS.

DR. J. RIDDLE GOFFE: I have here a specimen of multiple fibroid tumor of the uterus. It weighs nineteen pounds, and was removed by supravaginal hysterectomy on March 15th. The specimen consists of all of the uterus above the internal os, together with the tubes and ovaries which are attached to it, and six or eight large masses.

The history of the case is as follows: K. N., fifty-three years of age, unmarried. The patient first noticed some enlargement of the abdomen fifteen years ago when she was thirty-eight years old. The enlargement steadily increased since that time until her abdomen was as large as that of a woman at full term. Menstruation had always been regular and normal in all particulars with the exception that eight years ago she had a severe hemorrage during one of her monthly periods. For this there was no special treatment, and since then she has menstruated regularly. She has never had pain, but during the past year has suffered a great deal from flatulency and bloating, which at times has been so severe as to indicate more or less obstruction of the bowel from pressure of the tumor. Her bowels have been constipated, and she has had annoyingly frequent micturition both day and night. Upon examination I found the abdomen distended by a large irregular mass, part of which was firmly impacted in the pelvis. This rounded prominence filled up the right iliac fossa and reached as high as the umbilicus upon that side. The larger and most irregular mass was located upon the left side and reached to the lower border of the ribs. The cervix of the uterus was crowded forward over the symphysis pubis. Operation was advised, and the patient readily consented, as I had four years previously removed a symmetric fibroid of the uterus from her sister. She therefore entered my private sanitarium on March 14th, and I operated upon the following day.

Upon opening the abdomen, it was apparent that the fibroid mass arose almost exclusively from the posterior wall of the uterus, and that by pressure the entire tumor had been rotated through an arc of 90° from left to right. As the anterior wall of the uterus had not been greatly enlarged, the broad ligaments were not stretched up over the tumor as is frequently the case, but were short and concealed low down in the pelvis, the appendages of the left side being carried by the rotation of the tumor to the front, while those upon the right side were carried posteriorly and so low in the pelvis that they could not be reached. My method of procedure was as follows:

With the tumor still *in situ* but strongly carried to the right side, I was able to sufficiently expose the left broad ligament, to apply a ligature on the proximal side of the appendages so as to remove them with the tumor. With a Deschamps needle threaded with heavy catgut I transfixed the broad ligament from before backward about one-third of the distance down its face and tied the ligature over the free border of the ligament. Threading one end of this same ligature in the eye of the needle I again transfixed the ligament at a point just above the uterine artery and very close to the tumor, ligating as before.

My object in using the same ligature was to pucker up the broad ligament and carry it down near enough to the cervix so that its cut section could be easily covered over with the peritoneal flaps which are yet to be described. The ends of the ligatures were left long and held in an artery clamp to preserve their identity. After applying a temporary ligature near the horn of the uterus to prevent the escape of blood from the tumor, I cut down the broad ligament from its free border as far as it had been ligated. This gave more freedom of motion to the tumor, and, although I was unable to rotate it so as to reach the broad ligament of the right side, I quickly found that it permitted the tumor to be delivered through the incision.

By persistent manipulation the fibroid masses at the lower end of the tumor were disengaged from their impaction in the pelvis and lifted out of the wound, still attached at every point except where the tumor had been cut free from the left broad ligament. While the tumor was held by an assistant, a catgut ligature was applied to the right broad ligament and it was cut as upon the opposite side. The ends of the two incisions in the broad ligaments were then united with a circular incision through the peritoneum only, across the face of the tumor and extending over the upper border of the bladder. This flap of peritoneum with the bladder was then dissected from the anterior face of the uterus and cervix. A similar circular incision was then made on the posterior face of the tumor and the peritoneum dissected down, making a posterior flap to correspond with the one made in front. One end of the original ligature was again threaded in the Deschamps needle and the broad ligament transfixed inside of the peritoneal flaps already described, close to the cervix and below the uterine artery. When ligated this controlled the circulation in the uterine artery, and a similar procedure was carried out upon the right side. The tumor and uterus were then cut away at the level of the internal os.

The four principal sources of blood-supply having been controlled, there was no hemorrhage from the stump, and, after disinfection of the cervical canal with carbolic acid, the two flaps of peritoneum were brought together over the stump and stitched with a running catgut suture. By this last maneuver all cut tissue was buried beneath the covering of peritoneum and there was no raw surface left to favor adhesion to the intestines or omentum. The abdominal wound was stitched with a through and through silver wire suture, according to my usual custom. The patient to-day (twenty-four hours after the operation) is in a most excellent condition and all signs point to an uninterrupted convalescence.

This method of disposing of the pedicle after supravaginal hysterectomy for fibroids is one devised by me in the spring of 1888, and, although it has gone through some slight modifications since it was first employed, it is practically the same operation. The two operations which claim recognition at the hands of gyneologists in cases of fibroid tumors in which it is necessary to do a bysterectomy are: (1) complete hysterectomy and (2) supravaginal hysterectomy as just described. The advantages claimed for the latter are that the natural supports of the vagina and bladder are still retained and the remaining parts are restored to as normal a position as possible. Moreover, the operation is much easier for the surgeon and can be performed in much less time than can complete hysterectomy.

DR MURRAY: The peculiarity of Dr. Goffe's operation is that he leaves a portion of the cervix and does not open the vagina. Baer of Philadelphia does a somewhat similar operation but does not sew the peritoneum over the stump. He has reported fifty cases with but one death. Martin takes out the whole uterus and drains through the vagina. There is less liability to prolapse of the vagina in Dr. Goffe's operation, and it is claimed that much less effect is produced upon the sexual feeling of the woman if the cervix is left.

REVIEWS.

TRANSACTIONS OF THE AMERICAN PEDIATRIC SOCIETY. Eighth session, held in Montreal, Canada, May 25, 26, and 27, 1896. Reprinted from *The Archives of Pediatrics*. Edited by FLOYD M. CRANDALL, M.D.

THE recently issued "Transactions of the American Pediatric Society" show some valuable reports. One of the most interesting of these is on the use of the diphtheria antitoxin. Behring's original claim that if cases "are injected on the first or second day the mortality will not be five per cent." has been found to hold good. When the injections are postponed until after three days the mortality rapidly rises. Considerable attention is given to lumbar puncture, but as a rule the subjects are quite general in their range. The morning and evening sessions for three days were devoted to reading and discussing twenty-four papers, receiving the reports of committees, and electing officers. All in all, the session seems to have been thoroughly successful and enjoyable.

TWENTIETH CENTURY PRACTICE. An International Cyclopedia of Medical Science. Edited by THOMAS L. STEDMAN, M.D. In Twenty Volumes. Volume XI., "Diseases of the Nervous System. New York: William Wood & Co., 1897.

FULLY one-half of Volume XI.—the second volume on diseases of the nervous system—is taken up by Dr. J. H. Lloyd of Philadelphia, who writes on "Diseases of the Cerebrospinal and Sympathetic Nerves." Dr. Charles K. Mills contributes a description of the trophoneuroses, exclusive of scleroderma, akromegalia, and adiposis dolorosa, which latter are from the pen of Dr. Dercum of Philadelphia.

The section on diseases of the spinal cord, by Professor Bruns and Dr. Windscheid is well worthy of careful perusal. Especially is the description of acute anterior polymyelitis to be recommended. The article by P. J. Möbius on tabes dorsalis is followed by a very short description of the "Combined System Diseases of the Spinal Cord," by Professor Strumpell of Erlangen, under which are included "Hereditary Ataxia" and "Hereditary Spastic Spinal Paralysis."

The volume ends with an interesting speculative discussion on pain by Dr. Witmer. This article, we think, should be found rather in a work on psychology than in one on the diseases of the nervous system intended for the general practitioner. Its presence does not, however, by any means detract from the value of the book, which is very readable and excellently scientific.

THERAPEUTIC HINTS.

For Tinea Sycosis.—

℞	Oleat. hydrarg. (five per cent.)	ʒ v
	Zinci oxid. } aa Amyli }	ʒ ii
	Vaselini	ʒ iiiss
	Ichthyol	gr. xv
	Ac. Salicyl.	gr. xx.

M. Sig. For external use.

For Phrenoglottic Spasm in Nursing Infants.—After immediate treatment of the spasm by the inhalation of a few drops of chloroform, the following is to be prescribed:

℞	Tinct. moschi	gtt. xx
	Tinct. belladonnæ	gtt. x
	Aq. laurocerasi	ʒ ii
	Syr. aurantii	ʒ v
	Aq. lactucarii	℥ iii.

M. Sig. Give five or six teaspoonfuls twice daily.

—*Vergniaud.*

For Fetid Perspiration.—

℞	Chloral hydratis	gr. xxxv
	Sodii boratis	gr. xv
	Ol. fœniculi	O i.

M. Sig. To be used as a wash, night and morning.

Buckskin Dressing for Eczema.—*Davesac* recommends the application of buckskin over the ointment, which is then kept moist and not absorbed by the covering. It does not cause irritation, is easily cleansed, and, while fitting smoothly over the protected part, it readily yields to every movement.

For Chronic Gonorrhea.—

℞	Airol } aa Acaciæ }	ʒ ss
	Aq. dest.	℥ ii.

M. sig. To be used as a urethral injection once daily.

Powder for Infantile Eczema.—

℞	Menthol	gr. viii
	Ac. salicyl.	gr. xv
	Bismuthi subnit. } Lycopodii } Talci veneti } aa Amyli }	ʒ v.

M. Sig. For external use.

THE MEDICAL NEWS.

A WEEKLY JOURNAL OF MEDICAL SCIENCE.

VOL. LXXII. NEW YORK, SATURDAY, APRIL 23, 1898. NO. 17.

ORIGINAL ARTICLES.

PULMONARY ACTINOMYCOSIS; RECOVERY UNDER THE USE OF OIL OF EUCALYPTUS.

BY GLENTWORTH R. BUTLER, M.D.,
OF BROOKLYN, N. Y.;
ATTENDING PHYSICIAN TO THE METHODIST EPISCOPAL (SENEY) HOSPITAL.

THE following case seems of sufficient interest to be worthy of record:

W. S., Male, thirty-seven years of age; married; Swede; rigger by occupation. On October 3, 1888, while working on a vessel, he was struck upon the head by a falling plank and thrown into the water. When rescued he had lost consciousness. He was immediately brought to the hospital and admitted to the surgical service. Upon examination he was found to be suffering from a wound of the scalp and a compound fracture of the nasal bones. His temperature on the evening of that day was 104° F.; pulse, 140; and respiration, 65. There were no physical signs which could be considered indicative of water in the bronchial tubes. The next day, October 4th, his temperature was down to 99.5° F.; pulse to 72, and respiration to 20. The second day after (October 5th) the temperature was normal, and it so continued until October 10th, seven days after the accident. During this time, having received proper surgical treatment, the scalp wound healed and the fractured nasal bones were rapidly uniting. On the evening of October 10th, the temperature rose to 101.5° F.; his pulse was quickened, and his respirations reached 30 per minute. This condition continued during the next two days, October 11th and 12th. During the night of the 11th, he complained of pain in the right side and began to have a slight cough. On October 13th, the temperature was somewhat lower and he was very weak. Signs of pulmonary inflammation becoming evident, he was transferred to the medical service.

The medical examination showed a fairly well-nourished man, who stated that he had always enjoyed good health, with the exception of two attacks of rheumatism in the feet, ankles, and knees. He admitted an attack of gonorrhea several years before, but denied syphilitic history. He alleged only a moderate use of alcoholic beverages. At seven years of age he had an attack of illness, nature unknown, which left him with an otorrhea continuing at intervals until the time of admission. He had been troubled some weeks with cough and dark-colored expectoration before coming under observation. Physical examination of the chest showed some dulness, subcrepitant râles, weak respiration, and unaltered voice sounds over the right base posteriorly. The urine was acid; specific gravity 1016; no albumin, sugar, or casts. From this time on, during six or seven weeks, the temperature rose and fell remittently, and was accompanied by profuse sweatings, presenting a close approach to the pyemic type.

About October 16th, he began to have violent and prolonged paroxysms of coughing, with the discharge of an extremely offensive dark-brown sputum. The coughing attacks were frequently precipitated by change of position. The breath also become continuously offensive, though not always to the same degree.

October 25th, the physical examination of the chest showed nothing save a few bubbling râles at the right base and left apex.

November 1st, an examination of the sputum, by Dr. E. Hodenpyl, then pathologist to the hospital, was negative.

November 6th, in order to lessen the intolerable fetor of the breath and sputum, oil of eucalyptus was prescribed, five minims in capsules every four hours day and night, and spray inhalations of the same oil were given three times daily.

November 8th, the fetor of the breath and sputum was noticeably diminished. The oil being well borne the dose was increased to ten minims every four hours, and the inhalations were given every two hours

November 12th, it was noted that the patient coughed less frequently and that the sputum had only the odor of eucalyptus. On this day another examination of the sputum by Dr. Hodenpyl resulted in the discovery of the specific organism of actinomycosis in "considerable numbers." Examination of the chest on this day showed dulness at the left apex extending down to the level of the nipple, with tubular breathing above the clavicle, and a weak respiratory murmur with prolonged and low-pitched expiration over the infraclavicular area. Over the dull area there were numerous large and small moist râles on both inspiration and expiration. There was dulness over the right base posteriorly; here the respiratory murmur was weak and accompanied by moist rales.

The patient now gained steadily in flesh and strength, and by December 11th, sleep, appetite, and digestion were all that could be desired. The cough and expectoration had entirely disappeared. The pulse, temperature, and respiration were normal. The use of eucalyptus was discontinued, and he was soon after discharged cured. At this time there was still slight dulness over the left apex, with high-pitched breathing and prolonged expiration in the infraclavicular space, and a similar dulness, with a feeble respiratory murmur and prolonged expiration, at the right base, but no râles in either locality.

The entrance of the actinomyces (ray-fungus,

streptothrix actinomycotica) into the bronchioles results in the formation of areas of pneumonia, or peribronchitis, which may ultimately break down and form abscesses of varying sizes. The disease may, and in fatal cases usually does extend to other parts of the body. It may invade the vertebræ, passing down and forming a psoas or lumbar abscess, or involve the anterior mediastinum, sternum, and pericardium. The ribs and costal tissues may become infected, and an abscess point externally in the same manner as in empyema necessitatis. Perforation of the diaphragm and subphrenic abscess may result, or the liver, spleen, and other abdominal organs become involved. Ordinarily, the affection, when pulmonary, is unilateral and basic, but, as in the case here reported, may extend to the apex of the opposite lung. Indeed, there is no part of the body in which metastases have not been found.

The clinical course of pulmonary actinomycosis is essentially that of a chronic pyemia, with symptoms pointing toward the lungs as the seat of infection. The pulmonary symptoms and signs resemble either tuberculosis or a fetid bronchitis such as occurs in connection with pulmonary gangrene, pulmonary abscess, bronchiectasis, or empyema perforating the lung. Like other diseases of a pyemic type it may be mistaken for typhoid fever. The diagnosis is only to be made by the finding of actinomyces in the sputum or in the pus of abscesses and ulcerations. The tufts of the actinomyces may sometimes be seen with the unaided eye in pus or sputum as sulphur-colored particles, resembling grains of iodoform. In view of the increasing number of instances in which this disease has been demonstrated it is desirable that in all patients presenting fetid breath and expectoration as a symptom, an examination should be made for the presence of the ray-fungus. A similar precaution should be taken in cases, apparently of pulmonary tuberculosis, but in which tubercle bacilli cannot be found.

The prognosis of pulmonary actinomycosis is very unpromising. Of thirty-four cases reported up to 1890, thirty-two died, a mortality of nearly ninety per cent., and in a very recent volume, Wood and Fitz consider the prognosis to depend upon the site of the disease. If this be such that surgical treatment cannot be applied, death is the almost certain termination.

Treatment.—Among remedies, potassium iodid, in doses of 40 to 60 grains daily, has received favorable mention, although most of the successful cases were those which were also amenable to surgical treatment. Jurinka, in reporting three cases in which cure followed the use of the iodid (one of which was perityphlitic, and, with the other two, seems to have been surgically treated), states, as the result of experiments with cultures made in media containing the iodid, that the latter did not act as a parasiticide, but hindered the growth, and thus aided in the elimination of the organism from the system.

As a rule no reliance should be placed upon the results of a remedy employed only in one case. But if, as in this instance, a patient having a disease in which the prognosis is extremely bad, and further, which previous to the administration of a certain remedy is steadily advancing, begins to show improvement within three or four days after the new therapeusis is begun, and in a little more than one month has quite recovered, it is not a stretch of the imagination to attribute the arrest of the disease to the remedy employed. If the properties of the agent used in this case and the characteristics of the organism concerned are examined, it becomes still more likely that the conclusion reached is not an instance of *post hoc, propter hoc.* Leaving out of consideration the physiologic action of the oil of eucalyptus (which does not concern its value in this case), there is good evidence to prove that it has distinct antiseptic qualities. Binz finds that it acts more promptly than quinin upon the lower infusoria, and Wood endorses the statement of Gimbert, that its antiseptic power is very great. That it has a similar destructive action upon the Laveran organism must also be granted, although the majority of the observers to be mentioned made their reports before the possibility of accurate diagnosis by the blood examination became an accomplished fact. In spite of a lack of the demonstrated presence of the plasmodium, the testimony of Bohn, Carlotti, Gimbert, Haller, Lorinser, Musser, Tristany, and others, in reference to its curative power in malarial fever, is indisputable, and it is admitted to be useful in cases in which quinin is not tolerated.

The oil of eucalyptus after absorption from the stomach is eliminated by the lungs, skin, and kidneys. Its odor is usually very perceptible in the breath of those to whom it is administered. The perspiration and the urine may also have the odor of the drug. Bearing in mind its antiseptic action upon the lower infusoria and the plasmodium malariæ, and its easily perceived elimination through the lungs, I desire to call attention to the fact that the actinomyces are decidedly vulnerable to the action of germicidal agents. Hodenpyl, in his monograph upon this subject, states, as others do, that the actinomyces do not withstand even weak antiseptics, and to a certain extent seem prone to die and undergo absorption or calcification in the tissues.

These facts render it extremely probable that recovery in the case here reported was due to the antiseptic action of the oil of eucalyptus exerted upon the fungus during the elimination of the drug by way of the pulmonary circulation, the air-cells, and the bronchioles. The question whether or not the curative action of this oil, if such action be proved to exist, will be exerted upon other tissues than those of the lungs, remains to be solved by further investigation.

THE TREATMENT OF DELIRIUM TREMENS.

BY T. D. CROTHERS, M.D.,
OF HARTFORD, CONN.;
SUPERINTENDENT OF THE WALNUT LODGE HOSPITAL.

DELIRIUM TREMENS, as described in the text-books, is literally only one form of a great variety of mental disturbances which follow the use of alcohol and other poisons. Many widely differing states are called by this name simply because they have common hallucinations and delusions and at times muscular tremblings. Alcoholic mania, chronic inebriety, traumatic delirium, febrile delirium, convulsive delirium, delirium from meningeal and cerebral inflammation, are the names of some of the conditions to which the general term delirium tremens is applied. In many of these affections the muscular tremblings are absent, though they all have similar hallucinations and delusions.

In the consideration of treatment some discrimination between causes should be made. The continuous or paroxysmal use of alcohol, directly or indirectly associated with the affection that is being considered, the remote use of spirits, with an immediate history of injury or of febrile states, of exhaustion and nutritive poisoning, all have a similar meaning. The nerve-centers are seriously disturbed, and sensorial hyperesthesia and exaggerated functional activity are present up to irritation and inflammation.

Jacobson says: "In many cases delirium tremens is due either to the action of bacteria or to intoxications from diseases of the digestive tract, the kidneys, or the liver. The symptoms indicate the same toxic agent, which in many respects resembles the poisons of infectious diseases. Injuries of the nerve-centers from blows, shocks, and violent pertubations are not infrequently followed by delirium tremens. Often an incubatory period precedes its development, and a marked self-limited duration of the case follows. In most cases a rise of temperature with acute albuminuria occurs, and when a fatal termination results, it is preceded by parenchymatous degeneration of the liver, kidneys, and heart. In all cases there are toxemic states, indicating the presence of some poison whose elimination is encouraged by profuse action of the skin."

The treatment of delirium tremens requires careful study of the history of the patient and recognition of general causes, and then, removal of all conditions which seemingly have been active in the causation of the disease. In most cases the use of alcohol is the first question to determine. Formerly the slow withdrawal of spirits was considered essential. In 1855 Dr. Peddie of Edinburgh treated a number of cases by the sudden withdrawal of all spirits and the use of antimony. His results were favorable. Then others followed, using various substitutes. Dr. Kerr of London at once withdraws spirits and uses aromatic spirits of ammonia. During more than thirty years the question of sudden or gradual withdrawal of alcohol has been agitated. While the mortality has decreased in cases in which spirits were at once removed, the opponents of this method have explained it as due to other causes.

In many large hospitals the practice is to continue the use of spirits in slowly diminishing doses in all alcoholic cases in which there is delirium. When the delirium is violent, alcohol is administered as an essential in maintaining the strength, and thus in avoiding a fatal issue. This teaching a careful study proves to be without the slightest support from clinical data. In the cases of thousands of criminals and paupers suddenly incarcerated in jails and prisons and deprived of all spirits, the best results follow. Most of these cases are in chronic inebriates very much debilitated by alcohol, many of them delirious, and the sudden withdrawal of spirits is the beginning of restoration to health.

Dr. Kerr says: "Delirium tremens is a toxemic condition induced by alcohol, and to continue the use of this poisonous agent is to prolong its toxic action; each patient is weakened by the excessive and prolonged discharge of nerve energy and by muscular restlessness and convulsions. The more alcohol supplied, the greater the muscular restlessness and the greater the expenditure of nerve energy. Reaction with enfeeblement is inevitable, and the recovery of the patient is prolonged, and his peril increased."

My personal experience, consisting of several hundred cases, supports this view and sustains the assertion that sudden and complete withdrawal of spirits is the first assential in the treatment of delirium tremens. In my experience in asylum treatment, a hot bath, either hot air as in a Turkish bath with hot showers and free rubbing, or hot water alone with massage, are the first and most essential therapeutic measures. In private practice, hot tub-baths, free sponging with hot soap-water, and daily rubbings are required. Sequestration and full control of the patient, either in the home or in an asylum, is of course an essential part of treatment, and may be best accomplished with the aid of strong attendants who will prevent the patient from injuring himself. Next in importance to free bathing is catharsis, with calomel and salines. This should at first be free irrespective of all weakness and apparent prostration which may follow.

The insomnia and muscular agitations are limited and will end in sleep and rest after the fourth or fifth day. After free catharsis and bathing sleep follows within twenty-four or thirty-six hours. This delirious period cannot be cut short by narcotics, and no remedies of this class should be used. The hallucinations and delusions may continue a week or two, with lucid intervals, which constantly increase in length.

The first and most important object of the treatment is the elimination through the skin, bowels, and kidneys of the toxic poisons which are present, either from the alcohol or the bacteria formed within the body.

The primary causes of delirium tremens are in all probability irritative poisons, rather than nerve exhaustion or profound anemia. Hence, feeding is secondary in importance to elimination, and no food should be given until free action of all the eliminatory organs is established. Then, hot and easily assimilable liquid foods are required. In most cases such foods given at long intervals of four or five hours are better borne than when given at shorter intervals. No drugs, such as tonics or stimulants are given until after the subsidence of the delirium and the period of sleep and exhaustion is fully established.

Then nitrate of strychnin or cinchona can be used; the former in $\frac{1}{30}$-grain doses four times daily, and the latter in doses of ʒ i of the infusion every four hours. The various combinations of ammonia, chloral, opium, digitalis, and the long list of coal-tar preparations are dangerous and should not be used. In some cases where bathing is impracticable the use of diaphoretic drugs, of which ipecac is the best, is excellent.

The muscular agitation is often a question of much importance. Forcible restraint is in most cases dangerons to the patient, and followed by more profound exhaustion than if partial liberty were allowed. The rule is to permit the fullest exercise compatible with the safety of the patient and his surroundings. The delusions and hallucinations are rarely homicidal or suicidal, but always of fear and dread of injury, and the patients can usually be quite easily managed by attendants. If the patient is robust and well-nourished and the season permits, open-air exercise should be permitted several hours daily; if he is weak and emaciated, the freedom of a large room or hall in which the air is pure is preferable to a close room of any form. A clinical history of a few cases will bring out the plan of treatment found most effectual in my practice:

CASE I.—A builder who, after twenty years of moderate drinking, used spirits to great excess during two months. He became delirious, and had persecutory delusions and hallucinations, with muscular trembing. His family physician had freely administered chloral and opium without any results. On admission the patient was intensely agitated. He was forcibly held twenty minutes in the hot-room of the Turkish bath, and was freely rubbed and finally given a hot shower bath. He became calm and was placed in a large room where he could walk about freely. Four hours later he was given another bath with no resistance on his part, and this was followed by a quiet interval of three hours. Five grains of calomel, followed by sulphate of magnesia administered on admission, induced free action of the bowels five hours later, and was followed by a lucid interval. The third bath on the morning of the second day was followed by the first sleep, which continued three hours, and a distinct lucid interval.

The patient's muscular agitation was not restrained. He was taken out to walk in the yard twice daily, and always returned willingly to the asylum. The baths were also given twice each day; in the morning a hot followed by a cold shower bath, with free rubbing, and in the evening a Turkish bath which was followed by sleep. Hot milk and meat broths were given the second day at intervals of four hours. Recovery rapidly followed and the delusions disappeared completely alter the first week.

CASE II.—In a second case, a robust farmer was brought under restraint to the asylum; after a large dose of magnesia and a prolonged hot bath his excitement subsided; a few hours later a second bath was followed by sleep and the first lucid interval. On all occasions he was permitted to walk freely up and down the ward until exhausted. No solid food was given until the second day, the diet consisting of hot milk administered at intervals. After the second day convalescence was uneventful.

CASE III.—A third case of alcoholic mania, with irregular paroxysms of muscular excitement and persistent insomnia, occurred in a man who was said to be incurable. Free catharsis followed the administration of calomel and sulphate of magnesia, and this, with prolonged hot baths, broke up the insomnia on the second day. The mania disappeared after the first week and natural sleep became possible. Complete final restoration to health occurred after four-months' treatment. In this case baths produced a most marked relief of the mental disturbances, and restricted diet seemed medicinal.

While in hospitals and asylums many means can be commanded which are not accessible in private homes, still in general the same line of treatment can be applied in all cases.

CASE IV.—A summer boarder at a farm-house

was seized with alcoholic delirium, after destroying a room in which he was confined. By my advice he was put in charge of two men and permitted to walk two hours through the fields. Then he was forced into a tub of warm water and vigorously rubbed. Cathartics and cold water were given, also two doses of infusion of cinchona (ʒ i) to break up the craze for alcohol. After a third dose of cinchona all desire for spirits left him, and after the third bath he slept two hours and woke up with a lucid interval. From this time he became convalescent.

In my hospital, after the first bath, patients never object to its repetition, and usually look forward to it with pleasant anticipation. In private practice these cases can be treated with but little difficulty, with the aid of strong capable attendants who will compel the patient to follow directions. In many cases the forcible removal of such patients to hospitals and asylums is associated with difficulties not free from peril. With good nurses, bathing facilities, space for exercise, and with absolute withdrawal of spirits such patients can be successfully treated at home. The old method, consisting of gradually decreasing doses of spirits, with various compounds of narcotics to produce sleep, is full of peril to the patient and most seriously complicates recovery in all cases. It may be assumed that in all cases of delirium following alcoholic poisoning the treatment must be eliminative, by natural means and hygienic measures; also, that muscular and mental exhaustion, with diaphoresis, are efforts of Nature to throw off the poison. Baths and free exercise follow the line of Nature's suggestion.

In the almost endless complications which are likely to follow and be associated with alcoholic toxemia, widely varying therapeutic indications may be present, but baths and elimination are practical in all cases. In many cases the removal of alcohol is followed in a short time by delirium, particularly when opium and chloral are freely given.

That the delirium is due to the withdrawal of alcohol is not true, but it is due rather to the narcotic drugs which have checked excretion. The delirium rarely ever subsides until the use of spirits is abandoned unless followed by catharsis and withdrawal of narcotics. The withdrawal of alcohol should always be followed by drainage through the skin, kidneys, and bowels.

The D.-T. prescriptions of public hospitals, so often mentioned as practical, absolute, therapeutic measures, are both dangerous and misleading, as the mortality reports prove. The practice in the Berlin military hospital of treating all alcoholics with salines, shower baths, and meat broths, with a very low mortality, is much nearer modern therapeusis in these cases.

TREATMENT OF PLEURAL EFFUSIONS.[1]

BY W. M. PIRT, M.D.,
OF BARRIE, ONTARIO.

SEROUS effusions are frequently classified as (*a*) small, (*b*) moderate, and (*c*) large.

A small effusion is generally defined as one of two to four finger's-breadth at one base. In these effusions some authors claim there should be no active medication except that which is directed to restoration of the functions of the organs deranged by the fever. The patient should be kept in bed and a substantial nourishing dry diet prescribed, with occasionally a mild laxative, but there should be no purging, as such is not necessary, and only harasses the patient. Morphia may be of value, as it not only controls pain but "splints the pleura," places the patient in a better subjective condition, and is less constipating than opium. In vigorous patients hydragogue cathartics are useful, and under such circumstances Dr. P. Blaikie Smith of Aberdeen advocates the use of magnesium sulphate after Hay's method, *viz.:* give from 2 to 4 drams of the above-mentioned drug in the least possible quantity of water three times daily. Such medication is contraindicated when there is (1) urgent dyspnea, (2) phthisical tendency, (3) poor physique, and (4) purulent effusion.

To stimulate the action of the skin hot or vapor baths or small doses of pilocarpin may be tried. Regarding the use of salicylates, authors appear to differ. Talamon claims that sodium salicylate has a specific action in pleuritic effusions; others say it has a sudorific action, and others again, a diuretic effect, and nearly all agree that it is mainly useful on account of its power of increasing the elimination of uric acid and urates. Aufrecht, who introduced the use of salicylic acid in the treatment of pleuritic effusions, claims that it and not the salicylate of soda should be used, as he says the salicylate is weaker and produces marked secondary effects. He employs salicylic acid as follows: "Give the patient 90 grains per day, and advise, if within the first eight days there is no reduction in the amount of the effusion, that the physician should not despair, but stop the use of the drug one or two days, and then begin it again and continue several days longer with occasional interruptions of one or two days."

Rosenbach and Pohl discovered that salicylates introduced into the system were later found in all the healthy serous cavities as well as in those which were diseased. A number of authorities agree that sodium salicylate is useful as proving the nature of the effusion, *viz.:* if there is no decrease in the amount of the effusion under treatment with this drug, the fluid

[1] Fourth Prize Essay, MEDICAL NEWS' Prize Contest.

in the pleural cavity is purulent in character. Others again, hold that it is useful in all cases in which there is a rheumatic element, especially when combined with iodid of potassium, and may even do harm in non-rheumatic cases, in which digitalis or alcohol acts better. During the salicylate treatment the patient should be kept in bed, and the quantity of urine daily passed should be measured and recorded.

Koster gives sodium salicylate in 22-grain doses t. i. d., and also salicylic acid in 15-grain doses. One writer recommends liquor ammonia acetatis (ʒ ii to iv in milk every four hours with an alkalin effervescent), and claims that "it lessens the vascular tension and promotes the action of the skin and kidneys, and therefore lessens the amount of fluid."

Massage of the chest has been useful in some hands, as has also compression of the chest during expiration, five to ten minutes twice daily, and, when tenderness has disappeared, massage of the intercostal spaces should be applied.

An old formula consisting of potassium iodid, 5 grains, with syrup ferri iodidi, 10 minims, three times daily, has been found useful to promote absorption. In small effusions, if the fever has subsided and still the dulness persists, counter-irritation may be tried by means of the application of a fly-blister, unguentum rubri iodidi, or tincture of iodin.

As a local application the following is said to be beneficial:

℞ Guaiacol (pure) . . . . ʒ i
Tr. iodi . . . . . . ʒ vii.
M. Sig. Paint all this liquid upon the affected side every evening.

Following this application the temperature will fall, there will be profuse sweating, and the effusion will gradually subside.

Dr. Bowditch of Boston uses the following as a local application:

℞ Tr. iodi . . . . . . ʒ ss
Spts. ætheris sulph. . q. s. ad. ℥ i.

He directs that this should be painted upon the affected side once or twice, or until burning is produced.

Phenol vesication is recommended by Dr. Ollivier for children on account of their intolerance of cantharides and its preparations. The thirst cure is used by few, and consists of withdrawal of all fluids from the diet during two days, the use of lean meat, stale bread, and one-half pint of fluid on the third day, one pint on the seventh, and one pint on the eighth day. The jaborandi cure, which consisted of the administration of small doses of the fluid extract of jaborandi every three hours, is very rarely used.

In moderate effusions counter-irritation should be given a fair trial. Neuman uses simple blue ointment (a piece the size of a hazel-nut) rubbed well in twice a day on the affected side. If the fluid is being slowly absorbed, restrict the patient to a dry diet and administer diuretics, such as digitalis and acetate of potassium, during three or four days, and then substitute caffein (2 to 5 grains) with sodii benzoate (10 to 20 grains). This should not be given during the afternoon, or the patient will not sleep well. Dr. Howard considers that the administration of 1 grain of calomel three times daily, added to a pill of digitalis and squill, is excellent treatment. It is hardly necessary to add that care must be taken that the patient is not salivated.

It is held by some that the use of antipyrin occasionally leads to absorption. If the effusion does not diminish after the institution of some of the above measures, if after a two- to four-week's trial the affection remains stationary, then the question of paracentesis of the chest arises. In moderate effusions there is only one reason for aspiration, namely: to remove an effusion which Nature, after a fair trial, seems unable to do In small effusions all fluid may be withdrawn, though the same teaching does not hold good when there is a large quantity of fluid in the chest. Here, if diuretics and purgatives have been of no value within three or four days, their use should be discontinued, and potassium iodid and the salicylates should be given instead. An iron tonic is indicated throughout the whole course of the disease.

Before aspirating an exploratory puncture should always be made under strict antiseptic precautions to ascertain the nature of the effusion. The objects to be gained by tapping are: (1) the relief of pressure on the lung; (2) the prevention of death from compression of the lung, and (3) the removal of purulent fluid. It has been found that removal of a portion of the fluid relieves the pressure on the lymphatics, and thus aids absorption.

Aspiration should be performed during the acute stage, and (1) when one pleural sac is completely filled, as shown by dulness reaching up to the clavicle; (2) if there is marked displacement of the heart, or if one or more murmurs are developed in the heart; (3) in double pleurisy, if both sides are one-half filled by fluid; (4) if serious symptoms, such as orthopnea or a tendency to syncope, supervene.

In the afebrile stage, when Nature apparently makes no attempt to, or cannot reduce the amount of fluid, aspiration should be performed. Allow a period of from one to three weeks to pass before so doing (unless there are serious symptoms), but delay should not be too protracted, for if the lung is compressed too long its elasticity may be destroyed and it may not regain its functions. Delafield, Osler,

Bristowe, Pepper, Peabody, and others are all decisive in commending the timely removal of fluid from the pleural cavity.

Some claim that aspiration causes the formation of adhesions by bringing the inflamed layers of the pleura together. As soon thereafter as the strength will permit, we are advised that hill-climbing and pulmonary gymnastics are useful, as is also the use of the pneumatic cabinet.

Paracentesis of the Chest.—Not very long ago this operation was greatly dreaded, and only performed as a sort of last resort, principally in purulent effusions; but now, with our almost perfect aspirators, it is one of the simplest procedures and may be successfully performed by any one possessed of ordinary skill.

The patient should be placed in a lateral position with the hand of the affected side on the opposite shoulder to widen the intercostal spaces. Previous to the operation administer a stimulant to the patient, such as whisky, with 3 to 5 minims of tincture of strophanthus, or a hypodermic injection of strychnia. Make the skin of the affected side and the needle of the aspirator thoroughly aseptic. Spray the site of puncture with ether or ethyl chlorid. The site of puncture usually chosen is the axillary line (sixth interspace), for the reason that here (1) the chest-wall is thin; (2) the ribs are fairly well apart; (3) the patient cannot see what is being done, and (4) there is no risk of wounding any important organ.

Never puncture over the site of a resonant percussion-note. Make a valvular puncture by drawing the skin upward as the needle is introduced. The needle should penetrate just over the upper border of the rib in order to avoid wounding the intercostal artery. Withdraw the fluid very gradually, and thus (1) cough will not be likely to start; (2) there will be less disturbance of the circulation in the veins, and the patient will not be likely to expectorate, and (3) pressure will not be taken off the lung too rapidly. When the visceral layer of the pleura is felt to touch the needle the latter should be withdrawn a little, or it may cause cough.

If there should be pain or cough the aspiration should be stopped. In this connection Bowditch's precept should be remembered: "Suspend the withdrawal of fluid the moment the patient begins to suffer in breathing, even in the slightest degree."

If there should be signs of syncope, the reinjection of part of the fluid by reversing the action of the instrument is said to be useful. In moderate effusions remove all the fluid that is possible. In large effusions remove only part at once; for if all is removed collapse of the chest-wall may result. In large effusions be on the watch for edema of the lungs, and, if it is present, apply dry cups to the back and give alcoholic stimulants. Under these circumstances nitroglycerin or atropia is said to be useful. Follow the operation by a hypodermic injection of from 1/6 to 1/4 of a grain of morphia to relieve the pain and cough which results from sudden expansion of the lung.

The contraindications to aspiration are: (1) shock and collapse, (2) general prostration, (3) complicating croupous pneumonia. The dangers are syncope and cerebral embolism. Sudden death has occurred during the withdrawal of fluid from the chest, and is said, by Dr. Andres of Philadelphia, to be caused as follows: "During the displacement of the heart the circulation is depressed, but as the fluid is removed the heart returns to its original position, and the increased current washes an embolus into the circulation which lodges in the pulmonary artery, thus causing instant death."

The same author recommends aspiration if the fluid reaches to the clavicle (as shown by percussion), even though the patient be comfortable and present no sign of pulmonary distress, and in these cases the presence of fever does not contraindicate the operation. After evacuation of the serum, Dr. Jubel-Renoy uses an injection of a sterilized solution (one per cent.) of zinc chlorid. He very slowly injects a small quantity of this, and then withdraws it within ten or fifteen minutes. Dr. Levascheff of Kazan recommends the withdrawal of a certain amount of intrapleural exudate and at once replacing it with an equal quantity of sodium chlorid solution. This is repeated, and after awhile the cavity contains nothing but a neutral saline solution, which is rapidly absolved.

Gilbert of Geneva claims that in tuberculous cases the exudate contains a material analogous to Koch's tuberculin, and he withdraws into a syringe a cubic centimeter of the pleuritic fluid. He then partially withdraws the needle so that he can inject the fluid into the subcutaneous cellular tissues. The injection is followed by an active febrile reaction, and the exudate is gradually absorbed. He employed this procedure in twenty-one cases, and in nineteen there was recovery within two or three weeks. He says that "it is easy to perform and free from danger, but its mode of action is somewhat unexplained."

In multilocular pleurisy operate early, and puncture as low down as is compatible with safety in order to ascertain if there is a communication between the cysts, as is evidenced by a lessening of the fluid in the upper part of the chest. If not connected the cysts will require tapping at various points.

In hemorrhagic effusions, weak iodin injections into the pleural cavity may be tried. The patient should be kept absolutely at rest in the recumbent position until the temperature has been normal eight days, the heart and respiration being the guides as to increase or decrease of the effusion.

Aspiration is not always successful in causing cure in case the effusion is purulent. Incision and drainage and irrigation with a solution of salicylate of soda or thymol have given satisfaction in some cases. Irrigations with solutions of phenic acid are dangerous on account of their poisonous effects. The indications are to get rid of the purulent effusion as early as possible, and in the easiest, safest, and most thorough manner.

The advantages claimed by the advocates of aspiration over incision are: (1) that it is simple; (2) that it is free from danger with ordinary skill; (3) that it does not remove the fluid too rapidly, and thus allow a gradual expansion of the lung; (4) that it does not require general anesthesia; (5) that following it there is no confinement to bed, and (6) that aspiration alone sometimes cures, as the effusion after one or two aspirations becomes serous and is then rapidly absorbed.

Of course, in aspiration in purulent cases, a larger needle must be used than is necessary in cases in which the effusion is serous. Laffan aspirates as soon as he finds a purulent effusion, and he believes that seventy-five per cent. of the pleuritic effusions in children are purulent, and also that death is sometimes caused by pleural injections. It is thought that septic hypodermic or aspirating-needles often cause a serous exudate to become purulent.

Osler states that he never observed a case of conversion of a serofibrinous fluid into a purulent one.

THE ASEPTIC TREATMENT OF RETENTION OF URINE.

BY CHARLES S. HAMILTON, M.D.,
OF COLUMBUS, OHIO;
PROFESSOR OF PRINCIPLES OF SURGERY IN THE STARLING MEDICAL COLLEGE, AND LECTURER ON CLINICAL SURGERY IN MT. CARMEL HOSPITAL.

THE glans penis and the urethra are the habitat of several varieties of micro-organisms, some of them capable of producing pathologic effects when carried into the bladder, or when invading the peri-urethral tissues through a trifling wound. While a healthy bladder has a certain power of resistance which may enable it to successfully cope with an infection of moderate intensity, quite the reverse is true of one habitually distended, such as may be encountered in cases of enlarged prostate. The deposit of micro-organisms in a bladder, the resistance of which is impaired, may prove the starting-point of a septic process which terminates only with the death of the affected individual.

Simple urethral fever, prostatitis, epididymitis, ureteritis, pyelonephritis, and pyemia are probably only varied manifestations of the same group of bacterial poisons. It is therefore a matter of the greatest importance that the use of instruments in the urethra and bladder should be accompanied by the most careful antiseptic and aseptic precautions. It must be admitted that no germicide, no aseptic method, will acccomplish the result required, *viz.*: complete removal of pathogenic organisms from the field of operation. Though perfection is impossible, it should be our aim, and fewer disasters will then follow instrumentation.

When the physician is about to empty a bladder by mechanical means he should have in mind a certain definite routine to be followed, the object of which is three-fold: (1) Sterilization of the penis and urethra of the patient. (2) Sterilization of the instruments and hands of the physician. (3) Maintenance of the sterile condition until the operation is finished. Sterilization implies both cleanliness and the use of germicides—the former being probably the more important and essential of the two. One principle—a *sine qua non* to success—must be kept constantly in mind. No object, when once sterilized, should be allowed to come in contact with any unsterilized object. If such contact does occur, immediate re-sterilization is necessary. It is with reference to this point more than any other that we fail in carrying out the details of a perfect aseptic technic. For example, our precautions are in vain if we lay a sterilized catheter upon the bed or table until ready to use it; or if with well cleaned hands we draw the cork from an unsterilized bottle and proceed at once to handle sterilized articles. It would be well to remember that cleanliness in dealing with the bladder is just as imperative as in the lying-in chamber; for the possibility of infection is quite as great, though fatal results may not be so frequent. That which has been said applies quite as forcibly to the hands of the operator as to the instruments employed.

The following might serve as a description of one method of aseptic catheterization, the steps being, of course, subject to variations to suit circumstances:

The necessary articles will be:

1. Scrubbing-brush.
2. Catheter (rubber, woven, metallic, glass).
3. Lubricant. (Boroglycerid in glass-stoppered bottle, or vaselin, sterilized, in soft metal tubes).
4. A small glass syringe.
5. Towels, basin, and dish.
6. Bichlorid of mercury or carbolic acid.

Let some member of the family throughly scrub and repeatedly rinse a granite-ware basin and a vegetable dish, each holding one pint or more. I assume that these two articles or their equivalents can be found in any household. Put in the basin one pint of water from the kettle and a teaspoonful of carbonate of soda. Boil the catheters and an ordinary glass syringe in this solution five minutes, both having been cleansed before being placed in the soda solution. Mix ordinary weak carbolic or bichlorid solution in the vegetable dish, using by preference water from the kettle.

Now, the physician should scrub his own hands, being sure as to the condition of his finger-nails. Rinse them well and dip them in the antiseptic solution. Put a small clean towel to soak in the solution. The penis is now to be cleansed by scrubbing and rinsing, devoting particular care to the meatus. Lay the antisepticized towel over the thighs and abdomen in such manner as to leave the penis exposed. If there is some urethral discharge, repeatedly wash the anterior urethra with the syringe and antiseptic urethra solution. Take the catheter from the basin in which it was boiled and lubricate it with boroglycerid, poured on it from the bottle by an assistant or a member of the family, and then introduce it.

After using the catheter, scrub and rinse it, and inject antiseptic solution through it. Put it away in a clean towel, or boil it again and put it away in carbolic solution, in which case it will be again ready for use. A one- or two-per-cent. solution of carbonate of soda is especially appropriate for boiling glass or metallic instruments. It would probably prove rapidly destructive to soft catheters. The ordinary rubber catheter may be boiled in clear water, though such treatment undoubtedly shortens its period of usefulness. Woven catheters will not tolerate boiling, with exception of a special variety which is rather expensive.

In lubricating the catheter, as little of the lubricant as possible should be allowed to get into the eye of the instrument; for it is apt to accumulate in that portion of the catheter distal to the eye and constitute a trap for filth. A three- or four-per-cent. carbolic-acid solution is the best antiseptic for the preservation of either soft or hard catheters, as corrosive sublimate very rapidly hardens rubber and tarnishes metallic instruments.

Aseptic catheterization of the female can hardly be accomplished without exposure of the patient. The same routine must be followed as in the male. Every medical man has encountered cases illustrating the persistent cystitis which may follow unclean catheterization in women. In many cases of retention repeated catheterization is necessary, sometimes at hours when the physician cannot be present. Generally the nurse, or a relative, can be trained to pass the catheter in a clean, safe manner. Doubtless some objector will say that this proceeding is tedious and cumbersome; that life is too short for so much pains in so trifling a matter. I admit that the rules of surgical cleanliness may be violated, possibly seven or eight times out of ten, with impunity. The other two or three cases, however, may be very unfortunate. We should bear in mind that it is to such cleanliness as that described that modern surgery owes its advancement.

In a paper of this scope but little attention can be given to the mechanical features of urinary retention and their influence upon the aseptic progress of a case. In stricture of the urethra it is well to remember that no instrument which *can* pass an obstruction in the urethra requires the exertion of any force to *make* it pass. Urethral instruments should be introduced without the exertion of force or they should not be introduced at all. When resistance is encountered, either the instrument is too large or it is not in the right track; and when it is not in the right track, the slightest force may cause a wound of the unhealthy mucous membrane near the stricture with consequent extravasation and peri-urethral suppuration.

In the treatment of retention from enlarged prostate, the soft catheter is indicated whenever it can be used, on account of distortion of the urethral canal and engorgement of the mucosa in the prostatic region. Hemorrhage into the bladder is very common even after gentle instrumentation, and the resulting clot, if not evacuated, constitutes a nidus for the growth and multiplication of bacteria. The first catheterization in these cases is attended with great responsibility; for the bladder at first lacks the tolerance of catheter life and septic organisms which it acquires when the catheter has been used during months and years. This is well illustrated in cases of long-standing inability to empty the bladder voluntarily; these patients disregard all rules of cleanliness and for a long time at least, escape the consequences. However, eventually, they too acquire and succumb to the aggravated cystitis and surgical kidney which we find as a final stage of this and other incurable inflammatory conditions of the genito-urinary tract.

Baby Incubators at the Circus.—In speaking of Dr. Lion's incubators, *The Lancet* (London) passes severe strictures on the custom now prevalent in London of making a commercial speculation of incubators, and says anent their exhibition at Barnum and Bailey's show, "What connection is there between the serious matter of saving life, and the bearded woman, the dog-faced man, the elephants, the performing horses and pigs, and the clowns and acrobats which constitute the chief attraction at the Olympia."

HOSPITAL REPORT.

THE TUBERCULIN TEST FOR THE PRESENCE OF TUBERCULOSIS.[1]

BY W. P. NORTHRUP, M.D.,
OF NEW YORK.

THE following tests of the value of tuberculin for diagnostic purposes were undertaken in the medical wards of the Presbyterian Hospital in the spring and fall of 1897. With one exception the cases tested were all in adults.

A paper by Dr. Trudeau, appearing at that time (MEDICAL NEWS, May 29, 1897), served as a working guide, and certain oral communications from Dr. Trudeau assured the beginning of these investigations on mature lines. First of all it was necessary to have a reliable preparation of tuberculin and a uniform, diluted, injecting solution. The tuberculin used, made according to Koch's original standard, was furnished by Dr. E. L. Trudeau from the Saranac Laboratory, and kindly contributed for this work.

The diluted solution was prepared by Dr. George A. Tuttle in the pathologic laboratory of the Presbyterian Hospital, of a uniform strength, 1 milligram to 1 cubic centimeter of distilled water with carbolic acid, one-half of one per cent.

This solution was frequently made fresh; it was kept in a cool place, and never used after it was more than two weeks old; it was always made in the same way, and injected with the same syringe, by the same assistant, and in the same part of the body, at the same hour of the day. In other words, a standard grade of tuberculin was used, in constant dose, and under uniform conditions.

Dose and Administration.—The initial dose used was at first half a milligram; later it was thought just as well to begin in adults with 1 milligram. This was injected subcutaneously in the dorsal region, between the scapulæ, at midnight. The reaction was expected to begin from eight to twelve hours later, the temperature returning to normal from twenty-four to forty-eight hours thereafter. Injected at the above hour, the patient was under close observation during the hours of expected reaction, the temperature-chart showing its characteristics at the usual time of afternoon rounds. If there was no reaction from 1 milligram, two or more, often three, days were allowed to elapse, and a second dose of 2 milligrams was similarly administered. If this dose gave no reaction, 3, then 4, milligrams were administered after equal intervals.

Selection of Cases.—In order to judge correctly of the degree of reaction it was necessary that the patient

CASE XI.

Name [illegible] Date November 19th 1897

Temp.
109
108
107
106
105
104
103
102
101
100
99
98
97
96

Reaction from 5 milligrams of tuberculin.

[1] An extract from the forthcoming Annual Report of the Presbyterian Hospital for 1897–98.

should have been some days without fever (temperature taken every four hours), or should have a chart showing a small daily uniform variation, its average being not above 100° F. Such patients were selected from their charts, without regard to the lesions from which they were convalescing, excluding only cases of cardiac lesions sufficiently severe to cause symptoms, over-nervous persons, and convalescents from typhoid and other exhausting diseases.

Among these may be mentioned cases convalescent from acute articular rheumatism, malaria, acute bronchitis, lateral sclerosis, anemia, postdiphtheritic paralysis, cerebrospinal meningitis, chronic nephritis, varicose ulcer of the leg, etc. These, it will subsequently appear, were among the class of "unsuspected cases," as regards tuberculosis.

Local Irritation.—Swelling, tenderness, and redness about the point of injection, lasting one to two days, were the features noted; no suppuration. Local irritations were only occasional. Pain in the joints, suspected to be tuberculous, was frequent but not constant. Pain in the chests of patients reacting led to the suspicion of localized tuberculosis, but physical signs did not usually make it certain.

It was thought that the carbolic acid used to preserve the solution might be the cause of the local irritation at site of the injection when large doses were given. In several cases, to test this, the solution was made up fresh and used at once, without the addition of carbolic acid. Local irritation followed in the same patient to the same degree when no carbolic-acid preservative was used. Also, a control test was made by injecting an equal volume of distilled water, holding in solution an equal amount of carbolic acid—no local reaction.

The points of greatest interest are:

1. Is there any harm to the patient in the test?
2. Is it of practical value?

The answer to the first inquiry is: In sixty-one cases tested, with doses varying from ½ to 8 milligrams, there was no evidence of any resulting injury, nor is it the opinion of the writer, or of any observer, that there was the slightest evidence of injury to any individual. Indeed, the patients after recovering from the reactions usually believed they were improved by its administration, and believed themselves objects of especial care, profiting by new and improved methods of advanced medicine. Repeatedly the staff and myself, in our rounds, had occasion to say that if we could come to these patients with the mental preoccupation that Koch's was a sovereign tonic remedy, we would feel assured of this correct judgment from what we saw and from what these patients told us. They avowed themselves much im-

CASE XVI.

Name ______ *Date* 3rd 1897

Temp. 109° 108° 107° 106° 105° 104° 103° 102° 101° 100° 99° 98° 97° 96°

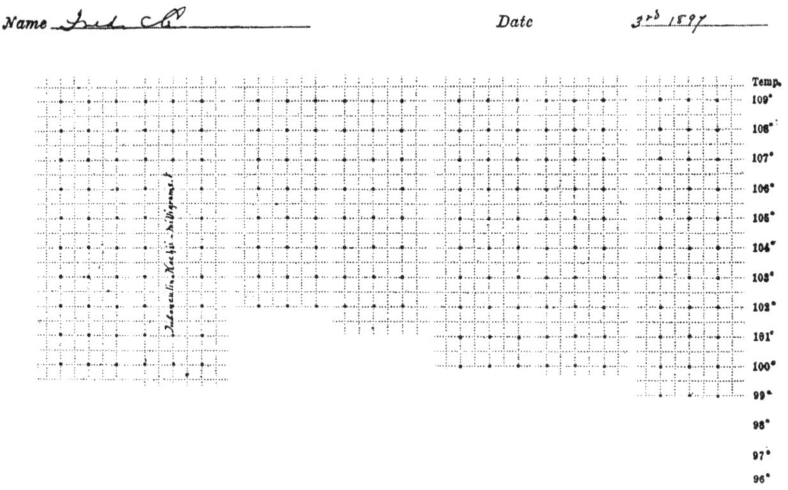

Reaction from 1 milligram of tuberculin.

proved, and were willing to remain in the hospital four days longer for the purpose of receiving another injection, however pronounced the reaction may have been, and however much they wished to go home.

General Reaction.—A characteristic reaction constitutionally manifested itself, usually, by rise of temperature above its habitual line, either the normal or the line of daily variations, the rise taking place six to twelve hours after the injection of tuberculin, the temperature continuing twenty-four hours or more above normal. In other words, the temperature-curve on the chart is characterized by a rather sudden rise, a continuance for a variable time at a high level, and a rapid decline. The patient has been carefully observed and faithfully recorded they will be accepted as a contribution to the discussion of tuberculin as an aid to diagnosis.

In the following cases no tubercle bacilli were found and no local reaction occurred unless mentioned:

I. Cases (sixteen in number) reacting in which clinically a diagnosis of tuberculosis could be made from: (a) Presence of tubercle bacilli in sputum; (b) physical (chest) signs; (c) previous history, bone lesions, and general condition.

CASE I.—Male, aged twenty-four years. Tuberculosis of hip-joint. Diagnosis confirmed by Dr. N. M. Shaffer. Treated several months by extension. Reacted

CASE XLIV.

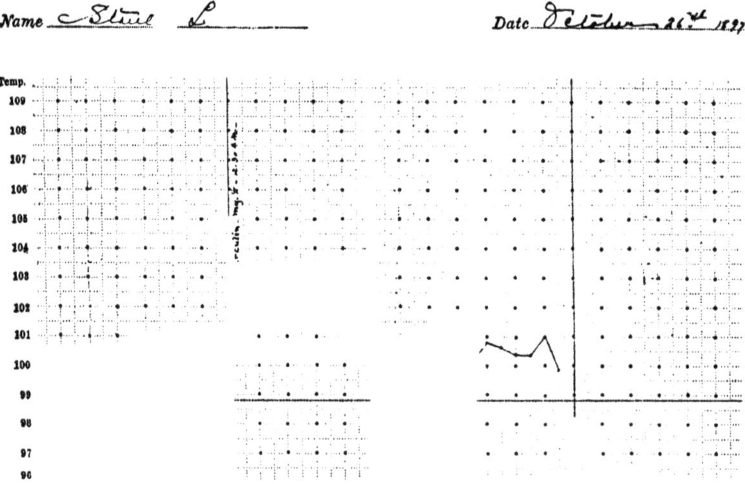

Reaction from 2 milligrams of tuberculin.

a flushed face, headache, sometimes local pains in the joints or chest, sometimes nausea, seldom chilliness, seldom vomiting, usually malaise. These symptoms appear with the fever, and continue and depart with it, the patient feeling quite as well as usual thereafter and, one could be easily convinced, feeling better.

The cases to be considered are sixty-one in number. To answer the two questions proposed, a large number of patients must be injected; those believed to be free from tuberculosis, and having different ailments, as well as those suspected and those known to have tuberculosis. No definite conclusions can be drawn from so limited a number as here given, but if they bear internal evidence of having

to tuberculin, 3 milligrams; no reaction to less amounts. No evidence of tuberculosis elsewhere. Usual temperature ranged from 98.8°–99.8° F. Temperature, 6 to 12 hours after injection, 99°–101.8° F.; from 12 to 24 hours after, 101.8°–98.2° F. Thereafter temperature pursued its usual course.

CASE II.—Female, aged twenty-seven years. T. B. in sputum. Reaction from one-half milligram of tuberculin: Temperature before injection, 98.8°–99.8° F.; after 6 to 12 hours, 100°–101.4° F.; after 12 hours, 101.4°–100.4° F.; after 24 hours, 100.4° F. Malaise.

CASE III.—Male, aged thirty-six years. T. B. in sputum. Reaction from one-half milligram of tuberculin:

Temperature before injection, 98.4°–99.3.° F.; after 6 to 12 hours, 101.3°–103° F.; after 12 to 24 hours, 103°–103.4° F.; after 24 to 48 hours, 100°–99° F. Pain in left chest.

CASE IV.—Male, aged nineteen years. T. B. in sputum. Reaction from one-half milligram of tuberculin: Temperature before injection, 98.4°–99.3° F.; after 6 to 12 hours, 99°–101.4° F.; after 12 to 24 hours, 101.4°–98.2° F.; after 24 to 48 hours, 98.2°–99.6° F. Malaise.

CASE V.—Female, aged twenty-six years. T. B. in sputum. Reaction from 2 milligrams of tuberculin: Temperature before, 99°–100.4° F.; after 6 to 12 hours, 100.4°–101.2° F.; after 12 hours, 101.2°–102.6° F.; veloped, emaciated. No physical signs of pulmonary disease at present, no sputum.

CASE VII.—Female, aged twenty-four years. Dulness, exaggerated breathing, and râles, front, right upper; night-sweats, loss of flesh, "white swelling" of knee. Reaction from 3 milligrams of tuberculin: Temperature before, 99.6°–98.4° F.; after 6 to 12 hours, 98.4°–102° F.; after 12 hours, 102°–102.4° F.; after 24 hours, 102°–100° F. Nausea, headache, muscular pains. Four milligrams, reacted in 16 hours, 103.6° F., with malaise returning to normal within 24 hours.

CASE VIII.—Male, aged eighteen years. T. B. in sputum; pulmonary and laryngeal phthisis. Reaction from

CASE XLVII.

Name Hcue. S 5 I 9 *Date* August 30th 1897

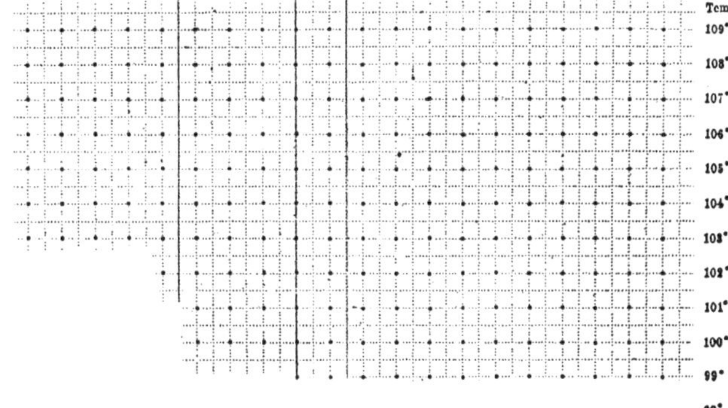

Reaction from 4 milligrams of tuberculin.

after 24 hours, 102.6°–99° F. Malaise.

CASE VI.—Male, aged sixty years. Arthritis; pronounced tuberculous by Dr. Shaffer. Slight reaction from 1 milligram of tuberculin; marked after 2 milligrams: Temperature before, 99°–100° F.; after 6 to 12 hours, 99°–102.4° F.; after 12 to 24 hours, 102.4°–102.8° F.; after 24 to 48 hours, 102.8°–99° F. Headache, pain in ankle, malaise. Subsequently 2 milligrams were given again without reaction. The question arose as to the establishment of tolerance by repeated doses. A year previously this man had had a similar attack in the same ankle, lasting two months. Thickening about bones of left ankle. Chest asymmetric (retracted?), poorly de-

5 milligrams of tuberculin: Temperature before, 100°–98° F.; after 6 to 12 hours, 98°–101.4° F.; after 12 to 24 hours, 101°–99° F.; after 48 hours, 99° F. Chilly, headache, malaise. After 1 milligram, chilliness, local irritation, pain in throat.

CASE IX.—Male, aged twenty years. Cavity, right apex, sweating, anemia. Reaction from 1 milligram of tuberculin: Temperature before, 100°–99° F.; after 6 to 12 hours, 99°–102.2° F.; after 12 hours, 102°–99.4° F.; after 24 hours, 99°–101.4° F. This reaction not being fully satisfactory, 3 milligrams were given nine days later. Temperature before, 101°–99° F.; after 6 to 12 hours, 99°–103.5° F.; after 12 hours, 103.5°–99.2° F.; after

24 hours, 99.2°–102° F. Temperature as observed on the chart is convincing that it was a reaction.

CASE X.—Male, aged thirty-six years. T. B. in sputum. Cavity. Reaction from 1 milligram of tuberculin: Short duration, 101.3° F. at the end of 16 hours. A week later, reaction from 2 milligrams: Temperature before, 98°–98.6° F.; after 6 to 12 hours, 98.6°–103.2° F.; after 12 hours, 103.2°–101° F.; after 24 hours, 101°–99.6° F. Vomiting, headache, malaise.

CASE XI.—Female, aged twenty-three years. T. B. in sputum; cavities both apices. Reaction from 5 milligrams of tuberculin: Temperature before, 96.6°–98° F.; after 6 to 12 hours, 98°–102.2° F.; after 12 hours,

ipheral neuritis. Not tuberculous in general appearance; no cough. Slight reaction from 1 milligram of tuberculin: Temperature before, 98.5°–99° F.; after 6 to 12 hours, 99°–100.4° F.; after 12 hours, 100.4°–99° F.; after 24 hours, 99°–99.2° F. Slight reaction from 3 milligrams; highest, 100.2° F., returning to 99° F. within 48 hours.

CASE XIV.—Male, aged forty years. Pleurisy with effusion two years before. Emaciated, looks tuberculous; dulness, exaggerated voice and breathing in apex, rales; irregular temperature, no expectoration. Reaction from 2 milligrams of tuberculin: Temperature usually 100°–101.5° F.; before injection, 99.8°–100.4° F.; after 6 to

CASE LVIII.

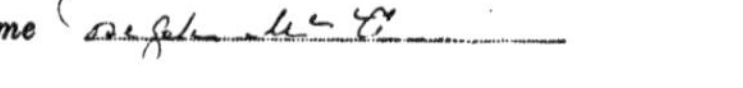

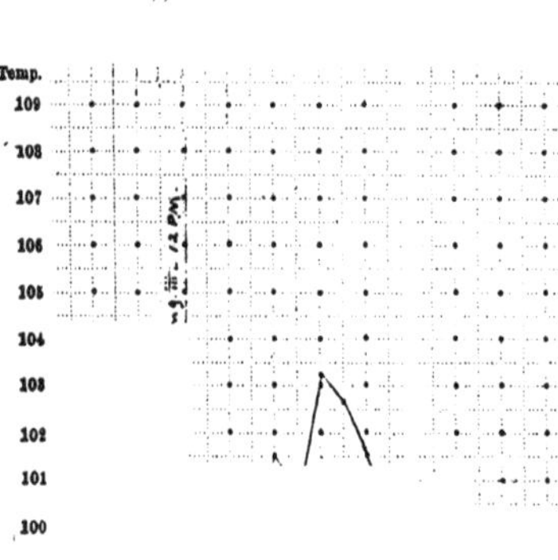

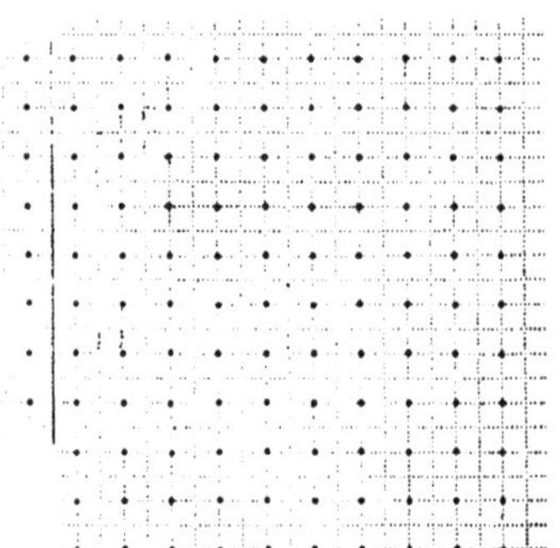

Reaction from 3 milligrams of tuberculin.

102.2°–100° F.; after 24 hours, 100°–98° F. Malaise. No reaction after 1 milligram; slight after 3 milligrams, with apparent increase of cough. Temperature reached 99.5° F. after 12 to 24 hours.

CASE XII.—Male, aged twenty-seven years. Cough, râles, emaciation, hemoptysis, pneumothorax. Reaction from 4 milligrams of tuberculin: Temperature before, 97.5°–98.6° F.; after 6 to 12 hours, 98.6°–100° F.; after 12 hours, 100°–101.6° F.; after 24 hours, 101.6°–100° F. Headache and local irritation. Five days later was given 5 milligrams, without reaction.

CASE XIII.—Female, aged twenty-eight years. Crepitant rales at apex and slight dulness; entered with per-

12 hours, 100.4°–104.4° F.; after 12 hours, 104.4°–103° F.; after 24 hours, 103°–99.8° F. Pronounced malaise.

First dose administered was one-half milligram, no reaction; second dose, 2 milligrams, reaction as above; third dose, 1 milligram. Temperature reached 103.4° F. Typical in all respects. Tolerance not established.

CASE XV.—Male, aged thirty-six years. Small cavity in right apex, and consolidation. T. B. found after long searching. Reaction from one-half milligram of tuberculin: Temperature before, 98.4°–99.3° F.; after 6 to 12 hours, 101.3°–103° F.; after 12 hours, 103°–103.4° F.; after 24 hours, 100°–99° F. Pain in chest, malaise.

CASE XVI.—Male, aged twenty-four years. Hemoptysis, loss of flesh, night-sweats, cough, expectoration, irregular temperature, crepitant and subcrepitant rales over left lung, with dulness at apex. No T. B. after repeated examinations. Slight reaction from one-half milligram of tuberculin, 101° F. in 24 hours. Reaction from 1 milligram: Temperature, 102° F.; 12 to 24 hours after injection, chilly, slight local swelling and tenderness. Reaction from 2 milligrams characteristic and well marked: Temperature before, 99.7°–98.7° F.; after 6 to 12 hours, 98.7°–103.5° F.; after 12 hours, 105°–103.5 F.; after 24 hours, 103.3°–100° F. Headache, chilly, nausea, general malaise, pain in left chest. Temperature returned to normal, and patient left hospital improved, having gained eight pounds.

2. Cases (nineteen in number) not reacting, in which there was no reason to suspect tuberculosis.

CASE XVII.—Female, aged thirty-two years. Cerebral tumor. On fifth injection of 4 milligrams of tuberculin, temperature after 16 hours, 101.4° F. No general symptoms. On sixth injection of 5 milligrams, temperature after 14 hours, 101.2° F. No general symptoms. Temperature normal after 24 hours. Patient left hospital. Diagnosis: Brain tumor. From the course of temperature observed on the chart this was not regarded as a reaction.

CASE XVIII.—Male, aged thirty-eight years. Lobar pneumonia. Previous to entrance cough during three months, and loss of flesh. Wife had phthisis. A child died of "meningitis." No T. B. found. No reaction from 5 milligrams of tuberculin. Recovery complete. Appearance such as not to create a suspicion that he was tuberculous.

CASE XIX.—Male, aged fifty-four years. Syphilitic pachymeningitis. No reaction from 2 milligrams of tuberculin.

CASE XX.—Female, aged twenty-six years. Gastro-enteritis, anemia. Brother died of phthisis. Fairly strong and healthy appearing. No reaction from 1, 2, or 3 milligram of tuberculin.

CASE XXI.—Male, aged thirty-nine years. Sciatica. Large, healthy-looking man. No reaction from ½ to 1 milligram of tuberculin. Slight local irritation.

CASE XXII.—Female, aged forty-five years. Gastritis. No suspicion of tuberculosis. No reaction from 1, 2, 3, 4, or 5 milligrams of tuberculin, either constitutional or local.

CASE XXIII.—Male, aged sixty-five years. Cerebral hemorrhage, hemiplegia. Large, robust man, engineer. No reaction from ½, 1, 2, or 3 milligrams of tuberculin, at intervals of three days, till 8 milligrams were given. No reaction, local or constitutional.

CASE XXIV.—Female, aged one and one-half years. Chronic spinal meningitis; recovered. Lumbar puncture; fluid negative on guinea-pig inoculation. No reaction from $\frac{1}{10}$-milligram of tuberculin, grading up to 1 milligram.

CASE XXV.—Male, aged forty-one years. Multiple neuritis. No reaction from ½ to 1, 2, 3, and 4 milligrams of tuberculin.

CASE XXVI.—Male, aged thirty-five years. Diagnosis on entrance: Constipation. Well-nourished; negative history. No reaction from 1 milligram of tuberculin.

CASE XXVII.—Female, aged thirty-five years. Puerperal sepsis. Negative history. No reaction from one-half milligram of tuberculin. Left hospital.

CASE XXVIII.—Male, aged forty-nine years. Dyspepsia. No evidence of tuberculosis. No reaction from 1, 4, or 6 milligrams of tuberculin, local or constitutional.

CASE XXIX.—Female, aged thirty-three years. Malaria (plasmodium found). No reaction from 1 or 2 milligrams of tuberculin. Malarial chill set in forty-eight hours after last injection.

CASE XXX.—Male, aged fifty years. Cirrhosis of liver; pleurisy, serofibrinous. No T. B. found in sputum or fluid. No reaction, local or constitutional, from 1, 3, 5, or 7 milligrams of tuberculin.

CASE XXXI.—Female, aged fifty-five years. Malignant tumor of the kidney (sarcoma), confirmed by exploration. No reaction from 1 or 3 milligrams of tuberculin.

CASE XXXII.—Female, aged fifty-one years. Gastric ulcer, abscess of pancreas (autopsy). Slight rise of temperature after 3 milligrams of tuberculin. No malaise, uncertain reaction.

CASE XXXIII.—Female, aged thirty-six years. Right kidney enlarged; leucocytes in urine, moderate amount. No T. B. found. Well-nourished, no loss of flesh. No reaction from 1, 2, or 3 milligrams of tuberculin.

CASE XXXIV.—Female, aged fifty-six years. Tertiary syphilis. Poorly nourished; slight cough; slight dulness, breathing harsh, few rales, not constant, in upper right lobe. Continuous temperature for eleven weeks. History negative; no sputum. One, 2, 3, and 5 milligrams of tuberculin given. No malaise; slight elevation of temperature, not considered a reaction.

CASE XXXV.—Male, aged forty-two years; maltster. Cirrhosis of liver. No reaction from ½ or 1 milligram of tuberculin. Died. No autopsy.

3. Cases (sixteen in number) reacting, in which tuberculosis was clinically suspected.

CASE XXXVI.—Female, aged twenty-four years. Diagnosis: Tuberculosis of ovaries or peritoneum; general abdominal pains and tenderness during five months; loss of flesh. Reaction from 1 milligram of tuberculin: Temperature before, 98.2°–99.6° F.; after 6 to 12 hours, 99.6°–99.4° F.; after 12 hours, 99.4°–102.6° F.; after 24 hours, 102.6°–100° F. Headache, malaise, increased abdominal pain. Nine days later, 1 milligram again given: After 12 to 24 hours, temperature, 101°–100.5° F., with malaise. Six days later, 2 milligrams: Temperature, 12 to 24 hours after, 102.8°–101.6° F. One week later, 2 milligrams: Temperature before, 98°–98.2° F.; after 6 to 12 hours, 98.2°–102.8° F.; after 12 hours, 102.8°–101.5° F.; after 24 hours, 101.5°–98.8° F. Malaise, moderate local irritation.

CASE XXXVII.—Male, aged forty-five years. Diagnosis: Tuberculous ankle. Father and sister died of phthisis. Ankle swollen, muscles of leg atrophied. Reaction from 5 milligrams of tuberculin twice: Temperature before, 99.2°–97.8° F.; after 6 to 12 hours, 97.8°–

100.5° F.; after 12 hours, 100.5°-101.8° F.; after 24 hours, 101.8°-99° F. Pain in foot, general malaise.

CASE XXXVIII.—Male, aged eighteen years. Tuberculous arthritis of knees and elbow, opinion of Dr. N. M. Shaffer. Negative family history. Duration, five years. Slow reaction from 2 milligrams of tuberculin: Temperature before, 98.4°-100.5° F.; after 6 to 12 hours, 100.5°-100.2° F.; after 12 hours, 100°-101.6° F.; after 24 hours, 101.6°-100.2° F. At a subsequent injection of 2 milligrams, temperature rose to 100.6° in 14 hours, and in 70 hours to 102° F.; then fell to normal, and so remained.

CASE XXXIX.—Female, aged fifty years. Abdominal nodular masses. Bloody fluid aspirated from peritoneal and right pleural cavity. Loss of flesh, anemia, sputum. No T. B. found. Moderate reaction from 1 milligram of tuberculin. Malaise, nausea. Greater reaction from 2 milligrams three days later. Five days later, temperature before, 98.8°-99° F.; after 6 to 12 hours, 99°-101.8° F.; after 12 hours, 101.8°-99.2° F.; after 24 hours, 99.2°-99.8° F. Vomiting, malaise, abdominal pain, and pain in right side.

CASE XL.—Female, aged thirty-six years. Diagnosis: Lobar pneumonia and pleurisy (tuberculous?). Consolidation persisting for weeks; râles for two and one-half months; profuse night-sweats; temperature varying from 103°-98° F. Negative family history. Moderate reaction from 1 milligram of tuberculin. No malaise; reaction slight and not characteristic from 2 milligrams. Reaction from 3 milligrams: Temperature before, 99.8°-98° F.; after 6 to 12 hours, 98.8°-99.4° F.; after 12 hours, 99.4°-102.4° F.; after 24 hours, 102°-100° F. Pain in back and general. Patient left hospital in improved general condition; slight dulness and few râles. Eighteen days later returned for examination: Slight dulness, no râles; condition good; improved in flesh and strength; does her own washing.

CASE XLI.—Female, aged twenty-three years. Hemiplegia (hemorrhage), and malaria (plasmodium found). Small frame; looked tuberculous; expectoration (no T. B. found). Reaction from 1 milligram of tuberculin: Temperature before, 100°-99° F.; after 6 to 12 hours, 99°-99.5° F.; after 12 hours, 99.5°-103.8° F.; after 24 hours, 103.8°-99° F. Chill 6 hours after injection; sudden rise of temperature, and sudden fall; spleen large, plasmodium found. Five days later, 1 milligram of tuberculin: Temperature before, 98°-99.4° F.; after 6 to 12 hours, 99°-102.8° F.; after 12 hours, 103.6°-101° F.; after 24 hours, 101°-99° F. Malaise, local irritation. Guinea-pig did not develop tuberculosis.

CASE XLII.—Male, aged forty-five years. Chronic lead-poisoning (painter) and chronic nephritis. Dulness, right apex anterior, subcrepitant râles. Poorly nourished. Reaction from 3 milligrams of tuberculin: Temperature before, 100°-99° F.; after 6 to 12 hours, 98.2°-101.4° F.; after 12 hours, 101.4°-101.7° F.; after 24 hours, 101.7°-99.5° F. Headache, nausea, malaise.

CASE XLIII.—Female, aged seventeen years. Arthritis of right ankle; edema, pain, redness. Hemoptysis once in life. Slight dulness and exaggerated voice at apex. Does not look tuberculous. Slight reaction from 2 milligrams of tuberculin. Pain in chest. Reaction from 3 milligrams (twice): Temperature before, 97.2°-98° F.; after 6 to 12 hours, 98°-102.2 F.; after 12 hours, 102°-102.8° F.; after 24 hours, 102.8°-99.4° F. Vomiting, malaise. After five weeks, still pain and tenderness in joint.

CASE XLIV.—Male, aged thirty-three years. Alcoholic. Dry pleurisy. Irregular temperature for ten weeks—98.6°-103° F. Loss of flesh. Reaction from 1 milligram of tuberculin: Temperature before, 99°-101° F.; after 6 to 12 hours, 101.4°-103.6° F.; after 12 hours, 103.6°-102° F.; after 24 hours, 102°-100° F. Malaise, slight local reaction. Subsequently characteristic reaction from 2 and 3 milligrams, with malaise. On a graphic chart this was believed to be a characteristic curve, a reaction.

CASE XLV.—Male, aged forty-two years. Pleurisy with effusion, persisting six weeks; loss of flesh. Does not look tuberculous. Slight reaction from 2 milligrams of tuberculin. Reaction from 3 milligrams: Temperature before, 99.2°-98.5° F.; after 6 to 12 hours, 98.5°-102.3° F.; after 12 hours, 102.3°-102.8 F.; after 24 hours, 102.8°-99° F. Marked local reaction.

CASE XLVI.—Female, aged twenty-three years. Convalescence from suspected irregular typhoid fever. Slight dulness at apex, few râles. Reaction slight from 3 milligrams of tuberculin: Temperature before, 99°-98° F.; after 6 to 12 hours, 98°-100° F.; after 12 hours, 100°-101° F.; after 24 hours, 101°-99.2° F. No malaise. Reaction considered fairly characteristic.

CASE XLVII.—Female, aged twenty-three years. Neurasthenia, with an uncertain history of pleurisy. Father died of phthisis. Râles; anemia; one hemoptysis (uncertain). Reaction from 4 milligrams of tuberculin: Temperature before, 98°-99° F.; after 6 to 12 hours, 99.2°-102.5° F.; after 12 hours, 102.5°-100.5° F.; after 24 hours, normal. Malaise.

CASE XLVIII.—Female, aged twenty years. Anemia; right apex, post. expiration prolonged and high-pitched. Negative family history; well developed. Slight reaction from 1 milligram of tuberculin. Reaction from 2 milligrams of tuberculin: Temperature before, 98°-98.4° F.; after 6 to 12 hours, 98.4°-100° F.; after 12 hours, 100°-101° F.; after 24 hours, 101°-99° F. Headache, nausea, and vomiting. Two milligrams again injected gave no reaction. Three milligrams gave 100.4° F. within 24 hours, with pains in back. Four milligrams gave a marked reaction—102.5° F. in 12 hours, falling to normal in 72 hours, with pains.

CASE XLIX.—Female, aged twenty-eight years. Small, poorly developed; cough mornings with expectoration. Reaction from 3 milligrams of tuberculin: Temperature before, 98.5°-99.3° F.; after 6 to 12 hours, 99.3°-100.2° F.; after 12 hours, 100.2-100° F.; after 24 hours, 100°-98° F. Malaise. On fifth injection of 4 milligrams, temperature reached 103.4° F. in 17 hours. Headache and nausea.

CASE L.—Male, aged twenty-nine years. Bronchitis, dulness, right apex. Six months before had a "cold," lasting one month. Said he was always healthy; light frame. Slight reaction from 3 milligrams of tuberculin, with pain in back. Reaction from 4 milligrams: Temperature before, 99°-98.6° F.; after 6 to 12 hours, 98.6°-99° F.; after 12 hours, 99.4°-102° F.; after 24 hours, 102°-101° F. Very marked local irritation, indurated swelling and tenderness, chill. Question—whether local irritation could not account for temperature.

CASE LI.—Female, aged twenty-four years. Acute rheumatism. Poorly nourished; anemia; losing flesh; cough with expectoration; "looks tuberculous." No chest signs. Reaction from 1 milligram of tuberculin: Temperature before, 98.5°-98° F.; after 6 to 12 hours, 98°-98.6° F.; after 12 hours, 98.6°-102° F., after 24 hours, 102°-99.5° F. Malaise, pains in legs.

4. Cases (seven in number) reacting, in which tuberculosis was not suspected or was clinically doubtful.

CASE LII.—Male, aged thirty-two years. Acute articular rheumatism. Brother died of tuberculous laryngitis. Reaction from 3 milligrams of tuberculin: Temperature before, 98.4°-98.6° F.; after 6 to 12 hours, 98.6°-102.8° F.; after 12 hours, 102.8°-103.6° F.; after 24 hours, 103.6°-99.5° F. Malaise. Three milligrams of tuberculin repeated after four days gave: Temperature before, 99.2°-99° F.; after 6 to 12 hours, 99°-104.2° F.; after 12 hours, 104.2°-104.3° F.; after 24 hours, 104.3°-98.3° F. Reactions marked and characteristic, and no foci found.

CASE LIII.—Male, aged twenty-one years. Post-diphtheritic paralysis of legs. Healthy-looking, not strong frame. Negative family history. Slight reaction from ½ milligram of tuberculin; greater from 1 milligram. Reaction from 2 milligrams: Temperature before, 99.4°-99.4° F.; after 6 to 12 hours, 99.4°-101.6° F.; after 12 hours, 101.6°-102.6° F.; after 24 hours, 102°-99.8 F. Headache.

CASE LIV.—Male, aged two and one-half years. Cerebrospinal meningitis. Convalescent. One-fifth, ⅓, ⅗ milligrams, up to 1 milligram of tuberculin, with no reaction; $1\frac{4}{15}$ milligrams gave reaction. Temperature reached 101° F. within 12 hours, 100.8° F. within 14 hours. Fair reaction. Recovered from chronic spinal meningitis, but deaf.; double optic neuritis. Spinal puncture; no tuberculosis in injected guinea-pig.

CASE LV.—Male, aged twenty-two years. Poor development; chronic hydrarthrosis; fluid clear; no growth on blood-serum. Reaction fair (101.9° F.) from 2 milligrams of tuberculin. Second injection of 2 milligrams: Temperature before, 98°-99.6° F.; after 6 to 12 hours, 99.6°-102° F.; after 12 hours, 102°-100° F.; after 24 hours, 100°-99.6° F. No symptoms. Patient under observation three months; condition unchanged.

CASE LVI.—Male, aged thirty-four years. Malaria; negtive personal and family history. Three milligrams of tuberculin gave good reaction, and no malarial organisms found: Temperature before, 98.2°-98° F.; after 6 to 12 hours, 98°-100° F.; after 12 hours, 100°-102.2° F.; after 24 hours, 102.2°-99.2° F. Subsequently did not react to 4 milligrams.

CASE LVII.—Female, aged sixty years. Varicose ulcer of leg. Subcrepitant râles in both bases on entrance. Reaction from 3 milligrams of tuberculin (temperature 103.4° F.), local and constitutional. Reaction from 4 milligrams: Temperature before, 97.4°-98.5° F.; after 6 to 12 hours, 98.5°-102° F.; after 12 hours, 102°-103.2° F.; after 24 hours, 103.2°-100° F. General malaise, vomiting. Subsequent injection of 3 milligrams gave 104.6° F. within 12 hours. Malaise, vomiting, and local irritation. Six injections given, reactions from 3 and 4 milligrams.

CASE LVIII.—Male, aged forty-six years. Lateral sclerosis. No evidences of tuberculosis. Reaction from 3 milligrams of tuberculin: Temperature before, 99°-99.4° F.; after 6 to 12 hours, 99.4°-101.4° F.; after 12 hours, 101.4°-100° F.; after 24 hours, 100°-99° F. Three milligrams subsequently produced no reaction. Question—whether tolerance was established.

5. Cases (two in number) not reacting, in which tuberculosis was clinically suspected.

CASE LIX.—Male, aged fifty-two years. Pleurisy, serofibrinous (pneumonia eleven years before); loss of flesh. Dulness, persisting four weeks after aspiration, with moderate irregularity of temperature. Thirty ounces of fluid aspirated; no growth on blood-serum. No reaction after ½ or 1 milligram of tuberculin; after 2, uncertain. Patient left hospital.

CASE LX.—Male, adult. Emphysema; hemoptysis. Sister died of phthisis. Winter cough, expectoration, sweating. Two hemorrhages, bright blood, on day of admission. Râles over upper right front and back. No T. B. found. No loss of flesh. Left hospital with lungs clear of râles. No reaction from 1, 2, or 3 milligrams of tuberculin. Dr. James felt certain this patient had tuberculosis.

6. No reaction. One case afterward proved tuberculous (autopsy).

CASE LXI.—Female, aged twenty-six years. Brain tumor, which on autopsy proved to be spindle-cell sarcoma—pressing upon the pons sufficiently to deform and displace it. In addition to this there were found at one apex a few adhesions, a number of old caseous nodules, and a few recent tubercles in near proximity. This case was never suspected to be tuberculous; examination of lungs negative. No reaction from 1, 3, or 5 milligrams of tuberculin: Temperature before, 96°-100° F.; with 1 milligram after 6 to 10 hours, 98° F.; after 12 to 24 hours, 100° F.; from 24 to 48 hours, 97° F. After 3 milligrams, highest temperature was 98.4° F. After 5 milligrams, 99.8° F. was the highest temperature 12 hours after injection. Question—Did pressure upon thermic centers cause the fluctuation of temperature and interfere with the test?

TOTAL, SIXTY-ONE CASES.

Group 1.—Reacting, tuberculous, 16 cases.
Group 2.—*Not* reacting, *not* tuberculous, 19 cases.
Group 3.—Reacting, clinically suspected, 16 cases.
Behaving as *expected*, Groups 1, 2, 3, total 51 cases; eighty-four per cent.
Group 4.—Reacting, clinically doubtful, 7 cases.
Group 5.—Not reacting, clinically suspected, 2 cases.

Group 6.—Not reacting, proved tuberculous, 1 case.

To return to the two principal inquiries of the paper, *viz.*, in this test (1) is there any harmful result to the patient and (2) any help to the diagnostician?

1. There was no possible injury observed in any case.

2. Of the total 61 cases, 51, or eighty-four per cent., did what was clinically expected, *i. e.*, the diagnosis was sustained.

The figures say that but 5 out of 6 tests confirmed the clinical diagnosis. Here let the answer to the second inquiry stand.

In this contribution to the discussion we have not brought forward the experiences in animal tests for tuberculosis, nor referred to the frequency with which small, unsuspected, tuberculous lesions are found at autopsies. The practical value of the test is to be worked out on the lines employed in this investigation. We have sought, so far as a limited number of cases can serve, to put forward answers to two practical inquiries and await an accumulation of experience to furnish the answer as to the practical value of the test.

If the tests were to be made on a second 61 patients, using the same strength solution of tuberculin, I would avoid slowly increasing doses. Tolerance may have been established in certain cases. These points have, however, been interrogated without definite results. For instance, after slowly increasing doses, patients have reacted to 5 milligrams of tuberculin. Again, patients have reacted to 2 milligrams, and have not subsequently reacted to 4 milligrams. Patients occasionally reacted again to 4 milligrams. Patients occasionally reacted to a small dose, failed on intermediate, and reacted again to larger doses. These reactions and failures have thrown doubt upon certain cases, and all doubt has been testimony against a favorable judgment on the action of tuberculin. In an effort to secure judicial fairness, the tendency has been to make the results less favorable than perhaps they should be. Again, the last case (61), proved tuberculous, the presence of "a few recent tubercles" about old cheesy masses, surrounded by firm adhesions—this can be assumed to correspond to the cases reported by veterinary commissions. Cattle having small recent tuberculous masses or glandular tuberculosis most commonly show more pronounced reactions than those having advanced tuberculosis. Just how active the "few recent tubercles" may have been one cannot say, but here is a case, proved tuberculous (beginning?), in which the test failed. Yet it must not be forgotten that the patient's temperature was fluctuating, and the lesion, brain tumor, sufficient to seriously disturb the physical economy. The effect of this upon the test no one can state in the light of present experience.

As a result of the experience here recorded it is to be advised:

1. To be sure of the quality and strength[1] of the tuberculin used.

2. To begin, in adults, with 1 milligram; if there is no reaction after an interval of two or, better, three days give 3 or 4 milligrams.

[1] Dr. Trudeau in a subsequent communication expresses a doubt as to the possibility, at the present time, of producing tuberculin of standard strength.

SUMMARY.

The present list comprises sixty-one cases.

Sixteen patients believed to be tuberculous all reacted to the test.

Nineteen patients believed *not* to be tuberculous all failed to react.

Sixteen patients clinically believed to be, but never proved, tuberculous, all reacted.

Fifty-one patients, eighty-four per cent. (the above), behaved clinically as was expected.

Seven patients, clinically doubtful, reacted.

Two patients, clinically suspected, failed to react.

One patient, subsequently proved tuberculous (autopsy "a few recent tubercles"), failed to react.

No harm to any patient from the test.

Local irritation (never suppuration) occurred in both tuberculous and non-tuberculous patients at the site of injection; no significance.

Constitutional reaction has a fairly characteristic temperature curve, with headache, local pains, malaise.

It is the personal conviction of the writer that with further study of dosage and methods of administration, the tuberculin test will prove to be a material aid in diagnosis of latent tuberculosis.

To Dr. H. S. Carter, house physician, I wish to express my appreciation of his never-ending devotion to the details in connection with this investigation, and of his good observation and judgment.

MEDICAL PROGRESS.

Treatment of Wounds by Steam.—BEYER (*Deutsch. Med. Wochenschr.*, February 24, 1898), observing the satisfactory results which follow the use of steam as a disinfectant for surgical dressings, has applied it to granulating wounds, abscesses, etc., to facilitate cicatrization, directing upon them at a distance of 50 cm. (20 in.), a jet of steam at a temperature of 53° C. (127° F). The results were most favorable, and ulcerations which were resistant to treatment rapidly healed under the influence of the steam.

Concussion of the Brain and the Use of the Seton.—This is a time when physicians are again trying the famed remedies of olden times, blood-letting for instance, and it is therefore of interest to read (*Berl. Klin. Wochenschr.* February 21 1898) that HEIDENHAIN has employed a seton with success in six cases of concussion of the brain with resulting complications such as dizziness, pain, etc. In all of the cases mentioned, remedies of various sorts had been tried without effecting a cure, while the introduction under aseptic precautions of a seton of linen, through the thick skin of the back of the neck, did not fail in a single instance to bring about a cure. The seton was daily removed and a fresh piece of linen, smeared with an irritating salve was introduced, while the whole was covered with a light dressing.

THE MEDICAL NEWS.

A WEEKLY JOURNAL

OF MEDICAL SCIENCE.

COMMUNICATIONS are invited from all parts of the world. Original articles contributed *exclusively* to THE MEDICAL NEWS will after publication be liberally paid for (accounts being rendered quarterly), or 250 reprints will be furnished in place of other remuneration. When necessary to elucidate the text, illustrations will be engraved from drawings or photographs furnished by the author. Manuscripts should be typewritten.

Address the Editor: J. RIDDLE GOFFE, M.D.,
No. 111 FIFTH AVENUE (corner of 18th St.), NEW YORK.

Subscription Price, including postage in U. S. and Canada.

PER ANNUM IN ADVANCE	$4.00
SINGLE COPIES	.10
WITH THE AMERICAN JOURNAL OF THE MEDICAL SCIENCES, PER ANNUM	7.50

Subscriptions may begin at any date. The safest mode of remittance is by bank check or postal money order, drawn to the order of the undersigned. When neither is accessible, remittances may be made, at the risk of the publishers, by forwarding in *registered* letters.

LEA BROTHERS & CO.,
No. 111 FIFTH AVENUE (corner of 18th St.), NEW YORK, AND NOS. 706, 708 & 710 SANSOM ST., PHILADELPHIA.

SATURDAY, APRIL 23, 1898.

SOME MEDICAL ASPECTS OF THE APPROACHING WAR.

"YOU know it is four killed to one wounded since the new ammunition came in. It is better so. I don't want to be wounded; and hate to think of being dreadfully mangled, and then patched up, with half my limbs and senses gone, yet 'a triumph of surgical skill.' No! I prefer to step down or up, and out of this world."

These are the words, penned to his brother by the American hero, Captain McGiffin of the Chinese battleship Chen Yuen, in the fight at Yalu with the Japanese, September 17, 1894. Such is the sentiment that will doubtless animate many a brave man in the contest that seems now so imminent, and such too will doubtless be his fate. It is estimated that in a naval engagement the torpedo-boat is least likely to escape destruction, and that in an attempt to accomplish its deadly work its crew is destined to certain death. Says a prominent daily: "A tiny torpedo-boat may wipe a five-million-dollar battleship off the sea and send five hundred men to the bottom, but the likelihood that any one on board the former will live to boast of the feat is very scant." Death will doubtless come either instantaneously by explosion, or by drowning the imprisoned men going down with the ship.

To men who meet this sad fate the medical arm of the service can be of no avail, but to the sick, the wounded, the suffering, the medical and surgical corps hold out assurance, by active scientific and efficient preparations, that reparative surgical skill is keeping abreast of the destructive agents of war. Improved methods in the conservation of life and limb are keeping step with modern weapons. Hygienic and sanitary measures, too, are surrounding the unfortunate sick and wounded with conditions most favorable for their comfort and recovery. Some weeks since the MEDICAL NEWS recorded the fact that the Navy Department had purchased the fast steamer Creole of the Cromwell line, and was fitting her up as a hospital ship to accompany the squadron and be present at engagements.

Anent the new conditions surrounding a modern naval engagement the *Boston Medical and Surgical Journal*, in a recent editorial, speculates upon the more or less permanent but subordinate injuries which the participants are likely to carry away from a conflict, especially the effects of concussion upon men confined in a limited air space, as deafness, and the effect upon the nervous system generally. In this connection the writer makes prominent the difference in the shock experienced in a naval engagement and that produced by the sudden and unexpected accident in a railway train, although in the enormously destructive effects of the torpedo and submarine mine the unexpected is becoming a large factor in the shock of warfare. Neuroses of a most varied sort are born of the traumatisms of the gas explosion and the railway accident, as well as the traumatisms of war, and grow to quite hopeless proportions as the years go by. The analogy is so intimate that each may throw some light upon the other.

CORNELL'S MEDICAL COLLEGE.

IN accordance with the anticipatory announcement in the columns of the MEDICAL NEWS, the Board of Trustees of Cornell University has formally established a medical department to be located in New York City, and has accepted the retiring members of the Medical Department of the New York University as its faculty. This medical school will be known as the Cornell University College of Medicine. The establishment of the medical department at this time was made possible by the munificent gift of Colonel Oliver H. Payne amounting to half a million dollars. The location of the buildings has not yet been definitely determined but will be in the vicinity of Bellevue Hospital.

The requirements for graduation will be a four-years' course of study. Two full years of the medical curriculum will be credited to the student who has gone through the literary department of Cornell University. This is in conformity with the rule which obtains in the Law Department. In accordance with the charter of Cornell University the holders of State scholarships will receive free tuition in the medical school as well as in other departments of the University. This department will also come under the uniform regulation of being open to women as well as men. The following is the roster of the faculty as far as it has been appointed:

William M. Polk, Dean and Professor of Obstetrics and Gynecology; Lewis A. Stimson, Professor of Surgery; Rudolph A. Witthaus, Professor of Chemistry, Physics, and Toxicology; W. Gilman Thompson, Professor of Medicine; George Woolsey, Professor of Anatomy and Clinical Surgery; Henry P. Loomis, Professor of Materia Medica, Therapeutics, and Clinical Medicine; J. Clifton Edgar, Professor of Obstetrics; F. W. Gwyer, Professor of Operative and Clinical Surgery; Irving S. Haynes, Professor of Practical Anatomy; Joseph E. Winters, Professor of Diseases of Children; Newton M. Shaffer, Professor of Orthopedic Surgery; Gorham Bacon, Professor of Otology; Irvin Sickels, Assistant-Professor of Chemistry and Physics; W. F. Stone, Instructor in Anatomy; Assistant-Demonstrator in Anatomy; George D. Hamlen, Instructor in Obstetrics and Gynecology; Lewis W. Riggs, Instructor in Chemistry; Percival R. Bolton, Instructor in Surgery; Warren Coleman, Instructor in Clinical Medicine; Edmund P. Shelby, Instructor in Materia Medica and Therapeutics; John Rogers, Assistant-Demonstrator in Anatomy; S. Connors, Instructor in Medicine.

In connection with the resignation of the members of this faculty from the University of the City of New York, the question arose whether the hospital positions occupied by them would be vacated by their resignation or whether they would carry the hospital position with them into the new school, thus securing the opportunity for clinical instruction in the new field. This has been definitely settled by the recent decision of the Commissioner of Charities, in which he decrees that no member of the visiting-staff loses his hospital position by resigning his professorial chair in a medical school. If this ruling holds, and at present there seems no reason to doubt it, the new school will spring full-fledged into existence and active clinical work.

TWO WAYS OF REGARDING CARBUNCLES.

PHYSICIANS of New York and its vicinity, and probably of a much more extended area, have recently received reprints of two articles upon the treatment of carbuncles; one written by a well-known surgeon, and the other by an equally celebrated dermatologist. The methods of treatment advocated in the two articles are so radically different that a comparison of them is most instructive, the more so as the writers agree upon the causes which produce a carbuncle, and both affirm that the customary treatment by poultices and incisions is painful and dangerous. The surgeon says: "If all such (fatal) cases were enumerated they would represent quite a respectable figure." The dermatologist says: "The last patient incised (by him) died from this and other complications, but there has not been a single case with such result in my practice since."

If treatment by incision is so unsatisfactory, how shall it be improved? In their answers to this question our friends take opposite views. Says the surgeon, "the affected area is filled with deadly bacteria which will cause a slough of the immediately surrounding tissue, and may even spread further. Therefore, to avoid this risk as well as to save time, let us take out the whole thing." He makes a circular incision down to the deep fascia, and removes the carbuncle in toto. "The results" he adds "have been extremely gratifying."

The dermatologist declares that "the power of resistance of the body must have been at a low ebb, or the germs would not have found its tissues a favorable soil." He, therefore, gives a mercurial purge to relieve the torpidity of the liver, iron to tone up the system, and perfectly fresh sulphid of calcium, ¼-grain every two hours, to keep suppuration in check. The carbuncle is covered with a salve of rose-water ointment, into 2 ounces of which there has been rubbed 10 drops of carbolic acid, and

2 drams each of fluid extract of ergot, starch, and oxid of zinc. During fifteen years he has treated carbuncles and other suppurative lesions in this manner, and has never been compelled to resort to the knife. Sometimes the inflammation is aborted, but usually the pus and sloughs readily come away, and with a minimum loss of time and of tissue.

Attention is directed to this subject, not because of the novelty of the treatment suggested, but because two men, both of whom are well-read, and who have for years occupied important hospital positions, hold such radically opposite views upon the treatment of so simple a trouble as a carbuncle. "Who shall decide when doctors disagree?"

ECHOES AND NEWS.

Ernest Hart's Estate.—The late Mr. Ernest Hart, editor of the *British Medical Journal*, left an estate worth about $80,000.

Smallpox in England.—The epidemic of smallpox which has been prevailing in Middlesborough, England, is now said to be fairly under control, although more than 400 patients are still under treatment in the hospital. More than 1200 cases have occurred.

Presidency of the General Medical Council.—Sir William Turner, who holds the chair of anatomy at Edinburgh University, has been unanimously elected to the presidency of the General Medical Council of Great Britain made vacant by the death of Sir Richard Quain.

An Attractive Feature of the Coroner's Jury.—According to the *Scientific American*, twenty-two business men who acted as the coroner's jury in the investigation of the recent great fire in London, England, and served fourteen working days, received four pence (eight cents) each as compensation.

A Physician Victorious in a Malpractice Suit.—Dr. C. D. Palmer of Cincinnati, against whom a malpractice suit was brought in the name of a Mrs. Eiselein, may well feel relieved that the case has been decided in his favor. The suit was begun about eight years ago, and has been stubbornly contested.

Decrease in the Number of Medical Students.—According to the *Lancet* (London), there seems to be in England a decrease in the wild rush by young men into the medical profession, and figures in the Medical-Students' Register are quoted to prove it. In 1897 the smallest number were registered since 1871.

Up to the Standard in Medical Requirements.—The Western University of London, Ontario, has been admitted by the Council of the Royal College of Surgeons, England, to the list of institutions recognized by the board at which the whole curriculum of professional study may be completed, and whose graduates in medicine are admissible to the final examination.

The After-Care Association.—In London this association, the only one of the kind in England, does much good work in assisting poor persons who have been discharged "recovered" from insane asylums. During the year 1897, 147 cases were brought before the council as compared with 135 cases during the preceding twelve months. Of the 147 cases 105 were in females and 42 in males. Assistance was given by boarding them out in cottages in the country, by gifts of money and clothing, by the finding of occupations, and in other ways.

Imbecile Farm for Ohio.—The news comes from Columbus, Ohio, that the Legislature of that State has passed the Alexander bill, which provides for the establishment of an imbecile village near Columbus. The theory of the promoters of the bill is that agricultural pursuits tend to raise the standard of intelligence of imbeciles. The bill calls for the appropriation of $150,000 for the purchase of land upon which the imbeciles, who are to be divided according to intelligence, are to reside. The farm is to be an adjunct of the Asylum for Feeble-Minded Youths.

Leprosy in Crete and the Balkan Peninsula.—Dr. Ehlers of Copenhagen states that leprosy is widely disseminated in the Balkan Peninsula. This region has long been reputed a center for leprosy, but precise information has not hitherto been obtained on account of the lack of trustworthy statistics. Rumania alone has been noted for correct information and systematic investigation with regard to this question. Dr. Ehlers, in the course of a long journey in the Balkans, has come across lepers almost everywhere throughout the peninsula. Crete also seems to abound with them. "The Cretan lepers," he says, "present all the ordinary symptoms of leprosy as seen elsewhere, but the disease is less severe there than it is in the countries of the north. This difference is undoubtedly due to the climate."—*London Lancet*, March 26.

Personal Efforts in Opposition to the Antivivisection Bill.—Dr. Howard A. Kelly recently sent out a circular letter asking various members of the profession to use their personal influence with senators and congressmen to secure their opposition to the Antivivisection Bill now before Congress. Pursuant to this request, the editor of the MEDICAL NEWS sent urgent letters to both of the New York senators. In response thereto Senator Platt replied that he is committed to a policy of opposition to that measure, and will do all he can to defeat it. Senator Murphy promises that the matter will have his very earnest attention. Is it not possible that a sufficient number of influential letters may secure a more positive statement from the latter official? Letters should be at once written to the various representatives as well as to the senators.

Night Duty for Adolescents.—Under this heading the *Medical Press and Circular* (London) says: "It would be difficult to exaggerate the services rendered to the public by the admirable organization which provides for the prompt services of messengers at all hours of the day and night. Nevertheless, one cannot but commiserate the fate of the lads who are called upon to pass the night on this fatiguing duty, especially when, as is often the case, they are of microscopic dimensions, and, therefore, presumably of very tender age. It cannot be doubted that the employment on night duty of undeveloped and still growing boys must be fraught with grave danger to their future careers from a physical point of view, and we would suggest to the managers of these institutions the propriety of restricting night duty to youths not less than sixteen years of age. Otherwise, it may be necessary to agitate for an amendment of the existing laws on the employment of labor, in order to protect these willing little workers against themselves.

Obituary.—Dr. George Hoppin Humphreys died on the 15th inst. at his residence in New York City. He was born in Philadelphia in 1834. He studied in the University of Pennsylvania, and was graduated from Jefferson Medical College. He completed his medical studies in Paris and Vienna, and came to New York in 1859. When the war broke out he joined the Ninth Regiment, Hawkins' Zouaves, as surgeon. After the war he settled in New York as a general practitioner. Dr. Humphreys was a member of the Academy of Medicine and the County Medical Society, and also of the Loyal Legion, and the Century and Union League Clubs.—Dr. Joseph F. Colgan of Brooklyn, died April 8th of acute tuberculosis. He was a native of that city, born there about thirty-two years ago, and has been in the practice of his profession there since March, 1890, which was the date of his graduation at the Long Island College Hospital. He was a young man of excellent attainments, and of high promise. The duration of his final illness was about four months. He was unmarried.

The American Orthopedic Association.—The next annual meeting of this association will be held at Boston, May 17, 18, and 19, 1898. In addition to a very complete and interesting scientific program, the local members of the association have evidently prepared an unusual variety of entertainment. A visit has been planned to the Industrial School for Cripples and Deformed Children, where the methods of instruction will be explained and the school inspected. A clinical session will be held on the afternoon of the first day of the meeting at the Children's Hospital. Cases of interest will be shown and the work-shop and museum will be inspected. In the evening an extra session will be held at the Harvard Medical School, and a paper and demonstration on "Tuberculosis of Bones and Joints" will be given by Dr. Edward H. Nichols, of Boston. Drs. Warren and Councilman will discuss this paper. Members are also invited to visit the Boston Normal School of Gymnastics (founded by the late Mrs. Hemenway for the purpose of physical training and massage). A carriage drive will be taken through historic Boston, including Cambridge.

Smallpox in North Carolina.—The most recent cases of smallpox in this State were in Clay county, and Dr. Sanderson, Superintendent of Health of that county, writes that the patients are all well. Considering the unpromising surroundings of the imported cases, the local authorities have done well. In Wilmington two cases occurred, both individuals being infected in South Carolina; no deaths; no extension. In Charlotte, total number of affected persons was five, three infected in South Carolina and two (children of one of the three) taking the disease from the father; two deaths; no further extension. One case, from Birmingham, Alabama, occurred in Alamance county, near Gibsonville. This was the only case there; recovery. A young man returning from North Georgia to his home in Clay county brought the infection with him and gave the disease to his family, every one of whom—ten in all—were attacked, but none died. While the color in these last-named cases was not given, it is more than probable that the patients were white, as negroes are scarce in the mountains, but all the other cases occurred in negroes.—*N. C. Bulletin* for March.

Permanent Blindness Not Due to Belladonna—a Physician Wins His Case.—The effect of belladonna upon the human vision was considered in a libel suit which has recently been reviewed by the Appellate Division of the Supreme Court at Albany, New York. The plaintiff in the action was a physician who treated the defendant's daughter for some ailment of the eyes, and in the course of the treatment administered belladonna. The girl subsequently became blind, and her father attributed the loss of her eyesight to the unskilfulness of the plaintiff and his ignorance in giving her belladonna, and thus producing her blindness. The doctor sued him for libel for publishing statements of this purport, and upon the trial a material inquiry was what were the actual effects of administering belladonna in like cases. Every medical witness testified that belladonna would not, and indeed, could not cause blindness in any person. They all agreed that the drug produced a dilation of the pupil, accompanied by a partial loss of vision, but that this was only temporary and the effect would gradually pass away. The proof on this point was so clear and conclusive as to leave no doubt in the mind of the Appellate Court that the unhappy father was mistaken in holding the doctor responsible for the misfortune of his child.

A Modern Aseptic Hospital Department.—The following are some of the details which come to us in a description of an ideal aseptic "ward" or room for one patient at the Temperance Hospital on Hampstead Road, London. The walls and ceiling are made of enameled glass tile, having a pale pink hue, with all the angles rounded. The floor is of marble mosaic, the angles also being rounded. Almost the whole of the wall facing west is plate-glass window. By this means a splendid light is obtained, which can on occasion be screened by an external blind. Below this large window is the fireplace, the flue being diverted to either side. The upper fifth of the window is so contrived as to open valvewise inward, this result being obtained by mechanism external to the ward. A small area of the glass-tiled east wall is correspondingly made to open, but when closed it is flush with the wall. Thus, free aeration can be insured. For ordinary ventilation a glass-lined air-shaft is provided delivering obliquely upward; in this shaft is placed a fan worked by electricity. The air-supply for this is drawn from high above the hospital buildings, being also filtered through cotton wool in its passage down the shaft. Artificial lighting is effected by electricity by means of a sunlight in the center of the ceiling. In a small glass-tiled recess are additional electric lights; when not required, this recess is closed by a glass door fitting flush with the wall. The furniture is entirely of metal, and can be washed with boiling water without fear of injury.

CORRESPONDENCE.

SMALLPOX AGAIN.

To the Editor of the MEDICAL NEWS.

DEAR SIR: I read Dr. Parke's letter on "Smallpox in Alabama" in the MEDICAL NEWS of March 26th with much interest, but I must confess that I cannot see any grounds for his belief that compulsory vaccination would have eradicated the disease. He declares that "the present epidemic has been characterized by the mildness of the cases, indeed, so mild that the colored people prefer it to vaccination." Will he please inform us why it has been so mild? It cannot be because of vaccination, for he tells us that the people would not submit to that. Then why was it mild? We should like to know, also, why he feels so confident that vaccination would have ended the epidemic? Does he know that it is a specific for smallpox? If he does, why then has it not proven to be so heretofore? I have never known it to be a specific with any one except those whom it has killed, and, therefore, is this not why so many refused to be vaccinated, preferring to risk the smallpox? If it is not a specific why does the doctor want to force it on the people? Is not strict isolation of patients and strict sanitation the safest and best exterminator of this affection? Let us hear from the doctor again.

ISAAC L. PEEBLES.

HATTIESBURG, MISS., April 16, 1898.

REPORT OF AN OPERATION FOR SPINA BIFIDA.

To the Editor of the MEDICAL NEWS.

SEVERAL of my professional friends have asked me to report an operation for spina bifida, which, with the able assistance of Dr. J. M. Davis, was performed October 3, 1896. Not thinking the work of a country surgeon would be of interest to the readers of the MEDICAL NEWS, the operation was never reported. However, a short time ago, in looking over "Pepper's System of Medicine," vol. v, Edit., 1886, it was noted that only twenty-three cases of excision, with separate suture of the sac (the operation we did), with sixteen successful results, had been reported. This encouraged me to report my own case, which, if it gives no other information, will show what we country fellows sometimes do.

The patient was first seen when he was about five or six hours old, and was found to be a healthy-looking child, with the exception of a large tumor over the spine at the lumbosacral junction, and a most remarkable absence of bone in the composition of the cranium, the anterior and posterior fontanels being very large, and the sutures plainly demonstrable.

Noting that the child kicked in a lively manner, which was taken as a criterion favorable to treatment, the parents were advised of possibilities and an operation recommended. They consented, and Mayo-Robson's operation was decided upon. Delay was deemed advisable, that the child might become accustomed to being outside the uterus, so we did not operate until he was seven weeks old.

The tumor was pedunculated, round, tense, slightly flattened, slightly transparent, and fluctuated. It was 13¾ inches in circumference at the largest part, and was covered by thin skin. There was a peculiar, reddish, crusty spot, about the size of a half-dollar, near the fundus of the tumor, from the center of which leaked a few drops of serum. Continuous pressure would cause the growth to relax, and would produce stupor of the child.

We made injections of a two-per-cent. solution of cocain about every half inch around the base of the tumor, on one side of the spine, then, making an incision, we worked a grooved director along and divided the integument. A copper uterine sound was pushed between the sac and the skin, and bent from one angle of the incision out at the other. Looping on a ligature, it was drawn around the tumor and tied. A cannula was now introduced, and and about half the fluid allowed to flow out. We found it very difficult to separate the flap from the sac, and the child began to show symptoms of shock. Dr. Davis advised and gave a hypodermic injection of diluted whisky. After the patient revived we finished separating the adhesions and laid open the sac.

I now discovered that I had failed to draw the ligature sufficiently tight to constrict the pedicle, and that a cord-like process, about three lines in diameter, came through the aperture in the spinal column and attached itself to the reddish spot above mentioned. This was later found to be a bundle of nerves, vessels, and connective tissue. Another ligature was placed on the pedicle and tied, after which the sac and cord were cut away. Almost at once the ligature slipped and a hemorrhage occurred from the stump of the cord, which was controlled by pressure with the finger. The bony ring was ⅞-inch in diameter. Thanks to my assistant the spinal fluid did not pour out. The sac was brought together transversely with a continuous silk suture. The periosteum should have now been grafted, but the patient being again in a condition of shock, we thought best to at once close the wound. The flap reached well around the internal wound.

Dr. Davis suggested that it would not be well for the child to nurse from his mother's breast because of her undue excitement, so a neighbor kindly consented to act as wet-nurse.

There is only one point in the dressing which should be mentioned, *viz.*, an improvised truss, consisting of a disk of lead about two inches in diameter, backed with a ball of cotton, and a pad of the same material in front. Four days after the operation the dressing was changed and the wound was found to be doing well. By the eighth day two-thirds of the wound had healed; and at this time the external stitches were removed. The temperature was not at any time over 101.5° F.

The patient continued to do well about four weeks, when a fistulous opening formed and the internal suture made its way out. The use of the truss was continued until about three months ago, when the bones were seemingly in such close proximity as to make its use no longer necessary.

In May, 1897, the child had hydrocephalus. For this the usual treatment was instituted. The circumference of the head was 20¼ inches.

The patient was recently again seen, and at this time, the last visit, the vertebra seemed to have approximated. The circumference of the head (with long hair) was twenty-one inches. The anterior fontanel still remained large. The patient does not use his left leg as well as the right.

A. DAN MORGAN, M.D.

WITT'S MILLS, AIKEN COUNTY, S. C.
MARCH 22, 1898.

OUR BERLIN LETTER.

[From our Special Correspondent.]

AN EDITOR IN CRIMINAL ANTHROPOLOGY PROVES TO BE A SWINDLER — DRUNKENNESS, UNCONSCIOUSNESS FROM OTHER CAUSES, AND IMPRISONMENT—SPRAINED ANKLES UNDER ROENTGEN-RAYS —CYCLOTHERAPY AND THE BICYCLE IN SURGICAL THERAPEUTICS.

BERLIN, April 14, 1898.

GERMAN medical men are having a quiet laugh at a novel bit of practical experience which some distinguished experts in criminology have had, the details of which are just coming to light in the course of the trial of a swindler. About a year ago a new medical journal was started here, the publisher being a well-known Leipzig medical publishing-house, with the title *Journal of Criminal Anthropology, of Prostitution, and of the Prison Question.* The names of some distinguished German and foreign, notably Italian, criminal anthropologists appeared among the co-editors. The editor had never been heard of before; however, this did not count for much as editors are sometimes obscure, overworked beings about whom few people bother their heads. The "journal" apparently successfully reached the end of its first year, and in several prominent journals of neurology and mental diseases there appeared complimentary comments on the publication in question, and congratulations on the fact that at last Germany, which has not accomplished much in the field of criminology, had an organ of its own for the expression of its opinion on these subjects,

Then there was a period of silence for awhile, followed by the arrest of the editor, who proved to be a swindler well known to the police, and who had been imprisoned for swindling some four times during the past fifteen years. This time he masqueraded under the title of a Doctor of Philosophy, and he would seem to have been in a better position to know practically the ground facts in criminology and the "ins and outs" of the prison question even more thoroughly than his contributors, though some of them were very distinguished criminologists.

His exposure came as a result of an attempt to transfer the publication of the magazine to another publisher, and it is the publishers who are prosecuting. Just how much the distinguished criminologists have paid for their bit of practical experience in criminology is not known. The ex-editor is evidently an illustration of the proneness of genius to perversion—a principle upon which modern criminal anthropologists have been insisting. A brochure from the defendant and the plaintiffs in the case would, it is thought, make interesting reading, and throw some new light on certain problems in social criminology, which the incomplete observations of interested parties on the American genus—the bunco-steerer (habitat, United States) —have unfortunately left obscure.

The lesson of the case for the medical public would seem to be the ease with which a new and pretentious journal may be started, find a publisher and co-editors without any responsible sponsors, and this without the formality of an introduction. In the flood of matter issuing from the press little heed is paid, even in supposedly scientific matters, to the scientific value, or authenticity of the material. The only question, in many cases, seems to be: "Will it sell?"

Three arrests of persons in coma, with the detention of the individuals over night in prison because drunkenness was suspected, have taken place during the winter in Berlin, and have led to some vigorous protests on the part of medical men. As practically all Germans take some alcoholic liquor with their meals, vomiting in case of unconsciousness is always accompanied with some alcoholic odor, and easily awakens the unfounded suspicion of intoxication. In one case, a short time ago, the detention in a cell over night, without medical care, of a young man whose unconsciousness came on suddenly as a result of epidemic cerebrospinal meningitis, would seem to have been an important factor in the fatal termination of the case.

Lively protestations were made at a recent meeting of the Berlin Society for Internal Medicine against detention in prison of persons in coma, and the opinion was practically unanimous that "in no case of unconsciousness should the judgment of the cause of the state be left to non-medical police officials and prison wardens." The condition of affairs which lead up to these protests, which here are to have some effect as the police authorities have already taken cognizance of them, practically exists all over and some remedy must be found in the interests of true humanity. In the meantime, what is "everybody's business is no one's business" and until some philanthropist specially devotes his attention to the subject the abuse is likely to continue.

Most doctors have had experience with troublesome sprains of the ankle, painful and inconvenient for the patient at the moment and with tendencies to recur which no care seems to be able to prevent. A German army-surgeon who has had the bothersome treatment of a number of such cases in the young soldiers of the infantry regiments, has found that they are not simple sprains. He has been taking Röntgen-ray photographs in every case, and has found that in nearly all some complication like fracture or dislocation of the little bones of the ankle was present.

The number of cases in which a simple rupture of ligament or capsule of the joint was the cause of the trouble, and in which, therefore, the Röntgen-rays would show the presence of no bony lesion or at most a pushing of the bones apart by the collection of fluid in the intra-articular spaces, was extremely small, while the number of fractures of little bones was very large, forming the real lesion in the majority of the cases.

He suggests that the only rational treatment is fixation of the foot in plaster, as for fracture, and the careful examination with the X-rays for a break. Otherwise false joints, bony overgrowths from irritation give rise to a condition which easily leads to recurrence of the symptoms whenever the slightest strain is put upon the foot. Besides, the breaking of one of these small bones and its delayed or incomplete union, make a point of "least resistance" of the most delicate kind. The chronic inflammatory condition makes it an especially favorable culture-medium for the bacillus tuberculosis, which does not take hold easily where there is rapid metabolism of healthy tissues; hence, the large number of cases of tuberculous arthritis of the ankle — a frequent sequel when there is the history of an old sprain.

Some modifications of bicycle frames, of the length of pedals, and of gears, so as to adapt the bicycle to therapeutic purposes, were exhibited at the Verein für Innere Medicin at its April meeting, and attracted a good deal of attention. Some of them were models that had actually been employed in surgical therapeutics in the treatment of ankyloses of various joints. Patients in whom gonorrheal and septic arthritis had left practically complete ankyloses and who had gradually acquired the power to bend their limbs again by the exercise on the bicycle, were also exhibited. The pedals may be so arranged and the gear so fixed as to use only the limited movement possible for a particular patient. The practical application of certain physical principles takes the new methods out of the realm of mere empiricism and gives the surgeon a very pleasant and efficient way of encouraging his patient to that use of the limb which obviates contractures.

TRANSACTIONS OF FOREIGN SOCIETIES.

Paris.

ARTHROTOMY FOR IRREDUCIBLE DISLOCATION OF THE SHOULDER—TREATMENT OF ABSCESS OF THE LIVER—GASTRECTOMY AND GASTROTOMY—THE PREVENTIVE AND VACCINATIVE POWERS OF ANTIVENOMOUS SERUM—INFECTION FAVORED BY DISABILITY OF THE KIDNEYS—THE USE OF BLISTERS IN PULMONARY TUBERCULOSIS — LOCAL APPLICATION OF SALICYLATE OF METHYL IN RHEUMATISM—VOMITING OF PREGNANCY RELIEVED BY OXYGENATED WATER.

AT the Surgical Society, March 2d, RIÇARD said that arthrotomy is the preferable treatment in recent irreducible dislocations of the shoulder, for in such cases there is always an interposition of tendon ligament or some other tissue which prevents the return of the head of the bone to its socket. An incision is less dangerous in such cases than violent attempts at reduction. If the dislocation is of several weeks' duration it is justifiable to make several quick turns of the head of the bone, combined with traction, in order to break up adhesions and to replace the bone in its capsule. If such movements are unsuccessful arthrotomy is indicated.

LUCAS-CHAMPIONNIERE spoke of the good results which follow resection, though it was his opinion that old dislocations with a fair amount of motion had better not be disturbed. If operation is undertaken, and it is found impossible to replace the head of the humerus in its socket, resection should be performed.

WALTHER, at the session of March 16th, discussed the subject of "Abscess of the Liver," pointing out the delicacy of a differential diagnosis between this affection and typhoid and malarial fevers. Exploratory puncture is a valuable aid to diagnosis. Loison reported the results of operation upon fourteen patients with abscess of the liver. Eight of them recovered. In eleven cases the transpleural route was chosen. In the other three, laparotomy was performed. A bacteriologic examination of the pus showed it to be sterile in three instances, while in three others it contained staphylococcus aureus, once a mixture of streptococcus and coli bacillus and once a mixture of coli bacillus and a diplococcus.

ROBERT said that exploratory puncture with him had become a routine practice, to be immediately followed by an incision if pus were found.

MONPROFIT removed a large tumor from the abdomen, including about one-third of the stomach wall. Finding it impossible to suture together the remaining portions of the stomach without too much strain upon the sutures, he divided the jejunum and performed post-colic gastro-enterostomy in the form of a Y, stitching the upper cut end of the jejunum into the side of the lower portion. No buttons or other artificial aids were used. The patient was two hours under chloroform and recovered without severe symptoms. Monprofit expressed himself as heartily in favor of gastrectomy when the tumor is accessible.

PHISALIX addressed the Biological Society, March 5th, upon the "Preventive and Vaccinative Powers of Antivenomous Serum." He had learned from experiments that these two properties are distinct. The vaccinative reaction is sufficient to protect the organism, but is not strong enough to generate in the animal antitoxic substances which will render other animals immune. There are, therefore, two different degrees of immunization. In the first case, we have simple vaccination, in the second case hypervaccination.

RICHE said that he had been able to clinically verify a fact that is well known from experiments upon animals, *viz.*, that interference with the action of the kidneys favors infection. A light epidemic of measles broke out in an infants' hospital. The only adult who contracted the disease was a woman who three months before had passed through a severe attack of nephritis with uremic symptoms requiring blood-letting. She had previously had measles. Notwithstanding this fact she contracted the disease again and in a very serious form, associated with pulmonary edéma requiring the withdrawal of thirteen ounces (400 grams) of blood. Convalescence was slow.

CHARRIN called attention to the fact that while certain forms of nephritis favor infection there are other forms in which just the opposite condition seems true, at least to infection with particular kinds of virus. In the case referred to, the weakened condition of the patient favored contraction of the disease and also favored the production of pulmonary edema. At no time during the illness was the toxicity of the patient's blood-serum much increased, nor was there much retention of urinary products in the system. The methyl-blue test showed the kidneys to be normally permeable, although, of course, portions of these organs might have been diseased.

At the Academy of Medicine, March 15th, VALLIN spoke of the "Indications for the Use of Blisters in Pulmonary Tuberculosis." They ought not to be employed if the disease is advancing very rapidly, or if there is a high fever and hemoptysis, or extensive tuberculous bronchopneumonia. On the other hand they are of great service in slowly progressing cases with a limited area of pleural, pulmonary, or bronchial congestion, and a temperature not exceeding 38.5° C. (101.3° F.) In such cases the application of a small blister, repeated three or four times, gives an excellence result. It also affords relief in cases of bronchopneumonia limited to a small area, without hemoptysis and with fever ranging from 39° to 40° C. (102° to 104° F.) Before prescribing blisters the afternoon urine should be examined, as the urine of a phthisical patient rarely contains albumin in the morning. Blisters should never be prescribed for old people.

At the session of March 22d, LINOSSIER spoke of the good results to be obtained by local application of salicylate of methyl in the treatment of rheumatism. Certain authors have mixed the drug with vaselin and applied it in the form of a salve, but when applied in this way it is far less efficacious, only one-half the amount being recoverable in the urine that is recoverable when the pure drug is applied. In either case it must be covered with some imperious material or it will not be absorbed at all.

GALLOIS addressed the Therapeutic Society, March 9th, upon "The Use of Oxygenated Water in the Vomiting of Pregnancy." He had only two failures to record. This treatment is without effect in vomiting due to gastric diseases, but it appears to be efficacious in the vomiting of consumptives. The mode of its action is not determined; perhaps it is a mechanical one, due to the presence in the stomach of the liberated gas; perhaps the oxygen in some way affects the digestive processes, and, perhaps it counteracts the influence of some ptomain.

Vienna.

PROLONGED USE OF ARSENIC FOLLOWED BY THE DEVELOPMENT OF ULCERS AND EPITHELIOMA—RELIEF OF PES EQUINUS BY A PLASTIC OPERATION UPON THE ACHILLES TENDON.

At the Imperio-Royal Society of Physicians, Feb. 25th, ULLMANN showed a patient, thirty-four years old, with keratosis and epithelial carcinomata from the prolonged use of arsenic. At the age of fifteen the patient had suffered from acne, and she took arsenic internally during seven consecutive years. In the course of time the palmar surfaces of the hands and feet and the skin of her face began to burn and smart. The skin became thick, uneven, and pebbly, and was darkly pigmented in spots; moreover, there was well-marked local hyperidrosis. The arsenic was discontinued and all symptoms disappeared except a certain amount of tenseness and a disposition to the formation of slowly healing ulcers. Some years later there appeared on her forehead a brownish-red spot, which was excised. It proved to be a non-ulcerating, subepidermoidal carcinoma. An ulcer upon the heel which resisted treatment a long time finally developed a tumor which was found to be an epithelioma with a tendency to cornification.

HEBRA said that he had once taken arsenic three months on account of an influenza-neuralgia, and that the soles of his feet became thickened and so painful that walking was impossible. The symptoms disappeared two or three weeks after the use of the drug was discontinued. There was no hyperidrosis.

At the session of March 11th, FRANK showed an adult patient upon whom he performed a plastic operation to lengthen the Achilles tendon and relieve the deformity of pes equinus produced by an osteomyelitis. An incision two and a half inches long was made on the inner side of the tendon and the latter was obliquely divided throughout the whole length of the skin incision. The ends of the tendon were sutured and the foot was placed in plaster of Paris in a corrected position. Within fourteen days exercises were begun, and in five weeks the patient could walk without a bandage. This operation permits the earlier use of gymnastic exercises and facilitates recovery. Recurrence of the difficulty is not to be feared. It is therefore preferable to subcutaneous tenotomy.

SOCIETY PROCEEDINGS.

NEW YORK NEUROLOGICAL SOCIETY.

Stated Meeting, Held March 8, 1808.

THE President, B. SACHS, M.D., in the Chair.

DR. WILLIAM HIRSCH presented a baby, aged fifteen months, who had been referred to him about one week ago because of certain movements of the head. The child had been perfectly healthy up to about two months previously, when it had fallen from a chair and struck the back of the head. Vomiting set in immediately afterward, and continued about a week. The mother then noticed the peculiar shaking of the head, which has continued ever since. Examination of the nervous system is absolutely negative. On examining the eyes one observes that there is a nearly absolute unilateral nystagmus. There is a horizontal nystagmus of the left eye, while the right eye shows the same condition, though very much less marked. The speaker said that it has been claimed by some that these movements in children are brought about by an effort at compensation for the nystagmus. A point in favor of this theory is that the movements cease during sleep. Others have claimed that the movements of the head and the nystagmus have a common cause, *e.g.*, a cerebellar lesion. None of the reported cases shows the difference existing in the two eyes in this case.

DR. W. M. LESZYNSKY said that he had seen quite a number of these cases. A great many of them had been found to also present ocular defects. In this case, the injury was probably only a coincidence. When the child gets old enough to fix the eyes these movements are prone to occur. Some years ago he had seen such a case at the Manhattan Eye and Ear Hospital. It was thought that the child was blind and had optic atrophy. He had kept the little patient under his observation seven or eight months, and improvement and ultimate recovery followed the application of tonic treatment. He did not believe, therefore, that there is any actual morbid anatomy in these cases.

DR. GEORGE W. JACOBY said that he had not found these cases uncommon, and he believed that they occur directly as a consequence of traumatism. There are two distinct classes of cases, *viz.*, those in which there is nystagmus, and those in which it is absent. In the majority of cases, by excluding vision, it would be found that the movements of the eyes cease. In this child there seemed to him to be some up-and-down movement complicating the other movements. Some years ago he had seen an interesting medico-legal case, occurring in an adult, a man who had been struck in the eye by an electric light wire. The eye had been perforated. After losing the eyeball he presented certain psychic symptoms, together with some head-nodding which had continued ever since. He was now rather feeble-minded. Inasmuch as in this man there was nothing pointing to injury of any other part of the brain except the frontal lobe, the question arose as to whether there was any possible connection between injury to this lobe and the movements.

DR. FREDERICK PETERSON said he believed Henoch first described these movements many years ago. He had himself described ten cases some years ago, representing all the different varieties. Most of the cases have a lateral movement, but some have the head-nodding. Henoch thought the condition was reflex from dentition, as the majority of the cases developed at about the age of eight or ten months. The theory which he had adopted is that these cases are almost always the result of a trauma or concussion. A point worthy of note is that there cannot be any marked pathologic lesion, as there is recovery in all such cases. The lateral movement of the head and the movement of the eyes seemed to him to be due to functional troubles in different parts of the brain. Many of these patients will temporarily stop the movement if the eyes are fixed upon an object. If the lateral movements are due to a nystagmus, it is curious that the nystagmus should be complicated by the head-nodding.

DR. MARY PUTNAM-JACOBI said that many years ago she had seen a case coming on spontaneously in a child two years old. It was peculiar in that a rotary movement occurred every night at bedtime.

DR. FRAENKEL said that he had recently seen a child nine months old, who, according to the mother, had exhibited a rotary movement of the head and a vertical nystagmus since it was three months old. This nystagmus occurred when the nodding movements ceased. This would seem to support the view of Dr. Leszynsky that it is dependent upon some refractive condition of the eye.

DR. HIRSCH said that the objective examination by Dr. Koller showed the eyes to be entirely normal. All the theories offered would not hold good in a case of unilateral nystagmus. That the condition in the present instance was caused by traumatism alone seemed almost certain from the history. The movements of the head are entirely separate from those of the eyeball. The fact that most of the children recover is sufficient to exclude an organic lesion, though slight pachymeningitis in the region of the cerebellum might result in resolution.

DR. FRAENKEL presented a child, two and a half years old, born of healthy parents. The family history was negative. The child was born at full term, the breech presenting. The labor was rather difficult. Immediately after birth the abnormal condition of the lower extremities was noted. The mother insists that the child has improved. Examination shows a moderate lateral curvature, and the child is unable to sit, walk, or stand. Electric examination shows extensive degeneration of all the muscles except those of the calves. The knee-jerks are absent, but there is an ankle-clonus on both sides. At first sight, the case seemed to be one of poliomyelitis, but it is conceivable that the condition is the result of a dropsy, or of a hemorrhage from rupture of the anterior spinal artery. As this vessel almost exclusively supplies the anterior horn, it is possible that a traumatic poliomyelitis had developed, extending from the mid-dorsal to about the third lumbar segment; further, there might be a localized cavity formation. He explained the existence of the ankle-clonus by the theory that, as the calf-muscles are in a state of increased tonus due to the fact that the antagonistic muscles are absent, the moment a sensory stimulus is applied and enters the cord, the latter being in a state of increased receptivity, the evidence of its having received this stimulus is shown by an additional motor discharge. The spinal curvature is to be explained by the unilateral involvement of the spinal muscles. The posterior muscles below the knee give an exaggerated response to both electric currents, while there is no reaction in the muscles above the knee.

DR. PETERSON asked why this explanation of the ankle-clonus would not apply to all other cases of poliomyelitis in which, it is well known, there is no ankle-clonus.

DR. FRAENKEL replied that the presence or absence of ankle-clonus is dependent upon quantitative changes in the tonus of the muscles. The increased tonus of the calf-muscles he did not think ordinarily existed in cases of poliomyelitis.

DR. JOSEPH COLLINS accepted the pathologic explanation given by Dr. Fränkel. The fact that ankle-clonus does not occur in ordinary cases of anterior poliomyelitis does not negative the explanation given. This case is, in reality, a unique substantiation of the theory proposed by Dr. Fränkel last winter, and adopted by Hughlings Jackson in his lecture this year. In no case of complete anterior poliomyelitis which he had seen had there been any hypertonus of the calf-muscles.

DR. B. SACHS thought there is at least one other view to be put forward. He did not think that there is this amount of spasticity in a very large number of cases of ordinary poliomyelitis. He had seen a single instance of ankle-clonus in an ordinary case of poliomyelitis; the unusual spastic condition in the present case must be due to some special lesion. It is fair to assume that in this case there is some developmental defect. The entire appearance of the leg reminded him very much of cases in which children had been born with defective limbs. On the supposition that the gray matter in the spinal cord is defective, chiefly in the region of the lumbar segments and in the lateral columns, one can understand how the knee-jerks might be absent and the ankle-clonus present.

DR. JOSEPH COLLINS presented a boy, thirteen years of age, with lateral curvature of the spine, atrophy of the muscles of the right upper extremity, and the condition of the face known as the Schultze eye, and a history of attacks of diarrhea which had no apparent relationship to ingesta or indigestion. The symptoms were of two- or three-years' duration and had slowly developed. He regarded the case as one of syringomyelia, despite the fact that there are no sensory disturbances. The lesion chiefly involves the anterior horns and the group of cells adjacent to Clarke's column, which have been shown in an investigation recently made by Dr. Onuf and himself to stand in developmental and functional relationship to the sympathetic.

DR. G. W. JACOBY said that to base the diagnosis on these three symptoms alone required considerable assurance. In his opinion, such a diagnosis is not warranted unless there are marked sensory disturbances accompanying the atrophy.

DR. WILLIAM HIRSCH said that he had recently shown two cases of syringomyelia in another society, which showed the same condition of the muscles and of the eye —the narrowing of the fissure of the eyelid and the contraction of one pupil. There were also present the typical sensory symptoms, but the atrophy of the ulnar group and the condition of the eye had led him to believe that it was a typical form of syringomyelia located between the last cervical and first dorsal segment. He had also recently seen in private practice a lady with the same condition of the eye, and with a herpes zoster in the trigeminal region, and who also showed, instead of an atrophy, a tremor of the left arm and a slight analgesia. The diagnosis made by Dr. Collins seemed to him perfectly justifiable. The more characteristic symptoms will probably develop later.

DR. L. STIEGLITZ concurred in the diagnosis of syringomyelia, and remarked that at the last meeting he had presented a counterpart of this case, in which no sensory symptoms were present, and also a typical case of syringomyelia. He thought it was not uncommon to find these cases without sensory symptoms.

DR. ONUF said that in a joint investigation, made by Dr. Collins and himself, they had found that the zone situated between the central ganglia on one side and the end of the lateral horn on the other, and between the base of the posterior and anterior horns, is intimately connected with sympathetic functions. They had found that atrophy of the cells of the lateral horn occurred in a certain group (the lateral, the central ganglia, and in the whole zone between), and that this atrophy was partly due to sensory and partly to motor fibers. The motor-fibers originate from the smaller cells of the zone mentioned. This being the case, it is evident that syringomyelia could present very different pictures, depending upon the particular locality affected. In the case under discussion the sympathetic symptoms are very marked in connection with the eye, and the diarrhea and the lateral curvature may also be considered as belonging to the same class. In three instances they had extirpated the stellate ganglion in cats. This was usually followed after some weeks by a diarrhea which was most persistent and exhausting. This ganglion is supplied chiefly by the upper dorsal nerves.

DR. M. ALLEN STARR said that the combination of the sympathetic paralysis with ulnar-nerve paralysis he had known to occur in one case of undoubted gumma on the anterior surface of the cord. The gumma was absorbed after a time. The condition had been undoubtedly produced by pressure on the anterior nerve roots.

DR. COLLINS said that he had been largely led to make the diagnosis of syringomyelia in this case by the experiments that he had conducted in conjunction with Dr. Onuf. There was nothing else which would produce the four prominent symptoms, *viz.*: the diarrhea, curvature of the spine, atrophy of the hand muscles, and the Schultze eye.

DR. HIRSCH presented a young woman who was an example of total unilateral congenital sweating of the face. She complained that half of the face would become red and moist while the left half remained dry and of normal color. She never sweats on the left side of the face. He had experimented with hypodermic injections of different drugs. Physostigmin had had no effect at all. Pilocarpin, injected hypodermically, caused perspiration all over her face, for the first time in her life, but, of course, this was only transient. The fact that in this case absence of perspiration is associated with vasomotor symptoms seemed to be in favor of the view that the vasomotor-centers and the sweat-centers are at least intimately connected. The condition is confined to the face.

DR. STARR remarked that a case of this kind, occurring in a man twenty-three years of age, had been entirely cured in his clinic by boring out the turbinated bones.

DR. FRAENKEL presented a young boy, who had come under his observation about three months previously, with a diagnosis of pulmonary tuberculosis, because of an attack of hemoptysis. He had been well up to two years before; then he began to suffer from shortness of breath. On admission to the Montefiore Home, the head was turned to one side, there was inspiratory stridor, a moderate amount of exophthalmos, swelling of the neck, and tachycardia. The physical examination of the chest was practically negative. The tumefaction in the neck was lobulated and moved up and down during deglutition. Under treatment with thyroid extract he had decidedly improved subjectively, and had gained fourteen pounds in body weight. The tachycardia had disappeared. The case was interesting as showing the difference between genuine Basedow's disease and the secondary or symptomatic form.

DR. C. E. NAMMACK asked if Hodgkin's disease had been excluded.

DR. FRAENKEL replied that a brother of this patient had twice had tuberculous glands removed, and there had been good reason to believe that this might be a case of Hodgkin's disease, but it had been excluded: (1) by the absence of other evidence of lymphatic involvement; (2) by its long duration; (3) by examination of the blood; and (4) by the mobility of the swelling in the neck on deglutition, showing its connection with the thyroid gland.

DR. B. SACHS presented a man, fifty-one years of age, whom he had first seen about one week before. The patient had been married twenty-seven years. Six years ago his first wife had been afflicted with the same affection as the one from which he now suffers. The patient himself had been in good health in former years, and he still weighs 230 pounds. He had been an extremely heavy drinker, chiefly of beer, taking at times as much as fifty or sixty glasses daily. Syphilitic infection could not be determined. He had been in good health up to January 12, 1898, when, while attending the funeral of a friend, he says he saw a flash of light, and this was immediately followed by double vision and intense photophobia. At first glance, there is apparently a double ptosis, but the eyelids can be moved upward. Ordinarily they droop in an effort to protect the eyes. There is slight nystagmus and a decided paresis of the left rectus externus muscle. The pupils are irregular; they do not react to light, and but slightly to accommodation. The case had been referred to him by Dr. Marple, who had found nothing, on ocular examination, to explain the photophobia. Further examination showed a very widespread and marked hemi-analgesia, but no impairment of tactile sensibility. He had arrived at the conclusion that there is a large hysteric element in the case. The visual fields are normal, the reflexes are normal, and there is no evidence of loss of power in the extremities. His diagnosis was hysteric ophthalmoplegia.

DR. FRAENKEL said that in a recent monograph hysteric ophthalmoplegias of this character had been described. Aside from the clinical aspect of the case, its development after emotional disturbance is particularly significant. About six months ago a man, in very simiilar condition, had applied for admission to the Montefiore Home. He presented ataxia, loss of knee-jerks, ptosis, and ophthalmoplegia. After admission, his ptosis and ophthalmoplegia disappeared, and the case clearly proved to be one of locomotor ataxia, the other symptoms having been hysteric, and added to the ataxic symptoms with a view to securing admission to the hospital.

DR. LESZYNSKY said it is important to distinguish between ptosis and blepharospasm. In the case under discussion there seems to be a certain amount of blepharospasm. With photophobia, tonic blepharospasm is much more likely to occur than ptosis. He had seen a number of such cases in hysteric individuals, and quite recently one in a young girl who responded promptly to hypnosis.

DR. SACHS then presented another case of ophthalmoplegia, in a boy seventeen years old. In October, 1894, at 9 A.M., the patient had found himself unable to utter words. This had passed away, but had been repeated at noon and at 4 P.M. the same day. He then had a convulsion, lasting ten minutes, after which the left eyelid had been noticed to droop. There had been no convulsions since then. He had been perfectly well previously. Examination showed complete ptosis of the left and slight ptosis of the right eye. The outward and inward movements were limited in single and conjugate action; both pupils reacted well to light and accommodation; the sensation of the face was normal. There had been comparatively little change in the past three years. There is now diplopia, chiefly when looking to the left. The diagnosis lay between thrombosis or embolism in the basilar artery. The heart action is irregular and rather rapid, but no murmur is audible.

DR. SACHS also presented a man, thirty-nine years of age, who had been admitted to the Montefiore Home some time ago. There was no evidence of syphilis. At the age of twenty he was weak in the knees and frequently made missteps. In 1887 he had sought medical advice because of difficulty of locomotion, noticed especially in climbing stairs. When examined in March, 1895, he complained chiefly of difficulty in walking, weakness in the extremities, and slight difficulty in speech. At first, the case was supposed to be one of locomotor ataxia. He now has an ataxic spastic gait, and also has static ataxia; the pupils react to light and for accommodation; the patellar reflexes are absent. There is no Argyll-Robertson pupil. There is distinct ataxia of the right upper extremity. He has a form of speech which is between a slow speech and a bulbar speech. The diagnosis lies between a bulbar form of multiple sclerosis and the possibility of a Friedreich's ataxia instead of an ordinary tabes. The great point against the latter is its occurrence rather late in life. There is no disturbance of sensation. The jaw-jerk is absent.

DR. FRAENKEL said that although the lack of coordination was first noticed when the patient was nineteen years of age, when his attention was naturally directed to it by entering the army, it was not improbable that it had been present long before. There was also slight atrophy of the optic nerves. The absence of sexual and sphincteric disturbance, and the peculiar thick and scanning speech seemed to point rather to the diagnosis of multiple sclerosis.

DR. COLLINS said that when he had first seen the

man, three years ago, the intention-tremor and the optic atrophy had not been present, and it was then thought that the man had Friedreich's disease. In the last two years the speech had become very much more bulbar in quality. He was inclined to believe that there was a diffuse insular sclerosis, bulbar and spinal.

DR. HIRSCH said that even at the present time there is not a perfect agreement as to what constitutes the pathologic basis of Friedreich's disease. The case seemed to him like the *spinal* form of Friedreich's disease.

DR. SACHS said that the term "Friedreich's disease" is at the present time usually applied to the ordinary hereditary ataxia, the disease located partly in the posterior, and partly in the lateral columns of the cord.

REVIEWS.

THE PRINCIPLES OF BACTERIOLOGY. A Practical Manual for Students and Physicians. By A. C. ABBOTT, M.D., Professor of Hygiene, University of Pennsylvania. Fourth edition, enlarged and thoroughly revised. Philadelphia and New York: Lea Brothers & Co., 1897.

A GOOD proof of the value of this book and the demand for it lies in the fact that the fourth edition has been reached within six years. Since the publication of the last edition some important advances in bacteriology have been made, and we find them fairly well reflected in the present revision.

We are more than surprised, however, to find that the bacillus of syphilis is still mentioned as one of the bacilli likely to be confounded with the bacillus of tuberculosis, and the differential points in the technic of staining are mentioned to guard against errors, but the author fortunately states later on that in the examination of sputum and pathologic fluids the syphilis bacillus will most likely not be encountered. We feel assured that on this point most observers will agree at the present time. We are pleased to note that in discussing the differential features between the typhoid bacillus and the bacillus coli commune the author lays stress on the characteristic reaction of the former when serum from a typhoid-fever case is added (Widal). Heretofore the diagnosis between these organisms has always been a source of much anxiety and annoyance.

The book has been so often reviewed and so much said in its favor that we must be pardoned if we content ourselves by simply adding that it still holds its own with any of the manuals on the subject and that it is deserving of the highest praise. A more extended index would, however, be much appreciated by the student. The book is well bound and printed, and several new illustrations have been added.

A MANUAL OF MEDICAL JURISPRUDENCE. By ALFRED SWAINE TAYLOR, M.D., F.R.S. Revised and edited by THOMAS STEVENSON, M.D., London, Fellow of the Royal College of Physicians of London, etc. Twelfth American, edited, with citations and additions from the Twelfth English, Edition. By CLARK BELL, Esq., of the New York Bar. New York and Philadelphia: Lea Brothers & Co., 1897.

THIS work follows the same general plan as did the eleventh edition, which was published some five years ago. Some of the sections have been extended and revised, notably the chapter on the examination of blood-stains. This chapter includes the valuable tables of measurement of blood-corpuscles by the late Dr. Treadwell of Boston and Professor M. C. White of New Haven, together with light plates from photomicrographs of human and other red blood-corpuscles in various grades of amplification. The entire question of blood-stains in its medico-legal bearing is of such vital importance that each contribution to this subject is of the greatest value to every microscopist.

In the chapter on death from electricity the autopsy notes in the cases of four criminals executed by electricity are given. So many observations in fatal cases of sunstroke have been made in the past two years that the chapter on this subject should have been revised. Hypnotism in its medico-legal bearings does not receive the consideration which its importance demands.

The book contains a vast amount of valuable information, and its shortcomings are few. For physicians, lawyers, and teachers of forensic medicine the work is admirably suited, and the highest credit is due to the editor and the publishers.

SPINAL CARIES (SPONDYLITIS OR POTTS' DISEASE OF THE SPINAL COLUMN). By NOBLE SMITH, F.R.C.S. Ed., L.R.C.P., London. Second edition. London: Smith, Elder & Co.

IN this monograph of 150 pages the author desires to confirm the conclusion expressed in a former edition that spinal caries is generally a curable disease, but that success in treatment depends, above all things, upon accurate support of the spine.

An account of the pathology and symptomatology of the disease, together with its differential diagnosis, is presented. The various types of deformity are demonstrated by numerous outline drawings, and the phases and peculiarities in the course of the disease as interpreted by different physicians are exemplified by the citation of cases from hospital records and from medical journals at somewhat tedious length.

An account of cases in the author's practice fills twenty pages of the book. Some of these are of interest as showing the course or outcome of the disease and others are quoted to prove the superiority of the "adjustable splint" as a means of treatment contrasted with the plaster jacket, which had been previously applied at other institutions.

The brace used by the author and the method of adjustment are practically identical with the original appliance of Taylor, which was described by him in 1863.

The book presents nothing new, either in form or substance, unless it be the practice of boring into the spinal processes to relieve local pain, on the theory that it is due to tension, the result of the disease of the adjoining vertebral bodies.

The principles and the details of treatment are, however, presented in a satisfactory manner, and if, as the author hopes, it may serve to impress upon the surgeon the importance of personal attention to the proper adjustment of support in contrast with the practice of leaving such details in the hands of mechanics, its publication will have been justified.

THE EYE AS AN AID IN GENERAL DIAGNOSIS. A Hand-book for the Use of Students and General Practitioners.. By E. H. LINNELL, M.D. Philadelphia: The Edwards & Docker Co., 1897.

THE author has given us a valuable compendium, well arranged, clearly written, and exact. After a short chapter on the general eye symptoms of nervous and constitutional disease, the affections of the individual structures of the eye and of its appendages are discussed successively. The chapter on the field of visions and the visual disorders due to lesions implicating the intracranial course of the optic-nerve fibers is particularly thorough, while necessarily brief. There are special divisions on "Reflex Neuroses," on "Ocular Affections of Toxic Origin," "Toxic Amblyopia," and, finally, a most important summary of the ocular symptoms attending and following general anesthesia. The work is printed in large, clear type on excellent paper. Unfortunately, its appearance is marred by numerous typographic errors. "Myosis" is a spelling which should no longer appear in scientific works. It has no philologic relationship to "myopia," and should be "miosis," or, better, "meiosis."

"THE EDINBURGH MEDICAL JOURNAL," Edited by G. A. GIBSON, M.D., F.R.C.P., Ed. New Series. Vol I. Edinburgh and London: Young J. Pentland, 1897.

IF every succeeding volume in the new series of this famous journal equals in interest the present one, it will undoubtedly have its full share of public recognition. The bound volume before us contains numerous articles of scientific interest written by men eminent in medicine. There are lengthy book reviews, reports of societies, and, in each number, a department of recent advances in medicine. The editing is carefully done, and altogether this volume of the *Edinburgh Medical Journal* is a thoroughly up-to-date, progressive publication.

TWENTIETH CENTURY PRACTICE: AN INTERNATIONAL ENCYCLOPEDIA OF MODERN MEDICAL SCIENCE. By leading Authorities of Europe and America. Edited by THOMAS L. STEDMAN, M.D. In Twenty Volumes. Volume XII. *Mental Diseases, Childhood, and Old Age.* New York: Wm. Wood & Co., 1897.

DR. G. F. BLANDFORD of London contributes the article on insanity, and begins by emphasizing the truism that "disorders of the mind mean disorders of the brain, and that the latter is an organ liable to disease and disturbance; like other organs of the body, to be investigated by the same methods and subject to the same laws."

Among the causes of insanity we fail to find even a mention of poisoning by cocain, ergot, tobacco, mercury, salicylic acid, iodoform, and the bromids; we miss, as well, a description of many other causes of insanity, all of which one would expect to find in an "Encyclopedia of Medical Science." It is much to be regretted that in an article so ably written we should be forced to note these and other omissions. The chapters on the prevention of insanity and on the "Insane and the Law" are, however, very complete and well written.

The section devoted to idiocy comes from the pen of Paul Soilier of Paris, and is as complete and comprehensive an account of the subject, for its size, as we have ever read.

Professor Lombroso contributes a short article on criminal anthropology, written in his usual interesting style.

The causes and symptoms of old age are discussed by Dr. J. Boy-Teissier of Marseilles, while Jules Comby of Paris writes on the diseases of children, exclusive of the infectious diseases and rachitis. The article is concise and comprehensive, but is written as if for medical students instead of for medical practitioners. We regret that the eminent Physician-in-Chief to the Hôpital Trousseau has not contributed more from the great fund of knowledge that we know he possesses.

DISEASES OF THE STOMACH.—Their Special Pathology, Diagnosis, and Treatment, with Sections on Anatomy, Physiology, Analysis of Stomach Contents, Dietetics, Surgery of the Stomach, etc. By JOHN C. HEMMETER, M.B., M.D., Ph.D. Philadelphia: P. Blakiston, Son & Co., 1897.

THIS volume, notwithstanding the avowed purpose of the author to treat his "subject concisely," is expanded into a work of large magnitude. The author either must have lost sight of his purpose or have found that the material at his command exceeded his expectations.

The reviewer takes decided exception to the statement of the author that in this special field of clinical medicine "the names of Austin Flint, Pepper, Osler, and Delafield are as well known as those of Kussmaul, Senator, Nothnagel, Leube, Ewald, and Boas in Germany, or Hager, Bouveret, Debove, and Mathieu in France. No one will detract from the eminence of the American authors mentioned, their fame having been attained by the brilliancy of their work in the general field of clinical medicine; but what work in the special line of gastric diseases, may we ask, has justified the author in placing these names on the same pedestal as Kussmaul, Leube, Ewald, and Boas? Why has the author not added to the latter the name of Riegel of Giessen, whose work on "Die Erkrankungen des Magens" in Nothnagel's system is perhaps one of the best, if not the best, work on the subject of stomach diseases in any language? Professor Riegel has done as much original work in this special field as any of the men abroad who are so specifically indicated by the author.

As to the present work, the reviewer desires to call attention to the fact that if the purpose of the author to be concise were followed, much could be abstracted, much could be condensed, and still the value of the book would not suffer. The book contains, indeed, much of real worth, and its contents are presented in a very fluent, agreeable, and pleasant style. Part I. deals with the anatomy and physiology of the digestive organs and with the methods and technics employed in diagnosis. Part II. contains the therapy and materia medica of stomach diseases, and could be very well condensed into a much smaller compass without detracting from the dignity and importance of the subject. Part III. is called "The Gastric Clinic," and presents the subject of diseases of the stomach. Even this part will admit of condensation.

A very complete bibliography accompanies the various chapters, and still we miss the names of some American writers on stomach diseases. The author, it is true, correctly states that there are but few American laborers in this field, but mention of some of the few has been neglected. The work deserves careful reading, as it presents its facts clearly, and represents the status of knowledge in this special field up to date.

The book is handsomely printed, reflecting credit upon the publishers.

A HANDBOOK OF MIDWIFERY. By W. R. DAKIN, M.D., B.S. (Lond.), F.R.C.P., Obstetric Physician and Lecturer on Midwifery and Diseases of Women to St. George's Hospital. Illustrated. New York, London, and Bombay: Longman's, Green & Co., 1897.

IN this book the author presents a work intended for students and junior practitioners. He has arranged the subject in two parts—physiology and pathology—each of the elements of pregnancy, labor, and the puerpery being considered in detail in each division. In the first part the development of ovum and decidua and the diagnosis of pregnancy are particularly dwelt upon. We note that the author prefers making a diagnosis of the duration of pregnancy from the instrumental measurement of the fetal ovoid rather than from the height of the fundus uteri. His peculiar terminology, the "lie" of the fetus, refers to the relation of the long axis of the child to that of the mother. He thus distinguishes longitudinal, transverse, cephalic, and pelvic "lies."

The physiology and management of labor are next considered, chloroform being the anesthetic of choice. The physiology of the puerperal period and of the new-born child occupy the succeeding seven chapters. Under the pathology of pregnancy the author recommends induction of labor if an existing albuminuria does not diminish or disappear under appropriate treatment. His treatment of eclampsia consists in emptying the uterus by a preliminary puncture of the membranes, awaiting the advent of pains, and, if these are delayed, the application of the forceps if the child is alive; craniotomy if it is dead. Diaphoretics, cathartics, sedatives, and venesection are the additional measures advocated. The immediate removal of the sac is advised as the only satisfactory (and the author might have added rational) method of dealing with an ectopic gestation. Chapters on the obstetric operations, the pathology of labor, the puerperal period, and the new-born child complete the book. Walther's position, which is advised when it is necessary to increase the conjugate diameter for the use of the forceps in flat or generally contracted pelves, and thrombus vaginæ and hematoma of the vulva are considered in appendices. The work is a thorough review, and is a safe modern guide for the student and practitioner. It is conservative, as, for example, in the treatment of puerperal septicemia, but it is thoroughly digested and comprehensive. The illustrations are more than usually profuse, and, for the most part are original. The heavy paper and fine typography aid in making this one of the most attractive of recent works on obstetrics.

THERAPEUTIC HINTS.

Iodo-mercurial Treatment of Nephritis.—CAMPBELL BLACK has treated a number of patients having acute or subacute nephritis by the administration of the following mixture. This effected a rapid subsidence of the renal congestion, with the gradual disappearance of the albuminuria and other symptoms:

℞		
	Hydrarg. chlor. corros.	gr. i–ii
	Potass. iodid.	ʒ iii
	Syr. simpl.	℥ i
	Inf. gentian.	℥ vii.

M. Sig. A tablespoonful three times daily.

For the Urethritis Caused by Injections of Potassium Permanganate.—The use of large quantities of a solution of this drug in the treatment of gonorrhea frequently causes an irritation of the mucous membrane of the urethra, with the appearance of a thick mucous discharge not containing gonococci. For this condition STERNE recommends the following injection:

℞		
	Zinci sulphat.	gr. iv
	Glycerini, Aq. dest. } aa	℥ ii.

M. Sig. For injection into the urethra three times daily.

Treatment of Amebic Enteritis and Dysentery.—In this condition it is recommended to keep the patient in bed and upon a liquid diet, to apply hot compresses to the abdomen, and to give enemata of a one-per-cent. tannin solution. The internal medication should consist of a strong infusion of ipecac or of the following mixture (formula of Gelpke):

℞		
	Cort. simarubæ, Cort. granati } aa	ʒ iiss
	Vini gallici albi	Oiss.

M. Macerate twenty-four hours and then filter. Sig. A tablespoonful every two hours.

For the Cough of Phthisis VERSTRAETEN has found the action of Hydrastis Canadensis to be favorable. If the sputum is mucopurulent, its character rapidly improves, and the quantity diminishes. He prescribes pills containing from $\frac{1}{16}$- to $\frac{1}{8}$-grain of the dry extract. Of these five are to be taken during the twenty-four hours.

For Chlorosis.—HAYEM advises the employment of the protoxalate of iron, administered in cachets just before or during each meal. The dose is at first 1½ grains, and is gradually increased to 3½ grains, which is not to be exceeded. After a month the use of the iron is stopped a short time. Hydrotherapy and change of air are also recommended.

THE MEDICAL NEWS.

A WEEKLY JOURNAL OF MEDICAL SCIENCE.

VOL. LXXII. NEW YORK, SATURDAY, APRIL 30, 1898. No. 18.

ORIGINAL ARTICLES.

THE UNITED STATES AMBULANCE-SHIP "SOLACE."

BY CHARLES F. STOKES, M.D.,
PASSED-ASSISTANT SURGEON UNITED STATES NAVY.

IN discussing, with a large number of medical men, various topics in connection with duty on board the United States Ambulance-ship "Solace," I was struck with the great interest manifested by them in the ship, and with the vagueness of their ideas as to her equipment and mission. In view of the foregoing I suggested to Surgeon-general W. K. Van Reypen, United States Navy, who first advocated the fitting out of an ambulance-ship as a part of the fleet in naval contests, that the publication of his paper, "Handling and Care of the Wounded in Modern Naval Warfare," read before the Twelfth International Medical Congress, held at Moscow, Russia, August 19, 26, 1897, would be of immense value and absorbing interest to medical men in civil life.

He has delegated to me the duty of giving some account of the "Solace," the necessity for her existence, and her mission, and has allowed me to make use of such of his paper as may be necessary for the purpose. Dr. Van Reypen's paper is published in full in the Report of the Surgeon-general of the Navy, 1897, and from it I take the following:

How best to handle and care for the wounded in modern naval warfare is a problem that now confronts naval surgeons. It is thrust upon us by the energy and accomplishments of experts in construction, ordnance, and engineering. While they have so successfully fulfilled their mission of destruction, we must not be laggards in our still more important work of succor to the wounded and helpless. It is theirs to destroy; it is ours to save.

The conditions under which we find ourselves in the present day of battle-ships necessitate a radical departure from our former methods of treatment of wounded men in action, and their subsequent care. In the days of wooden ships, with flush gun- and spar-decks, admitting of comparative easy transportation of wounded, there was very little difficulty in moving men injured in action to the sick bay, where they could receive every needed surgical attention. The surgical staff was a unit, exercising its function in a circumscribed sphere. Its work was brought before it; now it must seek it.

A modern battle-ship is a honeycomb of steel, each cell containing its quota of workers, all acting harmoniously and in concert toward the accomplishment of the desired end, the overthrow of the adversary. Separated from their fellows by steel decks and water-tight doors, some means for their assistance in time of distress must be devised by naval surgeons; means that will not interfere with the fighting efficiency of the whole, and yet sufficient to assure the combatants that if disabled in the performance of their duty they will not be cast aside as useless incumbrances.

Any one familiar with the construction of a modern battleship will readily see the impossibility of caring for wounded men as in the days of wooden ships. The object of making closed compartments is to have them closed in time of action. The object of battle-plates is to have them screwed on in time of battle. By as much as these precautions are neglected, by so much is the efficiency of the fighting machine decreased. In the tops, in the superstructure, and in some of the living spaces men may be reached and cared for, but never again in modern warfare will the sick bay be the place where all the wounded will be brought during an action, and where the surgical staff will expend all of its energies.

It is more than probable that future sea fights will be short and bloody, and be fought at short range. With modern rapid-fire guns, all exposed parts of a vessel would soon be cleared of the living occupants and heavy armor would be the only protection.

Further on Dr. Van Reypen says:

Meanwhile the importance of first aid is clearly manifest. This first aid can only be rendered by comrades. The thorough instruction of the whole ship's company in the efficient manner of thus administering first aid cannot be too strongly urged. One of the first duties of the surgical staff of a newly commissioned vessel should be the drilling of the crew in the proper methods of controlling hemorrhage from different parts of the body, the removal of foreign bodies from wounds, and the placing in positions of injured or broken limbs. They should also be taught how to carry a man up or down through narrow hatches, over obstacles, or through contracted or tortuous passages with the least fatigue to themselves and the greatest comfort to the wounded. In many instances it would be impossible to use a cot or any form of stretcher; under these circumstances the only alternative is that the disabled should be carried.

The fighting space allotted, especially in turrets, is so contracted that the immediate removal of a disabled or wounded man is of the utmost importance. There is no unoccupied space in the turret where he could be laid aside, out of the way of the gun-workers, until action is over. His presence would temporarily disable the gun. The only practicable method of caring for him is to lower him to the partially cleared space at the base of the turret, either by the ammunition-hoist or lashed in a hammock; even here he would receive only temporary aid, as the space is too limited for the performance of any operation. Here he must remain until a favorable opportunity arises for his transfer to the central station.

On the vessels that remain afloat after a modern naval engagement, the decks will be much encumbered with wounded, such first aid as was possible will have been given to them, but their comfort and well being will by no means be enhanced by retaining them on board the vessel. Naval engagements will not be likely to take place under the lee of a shore hospital, and humanity demands that wounded men shall have speedy transfer to the place where they can be best cared for, and that place can be none other than an ambulance-ship. Such a vessel should be as much a component part of a fleet as the admiral's flagship. It would greatly add to the morale of the men behind the guns, when they went into action, if they saw near at hand a commodious hospital, with all the appliances for their care and comfort, and under the superintendence of skilled medical officers. This vessel should be solely and entirely an ambulance-ship, with a crew only sufficient to work the ship, and all her available deck room given up to quarters for sick and wounded.

Such a ship is the "Solace" which has been arranged to include as many conveniences as is practicable. She is primarily a vessel adapted for the care and welfare of sick and wounded men, and all other considerations are made subservient to this end. She has a displacement of 3600 tons, and an average speed of 14 knots; is 352 feet on the load-line and about 370 feet over all. Forward, below is a tank of 27,000 gallons capacity. The ship carries powerful steam-launches and barges for transferring the sick and wounded at sea. On the upper deck on both sides there are steam-winches for hoisting and lowering the wounded, or boats, which can be used simultaneously. On the uppermost deck are some of the officers' quarters and offices; on the next deck, forward, is an operating-room, 30x30 feet, well lighted, and magnificently equipped with aseptic hospital furniture of the best pattern, and the outfit of instruments, sterilizers, dressings, etc., is complete in every detail. The floor is so tiled that it can be easily cleaned and slipping avoided. A dressing-room and a dispensary adjoin the operating-room. On this deck are mess rooms for the officers of the ship, for wounded officers able to be about, and for the petty officers of the ship. There is a lounging- and smoking-room for those able to be on deck.

On the engine-room deck is a fully equipped steam laundry, with a drying-room, and a disinfecting-chamber for wash clothes. An ice-machine has been set up, and a cold-storage room of good size is ready for use. The ship is equipped with three large formaldehyd generators.

There are numerous staterooms for wounded officers, and the men will be berthed in spacious wards in the forward and after parts of the ship, below, which will be ventilated by powerful blowers and supplementary electric fans. The vessel is heated by steam and lighted by electricity throughout. There will be accommodations for about 350 patients.

There are four medical officers attached to the ship; three apothecaries, one of whom is a trained nurse and an embalmer; eight graduated nurses from the Mills Training School, Bellevue Hospital; two laundrymen; a cook, and four mess attendants for the sick and wounded, complete the medical department of the ship.

As soon as an action is over the steam-launches of the "Solace" will tow their barges alongside the ships that have been in action, and the wounded will be lowered into them, and the boats will return to the ambulance-ship, when the wounded will be brought on board and placed in the surgeons' care for treatment. With the facilities at hand the results ought to be excellent.

In no sense is the "Solace" a hospital ship. When it is found that a second action is not impending she will steam to the nearest hospital and place her sick and wounded on shore for treatment, and will then rejoin the fleet. Should the army invade Cuba, it will probably fall to her lot to transfer its wounded to Key West. The vessel is more properly designated an "ambulance ship."

The ship will fly the Red Cross and will be protected by the articles of the Geneva Convention.

COMMUNICATION WITH A TOWN INFECTED WITH YELLOW FEVER.[1]

By H. R. CARTER, M.D.,
SURGEON, MARINE HOSPITAL SERVICE.

AN infected town is a source of danger to its neighbors, whether it be declared in a state of quarantine or not, because a certain amount of illicit communication will occur, especially if the epidemic be prolonged. In my experience, the rigid non-intercourse rule, if continued for considerable periods, is less safe than carefully regulated communication. The object then is to formulate general rules under which commerce through and from infected places can be carried on (1) with the greatest safety to other communities, and (2) with the least inconvenience. The measures to be taken to some extent vary from a sanitary standpoint with the degree of infection of the place and from a commercial one with the extent of the interests involved and the way in which these interests are involved. The problem, even considering only the risk of conveying infection, which naturally is the first consideration, is of extreme intricacy and only a general outline, to be varied in particular cases, can be given here.

Railroad Traffic through an Infected Town.—(1) A passenger train shall not stop in an infected town nor shall the windows or doors be allowed open while the train remains in the affected locality; and no communication shall be allowed between the passengers or train-crew and the town. (2) Freight traffic through such a town shall be without stopping. (3) In cases where stopping in town is absolutely necessary for freight traffic, and also when the town is large and the infection general, a special crew shall take the train through the town. The relay stations where these changes are made

[1] Read at the Meeting of the Interstate Quarantine Convention, Held at Atlanta, Ga., April 12, 1898.

shall be under sanitary supervision. (4) Sanitary inspectors shall be stationed in the town.

Railroad Traffic from an Infected Town.—(Through traffic, *i. e.*, to points incapable of receiving yellow-fever infection, to be designated hereafter as "points North." The places capable of receiving infection being designated as "points South.") (1) *Freight.* Freight of any usual kind in sealed cars can go without hindrance through to destination. (2) *Empties.* Empties must not stay in an infected town or if parked in such a locality, must be disinfected. Flat cars must be swept clean. Box cars made mechanically clean and dry must be sent open to the relay station where they are to be inspected for tramps. All fruit cars must be disinfected. (3) *Mail.* Through mail, not distributed South, needs no quarantine restrictions save disinfection of bags. Parcels, except mercantile sample packages, shall be barred. (4) *Passenger.* Traffic to points North can be allowed by preventing all chance of such passengers conveying infection *en route*, either by themselves leaving the train *en route* or by returning to points South, or by fomites mainly contained in their clothing. This traffic must be on special cars reserved for these passengers and preferably on a special train. A sanitary inspector must accompany them through the quarantined territory, under whose absolute charge the train is. The coaches which carry these passengers must be disinfected before they return South.

Duties of Inspectors.—Train inspectors must be properly relayed,and those running from the infected town should be immune. If they sleep in other than clean territory they *must* be immune.

Passenger Traffic.—(1) Direct passenger traffic from an infected town to points capable of receiving infection must not be allowed. (2) Immunes may go to such territory after disinfection of baggage without detention. (3) Others must pass a time sufficient to cover the period of incubation of yellow fever, ten days, and not be exposed to any infection during this period, before being allowed to enter this territory.

Relays of Trains.—(1) All train crews from an infected town must be changed, and not allowed to have direct communication with certainly clean territory. This should be done at a non-infected place as isolated as possible, a siding rather than a station and certainly not in a town. (2) Every man, mail-agent, expressman, and train-butcher must make this relay, unless we know he is going North not to return to points South, in which case he is like a through passenger. Pullman crew to be relayed. (3) None of the merchandise of the train-butcher, unless disinfected papers be excepted, must pass the relay. No possible fomites must pass the relay to the crew bound North, and as little communication as possible, none save such as is necessary for the run of the train, is allowed. The relay must be under the supervision of a sanitary officer or officers (two are generally required) whose position is one of great responsibility. At these stations a very careful search for tramps must be instituted. (4) The camps for the North and South crews must be at a considerable distance from each other, and the run of trains should be arranged so as to have the crews in camp as little as possible. For passenger trains there need be no delay; for freight trains generally there must be relays and their crews must go into camp. (5) Occasions may arise where it is necessary to guard the Southern relay camp by a number of guards, as if it were a camp of detention. It must never be allowed to become infected. If it does the camp must be moved. (6) *Laundry* of Pullman cars must not be done in infected places.

Steamboat Communication.—This can be carried on: (1) By relays like railroad trains. (2) By supervision of the landing of freight and loading of same so as to prevent communication between the people ashore and the boat. This is confessedly difficult, but possible.

THE USE OF QUININ IN MALARIAL HEMOGLOBINURIA,

By ALBERT WOLDERT, M.D.,
OF PHILADELPHIA.

For many years the discussion regarding the use of quinin in malarial hemoglobinuria has lain almost dormant, the majority of physicians of large experience being in favor of the administration of quinin in this condition, but Bastianelli again brings forward testimony of physicians who are still under the impression that there is a certain form of hemoglobinuria in which quinin is the causative factor and in which its administration is distinctly productive of harm. Tamaselli, Spyridon, Canellis, and Pasquale Muscato have recorded cases of hemoglobinuria occurring during an attack of ague and caused by quinin, and Karamitza speaks of a case in which hemoglobinuria could be produced in a student upon the exhibition of five grains of this drug.

Laveran tells us that Tamaselli maintains that quinin is capable of producing not only hemoglobinuria, but also an icterohematuric fever, which can be easily confounded with a similar form of fever occurring in hot countries. Plehn, Richardson, and others also hold to the opinion that quinin may cause hemoglobinuria.

Bastianelli admits that these cases are extremely rare in Italy and that no case has ever been reported from the Campagna. He states that the instances of spontaneous hemorrhages due to the use of quinin occur in those individuals who have recently had an attack of malarial fever, although the plasmodium cannot be found in the blood at the time of the onset of the hematuria. This observer divides the spontaneous hemoglobinuria into three classes: (1) Those in which the blood contains estivo-autumnal parasites or young hyaline forms; (2) those in which the blood contains only crescentic or ovoid bodies and pigmented leucocytes; or, (3) those in which the blood examination is entirely negative and the only evidence of there having been an infection is the presence of endothelial perilobular melanosis. Here the attack of hemoglobinuria does not depend upon the presence of parasites, but begins without apparent cause.

Bastianelli finally takes up the quinin hemoglobinurias, and asserts that: (*a*) It occurs only in individuals in whom a malarial infection has been recently present; (*b*) the hemoglobinuric attack is constantly produced every time quinin is administered, whether it be given while the malaria is in progress (Tamaselli), or when the malarial infection has run its course (Murri); (*c*) extremely small doses of quinin are capable of bringing on an attack; (*d*) quinin hemoglobinuria has been observed in patients who have already suffered from hemoglobinuria (Murri).

The *quinin* hemoglobinuria he divides into two forms: (1) That occurring during the paroxysm, or paroxysmal hemoglobinuria, and (2) postmalarial hemoglobinuria. In these varieties, through a considerable length of time quinin will produce hemoglobinuria whenever it is administered. The course to be pursued depends upon the blood examination. If hemoglobinuria occurs during a malarial paroxysm and parasites are found in the blood, quinin should always be given. If, however, no parasites are found, either as a result of previous administration of quinin or on account of the spontaneous disappearance of the organisms, Bastianelli says that quinin should not be given, owing to the possibility that the paroxysm may have been due to its previous administration.

It will be observed that this report of Bastianelli has been quoted at some length and it is hoped that the reader will keep in mind his classification of "quinin hemoglobinuria."

In this connection it might be well to first briefly explain the physiologic action of quinin.

Local Action.—When applied upon the mucous membrane quinin exerts a very perceptible stimulant or irritant action. It has the same effect when applied to a muscle.

Circulation.—Wood states that he has never been able to perceive any depressant action upon the circulation in man after ordinary (3 to 5 grains) doses of the drug. In large doses it lowers the arterial pressure, due to action on the heart and its paralyzant effect upon the vasomotor system. Laveran says that it cannot be classed absolutely either among the stimulants or among the depressants, as its effects differ according to the dose employed. In small doses quinin in healthy men and in rabbits causes an acceleration of the heart's action, and an elevation of the blood-pressure. In large doses it slows the action of the heart.

Effect of Quinin on the Blood-Corpuscles and Plasmodium Malariæ.—Binz and Schutte have investigated its action upon the red blood-cells, and reached the conclusion that it lessens the power of the hemoglobin to convert oxygen into ozone, therefore it lessens the ozonizing action of the blood. The experiments of Binz go to show that the action of quinin is poisonous to the protoplasm of the organism which causes the disease, in other words, that it is antiparasitic. In his experiments, he showed that in a dilution of 1:20,000 it killed infusoria—paramecium—beginning within five minutes, and at the end of two hours there was complete dissolution of the organism. Five grains of quinin circulating in the blood of a man of average size represents a dilution of 1:16,000 which is stronger than that with which Binz paralyzed the colpoda within five minutes.

Rossbach believes that it deprives the protoplasm of the power of absorbing oxygen, thereby forming a combination less easily oxidized than either substance alone.

Quinin, having this effect upon protoplasm, it has been supposed that it might limit or destroy the phagocytic action of the white blood corpuscles, but Laveran believes that instead of their action being diminished it is actually increased after its administration.

Effect of Toxic Doses of Quinin.—According to the experiments of Schlockow, Eulenberg, Briquet, and Cerna there is a lowering of the arterial pressure and the pulse is almost imperceptible at the wrist. The evidence is therefore clear that both in man aud in the lower animals quinin in toxic doses is a powerful depressant to the heart-muscle and ganglia.

Cases in Which Large Doses of Quinin Have Been Given without Producing Hemoglobinuria.—Guersent cites a case in which a lady became deaf, dumb, and blind from taking 10 drams of quinin sulphate within the course of a few days. Guiacomini spoke of a case in which a man took 3 drams of quinin and who only suffered from symptoms of depression of the heart and nervous system. Briquet records a death following the enormous dose of 55 drams taken within a period of ten days.

Laveran quotes from Baillio, who reports the instance of two soldiers, who, intending to take a purgative, but instead of taking sodium sulphate, by mistake, drank a solution of quinin, so that each received about 3 drams of the salt. Half an hour after taking the medicine the men were seized with cramps in the epigastric region and with vomiting. They presented paleness of the face, dilation of the pupils, hurried respiration, chilly sensations, a small, irregular, and slow pulse, sometimes hardly perceptible, together with ringing in the ears, and symptoms of syncope. In the case of one, the symptoms gradually disappeared; the other died of heart-failure. It may be said that in these cases the persons affected were in good health and that there was no concomitant poison, such as a toxin, present to aid in the production of hemoglobinuria. To this the writer can say that in nearly fifty consecutive cases of typhoid fever treated at the Mercy Hospital, Pittsburg, in which quinin was given, no case of hemoglobinuria developed. Thousands of cases can be added by others.

Absorption and Elimination of Quinin.—Under ordinary circumstances absorption takes place very quickly, and Kerner found it in the urine within fifteen minutes when given by the month. Carofolo has confirmed this investigation. Binz has found quinin in the saliva of a poisoned dog, and Landerer in the urine, sweat, tears, milk of nursing mothers, and in dropsic effusions, while De Renzi and Albertoni found it in large quantities in the bile, when it had been ingested by the mouth.

Baccelli, Briquet, Binz, Dielt, and De Renzi all agree that while the excretion of quinin through the kidneys begins early, yet at the same time it continues very slowly, Dielt and De Renzi having found it in the urine six or seven days after its administration. Baccelli agrees with the statement of Manossci, strengthened by the experiments of Welitchkowski, that fever retards the action of quinin.

Quinin Idiosyncrasies.—Ringer speaks of a case in which the administration of quinin always caused a uniform red rash over the whole body, most marked on the back of the neck, accompanied by very severe stinging pain, especially in the back of the neck, and in the clefts between the fingers. Desquamation as free as after a sharp attack of scarlet fever always followed the rash. Quinin sometimes produces large erythematous patches, urticaria, swelling of the face and hands, tingling of the end of fingers and toes, a sense of warmth, acceleration of the pulse, and often great gastric irritability, with nausea and vomiting. Wood reports a case of amaurosis produced by a dose of 12 grains.

Schamberg notes a case in which a man fifty-five years of age, who, when taking quinin, always suffered from violent balano-urethritis, the meatus urinarius being occluded by a pseudomembranous exudate.

It will therefore doubtless be observed that in all these cases of idiosyncrasies due to quinin, that the drug seems to spend its force upon the nervous system and mucous membranes, rather than having any notable effect upon the renal organs or red blood-cells; further, that in small, large, and toxic doses, both in man and in the lower animals, in health and in disease, quinin has no tendency to produce hemoglobinuria.

Varieties of Hemoglobinuria.—Possibly the most logical classification of hemoglobinuria is made by Osler, as follows: (1) Paroxysmal hemoglobinuria, (2) toxic hemoglobinuria. The latter includes those due to (*a*) carbolic acid, (*b*) chlorate of potash, (*c*) napthol, (*d*) carbon dioxid, (*e*) poisons of infectious fevers, such as scarlet fever, yellow fever, typhus fever, and malarial fever.

How Hemoglobinuria Is Caused in the Infectious Fevers.—Owing to the action of the toxin upon the red cells, a process of necrobiosis begins, leading to disintegration and degeneration, setting free the hemoglobin (hemocytolysis), which dissolves in the blood plasma and, with a certain proportion of serum albumin, is excreted by the kidneys. No doubt this is the process set up in all the infectious fevers in which hemoglobinuria is observed, and we have no right to believe that the congestion and the hemoglobinuria (or hematuria) arising from the malarial fevers differs in its mode of production from this observed in any of the other varieties of infectious disease.

Dawson and Davis maintain that the real underlying condition which leads to hemoglobinuria is essentially a renal congestion, the latter holding to the belief that there is also some alteration in the nutrition of the vessel-walls, which may be due to an obscure hereditary influence.

Bemiss believes the condition to be due to a combination of altered blood-pressure, impaired nutrition of the vessel-walls, and changes in the vascular pressure in the various congested organs.

Morbid Anatomy of the Kidney of Acute Malaria.—Thayer states that the changes in the kidneys in acute malaria are usually much less marked than in the liver and spleen. The gross appearance of the organs varies but little from the normal. The glomeruli, however, are considerably pigmented, the pigment at times being seen within the large white cells within the vessels, and sometimes in the glomerular endothelium.

The Kidney of Malarial Hemoglobinuria.—These changes in the kidneys when hemoglobinuria has supervened have been described by Thayer, Pellarin, Kierner, and Kelsch as follows: The kidneys are somewhat enlarged, the color varying from a deep reddish-brown, to a light yellowish-brown coffee color, often the color is distributed in pale, irregular, pin-head points, and blotches of a maroon-color are to be seen upon the surface, some several millimeters in area. The pyramids are of a deep red color from intratubular hemorrhages. The capsule is easily detached; the consistency of the organ is normal.

The epithelium of the convoluted tubules and of the large branches of Henle's loops is very opaque, the nuclei being scarcely visible. The epithelial cells are swollen and bulge into the lumen of the canal. The lumen of the tubule is filled with clumps of amorphous material or casts mixed to a greater or less extent with pigment. The epithelium and lumina of the tubules are filled with large granules often resembling casts. Between the glomerulus and capsule, usually near the mouth of the tubule, there is often quite a collection of granules, which are also occasionly found in epithelial cells, and sometimes free. In some cases there are small interstitial hemorrhages. The pyramids show few changes. The epithelium is usually intact, though sometimes protruding and vesicular cells suggest that this may take part in the formation of hyaline material. Almost invariably the tubes are filled with blood-corpuscles.

Having before us this vivid description of the morbid anatomy of the kidney of hemoglobinuria (hematuria) one cannot but see that it is a high grade of congestion due to some poison in the system having a profound influence upon the internal organs.

What Is the Cause of the Hemoglobinuria?—The law of causation involves the three following affirmations, each of which is the groundwork of a process of elimination: (1) Whatever antecedent can be left out without prejudice to the effect can be no part of the cause. (2) When an antecedent cannot be left out without the consequent disappearing, such antecedents must be the cause or part of the cause. (3) An antecedent and a consequent rising and falling together in numeric concomitance are to be held as cause and effect.

Possibly the first one of these affirmations is most applicable to this question: Having concurrently a dilute solution of quinin circulating in the blood, together with that of a powerful toxin, such as that formed by the plasmodium malariæ, can it be supposed that the former will gain the ascendancy and lead to the production of a condition which the largest doses have *always* failed to do?

Clinical Experience against the Theory of Quinin Hemoglobinuria.—Bastianelli admits that cases of hemoglobinuria following the administration of quinin in malarial fever are very rare in Italy, and that no case has ever been reported from the Campagna, but he states that the cases of spontaneous hemoglobinuria due to quinin increase in number as one goes toward the South. Laveran says he cannot understand why such a condition should be so common in Greece and Italy and so rare in Algiers. In North America let us trace its occurrence as we go toward the South: Dr. Ashhurst recently told the writer that he had never seen a case of hematuria (hemoglobinuria) produced by quinin, and that he would give quinin for this condition. Anders has seen hemoglobinuria produced in some cases of malarial fever in which quinin had not been taken, and states that it disappeared upon the administration of this remedy. Osler says that the condition does not exist in the latitude of Baltimore. Thayer, also of Johns Hopkins, in a recent private communication says that he has never seen a case of hemoglobinuria due to quinin. Dawson of South Carolina says: "I have avoided mentioning the theory, again recently discussed by Italian physicians, that quinin may of itself produce hematuria. This theory I believe to be wholly groundless, and it certainly is not maintained by physicians of to-day." Dr. Guiteras says that in his experience in Cuba he met with no such cases.

Dock, formerly of Texas, but now of Michigan, says that within the last few years, the subject of hematuria from quinin has been brought up again by physicians in Greece and Italy, but the unusual consequences of quinin in the hands of these men make it almost certain they did not have to do with malarial hematuria.

Consensus of Opinion Regarding the Use of Quinin in Malarial Hemoglobinuria.—Dock (1892): "The treatment of malarial hematuria, which also includes hemoglobinuria, belongs really to the treatment of acute and chronic malarial poisoning. No American physician at the present time has any doubt about the propriety of giving quinin in these cases, so that a consideration of that vexed question is unnecessary."

Thompson (1893) advises that quinin be given hypodermically in this condition.

Osler (1895): "In quinin we possess a specific remedy against malarial infection. In cases of estivo-autumnal fever with pernicious symptoms it is necessary to get the system under the influence of quinin as rapidly as possible. In these instances the bisulphate or muriate of quinin and urea should be administered hypodermically."

Laveran (1896): "It should be insisted upon that in grave forms of malarial fever, and in the continual types of malarial fever one should not wait for the intermissions or even the remissions for the administration of quinin." Laveran uses quinin by the mouth and hypodermically, preferring for the latter on account of its solubility the chlorhydro-sulphate (5 grains of which can be easily dissolved in 15 minims of water).

Dawson (1896): "The treatment of the different forms of malarial hematuria may vary somewhat as to detail, but our first effort should be to bring the patient as rapidly as possible under the influence of quinin in some form, so as to control the destructive power of the malarial germs, thereby holding the cause of the hemorrhage in abeyance, if not able to remove it completely." Dawson further states that he has used quinin in very large doses in malarial fevers, and has continued its use for long periods, and has never seen it produce hemoglobinuria.

Tyson (1897) recommends quinin in malarial hematuria, and believes that this symptom is due to another cause than quinin.

Anders (1897) says that he has observed several instances of hematuria in the milder forms of malaria in which no quinin had been taken and in which it had subsequently been given (16 grains daily) with the result that the hemoglobinuria had been relieved.

Since 1887, at the St. Louis Southwestern Railroad Hospital of Tyler, Texas, several hundred cases of malarial fever have been annually treated. It is the routine practice there to administer quinin both in *small* and *large* doses (2 to 30 grains) by the mouth and hypodermically, as the case may demand, and it is not known that any case of hemoglobinuria developed from its use. Further, since the year ending June 30, 1893, there were five cases of malarial hemoglobinuria admitted to the wards—in all of which the patients received quinin; in no case was the condition made worse by quinin, and all of the patients recovered.

THE USES AND LIMITATIONS OF NUCLEIN AS A THERAPEUTIC AGENT.

By J. H. BURCH, M.D.,
OF BALDWINSVILLE, N. Y.

PERHAPS nothing can demonstrate more fully the heterogeneous tendency of the medical thought of our age, than a careful perusal of current literature upon the action and uses of nuclein. While a few patient and careful observers like Vaughn, Metchnikoff, and Ames are earnestly working to demonstrate its sphere of usefulness as a therapeutic agent, scores of others, with no guide or aim than that of the grossest empiricism, are extolling its application in the most diversified and conflicting conditions. I well remember the hopes which some of these gushing opinions inspired in me, and the several failures which resulted from my early exhibitions of this agent, but, although I had several startling failures, I was often rewarded with signal success, and it was a careful review of these several successes and failures which led me to believe that nuclein, like every other remedial agent, has it uses circumscribed by clear-cut limitations. In this connection, I record the following case:

CASE I.—Mrs. S., aged forty-nine years, came to me presenting the appearance of an emaciated, overworked woman. She was the mother of seven children born in rapid succession. She had always attended to her household duties, working from early in the morning until late at night. While her family and personal history were all that could be desired, her sunken eyes, anemic and pinched face, bloodless lips, cold hands, and irregular heart-action, with its hemic murmur, all bespoke the impoverished condition of her blood. I examined her urine, and found that she daily passed about 1500 c.c. of urine, which was pale and clear with no other abnormality than that the phosphates were increased to sixteen per cent. Examination of the blood revealed the red corpuscles reduced to 3,200,000 to the c.m. (Thoma-Zeiss), poikylocytosis well marked, the red cells taking the stain badly (Ehrlricke), and leaving round hyaline spaces within the corpuscles. There were no nucleated red cells or other abnormal cell formation; hemoglobin seventy-five per cent.; the number of leucocytes was 8400 to the c.m., and they were normal in every respect, except, perhaps, a slight increase in the number of eosinophiles. With this history and clinical finding I prescribed nuclein, with the result that I allowed this poor woman to remain six weeks in this condition, carefully examining her blood three times weekly, with no other result than a marked leucocytosis which in no way relieved the anemia. A six-weeks' course of iron and arsenic almost completely restored her health.

After this failure I made a number of blood-counts, fifty in all, exhibiting nuclein in each case with the idea of determining its action upon the red blood-cells, and not in one instance, after repeated countings, did I find any abnormal change either in character or numbers except a slight variation which might be expected. Thus, I came to the conclusion that nuclein in simple anemia, or in fact pernicious anemia, *unless complicated* either by *qualitative* or *quantitative alteration of the leucocytes*, has no influence whatever. Yet, almost daily I read reports of all forms of anemia in which treatment with nuclein has been successful, and one writer even goes so far as to claim poikylocytosis as a special indication for its use. Still I have found instances of complicated anemia in which great benefit resulted from its administration, as the following case will illustrate:

CASE II.—Bertha D., age twelve years; previous

health and family history excellent. Her general appearance was bad; face, pale and wan; lips, colorless; deep circles under her eyes; hands and feet cold, etc. There was a hemic murmur. The cervical glands were swollen, one being in a process of suppuration, discharging thin pus, and showing little tendency to heal. Examination of the blood showed hemoglobin 49 per cent., red cells 3,600,000 c.m., normal in shape, but presenting end-globular changes characterized by hyaline spaces within the cells, as described by Maragliano. I also found a deficient leucocytosis; there were but 4000 white cells to the c.mm., the reduction being more appreciable with respect to the polymorphonuclear leucocytes. In this case the anemia was evidentily the result of a ptomain toxemia, and on this belief I prescribed nuclein; and whether future investigation proves the phagocytosis theory of Metchnikoff to be true or false, the fact remains that the number of polynuclear and mononuclear leucocytes increased to such an extent that at the end of one week the blood-count showed the red cells to be 4,300,000 to the c.m., and the white cells 10,000 to the c.m., the increase being manifested in regard to the polynuclear and mononuclear leucocytes. The suppuration ceased, and the little patient made a good recovery.

The next case presents to my mind a clear-cut picture of the indications for the use of nuclein.

CASE III.—John G., aged twenty-five years; occupation, clerk in the post-office; family history good; general appearance fair. Two years before he had had laryngitis from which he had recovered. His health had been good since, with the exception of slight attacks of bronchitis. April 8, 1897, he became ill with measles, which ran its usual course up to April 16th, when he had a chill followed by fever and pain in the side; in fact, he presented the usual clinical picture of pneumonia. The area of dulness extended from half an inch below the right nipple downward. His temperature was 103 F.; pulse, 120, weak and compressible; urine, normal, there being no appreciable diminution of the chlorids. Blood examination: red cells normal, 5,000,000 to the c.m.; leucocytes 7000 to the c.m., the tongue was dry and the bowels constipated. The expectoration was rust-colored, containing streptococci and pneumococci. I prescribed $\frac{1}{30}$-grain of strychnin every three hours. The condition remained practically the same until April 21st. The temperature was now 104° F. (evening), and the pulse was soft and compressible and oscillated from 100 to 130 per minute. The heart-action was weak and not very regular, and the local condition remained unchanged. The tongue was dry and brown. There was muttering delirium. The urine contained a slight trace of albumin and a few denuded, round epithelial cells and blood shadows; there was a very slight decrease of the chlorids. The urine was strongly acid in reaction and swarmed with very motile bacilli.

I made an inoculation from the urine on agar-agar, and after twenty-four hours obtained a culture. The culture and morphology of the bacillus resembled that of the bacillus coli communis, and upon further investigation I found that it caused fermentation of glucose, coagulated milk, clouded bouillon, and produced indol. I therefore felt safe in pronouncing it the coli bacillus. Blood-count: red cells, 5,000,000 to the c.m.; white cells, 6800; hemoglobin, forty five per cent. The general appearance of the patient was bad. There was diarrhea, the bowels moving four times within twenty-four hours. There was also iliocecal gurgling and tenderness; Widal-test negative. I prescribed strychnin, 1/20-grain every four hours.

April 22nd. Temperature, 104° F.; pulse, 120, very weak and somewhat irregular; tongue, dry and brown; patient delirious and restless through the night; local condition unchanged; urine contained albumin and a few more round, denuded epithelial cells than the day before; chlorids somewhat diminished; reaction acid, and coli bacilli still present. Blood-count: red cells, 4,000,000 to the c.m.; white cells, 6780 to the c.m.; the polymorphonuclear cells presented a very peculiar appearance. The nuclei were pale, granular, and not well defined, the the protoplasm of the cell being filled with granular dots and the limiting membrane broken in places. In some of the cells the protoplasm was altogether deficient. Others again were deficient in limiting membrane, amorphous in appearance, and contained degenerated nuclei and protoplasm, resembling a cross between a myelocyte and an eosinophilocyte, but still not like eosinophilic-myelocytes.

I prescribed Auld's nuclein, two tablets every two hours, and the strychnin as before.

April 23rd. There was but little change in the patient's condition, except that his pulse was more regular; the diarrhea still continued, the stools being yellowish. The condition of the urine was unchanged. Blood-count: hemoglobin, fifty per cent.; red cells 4,500,000 and leucocytes 7500 to the c.m.; the polymorphonuclear cells presented the same appearance as the day before, but there were several very large polynuclear cells containing degenerated nuclei, and presenting somewhat the appearance of eosinophiles, and on this day, for the first time, I noticed very numerous granules scattered throughout the blood plasma. These were round refractive bodies similar to those described by Müller, and the addition of a one-per-cent. solution of acetic acid did not destroy them. After observing a fresh specimen of unstained blood for over an hour I felt very sure that I saw one of these granules escape from a polynuclear leucocyte.

April 25th. Patient's general appearance better; he rested much better through the night; the pulse was 100 per minute and regular; temperature, 102° F.; urine, free from albumin, and the coli bacilli was rapidly disappearing; tongue more moist; no diarrhea. Blood-count: red cells 4,800,000 to the c.m.; white, 8500 to the c.m., being mostly mononuclear leucocytes. The polynuclear cells were very small, and had distinct nuclei. The granules of Müller were more marked than the day before.

The local condition was beginning to show signs of resolution.

April 30th. The temperature was normal; pulse, 80, regular and steady; urine normal; tongue clean; dulness still continued, but subcrepitant râles were heard over the affected area. Blood count: 4,900,000 red cells to the c.m.; white, 12,000 to the c.m. Nuclein and strychnin were the only medicines employed. The patient made an uninterrupted recovery.

From a careful study of nuclein, *per se*, its origin, chemistry, and physiologic action, and from careful blood examinations in not a few cases, I am convinced that the one great indication for the exhibition of this agent is *deficient leucocytosis*, and that its only therapeutic property is its power to augment the number of leucocytes, thereby producing a protective leucocytosis, and, therefore, the only sure and safe guide for its exhibition is a careful examination of the blood in each and every case.

THE PRELIMINARY CONDUCT OF INTESTINAL OPERATIONS.

BY R. HARVEY REED, M.D.,
OF ROCK SPRINGS, WYOMING.

AMONG the many details essential to success in intestinal surgery are the preliminary preparations, and in regard to these it may be said that custom makes law, and law is binding because nearly every one conforms to it. I think this applies to intestinal operations, and at the same time I think that many of us have respected a particular law, the result of custom, without ever stopping to consider the relations between the physiologic effects of certain drugs used in these preparations and the pathologic conditions for the relief of which operative interference is proposed. For example, in intestinal obstructions, there are few diagnosticians who are able to tell prior to an exploratory incision the exact condition which has caused the trouble. The symptoms may indicate obstruction beyond any question, but who can say whether it is the result of an enterolith, cicatricial constriction, invagination, volvulus, or even paralysis. It is a common custom not only to resort to the use of cathartics in intestinal obstructions, but to continue their use until not only the entire alimentary tract above the obstruction is intensely irritated, but also until the muscular and serous coats are congested. As a result the intestines are oftentimes found in an acute inflammatory condition, with the presence of exudates and transudates in abundance.

Experience has led me to believe that the continued use of cathartics in any form of intestinal obstruction, not even excepting impaction, is injurious and unfits the patient for the ordeal of operation. The mildest cathartic is a stimulant to the glands of the intestinal mucous membrane, and as such is intended to increase the secretions and at the same time exaggerate the peristaltic action. If the use of cathartics is persisted in we are bound to set up a *vis a tergo*, resulting in stercoraceous vomiting, and whenever that occurs, we know we have reverse peristaltic action, together with an obstruction of some kind, prohibiting the onward movement of the intestinal contents through the natural channel. This being the case, what reason is there, either from a physiologic or pathologic standpoint, for increasing this peristalsis by administering drugs intended for that very purpose?

The use of opiates may allay the pain, but will surely mask the symptoms, and thus not only lead the patient and his friends astray, but the physician as well. Again, false hope may be engendered when the obstruction has continued sufficiently long to produce paralysis or gangrene; in either case, the pain subsiding, the patient imagines he is better, and not infrequently the attending physician is similarly misled by these very serious and usually fatal symptoms.

I am sure there is not a general surgeon who has not repeatedly operated for intestinal obstruction and found the bowel congested or possibly necrotic and distended with secretions. This, of course, may occur in cases in which there has been no irritation of the mucous membrane by medication, but in my experience, I have found less congestion, less secretion, and less dilation when cathartics have not been used. If this is true in the experience of others, we should be guarded in the use of laxatives, and especially in the use of drastic cathartics in all cases of intestinal obstruction.

I recall three cases of fecal impaction, in one of which the intestinal tract was obstructed by cherry stones to such an extent that nothing but mechanical interference could give relief. In the other case the obstruction was caused by hardened feces, necessitating operative interference, and in a third case there was an obstruction by a large enterolith which had lodged at the ileocecal valve and produced complete obstruction. According to text-book teaching and "custom," in the cases referred to, patients were all given cathartics irrespective of stercoraceous vomiting and intense intestinal pain. From irritation by these drugs the bowels were distended with secretions and were congested to such an extent as to produce profuse transudations, in several instances exudations, placing each patient in a perilous condition without in the least relieving the obstruction.

The argument against the use of cathartics also holds

true in circular constriction of the bowel, whether of malignant or cicatricial origin. It also holds true where there is an obstruction by adhesive bands, volvulus, or invagination, and I wish to enter my protest against the persistent use of cathartics in any and all of these conditions: (1) for the reason that as a rule they fail to relieve intestinal obstruction; (2) because they produce unnecessary congestion and irritation of the intestinal tract and thus place the patient in still greater peril, and (3) for the reason that operative interference becomes more dangerous, because of the irritation produced by their use.

There are exceptions to all rules, but these exceptions only tend to prove the rule, and, while I believe that the persistent use of cathartics is usually injurious to the patient and as a rule fails to relieve the obstruction, it is true that occasionally there are cases of severe obstruction in which recovery follows their use. Among these exceptions, I might mention two cases in which the obstruction was caused by invagination and in which, after from fourteen to twenty days of absolute obstruction, the invaginated portion of the gut became necrotic, sloughed out, and escaped with a gush of feces, the patients ultimately recovering. Notwithstanding occasional exceptions, I am still of the opinion that it is not to the advantage of the patient with obstruction to continue the use of laxatives, and much less the use of drastic cathartics.

The fact that when given continuously cathartics produce irritation and oftentimes inflammation of the intestinal tract, even in patients who are not suffering from obstruction, is to my mind sufficient evidence that they should not be so employed, especially in the affection under consideration. Such a course adds a serious complication to the existing pathologic condition, which we, as physicians and surgeons, should strive to avoid.

It must be conceded by every operator that the less the irritation of the intestinal tract, as well as of the intestinal and parietal peritoneum, the more favorable the prognosis. This being true, it is quite evident that a patient who must submit to an operation for the relief of intestinal obstruction is placed in a position of greater danger when the entire intestinal tract above the obstruction is irritated by laxatives and especially by drastic cathartics. Under these circumstances, the surgeon must contend not only with inflammation, but also with the increased amount of material in the intestines which has resulted from the use of cathartics, to say nothing of the increased peristaltic action, which, of course, must interfere with any operation that necessitates incision of the intestine. It is an indisputable fact that increased peristaltic action has a tendency to retard repair of intestinal wounds, as the continued shaking up of a fracture retards the repair of the bone. With this in mind, it is highly important that the intestinal tract should be as nearly immobilized as possible after an operation, and kept so until the process of repair have sufficiently advanced to make it certain that there will be no extravasation of intestinal contents into the abdominal cavity.

For the reasons given I feel that I am justified in protesting against the use of cathartics prior to operations upon the intestinal tract, and also in insisting that only remedies should be used which have a tendency to empty the intestinal canal without leaving the bowel in a state of irritation to complicate the dangerous operation which may soon be necessary.

To reiterate my position I maintain that in all cases in which intestinal obstruction is suspected and in which the use of mild laxatives, together with enemas and massage, fails to give relief, the employment of drastic cathartics should be guarded against. I believe it is much safer to make an early exploratory incision, if need be, to determine the diagnosis than to continue the administration of drugs which may cause inflammation, a serious complication we should always seek to avoid.

RHINITIS FIBRINOSA, INCLUDING A BACTERIOLOGIC AND HISTOLOGIC EXAMINATION OF CASES.

BY GEORGE L. CHAPMAN, M.D.,
OF CHICAGO;
ASSISTANT IN PATHOLOGY AND IN LARYNGOLOGY IN THE CHICAGO POLYCLINIC.

THE subject of rhinitis fibrinosa is as a rule very briefly if at all, treated, in such text-books as might be expected to contain a detailed account of it. This disease was recognized and described by B. Fränkel, Hartmann, Seifert, and others. It is referred to under a variety of names, *viz.*, croupous, membranous, fibrinous, primary pseudomembranous, plastic and fibrinoplastic rhinitis, and nasal diphtheria. Rhinitis fibrinosa is not a common disease; therefore, when observed, it deserves more than passing notice. It is characterized by an acute inflammation with a fibrinous exudate limited to the nasal cavities. The symptoms are usually benign, the most distressing being sudden nasal occlusion, necessitating almost constant oral respiration, mucopurulent discharge, and a somewhat chronic course.

The etiology of this form of nasal disease, as has been demonstrated by careful study, is not uniform. A few years after it had been generally recognized that the cause of a certain form of primary faucial diphtheria was the Klebs-Löffler bacillus, this micro-organism was looked for, and found to be present in a large percentage of the cases of rhinitis fibrinosa in which a bacteriologic examination was made. Concetti was the first to call attention to the contagions nature of the disease, and he recommended isolation and disinfection. The first authors who undertook the bacteriologic examination of cases of rhinitis fibrinosa were Gradenigo and Maggiore. They claimed that the staphylococcus pyogenes aureus was the cause of the affection. Lieven isolated a staphylococcus which he claims is similar to the staphylococcus pyogenes aureus, but not identical with it. It is distinguished from the staphylococcus pyogenes aureus by some cultural features and by its lesser virulency. Abel did not find the diphtheria bacillus, but isolated pneumococci having a very mild degree of virulency.

Abbott reports three cases in which he found the diphtheria bacillus. His work is of special interest because of its thorough character. In two of his cases he found a bacillus similar to that of true diphtheria, but of lessened vitality. In the other case the bacillus found could not be differentiated from the typical diphtheria bacillus. M. Ravenel, in an investigation of ten cases, followed Abbott, and found in all but one a bacillus similar to the Klebs-Löffler bacillus, except for a lessened vitality and virulency. In one case, he found a bacillus which could not be differentiated from the true virulent, diphtheria, bacillus. Bluder examined six cases, finding the diphtheria bacillus in all. Buys examined one case, finding the diphtheria bacillus. D. Braden Kyle reports two cases in which he found the staphylococcus aureus; he described the exudate as organized, laminated, fibrinoplastic.

The most extensive bacteriologic study of rhinitis fibrinosa was made by Meyer, who investigated thirty-one cases. He found that rhinitis fibrinosa may be caused by the diphtheria bacillus, but also by streptococci and staphylococci. In spite of the difference in the bacteriologic findings there was no material variation of the clinical course in his cases. In his excellent paper he calls attention to the fact that "a bacteriologic examination with reference to an exudate found in the nose must of necessity be frequently misleading, since the nasal cavity is normally the habitat of a variety of micro-organisms, among which is also found, occasionally in health, the diphtheria bacillus, which then may be obtained in culture without being the true cause of the disease."

Somers reports an interesting case in which the first culture did not show the diphtheria bacillus, though a subsequent culture revealed its presence. In this instance the disease was characterized by mild symptoms, although two other members of the same family became severely infected, one with laryngeal and the other with faucial diphtheria.

As is well known, a fibrinous exudate is frequently found after operations in the nasal cavity, especially after cauterization of the turbinate bodies.

Experiments to artificially produce rhinitis fibrinosa in man have been made only by Lieven, who, as stated before, claims that a specific staphylococcus is the cause of this affection. His experiments, while carefully made under the supervision of Seifert in Würzburg, have not yet been confirmed by others.

In view of the uncertain character of a bacteriologic examination in rhinitis fibrinosa, it has not been made the main feature of investigation in the cases to be reported in this paper. It may be at once stated that the diphtheria bacillus was not found in any one of them. Recently the nature of the exudate in bronchitis fibrinosa has become a matter of controversy. Beschorner, and also Grandy, have lately claimed that in bronchitis fibrinosa the casts consist of mucin, while in two cases examined by Herzog, the fibrinous nature of the exudate was demonstrated. It therefore appeared of interest to study the exudate in rhinitis fibrinosa to determine, if possible, its true nature. A satisfactory histologic examination cannot be easily made in each and every case; since it is difficult to obtain from the nasal cavity a piece of the pseudomembrane without crushing it in such a manner that it becomes useless for examination purposes.

CASE I.—R. J., male, aged six years, was brought to the nose and throat department of the Chicago Policlinic, Dr. M. R. Brown's clinic, October 4, 1897, complaining of nasal stenosis. The patient's temperature was normal. On examination, a dirty-white membrane was found, occluding both nasal cavities. The membrane extended over both the turbinate bodies and septum, beginning anteriorily about the mucocutaneous margin, and extending posteriorly, but limited to the nose. The boy's mother stated that he was restless and feverish at night, and had some discharge from the nose. On further inquiry it was found that the patient had had diphtheria some two years before, and that an older child was just recovering from an attack of sore throat—in all probability a follicular tonsillitis. The family was a large one, but there was no further contagion. A raw and bleeding surface was left upon the removal of a portion of the membrane for cultural purposes. A clinical diagnosis of rhinitis fibrinosa was made, and the following treatment instituted: Internally, an iron tonic, and locally, an alkaline cleansing wash, followed by insufflation of nosophen. The disease continued about three weeks, with more or less mucopurulent discharge. On examination of the culture a large staphylococcus was found. Its growth on agar-agar at ordinary room temperatures was dry, having a ragged margin and a distinct fetor; on gelatin; liquefaction was produced.

CASE II.—M. M., male, aged ten years, came under observation, October 11, 1897, suffering from nasal trouble. On examination a dirty-white membrane was found, anteriorily covering the septum and turbinate bodies. The posterior rhinoscopic image showed a similar condition, with a moderate hypertrophy of Luschka's tonsil. The membrane was confined to the respiratory region of the nasal mucous membrane as in the former case. A raw and bleeding surface was left upon the removal of a portion of the membrane. The submaxillary and cervical lymph-glands were swollen, simulating the collar of brawn of scarlet fever, but were not tender. The swollen condition of the glands continued about three weeks. The temperature was slightly elevated (99° F.), and the mother of the patient stated that he had been feverish and restless at night and had complained of some frontal headache during the previous three or four days. Most of the distress was caused by the nasal stenosis. The history revealed no immediately preceding sickness which would account for the trouble. The illness continued benignantly, with a mucopurulent discharge, for about four weeks. No history of contagion could be obtained, although the patient was in almost constant contact with a brother. A clinical diagnosis of rhinitis fibrinosa was made, and treatment instituted as in the former case. The following day the patient returned for a bacteriologic examination. The membrane in this case was fortunately very readily removed with very slight hemorrhage, and cultures were made. The culture on agar-agar showed a staphylococcus and a species of saccharomyces. The growth on gelatin did not cause liquefaction.

Of the membrane obtained in this case, part was at once transferred to absolute alcohol; another part, without being subjected to any other treatment, was exposed to the action of dilute acetic acid, and a third portion,to that of artificial gastric juice. Dilute acetic acid caused the membrane to become almost perfectly transparent; at the same time there occurred on carefully shaking the test-tube without breaking up the membrane a very slight turbidity in the fluid. The result of this experiment showed that the membrane largely consisted of fibrin mixed in some way with a small amount of mucus. Exposed to the action of artificial gastric juice, the membrane within a few hours was almost completely digested. There remained only a very small, hardly appreciable, amount of undigested residue. This likewise proved the fibrinous nature of the exudate. The piece of membrane hardened in alcohol was subsequently embedded in paraffin and sectioned. The sections were studied with Gramm's, Weigert's, Altmann's, and a hematoxylin stain. The mass of the exudate, as shown by the study of the sections, consisted of numerous, mostly polymorphonuclear leucocytes, a few epithelial cells, some cocci, and some indefinable débris; all of these elements were embedded in a dense fibrillar network. This network stained violet with hematoxylin, a beautiful blue with Weigert's fibrin stain, and red with Altmann's acid-fuchsin-picric-acid stain.

CASE III.—T. C., male, ten years, presented himself for treatment, November 26, 1897; temperature normal. On examination a dirty-white membrane was found covering the septum and turbinate body of the right nasal cavity only; there was also present a deflection of the septum to the right. The patient's mother stated that he complained of some nausea and had a slight fever three days before, and was also greatly distressed because of the limited amount of nasal respiration permitted, which made him restless at night. Pieces of the membrane were removed, leaving the characteristic raw and bleeding surface. There was no history of contagion and no further symptoms of importance developed except a more or less mucopurulent discharge, the case continuing benignantly. A clinical diagnosis of rhinitis fibrinosa was made in this case, and similar treatment applied as in the previous cases. From the membrane removed cultures were made and a staphylococcus found. The growth of the staphylococcus on agar-agar was moist and somewhat yellow. On gelatin, an extensive liquefaction was produced. Only small pieces of the membrane could be obtained in this case, but enough was secured to make the chemic tests, and a small part was hardened for sectioning as in the preceding case Dilute acetic acid caused the membrane to become almost transparent. Artificial gastric juice caused an almost complete digestion within a few hours, with only a small amount of residue. The mass of the exudate was again proved to consist of numerous polymorphonuclear leucocytes, a few epithelial cells, cocci, and some indefinable débris, all embedded in a dense fibrillar network. This network stained blue with Weigert's and red with Altmann's stain. The stains employed, as well as the chemic tests, proved beyond a doubt that the great bulk of the exudate, as in the previous case, consisted of fibrin.

In conclusion, it is my agreeable duty to sincerely thank Dr. M. R. Brown for permission to publish these cases from his clinic, and also to thank Dr. Maximilian Herzog, director of the Pathologic Laboratory of the Polyclinic, for his assistance and direction in the examinations.

OROPHARYNGEAL MYCOSIS.[1]

BY R. P. LINCOLN, M.D.,
OF NEW YORK.

OROPHARYNGEAL MYCOSIS is a parasitic disease which is not infrequently found in the deep parts of the oronasopharyngeal cavity, and was first described by B. Fränkel of Berlin in 1873, under the name "mycosis tonsillaris benigna," and later by Hening as "pharyngomycosis leptothrica."

I have selected this subject for discussion be-

[1] Read at a meeting of the Harvard Medical Society of New York, March 26, 1898.

cause it is more likely to be observed by the general practitioner than by the specialist. The now well-known nature of the disease proves it is not of recent origin. That it has so long been overlooked is evidence that its consequences are not often serious, that it has been confounded with another affection, and that it must frequently disappear spontaneously. That it is not very uncommon is evidenced by three cases which came under my care about three months ago.

Of these cases, two were in males and one in a female. The patients were in middle life, in excellent general health, without constitutional taint, and free from other disease, being neither dyspeptics nor having rheumatic or gouty diatheses, and being free from catarrhal troubles. Two of the patients were residents of this city. In neither of these, so far as I could determine, had a correct diagnosis been previously made. The female patient had been treated in Paris last summer for what she was told was follicular tonsillitis, but without relief of her trouble, which she first noticed when in Italy last June. One of the male patients had been treated locally with sprays and gargles, and had himself used them six months without result; the other had depended upon internal medication and gargles irregularly for a year and a half, having spent a greater part of that time in Asheville and the Adirondacks, caring for an invalid wife, and thus under favorable climatic conditions.

I know of no definite statistics of the duration of this disease, but we must accept in one of these patients a period of a year and a half. Dr. Wright cites a case of two-and-a-half years' duration, and Dr. Mulhall had one under observation six years.

There were certain objective appearances common in all the cases and characteristic of the affection. These are included in the following description: The disease involved the tonsils and the base of the tongue, the latter being the site of many tufts of the growth, at least thirty or forty. In one case, the growth was present on the soft palate and the post-pharyngeal wall, with two or three tufts in the inter-arytenoid space, and on the epiglottis. On inspection there were observed, apparently covering or protruding from the orifices of the mucous follicles, yellowish-white patches or plugs, fungoid in appearance, which are literally a collection of growths. They vary in size from a thread in diameter to perhaps a line, and sometimes, by coalescing, form patches as large as one's finger-nail. They are moist and soft to the touch, and usually removed or broken off on a level with the mucous membrane by moderate friction, to be reproduced during the following twenty-four or forty-eight hours. When the superficial or protruding mycotic growths are thus removed, there is not left behind that clean, smooth surface which we find when we express a cheesy, cretaceous mass from a mucous crypt; on the contrary they are more or less adherent, and it is frequently necessary to seize the projecting fimbriate mass with forceps and exert considerable force, as evidenced by a few specks of blood at the seat of implantation.

The study of a single case, even without the microscope, ought to convince one that the growth is implanted, not upon the superficial mucous membrane, but upon the lining of the canicular and mucous follicles and in the depressions between the folds of nasopharyngeal lymphoid tissue. Often where the point is favorable for examinatian a lacuna can be seen distended with the growth beyond its normal caliber.

There is not yet a uniformly accepted opinion as to the etiology of mycosis; its origin and specific nature are *sub judice*. Different fungi are found in the extruded masses, but leptothrix buccalis is acknowledged to be always present. Besides this leptothrix, we also find oidium albicans, the micro-organism of nigrities linguæ, a sarcina, and the aspergillus fumigatus, and others. Among predisposing causes the following have been claimed by almost as many different investigators: catarrhal inflammations; mouth-breathing; rheumatic diatheses manifested by tonsillitis, dyspepsia, acidity of the saliva; damp habitations; unhealthy skin; dental caries; neglect of mouth cleanliness thus favoring calcification in the presence of alga leptothrix—leptothrix buccalis seems to be always present in the mouth. Considering that leptothrix buccalis predominates in the morbid product, it may be not irrational to conclude that as the soil has become favorable by a certain degree ot inflammation, the spores of the leptothrix find lodgment in the mucous crypts and develop more rapidly than under ordinary circumstances; and that these bundles with their products, though other fungi may be associated with them, constitute the disease.

The subjective symptoms are almost never pronounced. They consist of a tickling or rough feeling, sometimes causing a cough or choking, which in turn results in an unavailing effort to clear the throat. There also may be a sense of dryness or burning. Pain, from a consequent inflammation is said to be sometimes present. I have never seen an instance. The affection is more often annoying than dangerous, through E. Fränkel claims the fungus may be destructive to the tissue upon which it grows, and reports a case of penetration of the tonsil to a depth of several millimeters.

If there is any doubt in diagnosis, the microscope should be used. My friend, Dr. Jonathan Wright, whose painstaking investigations are well known, has generously furnished me with the following account of the result of his recent microscopic work on this subject:

"Sections of the piece of lingual tonsil submitted to me for examination were made in such a way that they fell through the lacunæ containing the mycelial tufts. Staining with hematoxylon-eosin shows the mycelial threads or straws lying in close apposition with the thickened epithelial lining of the crypts. Desquamated epithelial cells are seen among the straws. With this stain the spores are not differentiated. I cannot discover in this specimen or in others which I have hitherto examined any evidence of the mycelial threads penetrating the subjacent tissues, or even of being fairly within the epithelial layer. With the eosin stain, however, may be seen, close to the crypt, fibrous tissue with long straight fibers which resemble somewhat the mycelial threads, but when the gentian-violet stain with the Gram-iodin decoloration is used, it is seen that the epithelial straws are sharply defined from the tissues, and there is no appearance of their having penetrated into them. Kelly claims, however, that in some cases this is noted. It is possible, though I will not venture a positive assertion on this point, that his stains have deceived him as intimated above.

"Both Kelly and Siebenmann assert their belief that the thickening of the epithelial lining of the crypts is the initial lesion and the mycelial growth a secondary phenomenon. This assertion I am also not at present in a position to positively controvert, but I am strongly of the opinion that this so-called 'keratosis' is merely the result of the irritation of the presence of the mycelium As for the assertion that no evidence of inflammation is found in the lymphoid tissue, this I am still more disinclined to accept. Not only is this not in accord with the usual clinical appearance and history, but hypertrophied lymphoid tissue is itself evidence of, and the product of inflammation, while the existence near the crypts of the extra amount of fibrous tissue spoken of above is a still further evidence of the chronic inflammatory process. Such a 'keratosis' we get upon the mucous membranes wherever friction or other irritative influences are at work. Nasal polypi at the point where they rub the septum, atrophic rhinitis with crusts, the nasal mucous membrane when it is bathed in the ichorous pus which flows from the suppurating accessory sinuses, the pachydermia verrucosa of the posterior wall of the larynx in drinkers and in phthisical patients, the tips of the lingual lymphoid hypertrophies in adult patients—all these show quite as much 'keratosis' as does the epithelial lining of the crypts filled by the threads of the leptothrix buccalis.

"The specimen stained with gentian-violet and Gram's iodin shows among the leptothrix threads the presence of another fungus, the so-called 'bacillus maximus buccalis.' The gentian-violet stain also brings out enormous numbers of spores, grouped in irregular masses outside of the mycelial straws, but also here and there they are seen enclosed within the lumina at irregular intervals. They are very minute, some of them much smaller than the smallest micrococcus. Now, between these two forms, the minute spores and the full-grown mycelial threads or straws, are all degrees of involutionary forms, including those indistinguishable in size and appearance from various bacilli—all deeply stained with the gentian-violet. The same may be noted of the 'bacillus maximus' and its spores stained with the iodin."

Treatment. — Mycosis may disappear spontaneously, though its usual course is very persistent. As is usually the case when no treatment is satisfactory, many methods are advocated. I will enumerate a few: Attention to the general health; local use of chlorate of potash, borax, absolute alcohol, lactic acid, chlorid of zinc, perchlorid of iron, iodin and its compounds, bromid of iodin, chromic acid, nitrate of silver, solution of bichlorid of mercury; curetting or forcibly pulling out the filaments, followed by the use of some astringent, as nitrate of silver; excision; a course of sulphur waters; application of pyoctanin, and last, the galvanocautery. Each has had its advocates; none is satisfactory, but the last is probably the most useful. At present I rely upon the galvanocautery and pyoctanin. With these two means, and perseverance, patients will recover, but perhaps as my friend Dr. Wright says, "not because of them." I must confess, however, I am not now willing to accept his conclusion.

A few words about the application of these remedies. The treatment must be radical—all the deposit must be destroyed and the surface from which the leptothrix develops changed. If the points of disease are few and favorably located, as on a tonsil, they may be excised and the trouble at once eradicated. The galvanocautery is also applicable in such cases; even when a considerable number of growths are present it is effective, the objection to it arising, when too freely used, from the degree and extent of inflammation it may cause.

The following extract from a paper on "The Uses of Pyoctanin," read by me before the American Laryngological Association in 1891, still expresses my opinion of its advantages: "Pyoctanin is a powerful germicide. It is odorless, almost tasteless, non-poisonous, slightly anodyne, and non-irritating. It does not coagulate albumen, has great penetrating and disseminating power, and hence, does not form a protecting shield about diseased germs. It rapidly destroys bacteria." In using it, after freeing the points to be treated as far as possible of mucus and protruding filaments of growth, the pure powder should be rubbed thoroughly for several minutes upon and into the lacunæ. This process should be repeated at short intervals, daily for a while, until the reappearance of the growth ceases. An intelligent patient can without danger contribute to the success of the treatment by spraying a solution of the remedy upon the diseased surfaces.

MEDICAL PROGRESS.

Venesection in Uremia.—LAACHE (*Deutsch. Med. Wochenschr.*, March 3, 1898) is an advocate of simple venesection without infusion of saline solution in cases of uremic intoxication with increased arterial pressure. The quantity of blood withdrawn by him has been in general from 500 to 600 grams (16 to 20 ounces). In some instances of anuria he has withdrawn twice this quantity.

Extraction through the Mouth of a Plate Lodged in the Esophagus.—WHITE (*Vir. Med. Semi-monthly*, March 11, 1898) was asked to see a patient who two months previously had swallowed a plate bearing one central upper incisor tooth. The plate had lodged opposite the cricoid cartilage, and the man was unable to swallow anything but liquids. At first White was unable to pass any instrument, but on the second day a slender uterine probe passed the plate, and by applying cocain to the esophagus on a swab, it was possible to pass a bougie 4 mm. in diameter. This treatment was continued daily, as esophagotomy was rejected on account of its considerable mortality. After four-days' trial a forceps was passed beyond the plate and the latter was turned partially around, though not extracted. On the seventh day a bristle-probang was passed and by its withdrawal the plate was extracted. The symptoms due to the long presence of the plate seem to have been very slight, and they quickly subsided after its removal.

Recurring Attacks of Vomiting of Eighteen-Years' Standing Cured by Division of Adhesions.—NAYLOR (*Indian Med. Rec.*, February 1, 1898) gives an account of a case of recurring attacks of vomiting in an unmarried woman aged forty-four years, which had continued eighteen years in spite of all treatment. As food was frequently ejected after some hours' retention in the stomach, the diagnosis of pyloric stenosis was made and a laparotomy was performed, the operator expecting to relieve the stricture by a pyloroplasty. The pylorus was not constricted in any way, but there were adhesions between the stomach and the colon, as well as between the pylorus and the liver. The former were divided, but the latter were too deep down to permit of easy division, and through fear of hemorrhage they were left. The patient made a complete recovery, and was not thereafter troubled with vomiting. While adhesions may not be a common cause of uncontrollable vomiting, yet they are sufficiently common to receive consideration.

Hemorrhage from an Atonic Uterus.—ARENDT (*Therap. Monatsheft.*, January, 1898) says that in post-partum hemorrhage from an atonic uterus, tamponade of the organ is the most rational treatment. It has without doubt saved many lives since the directions for its employment were first given by Duhrssen. It carries with it, however, a certain risk of infection, and there is of necessity a slight delay in its application which is harrowing to the patient. He therefore advises in all cases of alarming hemorrhage, that the cervix be grasped with a couple of strong forceps and pulled firmly down. The traction alone is often sufficient to completely shut off the blood-supply, so that one might split the uterus without there being a loss of any more blood. Moreover, the irritation causes even a very soft uterus to contract to a hard ball. As it will again relax, all danger is not over and the clamps should be left in position a few minutes, to be pulled upon again if necessity arises. If a tamponade is employed, it is rarely necessary to leave it in position more than an hour if it soaked with some irritating substance, such as carbolic acid (five per cent.). The advantage of rubbing and kneading the fundus uteri should not be forgotten. In milder cases this is all that is required to produce contraction and so stop the hemorrhage.

Widal's Reaction in Yellow Fever.—LERCH (*Journal of the American Medical Association*, February 26, 1898) says that the blood of a patient who was suffering from yellow fever when tested by Widal's method with the bacillus icteroides of Sanarelli, gave the following results: In a dilution of one to ten arrest of motion of the bacilli and agglutination were complete within a few minutes, and in a dilution of one to forty, the agglutination and arrest of motion of the bacilli took place within twenty minutes.

The prompt agglutination of the bacilli and their arrest of motion in the hanging-drop culture, contaminated with the blood of the patient, may prove of the highest value in the future, and allow an early recognition of the disease while yet there is time to prevent its spread.

Palpation and Auscultatory Percussion.—MAGUIRE (*Medical Press and Circular*, February 23, 1898) asserts that palpation of the chest is for most purposes more delicate than percussion, and after a little practice, it is freer from fallacies. In the beginning it is recommended that one press alternately with the first and second fingers of the right hand, but after a little practice it will be enough to pass the hand slowly over the chest wall pressing lightly, as is done in examining the eyeball in a case of suspected glaucoma. Differences of resistance will be observed not only when pressing upon the soft parts, but almost as plainly when pressing over the ribs or sternum. Palpation practised in this way will define more accurately than percussion the exact areas of the heart, liver, and spleen. Spots of thickening, probably due to a previous pneumonia or pleurisy, have often been made out by the writer, who strongly recommends this method, which he has tested in every possible way, including experiments upon the dead body.

Auscultatory percussion is a valuable method of physical examination, but too much has sometimes been claimed for it. If the stethoscope be placed over some organ in contact with the chest, and a finger used to make light taps in the vicinity, the exact size of the portion of the organ in contact with the chest can be accurately determined, not, as has sometimes been claimed, the size of the whole organ. The limits of a dilated stomach or intestine may be made out, or the fissures between the lobes of the lungs, a point often of importance in phthisis, as the spread of the tuberculous process to the middle lobe is a serious matter and always indicates a late stage of the disease. The retraction of the apex of one lung and the level of the fluid in pleurisy are easily made out by means of auscultatory percussion, while they can only be determined by the acute and practised ear, by simple percussion. Hence, this method of examination, which was advocated long ago by Laennec, should not be allowed to fall into disuse.

THERAPEUTIC NOTES.

Hydrocyanic Acid as an Antidote to Chloroform.—HOBDAY (*Lancet*, January 1, 1898), having observed the different effects of hydrocyanic acid and chloroform when used to produce death in animals, conceived the idea that the former drug might be used as an antidote to the latter in case of an overdose. So successful has it proved in experiments upon animals, that in the Royal Veterinary College in London, when operations upon animals are performed, there are kept on hand no other stimulants than ammonia and Scheele's acid. If the animal goes into collapse the tongue is drawn well forward, and a full medicinal dose of the acid is placed well back upon it. Artificial respiration is performed with the animal in the horizontal position on the side, and when respiration commences the ammonia is held under the nostrils. The stimulating effect of the acid upon respiration is almost instantaneous, and continues about twenty minutes. The dose required for a dog or cat is about 1 minim for each eight pounds of body weight. If an overdose is given the fumes of chloroform will readily control the spasms until the effect passes off.

Scientific Treatment of Chronic Gonorrhea.—VALENTINE (*Clin. Recorder*, January, 1898) has published an article upon "Chronic Gonorrhea," of which the following is a summary:

1. There are no incurable cases of chronic urethritis.
2. All drugs suggested for the treatment of chronic gonorrhea are soon relegated to merited oblivion.
3. The only efficacious method of treating chronic gonorrhea is by dilations, as proposed by Oberlander, followed by irrigations, without a catheter, of the urethra or bladder or both.
4. Urethral fever or other disturbance does not supervene after urethral instrumentation followed by irrigation.
5. Carefully conducted dilations and irrigations are not painful.
6. Gradual, careful pressure by dilators is preferable to the use of sounds in the majority of cases.
7. The effect of dilations is to stimulate absorption of the infiltrations.
8. Functional disturbance and nervous symptoms are improved very early in the treatment.
9. Chronic urethritis can be exceptionally diagnosed and successfully treated, but never pronounced cured without the aid of the urethroscope.

Antipyrin and Quinin in Influenza.—LANDOUZY (*La Presse Méd.*, January 29, 1898), has this to say of the treatment of influenza: "The pressing indication to be met in asthenic patients lies in the state of their forces which need sustenance. Stimulating remedies should occupy the first place. Thus, alcoholic liquors, diffusible stimulants, and tonics should be made the basis of medication. For a number of reasons antipyrin ought not to dethrone the salts of quinin in the treatment of influenza, but should march behind them or at their side to render assistance when needed. The salts of quinin, selected and administered with judgment, will not only control many of the pains of the disease, but will relieve the weakness and stimulate the patient. Without exaggeration one may almost say that quinin meets every symptom of influenza, being at once stimulating, tonic, and anti-infectious. The rule should be to make quinin the medicin of choice, antipyrin the medicine of necessity."

Treatment of Syphilis in the British Army by Injections of Mercury.—LAMBKIN (*British Medical Journal*, February 19, 1898), thus describes the advantages of the treatment of syphilis in the British army by injections of mercury: (1) The surgeon carries out the treatment himself, so that there is no chance that the negligence of the patient will interfere with its faithful application. (2) Diarrhea and indigestion are never produced. (3) It is of advantage to the State, in that the number of day's residence in hosipital is greatly reduced.

The results obtained by the writer in his six-years' experience were satisfactory. The healing of the primary lesion was always rapid. The patient was kept in the hospital only until the worst primary and secondary manifestations were past, and then he returned once a week for his injection. The preparation used was a mixture of equal parts of metallic mercury, pure lanolin and two-per-cent. carbolized oil. The maximum dose injected was 10 drops. Not a single abscess resulted in over 6000 injections. The injections were made into the muscles, and caused no pain worth mentioning, and never rendered necessary any interruption in the soldier's service. The buttock was invariably selected as the site of injection.

The weight of the patient, especially in tropical countries, is an absolute guide to the continuance of treatment. So long as it increases or remains stationary, the injection should be continued; if weight is being lost, the injections should be omitted for a time.

THE MEDICAL NEWS.

A WEEKLY JOURNAL

OF MEDICAL SCIENCE.

COMMUNICATIONS are invited from all parts of the world. Original articles contributed *exclusively* to THE MEDICAL NEWS will after publication be liberally paid for (accounts being rendered quarterly), or 250 reprints will be furnished in place of other remuneration. When necessary to elucidate the text, illustrations will be engraved from drawings or photographs furnished by the author. Manuscripts should be typewritten.

Address the Editor: J. RIDDLE GOFFE, M.D.,
No. 111 FIFTH AVENUE (corner of 18th St.), NEW YORK.

Subscription Price, including postage in U. S. and Canada.

PER ANNUM IN ADVANCE $4.00
SINGLE COPIES 10
WITH THE AMERICAN JOURNAL OF THE MEDICAL SCIENCES, PER ANNUM 7.50

Subscriptions may begin at any date. The safest mode of remittance is by bank check or postal money order, drawn to the order of the undersigned. When neither is accessible, remittances may be made, at the risk of the publishers, by forwarding in *registered* letters.

LEA BROTHERS & CO.,
No. 111 FIFTH AVENUE (corner of 18th St.), NEW YORK,
AND NOS. 706, 708 & 710 SANSOM ST., PHILADELPHIA.

SATURDAY, APRIL 30, 1898.

A GREAT STEP TOWARD QUARANTINE UNIFORMITY.

THE Health and Quarantine officials of the South Atlantic and Gulf States held a convention in Atlanta, April 12, 1898, Texas and North Carolina alone not being represented by delegates. Dr. H. B. Horlbeck of Charleston, S. C., presided. Although especially called to formulate a uniform system of inland quarantine procedure, the convention endorsed by the following resolutions, two important measures of international quarantine:

"Resolved, That this convention approves the plan of having medical inspectors attached to those consulates where yellow fever and cholera are epidemic, with a view of securing for our protection definite information as to the exact sanitary condition and the presence or absence of contagious diseases in such consular district. And that Congress be urged to make the necessary appropriations to carry the plan into effect.

"Resolved, That this convention is of the opinion that it is a duty devolving on all nations to take measures to eradicate any plague-centers from their territory, and that the existence of such plague-centers is a menace to all other nations, and that our State Department be requested to take measures though proper diplomatic channels for the conveyance of this opinion to the governments deemed obnoxious to the opinion as herein expressed."

The convention was harmonious thoughout, and unanimously formulated regulations which, if applied, will render epidemics of yellow fever wellnigh impossible.

These regulations provide for the timely establishment of disinfection and detention stations, or camps, on the lines of travel by rail or boat, to be erected and operated by the Marine Hospital Service. Twelve sections are devoted to the subject of handling freight and merchandize.

The resolution suggesting that manufacturers or shippers employ and pay a sanitary inspector appointed by the Marine Hospital Service may not meet with ready acceptance, but such action would redound to the profit of a business house, because of the confidence inspired by inspected and practically guaranteed goods. The regulations formulated for isolating and stamping out the disease, and those for preventing its spread by railroads, steamboats, or other means, seem possible and likely to prove efficacious. Particular care seems to have been exercised in obtaining the minimum degree of interference with traffic compatible with the maximum degree of protection. Uniform restrictions, though rigid, will be found much more tolerable than the erratic, despotic exactions of local quarantine officers, such as have characterized past epidemics. The methods of disinfection endorsed are simple and efficacious.

The following are considered efficient germicidal solutions:

1. Bichlorid of mercury, acid, 1-1000.
2. Carbolic acid, pure, five-per-cent. solution.
3. Trikresol, two-per-cent. solution.
4. Solution of formaldehyd, 1-500 (which is two parts of a forty-per-cent. solution of formaldehyd to twenty-five parts of water.
5. Solution of hypochlorid of calcium (chlorid of lime).

Reliance is not placed upon these agents alone but for special purposes sulphur dioxid, formaldehyd gas, steam or boiling are recommended.

The interstate quarantine regulations adopted by this convention are practically those formulated by the Marine Hospital Service, and it was largely due to the presence of Surgeon H. R. Carter of that service that the business of the convention was so scientifically conducted and speedily concluded. A more intelligent body of men has scarcely ever assembled in the South, and their work is bound to result in untold good to their own section and to the whole country.

THE DUTY OF THE STATE RESPECTING THE AFTER CARE OF VACCINATIONS.

DR. CALCOTT FOX, dermatologist to the Westminster Hospital, London, who has written previously on the best precautions against the occasional untoward results following vaccination, takes up the subject again in the *London Lancet*, as given below. He is also known as a consistent advocate of antiseptic methods in this procedure. His letter in the *Lancet*, for Feb. 12, says that " a distressing case of post-vaccinal erysipelas which has just come under my observation prompts me to ask once more whether it is not desirable and practicable to take some further steps to lessen the chances of similar disasters.

"The State ordains that for the good of the individual and the community a certain inoculation should be practised. The operator satisfies himself that the inoculation is successful, but alter that the State takes no further interest in the matter and the wounds are left to heal as best they may, subject to the chances of various contaminations. No doubt these disasters are infrequent, but when they occur they make an indelible impression upon a more or less considerable section of the community. It is useless to explain that the vaccination was not the direct cause but that the erysipelas might just as well have followed a cut or a scratch. It is these preventable accidents which are responsible for very much of the feeling against vaccination, and very naturally so too. Is it not the duty of the State, having carried out the operation, to see that the wounds heal under proper conditions?" Dr. Fox answered his own question very positively by saying that in the case of such operations the authorities are not quit of their responsibilities until each such operation has been conducted to a close. This proceeding undoubtedly does mean considerable additional trouble and care "but it is none the less the duty of the authorities to carry it through."

PATHOLOGIC DEPARTMENT OF COLUMBIA UNIVERSITY, N. Y.

IN the *Bulletin* of the University, for March, Professor Prudden has an entertaining lecture on the growth of pathologic teaching in the medical department of the College of Physicians and Surgeons. The number of teachers and assistants therein at the present time amounts to nineteen. It is the aim to provide at least one instructor for each fifteen to twenty students who take the practical course. Five special attendants care for the microscopes and other apparatus, for the cleanliness of the laboratories, and for the messenger service. Besides the undergraduate instruction in classes, the department affords each year facilities for the pursuit of special advanced lines of study in bacteriology and pathology, and in general microscopy to physicians, to candidates for the higher university degrees and to those preparing for expert careers in various lines. The number of such graduate workers has of late been about twenty each year. As to original work, Dr. Prudden states with gratification that his staff has not been idle; on the contrary, it has found opportunity to keep the fires at least alight upon the altars of research. Altogether, over one hundred and fifty original papers, embodying the results of special studies, have been published by those connected with the department since the founding of the laboratory of the Alumni Association. Reprints of these publications have of late been gathered into volumes for serial issue, the expense of publication having been borne by the Association of the Alumni. The scope of the work in pathology for the future is boundless, and the prospects of beneficent success is most alluring. The greatest danger in a department like this, in which the teaching functions are urgent and dominant, is that the research work may be swamped in academic routine. But it is confidently believed that the maintenance of high standards will be secured in the future, as it has been in the past, by the loyalty to science and the devotion to the department of the men who, year by year, make up its working force.

ECHOES AND NEWS.

New President of the General Medical Council.—At a recent meeting of the General Medical Council Sir William Turner was unanimously elected to its presidency, made vacant by the death of Sir Richard Quain.

International Association of Railway Surgeons.—The next meeting of this Association will be held in Toronto on July 6, 7, and 8, 1898. It is expected that between five and six hundred of the members will be present.

Tax on Proprietary Medicines.—In the war tax about to be imposed, it is proposed to place a tax of two cents on packages or bottles of patent medicine retailing at twenty-five cents or under, and four cents on those retailing at a higher price.

A State Medical Law Upheld. — The United States Supreme Court at Washington recently affirmed the constitutionality of the act of the New York Legislature of 1895 prohibiting persons who have been convicted of, and punished for a crime, from practising medicine in the State, the opinion being delivered by Justice Brewer.

Obituary.—Dr. Erasmus Garrett, during a quarter of a century Chief Medical Inspector of Chicago's Health Department and an eminent authority on smallpox, died of heart failure on the 19th inst. at his residence in Chicago. Dr. Garrett was born in Frederick County, Maryland, February 14, 1836, and was graduated from the University of Maryland.

Epileptic Colony for New Jersey. — A bill is before the New Jersey Legislature for the establishment of an epileptic colony. The commission of inquiry which recommended the bill stated that there are at the lowest estimate two thousand epileptics in insane asylums and almshouses throughout the State, neither of which are fit abodes for them.

The City Physician: Is He the Football of Fortune?—Dr. Johnson, in his "Life of Akenside," says very truly: "A physician in a great city seems to be the mere plaything of fortune; his degree of reputation is for the most part totally casual; they that employ him know not his excellence; they that reject him, not his deficiency. By any acute observer who had looked on the transactions of the medical world for half a century a very curious book might be written on the 'Fortune of Physicians.'"

Dr. Tarnier's Munificent Bequest. — Professor Tarnier has bequeathed to the Paris Academy of Medicine a yearly income of 5000 francs, 3000 of which are set aside for a prize to be given annually and to be called the Prix Tarnier. It will be awarded for the best work on a subject in obstetrics or gynecology. The prize will be given in one sum and will be allotted in the first year for obstetrics and in the second year for gynecology. The Academy can make what use it pleases of the remaining 2000 francs.

New Electric Discovery.—Rychnowski, the electrician of Lemberg, claims to have discovered an electric fluid which he calls "electroid." The discovery has caused a great sensation in Europe. The effects of the fluid are said to be startling, producing light and causing Geissler tubes to omit fluorescent rays. It works photochemically, rotates objects in midair, produces whirlpools in water, and kills bacteria. Metal and glass thereby can be charged with electricity, and the magnetic needle changes direction under its influence.

Plague in Bombay.—According to recent news from Bombay the plague is rapidly declining in that city. The death-rate from the disease is now less than a thousand per week, and that for each succeeding week is a little lower than for the one which preceded it. Dr. Galeotti, of the University of Florence, has arrived at Bombay with the curative serum produced by Professor Lustig and himself. Patients at the Arthur Road Hospital have been placed at his disposal, and some few have undergone the treatment and have recovered.

Homeopathy in the University of Munich. — At a recent meeting of the Financial Committee of the Bavarian Parliament, says the *British Medical Journal*, Herr Landmann proposed that a University Chair of Homeopathy be established in the University of Munich. The Minister replied that the university, to which the question had been referred, had replied that the need of such a chair was not felt, inasmuch as homeopathy was not a science. A similar incident, which ended in like manner, occurred not long ago in the Würtemberg Landtag.

A Fire Extinguishing Powder. — A public exhibition has been made in Brooklyn of the powers of a powder called 'kilfyre," to put out fires. A pine structure, with a sixteen-foot flue, was put up in one of the small parks; it was then well covered with kerosene and tar and set on fire. The exhibitor allowed the flames to gain good headway before he applied the powder. Four seconds after the latter was scattered over the pyre the roaring mass was a blackened ruin, every spark having been put out. It is claimed that this powder is especially adaptable for use in public meeting-places, as schools, churches, theaters, etc.

The Peabody Buildings of London.—A London newspaper says of the huge blocks of Peabody buildings, scattered in various parts of that city, that they are not to be considered among the pleasant sights of the streets; we can hardly associate with them the idea of a cosy home. Nevertheless, plain and indisputable figures show that they are healthier places than the average London home, and that is a high though not a final test of fitness. While the population in them is thirteen times denser than in London generally, the death-rate of infants is nearly twenty-two per thousand below the London average; the total death-rate is nearly three per thousand below the London average. The scheme is a paying one, as is also Lord Rowton's, which is working admirably. Would that no Londoner were worse housed than those in the Peabody buildings.

Photochromography for Pathologic Illustrations.—At a recent meeting of the Midland Medical Society in London Mr. Christopher Martin described the process of photochromography or trichromatic printing for the production of colored illustrations of pathologic specimens, etc., and showed a number of photochromographs made by himself. The process is as follows: Three photographs of the object are taken, on specially prepared films, through red, green, and violet glass screens. From the positives three process blocks are then prepared. The block made from the photograph taken through the red screen is used to print the blue tints, that through the green screen the red tints, and that through the violet screen the yellow tints. The yellow picture is printed first; in twenty-four hours the red picture is printed over it, and after another interval the blue. By the combination of the three-color pictures a perfect reproduction of all the tints and shades of the object photographed is obtained.

Decrease in the Death-rate from Diphtheria in Germany.—The Imperial Office of Statistics recently published the returns of the causes of death in the towns of Germany of more than 15,000 inhabitants from the year 1885 to the year 1895. These returns show that from 1885 to 1894 there were 119,038 deaths from diphtheria or croup, the average number thus being 11,904 per annum. The maximum was reached in 1893, there being in that year 15,860 deaths, and the minimum in 1888, with 9934 deaths. In 1895, when diphtheria antitoxin was first used on a considerable scale, the number of deaths went down to 7266. The diphtheria death-rate was 10.69 per 10,000 of the population in the preceding ten years, and only 5.4 in 1895, so that the mortality had fallen 49.48 per cent. Of 100 deaths 4.53 were caused by diththeria from 1885 to 1894, and only 2.53 in 1895. The decrease of the death-rate from diphtheria was almost uniform in every district of the empire; the prevalence of the disease was, however, about the same as it had been for the last twenty years, and it is therefore unquestionable that the serum treatment has had the effect of producing a remarkable improvement.—*Lancet*, February 19th.

A French Nurse Honored.—All Americans who have been privileged to visit Charcot's clinic at the Salpêtriére will remember his favorite head-nurse, Mlle. Marguerite Bottard; and they will not be surprised to learn that she has been decorated with the Cross of the Legion of Honor. It seems that this noble lady has been upward of fifty-six years in continuous service at the institution mentioned. It was in January in 1841 that Mlle. Bottard, who was then just nineteen years of age, commenced life there as a ward-nurse, and ever since, almost without a break, her time has been devoted to the care of the sick. An insatiable worker, she seldom quitted the premises, and it is reported that during a period of three years she never once crossed the threshold of the hospital. At first for some fifteen or sixteen years Mlle. Bottard carried on her duties under the successive direction of the elder Trélat, De Falret, and Legrand du Saulle. Then she was promoted to superintendent of the section for nervous affections under Charcot, with whom she remained until the end. He had the highest possible opinion of his faithful assistant, and often said that she richly deserved this very distinction which now has been awarded to her.

Responsibility of Hospitals for Injury to Patients.—A clear statement of the law relating to the liability of a charitable hospital corporation for the negligence of its servants, resulting in injury to a patient, is to be found in the opinion handed down a few days ago by Judge Cohen of the New York City Court, denying a motion for a new trial in the case of Ward *versus* the St. Vincent Hospital. The plaintiff was a pay-patient at the hospital. She was severely burned by an uncovered water-bag which a nurse had carelessly left in her bed. The evidence indicated that the hospital authorities had exercised due care in the selection of this nurse, and that she had been particularly instructed by the superintendent of nurses in regard to the proper use of water-bags. Indeed, there was no proof which would have justified the jury in finding that in selecting and employing the nurse the institution was in any respect negligent. Having fulfilled its duty in this regard, Judge Cohen holds, in accordance with the great weight of authority in this country, that the hospital is not liable for the subsequent carelessness of the nurse, unless notice of her unfitness had been brought to the attention of the corporation. The fact that the institution receives pay from some patients does not affect the application of the rule, inasmuch as St. Vincent's Hospital is a public charitable corporation, and is very far from being supported by the money received from patients.

Bogus American Doctors Abroad.—The following is from the *Medical Times and Hospital Gazette* (London): "Among the army of unqualified practitioners now operating in the metropolis of the British empire, the most audacious as well as the most successful financially, are the Yankee quacks. They fill the columns of our newspapers with the most wonderful stories of their cures of the blind, deaf, and halt, and they attract thousands of dupes who pay these pretenders large sums of money for their services, far beyond what they would think of paying hospital specialists for similar services. It is curious that these men never get into trouble for malpractice, notwithstanding that they often use risky operative methods of treatment, especially as they are unqualified and untrained when they arrive in England. We have learned recently that these men on arriving lose no time in visiting the wards of our special hospitals and attending the clinics of the leading physicians and surgeons. The presentation of a neatly printed card, describing the owner as Philadelphus Chicago, M.D., U. S. A., ensures the free run of the hospital wards and out-patient departments week after week, until they have picked up all that can be taught. Sometimes they attend post-graduate courses in special subjects, and in this way, although the most arrant knaves, they acquire a certain amount of skill which enables them to carry on their quackery with the minimum of risk. Unless properly introduced, hospital tramps hailing from the United States and calling themselves M.D.'s should be rigidly excluded from seeing hospital practice except as patients."

CORRESPONDENCE.

THE ARMY SURGEON'S EQUIPMENT.

To the Editor of the MEDICAL NEWS.

DEAR SIR: During the first year and a half of the War of the Rebellion each regiment was provided with a cumbersome wagon to carry its medical and surgical supplies. This "medicine wagon" when loaded weighed over 3000 pounds, and required four mules to draw it. The quantities of the materials carried were not well apportioned, being in the case of many articles excessive, and in a few instances insufficient. After Jonathan Letterman became medical director of the Army of the Potomac in 1862, the amount of material to be carried was largely reduced by judicious selection, a lighter wagon was introduced, and one wagon was allotted to each brigade instead of to each regiment as previously. This system continued in use to the close of the war. Since that time medical supplies have been reduced in bulk in various ways, and the regular army is now supplied with medical chests and surgical chests, each weighing about ninety-five pounds, and containing a complete equipment for a regiment. The medical chest contains an ample variety of medicines, from acetanilid to sulphate of zinc, all in tablet form except alcohol, ammonia water, chloroform, oil of turpentine, whisky, and brandy. There are also numerous miscellaneous articles, such as hypodermic syringes, rubber, self-injecting syringes, reagent case, stethoscope, mustard plaster, beef extract, candles, etc. The surgical chest contains antiseptic tablets, ether, chloroform, glycerin, tincture of opium, and whisky, various instruments, trays, and a supply of dressings.

Each private of the hospital corps when in the field carries a pouch containing aromatic spirits of ammonia, rubber bandages, first-aid packets, wire gauze for splints, surgical plaster, scissors, and dressing forceps.

Yours sincerely,

JAMES P. KIMBALL,
Surgeon United States Army.

GOVERNOR'S ISLAND, N. Y., April 23, 1898.

A PROTEST AGAINST QUACKERY.

To the Editor of the MEDICAL NEWS.

DEAR SIR: Much has been said and written of late on the subject of more thorough medical education. The writer will readily admit that it is possible to improve our methods of instruction. Not in more or longer terms at college, or in a greater amount of laboratory training, but in practical hospital work. It is very probable that the young sawbones entering upon his career has never dressed a fracture, reduced a dislocation, performed an an amputation, or even been called upon to diagnose and treat a case of measles. He has a diploma or license and if the people will give him an opportunity he is ready to begin his medical education. He has seen many brilliant surgical operations, and knows to what operator and to what hospital to send any particular surgical case. There are two parties to the practice of medicine, the profession and the people. The profession has its faults, but the imperfections of the laity do not seem to be so distinctly recognized. The town in which the writer lives is situated in a fertile spot in central Indiana. It has a population of about 8000 inhabitants, four railroads, numerous churches, and excellent schools. Travelers from the effete East say that it is a good town. It is nine years since the writer cast his lot in this community, and in that time he has learned many things he never heard of at medical schools. He has learned that a dry-goods clerk can go to a house where the wife is suffering from erysipelas, walk around the house burning something on a shingle and muttering some incantation in German, and that both the doctors and the disease will be put to flight. He knows a saintly old man in the country, who, by placing his hand on a person afflicted with erysipelas and repeating a certain verse from the Bible, restores the sufferer to health. He tells me that he has cured many cases of "St. Anthony's Fire." Recently Senator Foraker's pet, osteopathy, has been received into public favor. Last week the "Herbs of Life Co." filled the spacious Opera-House nightly, dispensing low comedy and "medicine." The latest, and to the writer the most flagrant instance of quackery which has come to his notice, are the exploits of a magnetic doctor from an Ohio city. He makes use of neither medicine nor instruments, and is not amenable to the law. He is dirty, ignorant, profane, obscene, and intemperate. His patronage is the best, and this is "no mean city." He charges good fees and collects them. It is said he has had 200 patients here. That is a matter of conjecture, but the writer knows that he has had a great many very excellent people as patients, ministers, lawyers, business men, their wives and children, and one man who in early life studied and practised medicine but afterward became a prosperous business man. It is needless to specify the many instances of credulity among people whom one would confidently expect to be more enlightened. It is an endless procession of disgusting deceit.

Before the writer attended medical school he was a student at two of the leading colleges in this interior valley. He found his class at medical college composed of men, who, in manly character, morals, and intellect were the equals if not the superiors of the students enrolled in the scientific and literary schools. His observation since is that with few exceptions the class of young men who enter upon the study of medicine is as intelligent as that engaged in the study of any other profession. The writer also thinks he knows, from a professional standpoint, something of the character of the people to whom these young men after graduation appeal for sympathy and support. It is casting "pearls before swine." The medical profession has its defects, but has more than discharged its obligations to the public. The leaven of reform should be spread among the people. If that does not bring about a change for the better it might improve conditions for each medical school to add to its curriculum a department of humbug, fraud, and deceit.

A CONSTANT READER.

April 7, 1898.

OUR BERLIN LETTER.

[From our Special Correspondent.]

SPECIAL HOSPITALS FOR POOR BUT NOT PAUPER PATIENTS WITH NERVOUS DISEASES—SPORADIC SCURVY AND BLOOD PATHOLOGY—AN EPIDEMIC OF TYPHUS IN THE BUKOWINA TRAMPS, AND THE SPREAD OF TYPHUS AND EPIDEMIC CEREBRO-SPINAL MENINGITIS—TWO RECENT GERMAN CONTRIBUTIONS TO APPENDICITIS.

BERLIN, April 21, 1898.

ALL the arrangements are completed for the establishment of a special hospital in the neighborhood of Berlin, in which patients suffering from nervous affections, and unable to afford the expense of treatment in private hospitals, will receive attention. It is in accordance with the idea sketched by Möbius of Leipzig some time ago that the new hospital is to be directed. There are to be some features which are very special to it and rather exceptional in Germany: For instance, the use of alcoholic liquors is to be forbidden, and special provision is to be made to furnish the patients the opportunity to do gardening and outdoor work of various kinds, as well as light work at various trades. This method of treatment in specially arranged hospitals and institutions, favorably located, represents the most popular thing in therapeutics in Germany at the present time. I have mentioned the similar institutions for tuberculous patients before. They are springing up all over Germany now. Philanthropy is to a great extent taking the form of endowment and foundation for such institutions. Most of them are not intended for the very poor—the paupers—who it is considered will be cared for, for the present at least, in public hospitals as they exist, but for that lower middle class who, though unable to pay much; are yet willing and ready to pay something, who are too sensitive to mingle with the paupers, and yet, who are eminently deserving of aid. The object of the charity is a most deserving one, and the manner in which it is offered most delicate, so that it may be expected that a great deal of suffering will be relieved.

As to the value of the therapeutic principle involved in the treatment of a certain class of patients, uniformity of life, diet, and habits being easily secured when all can be subjected to practically the same régime, this must wait further trial before it can be definitely accepted. Within the next few years it is to receive a most thorough trial here, and the Germans are assured that it will not be found wanting in its practical results. The outcome will surely be watched with a good deal of interest.

A very interesting case of sporadic scurvy (scorbutus) has recently been reported here. It is one of those isolated cases which sometimes occurs even in people in reasonably comfortable circumstances, when no possible reason can be ascertained for the serious nutritional disturbance that develops. This patient had never been on a sea voyage, and had no capricious likes or dislikes for certain articles of diet, which might lead to the conclusion that some important nutritional element was lacking in his food. The first symptom noticed was blood-stained semen. Sometime after this an intense tired feeling and absence of all desire for exertion developed. Not until eight months after the first symptom was noticed did the spongy, bleeding gums, and the subcutaneous hemorrhages lead to the diagnosis of scorbutus. Despite every effort of therapy the nutritional condition grew steadily worse, and a fatal termination ensued. This is the first time that a blood dyscrasia, of which, however, absolutely nothing could be seen by microscopic examination of the blood, has been known to cause bloody seminal discharges, and there is a suspicion that the symptom may occur oftener than is thought; but that its presence is not suspected, as usually opportunities for observation of it are extremely limited.

Meantime the blood dyscrasia itself is thought to represent one of those obscure pathologic modifications of the blood plasma, the study of which is the only hope of blood pathology at present; for, after all the work that has been done on the morphology of the blood, there is coming the realization that in this alone there is very little of promise for the future. One of the most distinguished blood pathologists in Europe, Ehrlich, here at Berlin, has practically given up the study of blood pathology as there seems to be so little to be gained from it. If the further study of blood plasma will illustrate these sporadic cases of scurvy, of which a number of cases have been reported, one of the modern medical mysteries will be solved.

An epidemic of typhus (spotted typhus, as they call it here, or hunger fever) is reported to be raging in the Bukowina, a province of the Austrian Empire bordering Hungary, Turkey, and Russia. The province is an extremely poor one, and the people live with the worst hygienic surroundings, so that the typical conditions prevail for the development of the disease. Typhus is so common in some of the outlying districts of Hungary that the affection is known in certain parts of Europe as the Hungarian disease. Special medical interest has been aroused in the epidemic, which is not a severe one, by the hope that improved bacteriologic methods may lead to the discovery of the etiology of the disease.

The health authorities of neighboring provinces are bestirring themselves to see that the disease does not spread beyond the district at present affected. Special care is being taken that tramps in their wanderings do not carry the disease with them; for it is becoming very clear that these homeless wanderers, who sleep any place where they may lay their heads, who are not finicky about their surroundings and food, who use cast-off wearing-apparel without a word as to what may have happened to its former owner, who huddle together in the winter and so spread any germs with which they or their clothing may be infected, are responsible for the dissemination of more disease than has heretofore been imagined. Of typhus, this seems particularly true, so that special regulation of tramps is to be instituted in the affected districts.

Though typhus is considered to be essentially an epidemic disease, every year there are occasional cases of it that turn up in the hospitals of Berlin. So that the disease is considered to have acquired a certain endemicity here, through the prompt intervention of the health authorities, and the immediate and thorough segregation of the cases, prevent anything like an epidemic.

Of interest in the matter of tramps and the dissemination of disease, is the fact that during a recent small epidemic of cerebrospinal meningitis epidemica, the diagnosis being made by the finding of the meningococcus intracellularis, the first case occurred in a tramp, a member of a very respectable family whose shiftless ways and love of wandering had brought him to this mode of life.

Two interesting articles on appendicitis from the pens of German surgeons, who treat the question much more from the American standpoint than is customary over here, have recently appeared. Professor Sonnenberg's article in *Communications from the Borderland of Surgery and Medicine* (the last number) contains an interesting discussion of certain points in the etiology and pathology of the disease. It forms an additional chapter to his book on the subject which appeared at the end of the year.

Professor Kummel's article in the *Berliner Klinische Wochenschrift*, April 11th, is of more practical import. Kummell's statistics of the mortality from appendicitis, according to the period of the disease at which treatment is begun, are interesting. In 15 cases in which treatment was begun on the first day, there were no deaths; of 44 on the second day, there were two deaths; 76 on the third and fourth days, with 4 deaths; 4 on the fifth day, with 2 deaths; 102 between the sixth and tenth days, with 9 deaths; 54 between the eleventh and fifteen days, with 4 deaths. Treatment does not necessarily mean radical surgical intervention, but coming under medical care in such a way that the course of the disease may be carefully observed, and unhampered judgment as to the best method to be followed in the case can then be made.

TRANSACTIONS OF FOREIGN SOCIETIES.

London.

CHRONIC GASTRIC ULCER AND ACUTE PERFORATING ULCER—AGE CHANGES IN PLACENTA AND MEMBRANES—PERFORATING WOUNDS OF THE KNEE-JOINT—AMMONIUM-CHLORID TEST FOR URIC ACID—NATURE OF KALA-AZAR—ASEPTIC OPHTHALMIC SURGERY—GASTRIC DILATION.

AT a meeting of the Medical Society, March 14th, TAYLOR read a paper on "Gastric Ulcer." He said he believed that chronic and perforating ulcer and acute ulcer are two different and distinct diseases. The former attacks males in seventy-two per cent. of the cases, and usually subjects between forty-five and sixty years or age. It occurs in those persons who live busy, energetic lives. It is irregular in outline, situated near the pylorus, and the proliferation of tissue which it produces usually prevents perforation before there has been formed an adhesion to some solid viscus. There is little doubt that such ulcers are chronic from the first. The patients are extremely prone to errors in diet. A clean punched-out ulcer is very rare in males, and in females it occurs almost exclusively, between the ages of sixteen and thirty years. The frequent association of chlorosis and ulcer is more than accidental, for in almost every acute ulcer there is a previous history of chlorosis. These ulcers have no proliferative zone, as do the chronic ones in men. He suggested that the lesion is of the nature of a neurotic dystrophy. Other theories which have been advanced are: (1) mechanical, which has not clinical evidence to support it; (2) vascular, which does not explain the occurrence of a single ulcer instead of many; (3) glandular, which does not explain the fact that these ulcers occur in women alone. In favor of the local neurosis theory is to be mentioned the fact that these ulcers occur in young women; that in appearance they resemble perforating ulcers of the foot, and that they are undoubtedly associated with chlorosis.

WILLIAMS said that the association between chlorosis and ulcer is not a very close one, since ulcer occurs in only a small proportion of chlorotic patients. In the treatment of these patients he prefers to feed by rectum, though that sometimes occasions biliousness, due apparently to the lack of the normal stimulus to the flow of bile which the presence of food affords.

BOWLES said that many of the patients are hard-worked servants, who did not get sufficient rest. Rest of mind and body and good hygienic surroundings are the essentials of treatment. He had observed good results from the use of bismuth and hydrocyanic acid, with or without small doses of opium.

At the Pathological Society, March 15th, EDEN read a paper on "Age Changes in the Placenta and Membranes." The life of the placenta is a short one. It grows rapidly, and as rapidly grows old, and is then shed like a withered leaf. The ripe placenta is a worn-out organ, and shows changes of senile degeneration which must be distinguished from real pathologic changes. It is because these alterations have often been mistaken for pathologic ones, and also because the placentas of macerated fetuses have been used for purposes of study that there is so much confusion about this subject. The following senile changes can be detected in the placenta at term: (1) Endarteritis obliterans affecting considerable tracts of the middle-sized umbilical arteries; (2) degenerative changes in the chorionic epithelium and in the decidual cells of the serotina; (3) the formation of "white infarcts"; (4) thrombosis of a certain number of the subplacental sinuses and serotinal vessels. The presence of these changes in placental tissue suffices to indicate that it belongs to the end of the gestation period.

At the Clinical Society, March 11th, WALLIS detailed three cases in which the knee-joint had been perforated. In one, seen twenty-four hours after the injury, the joint contained only blood. In two others, seen two and fourteen days respectively after the accident, there was already suppuration in the joint-cavity. In all of the cases the joints were washed out with a dilute solution of bichlorid of mercury and then sewed up. In the first, healing occurred without trouble; the continued suppuration in the other two required further incision and drainage, and in the last case excision of the knee was finally required. Though in the two cases of suppuration mentioned it had been necessary to reopen the joints for drainage, the speaker thought it better to attempt a cure without drainage, as this treatment is sometimes followed by success.

BARKER agreed with Wallis that drainage of the knee-joint is often overdone, though in septic cases it is sometimes unavoidable. He objected to the use of irritating antiseptics for irrigation. Those germs which are too deeply seated to be mechanically flushed out, can only be killed by antiseptics which are too strong for use in irrigation. He, therefore, flushed the suppurating joint with hot water. The success which has followed the extension of surgical procedures to the knee-joint in recent years has been due in no small measure to the practice of closing the joint without drainage.

HAIG gave the Royal Medical and Chirurgical Society, March 22d, a demonstration of some results which may be obtained by the use of the ammonium-chlorid process in the microscopic detection of uric acid in the blood. A minute drop of blood is mixed with a similar drop of a ten-per-cent. solution of carbonate of sodium, and then with a drop of a twenty-per-cent. solution of chlorid of ammonium, and finally placed on a cover-glass. Evaporation is prevented, and it is allowed to stand thirty minutes. If then examined with an ⅙-inch objective, pale spheric granules are seen all over the field. The proportion which these granules bear to the red blood-cells shows roughly the amount of uric acid that is being excreted with the urine.

LUFF said that uric acid cannot be shown to be present in human blood, even in minute quantities, and that the same reaction as that described can be seen in goose blood, which certainly contains no uric acid whatever, and also in a solution of a mixture of cheese and caustic potash.

In reply, Haig said that he did not pretend that this was a test for uric acid, but that the number of crystals, whatever they may be, varies according to the amount of uric acid secreted by the kidneys, as can easily be proved by any one who will take the trouble to carry out the necessary analysis. In a case in which the proportion of these granules to the red blood-corpuscles was 1 :8, it rose upon the administration of the salicylate of soda to 1 :2.

ROGERS gave an account of the investigation of an epidemic of kala-azar, or black fever, which has slowly spread up the Assam Valley during the past fifteen years, carrying off at least one-fifth of the population of some districts. It was at first thought to be malaria, but in 1889, after a special investigation, it was reported to be ankylostomiasis. Since then, however, it has been proved that the specific worms are as frequent in non-affected as in affected natives, and more recent and thorough examinations of those attacked have shown the disease to be a severe form of malaria, of an irregularly remittent type, resistent to the action of quinin, and producing progressive anemia, diarrhea, and often dropsy, with enlargement of the liver and spleen. The epidemic seems to have originated in an intensification of the ordinary malarial fever in a very malarious district during an extraordinary succession of unhealthy years, due to deficient rainfall.

At the meeting of the Ophthalmological Society, March 10th, MCGILLIVRAY read a paper on the "Aseptic Treatment of Wounds in Ophthalmic Surgery." Antiseptic solutions, however weak, have an irritating effect upon cut surfaces, and hence their use in eye surgery has been very largely superseded by normal salt solution, for the antiseptic solutions when employed could only have a mechanical power of cleansing a wound; since in a strength suitable for irrigation they require several hours' contact with bacteria to destroy them. A description of the operation for senile cataract was then given as an illustration of the best aseptic technic. No antiseptic is used at any time. The eyelashes are cut short to prevent them from coming in contact with instruments during operation, and to facilitate cleansing the margins of the lids. The face is washed with soap and warm water, especial attention being paid to the folds of the eyelids. The conjunctival cul-de-sac is then flushed with normal salt solution, the lids being everted one after the other, but no mop is used to cleanse them, as it irritates their surfaces and so increases secretion. All instruments, etc., are sterilized by heat. Before and after the operation, while the speculum is in position, the eye is again flushed with sterilized salt-solution. The dressing consists of a layer of moist gauze, covered by a thin layer of absorbent cotton which is held in place by a vertical and horizontal strip of adhesive plaster. The other eye is not covered.

ARMSTRONG read a paper before the Harverian Society, March 17th on "Gastric Dilation, speaking especially of idiopathic dilation. The chief causes of this were said to be: (1) Habitual distension from chronic dyspepsia; (2) the taking of too bulky meals; (3) bolting of food and drinking of much fluid with meals; (4) failure of power in the central nervous system; (5) neurasthenia; (6) worry, anxiety, and overstrain, mental or bodily; (7) debility, atrophy, or fatty degeneration of the muscular coat of the stomach itself, and (8) the after-effects of febrile diseases, especially typhoid fever. Among the various methods of making a diagnosis none is more reliable than "splashing." The rules for treatment should be: (1) To distend the stomach as little and as seldom as possible; (2) to promote evacuation of the lagging contents of that organ; (3) to keep down fermentation; (4) to regulate the dietary, and (5 to improve the tone of the general nervous system. Fuming hydrochloric acid, 6 to 12 drops in 6 ounces of water, calomel, arsenic, strychnia, and kola are remedies worth trying. While it is desirable to keep up the general nutrition, the patient should take as few meals as possible, giving the stomach time to empty itself. Bread, farinaceous foods, bulky vegetables, and milk were spoken of as being harmful in cases of dilation; what little bread is taken should be twice baked or cut very thin, and thoroughly torrefied. As little fluid as possible should be taken with meals, such fluid as is required for the purposes of the system being taken one hour before food.

HARE said that no one class of remedies does as much good in gastric dilation as emetics. Vomiting is a much more effective method of evacuating the stomach than the tube, since the violent contraction of the muscles squeezes out a great quantity of mucus from the cells. He has, over and over again, stopped a vomiting of several weeks' duration by a single dose of ipecacuanha, 20 grains being made into an ounce draught.

MORRISON said that dilation of the stomach should be treated on the same principles as that of any other hollow organ, for instance, the heart, by postural and functional rest, limitation of its contents, and the use of tonics to increase the muscular power.

GOODHART disputed the idea that dilation was the result of obstruction. How rarely in cases of obstruction due to pyloric cancer is there any dilation. The real cause of dilation is muscular weakness, and not stricture. He expressed himself as doubtful of the good effects to be derived from posture, but spoke highly of the relief which follows the application of a proper bandage.

SOCIETY PROCEEDINGS.

AMERICAN SURGICAL ASSOCIATION.

Nineteenth Annual Meeting, Held at New Orleans, April 19, 20, and 21, 1898.

FIRST DAY—APRIL 19TH.

MORNING SESSION.

DR. J. HOLT of New Orleans delivered an "Address of Welcome," after which the various committees made their reports. The President of the Association, DR. T. F. PREWITT of St. Louis, Mo., delivered his address upon "The Future of the Association."

After referring fully to the organization of the society and to some of its former presidents, especially to its founder, he dwelt upon the standing in the profession of its present and future members, and especially upon their contributions to the art of surgery. He also referred to the many signs of progress of the Nineteenth Century, among other things mentioning the railroad, steamboat, telegraph, telephone, and electric light, as well as the rapid strides made in surgery, and concluded by urging the hearty cooperation of all distinguished surgical practitioners, writers, and teachers in enabling the Association to occupy the proud position its founders destined for it.

AFTERNOON SESSION.

DR. CHARLES A. POWERS of Denver, Col., read a paper, entitled

THE QUESTION OF OPERATIVE INTERFERENCE IN RECENT SIMPLE FRACTURES OF THE PATELLA.

The author first referred to the writings of Dennis, Bull, Czerny, and Myles upon this important subject, and then commented on the two most important tests for this fracture, the structural and the functional. As to the mechanism, he believed that the majority of these fractures are due to muscular action, in that the patient endeavors to save himself from falling, and thus strongly contracts the quadriceps femoris. He showed, in treating the question of pathology, that there are but two fragments in the fracture due to muscular action. The upper one generally being the larger, the fractured surfaces are, as a rule, irregular, and the line of the break transverse or oblique. The author enumerated the conditions tending to cause imperfect union and the obstacles to union as follows:

1. Separation of the fragments, due to (*a*) retraction of the upper fragment from contraction of the quadriceps femoris and a slight drawing down of the lower fragment through shortening of the ligamentum patellæ, and (*b*) to the presence of effused blood.
2. Tilting of the fragments (this may be present to a marked degree, and unrecognizable without operation).
3. Rupture of the tendinous expansion of the vasti and of the lateral portions of the capsule of the joint.
4. Prolapse of prepatellar tissues into the break.
5. Atropy of the quadriceps femoris due to (*a*) disuse; (*b*) arthritis; (*c*) marked contusion of the muscle; (*d*) blood extravasated from the joint through the rent in the upper part of the capsule.
6. Arthritis of the knee-joint.
7. Adhesion of the patella.

Further, though of little value, may be added:

8. Natural poverty of the blood supplied to the bone (rendered negative by the fact that the vertical fractures healed satisfactorily).
9. Exceptional tendency to osteitis, seen in fat people, in the aged, and in certain conditions of the blood.

In reference to the non-operative management of fractured patillæ, the speaker considered that no better evidence of the unsatisfactory results need be adduced than the large number of devices and plans which have been resorted to from time to time. He then liberally quoted from numerous personal letters from prominent surgeons all over the United States, each giving his opinion and preference as to the treatment of this fracture. The results of various kinds of treatment by many different surgeons, and the comparative mortalities from the various methods were presented in elaborate statistics.

Dr. Powers then took up the subject at great length, under the headings of limitations attending the operation, selection of cases, time of operation, operative procedures, and, lastly, dangers and immediate and remote results of operative management and comparison of these results with those obtained without operation.

DISCUSSION.

DR. J. D. BRYANT of New York, speaking of the comparative value of the different methods of treating fracture of the patella, referred to the work of the late Professor Frank H. Hamilton on this subject, and called attention to the importance of the following determining factors: (1) The degree of physical injury; (2) the duration of confinement in bed, as bearing respectively on the comfort, health, and business demands of the patient; (3) the character and importance of the inherent and acquired complications of respective methods of action, and (4) the final burdens imposed by the sequel of different plans of treatment.

Dr. Bryant said that except in cases emphasized by a special indication he was not inclined to the practice of suture of the patella, but thought it a justifiable procedure in selected cases.

At present the technics of operations which he employs consist (1) in making a short vertical incision; (2) removing the blood-clots from the fractured borders of the bone along with the interposed fibrous tissue that is sometimes present, and cleansing the joint cavity; (3) draining the joint with a few strands of silk-worm gut at the outer side; (4) uniting the fracture with a small wire so placed as to cause retention and proper apposition of the fragments, and (5) closure of the wound, antiseptic dressing, and fixation in bed for two weeks, followed by plaster-of-Paris bandage, when the patient is allowed to be about on crutches.

In closing, he called especial attention to a mechanical method wholly or in part employed by himself during the past twenty years in the treatment of fifteen cases of simple fracture, for which he claimed (1) greater comfort and efficiency; (2) less danger and only a week's confinement in bed, and (3) results equal to the best attending the employment of other mechanical methods.

DR. H. M. RICHARDSON of Boston spoke of the importance of good surroundings, good health of the patient, and surgical experience in aseptic technic in the treatment of these fractures. He thought wiring should be seriously considered if, owing to extensive lacerations, complete control of extension cannot be obtained. He also thought that in ordinary cases the time of confinement should be six months. He considered that a wound of the knee-joint is especially liable to infection. When failure of the conservative methods has been demonstrated, wiring of the patella should be considered.

DR. JAMES E. MOORE of Minneapolis thought that the opinion of American surgeons of the present day was represented by Dr. Powers' paper, believing it to be better than the results reported from the use of non-operative methods. He believed that an open arthrotomy would be less fatal than the passage of ligatures around the patella, and strongly advocated asepsis, proper environment, experience in performing operations about the knee-joint, immediate operation, and he believed the approximation of the fragments would thus be made easier. So as to avoid over-distension and interference with circulation, he believed better results would be obtained by temporary drainage. However, he did not feel that the amount of separation is any index as to the future usefulness of the joint.

DR. W. S. HALSTED of Baltimore was in favor of drainage only when the tissues were themselves not able to take care of the infection. He advocated immediate opening of the joint with thorough washing, and also the use of rubber gloves during these operations.

DR. POWERS closed the discussion by stating that he had expressed the opinion in the body of his paper that if a surgeon felt able to perform one of these operations he ought to feel equally safe in dispensing with drainage.

DR. NICHOLAS SENN of Chicago read a paper, entitled

THE ETIOLOGY AND CLASSIFICATION OF CYSTITIS.

After speaking at length of the anatomicophysiologic construction of the bladder, and referring to its lack of absorptive power, he spoke of the etiology, which he considered under the following heads:

1. Predisposing causes: (*a*) Retention of urine; (*b*) abnormal urine; (*c*) tumors; (*d*) unrest of the bladder; (*e*) calculus and foreign bodies; (*f*) exposure to cold; (*g*) venous stasis and trauma.

2. Exciting causes: (*a*) Infection through the urethra; (*b*) infection by the urine; (*c*) infection from adjacent organs; (*d*) infection from the blood, etc.

After mentioning Guyon's classification, he next considered this part of the subject, dividing it into (1) the anatomic, (2) pathologic, (3) clinical, and (4) the bacteriologic. He subdivided the anatomic into paracystitis, pericystitis, interstitial cystitis, cystitis; the pathologic into suppurative cystitis, exudative cystitis, catarrhal cystitis, ulcerative cystitis, exfoliative cystitis; the clinical into chronic cystitis, acute cystitis; and the bacteriologic into streptococcus infection, staphylococcus infection, bacillus coli communis infection, diplobacillus infection, saprophytic infection, gonococcus infection, erysipelatous infection, tuberculous infection.

DISCUSSION.

DR. JOHN PARMENTER of Buffalo, N. Y., in reference to the bladder not possessing any power of absorption, mentioned his experiment of injecting eight drops of sulphuric ether in a dram of water into the bladders of twelve healthy men, and detecting the odor of ether on the breath one minute after the injection. He considered that infection is usually due to a combination of traumatism, with the presence of micro-organisms, and urged greater care in the disinfection of the urethra before the passage of sounds.

DR. W. S. HALSTED of Baltimore, referring to the work of Dr. Young, one of his assistants, mentioned that Dr. Young found the gonococcus occasionally present in neutral urine, sometimes in acid, and once in alkaline urine.

DR. ALEXANDER of New York said that there are lymph-nodules present in the bladder and ureters, and he took exception to Dr. Senn's statement that there are no glands in the mucous membrane of the bladder. He said that sometimes these lymph-nodules give rise to a peculiar inflammation which he termed "nodular cystitis." He thought that cystitis was usually caused by retention of urine, and that in moderate cases of stricture an appreciable amount of residual urine is found, and further, that sexual hyperemia results from a moderate prostatic congestion. In regard to traumatism, he thought it was often due to destructive diseases brought about by irregular catheterization, and said that when a patient with prostatic enlargement is catheterized with an absolutely clean instrument infection will still occasionally occur. He also said that if a patient is catheterized at nine o'clock in the morning, again at five or six in the afternoon, and not again until the next day at noon the resulting over-distension of the bladder will produce trauma, and consequently, the more rapid occurrence of infection.

DR. SENN, in closing the discussion, stated that he believed the smell of ether on the breath in Dr. Parmeter's cases was the result more of a process of diffusion than of absorption and that the vesical mucous membrane does not possess power of absorption, though the urethra and neck of the bladder do.

(To be continued.)

NEW YORK ACADEMY OF MEDICINE.—SECTION ON ORTHOPEDIC SURGERY.

Stated Meeting, Held March 18, 1898.

A. B. JUDSON, M.D., Chairman.

CONGENITAL DISLOCATION OF THE HIP CURED BY LORENZ METHOD OF FORCIBLE REDUCTION.

DR. ROYAL WHITMAN: This little girl, two and a half years of age, had a congenital dislocation of the hip. I operated upon her when she was eighteen months old by the Lorenz method of forcible reduction, and put her in plaster. This she wore six months, and for two months more she wore an apparatus. She now walks very well for so young a child. I have operated in sixteen cases by this method. The main point is to operate early. In this case the protruding abdomen led to the child being treated for rickets. There was a shortening of three-fourths of an inch in the affected limb, and now I doubt if any of you can tell which it was. I consider this a perfect result.

DISCUSSION.

DR. R. H. SAYRE: This is the first case I have ever seen in which a perfect cure has resulted.

DR. T. HALSTEAD MYERS: Last summer I saw a case in which a perfect cure was obtained. There was one-eighth of an inch of shortening, but the child could run, jump, and do anything that other children could do.

DR. A. M. PHELPS: This seems to be a case of dislocation occurring at birth in a child in whom the acetabulum was normal. I have treated thirty-one patients with congenital dislocation of the hip, and in only one have I found a normal acetabulum. There is a perfect reduction in this case, but it should not be placed before us as a standard; for in most cases there is no acetabulum in which to put the head of the bone. I do not believe that bloodless forcible reduction is a good method; for shortening will follow because there is usually no acetabulum in which the head of the bone can rest. The only way to treat these patients is to make an acetabulum with the chisel. Of course, I am in favor of making an attempt at reduction, especially if the X-ray shows the presence of an acetabulum.

DR. GEORGE R. ELLIOTT: In regard to the non-cutting operation for congenital dislocation of the hip, I wish to emphasize the fact that there is considerable acetabulum in young children when the joint is dislocated, say in children under four years of age, and this is readily appreciated by the operator at the time of reduction. The head of the femur can be distinctly felt as it is forced over the posterior border of the socket. It is felt to be retained, and can be easily dislocated again. Now, if the limb is fixed at the proper degree of abduction, there is no possibility of its getting out of position, being held by the ligamentous and muscular structures of the joint. If it is not felt to be in something at least partially performing the functions of a socket, I believe the probability of its being retained, and thus leading to more perfect acetabular development, is greater than after the cutting operation in which the ligamentous and muscular structures have been divided. The field for the operation is in young subjects.

DR. WHITMAN: This case is one of a series of sixteen in which I have employed the bloodless method of reduction. I think the head of the bone is capable of making an acetabulum. A rudimentary acetabulum exists in nearly all cases. I know this because when I push the head of the bone in place it stays there. When the dislocation is anterior, which is not usually the case, I twist the bone around.

POTT'S DISEASE.

DR. R. W. TOWNSEND: This little child is three years of age, and was brought to the Hospital for Ruptured and Crippled last week because of a swelling of the neck. The question of the causation of this tumor was investigated, and it was found that the child had Pott's disease of the upper cervical vertebræ. This condition had not been suspected, although the child had been seen by a number of physicians. It is rather unusual to see a Pott's abscess in this location; under these circumstances it is much more apt to be retropharyngeal. She was put on this temporary frame, and as yet nothing much in the way of treatment has been done for her.

DISCUSSION.

DR. PHELPS: When these abscesses occur in the cervical region they should be at once operated upon from without on account of their liability to rupture internally. I have seen cases in which such an abscess appeared and pushed the pharynx forward. If they rupture internally the child will die of pulmonary tuberculosis. Therefore, they should be incised from without.

ENLARGEMENT OF THE TIBIA; OPERATION.

DR. B. FARQUHAR CURTIS: You will remember that Dr. Ketch showed this little girl at one of the meetings last fall. She is twelve years old, and had an anterior bowing of the right tibia and some eversion of the foot. The right tibia was three inches longer than that of the sound leg and greatly thickened, the circumference of the affected leg being one and a half inches greater than that of the other. The child's general health was also poor, probably as a result of pain. A skiagram showed a thickened tibia with some irregularities in the enlargement, and an almost complete disappearance of the epiphyseal line, which was due to pressure. When the child was shown there was some discussion as to the exact nature of the affection. There was no ascertainable history of syphilis, but in order to give the patient the benefit of the doubt, she was given iodid of potassium. She was operated upon on January 6th, after a month of medical treatment and rest in bed. During this time the tenderness disappeared and her general condition improved. The tibia was then exposed and a wedge-shaped piece of the bone removed. This wedge, however, was not sharp at one end, and was sufficient to shorten the leg about an inch. The bones went into position very well, but the soft parts were so voluminous that the skin could not be made to cover the wound, and consequently it burst open. Later, it was necessary to do a plastic operation. Two long incisions were made on either side of the wound, the skin dissected up and drawn together over the wound. Thiersch grafting was performed on February 22d. She now has a fairly good leg. The bone is the same length as that of the sound leg, and there is absolutely no tenderness. As yet, she does not walk very well, because she has been out of bed only a week.

The bone was found to be roughened on the surface, and the central canal had entirely disappeared. It was much more solid than usual, although not as hard as cortical bone. My recollection is that the wedge measured over an inch at the narrowest part, which was posteriorily, and as much as two inches on the anterior surface. Only the fibula was fractured. I think the condition was due to syphilis.

DISCUSSION.

DR. WHITMAN: This case brings up the interesting question as to whether such hypertrophied bones should be shortened so as to make the two extremities of equal length. As I understand it, when bone becomes hypertrophied it becomes hard and does not grow. Therefore, I should not think it necessary in a young subject to shorten such a bone to make it the same length as the other, for the latter will grow as the child gets older and the hypertrophied bone will not.

DR. SAYRE: Last month I showed a patient before the Section on Surgery who had marked enlargement of the tibia, which developed rapidly after a traumatism. From the radiograph which was made in Dr. Curtis' case, it seems to me that there is a mottled appearance of the bone such as I have seen in syphilitic disease.

DR. THOMAS H. MANLEY: The case submitted by Dr. Curtis presents about all the gross features of malignancy—of osteosarcoma. This lesion, as in most forms of true malignancy, is limited to the cortical or compact diaphysis, the infiltration extending into and involving all the soft parts; in fact the evidence points to diffusion at the present time. The result from the osteoplastic procedure is all that can be desired in the way of reducing the length of the limb, but it is apparent that further trouble is certain to ensue. It will be interesting to note the future progress of the case.

OBSCURE DEFORMITY OF THE SPINE.

DR. TOWNSEND: This little girl is eleven years of age. She was brought to the clinic last week for the first time, with the mother's statement that two weeks previously, while giving the child a bath, she noticed a prominence of the spine. The child has absolutely no symptoms, no pain, and no history of illness. She can move her back in any direction without complaint, and stands any amount of jarring. It is a question if she ever had Pott's disease. If so, it is one of the mildest cases I have ever seen. Of course, we all know that Pott's disease can exist without pain and with a considerable amount of flexibility of the spine, but this child can bend remarkably well in any direction.

DISCUSSION.

DR. GIBNEY: This case reminds me of one I saw not long ago in which a child had a deformity very like the one present in Dr. Townsend's case. There was no pain and the disease seemed to me to be a rachitic deformity. I am going to try forcible reduction.

DR. TOWNSEND: It is a question in my mind whether such a sharp curve as is present in my case is a favorable one for Calot's treatment.

POLIOMYELITIS.

DR. TOWNSEND: This little boy is suffering from poliomyelitis. The spinal muscles are affected, and there is more or less bulging of the sides of the body. The child has not sufficient strength to stand erect. He was first seen in October, 1897, and has been treated with tonics and electricity. Pads were applied to the sides, and maintained in place by a belt round the body to prevent the bulging. There is no curvature or bending of the spine.

POTT'S DISEASE; TREATMENT BY FORCIBLE REDUCTION.

DR. V. P. GIBNEY: These are cases in which I have employed forcible reduction after the method of Calot. The first is in a boy twelve years of age. The disease has lasted ever since he can remember, and he has had no previous treatment. The kyphos in the dorsolumbar region was very marked, as is seen in this tracing. He had the girdle symptom of which Dr. Sayre speaks. On March 1st, 1898, he was put under the influence of an anesthetic, and forcible reduction was performed. A plaster-of-Paris corset was then applied in the prone position, beginning at the pelvis, because the deformity was low and reached up to the axilla. The head and neck were not fixed. There was absolutely no reaction. I employed only a moderate amount of force, but it was sufficient to reduce the kyphos to a large degree. The parts yielded easily. He was kept in bed three days, much against his will, and since then he has been playing about the wards.

The second case occurred in a boy six years of age, who was operated upon on March 8th. He had been treated by apparatus, jackets, etc., and the disease, which was also in the dorsolumbar region, was arrested. The tracing of the kyphos is shown in this drawing. The amount of force employed was not greater then in the first case. During the operation his respiration became rather labored, and the administration of the anesthetic was discontinued. The only reaction was a slight slowing of the pulse after the operation and again a few days afterward.

The third case, in a girl aged fourteen years, is one of marked curvature of the spine in which I was led to attempt a similar operation because her parents urged me to do something to correct the deformity and were even willing to have section performed. She took the anesthetic badly, and three attempts were made. I employed a twisting motion for some five or ten minutes and then put her in plaster of Paris. There was no reaction. She is now an inch and three-quarters taller than she was before the operation, and the back is in a much better position than it was previously.

I have presented these three cases merely to show that the operation can be done without bad results. I have a patient who has paraplegia due to pressure and upon whom I expect to operate by this method in the hope of relieving the paraplegia. Cases have been reported in which this has been done. While I believe, as do most of the Continental and English surgeons, that deformities can be materially reduced by this method, I am of the opinion that it is best to go slow and do it gradually at several sittings rather than all at once. I appreciate the objections which have been raised against the method, but the clinical facts must bear some weight in the discussion.

I have here also a rather obscure case. This boy came to the hospital during May last. In January, 1897, he complained of pain in the left knee, and walked lame. The mother was told that he had "consumption" of the knee, and the limb was amputated at Bellevue Hospital during March of that year. The history is rather confused, but it was said that he had had a fall. There is now an excoriation of the shaft of the left humerus upon which we have operated several times, and also one upon the right elbow. In the discharge from the latter streptococci, staphylococci, and some micro-organisms which resembled diphtheria bacilli were found, but no tubercle bacilli. Recently the house surgeon called my attention to the fact that the patient has some difficulty in opening the mouth, and there seems to be a beginning ankylosis of the jaw.

DISCUSSION.

DR. PHELPS: In connection with Dr. Gibney's cases of Pott's disease treated by forcible reduction, I have one which I would like to present. This little girl is seven years of age. Four and a half years ago she developed a curvature of the spine, and since then has worn a jacket. She had had some cough, but no evening temperature. She had a kyphos, which is shown in this tracing, between the sixth and ninth dorsal vertebræ. She entered the Post-Graduate Hospital, and I operated upon her there. I confess that I approached the case with fear and trembling, and when I began making pressure there was so much snapping and cracking that I desisted, for I thought the child's back was broken. However, the kyphos was somewhat reduced as is shown by this second tracing, made after the operation.

The operation seems very cruel, and, if I had not been fortified by the favorable reports of the French surgeons, I would not have dared attempt it; and yet there was no reaction following the operation. The child was up and about within less than four days. In one other case I succeeded, without anesthesia, in reducing a beginning kyphos by this method.

DR. TOWNSEND: It seems to be that we ought to go slow in advising the profession to employ this treatment. The dangers of the operation are many. For instance, the result would have have been disastrous if forcible reduction has been employed in a case we had at the hospital last week. A child three years old, with Pott's disease, was admitted and was put upon an open frame. She had some difficulty in moving the head. She had had an attack of bronchitis before admission; so when a slight cough developed it was ascribed to the bronchitis. I was called up one night by the house surgeon who said that the child's respiration was bad. I suggested some mild remedies, and the next morning asked Dr. Holt to see her. He advised the use of a croup kettle. At this time there was no pneumonia and no asphyxia. That night the child became asphyxiated and died. Autopsy showed a retro-esophageal abscess in the median line directly over the vertebral column and extending to the right. There was no pressure on the trachea, which was normal in size and not flattened. There were numerous enlarged glands, and these pressed upon the nerves. The second dorsal vertebra was much diseased, so much so that in examining it I pushed my finger clear through the spinous process. If I had attempted forcible reduction in this case I would have ruptured that abscess or caused damage to the bone. I am aware that we all realize the dangers of the operation. The difficulty will be to select the cases in which it may be safely performed.

DR. H. L. TAYLOR: I quite agree with Dr. Townsend that we ought not to let the impression go out that we advocate the method until we have had more experience with it. The operation has been much modified since it was first suggested. In his first article, Calot said that "the spine should be forced into place." In his next article he said that if any difficulty was experienced in forcing the spine straight, he took out a wedge-shaped piece of the bone. Chapeaux (7) considers it essential to wire the spinal processes. All these modifications of the operation have been adopted. The French surgeons also consider it important to encase the head and shoulders in a plaster-of-Paris jacket. It has further been suggested, and very sensibly, that the reduction should not be done at one sitting, but at several. The tendency is to make the operation very much less radical. Many surgeons say that it is wrong to use much force. Calot says he uses all his strength—"*toute ma force*"—while traction is made upon both upper and lower extremities. The operation has been so much modified that it remains to be seen how much of the original procedure will be left after it has been well studied. While it is in the hands of experts, we are safe; but it is not well to let experimentation extend into non-expert hands.

DR. SAYRE: "An ounce of prevention is worth a pound of cure." In Pott's disease the diagnosis should be made before the kyphos forms, and there will then be no necessity for correcting it. I would like to call attention to the fact that as far back as 1830, or thereabouts, this same procedure was employed, except that instead of the hands, they used a large windlass arrangement and a long lever with which to force the spine into position. This apparently met with disfavor, for it passed out of use. It seems to me that in a great many instances forcible reduction would be followed by very serious results. If we could only determine in advance the cases in which the spine could be safely straightened we would be able to proceed intelligently. Inasmuch as we cannot do this, it is difficult to know what to do. In some cases the bone is so diseased that any attempt to forcibly straighten the spine will result in producing gaps between the vertebræ; in other cases a psoas abscess will result.

When my father first applied plaster-of-Paris jackets, he stretched the patient as much as he could and still not cause discomfort. One of the celebrated German surgeons, probably on the ground that if a little of a good thing is good, more is better, stretched his patients by means of weights applied to their heels. Two or three of them promptly died, and the autopsies showed that in each an abscess had been ruptured. How much the relationship between perpendicular position and the anesthetic had to do with the deaths, I do not know. I believe there is now a surgeon who suspends his patients by the heels when he applies a jacket.

Forcible reduction has been employed in quite a number of cases, and the death-rate, I believe, is so far only one per cent. It is extremely doubtful, however, whether we should employ this method. The cases should be most carefully selected. There should be no elevation of temperature and no active pathologic process. I recall a case almost exactly like the one referred to by Dr. Townsend, in which the child died within two hours. Autopsy showed a large saddle-shaped abscess at the junction of the trachea.

DR. ELLIOTT: In a recent number of the *British Medical Journal* Murray reports two cases in which forcible reduction was followed by death. One patient died of acute tuberculous pneumonia and the other of acute tuberculous meningitis.

DR. PHELPS: As I said before, I confess that I undertook the operation in fear and trembling and against my convictions. After examining pathologic specimens and noting the bone changes which take place in Pott's disease and in analogous affections, it seemed a dangerous thing to do. I have studied the literature of the operation, and find that it is a very old one, although there is no question but that Chipault is the modern originator of the method. Calot followed him in the work. The latter presents deductions which seem to show that the bone is reproduced in cases in which there is wide separation after reduction. Regnault also reports reproduction of bone. Lorenz and others have had relapses and have reported them. Ménard had a case in which he reduced the kyphos and ruptured an abscess. In another case fracture of the vertebræ was produced. Calot reports 204 cases with no accidents and no deaths on the operating-table. Menod criticises him and says his results are too good and should not carry weight. Chipault says there are too many relapses, and contends that all cases will relapse unless the spine is wired. Lorenz reports paralysis and relapse following the operation. Jonnesco has reported three deaths in thirteen operations. Lorenz and Ménard are the chief critics and they denounce the operation. Chipault is conservative and cautious. Ménard is judicial and skeptic, and the majority are enthusiastic, says Lovett.

The patients presented here to-night are not the first to be operated upon by this method in this country. Ridlon of Chicago has performed the operation a number of times with excellent results. I believe there is a legitimate field for this method. The time to employ it is early in the course of the disease. In case of long standing, in which there is a large kyphos, ankylosis, and abscess, it is a dangerous procedure. I think we should go slow, and that this Section ought to discourage the general employment of the method. For the present it should be confined to experts in orthopedic surgery. Within a few years we will know more about it.

DR. GIBNEY: I think we all agree with what has been said. We should discourage the wholesale performance of an operation of this kind. Lovett has recently discussed the subject fully in a paper in the *Boston Medical and Surgical Journal*. Mr. Jones of Liverpool has also reported fifty or sixty cases in which he has performed the operation. I appreciate all the dangers connected with it, and I merely presented these cases this evening to show that it could be performed without reaction, and not for the purpose of advocating its general employment. The case referred to by Dr. Townsend is an exceptional one. Most of the cases we see offer no special contraindication to the operation.

In regard to what Dr. Myers has said about waiting for a cure by other means, if anybody waits longer for a cure than the orthopedic surgeon, I would like to know who he is. We treat our patients and kept them in braces for years, and I do not see why they should wear apparatus for these long periods if forcible reduction can cure them within a shorter time.

There is much difference of opinion in regard to the details of the operation. Mr. Jones and his colleagues in Liverpool criticise the French surgeons for putting their patients up in cotton. They also advocate the steel apparatus rather than the plaster-jacket. All of us know that there are great differences in plaster-jackets. We also know that if too much cotton is used, we do not get a good fit, for the parts recede and the jacket is then much too loose. If the plaster is properly applied and fitted over the hard parts, it will give no trouble. Lovett claims in his article that a certain proportion of patients with hip-joint disease treated by forcible reduction have died of tuberculous meningitis. I, for one, do not put much faith in this statement. I do not know how the reports of other operators read, but I do know that for years I have been forcibly correcting deformities of the hip, and that it is the rarest thing in the world to cause dissemination of the bacilli.

I do not find that patients with a deformity of the spine are willing to go through life with it. They are morose, and feel that Nature has treated them harshly, and it is very necessary to do something for them. I know that if I had a child with such a deformity I would welcome anything which promised relief. I think there is a way of treating these patients by studying them and making a proper selection of treatment and not trying to do too much all at once. I do not believe it is necessary to fix the head and shoulders. If we bring the plaster well up, we will not have any recurrence. Just what Nature will do in these cases remains to be seen.

MALIGNANT DISEASE OF THE SPINE.

DR. H. L. TAYLOR: This man is forty-seven years of age, a waiter by occupation. He tells me that a number of years ago he was kicked in the chest by a horse. The injury resulted in the formation of a tumor which was excised six weeks ago at Mt. Sinai Hospital. The exact nature of the tumor is not known, but the man tells me that it was the size of his head. About eight months ago he began to have very severe pain in the lower part of the back. Cough and expectoration also began at this time. Examination of the back shows it to be round, and on the left side of the median line there is a projection which appears to be an enlargement of a spinous process at about the first lumbar vertebra. There is marked stiffness and limitation of motion. In addition to this there is an area of sweating on the right side which points to the existence of a carcinomatous tumor. This is a pathognomonic sign of carcinoma, as proved by antopsy in cases in which the diagnosis was not made during life. This symptom is probably due to involvement of some of the sympathetic ganglia of the lumbar region, and is never seen in tuberculous disease of the spine.

APPARATUS FOR FORCIBLE EXTENSION.

DR. ELLIOTT: I have here an instrument which I have devised for forcible extention. It is especially intended for use in reduction of the congenitally dislocated hip. It can also be used for forcible reduction of the spinal column in cases of the angular curvature of caries. It can be adjusted to any table or bed, and the force employed can be regulated at will, and, if desired, measured in pounds. It is light and inexpensive and was made for me by John Reynders & Co.

REVIEWS.

A TEXT-BOOK OF MATERIA MEDICA FOR NURSES. By LAVINIA L. DOCK, Graduate of Bellevue Hospital Training-school. Third edition. New York: G. P. Putnam's Sons, 1897.

THIS little book has long been known in the field it so admirably covers. It is gratifying, therefore, to find that the demand for it is sufficiently strong to call for a new edition. In the present book the metric system has been added, and the newer drugs of the pharmacopeia have been considered. The description of the older drugs, too, has been revised. The work is neither too diffuse nor too limited, but seems to cover exactly the field allotted to it.

THERAPIE DER HAUTKRANKHEITEN. Von DR. L. LEISTIKOW, mit einem Vorwort von DR. P. G. UNNA (TREATMENT OF SKIN DISEASES. By L. LEISTIKOW, with a preface by DR. P. G. UNNA). Hamburg and Leipsic: Leopold Voss, 1897.

OF the great additions which have been made in recent years to the treasures of our materia medica, dermatology has certainly enjoyed her full share. It is, however, not only in the acquisition of new drugs, but especially in their mode of application and in the determination of precise indications for their use, as well as for their mode of application, that the greatest progress has been made. The scientific dermatologist finds some other indication than the convenience of his patient for determining whether a particular drug shall be used in the form of a plaster, a salve, a paste, a lotion, or a varnish. Among those that have contributed to the advancement of dermatology in this respect there are none greater than Dr. P. G. Unna of Hamburg, under whose eye the book before us has been published.

Dr. Leistikow is peculiarly fitted for the task of presenting the methods of treatment employed by Dr. Unna, having been associated with him in his private and public dermatological practice during the past seven years. As a rational dermatotherapy must ever aim at correcting the pathologic conditions which underly a particular lesion, it was but natural that in the arrangement of his work the author should follow the classification observed by Unna in his "Histopathology of Skin Diseases," and Leistikow's book, therefore, forms a perfect complement to Unna's great work.

The first part of the book is devoted to a review of the dermatologic materia medica. Among the subjects discussed are the uses and mode of preparation of baths, pastes, varnishes, gelatins, salves, mulls, soaps, etc. In the second, the major part of the book, the treatment of the various skin diseases is considered. The author is particularly to be congratulated on the perfect and complete manner in which he has covered the ground, while yet maintaining the concise form necessary in a compendium of this kind. Nor has he failed to observe a just proportion in the amount of space devoted to each subject. Thus, to the treatment of eczema, which constitutes so large a proportion of the diseases observed in dermatologic practice, fifty of the four hundred pages of the book are devoted.

On the whole, while there is naturally but little that is entirely new to the student of dermatologic literature, the book forms a perfect storehouse, rich in valuable suggestions in the line of the latest advances in dermatology.

ÉTUDE SUR LES MALFORMATIONS CONGÉNITALE DU GENOIE. Par le DOCTEUR G. POTEL. Lille: Imprimerie L. Dauel; 1897.

THIS monograph is an exhaustive study of the literature of the congenital malformations and distortions of the knee-joint. The author claims to have written practically a new chapter in orthopedic surgery in bringing together the detached cases of what were supposed to be examples of rare deformities and thus proving them to be not at all uncommon.

Nearly 300 cases of deformity or of defective development of the constituents of the joint, many of which are quoted in minute detail, prove the truth of the author's contention and testify to his industry. He has, for example, collected 50 cases of defective development or absence of the tibia, and states that the list of 97 cases of defective fibula recently published by Haudek might be easily doubled.

Seventy-two cases of genu recurvatum are presented. A proper distinction is made between this deformity of the leg, which is the result of an exaggeration of the range of extension, and true dislocation, in which the joint surfaces are actually displaced. Genu recurvatum and absence of patella (100 cases), which is often associated with it, are due to primary contraction or defective development of the quadriceps extensor muscle.

Malformations of the bones, aside from a small proportion caused by amniotic adhesions, are due to defective development of the fetus, the result of infection with some unknown poison.

The author quotes Morgagni, to the effect that the best way to ascertain the truth on any subject is to bring together as many observations as possible for comparison and study. If, therefore, one does not agree with the author's conclusions, he may study the cases in the search for a better theory of the cause of congenital deformities.

This monograph, which was written as a graduation thesis, is a valuable contribution to medical literature, and might well serve as a model for similar productions.

CLINICAL DIAGNOSIS: The Bacteriological, Chemical, and Microscopical Evidence of Disease. By DR. RUDOLF VON JAKSCH, Professor of Special Pathology and Therapeutics, and Director of the Medical Clinic in the German University of Prague. Third English, from the fourth German, edition by JAMES CAGNEY, M.A., M.D., Physician to the Hospital for Epilepsy and Paralysis, etc. London: Charles Griffin and Company, Limited, 1897.

IT needs but the perusal of Von Jaksch's monumental work, in the original or in English, to refute the statement so often made by surgeons, that surgery has advanced more than internal medicine within the past twenty years. The physician of the present day, if he would prove his diagnosis beyond cavil, must be master of the arts of the laboratory and of the revelations of the microscope. The author of the work under consideration is responsible for this in no small degree. He was not only among the first to teach the newer methods of diagnosis at the bedside, but he was the pioneer author in this field when he published his first edition of this book. Many of the clinical methods of diagnosis, too, here described and now universally employed, sprang from his initiative.

The present edition scarcely needs further notice here than to announce its appearance. There is nothing omitted from the work that belongs to it, and matter was inserted, seemingly, up to the hour of going to press. Even the serum diagnosis of typhoid fever is fully discussed; the announcement of Sanarelli's bacillus of yellow fever appeared too late for insertion here, it would appear. There is no work on the chemic and microscopic diagnosis of diseased states which can supplant this classic book. Others may copy from it, but Von Jaksch's will always be unique among books of its class.

As in former editions, the illustrations are profuse and finely executed. The translator has done excellent work, as comparison with the original reveals, and has given evidence of his wide reading by the numerous additions he has made to the original text.

INTERNATIONAL CLINICS. A Quarterly of Clinical Lectures. Edited by JUDSON DALAND, M.D., Instructor in Clinical Medicine in the University of Pennsylvania, etc., J. MITCHELL BRUCE, M.D., F.R.C.P., Physician to Charing Cross Hospital, London, etc., and DAVID W. FINLAY, M.D., F.R.C.P., Professor of Practice of Medicine in the University of Aberdeen, etc. Vol. III. Seventh series. Philadelphia: J. B. Lippincott Company, 1897.

THE third volume of these clinical lectures for the current year has appeared, and contains, as usual, some notable contributions. Prominent are: "Opium; Its Use and Abuse," by Dr. Herman D. Marcus; "The Treatment of Pulmonary Tuberculosis," by Dr. Norman Bridge; "Hematuria," by Dr. James Tyson; an article of striking merit by Dr. Byron Bramwell on epilepsy; "The Surgical Treatment of Gall-stones," by Dr. James F. W. Ross; "Bleeding in Pregnancy and Labor," by Dr. A. H. F. Barbour, and a timely lecture by Dr. Geo. M. Boyd on "The Desirability and Importance of Locating the Site of Infection in Puerperal Sepsis." With one or two exceptions, the lectures in the present volume are of very superior merit, and demonstrate the wisdom of publishing them in this form.

THERAPEUTIC HINTS.

For Amenorrhea.—

℞ Strych. sulphat. . . . . . gr. ii
Ac. oxalici . . . . . . gr. x
Mangani lactat. } aa . . . ʒ ii
Ferri peptonat. }
Ext. colocynth. comp. . . . ʒ ss.

M. Div. in pulv. No. XL. Sig. One powder twice daily after meals.

For Neurasthenia.—

℞ Ferri arsenas . . . . gr. iv
Ferri lactat. . . . . ʒ ii
Ext. nucls vomicæ . . . gr. viii
Ext. gentianæ . . . . gr. xlv.

M. Div. in pil. No. C. Sig. Two pills three times daily during meals.

Administration of Alcoholic Stimulants to Infants.—To avoid an irritating local action COMBY advises that alcoholic stimulants should invariably be diluted three to six times with sweetened water, milk, syrups, mucilages, etc.

Trional in the Treatment of Whooping-Cough.—This drug is reported as being very useful in the treatment of pertussis. A dose of from 1 to 8 grains, according to the age of the child, induces a peaceful sleep, only temporarily disturbed by an attack of coughing. It is also advised that the throat be sprayed or frequently swabbed with a one-per-cent. solution of carbolic acid in glycerin and water.

For Gastralgia.—

℞ Orthoform hydrochlorat. . . gr. xv
Aq. dest. . . . . . . ℥ iii.

M. Sig. One tablespoonful several times during an attack.

For Gastro-Intestinal Catarrh.—In cases in which opiates are not indicated, LIEBREICH recommends the following mixture for the diarrhea:

℞ Tinct. calumbæ } aa . . . ℥ ss.
Tinct. cascarillæ }

M. Sig. Twenty drops four or five times daily.

For Urticaria.—

℞ Menthol . . . . . . gr. xl
Chloroform. }
Ætheris } aa . . . ʒ ii.
Spts. camphoræ }

M. Sig. For external use as a spray or lotion. The affected part should then be dusted with powdered starch or oxid of zinc.

THE MEDICAL NEWS.

A WEEKLY JOURNAL OF MEDICAL SCIENCE.

VOL. LXXII. NEW YORK, SATURDAY, MAY 7, 1898. NO. 19.

ORIGINAL ARTICLES.

A GENERAL CONSIDERATION OF MASTOID DISEASE.[1]

BY SEYMOUR OPPENHEIMER, M.D.,
OF NEW YORK;
ATTENDING LARYNGOLOGIST TO THE OUT-DOOR DEPARTMENT OF BELLEVUE HOSPITAL; SENIOR ASSISTANT TO THE CHAIR OF LARYNGOLOGY IN THE UNIVERSITY MEDICAL COLLEGE.

DURING the past decade the study of inflammation of the mastoid process of the temporal bone has advanced with enormous strides. The various methods of accurate investigation as now applied to this portion of the body, in conjunction with the aseptic treatment of wounds and improved methods of operation, have combined to make what a few years ago was considered a very serious operation a matter of every-day experience, and this without fear of evil results following extensive removal of diseased bone from the mastoid process, or operative interference in the intracranial complications of purulent inflammation of the mastoid cells. With the symptomatology clearly defined by constant observation, it is only in exceptional cases that the trained aurist neglects to make the proper diagnosis early in the disease, and, upon early operation not only depends the restoration of the diseased portion of the cranium, but sometimes life itself.

In outlining proper means and efficient measures for the prevention of mastoid suppuration and necrosis, we are confronted with two problems, and depending upon the successful solution of these alone, will grave disease of mastoid be avoided:

1. The cure of chronic suppurative otitis media—from which the majority of mastoid cases originate.
2. The proper treatment of acute otitis media.

Burnett remarks, in a recent publication: "When every member of the profession is sufficiently impressed with the importance of inflammation of the middle ear and prepares to treat this disease efficiently in all its stages, the necessity for mastoid operation will probably seldom arise."

A few words will convey what is meant by the proper and improper treatment of acute inflammation of the middle ear.

In the majority of cases, ordinary antiphlogistic measures, as applied to any acute inflammation elsewhere in the body, will ameliorate the disease, but we frequently find that septic fluids have been injected into the acutely inflamed ear, or oils instilled which, as soon as perforation of the drum membrane occurs, give rise to secondary infection and mastoid involvement. When pus has formed in the tympanic cavity and Nature is not prompt in evacuating it, paracentesis should be performed without further delay. This operation should be done under strict antiseptic precautions. A safe rule to follow, in the treatment of acute non-perforative suppurative otitis media, is to regard the condition as we would an acute abscess elsewhere in the body and treat it in the same way, *i.e.*, by early evacuation and drainage. Possibly, during the past few years, otology has been placed more upon a scientific basis by the increased recognition of this cardinal principle than by any other method of treatment.

Without exhaustively entering into all the details of mastoid disease, it is the object of this paper to outline, in a general way, some of the points necessary to a proper appreciation of mastoiditis and its successful treatment. It is practically impossible to determine the percentage of frequency of involvement of the mastoid in relation to the number of cases of both acute and chronic suppurative otitis media. Since the severe epidemic of influenza several years ago there has been a large increase in the number of cases. From the topography of the temporal bone in children, with its numerous sutures and fissures, we find mastoid involvement to be much more frequent in young people than in adults. This is due not only to the anatomic peculiarity of the parts but also to the fact that frequently there exists in children a purulent discharge from the ear, which is not recognized until, from auto-infection and extension of the morbid process, severe symptoms, such as meningitis or sinus thrombosis, are manifested.

Mastoid disease may be divided into two classes, primary and secondary. True primary mastoiditis is rare, generally being due to traumatism of the parts. Beginning as a periostitis with damage to the overlying soft tissues, we later find the disease extending inward, osteitis and necrosis of the body of the bone resulting. This form may also be due to exposure, tuberculosis, or specific disease, in the last instance following the development of gummata. Recently a number of observers have studied this acute form and have elucidated many new and valuable points. Sheppard, in a very extensive review,

[1] Read at a meeting of the Society for Medical Progress of New York, February 9, 1898.

collected 114 cases, giving the history as far as ascertainable in each, and thus throwing much light upon the subject.

The common habit of indiscriminately blowing a so-called antiseptic powder into the auditory canal or middle ear is productive of much harm, the powder becoming impacted and preventing the discharge of the purulent material so that retention of pus with all its disastrous consequences results. Syringing the diseased ear, unless performed with much care and always under proper illumination, is to be condemned. It is a good rule, and one which should always be observed, that no instrument or solution should be applied to the tympanic cavity unless the parts are under the direct control of the eye.

Galette, in a recent article, conclusively shows that mastoiditis following acute tympanic suppuration is always due to secondary infection; therefore, it will be seen that the study of the etiology and prophylaxis of mastoid disease is in reality a study of middle-ear suppuration, and from the hygienic point of view the proper aseptic treatment of the latter affection alone will prevent the occurrence of a great number of mastoid cases. Gelle and Luc, from an exhaustive study of a large number of mastoid cases, arrived at the conclusion that direct infection may occur without middle-ear involvement.

Bearing in mind the sequence of events consequent to osteitis elsewhere in the body, we find that inflammation of the mastoid presents nothing unusual. At first there is an increased vascularity of the soft tissues lining the pneumatic cells, the lining membrane becomes thickened, and the bone shows inflammatory invasion. This process may cease, resolution taking place, or, if it continues, new osseous tissue is produced, causing the cells to become reduced in size with obliteration of the diploic spaces. Finally, a complete obliteration of the pneumatic spaces occurs, the bone becomes sclerosed and ivory-like in consistency. In other cases, from the extension of pathogenic organisms from the middle ear, suppuration ensues and the bone instead of becoming sclerosed, becomes necrotic. Should a large area of the mastoid process be involved in this destructive process a sequestrum is formed deep in the bone, while, should the inflammation affect a smaller area the parts will be found softened and disintegrated, small particles of dead bone, tissue-débris, and pus being presented in the operative field.

The anatomic characteristics of this portion of the temporal bone readily explain the occurrence of that most dangerous complication of mastoid suppuration, *viz.*, rupture of the abscess into the cranial cavity. This is faciliated by the thick wall externally and the very thin lamella of bone separating the pus collection from the brain cavity. In some instances this occurs—the outer or external table of the skull presenting a far greater resistance than the inner, and infection of the brain and its vessels is likely to occur unless prevented by early operation. In a few rare cases, especially in children, the pus breaks through the outer plate and spontaneous external rupture occurs.

Purulent matter escaping but rarely through the mastoid process, as just seen, it may make its exit in other directions much more serious to the patient. It may produce necrosis of the bone downward and backward into the digastric fossa, the pus burrowing underneath the sternomastoid muscles and infiltrating the tissues and fascial planes of the neck. This is the so-called Bezold's form of mastoiditis, and, although not as serious as when the purulent matter makes its exit from the mastoid cells in other internal directions, yet it requires more or less extensive operation and considerable time for the ultimate cure of the disease. In a case of Bezold's mastoiditis reported by Mendel, the patient was able to force pus from the tympanic cavity by pressure upon the swollen and tender region beneath the tip of the mastoid. Far more serious to the patient are the two remaining routes by which pus may escape: (1) through the tympanic vault into the middle cranial fossa, and (2) into the posterior fossa of the skull.

A few years ago the literature on the intracranial complications of mastoid disease was as meager as the knowledge of them, but at the present time, special attention having been directed to this subject, the literature presents the histories of many cases in which operations were performed for cerebral abscess or meningitis—with resulting cure of the disease.

Unlike a great many local affections, the symptomatology of infection of the mastoid process is accurately known, and, with a better understanding of the more prominent subjective and objective signs of the disease, the indications for treatment are clear in the large majority of cases. Pain over the affected mastoid, or on the same side of the head, is a valuable indication, but the absence of pain does not invariably mean that the interior of the antrum is not the seat of a morbid process. In a few cases pressure over the mastoid region will elicit pain even when the parts are healthy—and in studying this symptom we should always compare the suspected with the healthy side.

Bulging of the posterior-superior wall of the external auditory canal is a most valuable indication of the presence of pus in the adjoining mastoid cells. This projection forward of the wall into the lumen of the canal is in the majority of cases sufficient evidence to warrant immediate operative interference, even should other marked symptoms of mastoid involvement be absent. Pulsating tinnitus is sometimes present and indicative of vascular engorgement and, consequently, pressure upon the middle ear, and this, in conjunction with other signs, facilitates the diagnosis. Should otorrhea be present previous to the mastoid disease, the diminution in amount or sudden suppression of the discharge from the middle ear will, in a considerable number of cases, indicate involvement of the mastoid. This retention, although not always reliable, should be very carefully investigated, as it may mean that the pus is either accumulating or discharging in another less favorable direction.

The external signs of mastoid inflammation may be well-marked when a case is first seen, and then the diagnosis is readily made, the mastoid process being red, swollen, painful, and sometimes edematous. Should the case be seen before marked inflammatory changes are evident over the external surface of the bone, there are still many symptoms upon which to base a diagnosis. Of considerable importance, associated with bulging of the wall of the auditory canal, is the presence of a perforation of the flaccid membrane in its posterior-superior quadrant, indicating attic involvement. This is especially diagnostic when, projecting through the small perforation, is a teat-like fold of the internal mucous membrane.

The constitutional symptoms may not be in any way characteristic, it being a frequent experience to find considerable mastoid involvement with pus formation with but a moderate degree of fever and acceleration of the pulse. In other cases the constitutional symptoms are well marked, serious depression, high temperature, intense pain, and general distress being present. Should brain or sinus involvement occur in conjunction with the mastoid suppuration considerable information may be obtained from the constitutional manifestations. Probably the objective symptoms taken in all are of more value in correctly estimating a given case than the subjective symptoms alone.

In some cases it is necessary to accurately ascertain, not only that the mastoid is the seat of a morbid process, but also to define the amount of bony tissue involved. In cases of this class, Wild recommends percussion of the suspected mastoid with a metallic hammer, a comparative study of the affected with the healthy side showing a marked difference in the percussion-note, dullness, localized or general, indicating the seat and area of the osseous changes. As an aid in these cases, Gabritachewski uses the ordinary stethoscope applied over the suspected mastoid and at the same time strikes a tuning-fork on the cerebral vertex. If the suspected mastoid be the seat of morbid changes there is impairment of the sound waves as they are transmitted through the bones of the head.

Caldwell calls attention to the usefulness of transmitted light as a means of diagnosis in cases of suspected suppurative mastoiditis. An electric lamp of two- or three-candle power is placed well within the external auditory meatus, the room in which the examination is conducted is thoroughly darkened. The mastoid cells are thus illuminated with a ruddy glow. If suppuration exists, this glow will not be perceived, as the fluid will prevent the transmission of light.

The subject of treatment of mastoiditis may be conveniently divided into two parts, *viz.*, medical and surgical.

What may be designated as medical treatment consists of rest in bed and the application of antiphlogistic measures, as in the treatment of inflammation of other parts. The bowels must be opened, the patient should be placed upon a fluid diet, and attention given to the middle-ear and mastoid region. Should there be indications of fluid in the middle-ear, paracentesis of the drum should be immediately performed, thus providing free drainage. The parts may be irrigated with an antiseptic solution, and cold applied over the mastoid by means of the Leiter coil. This should never be used more than forty-eight hours, as by the long continued lowering of temperature the vitality of the tissues is impaired and in consequence the disease is aggravated. An incision through the soft parts over the mastoid and down to, but not entering, the bone, the so-called Wild's incision, was formerly recommended in practically all cases, but now has been discarded by the otologist as being of no value in aborting the inflammation, and at the same time it presents a new field for septic absorption: Should pain be excessive, anodynes may be employed in small doses during a short time, but this practice is dangerous, as important symptoms may be masked and indications for operative procedure thus not be recognized. Should the inflammation give no indications of lessening within forty-eight hours under the treatment mentioned, we should not delay operation for the appearance of the objective signs of mastoid involvement, such as edema and redness, but a safe rule is to operate as soon as there is bulging of Shrapnell's membrane and drooping of the posterior and upper cutaneous lining of the wall of the external auditory canal.

The most brilliant results in otology are those obtained by early and thorough operative interference in mastoid disease. This is especially evident at the present time, medical literature being filled with reports of successful cases in which the mastoid has not only been opened and the diseased tissues removed, but also in which surgical treatment of the serious complications has been instituted, the brain cavity being entered and abscesses evacuated and thrombi removed from the brain sinuses. The operation which has been received with the most favor in this country is known as the Stacké operation, and it is performed in the following manner:

The auricle is drawn well forward and detached along its posterior border. The cartilaginous auditory canal is then detached from the bony canal, laying open the posterior wall of the bony canal and antrum into one cavity. Granulations and necrotic tissue are removed and the resulting hollow covered with skin and periosteal flap from the external auditory meatus.

Bergman's operation is somewhat similar, while that advocated by Wolf and Kuster, in which the antrum is opened through the meatus, is more difficult and not as satisfactory, as it does not furnish sufficient space for the removal of all diseased tissue, and is indicated only when mastoid infection is limited to the region immediately between the middle ear and the mastoid.

AUTOHYPNOTISM.

BY STANLEY WARREN, M.D.,
OF WASHINGTON, D. C.

FROM the unusual increase in the number of suicides within the circle of refined, intelligent people of social position and wealth, and especially of young women who by the laws of heredity, sex, and the influence of their environments inherit and acquire refinement, gentleness, purity, and the highest conception of morality, with a natural horror of crime, pain, and death, it suggests itself to me as a cause of suicidal mania, that there must be present in such cases some auto-infection or self-hypnotism. Such a condition may result from a constant and persistent thought that is being daily suggested through the medium of certain special senses, at first occasionally, and then habitually, becoming automatic and finally auto-infective, resulting in emotional outbreaks, melancholia, hypochondria, hysteria, and suicidal mania.

All mental phenomena, as we know, are the result of education or habit, for example, thought, speech, emotions, dreams, love of music, art, and all things beautiful, artistic, dramatic, etc. Of course, the stimulus at first comes from without, and unconsciously from without at all times. These external things stimulate the mind to conceive while the mind commands the body to act, and so we see music, for instance, in the finger-tips, and hear it in the trained voice, although it is born within, and so all of the attributes of mind become material and active in the body.

The neurologist is often confronted with cases in which his intuition and experience warn him that the mental condition of his patient is serious while no symptoms are apparent, and in the majority of these cases the family history is good. In such the patients have often been heard to say in the most nonchalant manner that they, he or she, will kill themselves. This is most characteristic of suicidal mania, and to my mind the most conclusive evidence of autohypnotism—this one idea has become automatic. If at the time the patient makes this statement you ask him a question relative to the line of thought previously pursued, you will notice that he will take it up at once, showing that the statement "I will kill myself" is not the result of thought or that he is conscious of having uttered these words, but it is an example of purely automatic speech, the result of one idea becoming mechanically constant. Thus, the act of self-destruction becomes an unconscious one and, therefore, is not a crime in the eyes of law, or God, nor does it require courage, because there is no appreciation of pain; and so the delicate woman, refined as she is, will, when in this condition, inflict ghastly wounds upon herself or take the most deadly drugs and calmly lay herself down to die.

Autohypnotism is not necessarily a disease, and only becomes so when the dominant idea is a diseased one and is of such a character as to suggest the abnormal, either criminal or pathologic. Of course heredity and ill-health predispose the character of the idea. The only external cause to be considered is the suggestion, and I will discuss its relative importance later. As an example of autohypnotism in health let us take a child bodily and mentally normal and having no hereditary taint. If this child be a male, naturally, suggestions of manly habits and occupations will appeal to it, but if a female, suggestions of its mother's duties will be more readily accepted. So, we see the little girl becoming the mother of her dolls, or imitating the mother's duties about the home, while in the boy we see an embryo mechanic, if his father be one, or whatever the father's work is as a man, you will find reflected in the boy's play as a child. Thus, the father's occupation suggests the boy's, and the idea becomes dominant in the latter, to show its fruit later in life unless some counter-suggestion destroys it by becoming the stronger, when the mind and character change for the man's. What is thus demonstrable in the healthy mind is equally as true of the diseased mind. Autohypnotism as a disease resulting from unhealthful suggestions does not necessarily result in self-destruction, but the result of all unhealthful thought is mental disease direct, and bodily disease indirect. As the result of automaticity of suggested thought there may be almost any condition. Suicide is the result of constant suggested thought of self-destruction.

Hysteria sometimes results from the constant dwelling of the mind upon disease; and it is believed by some authorities that even organic changes result from this constant concentration of the mind upon disease. Then there are all kinds of simple manias, as the mania of self-adornment which leads the rich to kleptomania and the poor to steal; the mania for notoriety and publicity, which indirectly leads to crime, as men and women in the higher circles sometimes commit indecent and immoral acts for a little cheap notoriety, suggested by the acts of people who have no regard for morals. At present we have a most laughable mania which has become epidemic in political life, *viz.*, "The Jingo Mania," a mania the politician has for getting cheap newspaper advertising, which throws him into such a trance that he gets up in public assemblies and makes wild, incoherent, illogical, and sensational statements, and goes home to read his reconstructed and rewritten speech in some daily paper and is hypnotized into believing that he is a statesman. This is, unfortunately, an autohypnotism which never leads to self-destruction.

The publicity then, of acts and speech when criminal or inciting to crime is a suggestion to weak and receptive minds, whether hereditary or due to ill health, which results in imitation. As an illustration of this the following is interesting: A few months ago in the city of Washington and throughout the country there were a number of suicides among young women, following each other in rapid succession, and the telegraphic despatches invariably said: "That Miss——, having read with much interest an account of the suicide of Miss——, shot herself" or took her life in some other manner. As a strange coincidence they always used the same methods and went about the act in the same way as was suggested to them after reading the sensational accounts. This occurred in a circle of refined, educated women where no cause other than ill-health could be assigned, and it is logical to presume that if these women could have been guarded against these suggestions while mentally irresponsible they would have scorned such an idea after regaining their normal condition of health and such immunity as a healthy mind enjoys against such unhealthful imagery and its results. I give this only as an illustration of one of the many manias due to autohypnotism from suggestions arising from publicity of criminal "news."

In the therapy of all mental disease we recognize as the first and most important step, the general tonic and rest treatment, to bring physical conditions back to normal; and in addition it is desirable that the patient has a change of scene and occupation with mental rest. This is done with but one object in view, *viz.*, to eliminate the predominant thought or idea which is constantly suggesting itself to the patient—if it be suicidal mania, the idea of self-destruction, if it be hysteric, that he has some disease, and so on. Of course, we recognize the fact that the ideal treatment of all diseases is to remove the cause; but, unfortunately, the exciting cause here is known to be suggestion from without, and I maintain that the most potent cause is publicity given to the cases of these unfortunates in the daily press and also in problematic and suggestive books, cheap editions of which flood the country. Alcohol and narcotic poisons are responsible in a small way.

The first causes mentioned, which could be so easily remedied, we must endure for fear of infringing upon the liberty of a few persons and sensational journals. While the laws give us a right to fight bodily contagion and go to any limit in restriction of personal liberties when quarantining against contagious diseases, yet when an epidemic arises which threatens the morals of the nation and we offer any remedy which means death to the crime-producing "micro-organisms," a lot of selfish politicians and blood-thirsty journals arise and say "its unconstitutional."

In addition to the usual treatment of mental derangements which are purely functional, it has occurred to me that instead of accentuating the dull, morbid condition by the administration of large doses of depressing drugs, it is more desirable to give some form of mental gymnastics that will counteract as much as possible the dominant idea which in itself is the disease. This is of two-fold value; it destroys the automaticity and constancy of the predominating thought and produces a mental tire that is most conducive to natural sleep. For example: Suppose you have a patient who is bent upon self-destruction. Of course, as a matter of precaution, the patient is constantly watched. Here you can convey to this patient's brain a contrary idea by and through any of his special senses. In such a case I would take advantage of two senses, sight and hearing. Give for an exercise the word "life," which is to be repeated aloud a certain number of times during the day and can also be used as a written exercise. If the patient refuses to either speak or write, have the attendant speak aloud the word at intervals, and the same word should be displayed conspicuously about the room. Certain sentences can be substituted if desired. The object in this treatment is to start another line of thought, and the constant suggestion of this word to the mind will act as a stimulus. This will probably at first impress the patient as being absurd and ridiculous, then interest him and arouse his curiosity, and finally suggest to him that somebody is crazy and he will naturally infer that it is himself, and when you get a crazy man to realize that he is crazy you have made the first advance toward his cure. In selecting words or sentences, be careful to select such as will naturally cross and oppose the diseased idea.

I am compelled to offer this merely as a suggestion in treatment, not yet having tested its efficiency, and I trust some neurologist is in a position to give it a trial and make his experience known. As a proof of the value of this treatment we can all recall that in our experience we have had patients tell us, and especially hysteric patients, that when they have an almost insane desire to commit some folly, thoughts come to them which are entirely foreign to the act, and thus it seems that the cycle of thought which is constantly passing through the mind gives it some immunity from rash acts. Again we see the value of distraction of thought by suggestion, in the mother and the child, when the child pleads for something which the mother knows is not good for it. A wise mother does not oppose, but quickly changes its thought to another subject by suggesting something foreign to its present wants.

A REVIEW OF DR. SEGUIN'S CONTRIBUTIONS TO MEDICINE.[1]

By B. SACHS, M.D.,
OF NEW YORK;
PROFESSOR OF NERVOUS AND MENTAL DISEASES IN THE NEW YORK POLYCLINIC.

DEATH has removed from our ranks a man whose life was one of many trials, sweetened only by the satisfaction to be derived from serious professional labor. A review of Seguin's contributions to medicine furnishes some solace to those who, in the midst of a busy life and with that pessimism inherent in all of us, stop to ask, What profits it to toil incessantly merely to add a few stones to a building which others would or might build as well? It profits little indeed, unless one is fortunate enough to add so materially to the structure that its foundations become firmer and more enduring. The practice of medicine, and particularly of neurology, owes much to Seguin. Some of his suggestions have been so generally adopted that the majority of those following them do not remember or do not know that it was he who originated them.

Edward Constant Seguin was born in Paris in 1843. At the age of five years he was brought to this country by his father, Dr. Edouard Seguin, whose valuable and beneficent work on behalf of the idiotic and feeble-minded is well known on two continents. The early, and indeed the whole education of the younger Seguin was irregular until he entered the College of Physicians and Surgeons, from which he was graduated in 1864, then only nineteen years of age. Two years before his graduation he was appointed a medical cadet in the regular army, so that his medical training, too, was not of the ordinary routine character. The experiences gained in those stirring times made amends for deficient class-room instruction, and Seguin belonged to that fortunate class of men whose services in the Civil War gave them a particular distinction. It left them, moreover, with an increased love for their country and also a warm sympathy for those who had served in the same cause. I can testify to the fact, from personal knowledge, that however busy Seguin was in later years he was always and particularly willing to help any poor fellow who was suffering from wounds received during the late war.

Shortly after graduation he served as Acting Assistant Surgeon at Little Rock, Arkansas. In the spring of 1865 he was appointed Assistant Surgeon United States Volunteers. In this early period of his life he was hampered by ill-health, suffering from incipient tuberculosis, and on this account had himself transferred to New Mexico, where he acted as post-surgeon. On his return to New York (1869) he came again under the influence of Dr. Draper, under whose guidance, at the New York Hospital, he had done his first medical work. In 1866 he published a short paper on "The Use of the Thermometer in Clinical Medicine," in which he submitted the thermometric records of three cases of pneumonia, calling "attention to a means of diagnosis and prognosis not second in importance to any single one hitherto employed," and gave the first chart of vital signs published in this country. As though the method needed further endorsement, he stated that "Wunderlich and others make constant use of the thermometer in private practice." Seguin recognized at that early day that temperature observations were especially valuable, because "surface heat cannot be immediately affected by causes acting through the senses, which so disturb other subjective signs; for instance, the sudden arrival of a physician, of a friend, of news, etc." In 1867 he published two

[1] Read at a meeting of the Manhattan Medical Society, March 18, 1898.

other short papers—most of his papers have the great virtue of brevity—on subcutaneous injections of quinin in malarial neuralgia and in the treatment of malarial fevers. This special form of treatment was suggested by Draper. The entire method of hypodermatic injection was new at the time, and we must realize this to understand why it should have been necessary for him to state that the slight hemorrhage following the operation—that is, the injection—can easily be controlled by finger pressure. It is historically interesting to record the explanation given of abscesses following these injections of quinin "In each instance the result was attributable to the introduction of insoluble particles along with the fluid." In another place he insists upon the importance of keeping the needle clean. The difference between then and now is also accentuated by the reason which Seguin gave for the hypodermatic use of quinin, the first being "when economy is a desideratum."

Seguin's war training and his hospital experience were well calculated to prevent his becoming a mere specialist. As the son of the elder Seguin, it was natural for him to be interested in the study of mental and nervous diseases; but unlike some of our latter-day general clinicians, he felt that special knowledge does not come by intuition, but only after careful special study. In 1869 he went to Paris, where he became a student of Brown-Séquard, Charcot, and Ranvier, the master minds of the day. Neurology was still in its infancy. The question of cerebral localization, which is now well advanced toward a happy and final settlement, was in the air; it had been suggested by the teachings and investigations of Hughlings Jackson; by the long controversy over Broca's contention that the left third frontal convolution was the speech center; but the famous experiments of Fritsch and Hitzig had not yet been published. It was nine years before the appearance of Nothnagel's topical diagnosis. At that time the French school, under Charcot, was making wonderful strides in advancing the knowledge of the various forms of spinal disease and in the recognition of functional nervous diseases, but it was before the days of the modern German school, before the publication of Leyden's great work on spinal-cord diseases, and before the recognition of the reaction of degeneration. It was Seguin's good fortune to start in upon his life's work at a time when neurology presented innumerable problems, as every science does in its formative period.

He returned to America at a time when only two other men were prominent in the specialty: Weir Mitchell and Hammond—both excellent observers, and both men of exceptional intellect. Under the influence of Charcot and Ranvier, Seguin made every effort to promote the study of the morbid anatomy in spinal and cerebral diseases. In 1871 he recorded an autopsy on a case of mania—a disease on which further light is needed at the present day; also, an examination of the cervical sympathetic nerve in the case of unilateral sweating of the head, in which the finding was not conclusive. In 1878 Seguin reported upon the findings in a case of disseminated cerebrospinal sclerosis—one of the few autopsies of this disease recorded in this country. In this instance the spinal cord only was examined.

The duties of an active professional life prevented the continuance of work that must be done day after day in a laboratory. In this Seguin shared the fate of so many others in this country who deplore the lack of willing assistants. In Seguin's case we need not regret this particular defect, for he was thus compelled to turn his efforts to purely clinical studies, and, above all, to therapeutics, in which he stands preeminent. A mere enumeration of his clinical studies would take up more time than is at my disposal; but I will call attention to a few.

His first article on the aphasia question was not only a fine review of the arguments for and against Broca's theories, but contained a large number (50) of valuable histories bearing upon the subject. His discussions of anterior poliomyelitis helped to promote the understanding of this important disease of childhood. His lectures on cortical localization, delivered at the College of Physicians and Surgeons, were masterly expositions of the subject, characterized by extraordinary terseness of style and by a thorough understanding of the points upon which accurate information was needed. These lectures were delivered, in great part, before Nothnagel's work appeared, and must be recorded as contributions of vital importance to a subject which was then much in doubt. It will be unnecessary to review all of Seguin's papers in which the subject of cortical localization was treated. It is sufficient to say of one and all of them that they were prepared with the greatest care; that the histories were taken with a minuteness characteristic of Seguin's work, and that pathologic findings were recorded in such a way as to make them thoroughly serviceable. In the history of this important question of modern neurology Seguin's name must be classed with that of Nothnagel, Charcot, Pitres, and other clinicians of like fame. His most notable clinical contribution, however, was the recognition, in advance of Erb and of Charcot, of the condition of spastic spinal paralysis, to which he gave the very unfortunate name of "tetenoid paraplegia." The importance of this clinical discovery may be gaged by the fact that spastic spinal paralysis has led to the study and to the recognition of many different forms of diseases of the central nervous system, and has been more hotly discussed than, perhaps, any other clinical type. It is well to insist upon Seguin's merits in this controversy, for European writers have done him scant justice.

There are other valuable papers on cervical paraplegia, on cerebral syphilis, on optic neuritis with myelitis, each containing careful clinical observations. I hasten to pass from these to his contributions to the therapeutics of nervous diseases; for I believe that in the history of neurology Seguin's fame will rest largely upon his efforts in the treatment of a class of diseases which the general practitioner has always considered thoroughly unpromising. But let any one who is skeptical as to what can possibly be done for functional, and particularly for organic diseases of the nervous system, read over these various papers of Seguin, and he will acknowledge that neurologists may achieve victories in the treatment as well as in the diagnosis of the affections.

While the subject of this brief review had an unusual faith in drugs, he was by no means obtuse to other methods of treatment. The surgical furor seized him in his earlier years, as it has so many others. As long ago as 1873 he proposed the "excision of the cords which go to form the brachial plexus in "a case of traumatic brachial neuralgia." The history of this patient is given in masterly detail, and the case itself seemed to have interested the surgical lights of the day. The operation was carried out according to Seguin's idea, and though it failed of its purpose, I refer to it to show that Abbe's intraspinal section of the posterior roots for the relief of neuralgic pain performed a few years ago was carried out on the lines underlying Seguin's plan in this case. Unfortunately, Abbe's more radical operation was not more successful.

A lecture, still of great value, was delivered at the College of Physicians and Surgeons in 1874, on "General Therapeutics of the Nervous System." The author showed therein that he had not only unbounded faith in medicinal agents, but that he advocated the administration of drugs to their physiologic limits. In the lecture just referred to he advocates the free use of quinin as a spinal excitant, and the frequent use of the drug as a tonic in late years is to be attributed to Seguin's recommendation. The same is true of phosphorus, which he considered the restorative *par excellence* in diseases of the nervous system. Quinin is also considered as a cerebral excitant—a claim that might be substantiated; but one is apt to be a little skeptical as to the validity of his proof when it is merely stated that "Dr. Draper has given small doses of the medicine to two well-known clergymen, with the result of restoring their power of extemporaneous speaking." His suggestion regarding conium and the bromids have been followed by thousands, and were so thoroughly rational that they were adopted by many without hesitation. It is worth noting that in Seguin's opinion the bromids were not contraindicated in anemia. He insisted upon the absence of the palate reflex as a test of the drug, but I am not able to state positively whether or not this test originated with him.

Counter-irritation was warmly advocated, with special reference to the blister and actual-cautery. He believed that "counter-irritants almost always act through the spinal cord, and their mode of action is exemplified by a morbid process that takes place as a consequence of severe burns." Patients are endangered by visceral complications which occur in parts bearing a definite relation to the burn. "Brown-Séquard demonstrated that by cutting across the spinal cord above the region of the nerves going to the burned part no visceral lesions occurred, thus proving that these lesions were set up by a morbid state of the spinal cord, produced by the burn. The burn corresponds to our counter-irritation." This explanation may hold good for deep blistering, but for superficial irritation, caused by the actual-cautery, it is insufficient, and Seguin protested against any but superficial cauterization. Surface irritation must act upon the superficial nerve filaments. For my own part, I believe that the effect of counter-irritation has been much over-rated, in the treatment of spinal affections at least. It is often palliative, rarely curative.

In electricity, Seguin said that he had the greatest faith, within certain limits, in the power of faradism and galvanism as remedial agents, and to this faith I know he adhered in later years.

Excellent service was rendered the medical profession by the publication in 1877 of an article on "The Abuse and Use of the Bromids." If I had my way about it, this essay should be reprinted and redistributed at least once a year; for the bromids are still used altogether too frequently. Neurologists have limited the administration of these drugs to the cases in which depressant action is desired, but, I fear many medical men still use the bromids for the treatment of any and all nervous symptoms. It would be difficult to estimate the number of neurasthenics made worse annually by the use of bromids. It was Seguin's just dictum "that epilepsy is the only disease in the cure of which we are justified in deliberately producing bromism." His formula, combining bromid and chloral, is still in favor in this city.

His confidence in drugs was evidenced once more in his endorsement of cannabis indica for migraine. The recommendation was originally made, however, by Dr. Richard Green, an English physician. The drug was to be given for the cure of the disease, and not merely of the attack. It is to be employed during a long period, in doses of 1/3 to 1/2 grain of the alcoholic extract. "It should be given," said Seguin, "just as faithfully and regularly as bromids are in epilepsy." Though he extolled the treatment, it has not been universally adopted; and I take it, the chief reason for this was the difficulty of obtaining thoroughly satisfactory preparations; for any one who has seen cases of cannabis indica poisoning will be, as I have become, a little chary in the use of the drug.

Seguin's most signal achievement in the therapeutic line was his energetic advocacy of the use of the iodids in large doses, and his explanations regarding the proper mode of administration. The so-called "American method" is practically Seguin's own. It is to him that we owe the suggestion that the iodids should be given not in small quantities of 15 and 20 grains three times a day—the method which obtains almost universally in Europe—but, if the drug is to have any distinct effect, it must be given in quantities varying between 50, 100, or even 150 grains three times daily. It was Seguin who advised giving the iodids in alkaline waters, and in administering them before meals on an empty stomach, so that they could be rapidly absorbed without producing any gastric irritation. Doubts have arisen as to the rationality of this method; for it is claimed that the system cannot possibly absorb the amount of the drug thus administered. However, the fact remains that in many cases of cerebral and spinal disease in which there was no improvement when smaller doses were given, improvement quickly occurred under the use of larger doses. The good effects, moreover, were noticeable not only in specific disease, but in many forms of exudation and in some of the chronic disorders of the nervous system.

Without wearying the reader with further details, let me call to mind the fact that the use of aconitia in neuralgia has become general as a result of Seguin's writings, that the effect of hyoscyamia has been better understood, and that the treatment of chorea by large doses of arsenic is also to be attributed to the influence of Seguin's numerous papers on the subject. In the latter recommendation I believe he erred, and those of us who resort to other measures feel that a vast majority of cases of chorea can be cured without resorting to poisonous doses of a drug whose effect is apt to be lasting and injurious.

These numerous and important clinical and therapeutic contributions were put forth during a brief period of twelve years, until his services to medicine were suddenly arrested by the sad domestic tragedy of 1882. Believing, as he stated, that an unlimited interruption had taken place in his professional life, he had his various publications edited by Amidon, and published in book form, under the title of "Opera Minora," in 1884. I can well recall some of the remarks made by prominent medical men of the day, who thought it presumption on the part of any man to put minor contributions, as they were modestly called, in book form before the public. But as every man is entitled to have a just appreciation of his own work, I find it natural that Seguin felt within himself that much of what he had done would be of lasting benefit to medical science, and should be made a matter of careful record.

In later years, and after his return from his sojourn in Europe, Seguin, as you know, took up active practice and did considerable literary work; but nothing done at that time eclipsed the value of his former writings, although his article on Hemianopsia, in which the importance of the cuneus was established, his contributions to Pepper's and Keating's systems of medicine, and, above all, the last lectures which he delivered before the Medical Society of the University of Toronto in the spring of 1890, "On Some Points in the Treatment and Management of Neurosis," were characterized by unusual vigor of thought, by simplicity and clearness of expression, which all would do well to emulate, and by the ripened experience and reflection of maturer years.

Imperfect justice would be done Seguin if we did not make brief reference to his efforts on behalf of general medicine. As editor of *The Archives of Medicine*, which were too good to be long-lived, and in the creation of an "American Series of Clinical Lectures," the editor showed his wide medical sympathics and his desire to pass beyond the limits of any specialty, however broad. Add to these literary achievements, though they include a few failures, the good work that was done by him as a teacher of students and as the chief of his clinic, and you can well understand why his influence on the medical men of the present day and on the younger school of neurology has been so powerful.

It is greatly to Seguin's credit that he steered midway between the therapeutic nihilism of the German school and the extravagant claims made for various therapeutic measures by unthinking medical men in this and other countries. Hypnotism and metallotherapy interested him, but he was not led astray by them. It seemed only with reference to the relation of the ocular muscles to functional neuroses, that his former calm judgment forsook him. His acquaintance with German literature prevented his becoming an abject follower of the French, and he was too cosmopolitan in his views to be a disciple of any one school. He may truly be said to have been a leader of neurologic thought. Since 1890, little work emanated from his pen, but he still continued in active practice until 1894, when the first symptoms of his last painful illness appeared, which led to his death on February 19, 1898. It is entirely fit that we should do homage to a man who, in spite of some shortcomings, was an unusually capable worker in the field of medicine, and whose professional skill was of the highest order.

CLINICAL LECTURE.

DIET FOR CONSUMPTIVES.

BY REYNOLD W. WILCOX, M.D.,
OF NEW YORK;
PROFESSOR OF MEDICINE AND THERAPEUTICS IN THE NEW YORK POST-GRADUATE MEDICAL SCHOOL AND HOSPITAL.

GENTLEMEN:—You have just had an opportunity of examining a number of cases of pulmonary tuberculosis. If I were asked, in patients of this particular class, what was the most important thing to be done, I would say, "feed them." It is more important than climate. Feeding stands in the first place, but it presents more difficulties than perhaps any other phase of the treatment. You may talk as much as you wish about tuberculosis being an infectious disease; there is no doubt that any system of treatment which deals with tuberculosis as an infection and which ignores the patient, is going to fail. That has been the fault with the laboratory men, but it is a fault which they are fast correcting. The findings of the laboratory deal with the condition of the disease; we, as physicians, cannot afford to ignore the patient. Without going into the question of pulmonary antiseptics; without going into the questions in relation to the value of particular drugs in their direct action on the results of the activity of the tubercle bacilli, or upon the elimination of ptomains, we shall consider the question of prime importance, *i. e.*, the feeding of the patient.

Two years ago, a reporter from one of our disgraceful daily papers came to me and said: "Last Sunday we published an estimation of the number of bacteria that were in the different bacteriological laboratories of the city, and spoke of the great danger that would accrue to the city if the cholera bacilli were emptied into the reservoir, and the tubercle bacilli were spread in the street cars, and of the serious results that would occur if all these pathogenic bacteria in the various laboratories were put where they could attack human beings. We want in next Sunday's issue to publish statements from clinicians and physicians as to what would happen if this thing should take place." Replying categorically to the question as to what would happen, I said: "Nothing at all." You can sow all the wheat and corn and rye you like in the alkali desert of Arizona, and they will not grow because there is not the proper soil there for them. In the same way, you can sow all the tubercle bacilli you like in the lungs, and they will not grow unless there is a proper soil for them. If infection has occurred, you can discourage its progress by rendering the soil unfit for the growth of the bacilli.

A well-known physician who has, as his fad, a farm, told me that he had been having a great deal of trouble with some fine peach trees because they had been attacked with the "yellows"—a parasitic disease. He had applied all sorts of antiparasitic remedies to the trees, but they still had the "yellows." On general principles, I thought if he would dig around his trees and put in some fertilizer, he might see the "yellows" disappear. He did this, and the disease disappeared without any further use of the antiparasitic remedies, and he had an abundant crop of peaches the next fall. This is a homely illustration of what may occur in tuberculosis patients.

There are two old proverbs about the question of feeding. The first is this: "A patient who has but little appetite needs to be very carefully fed." The second is an old French proverb which, when translated, reads: "Appetite comes on eating." A great many patients will say that they cannot eat, yet if you encourage them to start, before they get through the meal they will have a very respectable appetite. Of all the systems that have been advanced for feeding tuberculous patients, any system which departs markedly from the proper proportion of proteids, carbohydrates and fats is not a wise one. The raw-beef and hot-water treatment has been applied to tuberculous patients in this city for many years. I have seen them before they went under this treatment, and I have seen them—or rather what has been left of them—after they have been through it. The treatment fails in a large proportion of cases because the amount of albuminous material is so great that it overtaxes the individual in its elimination. There is, however, a mode of treatment, with which I had a good deal of personal experience some years ago, and which I occasionally employ at the present time.

In 1882, when I was studying in Paris under Dujardin-Beaumetz, we tried the Debove method of treatment by overfeeding. We had under observation between fifty and sixty patients suffering from tuberculosis. We took lean meat, removed all the gristle and tendon and a good deal of the fat. It was then chopped finely and dried in an oven at a temperature of 150° until it was absolutely dry. When this had occurred, the temperature was raised a little, say to between 165° and 180°—pasteurized, if you will. When this meat had been made absolutely dry, which took a number of hours, it was ground up in a mortar and sifted. Six pounds of raw beef treated in that way would bring us about one pound of beef-powder. Then we would pass the stomach-tube into the patient and wash out the stomach. Beginning with three-quarters of a pound of the beef-powder, which represents about six times that amount of beef, we added three times as much milk. This was left in the stomach. At first, this meal was given twice a day, and the amount was increased until the patient took from one to one and a half pounds of beef-powder and four or five pints of milk in a day. If there was trouble in digesting this, we started out without the milk, and added a little diluted hydrochloric acid to the meat. We used to take apparently hopeless cases of laryngeal and pulmonary tuberculosis and feed them in that way, and they would gain flesh and the tuberculosis would remain stationary, on the other hand, it required a very active watchfulness on the part of the physician to prevent the disagreeable consequences of over-feeding. We had to consider the digestive powers of the individual, the occurrence of intestinal decomposition and the curdling of the milk.

In my practice at the present time, I reserve this Debove method solely for one class of patients, *i. e.*, those who suffer from tuberculous laryngitis, where every act of swallowing and of coughing is painful. By applying a small amount of cocain to the larynx the tube can be passed without pain, and enough of the prepared food can be put in the stomach to nourish the patient for twenty-four hours. In this way you will save a great deal of discomfort. This is the only class of cases in which I use this method of feeding at the present time. It has one advantage, and that is of inestimable value in certain cases. It is a curious fact, but where a patient suffers so much from tuberculous laryngitis that vomiting is an exceedingly distressing symptom, it is extremely rare that the patients vomit when the food is introduced with a stomach-tube. Why they should not vomit when the material is given through the stomach-tube and yet vomit when it is taken by the mouth in the ordinary way, I cannot say, but the observation is founded on large clinical experience. On the other hand, the care required in carrying on this treatment, and the disadvantages mentioned make me reserve it for the class of cases referred to.

The true diet of a patient suffering from pulmonary tuberculosis I believe should consist of meats, starches, and fats, with an excess of the last, and a certain amount of phosphates. There are several things to be considered. According to the English writers, patients who suffer from a slight infiltration at the right apex suffer frequently from vomiting, which apparently occurs without cause; hence, the majority of these patients are treated as dyspeptics. I have seen a number of those patients, and have always succeeded in demonstrating that there were physical signs at the right apex which warranted the belief that we were dealing with an interstitial pulmonary tuberculosis. Competent clinicians, however, tell me that there are patients in whom no physical signs can be demonstrated, and yet who suffer from this form of vomiting, which the English call "the pre-tuberculous vomiting," and they are of the opinion that the gastric irritability antedates the tuberculous infection. I believe they are wrong, but I am open to conviction. Why it should occur with consolidation at the right apex rather than at the left, I do not know, but the fact remains. These cases are often treated up to the time of the formation of cavities without a proper realization of the true condition.

We now have stomach specialists and I presume that we shall have scrotum specialists some day, and I see no reason why not—they are both "bags." The really important digestive processes take place in the intestine and, according to Carteret, in a statement published in 1870, and which I believe is as true now as then, in seventy per cent. of all patients suffering from digestive disturbance, the trouble is due to faulty digestion of the starches. This means that the difficulty is connected with the mouth and the small intestine, and not with the stomach, to any great extent. We see, therefore, why attention to a particular organ is very apt to mislead.

Again Schlatter's recent operation shows that the stomach can be excised and the patient gain weight and get along very well. His patient has been alive since the first of last October. A dog from whom the stomach was removed in Heidelberg, lived for five months, and never found out that he had no stomach. If he had been more intelligent, and had known that his stomach was gone, the chances are that he would have pined away, or consulted a stomach specialist.

I have been in the habit for a number of years of using food for a purpose which is not originally contemplated in the treatment of pulmonary tuberculosis. A great many patients awaken in the morning bathed in a cold, and clammy perspiration. If you go to the health resorts and sit at table with a colony of one-lunged people, the first question that they ask one another is, not regarding how much they coughed through the night, but "how about the sweating last night?" Nothing discourages an old tuberculous patient so much as to find that he is bathed in this cold, clammy perspiration. This can be done away with in a large proportion of cases. If you will awaken the patient at about four o'clock in the morning sufficiently to take a glass of warm milk, with a little alcohol in it, the sweating will be greatly reduced, and it will not have the same demoralizing effect upon him. In this way you get a little extra food into the patient, and at the same time prevent the prostration which is associated with this sweating.

The secret of feeding tuberculous patients is to give them light and nutritious food and food which is easily digestible, feeding them "early and often." I have been in the habit of separating the meals into those containing the bulk of the starchy food and meals containing the bulk of the proteids. I have always been in the habit of giving the patient three hours, or three hours and a half in which to digest the heavier meals, so as to be sure that the stomach is fairly emptied before the next consignment of food goes into it.

About seven o'clock in the morning the patient's day begins; and I give them first a glass of warm milk (not hot), and I put into this a tablespoonful of strong coffee, made according to the French method. Or, if the patient is exhausted from a bad night, I give instead of the coffee, a dessertspoonful of rum or other spirit. But you should first mix it with a little water, because if you place a spirit containing forty or fifty per cent. of alcohol directly into milk, it will cause a certain amount of coagulation, and render the milk more or less indigestible. It is, therefore, important to mix the rum with two tablespoonfuls of water before adding it to the milk.

In my medical student days in Boston, we were accustomed to go to hear that great theological acrobat, Reverend Joseph Cook, who used to deliver a talk on Mondays. In this audience there was always a large collection of short-haired women and long-haired men. One day, he came into Tremont Temple with an egg in one hand, a glass in the other, and a bottle sticking out of his pocket—in fact, he looked quite sociable. He proceeded to put the white of the egg into the tumbler, and to pour his absolute alcohol into the egg albumin. Of course, the albumin was coagulated. According to him, the albumin represented the brain of a drunkard. Without wasting time to go into all the details, I may say that he ended up by getting complete coagulation of the albumin in his tumbler, and then he announced that that was the stage when a sot beat his wife, turned her into the street, lay in the street himself, dead drunk, and later became a public charge. It was very dramatic and very interesting, and had just enough of truth in it to make it a first-rate lie.

It is true, however, that alcohol when insufficiently diluted does render albumin a little insoluble and a little more difficult to digest, but, as a rule, the stimulating effect of the alcohol outweighs that disadvantage. It is well enough to remember the practical point and forget all about the Rev. Joseph Cook, who is not a scientific authority.

Next, we come to the breakfast that is taken at about nine o'clock. The patient should have eggs, cooked in any way except fried. If the patient insists upon having them fried, fry them according to the Italian way, *i.e.* in olive oil. They are then much less indigestible than when fried in pig refuse, called lard. Butter is all right, but the melting temperature of butter being a good deal higher than that of olive oil, some of the fatty acids in the butter may be decomposed. However, butter is vastly better than lard. They may also be allowed some bread, and sometimes they like marmalade, as it is grateful to their parched mouths. Finnan haddie, tuberculous patients like pretty well, when it is cured by smoking and without salt, and although not the correct thing theoretically, it seems to agree with them. Toasted bread may also be given, or good rolls, but the latter must not be hot. Bread and butter, milk and coffee may be used for variety.

About eleven o'clock the patient has the second breakfast, which usually consist of a little cocoa from which the fat has been taken out. Cocoa butter is about the most indigestible fat there is, therefore it should be removed, or else predigested. The patient may also have coffee, a little bread, a little soup or a little beef-extract. An egg-nog is permissible, and kumyss or matzoon is often acceptable.

The dinner should be served about one o'clock in the afternoon, and should be *the* meal of the day. The patients may have any kind of meat they relish, except salted meat, but it must not be fried. Potatoes, fresh vegetables, fruits, and puddings may also be allowed. Coffee, tea, or possibly a bottle of light beer can be added.

About four o'clock in the afternoon they should have a little meat extract with toasted bread, and about five o'clock, a little more should be given. About seven o'clock in the evening comes supper, consisting chiefly of farinaceous food. Many of these patients like what is known in New England as "hasty pudding." It is made by putting corn-meal into a kettle with water, and stirring it while it is boiling, seasoning to suit the taste. Various jellies, beef-extracts, and gruels are useful at this time. If the patient is awake at eleven, a cup of milk or hot soup or gruel may act as a hypnotic.

In patients who are hectic I think alcohol should stop with dinner at one o'clock, because I am pretty sure from clinical observation that alcohol adds to the hectic. The alcohol should be in moderate amount, and well diluted. The only alcohol I allow in the afternoon is light beer or possibly stout at bed-time. The various degenerations which follow the inordinate use of alcohol must be avoided.

How are the starchy foods and sugars digested? If you take a seed that has been dried many years, and put it in water, it begins to sprout, but it does not do this until the diastase begins to act and digest the starches therein contained, producing maltose. I have been in the habit of giving my starchy foods, for it is upon these that we must depend to improve nutrition, with as little liquid as possible, and increasing their digestibility by malt extracts which really contain diastase, and also are nutritive.

I have spent about fifteen years in investigating this subject. All *liquid* malt extracts are utterly useless for the transformation of starch into dextrin and maltose, because they contain alcohol which inhibits the effect of the starch, and because they contain acids, generated in the process of fermentation, which also inhibit the action of the diastase. The semi-solid extracts of malt convert starch into sugar. This conversion commences to take place in the mouth. For the first thirty or forty minutes after food has been taken into the stomach, this process goes on. It later stops, but recommences in the duodenum and continues until all the starches are converted into dextrin, and finally into maltose. That this conversion continues in the stomach has been proven conclusively by Kellogg. The great disadvantage of most of the active preparations of malt is their viscosity, which renders them, after a little time, objects of disgust. I have objected to this year after year, and finally I have gotten some one to listen to me. It is now possible to obtain a preparation of malt which, as Professor Tucker of Albany assures us, contains from four to five per cent. diastasic converting power. With such a preparation as maltzyme I can assure my patients that the starches will be digested. The starches are for nourishment, for the generation of heat, and for the formation of fat. This is just what you want for a tuberculous patient. Further than this recent investigations tend to show that the sugars are important in the generation of force. That is to say: Under a constant diet more than a proportionately larger amount of energy is developed if sugar be added to the dietary.

This covers, I am sure, the important facts which you should keep in mind and in this way you can do your whole duty, not only in treating the disease, but what is more important, in treating the patient.

HOSPITAL REPORT.

OBSERVATIONS CONCERNING THE WIDAL TEST.

By ALBERT E. BLACKBURN, M.D.,
OF PHILADELPHIA.

THE following data, concerning the value of the Widal test in typhoid fever, were obtained from the medical wards of the Presbyterian Hospital in Philadelphia during my term as resident physician; *viz.*, May to October, inclusive, 1897.

The blood in all cases of suspected typhoid fever and in all cases in which the diagnosis was in the least obscure was subjected to this test until all doubt was removed. The specimen of blood was taken immediately on admission of the patients to the hospital, the object being to find the first day of the disease on which the test was positive. My list includes eighty cases of enteric fever as established by the clinical course, in all of which the test was positive, except in two, as shown by the table.

CASE XVII.—Female, white, 25 years of age, was admitted on the fifteenth day of the disease, had been a case of walking-typhoid. The prodromal history and the course of the case were complete. The symptoms on admission were typical of that stage of the disease. The patient died two days later of concealed hemorrhage. The test was negative as shown by the table. Post-mortem examination confirmed the diagnosis of hemorrhage, and numerous ulcers were found in the lower ileum.

CASE LXIV.—Female, white, age 5 years. The disease in this case ran a mild course with prolonged convalescence and ultimate recovery. As in the previous case the test was negative.

The following cases were proven not to be typhoid by the clinical course, the test being negative two or more times, except in one case to be noted:

Catarrhal fever 25 cases; uremia 6 cases; malaria 2 cases; pulmonary tuberculosis 2 cases; endocarditis 2 cases; peritonitis 2 cases; syphilitic pregnancy 1 case; Rheumatoid arthritis 1 case.

One case, in a female aged 20 years, admitted with fair prodromal history to typhoid, ended abruptly on the fifteenth day with the opening of an ischiorectal abscess. In this case catarrhal fever was diagnosed from symptoms present. The test was as follows: Seventh and ninth days negative; eleventh and thirteenth doubtful; fourteenth positive.

In one case of catarrhal fever the test was as follows: —Seventh and ninth days, negative; eleventh and thirteenth days, doubtful; fourteenth day, positive.

The following cases are worthy of note:—In one case of uremia on two occasions there were positive reactions, and the history showed that this patient had had typhoid five years before. In one case of catarrhal fever there was a positive reaction, typhoid three years before.

The following conclusions are drawn from these cases:

1. It is a good corroborative test.
2. In doubtful cases, early in the disease, it does not assist in diagnosis.
3. In severe cases the test is positive early.

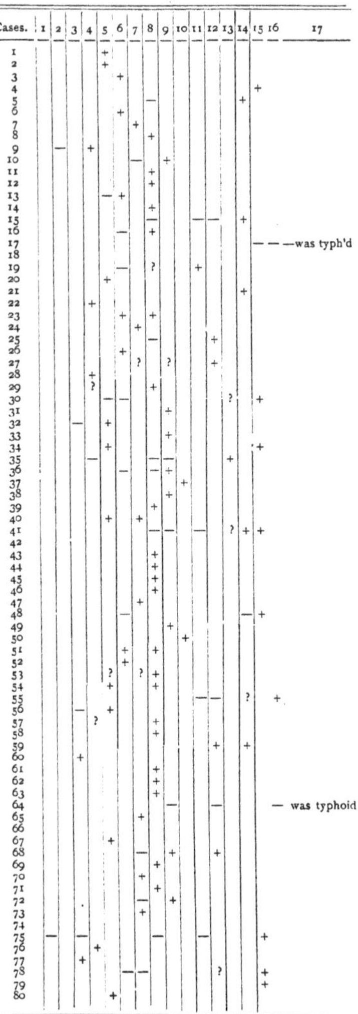

TABLE I.

Showing days on which tests were made; (+) indicates positive reaction; (—) negative, and (?) doubtful.

Day of Disease.

Cases.	1	2	3	4	5	6	7	8	9	10	11	12	13	14	15	16	17
1					+												
2					+												
3						+											
4															+		
5								—						+			
6						+											
7							+										
8								+									
9		—		+													
10							—		+								
11								+									
12								+									
13					—	+											
14								+									
15								—			—	—		+			
16						—		+									
17															—	—	—was typh'd
18																	
19						—		?			+						
20					+												
21														+			
22				+													
23						+		+									
24							+										
25								—				+					
26						+											
27							?		?			+					
28				+													
29				?				+									
30					—	—							?		+		
31									+								
32			—		+												
33									+								
34					+										+		
35				—				—	—				+				
36						—		—	+								
37										+							
38									+								
39								+									
40					+		+										
41								—	—		—		?	+	+		
42																	
43								+									
44								+									
45								+									
46								+									
47							+										
48						—								—	+		
49									+								
50										+							
51						+		+									
52						+											
53					?		?	+									
54					+			+									
55											—	—		?		+	
56			—		+												
57				?				+									
58								+									
59												+		+			
60			+														
61								+									
62								+									
63								+									
64									—			—				— was typhoid	
65							+										
66																	
67					+												
68							—		+			+					
69								+									
70							+										
71								+									
72							—		+								
73							+										
74																	
75	—		—					—			—				+		
76				+													
77			+														
78						—	—					?			+		
79															+		
80					+												

Totals.																	
+	0	0	2	4	10	7	7	22	8	2	1	4	1	5	8	1	0
—	1	1	3	1	2	6	4	7	3	0	4	3	0	1	1	2	1
?	0	0	0	2	1	0	2	1	1	0	0	1	2	1	0	0	0

4. In a few typical cases the test appeared to be negative.

WAR ARTICLES.

MEDICAL ORGANIZATION OF THE CAMP AT TAMPA, FLORIDA.

BY HENRY I. RAYMOND, M.D.,
CAPTAIN AND ASSISTANT SURGEON UNITED STATES ARMY.

THE past week has witnessed a mobilization of seven regiments of the United States Infantry—the 4th, 5th, 6th, 9th, 13th, 17th, and 21st—from the States of New York, Illinois, Ohio, Kentucky, and Georgia, over the distance, for the regiments most remote, of about 1500 miles, to rendezvous at this point and organize into one large body for future contingencies.

Our division numbers at present about 3500 souls, soon to be increased to more than double that number by virtue of the Army Re-organization Bill, whose passage by Congress informs our minds and cheers our anxious hearts.

Each regiment from its respective post was accompanied *en route* by one medical officer and the proper quota of hospital-corps men with a complete outfit for a field hospital. This latter consists of (1) one medical and one surgical chest, a list of the contents of which is stamped on the morocco pad which is carried, reversed, under the cover of its chest. This list reveals a medical and surgical armamentarium in so compact and easily accessible form, and of so unquestionable utility that these chests are regarded by the medical officer in the field as his big guns in his citadel of defence against disease and injury. The chests are made of hard wood with all edges brass-bound and with arrangements for strapping them, one on either side of a pack-saddle on the back of a mule, and the lid and front leaf are so adapted that access can be had to the contents in transit, without deranging the packs. Where roadways permit the use of a wheeled vehicle these chests are habitually carried under the seats of the ambulance. Their combined weight is about 300 pounds. I have particularized these chests for the reason that as soon as our Division Hospital is established, which will probably be immediately, our regimental outfits will be bereft of everything that has hitherto pertained to them except the two chests, one chair, and a small table. (2) The canvas of a regimental field hospital consists of three hospital tents and one common tent. The common, or "A" tent, serves the purpose of a field dispensary under charge of an Acting Steward. The hospital tent is 14 feet long, 15 feet wide, and 11 feet to ridge, the wall being 4½ feet high. This space will accommodate six hospital field cots, three being placed with heads against each lateral wall, leaving a center aisle or passageway from end to end. The canvas at each end can be swung back allowing of ample ventilation. By placing two hospital tents in line with each other, end to end, but separated by a distance of fourteen feet, this intervening space being roofed in by a hospital tent-fly, fastened with guy ropes, an ideal twelve bed field hospital can be attained, having a large central area or middle room for storage of medical and surgical field cases and other supplies, and for accommodation of desk, bedside tables and chairs. If this central rectangular space were flanked by an additional hospital tent, accommodation would be afforded for a mess-room, and a storage or general utility room. (3) Other appurtenances to a field hospital consist of a mess chest, food chest, commode chest, field desk, and folding field furniture (chairs, cots, and tables), litters, pack-saddles, Red Cross ambulances and animals. The flag for a field hospital is made of white bunting, six by four feet, with a red cross of bunting three feet high and three feet wide in the center, the arms of the cross being twelve inches wide. The flags for ambulances and guidons to mark the way to field hospitals are made of white bunting twenty-eight by sixteen inches, with a red cross of bunting twelve inches high and twelve inches wide in the center, arms of cross being four inches wide. Thus it will be seen that preliminary to consolidation into brigades and divisions each regiment as an organization has a complete field hospital equipment capable of consolidation into brigade or division hospitals, and of being expanded or contracted to suit every possible contingency.

A roster of the medical and hospital corps of the Tampa Division gives our present strength as follows: Eight commissioned medical officers, 1 hospital steward, 10 acting hospital stewards, and 39 privates. Our ranking medical officer, Major Benjamin F. Pope, has been assigned as chief surgeon of the Tampa Division. He enters upon his important functions with a ripened experience begotten of actual war service in the sixties as Assistant Surgeon, Tenth New York Heavy Artillery, and of field service in the West in numerous Indian campaigns and of other responsible functions in the regular establishment for more than thirty years past. Major Pope as chief surgeon of the Tampa Division, commanded by Brigadier-General James F. Wade and under instructions from Surgeon-General Sternberg, has arranged for the establishment of one division hospital with a present capacity of sixty beds to be placed under the management of a division surgeon. Brigade surgeons will also be appointed but without formation of brigade hospitals, and to each regiment will be assigned one surgeon, and from these regimental surgeons, details by twos will be made as assistant surgeons at the division hospital for specified terms (probably two weeks) without relief from their regimental duties. The division hospital will thus consist of 1 surgeon, 2 assistant surgeons and the whole personnel of the hospital corps of the seven regiments, and their several field hospital equipments, retaining at regimental headquarters, only one medical and one surgical field chest, one wall tent, and one folding chair and stand. In an emergency the services of any or all regimental and battalion surgeons may be required at divisional headquarters. A picket ambulance will always be in readiness at the division hospital to respond to any calls from regimental surgeons for the conveyance of the sick to the command in need of hospital treatment.

Many interesting problems will be presented for solution by the medical corps should this campaign be carried into Cuba. Such, for instance, as transportation of wounded on an island where roads do not exist for ambulance carriage, and where yellow fever is indigenous and where, according to asseverations of intelligent native Cubans now resident here the hospital flag and brazzard (or arm badge) will not be respected by the belligerents.

But these matters together with the sanitary arrangement of our present camp, where we may remain for some time will form material for a future article.

In regard to sending into Cuba with our forces civilian physicians who are immune to yellow fever or at least acclimated by long residence in hot climates it will be of interest to know that twelve native Cuban physicians, refugees and at present resident here, have offered their services to the surgeon-general, through Major Pope, and are willing to accompany us as acting assistant surgeons into their native clime.

THE MILITARY AND CIVIC HOSPITALS OF CUBA.[1]

By W. F. BRUNNER, M.D.,
SANITARY INSPECTOR, U. S. M. H. S.

THERE are in Havana five military hospitals, the largest being the Alphonso XIII., which has a capacity of 3320 beds. It is built of wood on the pavilion plan, and is situated on a high eminence in the outskirts of the city, and is well removed from all other buildings. Its equipment is almost perfect, having been constructed by a Spanish engineer who was educated in the United States. The surface drainage is complete, and if this building is not destroyed it could be utilized by the United States as a hospital for the troops occupying the City of Havana. The lightest mortality of all the military hospitals on the island was recorded here. Cases of yellow fever and smallpox are treated at this hospital, several wards being set aside for that purpose. Here, it may be said, that but few cases of smallpox have developed among the soldiers.

There is a second wooden hospital called Cuartel de Madera, having 1000 beds, and situated in the parish known as Jésus Maria. It is poorly constructed, and could only be used as a hospital for yellow-fever cases.

The Benificencia Hospital has 2000 beds; it is situated near the Gulf, and is built of stone. The building was formerly used as a foundling asylum, but was taken by General Weyler in 1896. It would be unwise to use this structure as a hospital. No surgical cases have been treated there.

San Ambrosia is an old stone structure situated near the Taliapiedra wharf, and beyond doubt is the filthiest building in Havana, and has always shown a heavy death-rate. It should not be used for United States troops. It has 900 beds.

There are two hospitals in Regla, but in the official reports they are made to appear as one, and will be so spoken of in this report. The buildings are old sugar warehouses. They are poorly equipped, and the administration is bad. They contain 3000 beds. No attempts to isolate cases of infectious or contagious diseases have ever been made. Yellow fever and smallpox have been treated in the general wards.

There are also in Havana the following civil or municipal hospitals: Reina Mercedes, Paula, Quinta del Rey, and Dependiente. With the exception of the first, all of them are filthy institutions, and were erected many years ago.

The Reina Mercedes was built in 1885; it is of stone, has ten pavilions, each holding twenty-four beds. During the past year it has been overcrowded, and a high mortality has resulted. There were from 400 to 500 patients treated at this hospital each month from August to December, 1897, and there were over 750 deaths during that time. Such a bad state of affairs existed that clinical lectures of the medical college were abandoned on account of the danger to the attending students. Many cases of smallpox have occurred there during the past five months. There are fifty-six military hospitals on the island, and with but few exceptions they cannot be used by the United States Government on account of their being badly infected.

[1] From advance sheets of reports to the Supervising Surgeon-General United States Marine-Hospital Service.

THE MORBIDITY AND MORTALITY IN THE SPANISH ARMY STATIONED IN CUBA DURING THE CALENDAR YEAR 1897.[1]

BY W. F. BRUNNER, M.D.,
SANITARY INSPECTOR U. S. M. H. S.[2]

THE following mortality from yellow fever in the five military hospitals in Havana is correct, it being taken from official figures and verified by careful investigation:

Deaths from yellow fever at Havana and Regla in military hospitals during the year 1897.

Months.	Havana.	Regla.	Total.
January	132	109	241
February	43	74	117
March	42	56	98
April	76	112	188
May	89	102	191
June	181	234	415
July	211	227	438
August	185	112	297
September	179	138	317
October	71	57	128
November	48	53	101
December	17	15	32
Total			2583

This death-rate represents about 10,000 cases of yellow fever. It will be noticed that deaths from yellow fever began to decrease in August, when they should have increased. This is accounted for by the fact that the Spanish Government, alarmed by the increasing death-rate from that disease, began to place their sick in Havana Province in two hospitals at places known as Mariel and San Antonio de las Vegas. The following table will show the deaths from yellow fever in the other cities on the island during the calendar year 1897:

Matanzas	238
Santiago de Cuba	658
Sagua la Grande	378
Cardenas	235
Cienfuegos	212
Manzanillo	230
Holguin, Guines, Remedios, Sancti Spiritis, etc.	1500
Total	3451
Deaths in Havana	2583
Total deaths from yellow fever in military hospitals, 1897	6034

This death-rate represents about 30,000 cases.

But few deaths have occurred in Havana and in the other cities during the present year, but as over 12,000 recruits have been sent from Spain to Cuba, during 1898, nearly all of whom disembarked at Havana, previous to June 1st, a heavy death-rate will result.

SMALLPOX.

While this disease did not cause many deaths among the Spanish soldiers, still every city and town in Cuba has been ravaged by it, and as a result many houses are infected, and troops sent there should all be revaccinated. I give here the deaths from smallpox from January, 1897, to March, 1898, inclusive, in the city of Havana, including soldiers and civilians:

January, 1897	57
February, 1897	581
March, 1897	319
April, 1897	93
May, 1897	44
June, 1897	9
July, 1897	4
August, 1897	1
September, 1897	5
October, 1897	7
November, 1897	10
December, 1897	15
January, 1898	31
February, 1898	62
March, 1898	58

Smallpox has prevailed to a considerable extent during the past six months at Sagua la Grande and at Matanzas.

ENTERIC FEVER.

The heaviest death-rate from this cause existed at Havana and Matanzas. In the latter place both civilians and soldiers died in large numbers during the last six months of 1897, and a conservative estimate of deaths from this cause among the soldiers throughout Cuba during the year 1897 is 2500.

MALARIAL FEVERS.

Under this head must be included what have been termed by the medical officers of the Spanish Army pernicious fever and "caquexia paludica." Fully 7000 men were lost to the Spanish Army from malarial influences.

ENTERITIS AND DYSENTERY.

These two diseases caused no less than 12,000 deaths, due to the lack of proper food, both in the field and in the military hospitals. Nearly 5000 deaths occurred in the five military hospitals in Havana alone, and the patients in these hospitals were better fed and cared for than at any other points on the island.

GLANDERS.

This disease rarely attacking men in this country, not infrequently occurs in Cuba; in Havana over 100 cases occurred among the soldiers. Glandered

[1] From advance sheets of the report to the Supervising Surgeon-General U. S. Marine Hospital Service.

[2] Dr. Brunner was assigned to Cuba April 1, 1897, as the representative of the U. S. Marine Hospital Service to keep the quarantine service informed of the prevalence of infectious diseases there and the sanitary measures employed to prevent their transmission to the United States. He resided there continuously from April 1, 1897 to April 15, 1898.

horses are seen daily on the streets of Havana and the other cities of the island.

LEPROSY.

While there is a lepers' hospital in Havana, there is no law compelling lepers to be confined in this institution, and they are seen on the public streets. There are presumably hundreds of persons with this disease living under no sanitary restraint in the city of Havana.

TOTAL MORTALITY OF SPANISH ARMY IN CUBA.

The following figures are approximately correct for the year 1897:

Deaths from yellow fever	6034
Deaths from enteric fever	2500
Enteritis and dysentery	12,000
Malarial fevers	7000
All other diseases	5000
Deaths from all diseases	32,534

This does not include hundreds of deaths that occurred among certain troops sent back to Spain on the 10th, 20th, and 30th of every month in the last stage of the different diseases enumerated above. Having observed those departures from Havana, I can safely say that ten per cent. of the 30,000 invalided home were destined to a certain and early death. These enormous death-rates, it must be remembered, occurred in an army which at no time was properly cared for; badly clothed and badly fed, exposed to all the dangers of a tropical climate, they succumbed easily.

MEDICAL PROGRESS.

The Importance of Physical Examination in Making a Diagnosis of Insanity.—DOWN (*Yale Med. Jour.*, April, 1898) emphasizes the importance of physical examination before passing judgment upon the sanity of the patient. Not only does such examination afford an easy opening for conversation, but in many cases of mental impairment the attention of the patient has been especially directed to one or more organs of the body in regard to which delusions may be found to exist. This is especially true of the genital organs. Not infrequently, too, there are physical defects or abnormalities which may throw considerable light upon the questions to be determined.

Stab Wounds of the Abdomen.—BUDINGER (*Arch. für klin. Chir.*, Bd. 56, S. 163) describes an interesting case of stab wound of the abdomen received by a young man, aged twenty-two years, in a drunken brawl. The wound, which was caused by a pocket-knife, was immediately below the left costal margin. The patient was absolutely without symptoms for one week, excepting that an old bronchitis made him cough a great deal. For several days he had received plenty of solid food, the bowels moved regularly, and the wound was looked upon as a superficial one. Suddenly, without apparent cause, he went into a state of collapse. The abdomen was at once opened, and it was seen that a wound in the stomach three-quarters of an inch in length had pulled away from the slight existing adhesions, and had allowed the escape of a small quantity of the contents of the stomach. This wound was promptly sutured and the patient recovered. The case is of particular interest on account of the long interval, 158 hours, interposed between the accident and the first sign of danger; for it is usual in such cases to say that if twenty-four or at most forty-eight hours pass without grave symptoms, the abdominal organs have probably not been injured. In spite of this experience, Büdinger believes that the treatment of stab wounds should be an expectant one, unless the injury to the abdominal viscera is a gross one. At any rate, the chances of a secondary laparotomy are no worse than a primary one. This treatment is, therefore, the opposite of that advocated in gunshot wounds of the abdomen. The latter, on account of the great probability of visceral injury, ought to be followed forthwith by an incision. Of course, if a stab wound produces vomiting, small pulse, meteorism, etc., operation should be at once performed.

A Striking Instance of Maternal Impression.—GARDINER (*Amer. Jour. of Obstet.*, February, 1898) gives an instance of maternal impression which is no less striking than it is well-authenticated. An American woman had, during her third pregnancy, an unbearable craving for sunfish. During the fourth month her husband brought home for her some of these fish alive in a pail. She stumbled against it on the porch, and one of the fish flopped over the edge of the pail and came in contact with her leg. It sent a cold chill through her, but the pregnancy was not disturbed, and nothing further was thought of the accident until the child was born, when, to her surprise, a nevus in shape and size closely resembling a fish was seen upon the leg of the baby in the part corresponding to that of her own leg with which the fish came in contact. Otherwise the child's health was perfect, and she lived to grow up into a healthy woman. The annoying craving for sunfish which was temporarily present in her mother existed in her throughout a long life. It much resembled a drug habit. Time and again she has eaten sunfish until from repletion she has vomited, and then again has eaten them with unabated appetite.

A New Symptom of Scarlet Fever.—MEYER (*La Presse Méd.*, March 5, 1898) describes a new symptom for the diagnosis of scarlet fever which he has observed in eighty per cent. of the cases of this disease in adults. The symptom appears at the time of the eruption, when the patient complains of a weakness or numbness of the extremities, and a sensation of tingling or a creeping feeling in the palmar surfaces of the hands and fingers. Associated with it is a certain amount of congestion, which may be the only thing noticed, until the patient makes some little exertion, such as an attempt to take a glass of water. No pain accompanies this symptom. It may easily be confounded with (1) the itching which often accompanies the appearance of the eruption; (2) the swelling of the extremities, which may also accompany eruption, and interfere with the free movements of the fingers; (3) the stiffness produced by scarlatinal rheumatism. This is, however, a painful affection, and has its maximum manifestation in the joints, so that the two should be readily separated.

In cases of supposed scarlet fever this symptom may aid in establishing the true diagnosis. It may also be of value in cases of delayed or scanty eruption. Meyer has never seen it in connection with other eruptive fevers. It is wanting, also, in the eruptions of the grippe, of tonsillitis either simple or diphtheritic, and in toxic and medicinal erythema, including that produced by mercury, in which the diagnosis is often perplexing enough.

THERAPEUTIC NOTES.

Medicinal Treatment of Rheumatoid Arthritis.—BANNATYNE (*Edinb. Med. Jour.*, Jan., 1898) has found guaiacol carbonate and creosotol valuable remedies in the treatment of rheumatoid arthritis. He selected these drugs rather than others of the phenol group on account of their freedom from caustic and albumin-coagulating powers. They can, therefore, be given without intestinal irritation. Of the two, guaiacol carbonate is more pleasant to take. Given in doses of 5 to 15 grains three times a day, rapidly increased to six times a day, its effect is soon marked. Pain and swelling of the joints diminish, the facies which is often pronounced in the disease changes, appetite and sleep become normal, and the patient feels quite different. If nephritis complicates the arthritis guaiacol should be given with caution. The advantages of a dietetic and hygienic regimen are emphasized.

Treatment of Hemoptysis.—A writer (*La Med. Moderne*, March 25, 1898) recommends the following prescription for use in hemoptysis. It may be given by the mouth or subcutaneously:

℞ Ergotin	. . . . . .	gr. lxv
Antipyrin	. . . . . .	gr. xxxviii
Spartein sulphat.	. . . .	gr. v
Morph. hydrochlorat.	. . . .	gr. j
Aq. dest.	. . q. s. ad.	℥ ijss.

Five drops of this mixture may be given every five minutes for two or three doses, or at longer intervals according to circumstances. If the hemoptysis is slight it will cease after the administration of the medicine and a more exact diagnosis can then be made. Hemorrhages of a persistent character are due to the rupture of some small aneurism, perhaps in a tubercular cavity. If such is the case medical treatment is generally useless, and in spite of the administration of hemostatics and injections of salt solution death usually follows in a short time.

A New Treatment of Syphilis.—LALANDE (*La Presse Med.*, March 12, 1898) states that he has obtained remarkable results in the treatment of syphilis by the use of a fluid obtained by mascerating young calves' horns, finely powdered in a one-per-cent. saline solution. These horns are especially rich in keratin. The fluid thus obtained is yellow, clear, limpid, with an odor suggesting burnt horn and contains small amounts of calcium and potassium sulphate, calcium phosphate, and larger amounts of sodium chlorid and gelatin. This liquid is injected subcutaneously in doses of 15 to 45 minims once or twice a week, or even every day according to the urgency of the case. There is a slight reaction at the point of injection which soon disappears. The curative effects generally are manifest as early as the third injection. Mucous patches fade away, cutaneous lesions become copper-colored in a few days and then disappear, while ulcerating lesions dry and their crusts fall away leaving a smooth skin underneath. In this manner there have been treated thirty patients, seventeen of them being women. In nine cases the treatment was begun with the primary lesion; in nineteen in the secondary period, and in two in the tertiary period. The author does not offer any theory to explain the action of this remedy, but the results were to him most satisfactory.

The Treatment of Fevers Complicated with Delirium.—LECTOURE (*Gaz. des Hôpitaux*, No. 141, 1897) says that there are three indications to be met in all fevers complicated with delirium. Treatment should facilitate the excretion of the poisonous material in the blood, reduce the elevation of temperature, and influence the anatomical seat of the complication in the brain. Cold or lukewarm baths are most beneficial. Beside reducing the temperature, they have a powerful diuretic influence and a paper to regulate the functions of the nervous system. Quinin is indicated only in malaria. In order to act favorably upon the brain, hypnotics must be employed, and of them none is better than the bromids.

A New Method of Applying Unguentum Hydrargyri.—HOGNER (*Boston Med. and Surg. Jour.*, March 31, 1898) recommends most heartily Velander's new pillow-case method for the administration of ointment of mercury. It is practical, effective, convenient, and clean. Velander was convinced some years ago that the mercury in an ointment is absorbed after being vaporized. He has, therefore, given up spreading the ointment upon the skin, and spreads it instead upon the inside of a small pillow-case, which is hung upon succeeding days alternately on the back and on the chest. It is kept in position by ribbons over the shoulders and around the waist. The pillow-case is made of cheap cotton cloth, and one of its external faces is smeared with the ointment. It is then inverted so as to bring the ointment on its inner surface, and is placed in position so that the layer of cloth upon which the ointment is spread is in direct contact with the body, while its unsmeared side protects the clothing. Every night fresh ointment is spread over the old without removing this, and at the end of ten days the pillow-case is thrown away and a new one is prepared. Baths should be taken twice a week, and the skin of the chest and back should be washed every night. The quantity of ointment used daily is 6 grams (90 grains). The effect of the treatment is very rapid, as more mercury can in this manner be absorbed with fewer unpleasant effects, such as stomatitis, etc., than when it is otherwise administered.

THE MEDICAL NEWS.

A WEEKLY JOURNAL

OF MEDICAL SCIENCE.

COMMUNICATIONS are invited from all parts of the world. Original articles contributed *exclusively* to THE MEDICAL NEWS will after publication be liberally paid for (accounts being rendered quarterly), or 250 reprints will be furnished in place of other remuneration. When necessary to elucidate the text, illustrations will be engraved from drawings or photographs furnished by the author. Manuscripts should be typewritten.

Address the Editor: J. RIDDLE GOFFE, M.D.,
No. 111 FIFTH AVENUE (corner of 18th St.), NEW YORK.

Subscription Price, including postage in U. S. and Canada.

PER ANNUM IN ADVANCE	$4.00
SINGLE COPIES	.10
WITH THE AMERICAN JOURNAL OF THE MEDICAL SCIENCES, PER ANNUM	7.50

Subscriptions may begin at any date. The safest mode of remittance is by bank check or postal money order, drawn to the order of the undersigned. When neither is accessible, remittances may be made, at the risk of the publishers, by forwarding in *registered* letters.

LEA BROTHERS & CO.,
No. 111 FIFTH AVENUE (corner of 18th St.), NEW YORK, AND NOS. 706, 708 & 710 SANSOM ST., PHILADELPHIA.

SATURDAY, MAY 7, 1898.

WAR NEWS IN THE MEDICAL NEWS.

THE MEDICAL NEWS is gratified to announce to its readers that arrangements have been made to devote a certain portion of its columns each week to interesting and instructive articles suggested by the preparations for the war and the experiences of the future campaign. Men who are taking more or less prominent and active parts in the medical and surgical preparations for the military events most eagerly and anxiously awaited, have courteously consented to keep their professional brethren informed, through the columns of the NEWS, regarding the medical, surgical, sanitary, and hygienic features that may come under their observation.

In the naval arm of the service the interest of the medical profession is centered upon the practical working and success of the hospital ship Solace. A hospital ship is not only an untried experiment, but is a wholly novel and original idea, and one which has eminated from the Surgeon-General of the United States Navy. The MEDICAL NEWS is fortunate in having as its representative on board this ship, one of the assistant surgeons, who has been especially designated by the surgeon-general to report events of interest to the profession. Occasional articles may also be expected from surgeons assigned to the battle-ships.

As a representative of the military arm of the service, Surgeon Raymond commences in this issue of the NEWS, a series of most instructive articles on the life of the surgeon in camp, camp hospitals, surgical equipments, etc. To the members of the profession, inexperienced in military life, who are now going out with the volunteer forces, these articles cannot fail to prove most timely and helpful.

In the surgical contingent of the Red Cross organization, which is preparing to extend its succoring arm to the needy of either friend or foe, will also be found a representative of the MEDICAL NEWS, while the work of the Marine Hospital Service, whose forces are now organized and equipped to forfend us from the dread scourge of infectious disease, will be promptly portrayed in these columns.

THE HYGIENE OF A CUBAN CAMPAIGN.

THE necessity of landing a large number of United States troops upon Cuban soil seems unavoidable, and the consequent danger to their health from endemic disease is exciting wide comment and is apparently delaying a move most essential to the speedy termination of barbarous warfare and inhuman starvation. Military invasion means disease as surely as it means traumatism, and the only thing to predetermine is what diseases must be faced and how their acquisition and fatality may be minimized. It is the opinion of those best able to judge that the prospective danger to our troops has been greatly overestimated, a fact much to be deprecated, as it has apparently engendered delay and surely tends to dishearten the soldier. Moderate apprehension redounds to the army's good by rendering the men more amenable to hygienic restraint; immoderate apprehension demoralizes the troops and undermines discipline.

The diseases to which troops invading Cuba will be exposed, as is well understood, are smallpox, malarial fever, typhoid fever, diarrheal diseases, and yellow fever. With the exception of the last they are all diseases incident to camp life. From smallpox, which Cubans foster because of their unhygienic methods of living, our troops are practically immune From typhoid fever and diarrheal diseases they can be saved in great measure by the intelligent enforcement of a few precautions as to food and drink. A certain amount of malaria must be expected and is unavoidable, but its ravages can be greatly curtailed by hygienic precautions and prophylactic doses of quinin, hygiene however being more potent than medicine.

Yellow fever is the bugbear which seems to terrorize all alike. Of course one ought not to speak slightingly of this disease, but the fact should be appreciated that, whatever be its origin, it is fostered by filth and made epidemic and malignant by unsanitary conditions of life. It has repeatedly been demonstrated that civic, domestic, and personal cleanliness lessens the liability to and the virulence of infectious disease, while not precluding the occurrence of sporadic cases. Such being the case we should be reassured by the physical perfection, the good morale, and the intelligence of our troops, all qualifications conducing to the avoidance of and resistance to disease.

It would be an unmerited insult to the medical officers of the regular army to hint that all details of camp sanitation are not well understood by them or that they will not be strictly enforced. It is no reproach however to suggest that unusual precautions are called for, under the present unusual conditions, with reference to the selection of camp sites on elevated land and to a frequent change of site. Boiled water, coffee, or tea should alone be drunk, and fruit, except lemons, avoided. A light farinaceous diet is better suited to subtropical regions and nibbling hardtack is safer than gorging with meats and green or overripe and unaccustomed fruits.

In short to go there clean and to remain clean and abstemious should be the resolve of every officer and man.

Dr. John Guiteras concisely states the case when he says:

"All Americans, by reason of their habits of personal cleanliness, are better fitted to withstand such a climate than almost any other people. The men to suffer first would be those who are especially strong and healthy, and have such faith in their constitutions that they would despise many small but necessary precautions. Fever naturally takes a stronger hold upon such men, and they suffer more in proportion. Such a thing as a great epidemic fever in an American Army is, however, a most remote possibility, in my judgment.

"Men should go thirsty in preference to drinking water before it is boiled. Soldiers on a march should all carry a lemon to sip. Other fruit should be strictly avoided, no matter how tempting it may seem. Another necessary precaution is to dress warmly despite the heat, keeping the stomach and bowels covered at all times.

"Plans should be laid for the quick removal from Cuba of men stricken with fever of any kind.

"The medical department would probably have to be increased ten fold, but, better than medicine, will be strict observance of a few simple rules by the men most interested."

With special reference to yellow fever, Surgeon-General Sternberg says:

"Every case of fever should receive prompt attention. If albumen is found in the urine of a patient with fever it should be considered suspicious (of yellow fever), and he should be placed in an isolated tent. The discharges of patients with fever should always be disinfected at once with a solution of carbolic acid (five per cent.), or of chlorid of lime (6 ounces to a gallon of water), or with milk of lime made from quicklime.

"Whenever a case of yellow fever occurs in camp the troops should be promptly moved to a fresh camping-ground located a mile or more from the infected camp. No doubt typhoid fever, camp diarrhea, and probably yellow fever are frequently communicated to soldiers in camp through the agency of flies, which swarm about matter and filth of all kinds deposited upon the ground or in shallow pits, and directly convey infectious germs attached to their feet or contained in their excreta to the food which is exposed while being prepared at the camp kitchens, or while being served in the mess tent. It is for this reason that a strict sanitary police is so important; also, because the water-supply may be contaminated in the same way, or by surface drainage.

THE DESTINY OF THE CASE-BOOK.

AN interesting question of professional privilege is suggested by a clause in the will of a late prominent physician of New York City. This clause directs that all the notes and histories of patients in his possession at the time of death shall be handed over to a brother practitioner, who, during the testator's life, was in no way connected or identified with him in practice. As the legator was not only a most indefatigable note-taker, but also a prominent specialist and consultant for many years, there are naturally within the covers of his case-book the voluntary, unrestricted confidences of members of many of the leading families of this country. It would seem that the dead physician's object in bequeathing his case-book was to insure the completion of many important family records and, to a large degree, contribute to the solution of questions of familous and hereditary disposition. This, at least, is our interpretation, as the legatee is instructed to donate them, on the cessation of his usefulness, to such a person as will, in the judgment of the giver, be competent and willing to carry out the original plan of following out and studying the manifestations of disease as they show themselves in the various branches of the families whose physical, moral, and intellectual shortcomings are therein recorded. From a utilitarian point of view, this seems very well, and unquestionably much light could be thrown on the intricacies of the laws governing heredity if the mandates of the original testator could be carried out. We are of the opinion, however, that such action would be decidedly subversive of the canons of professional conduct. The physician has no more right to share with another the confidences imposed upon, or granted to him by patients than has the confessor to publish for the benefit of an inquisitive and scandal-mongering world a volume made up of the sad stories with which his flock has burdened his ears.

The case-book should die with the doctor, so far as it is the record of individuals. This does not necessarily imply that the facts set forth by such histories may not be utilized, if expedient, for the solution of problems in etiology or symptomatology. But when they are used for such purposes, the individuality of the person should not be known.

We are convinced that this is right from a legal point of view, and we feel certain that it is sound morally. It is a presumption on the part of the physician to claim the right to lay before the eyes of any person or persons, secrets, family skeletons, evidences of moral frailty, perhaps even crimes, of which no one else had knowledge and which is granted to him only because the guild of which he is a member stands as the prototype of integrity and honor. There is a written law which states that the physician shall not disclose the confidences of the consulting-room and the sick chamber, but mandates of obedience to it are not so binding as is the unwritten covenant between every patient and physician that the trust shall be inviolate.

The destiny of the case-book should be cremation; consigned to the flames unopened and unread; thus will the physician avoid the opprobrium of a recalcitrant covenanter.

ECHOES AND NEWS.

Medical Women in India. — There are 163 hospitals in India officered by women practitioners only.

Ether Drinking in East Prussia.—According to a physician's report ether drinking is so prevalent among the men, women, and even the children in East Prussia that the roads and market-places are scented with the fumes of the drug.

Reception to Dr. Northrup of New York.—Dr. Northrup addressed the Philadelphia Pediatric Society on April 12th, the subject being the "Portal Entry of Tuberculosis in Childhood." The meeting was largely attended and after it a reception was tendered Dr. Northrup.

The Suicide of a Medical Woman.—A young woman, one of the externes at the Paris Hospital committed suicide, fearing that she had neglected the proper treatment of an immature infant, but a post-mortem examination revealed that the infant had died from natural causes.

A Holmes' Definition. — An important line of demarcation between receding barbarism and civilization, said Dr. Holmes, is the clothes-line. The evoluting man by it shows, and by it knows, that he has passed beyond the stage where he must wear clothing of some kind, to that other and higher stage where he must have a change of raiment.

Female Nurses Not to Be Employed by the Army or Navy at the Front.—Hundreds of female nurses are kindly offering their services at the Army and Navy Departments. It has been decided, however, that their services will not be accepted for the present. If it shall be found necessary to establish hospitals remote from the seat of war, the services of these patriotic and devoted women will doubtless be in demand.

Dr. Peck Made Professor of the N. Y. Post-Graduate Medical School.—Dr. Edward S. Peck has been appointed Professor of Diseases of the Eye at the New York Post-Graduate Medical School and Hospital. Dr. Peck holds the position of Senior Ophthalmic Surgeon of the City Hospital, Visiting Ophthalmic Surgeon at the St. Elizabeth's Hospital, and Ophthalmologist at the Montefiore Home.

Michigan State Board of Health. — The Secretary of the Board, Dr. Baker, is earnestly engaged in the preliminaries of the quarter-centennial celebration of that board's establishment. It is expected to hold a jubilation on August 9th to 11th at Detroit; and the sanitarians and physicians of that city are already holding committee meetings preparing for the sessions and the social arrangements of the convention.

Tuberculosis in Fishes.—The existence of this disease in animals has long been known. From reports recently made to the Academie des Sciences by Messrs. Dubar, Bataillon, and Terre, fishes are likewise affected by it. In an artificial pond in which the sputa and dejecta of a woman, far gone in consumption, were thrown, the carp seemed to swell and die. On examination tubercle bacilli were found in the intestines of the fish.

Dangerous Economy.—It has just been brought to the attention of the authorities in Naples that the ragmen have been in the habit of purchasing the wadding or charpie used for dressing in the hospitals, and after washing it, selling it to upholsterers for padding sofas; the railroad cars have also been using this discarded material. A vigilance service has been established to prevent such sales and this wadding or dressing is now destroyed in the sanitary furnace at Pasconcello.

Increase of the Naval Surgical Staff. — A large number of applications for positions as acting assistant surgeons have been received by the Board of Naval Inspectors at the Naval Hospital at Brooklyn. The bill for the employment of these extra men is still before Congress, and as soon as it becomes a law an examination of the six or seven hundred men who have already applied at the different stations will be held. Unfortunately, the bill provides for only twenty-six acting assistant surgeons.

The New York Board of Health Provides against Emergencies.—The Health Department of New York realizing that conditions may arise during the coming summer requiring the employment of a large number of experts who have had experience in its work ask that all persons who have been employed in the department during the past twenty years, be and are hereby respectfully requested to send their names and addresses to the Secretary at the office, Center and Elm streets, New York City; said names to be placed on a roll, to be known as the "Reserve Sanitary corps."

Pollution of the Passaic River.—The New Jersey courts have now before them a prosecution of the City of Paterson by Jersey City, to restrain the former from continuing to discharge its sewage into the Passaic River. An argument was recently made before Chancellor McGill which will, if decided in favor of the plaintiff, be the first step toward compelling Paterson and some other filth-contributors to provide a modern sewage-disposal plant. The importance of this pending litigation to the public health and property values in and for the entire State of New Jersey, as well as in certain of its great cities, is great and far-reaching.

Von Bergmann Declined to Operate.—At the Berlin Medical Society, Von Bergmann showed two patients with bullets in the brain. In both the wounds were healed and the patients presented very few symptoms at the time of demonstration. At first, however, there had been in one case, hemiplegia, hemianesthesia, one side deafness and total blindness, which had all passed away, leaving finally a slight paralysis only of the left leg. The projectiles were skiagraphed with the X-rays. Notwithstanding the urgent wish of both parents to have the bullets extracted, Von Bergmann had refused to operate, as there was no indication for such interference.

Revaccination of Our Troops Is in Order.—Although very little has been said in the public prints respecting the possible danger from variola that may affect those whose business will take them to Cuba, it should not be overlooked by our authorities that that disease has in recent years been prevalent throughout that island. A very considerable mortality from smallpox has been reported in both of the contending forces. We trust that none of our fellow-citizens will be sent to Cuba without all the protection against that scourge of armies that is afforded by revaccination. The present is the time to undertake this duty—let no valued lives be sacrificed by neglect in this direction.

Puerperal Fever at Berlin. — This fever which caused great mortality in the Charity Hospital at Berlin during 1801 and 1852 has been much decreased by taking precautionary measures, but the idea of exterminating it did not occur to the mind of any one till the antiseptic principles came into practice. The mortality decreased to five per cent. in 1883, when a greater improvement was made by substituting corrosive sublimate for carbolic acid. In 1888, the sublimate was used as a disinfectant for the hands, the vaginal and uterine injections being prepared with carbolic acid or lysol. Lately the practice has been to disinfect the external genitals with soft soap containing three per cent. of carbolic acid.

The Action of the Atlanta Quarantine Convention Endorsed by the American Surgical Society. — The American Surgical Society at its recent meeting in New Orleans in giving expression to its approval of the regulations formulated by the recent Quarantine Convention held at Atlanta, Ga., unanimously passed the following resolution: "WHEREAS, The American Surgical Association sympathized deeply with the South during the last visitation of yellow fever, it is, therefore, *Resolved*, That the Association earnestly hopes that all the interested States will adopt such uniform regulations as will prevent the recurrence and spread of the disease, and avert the baneful effect of shotgun quarantine and *Resolved*, That it approves of the quarantine regulations adopted by the Atlanta Couvention, which the Health Boards of the interested States and the United States Marine Hospital Service framed."

Assignment of Army Surgeons to Inspect Volunteers.—Secretary Alger has designated in the various States the following named medical officers to examine volunteer troops called out by the President's proclamation as to their qualifications for the service: Major Ezra Woodruff, surgeon, Connecticut; Captain M. C. Wyeth, assistant surgeon, Delaware; Captain H. R. Stiles, assistant surgeon, Maine; Major Louis W. Crampton, surgeon, Maryland; Captain G. E. Bushnell, assistant surgeon, Massachusetts; Major Charles B. Byrne, surgeon, New Hampshire; Captain W. C. Gorgas, assistant surgeon, New Jersey; Major Louis M. Maus, surgeon, New York; Captain F. A. Winter, assistant surgeon, North Carolina; Major J. D. Hall, surgeon, Pennsylvania; Major C. L. Heizemann, surgeon, Rhode Island; First Lieut. W. F. Lewis, assistant surgeon, South Carolina; Captain J. R. Kean, assistant surgeon, Vermont; Major G. W. Adair, surgeon, Virginia; Captain B. L. Ten Eyck, assistant surgeon, West Virginia; Colonel W. H. Forwood, assistant surgeon, District of Columbia.

American Medical Missionary Work in India.—In the land of India, where many lethal diseases flourish like plants in a hot-house, and which is a nursery of epidemics and the permanent abode of cholera, it is not unnatural that missionaries should have been led to establish hospitals for the relief of the sick and suffering living about them. The American Board planted a mission in Madura, South India, in 1835, and from the beginning of this mission has devoted much attention to medical relief. Among the doctors who have gone out to Madura as medical missionaries stand the honored names of Steele, Lord, and Palmer—the last a brother of Senator Palmer of Illinois. At Dindigul, the veteran, Dr. Chester, has for thirty-five years devoted his time to this department of missionary work. The medical work carried on by this mission has done much to win the way of the mission into the favor of the native people of that district.

Medical Examiners versus Coroners.—Some doubt concerning the superior excellence of medical examiners as compared with the coroner's system is suggested by an occurrence in the Massachusetts General Hospital, which was recently reported from Boston. It appears from reports in the secular press that a well-known resident of New York who was a patient in that institution, committed suicide there on the 13th inst. The return of his death made to the authorities declared that he died "from organic disease of brain, cirrhosis of liver, laceration of brain, and shock to nerves." The fact was that he shot himself in the head, but this circumstance was concealed until disclosed by the undertaker. Suicide is either a crime, the commission of which ought not to be hidden, or if committed under circumstances which negative criminality, is so important an occurrence that the concealment of cases of self-destruction is of very questionable propriety. Is it possible that such cases can be concealed by the medical examiners under the Massachusetts statute?

Obituary.—Dr. Cornelius Nevius Hoagland died at his home in Brooklyn, April 25, 1898. The cause of death was heart failure. Dr. Hoagland was born in Neshanic, Somerset County, N. J., November 23, 1828. In 1834 he removed with his parents to Piqua, Miami County, Ohio. He studied medicine, and was graduated from the Medical Department of the Western Reserve University, at Cleveland, about 1852. After his graduation he married Eliza Ellen, daughter of Judge David H. Morris of Miami County. In October, 1861, he was appointed surgeon in the Seventy-first Ohio. He served through the war, and was mustered out in January, 1866. He was a participant in many engagements, and was wounded at Nashville. Dr. Hoagland then engaged in mercantile pursuits, and removed to Brooklyn in 1868. He was a Fellow of the Microscopical Society of London, a life Fellow of the American Geographical Society of New York, the New York Genealogical and Biographical Society, and the Long Island Historical Society, Regent of the Long Island College Hospital, and a trustee of Syracuse University. Ten years ago the Hoagland Laboratory was erected, and equipped by Dr. Hoagland at a cost of $100,000. During the first four years of its existence he paid all the running expenses, amounting to about $10,000, and at the end of that time he endowed the laboratory with $50,000. Dr. Hoagland was also interested in the Brooklyn Free Kindergarten Society. One of its sixteen branches was named after him, and was maintained entirely by him at an expense of from $1000 to $1200 a year. It was opened in September, 1895. On January 1st last, he made a New Year's gift of $24,000 to the Hoagland Laboratory, $20,000 to the Kindergarten Society, and $14,000 to the Brooklyn Eye and Ear Hospital. He was president of the Board of Directors of the last-named institution. On January 27th Dr. Hoagland, finding himself in failing health, took a tour through the Mediteranean. He returned to America on April 5th, and soon afterward was stricken down. He leaves three children.

CORRESPONDENCE.

THE MEETING OF THE AMERICAN SURGICAL ASSOCIATION AT NEW ORLEANS.

[From our Special Correspondent.]

THIS meeting has proved to be one of the most notable in the history of the Association. The character of the papers, the interest in the discussions, the importance of the subjects under debate all conspired to make the gathering one of great importance. It was thought at first that the long distance, the prospect of hot weather, the erroneous report of the presence of yellow fever, and finally, the onset of war, would deter many from undertaking the journey. The large attendance, however, gave proof that even these serious obstacles received only momentary consideration.

Few realize how comfortably the trip to the Crescent City can be made. Those who went over the Illinois Central Railroad enjoyed a ride free from dust and heat, and over one of the best roadbeds in the country. The Louisiana division is a model of railroad construction and management. The members of the association were much interested in seeing the amount of perishable freight sent from this district to Northern cities. For example, at one station there are despatched daily during the season ten freight cars filled with strawberries, and at another over thirty-five freight cars are sent out daily with fresh vegetables for the North. At the Stuyvesant docks there are facilities for unloading in one day a freight train twelve miles long into steamers for European ports. This road, under the efficient management of Mr. Fish, its President, is making great progress in all matters pertaining to the comfort of its passengers, the rapid transportation of perishable freight, and the building up of commercial interests in all the Southern towns and cities.

On Tuesday Dr. J. Holt of New Orleans gave a most eloquent address of welcome, after which the President, Dr. Prewitt of St. Louis, read an admirable paper on the future of the Association. After an executive session the

Boston Club gave an elaborate luncheon, at which Judge Fenver presided. At three o'clock the meeting was called to order, and an interesting paper on "Cystitis" was read by Dr. Senn of Chicago. In the evening a banquet was given at the New St. Charles Hotel, at which a large number were present.

A lunch was given on Wednesday morning by the Committee of Arrangements, after which the meeting was convened and papers were discussed. In the evening a beautiful reception was given by Mrs. Richardson, the wife of the late Dr. Richardson, who was one of the most prominent members of the association. There were many physicians present, as well as many beautiful women, for whom New Orleans is famous. Dr. De Roaldes gave a very elaborate dinner to some members of the association. The Doctor is a most genial host, and entertains in a regal manner. It is rare to find one who is so cheerful and happy when suffering from an affection which is calculated to depress the most sanguine and courageous. The Doctor has recently lost his eyesight, but was as entertaining and as cheerful as he used to be when in possession of his vision. Thursday morning was occupied by a clinic at the New Orleans Hospital, and Dr. Halsted performed his operation for the radical cure of hernia. The operating theater was the gift of Dr. Miles, and is one of the best-equipped operating theaters in this or any other country.

Thursday a lunch was given by the Polyclinic at one of the celebrated restaurants. After the feast the meeting was called to order by the President, and a discussion took place upon the question of the treatment of fractures of the spine. In the evening there was a grand reception given by the Polyclinic to the physicians of New Orleans to meet the members of the American Surgical Association. Friday morning most of the members took their departure, and all with the greatest feelings of gratitude to those who had done so much to make the meeting a notable success. To Dr. Sonchon and to Dr. Matas, the Committee of Arrangements, the association feels deeply its sense of gratitude for all these gentlemen did to make the meeting a most interesting one.

Some of the members returned by the Yazoo & Mississippi Valley route, stopping over at Vicksburg. Here they were met by Mr. Murray Smith, the attorney for the Illinois Central road. Mr. Smith escorted the party over this historic town and explained to them the changes of the river bed, and gave a most interesting talk upon the incidents connected with the War. To him the entire party felt exceedingly grateful for the vivid description of the battle scenes with which he was familiar, and for the eloquent manner in which he portrayed the leading events of the War.

The Yazoo Valley is a wonderful farming district. It extends from the bluffs at Memphis to Vicksburg, a distance of 218 miles, and is bounded on one side by the Mississippi River and upon the other by the Yazoo Mountain range. In this belt of land the soil possesses inexhaustible fertility. This valley district is on the northern limit of the cotton belt, and the southern boundary of the wheat and corn belts. In addition to the fact that all crops that will grow in the temperate zone will flourish here in abundance, the climate is phenomenal. In this valley there is only a variation of 80 degrees the entire year, while in Illinois it is nearly 120 degrees, and in Dakota still greater. This even temperature enables the farmer to have his crops protected from frost 179 days in the year, and permits him to work out of doors the entire fifty-two weeks.

The death-rate in this valley is very low. In the State of Mississippi it is only 12.89 for each 1000, while in Missouri and Tennessee it is over 16 per 1000.

Fruits of all kinds are found to grow in rich profusion in this district. The Illinois Central Railroad is offering every facility to people to settle in this district, and no country offers such advantages to those who are agriculturally inclined and who desire a rich country, a uniform climate, and a healthful home.

The one great drawback which the South is laboring under is the shor-gun quarantine, but the Atlanta Convention has framed regulations which will do away with this barbaric method and give to the country immunity from the ravages of yellow fever. The American Surgical Association did a wise thing when it placed its stamp of approval upon the quarantine regulations recently formulated by the Atlanta Convention. This it did in the passage of appropriate resolutions offered by Dr. Souchon.

OUR PHILADELPHIA LETTER.

[From our Special Correspondent.]

PREPARATIONS IN MEDICAL CIRCLES FOR THE WAR —RESOLUTIONS OF THE MEDICO-LEGAL SOCIETY REGARDING DISPENSARY ABUSE—DR. MADURO OF NEW YORK ADVOCATES THE SCHLEICH METHOD OF ANESTHESIA BEFORE THE COLLEGE OF PHYSICIANS —FORMALDEHYD AS A MILK PRESERVATIVE AND ADULTERANT—BEQUESTS TO PHILADELPHIA INSTITUTIONS—DR. JOHN M. GUITERAS AT THE SERVICE OF THE GOVERNMENT.

PHILADELPHIA, May 2, 1898.

PREPARATIONS for the war are conspicuous in the medical circles of Philadelphia. Scarcely a hospital in the city has failed to offer the use of its wards and of its medical and nursing staffs to the Government, and hundreds of medical men and nurses are falling over one another in the mad rush to enroll their names in the list of volunteers in the medical departments of the army and navy. The Red Cross Society's headquarters is the scene of a similar scramble for places, and the list of nurses and hospital attendants who are anxious to see service "at the front," must be, by this time, sufficient for the needs of half a dozen conflicts between first-class military powers. The homeopaths, too, have joined in the contest of patriotism—and official positions in the country's pay. Altogether, what a pathetic commentary upon the vicissitudes of the lives of doctors and nurses this spectacle furnishes! As yet, no definite steps have been taken by the War Department for the care in local hospitals of the sick and wounded troops, but in the event of active hostilities, which now seem imminent, this city will no doubt be an important center for the care of invalided soldiers, just as it was during the Civil War. It is estimated that the various hospitals of this city possess facilities for the care of about 2000 troops. The only relief organization which exists here, with the exception of the Red Cross Society, is the Pennsylvania Sanitary Commission, which was formed this week at a conference of a number of prominent Pennsylvanians with Governor Hastings. This commission will be conducted along the lines which were so successful throughout the War of the Rebellion, and is intended to succor the sick and wounded during the war, and to bring home and bury the bodies of the dead. The organization is to be sustained entirely by voluntary contributions, which have already begun to be received in generous sums.

At the last meeting of the Medico-Legal Society, held April 26th, the committee on hospital abuses presented an exhaustive report of their investigations of this subject, which was adopted by the society as a basis for future procedure along this line. The report recommended, among other things, that the medical profession of Pennsylvania should use its influence to secure the passage of a legislative act regulating the government of hospitals and institutions of the State, and also regulating the appropriations of State money to such institutions; that the medical profession of Philadelphia should use its influence to limit to those unable to pay for medical attendance the free dispensation of medical treatment; that in all hospitals private pay patients should be allowed to designate their medical attendant irrespective of his connection with the medical staff of the hospital; that scientific clinical medical instruction should be fostered and enhanced by the conservation of established and rational charitable measures; that a rearrangement of the medical charities of Philadelphia is urgently demanded, and that this rearrangement should be effected with due regard to the topographical conditions which prevail. The society further recommended that the views thus expressed be communicated to the rural county medical societies and to the State Medical Society, and finally adopted the somewhat radical measure requesting the Philadelphia County Medical Society to pass a resolution pledging its members to refuse to accept any position with a charitable institution made vacant by the resignation or discharge of the former incumbent on account of adhering to any measures of reform endorsed by the local county organization.

At the last meeting of the Section on General Surgery of the College of Physicians of Philadelphia, Dr. M. L. Maduro of New York, whose article upon this subject in the MEDICAL NEWS was the first to appear in this country, gave a valuable account of his personal experience in the anesthetization of 100 cases with the petroleum-ether method of Schleich. In the formulæ given by him it has been the author's object to obtain mixtures whose boiling-points are about that of the body temperature, inasmuch as the experiments of Schleich have shown that the nearer the temperature of the anesthetic approaches the temperature of the body the more effective and the less dangerous is the narcosis produced.

W. C. Robinson, the chemist of the Philadelphia Board of Health, has recently called attention to the introduction of formaldehyd as a milk preservative, as a substitute for other more easily detected chemicals like boric acid or salicylic acid. This new adulterant is now being widely advertised in the local market, and it is presumed that it is extensively employed. The city milk inspectors have been ordered to be on the lookout for this latest adulterant, and have received instructions for detecting its presence in milk. They advocate that suspected samples of milk be treated with small quantities of a mixture of sulphuric acid and ferric chlorid, which produce even with a very weak solution of formaldehyd a distinct purplish-violet reaction. The test is an absolute one, Mr. Robinson claims, and should simplify the detection of this formerly considered undetected chemical.

By the will of late Dr. Oliver A. Judson, $1000 is left to the College of Physicians of Philadelphia, to be held in perpetuity, the interest of this sum as often as it amounts to $100, is to be offered as a prize for the best original essay on "The Practical Prevention of Disease."

The late Anne L. Garesche, who recently died in this city, has bequeathed to the Pennsylvania Hospital the sum of about $50,000, to be applied to the endowment fund of this institution. The donor also made a reversionary bequest of her residuary estate upon the death of three legatees.

The Chester County Hospital at West Chester has been tendered a gift of $10,000 by the Rev. W. L. Bull, for the purpose of founding a training-school for nurses. The building for this purpose will be immediately erected upon plans already in possession of the managers.

Dr. John M. Guiteras of the University of Pennsylvania has been called upon by the Government to take charge of the sanitary conditions of the camps and troops at Tampa, Florida. Dr. Guiteras has accepted the call, and is to have general charge of the safeguarding of the American troops from the infectious diseases to which they are exposed in Southern climates.

TRANSACTIONS OF FOREIGN SOCIETIES.

Berlin.

COMBINED CYSTOSCOPE AND URETERAL CATHETER—ELECTRIC LIGHT AS A THERAPEUTIC AGENT.

AT a session of the Medical Society, February 9th, FRANK showed a cystoscope adapted for irrigation of the bladder and catheterization of the ureters. A catheter designed for the ureter is passed through a tube in the instrument until its end appears in the lighted field. By means of a screw the tip of the catheter can then be bent in any direction so that it can be slipped without difficulty into the mouth of the ureter. The parts of the instrument designed for catheterization and irrigation may be sterilized by boiling, but the cystoscope proper will not stand hot water. It may be sterilized by formalin gas. Numerous trials of this instrument upon living patients have demonstrated that it can be introduced easily and painlessly. There is further no difficulty in the withdrawal of the instrument while leaving the ureteral catheter in position, if desired.

At the session of March 2d, BELOW discussed the present position of electric-light therapy. An institute in Berlin, arranged for this purpose, has apparatus of two kinds, that for giving light baths and that for exposing patients to rays of light. The idea rests upon the fact that artificial light like sunlight causes sweating. Patients suffering from muscular rheumatism, skin diseases, etc., when given an electric bath, that is when brought into a small chamber and exposed to about fifty incandescent lights, will lose by sweating in fifteen minutes about two pounds weight. The chamber is kept at a temperature of 45° to 50° C. (113° to 122° F.) and cold compresses are used to avoid cerebral congestion. A douche of lukewarm water followed by packing in cold wet cloths and kneading of the whole body completes the treatment. Sometimes the heat rays are extracted by letting the light pass through blue glass or through ice-water. At this institution there were treated in about a year 122 patients, of whom 67 were cured, 36 were improved, and 19 were not benefited. No effect was noted in the case of benign or malignant tumors, in alopecia, in atrophy of the optic nerve, nor in cataract. The best results were seen in lupus, in ulcers of various sorts, in syphilis, and in muscular rheumatism. Eczema was also favorably influenced. Considering the well-known influence of light upon plant life, it is surprising that so little attention has been paid to it in medicine. Experiments have shown that under the influence of light, animals discharge carbon dioxid and take up oxygen more rapidly than they do if kept in the dark. Furthermore, strong light is known to be possessed of marked bactericidal power. Koch has shown this to be true of sunlight in connection with the tubercle bacilli. Kitasato, in connection with the recent epidemic plague in India, found that the plague bacilli were destroyed in three or four hours by direct sunlight. The effect of the light bath is different from that of an ordinary sweating, such as that caused by steam. It is accomplished even without a high temperature of the chamber and with far less excitement of the heart than is the case in an ordinary Turkish bath. The freedom of dark races in tropical countries from many of the diseases to which fairer skinned people easily fall prey, is attributed to the favorable influence of the sunlight extending over many generations. It is mentioned that the natives of Haiti, if attacked by syphilis, bury themselves in the sand and lie for days exposed to the sun, drinking meanwhile a tea made from sarsaparilla and other herbs. After some weeks they entirely recover from the disease without other treatment than this sweat-cure produced by air, light, water, and sand. The institute established in Berlin is working to determine the amount of benefit which may be derived from the use of light as a therapeutic agent in various diseases.

From the discussion which followed the reading of this paper, it was evident that the subject is one which has excited a great deal of interest among physicians in Berlin, though they do not accept Below's views altogether regarding the usefulness of the light baths.

BEHREND said that he did not consider the lupus patients presented as by any means cured of their diseases, because no person could be said to be free from lupus, as long as there was any redness to be seen in the infected area when the skin was stretched or pressed. He also disagreed with the reader when he said that the severest forms of syphilis can be cured by light- or sweat-baths. Such experimentation with a disease of the gravity of syphilis when we possess against it the absolutely reliable remedies of mercury and iodid, should be denounced in the strongest terms.

SENATOR warned against the inference that electric lights can cure disease, because a tropical sun and hot sand baths do so. Such an instance is a recommendation for the use of sand baths, not electric baths.

MUNTER said that he had had a very large experience with patients treated by sweat-baths, etc., for a variety of troubles, and that he had never seen a case of undoubted syphilis, cured without the use of either mercury or iodid. The early symptoms will disappear without any treatment at all, in many cases, but it is in just these apparently light cases, that the severe, late, nervous symptoms appear, unless there is a thorough treatment with medicine in the beginning. He saw in electric baths a very decided advantage over the other methods of sweating, since they are able to accomplish their object without great increase of the pulse and temperature. In many diseases this is most important, especially so in nervous, cardiac, or nephritic affections.

SOCIETY PROCEEDINGS.

AMERICAN SURGICAL ASSOCIATION.

Nineteenth Annual Meeting, Held at New Orleans, April 19, 20, and 21, 1898.

(Continued from page 570.)

SECOND DAY—APRIL 20th.

MORNING SESSION.

DR. W. S. HALSTED of Baltimore read a paper, entitled

OPERATIVE TREATMENT OF CARCINOMA OF THE BREAST.

After fully discussing a large number of cases seen and operated upon and giving the statistics of the results for the past nine years at the Johns Hopkins Hospital, the author at length and in detail referred to the rare, undescribed, cancerous tumors of the breast, to the relative malignancy of the various breast cancers, to the frequency, significance and treatment of cancerous supraclavicular glands, after which he spoke in detail of the operations themselves as performed by him and his assistant.

DR. CHARLES B. NANCREDE of Ann Arbor said that he was impressed by the large number of cases of cancer of the breast occurring under thirty-five years of age, and that he had had a limited experience of between 200 and 300 cases. As an example, he cited the case of a young girl who was operated upon by him last winter, in the early part of her twenty-fifth year, and who unquestionably had the same tumor in her nineteenth year. He inquired if any one's experience coincided with his as to the large number of cases occurring under the age of thirty.

DR. ROSWELL PARK of Buffalo asked what Dr. Halsted's teachings were with regard to endothelioma.

DR. M. H. RICHARDSON of Boston spoke of the good work done by Dr. Halsted in the past on the above subject, and remarked that he had noticed and observed many cases where there had been no infection of the axillary glands. He referred to two cases in which he had made a diagnosis of a tumor merely upon the symptom of pain. He believed there was usually early recurrence of cases where the axillary glands were affected. In referring to the value of gross appearances he commented on a case where the microscopic appearance did not at all agree with the diagnosis although the clinical appearance proved its correctness. In his opinion he did not consider a case as cured in three years, as he had seen recurrences in from seven to ten years.

DR. J. D. BRYANT of New York stated that he had found enlarged glands in the axilla in some cases where the increase in size was not sufficient to warrant the belief that the glands were infected until a microscopic examination had been made. He strongly commented on the fact that patients possessing a morbid growth would not only keep the fact to themselves but were encouraged in so doing by their physicians.

DR. J. MCFADDEN GASTON of Atlanta spoke on the occasional spontaneous disappearance of carcinomatous formation, and concluded his remarks by inquiring if constitutional measures employed synchronously had been observed to have any effect.

DR. ROSWELL PARK continued his discussion by telling that he had for several years been collecting data on the subject of the spontaneous disappearance of tumors, and was quite anxious to get as much information as possible, and desired to hear different opinions expressed on the subject.

DR. RUDOLPH MATAS of New Orleans gave a full synopsis of twenty-seven cases operated upon for malignant disease of the breast or its immediate vicinity, which cases had come under his personal notice between the years of 1887 and 1898. All of these, with one exception, were in women, there were no fatalities from operative causes. Eleven of these patients are living and well, and there has been only three recurrences. In two cases death resulted from accidental causes not connected with the operation. In performing these operations two excisions were made, eight gross operations and seventeen complete (Halsted and Meyer) operations. One case which survived two years died finally from metastatic cancer of the uterus. The man operated upon is still living, eight years after the operation, and is free from local recurrence. The speaker then referred to fifteen complete operations performed since November, 1894, and spoke at length of the results bearing on all the details. In conclusion, he gave a history of five cases that are living without recurrences after complete operation.

DR. F. H. GERRISH of Portland, Maine, alluded to the excellent work done by Dr. Halsted, and referred to the fact that the text-books contain scarcely anything bearing on the subject of this paper. He then commented on the various operations that had been performed and showed how step by step the present method was arrived at. He considered as one of the most important points the necessity of the removal of all mammary tumors whether benign or malignant. He laid great emphasis upon the thoroughness with which operations should be performed and the length of time required to do them. After discussing the hopefulness of the prognosis in these cases at the present time, he referred to the fact that many cases alluded to in the author's paper would, until recent years, have been regarded as absolutely unfit for operation.

DR. HALSTED in closing said he had seen one case of cancer in a woman about twenty-eight or thirty years of age and one of cancer of the liver in a patient twenty-one years old. He was unable to give a very satisfactory answer to Dr. Park's inquiry as to the proper teaching regarding endotheliomata. He recalled one typical case of cancer of the breast and another of epithelioma of the face which had disappeared spontaneously.

DR. ROSWELL PARK of Buffalo then read a paper, entitled

AN INQUIRY INTO THE ETIOLOGY OF CANCER, WITH SOME REFERENCE TO THE LATEST INVESTIGATIONS OF THE ITALIAN PATHOLOGISTS.

He stated that to handle this problem successfully pathologists of the future must begin by studying tumor formation in the vegetable world, that is, the comparative method of investigation must be adopted. The xylomata or woody tumors are so exceedingly common that they have failed to attract the attention which they deserve.

The lipomata are the most frequent, often multiple, and usually symmetrical and of traumatic origin. The fibromata are usually of traumatic origin and the majority contain foreign bodies, which have acted as the exciting cause. Myofibroma of the uterus, according to Billroth, always commence by formation around a small blood-vessel. Chondroma is most common in infancy and childhood and is practically inseparable from rickets. Osteoma is often seen as an exostosis or as an ossification. Adenoma, as every surgeon knows, frequently becomes converted into carcinoma.

The only two theories worthy of consideration in reference to malignant tumors is the embryonal and parasitic. In the vegetable kingdom it is hard to distinguish between various grades of malignancy, nevertheless, that tumors kill a large proportion of trees and shrubs will not be disputed by those who have studied the subject. Cancer has been happily defined as an abortive attempt of an epithelium to reproduce itself and sarcoma is a similar process pertaining to mesoplastic cells. It used to be taught that cancer was confined to persons of more or less advanced ages, but the author stated that, living in a region where cancer is exceedingly prevalent, he had witnessed the ravages of the disease in many relatively young people. As to the influence of sex, Williams has found for every 100 males dying of cancer 223 females perish from the same disease. With regard to age the most prolific cancer-producing age is between fifty-five and sixty-five.

Williams has also found that at least among females the disease is twice as frequent in brunettes as in blondes, while Beddoe states that red-haired individuals are the most exempt of all. As to heredity opinions differ very much. Patients with large hearts and arteries but small lungs are often the subject of cancer, whereas in tuberculous patients the opposite is true. Speaking geographically cancer is certainly on the increase in certain parts of the world, and so true is this that the neighborhood of Buffalo, N. Y., has been termed the "tropic of cancer." The question has often risen as to whether cancer can be disseminated through the agency of insects and whether water, especially in the neighborhood of woods could act as a medium of transport, which is a belief at present conceded. Up to the present time experimental auto-inoculations have practically failed.

DR. J. MCFADDEN GASTON of Atlanta read a paper, entitled

REMEDIAL MEASURES IN OBSTRUCTION OF THE COMMON BILE DUCT.

He stated that although the physician usually treats and relieves cases of jaundice which result from the temporary closure or constriction of the common bile duct, yet these conditions are the precursors of derangements which frequently require the aid of a surgeon. Although at the beginning it may be only a functional disturbance the termination is usually in organic derangement.

He took up the subject of the treatment of jaundice by the use of pilocarpin upon which Murphy had laid such great stress, but he believed that the majority of practitioners relied more upon the use of the phosphate of soda. Very good results have followed the use of olive oil internally and probably this was the best remedy today. It was possible for a stenosis of the duct to exist, or a partial obstruction of its lumen, due to a gall-stone, without complete occlusion of the canal, so that a certain amount of bile would be able to pass. Fenger had demonstrated the possibility of a gall-stone being so located as to form a valvular closure, and though one may artificially provide a means of escape for the bile by opening the gall-bladder through the abdominal wall, yet relief to the cholemia is not always afforded and the condition may continue even to a fatal termination. He favors an incision an inch and a half below and on a line with the border of the costal cartilages in cases presenting no enlargement of the liver, which incision should be about three inches in length. It is not always possible to attach the gall-bladder to the edges of the parietal opening nor can one always suture the incision in the wall of the duct after the stone is extracted so that it is sometimes necessary to employ drainage and leave the ends of the gauze hanging out of the wound.

He had operated upon three white women for obstruction of the common bile duct, in which he made a fistulous opening for the bile externally, but the cholemia still persisted as long as the patient survived. Occasionally the attachment of the incised gall-bladder to the parietal opening, where there has been temporary impediment to the flow of bile through the duct, has relieved the obstruction and been followed later by restoration of the biliary flow. The author's experience has been that an artificial opening from the gall-bladder or the common duct into the alimentary canal has only been thought proper when other methods have failed to overcome complete occlusion of the duct.

Anastomosis may be effected with the duodenum or the small intestine, but the method with the colon which is sometimes employed is the least desirable of all. He then referred to his experiments upon dogs which demonstrated the feasibility of a fistulous communication of the gall-bladder with the bowel. From statistics he showed that the various methods are comparatively free from danger and are really attended with considerable success.

DR. H. W. CUSHING of Boston read a paper, entitled

TRAUMATIC RUPTURE OF THE PANCREAS; FORMATION OF HEMORRHAGIC CYST; OPERATION FOLLOWED BY A PANCREATIC FISTULA AND RECOVERY.

The rupture of the pancreas in this case was caused by a blow on the abdomen and was rapidly followed by the formation of a large pancreatic cyst closely resembling an abdominal aneurism. Five weeks after the injury the author evacuated the cyst through an incision in the abdominal wall and put in drainage. On the third day following the operation there was spontaneous evacuation of a subphrenic abscess through a bronchus, following which rapid improvement in the patient's condition was noted. Considerable pancreatic fluid escaped from the abdominal wound, the cyst rapidly became merely a small sinus and this healed seventy-seven days after the operation.

During the patient's convalescence the author took advantage of the rare opportunity to investigate the character of pancreatic fluid in the human subject. It was found to be strongly alkaline in reaction and was of a specific gravity of 1011 instead of 1030 as quoted by many authors. When this fluid came in contact with the epidermis it destroyed it, much to the patient's annoyance, but it did not effect the peritoneum or the granulation tissue. Upon measuring the amount of secretion it was found to vary from 5 to 60 cubic centimeters per hour, the maximum being during digestion. The total amount per day was quite double that generally stated by physiologists who claim about 300 cubic centimeters, whereas in this case it amounted to from 500 to 660 cubic centimeters.

The interesting features of this case were the peculiar character of the injury which caused the lesion, the difficulty of diagnosis, the complication of a double parotiditis, and its connection with the abdominal injuries, to say nothing of torticollis, a subphrenic abscess, and the exceptional opportunity afforded to investigate human pancreatic fluid. So far as the author knows on no previous occasion has the rate of flow and accurate measurement of this fluid been made. Fifteen months after the operation the patient was well and seemed none the worse for his experience.

DR. W. W. KEEN of Philadelphia referred to a case which came under his observation in which there was no wasting, no sugar in the urine, and no fatty stools. He inclined to the belief that simply opening and draining these cases was usually sufficient.

DR. HALSTED stated that he had seen four or five cases of pancreatic cysts.

DR. T. F. PREWITT of St. Louis referred to a case of enlarged spleen which he observed some fifteen years ago, and when operated upon a cyst of the pancreas was found connected with it. The woman made a perfect recovery. He also stated that he had seen a case which had lost much flesh while confined to bed for four months with a large tumor-like swelling in the median line. Upon opening this, much pus and fluid escaped and it was noted that the tumor extended to the backbone, making a counter-opening necessary. A calculus, believed to be of pancreatic origin, was found and removed and was probably the cause of the tumor.

DR. N. B. CARSON of St. Louis presented a paper, entitled

CEREBELLAR TUMORS.

He called attention to a much-neglected symptom in these cases, namely, the so-called "cranial cracked-pot sound." This sound is due to separation of the sutures from internal pressure caused by an accumulation of fluid in the brain cavities owing to pressure upon the veins of Galen. He had been able to elicit this sound in four cases but cautioned surgeons against mistaking it for certain high pitched sounds that are occasionally present in certain brain tumors. The sound, he claimed, may be present at any time of life before the sutures have become permanently united.

DR. KEEN mentioned a case in which this sound was first elicted by a patient himself when feeling his head one morning after having the night before fallen through the roof and fractured his skull. It was a valuable symptom and particularly where any doubt existed as to the fracture or the necessity for operation. He had observed hydrocephalus in the acquired form many times during the past few years. He did not believe it possible to get this sound where the edges of the bone had become separated, but he had seen a case where it was heard ten feet from the patient.

DR. DEFOREST WILLARD of Philadelphia referred to the case of a child less than one year old in which a cerebellar tumor was suspected and hydrocephalus was marked. Owing to the age of the child it was not supposed that the cracked-pot sound could be obtained. The rigidity of all the muscles of the body was very marked, and there was total lack of cerebral development.

DR. CARSON agreed with the speakers that it was only in cases of acquired hydrocephalus and extensive fracture of the skull that this sound could be elicted.

DR. W. W. KEEN of Philadelphia read a paper, entitled

A CASE OF APPENDICITIS IN WHICH THE APPENDIX BECAME PERMANENTLY ADHERENT TO THE BLADDER PRODUCING A URINARY FISTULA.

The case occurred in a young man twenty-four years of age from whose urethra, at the age of seven, a pin was removed, no history of the insertion of which could be obtained. Some years subsequent the patient suffered from a supposed abscess of the prostate from the spontaneous bursting of which a fecal fistula was established between the bladder and the rectum, and several attacks of cystitis followed. Numerous efforts were made to locate the two ends of the fistula, and the conclusion reached was that the rectal end was very near the surface. At the age of twenty-five years he was first operated on and a perineal section was done, but the fecal fistula still continued. The formation of an artificial anus was then decided upon, the result of which was not altogether satisfactory, fecal matter frequently passing into the bladder before any was passed out of the artificial anus, and after eating strawberries the seeds were found in the urine before they escaped from the anus. These facts seemed to indicate that the fistula was between the bladder and some point in the intestinal tract considerably above the site of the artificial anus. The third operation was consequently performed when a very long appendix was found dipping into the pelvis, the tip lying just behind the prostate and solidly incorporated in the wall of the bladder. A cuff of peritoneum was dissected from the appendix and used to cover the stump and the meso-appendix was then divided. The cecal end of the appendix was treated in the same way and the abdominal wall closed without anything being discovered in the way of a point of connection between the bladder and the bowel. Subsequently a fourth operation was performed to close the artificial anus and to destroy a spur which existed at the site of the anus so as to restore the entire caliber of the bowel. Shortly after leaving the hospital attacks of vomiting and constipation occurred, and twenty-four days after the last operation the patient died. At the necropsy, twenty-seven hours later, the one striking fact observable was the absolutely black color of the small intestines in the lower part of the abdomen, and an examination showed that seven or eight feet of the ileum had been rotated to the right in one vast volvulus. Its mesentery formed a band which stretched across the ileum just before it joined the cecum and this had evidently obstructed the ileum sufficiently to cause gangrene.

The diagnosis of a prostatic abscess was a very reasonable one as long as an appendix dipping into the pelvis and anchored by its meso-appendix immediately behind the bladder and the terminal appendical abscess so close to the prostate might well be mistaken for this condition. The possibility of the involvement of the appendix never occurred to those in attendance. Although appendicular abscesses bursting into the bladder are not at all uncommon, I know of no case in which the appendix has been so thoroughly united to the wall of the bladder as to form as it were a third ureter. While it may be said that a fifth operation in the form of an exploratory abdominal section should have been done the uncertainty of the diagnosis together with the fact that the patient had been operated on so much caused me to refrain.

DR. PARK mentioned two cases of pins in the urethra which had come under his observation and which he believed to have been swallowed, although there was no history in either case as to how the pins got there.

DR. CARSON had also found a pin in the urethra. In connection with Dr. Keen's case he also reported one in which a horseshoe-shaped appendix thirteen inches long had been found by him since.

DR. KEEN said that it was not at all unlikely that the pins in these cases were swallowed.

The rest of the papers on the program for this day were read by title.

THIRD DAY—MORNING SESSION.

This was devoted to council and executive sessions.

AFTERNOON SESSION.

DR. T. F. PREWITT of St. Louis read a paper, entitled

GUNSHOT INJURIES OF THE SPINE WITH REPORT OF A CASE.

A case illustrating this form of injury and resulting in recovery was described at great length by the author, who then referred to the writings of a number of prominent surgeons on the treatment of these conditions.

The author divided these injuries into three classes: (1) Those that simply fracture the arches, (2) those that invade the canal crushing the cord and damaging the vertebra, and (3) those complicated by serious injury to the abdominal or thoracic viscera. Details of cases with the result of treatment occurring in the practice were then given and the author stated that of forty-nine cases treated since the aseptic era twenty-four had been subjected to operation, resulting in eleven recoveries and thirteen deaths.

The author concluded his paper by stating that: (1) It is the duty of the surgeon to advise immediate operation in all cases of gunshot wound of the spine, provided the wound has involved the posterior or lateral parts of the spine at an accessible part, unless the condition of the patient is such as to indicate clearly that he is hopelessly crippled. (2) To wait to see whether Nature is competent to restore the damage is to wait until irreparable damage has been done in many cases and rapid degenerative changes, meningitis and myelitis, have resulted. The delay permits of the continuance of conditions the removal of which is the purpose of the operation. These considerations apply with greater force if possible in gunshot injuries than in others. (3) The presence of complications due to penetration of the great cavities and injury of the viscera will influence the question of operation but not necessarily forbid it.

DR. KEEN spoke in favor of operating for gunshot injuries of the spine in the absence of evidence of a total transverse lesion, the principal index of which would be the entire loss of the patellar reflexes. In looking up the question of the surgery of the spine some years ago he noted that although there were very few cases of suturing the spinal cord on record yet in no case did the result seem to be good.

DR. RICHARDSON expressed great hesitancy in operating on these cases on account of the difficulty of diagnosing the conditions present.

DR. BURRELL believed that the only way to arrive at a proper recognition of these cases was to first understand the pathologic condition existing in the cord and to do this all cases should be opened up and examined unless contraindicated by the presence of shock. He cited the case of a woman who died thirty-six hours after having jumped from a window, doubling the spine on itself and causing complete paralysis. At the autopsy it was noted that red softening had already begun although no compression of the cord was apparent. In his opinion this was evidence in favor of prompt operative interference for the removal of a clot, bullet, or fragment of bone.

He had presented a report to the British Medical Association in 1894 containing statistics on this subject which he divided into those extending from 1864 to 1886, and those from 1887 to 1894. The cases referred to in the first group were treated by immediate rectification of the deformity by force, and out of one hundred cases thus treated eighteen per cent. recovered. The second group contained those cases treated by immediate suspension and the use of a plaster-of-Paris jacket and as a result twenty-eight per cent. or an increase of ten per cent. recovered.

DR. CARSON was also of the opinion that there would be a considerable number of recoveries after operation. He referred briefly to an accident which happened to a man who, while trying to enter a low doorway riding on a load of hay, was caught by the neck and pulled forward, causing a complete dislocation of the spine followed by loss of sensation and paralysis of the bladder. He was immediately suspended with a Sayre's suspension-apparatus and by extension and counter-extension the dislocation was readily reduced. No sooner was this done than the patient immediately collapsed and lost consciousness, so that he had to be lowered at once and after being well padded was left alone. The further treatment consisted in the application of a plaster-of-Paris jacket. The patient made an excellent recovery.

DR. CONNER felt that it was well always to ascertain the exact character of the injury and remove any substance that might be pressing upon the cord, to do which he believed an operation both necessary and justifiable. The symptoms present in his opinion did not ordinarily act as an index to the real character of the lesion present. In spite of the fact that the mortality from operation would be considerable he believed it the preferable method of treatment.

DR. F. S. DENNIS of New York stated that he had published some time since a number of cases treated with the plaster-of-Paris jacket in which he obtained excellent results. A method which had found great favor with him was the administration of large doses of potassium iodid during the time the patient was wearing the plaster-of-Paris jacket as in his opinion this drug was of great benefit in absorbing the clot.

DR. CARSON continued his previous discussion by stating that he had been very well pleased with the results following the employment of the plaster-of-Paris jacket.

DR. CARMALT thought that in order to prevent infection in cases of gunshot wound one should operate without hesitation. He recalled, however, one case where operation was refused and the application of the plaster-of-Paris jacket brought about an excellent recovery. While in the second case presenting practically the same symptoms the same method of treatment was of no avail; the patient died in three days. He did not think surgeons were at present in a position to formulate any rules for the treatment of these injuries.

DR. BURRELL also continued the discussion by commenting on the cases reported by Drs. Carson and Carmalt, and stated that no doubt a reunion of the fibers of the cord by the formation of connective tissues often took place in cases of these injuries, this connective tissue subsequently undergoing absorption.

DR. HALSTED reported having bad one successful case of this kind in his experience. He agreed, however, in the main with what had already been said on this subject.

DR. PREWITT said that fractures of the kind referred to by Dr. Carson should be called simple fractures in the speaker's opinion especially as they oft times resulted from a displacement of the body of the vertebra itself. Pressure upon the cord can as well be caused by a dislocation as by a fracture and this is particularly true if there be a fracture of the lamina. He believed that gunshot wounds should always be considered as compound and local and considered that the inability to determine the method of procedure in these cases was due principally to the fact that one was not able to judge, from the symptoms present, what the exact condition of the cord was, thus making an operation necessary to determine this point. No harm could be done by opening up and disinfecting the wound, particularly when it has been proven that most of the cases die anyway. He was strongly in favor of giving the patient the benefit of whatever doubt might exist, especially as one might at least reduce the likelihood of meningitis, even though life might not be spared very long.

He drew especial attention to a case reported by Hawley of gunshot injury of the spine where the cause of death, which occurred 5½ years later, was due to irritation caused by a fragment of bone. He was confident of the opinion that this man's life could have been spared many years had an operation been performed at the time of the accident and the fragments removed.

With regard to the use of plaster-of-Paris jacket the author had been quite favorably impressed with the results obtained, and called attention to the statistics of Dr. Burrell. If, in cases of gunshot injury, one had good reason to believe that there was no pressure upon the cord, he would not urge immediate operative interference but he was of the opinion that in all these cases pressure, symptoms would be noted from the presence of spicules of bone and pieces of lead long after the accident. As stated by Erichsen, since little harm could be done by operation and a few cases would be rescued, the speaker believed operation advisable.

DR. JAMES E. MOORE of Minneapolis read a paper, entitled

HYSTERIA FROM A SURGICAL STANDPOINT.

Hysteria is so frequently met with in surgical cases that it is something one must always be looking for or grave errors in diagnosis and prognosis will result. Hysterical symptoms not infrequently occur as a complication of operation, while a rise of temperature after an operation may also be neurotic. To illustrate this fact, and also that persistent hiccough, cough, and emesis following anesthesia may be hysterical, a number of cases were cited in detail.

The author then referred to the peculiarities of some cases of phantom tumors and to one of hysterical aphonia following an operation on an adult male. He urged great care in operating, or even advising operation, upon neurotic females in whom the subjective symptoms are often out of all proportion to the objective, especially as these women not only are often willing to submit to grave surgical operations when their sufferings are entirely imaginary, but because they not infrequently derive considerable morbid pleasure from the procedure. In his opinion the osteopaths and Christian scientists rather than a surgeon should undertake the treatment of these cases.

The most skilled diagnosticians will often be misled by the mingling of real diseases with hysterical hyperesthesia, anesthesia, paresis, and seemingly complete paralysia. As a valuable aid to diagnosis the author referred to Patrick's method of diagnosticating hysterical hyperesthesia or anesthesia by means of the shifting border of the affected area. The surgeon most frequently meets with hysteria in joint and spinal ailments and a surgeon should always remember to avoid mistakes in diagnosis and prognosis in the case of hysterical joints, as they bear such a close resemblance to joints, the seat of disease. These hysterical joints often follow an injury and there will be slight atrophy but no local rise of temperature, in fact the temperature may be subnormal, no marked swelling but slight puffiness may be noted. There is usually marked restriction of motion which is voluntary in character however, and readily overcome when the patient's attention is directed to something else. The muscular spasm in these cases is more pronounced and different in character from that in tuberculosis and the deformty is often exaggerated and differs considerably from that which is present in disease. Hysterical joints are o course most prominent in hysterical persons, but have been observed in persons not in any way hysterical. The prognosis in the case of a hysterical joint is good and it is very rare that organic changes occur.

The author then dwelt at great length upon various valuable means of treating these conditions, among other correction under anesthesia, but did not consider any cutting operation necessary. Hysterical patients he observed may develop a tubercular joint, but changes in the cord do not occur from hysteria and besides, hysterical spine is easily diagnosticated as it bears no resemblance whatever to deformity as a result of disease.

The following officers were elected for the coming year:

President, Dr. W. W. Keen of Philadelphia.
First Vice-president, Dr. A. Vandeveer of Albany.
Second Vice-president Dr. C. H. Mastin of Mobile.
Secretary, Dr. H. L. Burrell of Boston.
Recorder, Dr. DeForest Willard of Philadelphia.

Treasurer, Dr. G. R. Fowler of Brooklyn.

Delegate to the Association of American Physicians and Surgeons, Dr. Wm. M. Mastin; Alternate, Dr. F. H. Gerrish of Portland, Maine.

Place of next meeting, Chicago, Ill.; date to be determined later.

REVIEWS.

TRAITÉ DE MÉDICINE ET DE THERAPEUTIQUE. Par P. BRONARDEL et A. GILBERT. Tome, 4me. Paris: J. B. Bailliere et fils, 1897.

THIS volume of the system of medicine, edited by Bronardel and Gilbert, deals with the diseases of the digestive tract and of the peritoneum. While in the main the articles are carefully written and show scientific research, there is very little uniformity in the method of treatment. This fault is, of course, to be ascribed to be a necessary consequence of system works. While some of the authors show a fair acquaintance with general scientific literature, a few show a wonderful lack of this, especially of work done by English and German writers.

Worthy of praise are the chapters on diseases of the stomach by Hayem and Lion, diseases of the intestine by Galliard, although the article on appendicitis in this chapter is quite primitive. Duprés chapter on the diseases of the peritoneum is classic and deserves special recognition, not only for the careful and painstaking historic introduction, but for the amount of critical observation and clinical experience which he brings to bear upon his work.

CONSTIPATION IN ADULTS AND CHILDREN; with Special Reference to Habitual Constipation and Its Most Successful Treatment by the Mechanical Methods. By H. ILLOWAY, M.D. New York: The Macmillan Co., 1897.

TO write a book of 500 pages with over 100 illustrations upon the commonplace subject of constipation, may appear to many as a waste of paper; but certainly, no one who carefully reads what the author has to say upon his subject will find fault with him for saying too much. Evidently there has been no attempt to condense the material, and cases are cited and illustrations used with the greatest freedom; but the end aimed at is accomplished, and the reader will lay down this interesting book with a much wider knowledge of the physiology and pathology of defecation than he ever possessed before. The treatment of constipation in the adult due to atony, occupies about one-fifth of the entire work, and in the chapters devoted to it are given in detail the various movements recommended by different masseurs to restore the normal peristaltic motion of the bowels. Some of these are decidedly fanciful, and at the close of this part of the subject the author himself says: "It will, of course, be readily understood that all the manipulations here described are not needed in all cases. . . . However, the physician—and I hold that massage is as much his province as the setting of a fracture or the application of electricity—should familiarize himself with most and, if possible, with all of the manipulations here described, and be prepared to make them. . . . With massage, just as with medicine, in chronic cases, a change from time to time in form and mode of administration is of the greatest advantage."

At the beginning three treatments a week are advised, and after six weeks or a longer time if need be, the number is gradually reduced. Swedish movements, both free and resisted, passive movements, hydrotherapy, and electricity are also described in detail.

The book is an eminently practical one, and ought to assist physicians to cure constipation by removing its cause. By reason of the profuse illustrations, it is easy to understand the performance of the different movements of massage and gymnastics recommended.

THERAPEUTIC HINTS.

Antineuralgic Powders.—

℞	Quininæ hydrobrom.		grs. xv
	Ext. nucis vom.		grs. iii
	Phenacetin	aa	grs. vi.
	Exalgin		
	Pulv. ipecac. et opii		

M. Ft. pulv. No. VI. Sig. Two powders a day before meals.

For Chilblains.—

℞	Sodii boratis	ʒ iss
	Glyceriti amyli	℥ i.

M. Sig. Inunction, apply after soaking the feet in hot water.

Formula for a Diuretic Powder.—

℞	Pulv. digitalis	aa	grs. xv
	Pulv. scillæ		
	Potass. nitratis		ʒ iiss.

M. Div. in pulv. No. XX. Sig. Four to six powders a day, to be taken in cachets.

An Antiseptic Dentifrice.—

℞	Ac. carbolici.	grs. vii
	Ac. borici	ʒ iiss
	Thymol	grs. iv
	Ol. menth. pip.	gtt. x
	Tinct. anisi	ʒ iiss
	Aquæ	Oi.

M. Sig. Dilute with equal parts of water.

For Asthma.—

℞	Sodii iodidi	aa	℥ iss–ʒ iii
	Tinct. Stramonii		
	Ext. glycyrrhizæ		ʒ i
	Syr. scillæ		℥ i
	Aquæ dest.		℥ viii.

M. Sig. One tablespoonful three or four times a day.

Destruction of Vulvar Papillomata.—MENCIERE advises the employment of flexible collodion containing forty to fifty per cent. of salicylic acid. A few drops are daily applied, at first to six or eight of the growths, the treatment being extended to all and continued until the cure is completed. It is claimed that this occurs within a fortnight, and that no cicatrix remains.

THE MEDICAL NEWS.

A WEEKLY JOURNAL OF MEDICAL SCIENCE.

VOL. LXXII. NEW YORK, SATURDAY, MAY 14, 1898. NO. 20.

ORIGINAL ARTICLES.

X-RAY IN MEDICINE.[1]

BY FRANCIS H. WILLIAMS, M.D.,
OF BOSTON.

THE X-rays as a means of studying anatomy, physiology, and pathology in the living body have many sides, but we, as practitioners, are chiefly concerned with what may directly promote the welfare of our patients. From our point of view, then, this new means may be considered simply as a method of examination, and it is my privilege to-day to briefly indicate to you some of the ways in which it may be of service to physicians, in contradistinction to surgeons. It is chiefly adapted to certain lines of study, and its limitations are drawn by pathologic conditions which involve a change in shape, as in cardiac enlargement; in chemic compositiou, as in rickets and calculi; or in density, as in pneumonia. I shall limit myself to a few words in regard to the method of making examinations and then take up, by way of illustration, some of the diseases in which they most readily find their application.

The apparatus required in making medical X-ray examinations is as yet expensive and difficult to manage. It should be of the best, and furnish a steady light, neither too strong nor too weak, and of a quality to differentiate well between different tissues, that is, adipose tissue, muscles, and tendons. It is important to be able to vary the intensity of the light while looking in the fluoroscope.[2]

The examination may be conducted with the patient in any position. Hospital patients who are too ill to sit or stand may be placed upon a stretcher and carried to the X-ray room. The stretcher may then be placed upon suitable supports and an examination made without disturbing the patient. In private practice, if the patient is too ill to come to my office, I send a portable X-ray apparatus to the house. The room should be darkened and the physician be careful to wait five or ten minutes in the dark room, or else wear dark smoked glasses a few minutes (if in the daytime) before making the examination, in order that his retinæ may be in a condition to use the fluoroscope. The tube should be placed below the stretcher, under the mid-sternum, on a level with the fourth rib and two feet or more from the patient; it should be brought to its exact position by plumb lines. The outlines, as seen in the fluoroscope, may be recorded by first dotting and then drawing them on the skin with a crayon[1] opaque to the rays, but the physician must bear in mind that the skin may be moved either by the crayon or by the movements in respiration or by changes in the position of the patient. These lines may be traced on tracing-cloth, or they may be measured off and transferred to a chart.

Among the scores of thousands of examinations which have already been made with this new agent by persons necessarily inexperienced it is not surprising that in some instances harmful effects have followed; but the number of such effects is so small, when all the circumstances are taken into consideration, as to prove that with the better knowledge furnished by experience, the rays are practically harmless. Untoward results from X-ray examinations are, I believe, unnecessary, and entirely avoidable. I have never seen any inconvenience follow their use in the more than one thousand examinations that I have made.

Among the many ways in which the X-rays assist us is that demonstrated by Dr. Fisk of New York, who has shown how gouty deposits may be recognized by an X-ray skiagraph; he has also pointed out that a differential diagnosis may be made between a gouty and a rheumatic process.

Examination of the Heart in Health.—The best view of this organ is obtained during full inspiration, as then the diaphragm is so depressed as to allow the apex to be seen; in some persons the heart is depressed during full inspiration about one inch and pushed toward the right so that the right ventricle may in some cases be indicated on the right side of the sternum. In expiration, the outlines of the heart are not so complete, as the diaphragm is then higher. The apex beat, as felt, does not always

[1] Read by invitation at the Ninety-Second Annual Meeting of the New York State Medical Society, January 25, 1898.

[2] This may be done with the static machine, by varying the length of the spark-gap or the speed of the machine; with the coil, by varying the spark-gap, changing the speed of the commutator, or using more or less condenser. I some time ago devised adjustments for thus varying the intensity of the light and have found them a necessary part of the apparatus. I have also arranged a brush for the commutator of the coil so that it now requires little or no attention. The static machine and the coil were devised by Messrs. C. L. Norton and R. R. Lawrence of the Massachusetts Institute of Technology and they are made by E. S. Ritchie & Sons, Brookline, Mass.

[1] This crayon is made by mixing vaselin with some heavy powder such as bismuth or oxid of lead, or mercury and a little lampblack; is about one-eighth of an inch in diameter, and covered with paper to give it stiffness.

correspond to the apex of the heart as seen in the fluoroscope; by means of this instrument we see that it is sometimes lower. On the left side of the sternum the outlines of the ventricles and the pulmonary artery may be seen; on the right side, what is seen depends upon the excellence of the apparatus and also upon the individual examined. Under favorable conditions both the right auricle and the border of the right ventricle are visible.

In disease the fluoroscope enables us to get a much more complete outline of the heart than can be obtained by auscultation and percussion, and even in size of the right auricle may frequently be estimated. In cardiac hypertrophy and dilatation the size and position of the heart may be more fully obtained with the fluoroscope than by any other means. The left border of the heart may sometimes extend beyond the nipple and approach so near the left wall of the chest that percussion gives an area of dulness, reaching, for example, to the anterior axillary line, whereas the fluoroscope may show that the heart is not so enlarged as the former method of examination seemed to demonstrate. The exaggerated idea of size, in such a case, is due to the fact that the heart

FIG. 1.

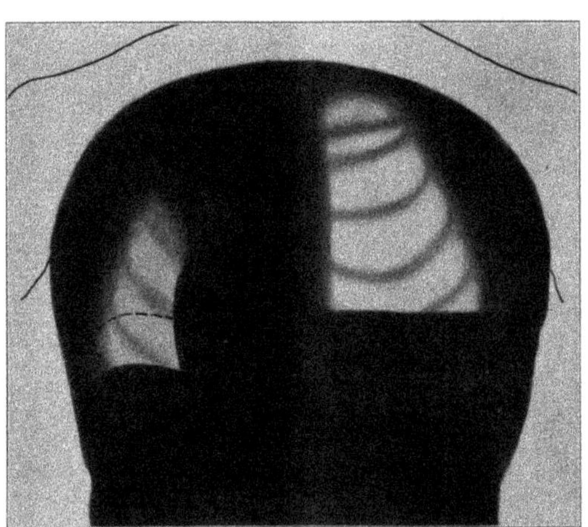

Diagram illustrating the appearances seen in the fluoroscope in a patient with tuberculosis on the right side and pneumohydrothorax or pneumopyothorax on the left side.

The right side is encroached upon by the displaced heart and by the dense tuberculous process at the top of the lung; the excursion of the diaphragm between expiration and inspiration is less than normal (the broken line indicates its position in expiration).

On the left side the appearances, when the patient is examined in a sitting position, remind one of a tumbler partly filled with ink. If the patient bends backward or forward the height of the fluid on the chest-wall changes; if to the left the beating heart is exposed to view; if the patient is shaken gently the surface of the fluid is seen to be agitated; it is also seen to be disturbed by the pulsations of the heart.

This diagram is made clearer by a comparison with Fig. 2, which illustrates the appearances seen in the fluoroscope in a normal chest.

health, although the difference here is not so marked, the advantage is with the fluoroscope. The size of the heart in disease is an important element in estimating its condition, and guides us in prognosis and treatment. It is not necessary to emphasize the cardinal value of this knowledge in cardiac disease. The fluoroscope enables us to determine the position of the left and usually the right border of the heart, whereas by percussion, in some patients, the heart may seem to be either larger or smaller than it is. By means of the fluoroscope the is so abnormally near the left wall of the chest that by percussion its lateral is not distinguished from its anterior portion. We may even obtain a better knowledge of the size of a distended heart by means of the fluoroscope than by an autopsy. If we look through the body from side to side, on a level with the diaphragm, during full inspiration, we see a light area triangular in shape, the lower side of which is bounded by the diaphragm, the anterior by the heart, and the posterior, which is less defined, by the spine. It is by means of this area, if the lungs are normal, that we are able to get a view behind the heart and between it and the spine, and this area will be found to vary in size under different conditions. With an enlarged heart it may be much smaller, or it may be nearly or quite obliterated. Enlargements of the heart may be detected not only by observing the right and left borders, but also by seeing the posterior and lower borders; a collection of pus or a growth behind the ventricles or a pericardial effusion, for example, would also alter the appearance of or obliterate this area. The whole of the anterior border of the heart, as well as of the posterior border, may also be made out in a few individuals when looking through the body from side to side.

ample, can sometimes be seen in the fluoroscope in this disease.

Displacement of the heart when there is pleuritic effusion, especially when the effusion is on the left side and the heart therefore displaced to the right, is readily seen in the fluoroscope, when often it is not demonstrated by means of percussion. In pleurisy of the left side with effusion, or when the heart is enlarged, the outlines of the right ventricle may be seen much to the right of the sternum. A dilated right auricle, especially in emphysema, may also be distinguished. In one patient during convalescence from pneumonia, the heart was adherent in such a way that the apex was tilted up at each full inspi-

Fig. 2.

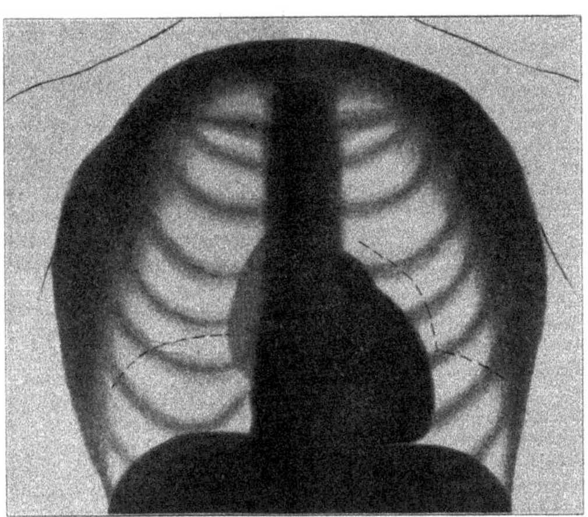

Cut showing the heart and diaphragm of normal chest as seen in the fluoroscope during full inspiration. The broken lines show position of heart and diaphragm in expiration.

In a much-dilated heart we can see that its volume is made smaller by deep inspiration, which shows that it is capable of being compressed by a forced inspiration. In a few cases we may thus be assisted to distinguish between a heart which is simply dilated and one which is hypertrophied. Enlargement of the heart in arteriosclerosis may be detected, as may also the unnaturally small heart which obtains in certain conditions. We may also find evidence of changes in the arteries in arteriosclerosis. I have taken an X-ray photograph which shows normal arteries, and those in arteriosclerosis are, of course, even more easily skiagraphed; the radial arteries, for ex-

ration instead of being forced downward.

The fluoroscope cannot always be employed to ascertain the size and position of the heart, as it requires for its use that the neighboring lungs be in a fairly healthy condition, otherwise these organs are less permeable by the rays and do not furnish the contrast with the more solid heart which is necessary in order that it may be brought clearly into view. As we shall see later, fluid in the pleural cavity or a dense lung may partly or even wholly obscure some of the cardiac outlines as well as displace the heart. The condition of the lungs may hide that of the heart in so far as it is obtained by direct view with the fluoroscope, but on the other hand the condition of the lungs may be an indication of disease of the heart, or of the kidneys. If the circulation of the lungs is such as to cause a passive congestion or edema, it is difficult for the rays to pass through them, and we find the pulmonary areas darker than usual. The practical value of this information may be illustrated by one or two cases.

CASE I.—A. B., was thought by his physician to be suffering from emphysema of the lungs consequent upon asthma, to which he had been subject for sixteen years. There was much dyspnea. I made an X-ray examination which showed that the lungs were darkened by passive congestion, or edema, and the heart enlarged. Auscultation indicated a mitral lesion. I advised rest, together with digitalis in suitably large doses. This treatment was soon followed by improvement and the disappearance of the dyspnea.

CASE II.—C. D., had chronic interstitial nephritis, but he was able to be at his business every day. An X-ray examination showed an opacity of the lungs due to edema, which suggested that the patient was in a more critical condition than had been indicated by any other sign or symptom and he was therefore cautioned to put his affairs in order and thus given an opportunity to advantage his family by many thousands of dollars. He suddenly died within two months.

In certain cardiac diseases we are now able to follow the improvement of the patient not only by the disappearance of the dyspnea, but also by watching the lungs in the fluoroscope and observing them gradually grow clearer and clearer, and sometimes, also, by seeing that the enlarged heart has become reduced in size.

Pericardial effusion may be recognized with the fluoroscope more certainly and readily than hitherto, and the outlines of the pericardial sac, when drawn on the chest, make an excellent guide when tapping the pericardium, should such a procedure be necessary.

Thoracic aneurism was among the earliest diseases recognized by the medical use of the X-ray, and now, an X-ray examination is the accepted way of making or confirming the diagnosis of this disease. Often an aneurism of the thoracic aorta may not be recognized in its early stages by ordinary means of examination and may be overlooked by several excellent diagnosticians; also, a very large aneurism may give no definite physical signs. In this connection the following case is of interest.

CASE III.—M. C., was thought by his physician to be suffering from a stricture of the esophagus, and a bougie had been passed every third day for several months. Three weeks before he was sent to me for an X-ray examination the bougie was not used and the symptoms improved. The X-ray examination showed that he had a small aneurism of the thoracic aorta.

Let us now briefly consider some of the applications of the X-ray in diseases of the chest other than those of the heart and aorta. In health the lungs are readily traversed by the ray and they appear in the fluoroscope as light areas on either side of the backbone and the heart. The lower portion of the lungs, bounded by the diaphragm, is seen to move up and down through a distance of about half an inch during quiet breathing, and to descend during full inspiration to a point about two and one-half inches below its level in expiration. There are three principal ways in which the fluoroscope may lead us to suspect disease in the chest: (1) The appearance of the dark areas which occur in tuberculosis, pneumonia, carcinoma, diaphragmatic hernia, gangrene of the lungs, and in echinococcus cyst, infarction, pleurisy, empyema, etc., due to the increase in density, which, by obstructing the passage of the ray, diminishes the normal brightness in the chest or changes its normal outlines; (2) the occurrence of abnormal brightness which is found in emphysema and pneumothorax consequent upon decrease in density, which makes the lung area appear lighter than in health as seen in the fluoroscope; (3) the restriction of the maximum excursion of the diaphragm and its altered position and curve from that observed in health.

The fluoroscope shows that certain changes are characteristic of special diseases. For example, in tuberculosis I observed nearly two years ago[1] that the consolidated portion of the lung appeared darker than normal in the fluoroscope; this consolidation usually beginning at the apex of one lung, The expansion of the lung is also reduced, either by changes in itself or in the pleura, and therefore the excursion of the diaphragm downward is diminished during full inspiration, but this muscle is carried up into the thorax as high, or it may be even higher than in health. If a patient with tuberculosis is examined from time to time with the fluoroscope the pictures presented are usually as follows: (1) The apex or one lung is darker, as already stated; the clavicle and upper ribs are less marked on the diseased than on the normal side; the darker area extends more and more as the disease progresses, and finally may cover nearly all the space occupied by one lung, so that no ribs or other outlines are seen on the affected side. Before this latter condition develops the apex of the other lung begins to darken and this area continues to extend. The diminishing excursion of the diaphragm, which is also a characteristic feature of this

[1] See "Notes on X-Rays in Medicine." *Transactions of the Association of American Physicians*, April, 1896.

disease, may likewise be observed, and sometimes may be the earliest sign of an abnormal condition of the lung. In this connection the following case is of interest:

CASE IV.—B. F., a woman forty-six years old, with bronchitis, was a patient in my service at the Boston City Hospital in February, 1897. The only evidence of other disease of the lung was the diminished excursion of the diaphragm. This moved only one and a quarter inches on the *left side* (which is much less than normal, and was higher in the chest than in health), but full two inches on the right side. She was discharged from the hospital March 4, 1897, but was readmitted into another service during December of the same year. At this time the signs on auscultation and percussion were indefinite, but bacilli were present in the sputum; on January 5th, 1898, I examined her again with the fluoroscope, which showed that the whole *left* apex, and to a less extent the right apex, was darker than normal and that the excursion of the diaphragm on the *left side* was less than half an inch, and on the right side one and one-quarter inches.

In some cases it is possible by means of the fluoroscope to anticipate, especially in acute tuberculosis, the knowledge gained later by auscultation and percussion, and also, to better appreciate the amount of lung-tissue involved in the different stages of the disease. I have detected signs of tuberculosis in the lungs by means of the fluoroscope after a physical examination had failed to show them. In cases in which the suspicions of the practitioner are aroused by the first examination, a second one should be made, after an interval, to verify or disprove the first.

It is essential in tuberculosis to use every possible means to determine the condition of the lungs in order to decide upon the course the patient should pursue, and, by the aid of the information obtained from the fluoroscope, a long and costly journey in a fruitless search for health may, in some cases, be avoided—that is to say, we may find by means of the fluoroscope that the lungs are more diseased than the usual physical examination indicate; or, on the other hand, we may detect, it is too soon to say in what proportion of cases, an abnormal condition of the lungs before it is suggested in any other way and so early that the best opportunity for arresting the disease is afforded. It is unnecessary to emphasize the value of early recognition in a disease often so amenable to treatment in the beginning. I advise young adults with a tubercular family history to have an X-ray examination from time to time, or immediately if they are out of condition. In other papers[1] I have discussed at length the appearances seen in the fluoroscope in pulmonary tuberculosis, and therefore will not go further into detail here.

In pneumonia the affected areas are easily recognized in the fluoroscope, and in a central pneumonia, may be seen when auscultation and percussion do not reveal them. The excursion of the diaphragm is also restricted, and the heart may be much displaced to the right, if the pneumonia is only on the left side. As the patient improves the dark areas are seen to disappear and the movement of the diaphragm to lengthen. A diminished respiratory movement and areas darker than normal may be seen after an abnormal condition of the lungs ceases to be detected by auscultation and percussion. An empyema, as is well known, may follow pneumonia, but may be overlooked for some time; we can, however, find evidence of its presence by means of the X-ray. The pleuritic effusion which sometimes accompanies pneumonia may be suspected in a given case and yet proved not to exist if a bright area and the outline of the diaphragm below the dark pneumonic portion are visible in the fluoroscope.

In pleurisy with effusion, or in empyema, the outlines of the lower part of the chest are dulled or obliterated, especially the diaphragm line. If the effusion is large, the whole chest is dark, and the heart and mediastinum are displaced. In a circumscribed pleurisy or empyema an exploring needle may fail to reach the desired spot, but we may sometimes, by means of the fluoroscope, exactly outline the limits of the fluid. In one patient I drew such an outline, and its correctness was confirmed at the autopsy.

If the lungs are less dense than normal, as in emphysema, the area is brighter than in health and the distended lung or lungs may reach lower in the chest than normal. The maximum excursion of the diaphragm is much less than in health, as this muscle does not rise so high in expiration. These two signs are characteristic of emphysema, and in the later stages the enlarged ventricles and also the dilated right auricle are seen; the heart also lies in a more vertical direction and its position is not much changed by a deep inspiration. In young people, especially, an emphysema may be overlooked on auscultation and percussion, but is readily detected in the fluoroscope. I recall a girl of fifteen years who had dyspnea on exertion, the result of an emphysema. An appreciation of this condition was obtained only by an X-ray examination. On the other hand, the fluoroscope may show that there is little emphysema when auscultation and percussion suggests that it is present to a considerable degree.

In pneumothorax, the diaphragm is very low, loses its normal curve and movement on the affected side,

[1] "A Study of the Adaptation of the X-rays to Medical Practice," *Medical and Surgical Reports of the Boston City Hospital*, January, 1897. "The Röntgen-Rays in Thoracic Diseases," *American Journal of the Medical Sciences*, December, 1897.

and the heart and mediastinum are seen to be displaced to the healthy side. The fluoroscope is also useful in pneumohydrothorax when the patient is examined sitting up. (See Fig. 1 and Fig. 2.)

It is unnecessary to further refer to special diseases; it is obvious that certain pathologic conditions involving change in density will make the lungs more or less opaque to the X-ray. It is of interest, in passing, to note that even in health the brightness of the pulmonary area varies. It is lighter in deep inspiration than during expiration. There must, therefore, be more blood in the lungs at certain stages of respiration than at others. Further, not all persons have the same pulmonary brightness. It is less in a stout, muscular man than in a thin man. We can learn to make allowances for these differences in individuals as we do in percussion, and further we usually have an opportunity to compare a healthy with a diseased side.

In the following four cases, the only ones in which both an X-ray and a post-mortem examination were made at the Boston City Hospital, there was complete correspondence between my X-ray examination and the autopsy, which occurred not long after:

CASE V.—G. H., was a young man whose lungs, as seen in the fluoroscope, were normal; the post-mortem gave the same result. It was interesting to note that the heart in death was somewhat higher than in life, and did not extend so far to the right.

CASE VI.—P. C., a patient with pneumonia. Both the fluoroscope and the autopsy showed that the whole of the right upper lobe and a portion of the middle lobe were involved.

CASE VII.—D. F.; this patient had an old encysted pleurisy extending vertically along the outer wall of the left chest from the third to the ninth rib. These outlines seen in the fluoroscope, and drawn on the skin, corresponded with what was found at the autopsy.

CASE VIII.—J. K., a patient with arteriosclerosis; observations and tracings made by means of the fluoroscope showed dark areas to the right of the sternum, and at the post-mortem a calcification in the aorta near the heart was found.[1]

The abdomen is a more difficult field for exploration, and nothing is seen as clearly there as in the thorax. The outline of the liver and of the spleen may be followed. I have also seen the outline of the lower portion of the left kidney.

Improved apparatus will doubtless enlarge the field of usefulness of this method of examination. Among recent improvements is a Crookes' tube in which the platinum is kept cool by a stream of water running through the hollow anode, which makes it practicable to use a light of far greater penetrating power than has hitherto been possible. This is the invention of Dr. William H. Rollins of Boston, and is only one among several excellent improvements made by him in the course of his investigation of X-ray tubes. Another is his method of lowering the vacuum after it has become too high by the continued use of the tube.[1] Dr. Rollins has also invented another appliance for surgical purposes. This is an aluminum camera, and consists essentially of an aluminum tube in the interior of which is a photographic film. The metal protects the film from light and moisture and yet allows the passage of the rays. Such an instrument may be put into any cavity of the body, for instance, the rectum, and then an X-ray photograph may be taken of a phosphatic calculus in the bladder.

In employing X-ray examinations; as in auscultation and percussion, many cases must be studied in order to recognize the conditions presented, and it is obvious that this method of examination is not so easily carried out as most others. It would be well, however, for the students in all our medical schools to be familiarized with the appearances of the chest as seen in the fluoroscope, while studying auscultation and percussion, for there is much that after having been demonstrated by both this instrument and the latter method will later be recognized more easily by auscultation and percussion alone. The eye having assisted the ear to make a more complete picture of certain conditions, the physician is enabled to get a better idea of these conditions in cases in which, for lack of an X-ray apparatus, he must use the ear alone. Further, the X-ray examination will teach him to better appreciate the limitations of auscultation and percussion as well as to interpret more correctly the information derived from them. X-ray examinations will be found useful to life-insurance companies.

In making a diagnosis, physicians will find that although much that the X-ray reveals can be recognized by other means it would often be an advantage to have this information confirmed by another method, and we must also appreciate that it can extend our knowledge into a field which was previously beyond our reach. A diagnosis may be made by an X-ray examination alone in certain cases, as in aneurism, emphysema, and pneumothorax, and in a few cases by it alone, but as a rule it is only one method and should be used in connection with others. The fluoroscope and stethoscope, for instance, supplement

[1] Since this paper was read a post-mortem has been made of a patient who died twenty-four hours after his admission to the hospital. He was not examined by the X-ray, but the autopsy showed how serviceable this examination would have been in prognosis. The patient was forty years old, had pneumonia of the whole of the upper left lobe, emphysema of the lungs, and a right auricle that was then so distended as to be equal in size to the ventricles. The pneumonia would have appeared in the fluoroscope as a very dark area, and in contrast with the bright emphysematous right lung, the right auricle would have been most conspicuous.

[1] These appliances are made by Kirmayer & Oelling, Bromfield street, Boston, Mass.

each other. X-ray examinations, in suitable cases, give earlier evidence of disease than the older methods. I daily find them indispensable in making a complete examination of patients who may have a disease of the chest, and can by them determine in some cases the presence of an abnormal condition, or more fortunately its absence, or sometimes completely change the diagnosis which had been previously made.

The X-ray is still too recent a discovery to have reached the limit of its usefulness, and its application in medicine deserves and will repay careful study.

TUBERCULOSIS OF THE UPPER AIR-PASSAGES.[1]

BY EMIL MAYER, M.D.,
OF NEW YORK;
ATTENDING SURGEON TO THE NEW YORK EYE AND EAR INFIRMARY (THROAT DEPARTMENT); INSTRUCTOR IN LARYNGOLOGY IN THE NEW YORK POLYCLINIC.

THE short time at my disposal for the presentation of so exhaustive a subject must be my excuse for brevity on many points which would ordinarily require detailed and elaborate description.

Tuberculosis of the upper air-passages may be either primary or secondary. In the primary forms the disease is presented either as an ulcerative or a hyperplastic process. These may be differentiated from lupus and syphilis by the presence of numerous bacilli, and, clinically, by the history.

Although many maintain that the presence of tuberculous disease of the air-passages is coincident with acute miliary tuberculosis, yet cases of primary lesion have been reported in which pulmonary tuberculosis supervened two years after the local manifestations. The early diagnosis of the primary disease in the nose, as also in the pharynx and larynx, is of inestimable value when we consider that thus we may prepare for the coming storm, and with eternal vigilance as to habits of life, great care in the selection of nutritious food, and salubrious climatic influences, postpone the evil day when the system will be overwhelmed, or, still more happily, avert it altogether.

Nasal Tuberculosis.—Tuberculosis of the nasal passages is very rare indeed. It may be primary or secondary. In the former variety, persistent ulcers, bleeding upon the slightest touch, may be present, or there may be hyperplasia. The latter form occurs usually from the septum, the floor of the nose, or upon the turbinates. They may have irregular surfaces and vary from four to ten millimeters in diameter. Their nature is readily determined by microscopic examination.

By far the most frequent condition of the two is the secondary variety. In this, the diagnosis of pulmonary tuberculosis having been made, nasal ulcerations and hyperplasiæ are promptly recognized as existing from the conditions that are present. In both forms the symptoms are the same: Excessive secretion, the formation of tenacious crusts, the removal of which is followed by some hemorrhage, or a degree of nasal stenosis may be present. Pain is usually absent. The treatment consists in the thorough removal of all crusts by means of alkalin sprays, or by a solution of eucalyptol or menthol in albolene, and wiping with pledgets of absorbent cotton, after which an application, under cocain, of a fifty-per-cent. lactic-acid solution may be made. An insufflation of powdered iodoform or of nosophen is of value. New growths are best removed with a cold wire-snare, and their bases should be thoroughly cauterized with the galvanocautery under cocain anesthesia. If treatment of this kind be instituted early in the primary forms of the disease the prognosis is apt to be better than in any other tuberculous manifestation in the upper air-passages.

In the secondary forms of the disease only such treatment can be instituted as will add to the patient's comfort.

Pharyngeal Tuberculosis.—It is worthy of note that microscopic examinations of the lymphoid tissue, commonly called adenoids, removed from the vault of the pharynx have demonstrated the presence of the tubercle bacillus in quite a few instances. Such a microscopic finding is, of course, an indication for careful observation and attention. In about one per cent. of all cases of tuberculous laryngitis there are pharyngeal symptoms. This form of tuberculosis also occurs primarily. Thus, cases are cited in which a single tuberculous ulcer was found on the tonsil; still, the disease is very rare in this location. The velum and soft palate are most apt to be affected, and under such circumstances a number of minute gray nodules, which eventually break down and ulcerate, are found in these parts.

The chief symptom of pharyngeal tuberculosis, secondary to the disease in the larynx, is pain, usually extending to the ear. No pain is so constant or so distressing as this. The suffering becomes very acute, the agony is pitiful, the patient refuses food, there is constant rasping to avoid swallowing the abundant saliva, and the physician hastens to relieve the symptoms with every means at his command. An examination readily reveals the condition. The uvula is usually intensely swollen and edematous, and, covering the whole of the soft palate, the faucial pillars, and the tonsils are grayish sloughs in separate patches. The surrounding local

[1] Read at a meeting of the Harlem Medical Association, March 14, 1898.

anemia aids in differentiating it from syphilis, as does the absence of great destruction. It is more difficult to differentiate from lupus, however, but here the microscope will show abundant tubercle bacilli in the tuberculous cases, only a very few being found in lupus.

The *treatment* must be heroic. There is no chance for recovery, and the physician must be sufficiently humane to liberally administer one of the more powerful anodynes, irrespective of the fear of the patient's becoming addicted to drug-habits. Morphin, in combination with cocain, freely given every hour, with cocain sprays used before deglutition, the application of lactic-acid (fifty-per-cent.) solution to the affected parts, incision of the edematous uvula, all these measures will relieve and call forth expressions of sincerest gratitude from the sufferer. One of the most practical suggestions for the treatment of these affections was made by Delavan. This consists in giving the patient nutritious enemata for several days and no medicine nor food by the mouth, resting the muscles of deglutition. By this short rest much relief is occasioned and deglutition becomes no longer painful, or very slightly so.

Tubercular Laryngitis.—Perhaps every writer on this subject mentions the case of a child aged four and one-half years, reported by Demme, who died of tuberculous meningitis, in which the tuberculous deposits were found in the larynx at the autopsy, while the pulmonary tissues were normal. Primary tuberculosis of the larynx does occur, but the vast majority of cases occur either simultaneously with pulmonary tuberculosis or as a sequel thereof. The latter forms are by far the most frequent.

The following is a brief history of a case of simultaneous pulmonary and laryngeal tuberculosis:

A girl of seventeen was referred to me by her family physician in July, 1897. She gave a history of having had a short cough with slight expectoration, and accompanied by huskiness for the past two months. Her voice was hoarse at the outset, and finally became less and less clear, and at the time of presentation the aphonia was almost complete, she was only able to whisper. Her family history was good, her father and mother being of strong physique. Her general condition was very good. There had been no attacks of hemoptysis, nor had there been any night-sweats. There was no perceptible loss of flesh. A laryngoscopic examination showed that both arytenoids were greatly infiltrated, so much so that it was only by repeated examinations that the vocal cords could be seen. There was no visible destruction of tissues, nor any evidences of acute inflammation. The swollen arytenoids met in the center, did not decrease on application of cocain, and the mucous membrane over them presented a perfectly normal appearance. It was apparent then that the aphonia was due to the mechanical presence of these arytenoids, which prevented action of the vocal cords. There was marked consolidation at both apices, and the sputum was full of tubercle bacilli. No improvement of the voice has occurred as the result of treatment. The latter has been non-surgical because of the extreme sensitiveness of the patient. The patient is still under observation, and in addition to other forms of treatment, is receiving Maragliano's serum hypodermically. This treatment was instituted by the parents on their own responsibility. No marked benefit has been noted from it; on the contrary, the pulmonary destruction is advancing.

In that most frequent form of tuberculosis of the larynx, secondary to pulmonary tuberculosis, the arytenoids are most often involved, next the ary-epiglottic fold, and the true vocal cords. The hypertrophy rapidly gives place to ulceration, which soon extends to other parts. An examination of the larynx shows the epiglottis greatly swollen in its upper and anterior border, assuming a crescentic or turban-like shape. The arytenoids are also swollen, and the narrow chink left for breathing is usually filled with mucus. Ulceration occurs in the inter-arytenoid space, and also in all parts of the larynx.

A point in diagnosis of this affection is the extreme pallor of the soft palate. Practically every case of tuberculous laryngitis shows this anemia to a marked degree.

The symptoms present are huskiness or complete aphonia, more or less pain on swallowing, severe cough, and occasionally dyspnea has been observed. The latter may become severe enough to require intubation or tracheotomy. Tuberculous laryngitis may be differentiated from all other affections by a microscopic examination of the sputum or of parts removed.

Treatment.—The treatment consists of the internal use of creosote or guaiacol; the local application of menthol in olive oil, lactic acid, iodoform, medicated steam; careful regulation of the diet, and, finally, the application of suitable hygienic measures. Surgically the arytenoids have been removed, and from this treatment Krause of Berlin, Heryng of Warsaw, and others in this country, claim gratifying results.

In all these cases the question of a change of climate must be very carefully considered. That these patients require local treatment, which is rarely attainable in the resorts sought out by them, is the main reason for keeping them under observation. Their physical condition often precludes an extended trip, and in advanced cases nothing is gained by sending them away. In cases in which the disease is yet at an early stage, the most important therapeutic remedy is a complete change of surroundings to a climate suited to the physical condition. Not enough stress is laid upon this, for we are apt to mention a locality on very broad general principles without carefully considering the needs of the patient. The physician should know where the proper climate is to be found, and then, having a knowledge of the nature of the disease and the demands of the case in hand, should render his opinion.

Generally speaking, a New Englander will thrive in the Green Mountains, the Adirondacks, or the Catskills, while his warm-blooded Southern brother will improve in the piney woods of North Carolina, or at Aiken, S. C. Others again, do well far away from the sea, and for these Phœnix, Arizona, or the mountains of Colorado seem to be the most salubrious. Southern California has much in its favor for certain patients. It is not enough to select a resort, but the habits of life should be carefully regulated. The average mountain home or boarding-house seems to be worse than useless. These places are usually styled "Inns," and are to be found in parts of the country where many tuberculous patients congregate. The patient is given a room but lately occupied by another unfortunate, himself in the last stages, and who has probably gone home to die. Nothing is done to destroy any remaining germs, and the new occupant is being constantly reinfected.

By far the most ideal mode of life is in a cabin made of wood and containing a single apartment, or a tent with wooden flooring, and the more solitary it stands the better. A bedstead is readily made by any woodsman from the limbs of trees, and a spring and hair-mattress, with appropriate bedding, complete this important part of the domicile. A few other articles of a primitive nature, such as chairs, basins, etc., will be required.

An enterprising company in one of the Southern resorts has small wooden dwellings or more pretentious ones on sale. Life in these little houses is not apt to be so very tedious, and especially if the invalid can arrange to be quite by himself except for a competent guide. The latter, in addition to being a very good cook, is huntsman, oarsman, and fisherman. He is often quaint and quite a philosopher. His home is in a smaller tent, and an adjacent boarded space gives shelter to his stove, refrigerator, and table.

Through the courtesy of one of our most distinguished citizens the writer was enabled to spend a few days in a camp and partake of the joys of outdoor life. I trust I may present a brief description for your benefit and also for that of your patients.

This camp is on the edge of a beautiful lake in the heart of the Adirondacks, two miles away from any human habitation, and reached by a row-boat after an hour's ride by coach from the station. The wooded hills have pines, firs, and hemlocks in vast numbers, the ground is thickly carpeted with moss and the débris of leaves, the accumulations of centuries. Here and there this carpet is trodden a little more firmly, and is then called a trail. Whether the day's outing be inland to some trout pond which is reached after a long walk through the woods, or a row on the lake with fishing for pastime, or even hunting for game, in season, it is bound to be one of pleasure. The guide knows where to begin to fish, and where the coolest spring of pure water is, and he knows where he may start a fire for dinner. He has brought the necessaries along, and we are called ere long to partake of the meal he has prepared, for which the appetite has become fully sharpened. While we miss many an essential to fine table service, we do ample justice to the tasty food supplied. Rowing back, and trolling the while for pickerel or bass, we reach camp thoroughly sunbrowned and delightfully tired.

Supper is soon served and night comes on. Except for the rustle of the leaves, the occasional hoot of an owl, the chirp of crickets or smaller insects, and the gentle lap of the waters of the lake as they strike the stones on shore, all is at peace. The moon shines on the water and a cloudless sky shows a myriad of stars; or, it storms. The rain beats down on the leaves and drips on the tent from which it rolls off to the ground, and to the soft music of its patter we lie down, and soon "Nature's sweet restorer, balmy sleep" comes to us and we awaken the next morning thoroughly refreshed. To an invalid how much this all means you know, and to many a one it brings a new lease of life in his own sphere of usefulness.

A CASE OF PRIMARY MULTIPLE SARCOMA OF THE STOMACH, FOLLOWING GUNSHOT WOUND.

By HARLOW BROOKS, M.D.,
OF NEW YORK;
ASSOCIATE IN BACTERIOLOGY, PATHOLOGICAL INSTITUTE OF THE NEW YORK STATE HOSPITALS; INSTRUCTOR IN HISTOLOGY IN THE BELLEVUE HOSPITAL MEDICAL COLLEGE; ASSISTANT CURATOR TO BELLEVUE HOSPITAL.

FOR the history of the following cases I am indebted to Dr. J. D. Brown, late House Physician, Fourth Medical Service, Bellevue Hospital:

Male, aged sixty-seven years; born in Germany; resident in the United States during thirty-five years. The patient was admitted to Bellevue Hospital October 26, 1895. The family history was negative. He had been a beer-drinker for the past forty years, usually taking four or five glasses daily. During the Civil War he received a bullet-wound in the region of the ensiform cartilage. The ball was not found, but his recovery was uneventful.

About seven months before entering the hospital the patient began to be troubled by pains in the abdomen. He steadily lost strength, and his appetite began to fail. He complained of headache and of spots before the eyes. The feet and ankles became swollen. He rapidly lost weight, and was finally obliged to give up his occupation of cabinet-maker. About six months previously he developed a cough with considerable expectoration which was occasionally bloody. At this time he suffered from dyspnea upon slight exertion. He complained of pain located in the left mammary region.

While in the hospital the patient's appetite remained fairly good. There was tenderness of the abdomen, but it was not localized. At times he vomited quantities of blood. In one of these attacks the nurse stated that he vomited as much as a pint of bright, red blood. The stools were occasionally tinged with blood. Shortly before death purpuric spots developed beneath the skin of the body and extremities. The physical examination, as far as tumor of the stomach is concerned, was negative. He died December 31, 1895. The autopsy was performed twenty-four hours after death.

Autopsy.—The body was fairly well nourished. The skin and mucous membranes were anemic. There were a few purpuric blotches over the sides and back of the body, over the forearms and backs of the hands. There was an oval scar half an inch long just to the left of the right nipple line and between the seventh and eighth ribs (bullet wound). There was a considerable mass of bony tissue thrown out from the ends of the seventh and eighth ribs, beneath this area. Rigor mortis was slight.

The panniculus adiposus was small in amount and highly colored. Muscles were fairly good in volume, but soft and anemic.

Pleura.—There were general old pleuritic adhesions over the apices of both lungs.

Heart.—Small, weighed eight ounces; the chambers were contracted; the heart muscle was firm, but light in color. The segments of both aortic and mitral valves were considerably thickened. The conus arteriosus showed endarteritis of moderate degree; the coronary arteries, a few diffuse areas of endarteritis.

Respiratory System.—The mucous membrane of the trachea and bronchi was considerably congested. The pulmonary artery contained a small amount of antemortem clot. The lung tissue showed extensive emphysema, with moderate congestion posteriorly.

Liver.—Weight, two pounds, seven ounces. The left lobe was very small, and was adherent on its inferior surface to the wall of the stomach. The capsule was smooth. There was an old scar situated on the superior surface of the left lobe. This area corresponded with the external scar mentioned above. The tissue was firm in consistence, and light brown in color. The interstitial tissue was apparently considerably increased, and fatty degeneration was marked.

Spleen.—Enlarged; weight, two pounds. Regular in contour. Capsule thickened. Tissue firm and solid, light purple in color.

Adrenals.—Negative.

Kidneys.—Weight, five ounces each. Capsules were rough and adherent. Cortex thin and irregular. Markings indistinct and irregular. Tissue firm. Cut surface somewhat granular. Perivascular connective tissue considerably increased.

Bladder.—Small; it contained a small amount of clear, light-colored urine. Mucous membrane normal.

Pancreas.—Small; the tissue was firm and light pink in color.

Stomach.—The stomach was small and its peri-

FIG. 1.

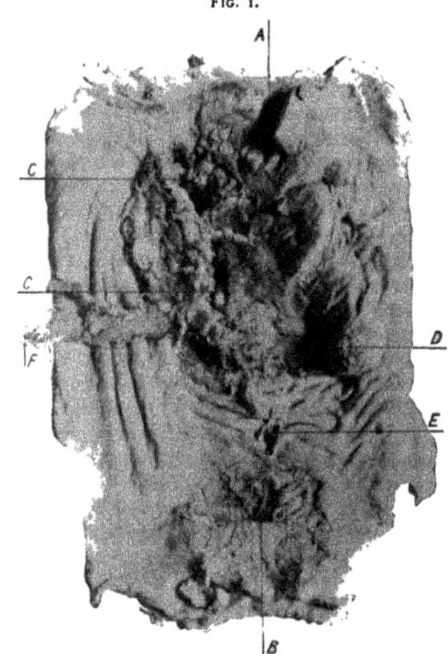

Showing the superior and anterior surfaces of the stomach mucosa. (*A*) Pyloris. (*B*) Entrance of esophagus. (*C-C*) Area adherent to and detached with the liver. (*D*) Large nodule, with ulcerated cap. (*E*) Small nodule removed for microscopic examination. (*F*) Strip detached from border of *C-C*.

toneal coat smooth. Just to the right of the esophageal entrance this organ was adherent to the inferior surface of the left lobe of the liver over an area about three-fourths of an inch in diameter. On attempting to separate these adhesions, the wall of the stomach over this area came away attached to the liver. The portion so detached was found to present simply an area of dense cicatricial tissue. On incising the stomach the area of adhesions was found to be surrounded on the internal surface by a circle of nodular masses, varying in size from half an inch to an inch and a half in diameter. Similar nodules were found scattered over the anterior and superior surfaces of the organ, and extending to the pylorus, where they nearly occluded the passage, into which they projected in large, fleshy masses, leaving only a narrow tortuous canal into the duodenum. These nodules were firm, and for the most part were covered by the mucous membrane of the stomach. In places the mucous membrane over these masses was eroded and ulcerated, and in such areas the dilated vessels showed evidences of recent hemorrhage; some of the nodules were surmounted by masses of blood-clot. The cut surface of the nodules was firm and somewhat granular, light pink in color, and showed numerous blood-vessels. Connective-tissue stroma was not evident. The mucous membrane remained intact over the majority of the masses, which evidently originated in the submucous layers. The posterior and inferior surfaces of the mucosa were mostly free from the growth. The capillaries of the mucous membrane were universally congested. The stomach contained a dark, greenish fluid, evidently largely composed of partly digested blood.

There was no enlargement of the lymphatics in the region of the stomach, and there were no evidences of inflammation save in the area of adhesions before mentioned, where the process was evidently a very old one.

The external scar, the cicatrix on the superior surface of the left lobe of the liver, and the adhesions uniting the stomach-wall to the liver, were in almost a straight line.

Intestine.—The mucous membrane of the duodenum was slightly congested. Both large and small intestine were collapsed, and their mucous membranes were anemic.

Cerebral Meninges.—Normal.

Brain.—The brain was well formed; the hemispheres were symmetric; the convolutions broad and well marked; the sulci deep. The cortical layer of gray matter was deep and regular. The brain tissue was firm, but somewhat edematous. No lesions were evident. Weight of encephalon, two pounds, eight ounces.

No new growth beside that in the stomach was found in any part of the body. Microscopic sections of the nodular masses demonstrated that they were composed of small, round-cells, very similar in appearance and size to lymphocytes. The tissue was very compact and cellular. Blood-vessels were numerous, but were mostly of the capillary type, so that the cells were found lying in direct contact with the thin walls. Connective-tissue stroma was present in small amount, but no regularity of arrangement was present. The new growth was found to be located in the submucous layers, and in most cases the mucous membrane over the nodules was normal, though in certain areas infiltration had occurred upward between the gastric tubules (see Fig. 2). Small fibrils of connective tissue were found passing between the cells in every direction. (See Fig. 3.)

The submucous lymph-nodes appeared, for the greater part, free, but in places they were surrounded by areas of small round-cell infiltration, apparently inflammatory, and not neoplastic. In all the sections taken from various portions of the anterior and superior surfaces of the stomach the submucous layer of connective tissue was found to contain masses of greater or less size, and presenting the same characteristic picture in each case. One small nodule taken from near the esophageal opening (*E*, Fig. 1) presented the usual submucous masses, but in this section the glands of the mucous fold were found to be dilated, and, in places, of an almost adenomatous character. The submucous vessels were very large, and filled with blood-cells. Similar appearances were not found in any of the sections taken from other portions of the stomach.

The growth appeared to be a typical round-cell sarcoma. Its point of origin, no doubt, was in the submucous connective-tissue layers of the stomach. Notwithstanding the great similarity of the growth in its structure to lymphosarcoma, it seems probable that if this were the case more involvement of

FIG. 2.

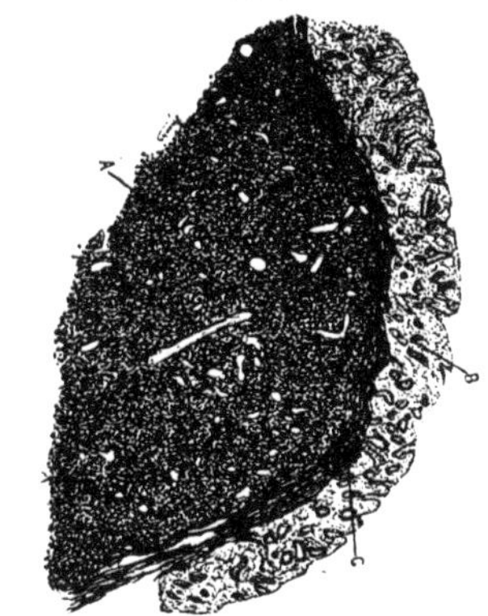

(*A*) Tumor growths. (*B*) Uninvolved mucous membrane. (*C*) Lymph-nodule.

the lymph-nodes would have been present, and also that the growth would not have been so strictly localized as it was found to be.

From the location of the external scar made by the entrance of the bullet, the position of the scar on the surface of the liver and the area of old ulceration in the wall of the stomach, it seems probable that the bullet, after piercing the parieties, perforated the left lobe of the liver and passed on into the stomach. Unfortunately, the symptoms immediately following the infliction of the wound were not minutely inquired into, but from the anatomic findings we were forced to conclude that such was the course of the bullet. That the new growth was primarily induced by the wound is negatived by the time elapsing between the infliction of the wound and the onset of symptoms indicative of gastric neoplasm. Yet it is probable that the irritation resulting from the old ulceration finally favored the formation of the growth, which evidently first developed near the seat of the old process.

Cases of sarcoma originating in such seats of irritation are commonly reported. From the character of the growth and from the clinical history it is evident that it developed quite rapidly.

Primary sarcoma of the stomach is an exceedingly rare disease. No, doubt, however, it is more frequent than the number of cases reported would seem to indicate, since microscopic examinations are not universally made in cases of gastric tumor, for the tendency is to rely upon gross appearances, which are extremely unreliable in differentiating between ordinary carcinoma and some of the varieties of sarcoma and endothelioma.

In most of the reported cases the growth has been located at the lesser curvature of the stomach, or its

FIG. 3.

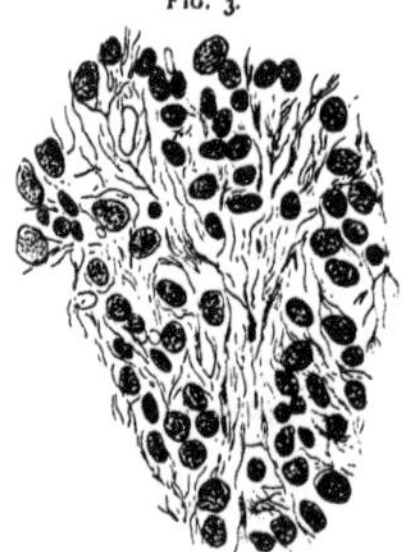

Growth sketched under one-twelfth oil immersion (Zeiss).

maximum growth has been in this region. It is somewhat unusual to find sarcoma originating after adult life, and the advanced age at which the growth developed, not only in this case, but also in several of the cases recorded in literature, is quite striking.

Of the 15 cases of primary, gastric sarcoma which the author has found reported, 6 have been round-cell sarcomas, 4 of the spindle-cell variety, 2 myosarcoma, and 2 of uncertain type. The case reported by Hadden as lymphosarcoma is beyond doubt one of perithelioma, as the author very perfectly describes the structure of this, at that time, unrecognized growth. In none of these cases did ulcer or traumatism of the stomach-wall precede the development of the growth, and in this respect the author believes the present case to be unique.

WAR ARTICLES.

CAMP SANITATION AS APPLIED AT "CAMP TAMPA HEIGHTS," FLORIDA.

By HENRY I. RAYMOND, M.D.,
CAPTAIN AND ASSISTANT SURGEON, UNITED STATES ARMY.

THE underlying principle of sanitation in the field is the preventability of camp diseases. For in this high-noon hour of sanitary science the presence of preventable diseases among troops on an active campaign is an opprobrium upon the sound sanitary sense of the present age and generation, and may be set down either to criminal negligence on the part of the sanitary officer of the command or to the overruling imperiousness of military necessity.

The selection of a site and the sanitary care of a camp constitute the responsible and paramount duty of the medical officer, as sanitary adviser of the commandant of the expedition, and upon his judicial acumen will largely depend the effectiveness of the army as a potential force. If the site of the camp is insalubrious, diseases incident to camp life cannot be prevented and evil consequences will inevitably result. Some of the essential factors that enter into the proper selection of a camp-site in southerly latitudes may be briefly summarized as follows: Convenience of water and wood, accessibility to food-supplies and forage, avoidance of prevailing winds from suspicious localities, protection from the sun's heat by woods, and last but not least, dryness of soil. Observance of this last precaution will eliminate a multitude of evils, for it should be constantly borne in mind that if one of the three factors that are essential to the origin and spread of infectious diseases—heat, moisture, and organic decay—can be eliminated, the vicious circle will be broken.

The military camp on Tampa Heights has been wisely selected from a sanitary point of view. The source of the water-supply is a spring in the vicinity of Tampa that furnishes clear, cool, potable water for the inhabitants of the town and the adjacent encampment of United States troops. The camp supply is abundant and is conducted by pipes into a large reservoir with capacity of one hundred thousand gallons, the reservoir being elevated one hundred and fifty feet on scaffolding.

This water contains magnesium and lime, and is, on that account, laxative for those not habituated to its use. Though there has been a number of cases of diarrhea and one or two of dysentery in camp the past week, I am inclined to attribute their causation not entirely or alone to the drinking-water, but largely to indiscretions in diet, iced drinks and cream, and to the marked diurnal range of temperature with chilling of the body surface at night. The heat of the sun's rays, while not excessive nor attended with much humidity of the atmosphere, has produced its quota of cases of ephemeral fever (thermic), superinduced by exercise at drill in a dust-laden atmosphere and upon a set of men not yet acclimated to this latitude, nor as yet provided with uniforms of suitable material for a tropical climate.

Camp Tampa Heights is located on a sandy soil covered in many places with a short growth of grass, which latter, however, soon becomes trodden down by the march of so many feet and the sand rises in dust-clouds and fills the eyes, ears, and nostrils with floating irritants and the imagination with clouds of battle smoke. One would have to dig many feet deep into this soil to come upon any solid substratum, and hence, the soil being so pervious to water and lying in an elevated locality the drainage is excellent.

Excavations for sinks and latrines are made in the sandy soil with so little expenditure of labor that pits have been constructed for these purposes in different parts of the camp and their daily accumulations of excreta are covered, night and morning, with the excavated soil. It is not unlikely that these vaults will be superseded by portable receptacles for the excreta so that their contents can be carted off, thus preventing any possibility of soil contamination and especially the conveyance, by flies and vermin, of disease-germs.

Second only to camp sanitation in importance is the personal hygiene of the soldier. Advise is cheap and the soldier like many of the rest of mankind learns many hard lessons by experience. But an effort is constantly made to impress upon each enlisted man who presents himself at sick call in the field that only by rigid adherence to the simple but salutary precepts of hygiene can he hope to avoid sickness in this climate, and imperatively so in Cuba. Avoid the use of alcohol in every form and in any measure, eschew the banana, crucify the luscious "mangrin," beware of the pastry and frozen cream that is vended so temptingly on the outskirts of the camp, be cautious of iced drinks, live abstemiously, bathe frequently, and sleep with some covering, however light, over you, and with as much covering as can be spared between you and the ground.

On the subject of prophylaxis, two measures are in contemplation on our departure from this comparative Eden to the disease-laden atmosphere of tropical Cuba. One relates to the use of quinin in doses of two to five grains daily as a preventive against malaria, and the other to the use of boiled water for drinking purposes to insure against paludal, typhoid, and yellow-fever (?) infection from that source. To insure the water being boiled, as well as to relieve it of its taste of flatness and insipidity, it would seem advisable to substitute for the plain boiled water a weak infusion of tea. The observance of this practice might be enforced by having the men fall in every morning just before marching and inspected as to their canteens being filled with hot tea; this liquid being hot on starting off would prevent the too early imbibition of fluids on the march.

In view of the possibility of spending a part of the rainy season in Cuba, where the tropical rainstorms descend as if the very windows of heaven were opened, I have busied myself to-day in rubbing a cake of paraffin over my blanket, trousers, shirt, felt hat, and other articles of apparel and then allowing the paraffin to soak in under the influence of the sun's heat until its presence cannot be detected by any outward appearance. This renders the garment water-proof as attested by actual trial and this quality of imperviousness is believed to be lasting. Many members of the medical and hospital corps have made use of the paraffin in a similar manner, having taken the cue from our chief surgeon.

TRANSPORTATION OF THE WOUNDED IN WAR.[1]

BY JAMES P. KIMBALL, A.M., M.D.,
MAJOR AND SURGEON, UNITED STATES ARMY.

THE first stage in the travels of the wounded man is from the ground on which he has fallen to the collecting or first-dressing station. This station, according to army regulations, is "the nearest place to the combatants where the wounded and those caring for them may not be unnecessarily exposed to fire." Formerly this was a distance of not more than 500 or 600 yards, but the increased range of the modern rifle now necessitates the establishment of the first-dressing station at least 1000 to 1200 yards behind the firing line. There is usually one such station behind each regiment engaged, or if the regiments be small, one behind each brigade. To these stations bearers carry on litters the seriously wounded, after they have received on the field the necessary first aid, such as the application of a tourniquet in cases of severe arterial hemorrhage, and of improvised splints to broken bones.

The bearers are a part of the sanitary force, which varies somewhat in strength in different armies, but is commonly equal to about four per cent. of the troops in line. In some of the European armies in which the proportion was less than four per cent. the rate has recently been increased, because of the general belief that in future wars the number of wounded will be larger than heretofore by reason of the greatly extended range of the new rifle. In our own army no definite plan has yet been formulated for fixing the ratio of the sanitary to the combatant force. If, however, we assume that the sanitary

[1] Abstract of article in the *Albany Medical Annals*, April, 1898.

force is equal to four per cent. of the command, a division—the administrative unit of an army, which in our service numbers, on a war footing, 12,747 men—will contain in round numbers a sanitary corps of 500 men. This corps in most armies is composed of two classes, about equal in number—the hospital corps, which consists of men specially enlisted for the medical department and permanently attached to it, and the company, or regimental bearers, who belong to the fighting force, and have been instructed in the duties of litter-bearers and in the methods of giving first aid to the sick and wounded. During an engagement these bearers are temporarily detached from their companies for sanitary service with their respective regiments; that is, to give necessary aid to the wounded on the battle-field, and to carry the disabled to the first-dressing stations. At the dressing stations and beyond the wounded are cared for by men of the hospital corps. The plan of taking men from the combatant ranks to serve as litter-bearers is disapproved by some authorities, and the question is still an open one.

The medical officers of the division number forty-four.

Having considered the personnel, we now turn to the means of transportation. The first conveyance used in carrying the wounded from the field is the litter. The

FIG. 1.

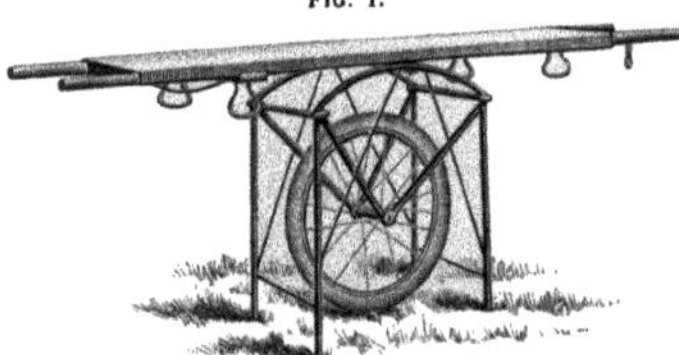

The Remington Hand Litter-Carrier.

evolution of the hand-litter is an interesting subject, but we shall consider only its recent development in the United States.

During the War of the Rebellion, and until lately in our regular army, the litter known as the Halstead was in use. This litter was eight feet in length, had folding wooden legs fourteen and one-half inches long, and weighed twenty-five pounds. It was a serviceable litter, and only when we contrast it with our present litter do we remember that the old one was heavy; that its legs were unnecessarily long, apt to become loose and unsteady, and to shut up unexpectedly; that its length and legs prevented its fitting into an ambulance, and that every wounded man on the way to hospital must therefore be lifted from litter to ambulance and from ambulance to litter, thereby wasting time and adding to the patient's suffering.

The present litter of the United States Army, model of 1895, weighs sixteen and one-half pounds. It folds compactly, and may be carried on the shoulder almost as easily as a rifle. The fixed wrought-iron stirrup-shaped legs, or rather feet, raise it four inches from the ground. The side-poles are seven feet six inches long, and the canvas bed six feet long by twenty-two inches wide. Two of the litters can be placed side by side in the regulation ambulance. Litter-slings—bands of worsted webbing to be passed over the shoulders and attached to the handles—are issued to the bearers as a part of their equipment, and are very valuable when the loaded litter is to be carried far.

The corps of trained men and the improved litter just described would seem to perfect the means of transporting the wounded to the first-dressing station. But there is still a weak point in the working of our scheme. Experieuce has shown that when the litters are wanted at the front in action, they are often far away in the rear with the ambulance-train, upon which they are carried. Troops, artillery, and ammunition-wagons have the right of way when battle is imminent, and ambulances and supply-wagons must not encumber the roads and must seek a place of safety. Thus it often happens that during an engagement, and perhaps for some time after, the litters are detained miles away from the battle-field.

It has been recommended that pack-mules be used to bring litters and medical supplies promptly upon the field. In the war with China, 1894 and 1895, the Japanese successfully used pack-horses for this work. The use of pack-animals seems the natural solution of the difficulty, for they can follow wherever troops go without obstructing the movements of the column. Yet, if for any reason pack-animals cannot be secured, men of the sanitary force

FIG. 2.

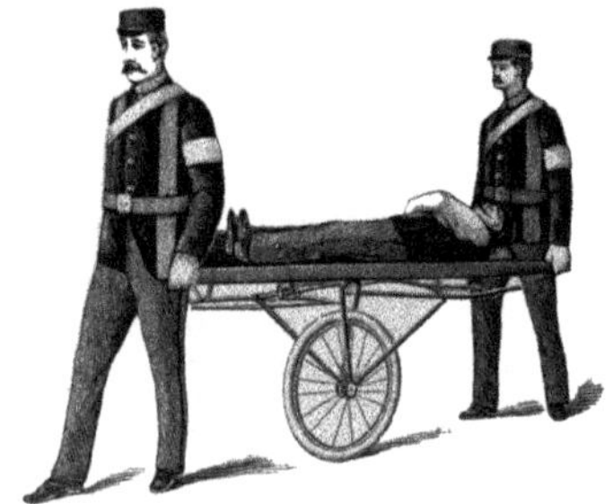

The litter-carrier in use.

could be required to carry the litters. Under these circumstances, when troops are in the vicinity of the enemy and battle is probable, the bearers should be ordered before leaving the ambulance-train to take the litters, one to every four men, and to carry them as they march in rear of the regiment. The light, compact litter now in use is easily carried by two men, and in fact is not an excessive burden for one man; and should the wheeled litter-carrier described below, or some similar device, be adopted, the work would be still further lightened.

At the first-dressing station dressings are applied,

urgent operations performed, and the wounded made ready for transfer to the ambulance station.

The ambulance-station is presumably 1000 or 1200 yards beyond the dressing-station, established "at some place of security in the rear, or in some convenient building near the field of battle." The site should have a convenient water-supply, and if possible it should be easy of access. To this station the wounded are brought in ambulances when practicable. If, however, on account of bad roads, or no roads, or the encumberment of the way by troops and wagons, the ambulances cannot reach the first-dressing station, then litters must be used for the intervening distance.

The ambulance, like the litter, has been evolved from more or less crude beginnings, but it is not yet as well suited to its purpose as is the hand-litter. The pattern now in use in our army, adopted in 1892, carries two patients lying down or eight sitting up. When required for recumbent patients, the removable seats are hung against the sides of the vehicle, leaving a floor space which just holds two litters. The patients are, therefore, carried in the ambulance upon the same litters on which they have been brought from the field.

FIG. 3.

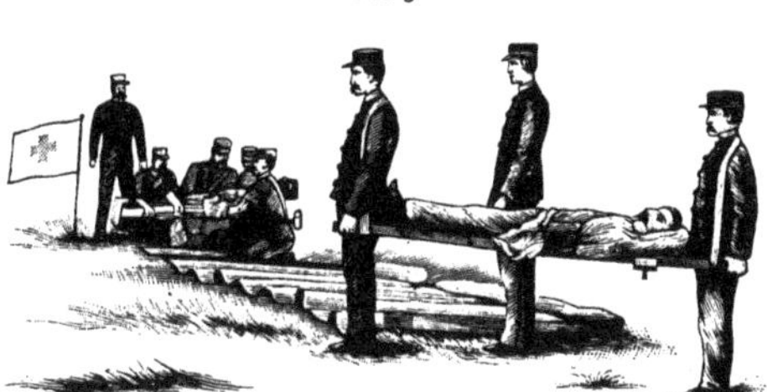

First-Dressing Station.

Wheeled litters, drawn or pushed by hand, have been modeled and remodeled from time to time, but on the chance ground of battle-fields, often rough and broken, these litters have hitherto been of little use. The "Cycle Ambulance" may prove valuable for use on city streets, but evidently it cannot be considered serviceable for rough and muddy country roads.

A recent invention by Mr. Frederic Remington, the artist, is by far the best adaptation of the wheel to the litter that has yet been made. Mr. Remington, in his campaign experiences with the army on the frontier, has had an eye for the needs of the wounded soldier, as well as for picturesque scouts and warriors. The invention, which he calls a "litter-carrier," consists of a single wheel, and of a framework to hold the litter. The wheel is twenty-four inches in diameter, and has a steel rim three inches in width, covered with a rubber band; within the rim is a V-shaped shield of wood, through which the spokes pass. The shield prevents the accumulation of mud or snow on the rim. The frame is made of steel tubing, upon which rest two three-leaved springs, placed twenty-two inches apart, so that the poles of the regulation litter may rest upon them. The litter is fastened to the carrier by a pin which is attached to the lower side of each litter pole, and passes through a hole in the spring, where it is made fast by a cross-pin. Folding legs are let down to hold the carrier firmly in position when the litter is to be put on or taken off. The litter-carrier thus adjusted, with the litter placed upon it, is about thirty inches in height, and could serve on occasion as an operating-table. When the carrier is in motion, the legs fold back, and are secured by a simple device to the litter poles. The wheel is readily detached from the frame, and the whole can then be packed in small compass. The model which I have tested weighs thirty-seven and one-half pounds, but Mr. Remington is confident that the weight can be reduced to about thirty pounds.

The litter-carrier is designed for two bearers, one of whom pulls, while the other pushes; but should one of the bearers become disabled, it can be moved by one man alone. Over even ground the loaded carrier is moved with little effort; over rough ground the labor is not excessive, and the broad tread of the rubber-covered wheel and the elasticity of the steel springs make the patient's bed at least endurable, if not wholly comfortable. In case of necessity the carrier and patient can be lifted over ditches or other obstacles. I have tried the carrier under a variety of circumstances, up and down steep slopes, along side-hills, on unpaved roads and across fields, and find it admirably adapted to its purpose. In one of these tests of the litter-carrier a patient weighing 160 pounds was carried without stopping a distance of one and one-twelfth miles, mostly over uneven meadow land, in twenty-two minutes, and without fatigue to the bearers. Over the same ground and distance the same patient was carried on a hand-litter in forty-six minutes; eleven minutes of this time were spent in necessary rest, and even then the bearers were very tired at the end of the course. For the long distances from the front to the dressing-station, Mr. Remington's litter-carrier promises to be of great value in lightening the labor of the bearers.

At the ambulance-station wounds are carefully examined and redressed if necessary, and operations performed as required. Record is made of every patient, and the wounded are fed and cared for until they can be sent on to the field hospital.

The division or field hospital is established at a distance probably two or three miles from the ambulance-station, sufficiently far in the rear to assure, if possible, its permanency undisturbed by the changing lines of battle. The water-supply and the character of the ground and roads are also factors in determining the site. From the ambulance-station to the division hospital the patients are transported in ambulances or by litter-carrier, and on occasion army wagons or other available vehicles are pressed into this service.

Owing chiefly to faulty organization, the removal of the wounded from the field has hitherto been the least satisfactory work of the army medical service. But conditions have changed, and we are now in position to remedy this defect. Formerly medical men performed their duties subject to the will and conveniences of other departments of the army. Now the medical department has full control of its men and material, enjoys complete autonomy in its own sphere. It has a corps of trained and disciplined men and improved appliances for transportation. As yet, however, a detailed plan for the organization of this force is wanting, and without definite regulations the best results are impossible. To settle the details of organization under the stress of battle requires executive ability which few men possess.

It is held by some authorities that in coming wars it will be impossible to carry away the wounded during the battle, since the bearers would all be killed by the wide and destructive fire of modern arms. Granted that at times this may be so, it does not do away with the need of preparation for the relief of the wounded at the first practical moment. The value of this preparation does not consist wholly in the actual work accomplished, but also in the confidence given the soldier, that, should he fall, he will be taken care of.

The work of the hospital corps will demand not technical skill alone. It will require military discipline, a training which develops courage, endurance, and self-sacrifice, teaches prompt and unquestioning obedience, which, in short, make a soldier. We have now followed the route of the wounded soldier from firing-line to hospital. Though such a journey may never be painless, yet the measure taken to relieve suffering and save life have at least kept pace with the inventions contrived to wound and kill.

CAMP SANITATION AT CHICKAMAUGA PARK, GEORGIA.

To the Editor of the MEDICAL NEWS.

DEAR SIR: THE troops included in the command now stationed at Camp Thomas, Chickamauga Park, Ga., the composition of which has been frequently changed during the last ten days, consist of the 2nd, 7th, 8th, 12th, 16th, and 25th Infantry, and the 1st, 2nd, 3rd, 6th, and 10th Cavalry, with detachments from the Hospital Corps, Quartermaster Department, Commissary Department, and Signal Corps, together with medical officers, headquarters, staff, etc., aggregating about 7000 men. These regiments have been collected from all parts of the country. The 2nd, 16th, 25th Infantry and 10th Cavalry from the high altitude and severe cold of Montana and Idaho; the 7th, 8th, 12th Infantry and part of the 2nd Cavalry, from the similarly environed but warmer regions of Wyoming, Colorado, and Nebraska; the 1st Cavalry from Kansas, Illinois, and Oklahoma; 3rd from Vermont and Missouri, and the 6th from Virginia, Kansas, and Nebraska.

Chickamauga Park, where we are all camped, is a beautiful spot; the ground is rolling with many small hills, and large open spaces, alternating with wooded ground without underbrush. At first sight it would seem to offer an ideal spot for a large encampment, but such is in fact not the case. The soil consists of a few inches of loam, with an underlying bed of dense impervious clay of variable depth, but extending everywhere to the bed-rock. After a rain the ground remains damp and cold even after prolonged exposure to the sun, the water running down to the low ground remains in pools, and is soon converted into a muck by the constant traffic. The climate is very hot during the day, and cold and damp at night. The conditions would indeed seem favorable for the development of colds, rheumatism, tonsillitis, and diarrhea.

The water-supply of the camp is excellent in quality and quantity for drinking purposes, being pumped from artesian wells and from freely flowing springs. There are practically no bathing facilities, the nearest creek being several miles distant, but personal cleanliness is effected as far as possible.

The closest attention is paid to sanitary matters, and thus far with good results. Sinks, suitably sheltered, are dug for each company, and a layer of fresh earth is thrown on the fecal evacuations twice daily. When the contents of the pit are within eighteen inches of the surface it is filled up, marked, and a new one dug. All organic refuse and liquid slops are placed in tight barrels and removed daily by the farmers of the surrounding country. All other refuse is collected in piles and burned. All tents are ditched and drained, and many of the company streets have been filled in with gravel, which soon becomes packed and gives a firm footing. Straw is issued to the men for bedding, and many of them have extemporized platforms to raise them from the damp ground. Tent walls are raised daily, and the floors with straw, blankets, etc., exposed to the sun and air for at least two hours. The food of the men is inspected by a medical officer both before it is cooked and afterward, and all defects immediately brought to the attention of the proper authority; at the same time, every opportunity is taken to impress upon officers and men the purpose and importance of sanitary regulations.

No drugs are administered as prophylactics, none being considered necessary here. There has thus far been little sickness. A few cases of malarial fever among soldiers coming from parts where that disease is endemic, and a small number of cases of diarrhea, the result probably of a variety of causes, such as the extremes of temperature, errors of diet, and imprudences of various sorts. No diseases have been thus far noted as attributable to changes of climate, though this has been extreme in many cases; but a few mild cases of heat exhaustion have occurred as the result of ordinary drills in unaccustomed heat. A careful inspection of the entire command has been made with a view to vaccinating those who are unprotected. Each regiment in camp has one or more surgeons on duty with it besides a detachment of the Hospital Corps, and a field-hospital equipment, ambulance, etc. Every effort is being made to supply each command with a completely equipped medical department, both as to material and personnel. The exact nature of the organization and of the higher organizations which must be evolved from it will form the subjectof a later communication.

CHARLES F. MASON,
Captain and Assistant Surgeon, United States Army.
CAMP THOMAS, CHICKAMAUGA PARK, GA., May 6, 1898.

MEDICAL PROGRESS.

Pains in the Lower Extremities. — METTENHEIMER (*Zeitschr. für rat. prak. Aerzte*, January 18, 1898) takes up the subject of pains in the lower extremities, and discusses it in a scientific manner. The expression *Schmerzen in die Fuesse*, is familiar to every one who has come into contact with the Polish population in dispensary work. The author says these pains are due to a plethora of the veins in the lower extremity, although they may also occur in other parts of the body. As special causes he mentions an undue amount of standing, or of walking, or the use of wine, especially sour wines, or standing in cold places, or working in a sitting position in cold rooms. In some patients there is not a trace of varicosity to be seen in the veins. Nevertheless, the pains are due to the insufficient circulation of blood in the skin. Such pains are often spoken of as rheumatic, an entirely misleading name. As treatment, are to be mentioned bandages, a horizontal position, rest, avoidance of over-exertion, etc. Unfortunately, it is impossible for most of those who suffer from these pains to comply with such directions. The author says he has obtained good results by cold applications, pouring cold water daily over the affected parts, or if time and opportunity permit, cold baths. Added to this there should be a dry friction of the skin. This should be superficial, and not a deep massage such as one gets from rubbing in a salve. Electricity will also be found to be of service, but the most practical remedy, both on account of its cheapness and its ready application, as above stated, is cold water, followed by dry friction with the hand.

Tuberculosis of the Spleen.—HAYDEN (*Jour. Amer. Med. Assoc.*, April 2, 1898) treated for several weeks a patient with swelling in the splenic region without benefit. In fact, the patient grew steadily worse and the swelling increased in size. An exploratory operation was performed, and a large cyst in the spleen was found and its contents evacuated. These examined microscopically were found to contain pus-corpuscles and tubercle bacilli. Soon after, secondary tuberculosis appeared in the other organs, and the patient died four months after operation. Very few cases of primary splenic tuberculosis have been recorded. The writer believes that had the spleen been removed at the time of the operation secondary tuberculosis would have been avoided, although the great risk attendant upon the removal of this organ inclined him to the opinion that it ought not to be attempted.

To Determine Very Small Effusions into the Knee-Joint.—FISKE (*Med. Record*, March 12, 1898) says that small effusions into the knee-joint are best made out if the patient stands with the knees fully extended and with both hands resting on the anterior surface of the thighs at about their middle. Any fluid present in the joint at once sinks and settles behind the patella, causing it to "float." This position of the patient is one of ease and anterior relaxation. The muscular rigidity often present in ordinary examination of the knee-joint is absent. Care should be taken to strike the patella exactly in its center. Otherwise, one may obtain a deceptive tilting.

THERAPEUTIC NOTES.

Lysol as a Disinfectant.—At its recent annual meeting the Illinois State Board of Health expressed concurrence in the following recommendation made by Dr. John A. Egan, its secretary: Although corrosive sublimate is a cheap and reliable disinfectant, great care must be exercised in its use. All the solutions named are poisonous, and a child might drink sufficiently of No. 3 (1 dram each of corrosive sublimate and muriate of ammonia dissolved in 1 gallon of water) to cause its death. Carbolic-acid solutions are also poisonous, and might be drunk by a child or adult, causing at least injury to the throat. Lysol has none of these objections, being toxic only in large doses, and having a pronounced taste, thus precluding the possibility of it being swallowed by mistake. A two-per-cent. solution of lysol equals a five-per-cent. solution of carbolic acid. This preparation can be used instead of the carbolic acid, in the strength of 2½ ounces to the gallon of water.

A Specific Galactagogue.—Dr. Thos. More-Madden (*International Medical Annual*, 1898) calls attention to an article by Dr. Richard Drews, who states that somatose exercises a specific action upon the mammary gland of nursing women in that it produces an abundant secretion of milk and rapidly removes the disorders of lactation. It is therefore recommended, when the quantity is insufficient, and when at the commencement of lactation the flow seems about to cease. Of course, the integrity of the gland must be perfect, and there must not be present any diseases which contraindicate nursing. The dose is 3 or 4 teaspoonfuls daily, taken in milk, hot bouillon, or cocoa.

THE MEDICAL NEWS.

A WEEKLY JOURNAL

OF MEDICAL SCIENCE.

COMMUNICATIONS are invited from all parts of the world. Original articles contributed *exclusively* to THE MEDICAL NEWS will after publication be liberally paid for (accounts being rendered quarterly), or 250 reprints will be furnished in place of other remuneration. When necessary to elucidate the text, illustrations will be engraved from drawings or photographs furnished by the author. Manuscripts should be typewritten.

Address the Editor: J. RIDDLE GOFFE, M.D., No. 111 FIFTH AVENUE (corner of 18th St.), NEW YORK.

Subscription Price, including postage in U. S. and Canada.

PER ANNUM IN ADVANCE	$4.00
SINGLE COPIES	.10
WITH THE AMERICAN JOURNAL OF THE MEDICAL SCIENCES, PER ANNUM	7.50

Subscriptions may begin at any date. The safest mode of remittance is by bank check or postal money order, drawn to the order of the undersigned. When neither is accessible, remittances may be made, at the risk of the publishers, by forwarding in *registered* letters.

LEA BROTHERS & CO.,
No. 111 FIFTH AVENUE (corner of 18th St.), NEW YORK, AND NOS. 706, 708 & 710 SANSOM ST., PHILADELPHIA.

SATURDAY, MAY 14, 1898.

GLOVES FOR ARMY SURGEONS.

IN each surgeon's chest which has gone to the front with the army there has been placed a package containing three pairs of rubber operating-gloves, sterilized, and wrapped in rubber tissue, ready for use. Whether they will prove a valuable part of the armamentarium of the surgeon in his effort to obtain primary union, remains to be seen; at any rate the Surgeon-General has shown himself alive to the advances in his department by thus promptly acting upon the opinions which have recently been expressed in this country and Europe in regard to aseptic operations. Within a short time this subject of operating-gloves has been brought before both the New York Surgical Society and the Surgical Section of the Academy of Medicine. In one paper preference was expressed for rubber gloves—in the other for cotton, or lisle-thread gloves. Both papers excited a vigorous discussion, which turned not so much upon the kind of glove to be worn, as upon the point whether or not gloves should be worn at all. Age is ever conservative, and it was not surprising to find that the majority of the advocates of gloves were young men, while their opponents were almost without exception past forty summers. The arguments were chiefly in favor of gloves. Those who opposed the use of the gloves were only able to say that they considered them clumsy. To this the answer was made that a little practice overcomes this awkward feeling, and the fingers soon gain sufficient dexterity for nearly all operative maneuvers.

The gain for asepsis by the use of gloves is clear and unmistakable. They can be absolutely sterilized, as the skin cannot, and in addition they protect the wound from possible infection from secretions of the sweat-glands of the operator's hands. These facts were brought out in a variety of ways in the meetings mentioned, and one young enthusiast set the standard for the future by declaring that surgical etiquette is no less real than that of good society; and that it is as bad form to put the naked fingers into a wound as it is to pull to pieces a bit of broiled chicken at luncheon with fingers and teeth.

There seems no reason to doubt that in the next few years gloves will become universal in the best operating-rooms—just as in the past few years head-dresses have become common; or, as in the years immediately preceding, gowns gained a general foothold. Whether the gloves will be of thread or rubber, or of some other material, it is too early to predict. Undoubtedly all surgeons who while operating use liquids, for wounds or instruments or sponges, will prefer gloves which are absolutely impervious to moisture. For those who operate by the dry method throughout, thread gloves, at least for extra-abdominal operations, have some decided advantages over rubber—in that they are thinner, and less elastic, and do not sweat the fingers. With them, however, a more complete preliminary scrubbing of the hands is necessary than is the case when rubber gloves are employed. This statement would probably be stoutly contested by the advocates of rubber; but unless human nature is going to change, a congenital inertia and a due regard for his digital epidermis, will, in the end, lead the surgeon who knows he has a germ-proof sterile film of rubber between his fingers and the wound, to omit altogether or greatly to modify the annoying ten minutes of hand-scrubbing which one has to go through with to render his hands even approximately sterile.

As may be seen in the report of the Congress of the German Society of Surgery, which appears in this issue of the MEDICAL NEWS, the German surgeons are almost unanimous in the opinion that the introduction of gloves into the technic of surgical procedures marks a distinct advance in asepsis.

To the army surgeon rubber gloves will be especially welcomed. His hands are usually rough from a varied occupation and are sterilized with great difficulty, while the conditions of war compel him at times to operate for many hours together, so that oft-repeated scrubbing might well nigh flay his fingers.

To prepare them for use rubber gloves are washed with soap and water, rinsed with mild ammonia, lightly packed with gauze, wrapped in a towel and boiled for fifteen minutes in a one-per-cent. solution of sodium carbonate. Since they are non-absorbant, if they come in contact with no source of infection they must remain sterile throughout the operation. During the operation they may be washed on the hands with a sterile solution as often as necessary.

A ROYAL ROAD TO MEDICAL KNOWLEDGE.

ONE by one time-consecrated aphorisms succumb to the irresistible Admirable Crichtons of our generation. It has been universally accepted that there is no royal road to knowledge; yet a plan of manufacture and commerce in this commodity is now being agitated by certain enthusiasts in the medical profession of this country which claims to negative such acceptation. This consists of an organization to supply medical societies in different parts of the country with "talent," who shall come unto them laden with wisdom which shall be imparted and extracted, even to the complete satiety of those who are hungering and thirsting for such ready-made knowledge. The fathers of this scheme flatter themselves that these occasions will be found so invaluable that every town and county medical society will insist upon having a regular monthly supply. The question of supply is an easy matter, however, as it has been hinted that all the specialists in the large cities will welcome this opportunity to exhibit their wares first hand to the untracked territory from which consultations spring, and that they will hasten to cast their bread upon waters that it may return to them a hundred fold.

We are assured by the press agents of this company that the plan has been tried on various medical societies whose membership is made up of country practitioners and that it has been found a flattering success. A neighboring city seems to have the distinction of supplying, thus far, the "stars" of these buccolic companies, and, judging from the reports, the actors are highly pleased with the success of their one-night stands. If the medical societies do not soon awaken to the fact that they are pursuing an *ignis fatuus*, and if the stars cannot be made to see that they are selling their birthright for a mess of pottage, we may soon discover the dead-fences and the forsaken barns of the country town and suburban village covered with posters and lithographs heralding the coming of the next medical attraction, as plays and circuses are now announced.

Why should reasoning physicians delude themselves that the advent, for an hour or two, into the range of their audition of a man who has given special study to some intricate, and very often laboratory branch of their profession can possibly be of any advantage to them comparable to that which may be obtained by their gathering together in a spirit of mutual betterment to thrash out the truth by a comparison of individual experiences. It is only by such methods that the sinew and marrow of the ideal medical society can be developed. What are medical societies for? Are they for the glorification and lionizing of the individual, or are they arenas to which may be brought the difficult problems in diagnosis; the intricate questions of pathology, the vagaries of therapeutic results, in order that they may be discussed and elucidated by the clinical experiences of many men studying the same diseases amid the same invironments and under similar conditions? No one can honestly say, after having listened to some great star who has indulged in glittering generalities and skipped lightly over a vast subject, within the hour, let us say, that he goes home better fitted to cope with the exigencies of his daily work. On the contrary, it is extremely probable that if a vote were taken to determine the influence of the ordinary medical meeting of county and State societies in maintaining professional tone and keeping up the character of medical work the result would be no uncertain answer in favor of the present system—without stars.

ECHOES AND NEWS.

War Premiums of Insurance Companies. — It is a gratifying circumstance that the various life insurance compauies of the country are granting to the holders of their policies without additional premium therefor the privilege of engaging in the military or naval service of their country for at least one year outside of the limits of the United States.

Patriotism of Medical Men.—Thirty American physicians who were studying medicine in Vienna have left and are now on their way home to enter the army and navy.

Can Sex Be Distinguished in Skulls.—After an examination of more than 1090 skulls, Dr. Paul Bartels announces that he cannot discover there any positive characteristic of sex.

Meetings of the Pennsylvania State Board of Examiners.—The Pennsylvania State Board of Medical Examiners will hold its next examinations in Philadelphia and Pittsburg, June 14th, at 2 P.M. The Secretary is Dr. W. S. Foster of Pittsburg.

Changes in the Department of Charities, New York.—The office of Assistant-Superintendent of the City Hospital has been abolished. Miss Mary S. Gilmore has been appointed Superintendent of the Bellevue Hospital Training School for Nurses, at an annual salary of $1200, in place of Diana C. Kimber, resigned, whose salary was $1800.

A Hospital Ship for the Army of Invasion.—Among the recent purchases of vessels by the Government is the Vigilancia belonging to the Ward line; this vessel will be used as a hospital ship for the army and fully equipped for that purpose. Surgeon-General Sternberg has decided to place on board this ship an X-ray apparatus for the use of the surgeons.

Hotels to Be Utilized as Hospitals.—If the war is prolonged so as to need extensive hospital accommodations, the two hotels at Fort Monroe, the Chamberlin and the Hygeia, will be taken for that purpose. Fort Monroe has been chosen as the best place for the purpose, because of its healthful surroundings, the defences of the garrison there, and the ease with which men can be transferred from ships to the shore.

Fast Train to Denver.—The Rocky Mountain Limited, over the Chicago, Rock Island & Pacific Railroad, left Chicago at 2.30 P.M., May 5th, and reached Denver at 1.30 P.M., May 6th, the distance being covered in twenty-four hours and two minutes. No such record has ever been made before by a regular train between these points. The time on the entire trip averaging 52.3 miles per hour. The fastest time was 84 miles per hour.

A Regiment of Mounted Riflemen to Be Recruited.—Captain Leonard Wood, Assistant Surgeon, has been ordered to proceed forthwith to the following named places, in the order designated, for duty in connection with the recruitment of mounted riflemen to be organized under the recent act of Congress: Guthrie, Oklahoma Territory; Salt Lake City, Utah; Santa Fé, New Mexico; Cheyenne, Wyoming; Phœnix, Arizonia Territory; Boisé City, Idaho; Carson City, Nevada.

The Marine Hospitals Put at the Service of the Army and Navy by Order of President McKinley.—The United States Marine Hospitals are made available for the reception of the sick and wounded of either the United States Army or the United States Navy, upon a written request of the proper military or naval authority, the Marine Hospital Service to be reimbursed the actual cost of maintenance. A number of patients have already been received in the Marine Hospitals at Key West and Mobile.

Physical Requirements of Recruits.—A list has been issued by the War Department regarding the physical proportions for height, weight, and chest measurements. For the infantry and artillery, the height must not be less than 5 feet 4 inches, and weight not less than 120 pounds, nor more than 190 pounds. For the cavalry the height must be not less than 5 feet 4 inches, nor more than 5 feet 10 inches, weight not over 165 pounds. No minimum weight is given for the cavalry, but the chest must be satisfactory.

Herbert Spencer as a Vegetarian.—It appears from a story related by a London correspondent that Mr. Herbert Spencer, who has been credited with vegetarian principles, only adhered to that system of diet for one year. An enthusiastic devotee of the vegetarian school, meeting the philosopher a short time ago, asked him if he still adhered to vegetarianism. "I was a vegetarian for one year," Mr. Spencer rejoined, "but at the end of that time I went over all that I had written during the year and consigned it *in toto* to the fire."

Stamp Tax on Proprietary Medicines.—It has been the general expectation that the price of all articles upon which war tax may be imposed would advance in price to the extent of the tax. The Maltine Co. announces that despite the increasing cost of barley, wheat, oats, cod-liver oil, quinin, and other commodities that enter into the composition of the Maltine preparation, they have decided that they themselves will bear this tax of four cents per bottle which is to be imposed upon their output, and no advance in price will be made.

Dr. Kelsey and the New York Post-Graduate Medical Schoo and Hospital.—The Appellate Division recently reversed an order which granted Professor Charles B. Kelsey a writ of mandamus compelling the Directors of the New York Post-Graduate Medical School and Hospital to rescind a resolution revoking his appointment as a Professor of Surgery, and restoring him to the professorship and all the rights and privileges incident thereto. Justice Barrett wrote the opinion, which held that the By-Laws of the Corporation authorized the Directors to remove a professor at pleasure.

Sanitary Condition of the Camp at Chickamauga Park.—The policing of the grounds is excellent. Rubbish of all kinds is strictly tabooed wherever it is possible to avoid it. The daily details, with their suitable implements, keep the entire camp in almost immaculate condition. The health of the men, as a result of favorable natural conditions, pure air and pure water, supported by the efficient sanitary precautions, leaves nothing to be desired, and enforces many hours of idleness upon the hospital corps.

Ample opportunity for recreation is furnished for the men when not on duty. Baseball is the favorite sport.

Medical Examinations at Camp Townsend, Peekskill, N. Y.—The physique of the New York State militiamen who are being examined for enlistment as volunteers proves to be remarkably good. Only about five per cent. are being rejected. This is in striking contrast to the reports which come from Camp Rogers, State of Washington, in which it is announced that so many are being rejected that the officers declare that they might as well disband their entire commands and go home. This favorable showing for the Eastern recruits is undoubtedly due to the rigid system of gymnastic exercises constantly enforced.

X-ray Apparatus for Field Hospitals.—Professor Reginald A. Fessenden of the Western University of Pennsylvania has just completed a portable X-ray apparatus for use by the surgeons in the field during the war. The apparatus is as large as an unabridged dictionary and will weigh about twenty-five pounds. It is to be operated by a gas-motor of like weight, and the generator will be one of the smallest ever employed in practical work. The apparatus will supply X-rays of sufficient quantity and intensity to enable the surgeons to see through the body, and should provide a valuable adjunct to the equipment of the field hospitals.

Appointments and Promotions in the Surgical Department of the Army.—Colonel Charles R. Greenleaf, Assistant Surgeon-General, recently stationed at San Francisco, has arrived in Washington for duty on the staff of Major-General Miles, as chief surgeon of troops in the field. To be Chief Surgeons, with rank of Lieutenant-Colonel, Majors Benjamin F. Pope, surgeon United States army; Robert M. O'Reilly, surgeon United States army; Alfred C. Girard, surgeon United States army; John Van R. Hoff, surgeon United States army; Louis M. Maus, surgeon United States army; Rush Huidekoper of Pennsylvania. To be Assistant Surgeon-General, with rank of Lieutenant-Colonel, Nicholas Senn of Illinois. The House Committee on Military Affairs has reported favorably the bill authorizing fifteen additional assistant surgeons in the army, ranking as first lieutenants, and as many contract surgeons as the War Department deems necessary.

Obituary.—Dr. Isaac N. Quimby, a well-known physician of Jersey City, died of pneumonia, on the 6th inst., at his home in Jersey City. He was born at Bernardville, N. J. He was a graduate of the Medical Department of the University of New York. He was appointed Surgeon during the Civil War and served with the Army of the Potomac until after the battle of the Wilderness, when he established himself permanently in Jersey City. He was a member of the American Medical Association.—David Wendell Yandell, a distinguished physician and surgeon of Louisville, Ky., died Monday, May 2, after several years illness. He was born September 12, 1826, near Murfreesborough, Tenn., and graduated in medicine from the University of Louisville; he also spent two years in study in Europe, returning to Louisville to practice. He was Professor of Surgery in the University of Louisville in 1859, and a Medical Director in the Confederate Army from 1861 to 1866; he was also President of the American Medical Association in 1871, and became Professor of Surgery in the Indiana Medical College in 1874. In 1870 he established the *American Practitioner*.

CORRESPONDENCE.

OUR PHILADELPHIA LETTER.

[From our Special Correspondent.]

THE CONTROL OF MEDICAL CHARITIES—WILLS' EYE HOSPITAL AND ITS CRITICS—BICYCLE AMBULANCE-CORPS—A FLOOD OF NAUSEATING "LITERATURE"—MEDICO-CHIRURGICAL COLLEGES OF DENTISTRY AND PHARMACY—PROTECTION OF THE WATER-SUPPLY FROM POISONING BY SPANISH AGENTS.

MAY 7, 1898.

THE much-talked of meeting of hospital physicians and managers to consider the subject of the abuse of medical charities, was held at the College of Physicians on May 3d. The majority of the speakers, while entirely agreed as to the urgent need of reforming the abuse and of finding a remedy without loss of time for the present objectionable state of affairs, were by no means agreed as to the best method to be employed for the correction of the trouble. Although numerous plans, some of them seemingly excellent in many ways, were advanced and freely discussed, no definite agreement was reached, and no compromise was effected by which a single plan could be made acceptable to all concerned; it was, therefore, finally agreed to entrust to a committee of five the further investigation of the whole subject, this committee being instructed to formulate a definite line of action, and to arrange for a permanent organization of those interested in the furtherance of the work. At present, the difficulties to be overcome are many and powerful, because of the decided disinclination of many institutions to "fall into line," and to send representatives to participate in the consideration of the subject. The members of the committee appointed are to direct their attention largely toward these institutions, to try to solicit their interest and cooperation, and to ascertain from them, if possible, definite statements of their attitude concerning the present agitation. As soon as this is accomplished, and when the other instructions of the committee have been carried out, another meeting will be called, at which it is hoped the course of the procedure agreed upon by those interested will be announced in exact terms. At the meeting held this week Judge Ashman was the presiding officer, and Willim B. Thompson, Esq., was secretary. Among those who participated in the discussion were Drs. Edward Jackson, Carl Frese, J. V. Shoemaker, J. W. Walk, C. H. Burnett, and W. W. Holmes.

Quite a warfare of criticism is at present being waged against that historic institution, the Will's Eye Hospital, for its innovation in contracting with a single firm of manufacturers of optical instruments for filling the prescriptions issued to dispensary cases at a price barely above cost to patients. Recently the Board of City Trusts, the governing body of the hospital, became dissatisfied with the manner in which the filling of oculists' prescriptions was conducted, and resolved that it would serve all interests best to have the work done by a single firm to which all the patients of the hospital must go for this purpose. Accordingly they invited bids from manufacturers, with the result that it was decided to award the entire contract to the lowest reputable bidder, which happened, in this case, to be one of the leading and most reliable firms in the city. Under the new rule the patients are furnished with an order for glasses on the firm specified, instead of with a prescription to be filled by any optician to whom they may choose to go; this firm then receives direct from the hospital the prescription for the patient in question, which is filled on receipt of the patient's order. The hospital authorities claim that the benefits of the new plan are a saving of expense to the patient, and the facility with which defects in the filling of prescription may be traced and remedied. The critics of the system cry "pauperization of the community," and intimate favoritism along commercial lines. Meanwhile the experiment must work itself out, and time alone can indicate the wisdom or the mistake of the innovation.

Two offers have been recently made to the city authorities to furnish bicycle ambulance-corps for park and for street service. The first offer comes from the League of American Wheelmen's Emergency Bicycle Corps, which has offered its services to the Fairmount Park Commissioners during the season, free of expense for the proposed ambulance patrol. This corps consists of twenty uniformed surgeons, mounted on wheels, and two bicycle ambulances, each ridden by four persons. The second offer comes from the Emergency Bicycle Corps of the Department of Public Safety, consisting of sixty-five physicians, each of whom is in direct connection with the central police bureau of the city. A small metal red cross is to be attached to the members' wheel during the day, and a small transparent red cross in front of the lens of the lamp at night will enable the public to recognize the corps at all times. It is said that the Department of Public Safety will accept both offers, and that the service will be inaugurated before the end of the present month.

Philadelphia has been literally flooded of late with patent-medicine booklets from a New England firm, setting forth in glowing terms the merits of its nostrum, which, according to its manufacturers, eradicates every feminine ill, from uterine fibroids to acne. To remark that these advertisements are vile and obscene does not begin to express the nauseating nature of their contents, which are of the stamp which a profound sexual pervert would devour with glee and appreciation; and to state that these booklets find a widespead circulation conveys but a faint idea of the freedom with which they are distributed, by mail, by carrier from door to door, and by personal distribution at the street corners. The front paper-cover of the advertisement bears a lithographic illustration of the most innocent nature imaginable, and gives no hint of the contents, which are filled with matter utterly unfit for promiscuous or any other kind of reading, either among the old or the young. Postmaster Hicks, who has been asked to investigate the matter with a view to suppressing the circulation of the booklets, has looked into the case, and has expressed himself as entirely unable to exclude the matter from the mail, for the reason that "it has been decided that the matter referred to comes within the classification of legitimate medical advertising!"

After months of litigation, in which a prominent dental college of this city figured against the Medico-Chirurgical College, the latter institution has been granted by the courts an amendment to its charter permitting it to grant degrees in dental surgery and in pharmacy, in addition to the work of its medical school. The plans for the establishment of the two new schools have already been announced in these columns.

A wholesale spirit of excessive caution seems to have taken possession of our city legislators in prompting them to prepare an ordinance providing for the appointment of fifty special guards to protect the several city water reservoirs against any possible attempts on the part of Spanish agents to poison the water-supply of the city. Unlike New York City, which receives its entire water-supply from a single source through an enormous aqueduct which might be polluted at any point along its course with immense damage to the entire city, Philadelphia receives its water from several stations, each serving a separate district; so that any attempt at pollution could be at once traced with ease, and the section of the city supplied from the polluted storage basin cut off until danger is past.

The total number of deaths occurring in this city for the week ending May 7th numbered 445, a decrease of 25 from last week, and an increase of 27 over the corresponding period of last year. There were 207 new cases of contagious diseases reported, as follows: diphtheria, 86 cases, with 22 deaths; scarlet fever, 61 cases, with 7 deaths; and enteric fever, 60 cases, with 9 deaths.

OUR WIESBADEN LETTER.

[From our Special Correspondent.]

A GERMAN MEDICAL CONGRESS AND ITS SERIOUSNESS—THE DISPOSAL OF "BORES"—SOME WATERING-PLACES AND THEIR WATERS—AN OLD FOUNDATION AND MODERN SCIENTIFIC WORK AT FRANKFORT.

WIESBADEN, April 30, 1898.

A GERMAN medical congress is a very business like affair. At least here at Wiesbaden there are very few distractions from the work of the congress itself. One of the evenings is given up to a dinner of course, but beyond that there are no formal public entertainments. There is a café in which a number of the doctors meet during the midday intermission to take what in Rhineland they have specially named "Frühschoppen." (A social morning glass is the nearest translation of it I can find.) The term is a favorite one with the students' guilds; the custom also a favorite. In the evenings there is a special rendezvous for a social glass, but to neither of these places do more than a very small minority of the doctors go.

Sessions begin rather promptly at 9.15 A.M., and last till nearly 1 P.M., though 12 o'clock is announced for the end of the session. They begin again at 3 P.M., sharp, and continue until about 6 P.M. The morning session, particularly when discussions are announced, is very well attended. As in medical societies generally over here, a great deal of interest is taken. German medical men are, I think, less considerate of the feelings of the reader of a paper than we are. When, for instance, the perennial bore, the special *bête noir* of medical societies, the man who has nothing to say and takes twenty minutes in which to proclaim the fact, bobs up, he is apt to feel in the hum of conversation that very soon begins that he might as well be talking to the stars, or that his voice might be the music of the spheres, so utterly oblivious seems his audience of it.

On the other hand when really good things are said, be it only a good bit of comparative literary abstraction, that makes clear the present position of a subject, there follows a series of most encouraging bravos. The other bore, the man who thinks he has discovered a new symptom or a new therapeutic method in some long since exploited expedient, is very apt to be laughed out of countenance at once. During one of the sessions a young man attempted to demonstrate a new symptom of early pancreatic diabetes, in a tenderness about the tail of the pancreas, to be felt in the eighth intercostal space in the anterior axillary line on the left; "*et risu soloebantur tabule; sic nos servabit Apollo.*"

The congress is over now and the members have gone, that is all except a few, who remain to take the waters for awhile. They are, as a rule, the older ones whose faith has never been rudely disturbed by too close observation of the therapeutic effect of a little hot salt water, or whose credulity has returned with advancing years, the later stages of evolution corresponding to the earlier stages of evolution, a harking back to the time when tales were true and facts unquestioned.

For the wonderful thing about all this region around here and in the Rhineland generally, is that a little common salt water, or carbonated water, comes bubbling up out of the bowels of the earth, and straightway it is invested with marvelous powers, and people afflicted with all the ills that flesh is heir to, and a few others besides, come flocking to it from all over, and, stranger than all, go away cured, or at least wonderfully relieved and benefited.

One has a chance to study here at Wiesbaden and at the recently more fashionable Homberg, not far from Frankfort-am-Main, the secret of the success of the cure. That it is due to the waters themselves with their plenitude of common salt, and minimal amounts of calcium and lithium salts, and traces of iron and even arsenic, scarcely any one now will affirm. It is true there are those like Professor Liebreich in Berlin, who insist that our chemical analysis of the constituents of these springs is anything but final. Even in the last few years it has been found that the waters of Wiesbaden contain much more lithium than was formerly thought, yet the laboratory of the famous analytic chemist, Fresenius, is in Wiesbaden, and its reputation has been fully maintained by his son and successor. Then the discovery within the last few years of argon in the air, has shown how defective are present chemic methods for the analysis of the most familiar materials, even when the very best and most exact scientific chemic means are used. Finally, even if we did know the exact chemic constituents, it would be but coarsely; of their relations one to another in certain physic and chemic combinations and the effects on complicated human metabolism of a series of such unstable compounds, we know next to nothing.

But all this is the argument of a man who holds a brief for pharmacology and will not see lightly slip from the realm of drugs into that of the so-called natural therapeutic methods, the number of ailments which yearly are benefited at watering-places. The practitioners themselves at the watering-places have been more frank in their acknowledgement of the benefit to be derived from physical methods, and so there are in the town and neighborhood hydrotherapic, vegetarian, fruit, grape, gymnastic, massage, and electrotherapic cures, one of which at least, is associated in nearly all cases with the taking of the waters. The baths include every variety imaginable, hot and cold, steam and compressed air, dry and moist hot air, mineral, pine, and aerated baths. Twenty thousand pounds of grapes are consumed in a year for the grape cure. Of course this condition easily glides into the realm of charlatanism, but in this respect the various establishments are well managed and seem to be perfectly under control.

The régime required while taking the waters is itself the best therapeutic measure in Wiesbaden. They are drunk first in the early morning between 6 and 8 A.M., during which hours the band plays at the spring, and again in the afternoon between 3 and 5 P.M., so that the temptation to those of sluggish circulation to oversleep, is removed at the two periods of the day when it is most alluring. A dietary is always insisted on during "the cure" and this is not hard to kept up as all around one at the hotels and pensions are people with restricted diet. Then the walks around the town are most pleasant, gentle mountain walks lead through beautiful grounds and those never before given to walking much are tempted out. When to those factors are added the fact that it is fashionable to take the waters, that so many have been benefited and so much written about the curative properties of Wiesbaden's waters—printers' ink is an important constituent of many a proprietary preparation, that does not reveal itself to the most exact chemical analysis—then it is easy to understand how a course of the waters does good. It must be good—the wonderful suggestive element of all therapeutics—and there is an end of it.

Of course at Homberg there is the additional factor that Royalty goes there every year; the Emperor and Empress of Germany, the Czar and Czarina of Russia, the King and Queen of Italy, and Albert Edward, Prince of Wales, to visit his sister the Dowager Empress of Germany, who has a house there every year during the season. When to these are added the Knights and Grand Dukelings of the little German monarchies, the suggestive therapeutic influence of the springs at Homberg can be confidently looked to, to be almost fabulously effective. It is to be remembered however that they really do do good, however we may analyze their effect, and after all at the end of the century it is coming to be very generally admitted, even here in Germany, that a doctor's main purpose is to benefit his patient even if the means employed are not always those that admit of exact scientific explanation, or the definition of their indications remains persistently obscure.

Progress in scientific medicine is cared for in the Rhineland at the two universities, Bonn and Heidelberg. Frankfort has no university but as the result of an old foundation, she has a central point around which science is cultivated quite as effectively and successfully as if there really were a university.

In the middle of the last century a Dr. Senckenberg of Frankfort, who was interested in anatomy and lectured on the subject with dissections to some kindred spirits in a small amphitheater in his garden just inside the city walls, left the grounds and building together with his private hospital not far away and an endowment for their support, to the city for the cultivation of science, especially anatomy and botany.

The trust has been excellently administered and now the grounds are very valuable, not far from the center of the town, and the endowment income considerable. Very commendable, however, has been the liberal way in which the board of trustees have interpreted the clause of deed of gift as to the cultivation of science. All the scientific societies of the city have been given a free perpetual lease of ground for their buildings and the trust has aided them in their establishment where possible. Now the library of the Senckerberg institute is the combination of the libraries of all these societies in a special building. The Anatomical Institute has ever been the special charge of the trust of course. Its director at present is Professor Weigert, and here of late years have been elaborated his staining methods for details of anatomical work. Here Edinger has been doing his recent work on the etiology of tabes, and for years on the minute anatomy of the nervous system. Here nearly always are to be found a certain number of Americans, for where there is a good thing here in Europe, even though it may be but little known outside of its immediate neighborhood, there you will find American medical students.

And so the old Doctor of the first half of the Eighteenth Century lives on in the work of the end of the Nineteenth, when the anatomical studies he was so much interested in have taken a direction of which he never could have dreamed, but fortunately which no shortsightedness of his, from too narrow restrictions in his bequest, was allowed to hinder.

TRANSACTIONS OF FOREIGN SOCIETIES.

Paris.

ETIOLOGY OF CIRRHOSIS — CONGENITAL GOITER CURED—X-RAYS AND THE BLIND—UNUSUAL PERFORATION OF SMALL INTESTINE — SUBPHRENIC ABSCESS LOCATED WITH DIFFICULTY—POST-OPERATIVE PSYCHOSES GROSSLY EXAGGERATED—ERYSIPELAS SUCCESSFULLY TREATED WITH IODOLE—APYRETIC SCARLET FEVER.

AT the Academy of Medicine, March 29th, HAYEN said that in his experience one could establish a parallelism between the increase in the consumption of liquors, particularly of absinthe, and the decrease of cases of *cirrhosis* of atrophic character. This fact is in accord with the theory that wine-drinkers, being usually hypopeptic, are exposed to atropic cirrhosis, while those who drink strong alcoholic beverages are almost always hyperpeptic, and are, therefore, prone to develop a hypertrophic cirrhosis. The speaker said that the action of the sulphate of potash in the production of cirrhosis scarcely merited serious consideration.

At the session of April 12th, GASSICOURT reported a case of *congenital goiter* of an infant of three months cured by thyroid fed to its mother, she herself being also goitrous. The dried equivalent of about 20 grains of thyroid gland was given the mother daily in divided doses for about five days. The treatment was then interrupted for four or five days, and later it was resumed as stated above. No symptom of thyroidism appeared as a result of this medication either in mother or child. At the end of six weeks of treatment the goiter of the mother had become somewhat smaller, while that of the child was more profoundly benefited, and at the end of four months it had entirely disappeared.

At the Academy of Sciences, March 21st, DE COURMELLES communicated the interesting fact that *certain blind persons can distinguish the X-rays*, although they must have at least a slight perception of ordinary rays of light in order to do so. A test was made of 240 young blind scholars, of whom 36 were at once eliminated, as they had partial vision. Of the 204 considered suitable for experiment, 81 had absolutely no perception of light. No one of these perceived at all any one of the three kinds of electroluminous rays produced by Crookes' tubes. Among those able to recognize in some faint degree the nature of light, there were nine who perceived the fluorescent and cathode X-ray, while others less delicate were unable to recognize the X-ray, although perceiving the other rays of the tubes. The retina of the blind eye seems, therefore, to play to a certain extent the rôle of a photographic plate when submitted to the X-ray. This property seems to be lacking in the normal eye.

At the session of the Surgical Society, March 16th, KIRMISSON reported that he had operated upon a boy aged eight years for what was supposed to be an attack of appendicitis. There proved to be, however, nothing wrong with the appendix, but the abdomen contained blood and purulent matter from a *perforation in the small intestine*, at about its middle. The opening was situated close to the mesenteric border, and was sutured in the usual manner. There was a discharge of fecal matter for some days, and then the patient entirely recovered. No explanation as to the origin of the perforation was offered.

MONOD, at the meeting, March 23d, said that he had operated upon two cases with similar symptoms. One of them died, and the perforation which had not been discovered at the operation, was found to be situated in the small intestine, close to the cecal end. The other patient after a long purulent discharge recovered, so that the site of the perforation of the intestine, if such existed, was not located. It is certain that a number of ulcerations of the small intestine occur, besides those due to tuberculosis and typhoid fever. Potain admits that ulcers similar to those of the duodenum may be found in other portions of the small intestine, and Letulle describes intestinal ulcerations occurring in connection with uremia. In default of any other cause, it is necessary to ascribe them to some traumatism.

PICQUE was called to see a patient who had been ill for three months with what was supposed to be purulent pleurisy, although two punctures had been negative in result, and the signs of empyema were absent. An intrahepatic abscess was diagnosticated, and a transpleural incision was made. Portions of the ninth and tenth ribs were resected. The pleural cavity was free, and two punctures of the liver failed to locate the trouble. Finally a small *subdiaphragmatic abscess* was found, which, as proved by the microscopic examination, originated in the lung, and had made its way through the diaphragm.

PICQUE said, at a previous meeting of this society, that *post-operative psychoses* were often ascribed to the operations which preceded them, especially if these were upon the genital organs. The facts in this connection have been grossly exaggerated, for in many instances it is true that the patients have either been insane before or that they have inherited an abnormal nervous state. Thus, if an ovariotomy has been performed in an interval of lucidity after several periods of confinement in an insane hospital, a further attack of the mental trouble is almost invariably blamed upon the surgical interference.

WALTHER emphasized the importance in all cases suspected of insane tendencies of a most exact record of the previous and present mental condition of the patient.

RICHELOT thought that some of the cases of post-operative psychosis were due to an association of ideas with the parts operated upon in persons already insane or disposed toward mental derangement. In other instances there was absolutely no demonstrable connection between the operation and the succeeding mental state. In the eleven cases of post-operative psychosis which had come under his notice the operative act could not be said to have created *de novo* the insanity in a single instance. Sometimes an operation is followed by temporary hysterical trouble, but he doubted whether that was more likely to be true of pelvic operations than of those in other situations.

REYNIER, at the session of March 30th, expressed himself in accord with the previous speakers, and again urged the desirability of an exact mental diagnosis before attempting any surgical operation. In these persons we are likely to have psychoses after operation; there is a disproportion between the amount of pain complained of, and the lesion which produces it.

SEGOND said that a careful study of the subject had forced him to the conclusion that the psychoses spoken of as post-operative, were in reality pre-operative. It is also of interest to notice that a disordered mind is sometimes cured by an operation, as was the case in a woman from whom he had removed both ovaries for cystic disease.

At the Therapeutic Society, March 23d, LOBIT said that he had obtained excellent results in the treatment of erysipelas and lymphangitis by the use of a ten-per-cent. solution of iodoform and, even better, by iodol in collodium. In twenty-five cases of erysipelas a cure had resulted from this method of treatment in three or four days. The presence in the urine of iodin, shows that the drug is absorbed, the absorption being favored apparently by the presence of the collodium. These applications are not at all painful, on the contrary, they often give an immediate relief.

At the Medical Society of the Hospitals, April 1st, RENON communicated an observation which he had made in connection with scarlet fever, in a patient whose temperature did not go above 37.4° C. (99.5° F.). There was no doubt as to the diagnosis, however, and scarlatiniform erythema of toxic or infectious origin could be absolutely excluded. In this as in similar cases there was a dissociation between the pulse-rate and the temperature. The patient had no complications and recovered perfectly.

LEMOINE said that the fact of an apyretic scarlet fever was to-day established without a doubt. The gravest results may follow in these cases, just because the physician is thrown off his guard by the absence of fever, and omits the customary precautions. He referred to the nephritis in the patient himself, and to the dissemination of the disease among his associates.

SOCIETY PROCEEDINGS.

THE SIXTEENTH ANNUAL GERMAN CONGRESS FOR INTERNAL MEDICINE.

Held at Wiesbaden, Germany, April 13 to 17, 1898.

[From our Special Correspondent.]

THE Sixteenth Annual German Congress for Internal Medicine was formally opened by its President, Professor Moritz Schmidt, the distinguished laryngologist of Frankfort, on Wednesday, April 13th and closed on Saturday, April 17th. Some idea of the interest taken in it in Germany may be gathered from the fact that over four hundred German doctors, including most of the distinguished professors of internal medicine at the various German universities, took part in its proceedings.

PROFESSOR VON ZEIMSSEN of Munich, after the president's address of welcome, read a paper, prepared by special invitation, upon

CLINICAL INSTRUCTION IN MEDICINE.

He is of the opinion that the present teaching of medicine needs improvement in many directions, but especially in the *technical clinical training* of the young physician. For that as a *preliminary condition* there is needed (1) a *lengthening* of the medical course to ten semesters, five years (it is now nine semesters). (2) practical laboratory work in chemistry, anatomy, physiology, pathologic anatomy, and pharmacology. (3) fundamental lectures covering the whole ground of special pathology and therapy.

For the *practical technical* training itself there is required: (1) practical courses in diagnosis, not only physical diagnosis so-called, but microscopic, chemic, bacterioscopic, neuro-electro-diagnosis, and rhinolaryngoscopic; (2) Systematic practice in the actual employment of the therapeutic methods, dietetics, hydro- and balneotherapy, mechanotherapy, electrotherapy, inhalation and climatotherapy.

For the clinical training, service in a dispensary for a given time under proper direction till the student has acquired such efficiency that the care of patients is practically in his hands is needed.

Finally, to complete and round up his practical clinical training, the student should have a year, or at least a half year of actual hospital service, where as an assistant he would have to assume personal responsibilities for his patients. This hospital experience should come after the examinations, as otherwise inevitably the thought of examinations to come would lead him to pay special attention, not to what he considered valuable for practice, but what would be liable to be asked in examination.

PROFESSOR VON JAKSCH was the other referee on

MEDICAL EDUCATION.

He also demanded a lengthening of the course. It is now ten semesters long in Austria and he proposes to make it twelve semesters (six years). The extra year he would take away from the nine-years' course in the gymnasia and would devote it to a preparatory course for medicine at the university. This year would be devoted to zoology, botany, minerology, and geology. This thorough grounding of the medical student in the natural sciences he believes absolutely needed. Practical medicine would be supplemented by courses, during this year, in photography, Röntgen skiagraphy, and the care of electric apparatus.

As to the improvement of present teaching he would secure it by modifications of the present medical course, so that clinical medicine and its scientific foundations, would be the principal study up to graduation. The student should go to specialists only to learn where these specialties touched upon general medicine. No details of specialization should be admitted into the course. For specialists he would institute an extra year, during which, in a dispensary, or under a specialist's care, they should learn the operative technic and appropriate diagnostic methods of their specialty, only such as had had such training being permitted (as is customary in Europe) to assume the title specialist.

Von Jaksch thinks that while von Zeimssen's proposal to have a complete series of lectures on the whole subject of special pathology and therapy, is the expression of an absolute need, yet these lectures must not be purely didactic. Even Billroth found that his didactic lectures would not draw students enough to make it worth his while to continue them. The day for didactic lectures has gone by. The substance of them must now find a place in the regular clinical lectures, which must be so varied as to introduce the various subjects. The same opinion as to purely didactic lectures was expressed in the discussion of the question and seemed to be the general opinion.

DR. MENDELSOHN of Berlin, at the afternoon session, spoke of the

THERAPEUTIC USES OF EXTREMELY HIGH TEMPERATURES.

He, later in the week, demonstrated Tallerman's apparatus for the treatment of chronic joint affections by the inclosure of the affected limb in an air-tight chamber, the air of which is heated to 140° to 180° F. The method attracted a great deal of attention.

DR. ROSIN of Berlin, treated of

THE GOOD TO BE DERIVED FROM HOT BATHS IN CHLOROSIS.

One of the most promising recent advances in the treatment of obstinate cases of chlorosis is diaphoresis. Better than the dry, hot-air baths for this condition are the hot-water baths. The idea is an adoption of a Japanese custom. The Japanese, when very tired, get into a hot bath up to 45° C. (110° to 115° F.) which proves very refreshing. Chlorotics are persistently tired. Their muscles are easily exhausted because badly supplied with nutritive material. A characteristic symptom that Dr. Rosin finds in most of his chlorotics, and which makes them come complaining of something the matter with their lungs, is pain between the shoulder-blades. The erector spinæ muscles suffer from the act of keeping the patient erect. Slight pinching of the muscles or tapping of them gives pain. The reflex action of the hot baths causes more blood to be brought to the muscles and relieves this muscular discomfort. The removal of water from the hydremic blood by diaphoresis, reacts on the nutrition of all the tissues and the blood-making organs take up their functions once more. A bath at 32° R. (105° F.) with a wet towel wrapped around the head, though Dr. Rosin has seen no inconvenience result when this precaution was neglected, is given for one-half to three-quarters of an hour. This causes plentiful perspiration during the bath. It is followed by a cold douche to prevent further perspiration which would be exhausting. A bath is given three times a week for three to four weeks.

DR. DETERMANN of St. Bastien demonstrated the

DIAGNOSTIC SIGNIFICANCE OF BLOOD-PLAQUES.

They are not pathognomonic of any particular disease. Their presence is an index of the isotonicity of the blood, of the lack of vital resistance of red blood-corpuscles to external influences. He demonstrated a series of blood preparations showing red cells in the process of disintegration, or at least of constricting off a portion of their protoplasm. This he considers the origin of blood-plaques. Their presence in any considerable number then, is indicative of a lowered state of vitality in the red blood-cells and so is of diagnostic significance, often before any other morphologic change can be noticed in the blood.

DR. ENGEL of Berlin demonstrated preparations of the

NUCLEATED RED BLOOD-CELL OF A SPECIAL KIND.

He had found this in fatal pernicious anemia cases. It

is a large, nucleated, red cell, differentiated from megaloblasts by its different reaction to the tri-acid stain. He has found the same cell in human embryos of three to six months and in the embryos of rats of eight to twelve days. He suggests for it, owing to its embryologic connections, the name metrocyte (mother cell).

It is another step, Dr. Engel thinks, in the substantiation of Ehrlich's theory, that genuine pernicious anemia is a thorough reversion to the embryonic state of the blood-making organs. The finding of this red cell makes the prognosis of the case extremely unfavorable and decides the question that it is not a severe secondary anemia which must be dealt with, but a true progressive pernicious anemia.

PROFESSOR LEO of Bonn read by invitation a paper upon

THE PRESENT-DAY TREATMENT OF DIABETES MELLITUS.

As regards prophylaxis he detailed some of his own recent experiments, in which he has been able to produce mellituria artificially in dogs by feeding them a ten-per-cent. solution of sugar, in a state of fermentation. It was not due to the ferments present, since it occurred also when the liquid had been previously boiled. Fermented liquors such as beer, he thinks, may be of some etiologic importance in the production of diabetes. Not that they are actual causes, otherwise notably more men than women would become diabetic, which is not the case. In people with a nervous or diabetic heredity, or in very stout people whose faculty for sugar metabolism is distinctly less than that of normal individuals, he thinks the prophylaxis of diabetes includes especially abstention from beer and fermented liquors generally.

Professor Leo is of the opinion too that the metabolic faculty for sugar when lessened may be restored by absolute physiologic rest for a time. All carbohydrates cannot be kept out of the food at all times, but even in the lighter forms of diabetes he requires his patients to pass three to four weeks, three to four times each year, on an absolute diet, from which all carbohydrates are excluded. While bread and the food stuffs rich in carbohydrates must be forbidden, he does not believe, as do Cantani and others of the Italian school, that all vegetables should be forbidden ordinarily. Some of them, as the green vegetables, contain comparatively small quantities of the carbohydrates, while it is probable that they also contain, as Naunyn thinks, certain salts that are absolutely necessary for the human economy.

MINKOWSKI of Strassburg, in the discussion of the subject, reported that in dogs rendered diabetic by the removal of the pancreas, he had found that the exhibition of pancreas had done good. Von Leube has been trying this clinically with some encouraging results, but with insufficient experience as yet to speak definitely of the value of this mode of treatment.

PROFESSOR VON JAKSCH thinks that, like fever some years ago, the importance of decreasing the sugar in the urine is overestimated. Every one a few years ago was bringing down his patients' temperatures with antipyretics, and congratulating himself on his success just inasmuch as he succeeded in keeping his patients' temperature down almost to normal in the course of an infectious fever. No one thinks of doing any such thing now, and it is very possible that we shall have after a few years something of the same feeling with regard to our present attitude towards the all-important problem of rendering the urine free from sugar in diabetes. It is not the excretion of the sugar in the urine that is so serious, but it is that Nature, finding no use for it, treats it as a useless substance, and eliminates it. We are not improving matters by giving her no further sugar to eliminate. There will be no glycosuria, but the nutrition will suffer. What we must do is find some form of sugar that Nature will use, though she has lost the faculty of making use of grape sugar. Professor von Jaksch himself has had some very encouraging results with carbohydrates of different molecular constitution from ordinary sugar. Arabinose-methyl pentose has been the most satisfactory so far. It may be obtained rather cheaply, and is very well borne by the system when other sugar is immediately excreted.

Practically, all the disputants were agreed that *saccharin* was not the merely indifferent sweetening material that it has been represented to be. Dr. Bornstein found that it seriously disturbed the digestion, a very serious result in diabetics, on whose good digestion everything as regards prognosis depends. Boas had found it useful *as a drug* in abnormal fermentative processes in the intestine. Professor von Jaksch was very much opposed to its use, and was glad to have Boas speak directly of it as a drug. Its inhibitory action on abnormal fermentation had often extended itself to normal fermentative processes, on which digestion depends. He had seen not a little gastro-intestinal disturbance which he could attribute only to its use.

The question of the effect of *subcutaneous sugar injection as a means of nutrition* in diabetes remains an open one. Gumpert of Jena has tried it, and with some encouraging results, but the inconveniences are sometimes great. Professor von Leuhe has tried it, but has given it up because the injections are painful, and it is impossible to avoid infiltrations, and at times suppuration at the point of injection. In Leyden's clinic the results have been somewhat the same, but their experiments are not concluded.

As to subcutaneous injections of nutritive material in general, olive oil is in use for the purpose at a number of clinics, and is giving very good satisfaction. Professor von Leube considers that it is beyond its experimental stage now, and is to be regarded as an acknowledged adjunct to therapy. The importance of albuminuria in diabetic cases and its frequency was brought out by Dr. Grube of Neuenahr. Between thirty-five and forty per cent. of all diabetics have albumin in their urine. In most of these cases it is merely a functional kidney disturbance, due to the excessive sugar secretion, but this functional disturbance may easily go on to degeneration, the tubules may show signs of glycogenic degeneration, and finally chronic parenchymatous, or more rarely interstitial nephritis may develop. The necessity for prophylaxis in the matter by having the food of diabetics such as is liable to cause least kidney irritation was pointed out.

PROFESSOR MINKOWSKI reported the discovery in the urine of dogs fed upon thymus glands of,

A HITHERTO UNDESCRIBED NITROGENOUS SUBSTANCE.

This new substance resembles in many ways uric acid, and its discoverer suggests the name urotic acid. It occurs in dog's urine fed on calf's thymus in twenty times the amount in which uric acid occurs. Professor Minkowski regards it as an incomplete stage of the evolution of uric acid in the system and considers that further study of it may throw light on the processes by which uric acid is produced in the organism, which is as yet an interesting mystery.

DR. EDINGER began Thursday afternoon's session very attractively reading a paper upon

EXPERIMENTALLY PRODUCED DEGENERATIONS OF THE POSTERIOR COLUMNS.

These resemble the lesions of tabes. Rats that had been made anemic were compelled to overexert themselves in a tread-mill run by a water-motor. After forty-eight hours of work the degenerations exhibited had been produced. Not the whole of the posterior columns are degenerated *en bloc*, but a large number of the fibers. The method of staining is that of Marchi. Beside these specimens were placed the cords of animals in whom anemia alone had been at work and a striking difference was evident.

Edinger considers that this makes clear the etiology of tabes. It is a degeneration of the sensitive sensory nerve-fibers from overexertion, when their vital resistance has been lowered by some general systemic condition, be it anemia, toxic influences, or attenuated syphilis. The much debated question as to where the degeneration begins, becomes then of secondary importance. At different times the resistance in the various parts of the nerve may vary, and so the degeneration need not necessarily begin always at the same point.

For prophylaxis and treatment Edinger considers these observations of the greatest practical importance. Syphilitics, anemic people, and those in a run-down condition, must be warned of the serious risk of overexertion, or of exposure to cold for a long time, etc. Those in the pre-ataxic stage of the disease must be warned about the danger of making the symptoms develop more rapidly than they otherwise would if they are indiscreet in the amount of physical exertion undertaken. The movement therapy of tabes must be carried out with the greatest regard to not overfatiguing the patient.

PROFESSOR PETRUSCHKY demonstrated preparations of

STREPTOTHRIX HOMINIS.

He has now found this for the second time under circumstances which make him certain that it is pathogenic for the human race. He considers that it is the microbic cause of an affection which the common people in Dantzig call malaria, but in which Laveran's plasmodium is not found. ¶ This disease is characterized by more respiratory symptoms than are usual in ordinary malaria.

PROFESSOR VON ZIEMSSEN has observed the same parasite in the sputum of certain pulmonary cases, where tuberculosis was suspected but no tubercle bacilli found. He too considers it pathogenic.

DR. SCHOTT of Nauheim demonstrated by Röntgen skiagrams, that the dilatation of the heart, which accompanies disturbed compensation in ordinary valvular heart lesions, recedes under the use of properly graduated exercises with resistance. That the heart occupies less space in the thorax than before Professor von Ziemssen of Munich had demonstrated a series of Röntgen skiagrams of various thoracic conditions Dr. Schott thought every one must admit. The results shown by the Röntgen method are only the same as those which careful percussion had demonstrated beforehand.

PROFESSORS MULLER of Marburg and BRIEGER of Berlin read specially prepared papers Friday morning on

AUTO-INTOXICATION AND INTESTINAL ANTISEPSIS.

Both agree that auto-intoxication is the result of chemical absorption, not of bacterial invasion, though this is the teaching of some prominent French clinicians. Except where there are coarse lesions of the mucous membranes, the intestinal bacteria cannot penetrate the intestinal walls and enter the circulation. The ordinary saprophytic bacteria of the intestine play no important rôle in the production of the toxins, which are the result of chemical dissociations, when the intestinal contents stagnate.

In the urotoxic coefficient as an index of the toxins in the circulation, they have no confidence. Where so much liquid has to be injected into animals the isotonicity of the blood is disturbed and the results are absolutely of no value despite the faith of the Italians and French in the method. The toxins are excreted in the urine, and the only sure way to decide their presence and amount is careful analysis of the urine.

PROFESSOR EWALD demonstrated a new amido-toxin that he had found in the urine in a case of acute intestinal auto-intoxication. As to intestinal antisepsis it is an illusion. The best way to treat acute intestinal autointoxication is by a purgative. If the absorption seems to take place from the stomach, then this should be washed out.

BOAS thought that enough attention has not been paid to the urine in these cases of autointoxication. He has found it in a number of cases reduced as low as 300-400 c.cm. (20–27 ounces) in twenty-four hours. He considers prompt diuresis always indicated and think it fortunate that the best intestinal antiseptic (calomel) is also a good diuretic.

PROFESSOR MATTHES of Jena called attention to the fact that the intestinal contents instead of being uniformly alkaline, as stated by the text-books, is really amphoteric. To litmus and other reagents it gives an alkaline reaction, but is acid to still other reagents. This peculiarity of reaction is due to the presence of certain salts, especially the phosphates, which are taken with the food.

DR. JACOB of Berlin encouraged by the success of the Quincke lumbar puncture as a means of diagnosis and regretting that the hopes of its inventor, that it would be of therapeutic value, have not been fulfilled, has been trying to widen its use in therapeutics by the injection of medicaments into the subdural space, after the evacuation of some of the cerebrospinal fluid. Animals stand such injections very well and where they have been tried in severe cases in men, they have caused no untoward symptoms. Potassium iodid injected thus is eliminated in the urine in fifteen hours. Jacob considers that the method may be of great practical value in acute syphilitic processes in the cord or brain where it is important to get the immediate action of specific remedies in order to avoid lasting injury of delicate nervous structures.

DR. VAN NIESSEN presented a demonstration of

BACTERIA IN SYPHILITIC LESIONS.

In primary sores, in the epiphyses of children with hereditary syphilis, and in the blood of tertiary syphilitics, he has found various micro-organisms. These include especially diplococci, staphylococci, and streptococci. He considers that the bacterial cause of syphilis is not unique, but that its various types are due to mixed infection. His microbes take the ordinary stains, notably, carbolfuchsin, and have undobtedly been seen hundreds of times before by previous observers, who have considered that they had to do with a chance infection, or with a faulty technic. The recent publication of Van Niessen's paper by Virchow in his *Archives*, and his call to St. Petersburg, as was noted some time ago, to work on syphilis in the Institute of Experimental Medicine there, gives his communication no ephemeral interest. Van Niessen claims to have succeeded in producing syphilis-like lesions in swine, by the inoculation of specific infectious material, and announces a paper on the subject for the next congress.

DR. KEUHNAN of Breslau claims that proteus is intensely pathogenic in human mucous membranes. Its etiological rôle in ulcerative enteritis and cystitis has long been suspected, and Dr. Kühnan thinks that he can trace the deeply destructive processes that sometimes occur in oral and pharyngeal mucous membranes in the tonsils and base of the tongue to the same cause. He exhibited pictures of two such cases in which the protens had been found. For the proper study of protens a new technic will be needed, as its transplantation to the various media now used in bacteriology gives rise to morphologic changes which led to the description of as many varieties as there are media.

The next session of the German Congress is to be held at Carlsbad in Bohemia. It has been the custom so far to hold the sessions every second year at Wiesbaden, and then on alternate years at Berlin, Leipsig, Munich, and Vienna. The change comes at the suggestion of Professor Von Jaksch, and was voted unanimously. It is considered to be an expression of protest on the part of German medical men against the progress of "Slavization" in Bohemia, and the favoring of any such process by the Government.

Besides Van Niessen's paper on Syphilis, Professor Nothnagel of Vienna announces a communication "On Local Blood-Letting and So-called Local Counterirritation."

THE GERMAN SOCIETY OF SURGERY.

The Twenty-Seventh Congress, Held at Berlin, April 13, 14, 15, 16, 1898.

[Specially Reported for THE MEDICAL NEWS.]

THE Congress was conducted in a most practical and scientific manner and was a complete success. Important subjects were taken up in succession and after two or three twenty-minute papers were read on each, they were discussed by the house generally.

The first subject introduced was

THE LATEST METHODS FOR THE IMPROVEMENT OF ASEPSIS.

PROFESSOR MIKULICZ of Breslau, who first introduced gloves in operations, opened the scientific work of the Congress by describing and exhibiting a new aid toward absolute asepsis. It is a mouth and nose mask made of gauze. It is simple and light and is held in place by wires extending over the ears after the fashion of spectacles. He made a series of experiments with and without the mask, talking, coughing, and sneezing before agar plates; without the mask the plates always showed innumerable colonies, under the protection of the mask the number was reduced to one or two, and sometimes even no colonies. He considers that like the gloves this or a similar mask will soon be indispensable to the surgeon. He never operates without it.

He also announced that the gloves he now uses are no longer made simply of cloth, but of an impermeable substance, or if of cloth they are first rendered impermeable.

DR. PERTHES of Leipsic advocated gloves made of silk and rubber. They were not too thick, and so did not interfere with the sense of touch as did rubber gloves, and at the same time they had the advantage of impermeability. The only objection to them was that they are somewhat costly.

PROFESSOR DOEDERLEIN of Tübingen was satisfied with the old methods and did not believe in changing them. He still thought he could sterilize his hands sufficiently for practical purposes. Yet he saw a distinct place in surgery for the gloves. In emergency cases such as sudden hemorrhage when time for sterilization of the hands was limited he thought the gloves might be extremely useful.

In the general discussion on gloves the majority seemed to advocate them, and all acknowledged their usefulness. When one member went so far as to thank Professor Mikulicz in the name of surgery for the discovery, from every part of the hall came cries of bravo! bravo!

PROFESSOR WOELFLER of Prague, who introduced rubber gloves to the profession, said that he was no longer wearing them, but had found a better substitute in buckskin gloves which were prepared by soaking several days in xylol.

The Congress then took up the subject of

BACTERIA AND FRESH WOUNDS.

PROFESSOR FREDERICK of Leipsic showed by experiments on animals that the infection of fresh wounds remains superficial for at least 6 to 8 hours, but not much longer. He concluded therefore that the proper treatment of a wound was, if the wound came to the surgeon within the limited time to freshen the edges and stitch the wound. But if the wound was older than this it should be treated after the open method.

DR. NOETZEL of Königsberg repeated Schimmelbusch's experiments and confirmed his results, showing that bacteria were absorbed very rapidly from fresh wounds. Ten minutes after infecting a wound with anthrax bacilli, they could be found in the body. Still he thought this rapid absorption might be Nature's means of self-protection.

DR. SCHLOFFER of Prague found bacteria in wounds which healed by first intention. He believed from experiments that the secretions of healthy wounds were toxic to bacteria.

The next subject for discussion was

LOCAL ANESTHESIA.

DR. HACKENBRUCK of Wiesbaden advocated one-fourth per-cent. cocain-eucain solution. It should be injected warm and the part should, if possible, be rendered bloodless by an elastic ligature. Schleich's solutions were not successful in his hands.

DR. BRAUN of Leipsic advocated Schleich's mixture with the omission of its morphia. He thought the subsequent edema so frequently seen to be due to the action of morphia on the blood-vessels of the part. There still remained much room for improvement in local anesthesia.

DR. RUBENSTEIN of Berlin said that he found Schleich's without additions or omissions the best solution. He has done with it a number of operations on joints, especially the knee. He has also done bone operations where the tuberculous process was not very extensive, and claimed that infiltration of the periosteum with the anesthetic was sufficient since the bone itself was not sensitive.

In the general discussion it seemed to be pretty well agreed that Schleich's local-anesthesia solutions were the best and most useful combinations yet suggested. They did not wish the morphia omitted, and eucain had but the one advocate.

The morning of the second day was devoted to

SURGERY OF THE STOMACH AND INTESTINES.

PROFESSOR KROENLEIN of Zürich detailed the now famous case of total extirpation of the stomach done by his assistant Dr. Schlatter. The speaker insisted that this case was so far unique, though the American journals did say the contrary. He announced that the patient was in excellent health, and had gained thirteen pounds since the operation. She can take any ordinary nourishment and her digestion seems not at all impaired. In sixteen resections of the stomach which he has done during the last ten years for malignant disease only two died as a result of the operation, though six died later from recurrence.

DR. SCHUCHARDT of Stettin described a case of almost total extirpation of the stomach in which he was surprised to find no disturbance of digestion. The patient lived for over two years, and then died of pleurisy. The post-mortem revealed complete regeneration of the stomach. The speaker exhibited the specimen of the regenerated stomach which looked like a normal organ.

DR. LOEBKER of Bochum stated that he had seen cases where operators thought they had removed the entire stomach, but on post-mortem within a few days they found most of it remaining. There were cases of hourglass contraction of the stomach and under such circumstances one might easily be deceived.

PROFESSOR KRONLEIN insisted that in the Zürick case there was no such error made, that the esophagus was actually attached to the duodenum.

PROFESSOR MIKULICZ said that in operating on malignant neoplasms of the stomach the surgeon must not be afraid of doing a radical operation. He must remove everything that seems to be involved. Consequently before attempting such an operation he should know his technic thoroughly, and be sufficiently grounded in anatomy and pathology to know where to look for involvement. His method of completing the operation in a case of resection is to close. the end of the duodenum by stitches, completely stitch the hole in the stomach and making a new opening in both, join them by a button.

DR. DOYEN of Paris exhibited something new in the technic of stomach and intestinal operations. In order to do a bloodless operation (it also renders the operation more aseptic) he uses a clamp by means of which he crushes the walls of the intestine or stomach before cutting into it. The clamp is the large instrument which is used by gynecologists for clamping the broad ligament.

PROFESSOR HAHN read his own statistics of 141 gastro-enterostomies and 28 of resection with gastro-enterostomy. Of these 28, 10 died as a result of the operation. In 4 cases in which the patients were past 60 years of age all died, while of 12 cases between the ages of 40 and 50 only 2 died. This led him to believe that in old people the prognosis was extremely unfavorable. He recommended in case the patient was extremely feeble the doing of the operation in two stages, first perform a gastro-enterostomy and later do the resection.

DR. STENDEL of Heidelberg gave the statistics of the Heidelberg clinic. He said that in cases of non-malignant stricture of the pylorus they did not dilate, but did gastro-enterostomy. This operation was also done if a cancer of the pylorus, or immediate region, was found to be inoperable. They noticed in these cases such a marked improvement after the operation, and oftentimes such a long life, in one case over three years, that they were led to believe that the simple removal of the irritation not only brought the growth of the neoplasm to a standstill for a time, but that possibly even a retrograde change for the better took place in the tumor.

In the discussion on

THE MURPHY BUTTON

Frank's coupler was brought up and described, and samples of it passed around the room.

DR. KOENIG, JR., of Berlin advocated the coupler for side-to-side interstinal anastomosis, but from one fatal experience thought that it was absorbed too quickly by the stomach juices for a gastro-enterostomy.

PROFESSOR WOELFLER of Prague exhibited a modification of the Frank coupler which he had made. It consisted of a tube with two rings on it which could be drawn slightly apart, and on pressure sprung fast together. The whole was made of the same absorbable material as the coupler.

PROFESSOR JORDAN of Heidelberg and DR. KUMMEL making use of the statistics from Czerny's Clinic of sixty-three successful cases (in none of which the instrument had failed to pass in the natural way) advocated strongly the Murphy button.

The afternoon session was devoted to

THE TREATMENT OF POTT'S DISEASE.

Calot's procedure of applying pressure while extension is made was the one that met with universal approval.

PROFESSOR LORENZ of Vienna described a screw by means of which the pressure could be regulated. DR. WULLSTEIN of Halle exhibited a complicated device for keeping up the pressure, and DR. VULPIUS of Heidelberg a table on which the plaster-of-Paris jacket could be more easily and better applied.

PROFESSOR HOFFA of Würzburg mentioned the following contraindications: (1) Very long standing deformity. (2) If many vertebræ take part in the kyphosis. (3). Purulent collections at the seat of the disease. He said that the most suitable cases were those in which the prominence was just appearing. Paralysis was not a contraindication; he had seen some paralyses of the legs cured where the operation was done early after its appearance. A simple method of finding out in advanced cases whether the procedure should be tried or not was to apply extension without the patient being anesthetized; if the kyphosis partly disappears the procedure may be attempted; if the prominence remains the same without giving the patient too much pain, the operation would probably be useless.

The morning of the third day began with a discussion of

EMPYEMA.

PROFESSOR JORDAN of Heidelberg advocated for old cavities a combination of the Schede and Delorme operations. He resects the entire chest-wall that covers the cavity, and with his fingers loosens the contracted and shrunken pleura. Twenty-three cases so operated on gave 9 complete recoveries, 6 have only a small fistula remaining, 4 died, and the others are still under treatment. Of four tubercular cases 3 died. The extent of the resection depends on the size of the cavity. He exhibited a case of a boy eleven years of age, on whom the operation had been done five years before. Five ribs had been resected, and had now been completely regenerated.

DR. PERTHES of Leipsic demonstrated a water-vacuum-pump which he had used successfully in a number of cases of empyema and pneumothorax.

In the general discussion cases were presented where the most extensive resections had been done, and DR. GERULANOS of Greifswald exhibited the specimens (unfortunately the patient died twenty-two hours after the operation) of an entire half of the thorax which he had resected in a child for sarcoma.

A most interesting discussion followed upon

THE SURGERY OF THE LIVER AND BILE-DUCTS.

DR. PETERSON of Heidelberg presented the Heidelberg statistics of 162 operations on the gall-ducts and bladder, with six deaths. In cases where they were obliged to resect portions of the liver they had controlled the hemorrhage by hot air.

PROFESSOR POPPERT of Giessen spoke of fifty-seven cholocystotomies in which the fistula was managed by inserting a rubber tube into the gall-bladder, holding it in place by a Nelaton stitch between the bladder-wall and the tube, and then bringing the tube out through the abdominal opening. The tube is stitched in the same way to the abdominal-wall, and the wound closed up to the tube. He claimed never to have had any leakage of bile.

PROFESSOR HEIDENHAIN of Worms detailed a case and showed specimen where he had resected the gall-bladder for carcinoma. The tumor was only the size of a cherry stone, and the surrounding structures at the time of operation seemed healthy, yet the patient died of carcinoma of the liver in a short time. He concluded that the operator could never be certain that he had eradicated the disease.

DR. HOLLAENDER of Berlin described a case operated upon by him a few weeks ago where he resected a large portion of the liver and controlled the hemorrhage by hot air. The patient is in excellent condition. He demonstrated his apparatus for making the hot air, and recommended it for control of hemorrhage from other organs.

In the general discussion Holländer's method of hemostasis seemed to meet with general favor.

There was a brief discussion upon

THE RESULTS OF SERUM-THERAPY IN DIPHTHERIA.

PROFESSOR KROENLEIN of Zürich presented his side of the question so thoroughly and strikingly, and the assembly seemed to agree so entirely with him, that the President called for discussion in vain. Professor Krönlein gave the statistics of diphtheria in Zürick clinic and in the Canton Zürick since 1880. Since the serum was introduced in 1894 every case of diphtheria in the hospital has been treated with it. Between 1880 and 1894 they treated in the clinic 1336 cases, with a mortality of thirty-nine per cent.; between 1894 and 1898,437 cases, with a mortality of twelve per cent. In the Canton Zürick in the same years the average mortality was sixteen per cent. before the introduction of serum; eight per cent. since 1894. He believed they found in the majority of cases an improvement as soon as the treatment was begun. They noticed a fall of temperature, a loosening of the membrane, a decrease in the glandular swellings, and no further extension of the process.

On the fourth day came a conglomeration of addresses that were included under none of the general subjects of the congress, and on account of their number they were rushed through rapidly.

PROFESSOR BRUNS of Tübingen exhibited parts of

cadavers on which he had tried the effect of what he called

INHUMAN BULLETS.

During the late Indian war the English troops found that the bullets created much more damage when the points had been filed off them, and so the soldiers filed them down on stones. The effect was, as he showed, to splinter the bones in all directions, and when they struck only soft tissues to tear these beyond all conception.

The speaker begged that at the coming St. Petersburg convention the German members would take action that in case of war in Europe such bullets would be forbidden; that they wished to disable the enemy but not mutilate him. The speaker was loudly applauded, and the daily papers quoted his address in full.

DR. KUMMEL of Hamburg spoke on

THE TREATMENT OF LUPUS BY ROENTGEN-RAYS AND CONCENTRATED LIGHT.

He presented some cases partially cured and still under treatment.

DR. DOYEN of Paris stated most favorable results in

HEMICRANIECTOMY.

A number of idiots or microcephalics distinctly improved or cured. In one idiot with Graves' disease the exophthalmos and goiter had disappeared four days after the operation. Epileptics were markedly improved; one case had not had an attack in five, another in six months. In two cases of Jacksonian epilepsy, having found no lesion, he cut out the epileptogenic center; the first was successful, the second is still under treatment. He had removed a large subcortical tubercle with cure, and opened several deep-lying abscesses, which would not have been discovered but for the extensive resection. A case of occipital meningitis, moribund at the time of operation, was completely cured. He had lately attempted to reach some tumors at the base of the brain, but the cases had been particularly unsuitable. He exhibited many new instruments.

PROFESSOR BARTH of Dantzic advised in empyema of the frontal sinus, trephining, enlargement of the passage into the nose, and immediate closure of the trephine wound.

DR. GROSSE of Halle presented the Halle Clinic statistics of 24 cancers of the face, with 16 complete recoveries. He exhibited several cases, one of a woman on whom an extensive radical operation had been done five years ago. They had removed the superior maxillary and malar bones, the eye, the zygoma, had chiseled away some bones of the orbit, and a portion of the temporal bone, as deep as the tympanum. The results were excellent.

PROFESSOR PARTSCH of Breslau exhibited a patient in whom he had made a temporary resection of the alveolar process, turning the flap back on the gum, and afterward replacing it.

PROFESSOR GARRÉ spoke of resection of the esophagus in its upper part, and DR. REHN of Frankfort-on-the-Main of resection in the thoracic portion. In one case the latter had successfully gone in from behind, though the patient died a short time after.

DR. KUTTNER of Tübingen reported two cases of syphilitic struma which had been diagnosed malignant and operated on. Microscopical examination of the tumors and later symptoms made the diagnosis certain.

DR. SPRENGEL of Braunschweig exhibited the specimens of two cases in which coxitis had been diagnosed from the symptoms and skiagraphs. Post-mortem proved them to have been traumatic separation of the epiphyseal head.

DR. HOFMEISTER of Tübingen presented a number of different Röntgen-ray photographs of a single normal pelvis, in which by moving the patient, or the apparatus, or both, during the procedure, almost every variety of deformity had been produced.

DR. WILMS of Leipsic described an apparatus by means of which the application of heat to inflamed joints could be regulated; DR. KRAUSE of Altona a hot-air apparatus for the same purpose.

PROFESSOR DUHRSSEN of Berlin advocated the employment of steam to control hemorrhage. He said it was particularly efficient in cases of excessive menstruation. He demonstrated his apparatus.

At the close of the Congress a vote of thanks was extended to the President, Professor Trendelenburg, for the efficient and successful manner in which the proceedings had been conducted. After balloting, it was announced that Professor Hahn of Berlin was elected President for the ensuing year.

THERAPEUTIC HINTS.

To Control Vomiting Caused by Cancer of the Stomach.—

℞		
Picrotoxin Morphin hydrochlorat.	aa	gr. i
Atrop. sulphat.		gr. 1/6
Aq. laurocerasi		ʒ vi.

M. Sig. Five to eight drops before meals.

For Rhinitis.—

℞		
Phenacetin Pulv. amyli	aa	ʒ i
Pulv. acaciæ		ʒ ii.

M. Sig. For insufflation several times a day.

For Anal Pruritus with Hemorrhoids.—

℞		
Ext. hamamelidis fl.		℥ i
Ext. ergotæ fl. Ext. hydrastis fl. Tinct. benzoini comp.	aa	℥ ii
Ac. carbolici		m. v
Ol. olivæ		℥ i.

M. Sig. For rectal injection, one or two ounces at a time, to be well shaken.

Ointment for Varicose Ulcer.—

℞	
Ac. carbolici	ʒ ss
Ac. borici	ʒ iiss
Camphoræ	ʒ ii
Ichthyol	ʒ v
Ol. amygdalæ dulc.	ʒ iiss
Ung. zinci oxidi	℥ iiiss.

M. Sig. For external use.

THE MEDICAL NEWS.
A WEEKLY JOURNAL OF MEDICAL SCIENCE.

VOL. LXXII. NEW YORK, SATURDAY, MAY 21, 1898. No. 21.

ORIGINAL ARTICLES.

THE DISINFECTION OF ROOMS.[1]

BY F. G. NOVY, M.D.,
OF ANN ARBOR MICH.;
MEMBER OF THE MICHIGAN STATE BOARD OF HEALTH;
AND
H. H. WAITE, A.B.,
OF ANN ARBOR, MICH.;
INSTRUCTOR IN BACTERIOLOGY IN THE UNIVERSITY OF MICHIGAN.

THE thorough disinfection of rooms and their contents, infected with disease-producing organisms, constitutes one of the chief means for the prevention of the spread of disease. The methods which aim to accomplish this result must stand the test of a thorough laboratory trial. It may be that the requirements exacted in the laboratory are more severe than those which occur in actual experience, and yet the results of experiment form the only safe guide as to the powers of any given agent. The laboratory can alone decide how much of the disinfectant is to be used, the length of time it is to act, the influence of the presence or absence of moisture, and how the contents of the room are to be arranged in order to insure disinfection. It is not sufficient to pile the bedding and clothing in one or more heaps upon the floor, to burn three or more pounds of sulphur during a few hours, and then assume that everything has been done that can be done. The proper disinfection of a room is a most delicate experiment and should be entered upon with full knowledge of the various conditions which are necessary to success.

There is no chemic disinfectant which will invariably yield the same result regardless of the organism to be acted upon and the surroundings or environment of that organism. Thus, while a mercuric-chlorid solution may destroy the cholera vibrio within a few seconds, it does not follow that it will also destroy anthrax spores. Again, the anthrax spores in water suspension will be destroyed by this agent much more rapidly than if suspended in a highly albuminous fluid such as blood. These and similar conditions are equally true for gaseous disinfectants. A gaseous disinfectant, even the most efficient, may fail simply because it is expected to accomplish too much. We may ridicule the attempt at disinfection of a privy-vault or cesspool by means of a few pounds of copperas, although this is no more absurd than many a so-called room disinfection. This or that gaseous agent is said to lack the power of penetration, and to be a mere "surface disinfectant." The latter property is an excellent one and constitutes about all that can be expected of any gas. While it is true that a gaseous disinfectant possesses little penetrating power, that is to say, it will not go through several mattresses or bundles of blankets, it should be remembered that this a deficiency which can easily be remedied if the disinfector will properly do his share of the work.

Sulphur fumigation is extensively employed for the purpose of room disinfection. Many doubts have been cast upon its efficiency, largely, perhaps, because it was expected to do too much. The causes of certain diseases, such as scarlet fever, measles, and smallpox, are still unknown, and it is purely gratuitous to assume that because sulphur fumes do not kill anthrax spores and other resistant organisms they are of no value for disinfection in such diseases as those mentioned above. The organisms which produce these diseases are probably as easily destroyed as those of cholera, diphtheria, and the black-plague. The Michigan State Board of Health, through its efficient secretary, Dr. Henry B. Baker, has always warmly advocated sulphur fumigation. When this method is properly applied there can be no doubt, as may be seen from the experiments to be related, of its efficiency in restricting the spread of certain infectious diseases.

Within the past few years formaldehyd has attracted considerable attention as a disinfectant. Various forms of apparatus have been devised for its generation and employment. In view of the strong claims for this agent and the grave doubts cast upon the efficiency of sulphur dioxid, it was thought desirable to make a comparative study of their usefulness. This investigation was undertaken largely at the request of the Michigan State Board of Health, and it is hoped that the results obtained will be directly useful to health-officers, physicians, etc., in this and other States. The report covers twenty-six distinct room-disinfection experiments. The number of specimens exposed to the action of disinfectants and then inoculated into culture-media exceeds 5000. It will be evident from these facts that the utmost care, regardless of time, was taken in order to insure practical results.

[1] A report to the Michigan State Board of Health, read at a meeting of the Michigan State Medical Society, held at Detroit, May 6, 1898.

The room employed for all but one of these experiments was especially suitable for the object in view. It was designed as a disinfection-room at the time the laboratory was constructed and it was intended to have a capacity of 1000 cubic feet. It really contains 1016 cubic feet (28.8 cubic meters). In order to make the room perfectly tight the cracks in the edge of the ceiling and in the corners of the room were filled with plaster of Paris. The plaster ceiling and walls were then coated with calcimine and glue and finally given a coat of paint. It should be said that two of the walls were brick and these were not painted. The spaces between the plaster and wash-boards, door, and window-frames were caulked with putty, as were also the spaces around the door and window on the outside of the room. The ventilator and waste-pipe opening into the room were tightly plugged. During the disinfection the cracks about the door were securely closed by caulking with strips of muslin. The room thus prepared was probably as gas-tight as possible. In the case of the formalin experiments there was no odor in the adjoining rooms, in which students were constantly at work. In sulphur fumigations the gas was at times noticeable in the adjoining room. This, it may be incidentally mentioned, is one disadvantage of sulphur as compared with formaldehyd. The latter does not tend to pass out of the room, unless, of course, gross cracks or openings exist; whereas, sulphur dioxid will always find an opening be it ever so small. Where the adjoining rooms are inhabited, as in crowded tenement-houses, formaldehyd possesses a distinct advantage over sulphur.

Twenty different organisms were exposed to the action of the disinfectant. The first six, as given in the tables, contained spores. These were the germs of anthrax, symptomatic anthrax, tetanus, and malignant edema, as well as the hay and potato bacillus. With the exception of the three anaerobic germs and the tubercle bacillus, the other organisms, sixteen in number, were grown on inclined agar at a temperature of 39° C. (102.2° F.). By means of a sterile pipette sterile bouillon (3 to 4 c.c.), about one dram was added to each agar culture. The growth was thoroughly whipped up and then pipetted off into a sterile Esmarch dish. The suspensions thus obtained were exceedingly rich in bacteria.

The spores of anthrax were very abundant and were obtained by growing the germs during several days on peptonless agar at a temperature of 39° C. (102.2° F.). The cultures of the hay and potato bacilli were likewise several days old and rich in spores. The three anaerobic organisms, those of malignant edema, symptomatic anthrax, and tetanus were grown in glucose bouillon in hydrogen for five to six days. The sediment, consisting chiefly of spores, was carefully drawn off by means of a sterile pipette with as little dilution as possible.

The names Sanarelli and Havelburg refer to the bacteria described by these men as the cause of yellow fever. The psittacosis bacillus is the etiologic factor in a parrot disease which is apparently communicable to man. The pus-producing bacteria are represented by the staphylococcus pyogenes aureus, streptococcus pyogenes and the bacillus of green pus.

Sputum containing many tubercle bacilli was employed in preference to pure cultures of this organism. The experiments with tubercle bacilli were not numerous but were very conclusive. After exposure in Esmarch dishes to the action of the disinfectant the tuberculous material was rubbed up with sterile bouillon and injected intraperitoneally into guinea-pigs.

Sterile silk threads, bits of muslin and cover-glasses were employed in these tests. The silk threads were about 1½ cm. (¾ inch) long. The bits of muslin were about 1 cm. (⅓ inch) square. Cleaned cover-glasses 20 mm. square were cut into halves and sterilized. The letters S. M. and G. in the tables refer to silk, muslin, and cover-glasses respectively.

The threads and muslin squares were thoroughly soaked in the bacterial suspension prepared as mentioned above. Care was taken to spread out each piece of muslin; eventually each piece was turned over so as to insure thorough soaking. The impregnated threads and muslins were then transferred to sterile Esmarch dishes. The cover-glasses were smeared, on one side only, with a large loop full of the bacterial suspension.

One set of specimens thus prepared was exposed during two and one-half to three hours at a temperature of 39° C. (102.2° F.) to dry. In order to insure drying the tops of the Esmarch dishes were left slightly ajar. Occasionally a muslin would not be completely dry in this time, and hence, when exposed to the disinfectant, was in reality a moist specimen, and as such would be readily disinfected. When dry the specimens were taken out of the incubator, and each piece of silk and muslin carefully loosened from the dish in order that the gas might act on all sides.

The second set of specimens, in order to prevent drying during the time that the first was undergoing desiccation, were placed in moist chambers. In spite of this precaution some specimens would become dry before the disinfectant had time to act, and in such cases the specimen became as resistant as a dry one. As might be expected, the cover-glass would be the first to dry, then the silk threads. When about to begin a disinfection both wet and dry sets were placed on a table in the room, and the tops of the Esmarch dishes were slipped to one side. The specimens were, therefore, in open dishes. Except

TABLE I.—SULPHUR DISINFECTION.

Amount used.		Three pounds.			Six pounds.		
Condition.		Dry.	Wet.	Control.	Dry.	Wet.	Control.
Anthrax.	S.	+ +	+ +	+	+ +	+ +	+
	M.	+ +	+ +	+	+ +	+ O	+
	G.	+ +	+ O	+	O O	+ O	+
Symptomatic anthrax.	S.	+ +	+ +	+	+ +	+ +	+
	M.	+ +	+ +	+	+ +	+ +	+
	G.	+ +	+ +	+	+ +	+ +	+
Malignant edema.	S.	+ +	+ +	+	+ +	+ +	+
	M.	+ +	+ O	+	+ +	+ +	+
	G.	+ +	+ +	+	O O	+ O	+
Tetanus.	S.	+ +	+ +	+	+ +	+ +	+
	M.	+ +	+ +	+	+ +	+ +	+
	G.	+ +	+ +	+	+ +	O O	+
Hay bacillus.	S.	+ +	+ +	+	+ +	+ O	+
	M.	+ +	+ +	+	+ +	+ O	+
	G.	+ O	O O	+	O O	O O	+
Potato bacillus.	S.	+ +	+ +	+	+ +	+ +	+
	M.	+ +	+ +	+	+ +	+ +	+
	G.	+ +	+ +	+	+ +	+ O	+
Cholera.	S.	O O	O O	O	O O	O O	+
	M.	O O	O O	O	O O	O O	+
	G.	O O	O O	O	O O	O O	O
Diphtheria.	S.	+ +	O O	+	O O	O O	+
	M.	+ +	O O	+	O O	O O	+
	G.	O O	O O	+	O O	O O	+
Glanders.	S.	O O	O O	+	O O	O O	+
	M.	O O	O O	+	O O	O O	+
	G.	O O	O O	O	O O	O O	O
Typhoid fever.	S.	+ +	O O	+	+ +	O O	+
	M.	+ +	O O	+	+ +	O O	+
	G.	O O	O O	+	O O	O O	+
Colon bacillus.	S.	+ +	O O	+	+ +	O O	+
	M.	+ +	O O	+	+ +	O O	+
	G.	+ O	O O	+	O O	O O	+
Sanarelli.	S.	+ +	O O	+	+ +	O O	+
	M.	+ +	O O	+	+ +	O O	+
	G.	+ O	O O	+	O O	O O	+
Havelburg.	S.	+ +	O O	+	+ +	O O	+
	M.	O O	O O	+	+ +	O O	+
	G.	O O	O O	+	O O	O O	+
Psittacosis.	S.	+ +	O O	+	+ O	O O	+
	M.	+ +	O O	+	+ +	O O	+
	G.	+ +	O O	+	O O	O O	+
Black plague.	S.	O O	O O	O	O O	O O	+
	M.	O O	O O	O	O O	O O	+
	G.	O O	O O	+	O O	O O	+
Staphylococcus pyo. aur.	S.	+ +	O O	+	+ +	O O	+
	M.	+ +	O O	+	+ +	O O	+
	G.	+ +	O O	+	+ O	O O	+
Pneumonia (Fraenkel).	S.	O O	O O	+	+ O	O O	+
	M.	O O	O O	+	+ O	O O	+
	G.	O O	O O	+	O O	O O	+
Green pus.	S.	+ +	O O	+	+ +	O O	+
	M.	+ +	O O	+	+ +	O O	+
	G.	+ +	O O	+	O O	O O	+
Streptococcus pyogenes.	S.	+ +	O O	+	+ +	O O	+
	M.	+ +	O O	+	+ +	O O	+
	G.	+ +	O O	+	O O	O O	+
Tuberculosis (see text).							
Total positive growths.[1]		79	32	51	64	24	55
Deducting hay bacillus.		74	28	48	60	24	52

[1] The total number of specimens exposed, in each column, was 114; the controls in each column number 57.

in the case of the sulphur experiments there were no dishes of water in the room.

At the close of the disinfection period the tops were rapidly replaced and the dishes then taken out of the room. Each specimen was transferred to a tube of bouillon. A sterile forcep was used for each specimen. The fifteen tubes of each anaerobic set were placed together in a Novy bottle, and hydrogen was passed through for from one to two hours. All the bouillon tubes thus inoculated were exposed to a temperature of 35° C. (95° F.) for from five to seven days, when they were examined and the results noted. As a result of careful, rapid work contaminations were exceedingly rare. Frequently an entire set of two or three hundred tubes would not show a single contamination.

In the tables "+" indicates that a growth had formed; on the other hand, "O" indicates that the tube remained sterile. It should be stated that frequently the growth when present was very slight, showing that marked attenuation of the germ had occurred as a result of the exposure. The specimens were invariably exposed in duplicate. Another set was kept in a cool, dark place for the same length of time as the exposed objects. These controls were then planted into bouillon at the same time as the exposed specimens.

SULPHUR EXPERIMENTS.

In these experiments the sulphur was placed in one or two iron water-baths on tripods which stood in shallow basins of water; 50 c.c. (1⅔ fl. oz.) or more of alcohol was added to each three-pound portion of sulphur, and then set on fire. The sulphur would burn three or four hours, and, as previously stated, some sulphur fumes would penetrate into the adjoining room in spite of the utmost precautions in closing up openings. The time of exposure was twenty hours. At the end of this time the room was entered and the articles were removed. When but three pounds of sulphur was used the air in the room at the end of that period was irritating, but tolerable; whereas, with six pounds of sulphur it was well nigh insupportable. The glass dishes, especially when six pounds of sulphur was employed, were coated with a white film, due to finely divided sulphur. On account of the presence of sulphurous acid the reaction of this deposit was intensely acid.

A maximum and minimum thermometer was placed in the room during each experiment. In the experiment with three pounds of sulphur the temperature varied from 19° to 28° C. (66.2° to 82.4° F.); while in that with six pounds it registered 16° to 29° C. (60.8° to 84.2° F.).

The exposed objects, as a rule perfectly dry when taken out, were planted directly into bouillon. The amount of sulphur dioxid adherent to the specimens was not sufficient to act as an antiseptic and inhibit the growth of the organisms, if any life was present. The absence of such inhibiting action was ascertained by repeated and prolonged washing of the specimens of one set in slightly warmed sterile water. No difference was observed between washed and unwashed specimens, and hence, in most of the experiments, the washing was omitted.

The suspensions used for the exposures in Table I. were the same as those used in the paraform experiments (Table II.). In order to prevent growth and consequent alteration of the suspension, they were kept in a jar immersed in melting ice. The results given in Tables I. and II. are, therefore, strictly comparable, since they were obtained with the same suspensions.

An inspection of Table I. will show what sulphur fumigation is capable of doing. In the first place, it will be seen that the dry specimens, as compared with the wet ones, are much more resistant to destruction. Furthermore, it will be seen that all the wet specimens were killed except those containing spores and tubercle bacilli. Sulphur, even in six-pound portions, cannot be used to destroy spores or tubercle bacilli. A comparison of this table with the one following will show that formaldehyd readily destroys wet spores and tubercle bacilli, and this fact demonstrates the relative superiority of formalin over sulphur. In actual practice the physician is not called upon, however, to destroy spores. With the exception of the tubercle bacillus only vegetating, actively growing, and weak forms of bacteria have to be destroyed. It will be noticed that the microorganisms of cholera, glanders, diphtheria, black-plague, and pneumonia are quite readily destroyed by sulphur.

With reference to the cholera vibrio it should be noted that even the control-tubes fail to develop. This organism is extremely weak, and mere desiccation for twenty-four hours usually suffices to destroy it. The bacillus of black or bubonic plague is almost as weak as the cholera vibrio.

Six pounds of sulphur are somewhat more destructive than three pounds. This is seen in the larger number of dried specimens which failed to develop after employment of the larger quantity. Out of 114 dry specimens only 64 gave a growth when six pounds of sulphur was burned; whereas, with three pounds of sulphur 79 specimens survived. As a rule, the cover-glass specimens were the first to die out. As stated before, the suspensions were spread only upon the upper surface of the cover-glasses, and this true surface distribution explains the fact mentioned.

If there is a considerable escape of sulphur fumes into the surrounding rooms the results are by no means as certain as those indicated above. Even the wet specimens of the germs of cholera, glanders, diphtheria, and typhoid fever may not be destroyed in such cases.

In order, then, to insure destruction of vegetating bacteria by means of sulphur fumes, it is necessary that these shall be in *direct contact with water*. It is not sufficient to have several pans of water in the room or to inject steam in order to saturate the atmosphere with aqueous vapor. In some experiments one liter of water was distilled into the room in which six pounds of sulphur was being burned. The previously dried specimens were not affected any more than if no steam had been introduced.

No experiments were made with sulphur fumigations for a shorter period than twenty hours. It is highly probable that exposures for from three to six hours, as practised in some cities, are not sufficient to destroy even wet specimens. In the *Biennial Report of the Department of Health of Chicago*, published in 1897 (pp. 85 and 250), a procedure is described which is intended to test the efficiency of sulphur fumigation. Inclined agar tubes are inoculated with the potato or hay bacillus (spores), and then exposed to the sulphur fumes in the room undergoing disinfection. The tubes are then taken to the laboratory and allowed to develop in the incubator, but more usually at the room temperature. If no growth develops the conclusion is drawn that potato or hay bacillus spores have been destroyed, and since these possess a marked resistance it is further assumed that the disinfection of the room itself has been thorough.

As a matter of fact, the control-test as outlined above is fallacious, for the simple reason that enough sulphur dioxid is taken up by the agar to act as an antiseptic but not as a germicide. Agar tubes prepared as above and exposed for twenty hours to the fumes from six pounds of sulphur are not disinfected. The agar becomes milky or opaque white in color, and becomes intensely acid on account of the presence of sulphurous acid. These tubes when placed in the incubator will invariably fail to develop, not because the spores are dead, but because their growth is inhibited by the presence of an antiseptic. If some of the material on the surface of such agar tubes is transplanted to a fresh agar tube, growth will invariably result.

This method of testing the efficiency of fumigation is therefore not to be relied upon. Moreover, the spores of the potato bacillus are vastly more resistant, as seen from the accompanying tables, than any of the common disease-producing organisms. This test, it may be added, is inapplicable even in formalin disinfection. One hundred and twenty grams of paraform volatilized in a room of 1000 cubic feet (4 gm. per cubic meter or 60 grs. per cubic yard) is not sufficient to disinfect agar tubes which have been inoculated with the two organisms mentioned. These tubes when placed in the incubator promptly develop, and if after the exposure transplantations are made to fresh agar tubes the growth will be perfectly normal. This result with agar streaks will be obtained even when most of the silk, muslin, and cover-glass specimens are destroyed.

Tubercle bacilli are known to possess considerable resistance, and this characteristic is well demonstrated in connection with sulphur fumigation. A specimen of sputum rich in tubercle bacilli was divided into three equal portions. These were placed in sterile Esmarch dishes. One of the dishes was exposed uncovered during twenty hours in a room where 6 pounds of sulphur was burned. Another dish was exposed the same length of time in the room in which 120 grams (4 oz.) of paraform was volatilized. After the exposure the contents of the dishes were still moist. Bouillon, however, was added to each dish, and the contents were then thoroughly stirred up and injected intraperitoneally into two guinea-pigs. The third portion of sputum was not exposed to a disinfectant but was injected into a guinea-pig as a control-test. The control guinea-pig died within fourteen days. The guinea-pig that received the sputum which had been exposed to sulphur fumes died within fifteen days. Both of these animals showed typical experimental tuberculosis. The guinea-pig that received the sputum which was exposed to formalin vapors was killed a month later and on examination was found to be absolutely free from tuberculosis. Sulphur fumigation is therefore of no value in destroying tubercle bacilli and hence, should not be depended upon in the disinfection of tuberculous material.

The sulphur experiments can be summarized as follows:

Sulphur fumes possess little or no action on most bacteria when in the dry state. If, however, the specimens are actually wet they will be destroyed except in the case of resistant forms such as the spore stage and tubercle bacilli. Sulphur is of no value in the disinfection of wet or dry spore-containing material, or of tubercle bacilli. It can be used for the disinfection of rooms which have been infected with ordinary disease organisms. To insure good results in these cases, from 3 to 6 pounds of sulphur must be burned for each 1000 cubic feet of space. The walls, floor, and articles in the room should be sprayed with water. The room should be made perfectly tight, and should be kept closed at least 20 hours.

PARAFORM DISINFECTION.

Schering's disinfector and paraform pastils were employed in these experiments. Paraform, or para-

TABLE II.—PARAFORM DISINFECTION.

Amount used.		60 grams.			120 grams.		
Condition.		Dry.	Wet.	Control.	Dry.	Wet.	Control.
Anthrax.	S.	+ +	O O	+	+ +	+ O	+
	M.	+ +	O O	+	+ +	O O	+
	G.	+ +	+ O	+	+ +	+ O	+
Symptomatic anthrax.	S.	+ +	O O	+	+ +	O O	+
	M.	+ +	O O	+	+ O	O O	+
	G.	+ +	O O	+	+ +	O O	+
Malignant edema.	S.	+ +	O O	+	+ +	O O	+
	M.	O O	O O	+	+ O	O O	+
	G.	+ O	O O	+	+ O	O O	+
Tetanus.	S.	+ +	O O	+	+ +	O O	+
	M.	+ +	O O	+	+ +	O O	+
	G.	+ +	O O	+	+ +	O O	+
Hay bacillus.	S.	+ +	O O	+	+ +	O O	+
	M.	+ +	O O	+	+ O	O O	+
	G.	+ O	O O	+	O O	O O	+
Potato bacillus.	S.	+ +	O O	+	+ +	O O	+
	M.	+ +	O O	+	+ +	O O	+
	G.	+ +	O O	+	+ +	O O	+
Cholera.	S.	O O	O O	O	O O	O O	O
	M.	O O	O O	O	O O	O O	O
	G.	O O	O O	O	O O	O O	O
Diphtheria.	S.	O +	O O	+	+ +	O O	+
	M.	+ O	O O	+	O O	O O	+
	G.	O O	O O	+	O O	O O	+
Glanders.	S.	+ O	O O	+	+ +	O O	+
	M.	O O	O O	+	O O	O O	+
	G.	O O	O O	+	O O	O O	+
Typhoid fever.	S.	+ +	O O	+	+ +	O O	+
	M.	+ +	O O	+	+ +	O O	+
	G.	+ O	O O	+	+ O	O O	+
Colon bacillus.	S.	+ +	O O	+	+ +	O O	+
	M.	+ +	O O	+	+ +	O O	+
	G.	O O	O O	+	+ +	+ O	+
Sanarelli.	S.	+ +	O O	+	+ +	O O	+
	M.	+ +	O O	+	+ +	O O	+
	G.	+ O	+ O	+	+ +	O O	+
Havelburg.	S.	+ +	O O	+	+ +	O O	+
	M.	+ +	O O	+	+ O	O O	+
	G.	+ O	+ O	+	+ +	+ +	+
Psittacosis.	S.	+ +	O O	+	+ +	O O	+
	M.	+ +	O O	+	+ +	O O	+
	G.	+ O	O O	+	+ +	+ O	+
Black plague.	S.	+ O	O O	+	+ O	O O	+
	M.	O O	O O	+	O O	O O	+
	G.	O O	O O	+	O O	O O	+
Staphylococcus pyo. aur.	S.	+ +	O O	+	+ +	O O	+
	M.	+ +	O O	+	+ +	O O	+
	G.	+ +	O O	+	+ +	O O	+
Pneumonia (Fraenkel).	S.	+ +	O O	+	+ +	O O	+
	M.	+ +	O O	+	+ +	O O	+
	G.	+ O	O O	+	O O	O O	+
Green pus.	S.	+ +	O O	+	+ +	O O	+
	M.	+ +	O O	+	+ +	O O	+
	G.	+ O	O O	+	O O	+ +	+
Streptococcus pyogenes.	S.	+ +	O O	+	+ +	+ O	+
	M.	+ +	O O	+	+ +	O O	+
	G.	+ +	O O	+	+ +	O O	+
Tuberculosis (see text under sulphur).							
Total positive growths.[1]		82	3	54	83	9	54
Deducting hay bacillus.		77	3	51	80	9	51

[1] See footnote to Table I.

formaldehyd is a polymerized formaldehyd. On gentle heating it breaks up and regenerates formaldehyd. The gas thus produced will remain in this condition if moisture is present in the atmosphere. In the absence of moisture the gaseous formaldehyd will repolymerize and hence will cease to be effective as a disinfectant. With Schering's disinfector it is maintained that sufficient water is formed by the burning alcohol to prevent this repolymerization. Owing to the great solubility of formaldehyd large vessels of water should not be kept in the room to be disinfected. When water is thus kept in the room scarcely any odor of formalin will remain in the room at the end of twenty hours, whereas in the absence of such water the odor at the end of the time mentioned will be intolerable. In the tabulated experiments with paraform and with formalin no vessels of water were allowed in the room.

The maximum and minimum thermometer in the room indicated a temperature of 23° to 27° C. (72.4° to 80.6° F.) in the experiment with 60 grams (2 oz.) of paraform, and a temperature of 19° to 28° C. (66.2° to 82.4° F.) in the experiments with 120 grams (4 oz.) of paraform.

Sixty grams of paraform for 1016 cubic feet corresponds to a little over 2 grams per cubic meter of air space. One hundred and twenty grams of paraform, therefore, represents a little over 4 grams per cubic meter. Two hundred to 300 cubic centimeters of alcohol were used in order to volatilize the paraform.

As stated under sulphur fumigation, the same suspensions were used for the tabulated paraform and sulphur experiments. From these suspensions, kept at the temperature of melting ice, the necessary silk thread, muslin square, and cover-glass specimens were prepared each day in the manner already described.

The exposed specimens were, as a rule, transferred directly to bouillon. In some cases they were previously washed with dilute sterile ammonium hydrate in order to neutralize any trace of disinfectant, but the results were in no wise different from those obtained with unwashed specimens.

A study of Table II. will show the same difference between wet and dry specimens as has been pointed out under sulphur. There is this striking difference, however, that wet spore material is thoroughly disinfected with formaldehyd, whereas such material is not affected by sulphur. Formaldehyd is, therefore, a more energetic disinfectant.

Practically all of the wet specimens were destroyed. It will be noticed, however, that 120 grams of paraform do not possess a greater action than 60 grams. Indeed, the results were not so good. It is possible that several of the wet specimens dried out before sufficient formalin was generated, and hence they acquired the resistance of dried specimens. As might be expected the cover-glass preparations would be the first to dry out, the silk thread next, and last of all the muslin squares. Of the nine positive growths seven were from cover-glasses and two from silk threads. In the first set all three of the survivals of the wet set were cover-glass preparations.

It will be further noticed that the weak disease-producing organisms, such as the germs of cholera, black plague, glanders, diphtheria, etc., are nearly all destroyed even in the dry state. Tubercle bacilli when in a wet condition are readily destroyed by formaldehyd vapors. Here, as in the case of spore destruction, is seen the superiority of formaldehyd vapor over sulphur fumes. The experiment in disinfection of tuberculous sputum has been described in connection with the sulphur experiments.

The results obtained with Schering's disinfector may be briefly summarized as follows:

Sixty grams of paraform pastils per 1000 cubic feet of space are sufficient to destroy within twenty hours all organisms regardless of whether they are present as spore or vegetating forms, *provided they are wet*. It is not sufficient to inject steam into the room. At least steam generated from one liter of water and injected into the room containing dry specimens will not alter the results. The walls and floor of the room, and whatever articles are present (previously spread out as much as possible) should be thoroughly sprayed with water before exposure to the formalin vapors.

FORMALIN DISTILLATION.

In Table III. are given the results obtained in the first trials with distillation of formalin. Formalin solutions on heating are said to readily polymerize, giving rise to paraform, which is supposed to interfere with further evaporation. Obviously, the cheapest and best way of employing formaldehyd as a gaseous disinfectant will be the distillation of formalin solutions. It is a matter of unnecessary expense to convert formalin into paraform and then from this regenerate formaldehyd vapors. The autoclave employed by Roux and Trillat in their experiments with formalin gave excellent results. Unfortunately, the size, weight, and expense of such an apparatus precludes its general use, and limits it to the health boards of large cities and to large hospitals.

The fear of polymerization of formalin on boiling is not well grounded. Certain it is that formalin can be distilled from its aqueous solution without polymerization, and that the results obtained are in every way equal to those obtained from paraform, and decidedly superior to the so-called formalin lamps. We have made no tests with formalin lamps, being convinced that they were but ephemeral playthings which would not fulfil the requirements of practical disinfection.

The results given in Table III. were obtained by

TABLE III.—FORMALIN DISINFECTION.

Amount used.		60 grams rapid distillation.			120 grams slow distillation.		
Condition.		Dry.	Wet.	Control.	Dry.	Wet.	Control.
Anthrax.	S.	+ +	O O	+	+ +	O O	+
	M.	+ +	O O	+	+ +	O O	+
	G.	+ +	O O	+	+ +	+ +	+
Symptomatic anthrax.	S.	+ +	O O	+	+ +	+ +	+
	M.	+ +	O O	+	+ +	O O	+
	G.	+ +	+ +	+	+ +	+ +	+
Malignant edema.	S.	+ +	O O	+	+ +	+ +	+
	M.	+ +	O O	+	+ +	O O	+
	G.	+ +	+ O	+	+ +	+ +	+
Tetanus.	S.	+ +	O O	+	+ +	O O	+
	M.	+ +	O O	+	+ +	O O	+
	G.	+ +	O O	+	+ +	+ O	+
Hay bacillus.	S.	+ +	O O	+	+ +	O +	+
	M.	+ +	O O	+	+ +	O O	+
	G.	+ O	O O	+	+ +	O O	+
Potato bacillus.	S.	+ +	O O	+	+ +	+ +	+
	M.	+ +	O O	+	+ +	O O	+
	G.	+ +	O O	+	+ +	+ +	+
Cholera.	S.	O O	O O	+	O O	O O	+
	M.	O O	O O	+	O O	O O	+
	G.	O O	O O	O	O O	O O	O
Diphtheria.	S.	+ +	O O	+	+ O	O O	+
	M.	+ +	O O	+	O O	O O	+
	G.	+ +	O O	+	+ +	O O	+
Glanders.	S.	+ O	O O	+	+ +	O O	+
	M.	+ O	O O	+	+ +	O O	+
	G.	O O	O O	O	O O	O O	O
Typhoid fever.	S.	+ +	O O	+	+ +	+ O	+
	M.	+ +	O O	+	+ +	O O	+
	G.	O O	O O	+	+ −	+ +	+
Colon bacillus.	S.	+ +	O O	+	+ +	+ O	+
	M.	+ +	O O	+	+ +	O O	+
	G.	+ +	+ +	+	+ O	+ O	+
Sanarelli.	S.	+ +	O O	+	+ +	+ +	+
	M.	+ +	O O	+	+ +	O O	+
	G.	+ +	O +	+	+ +	+ +	+
Havelburg.	S.	+ +	O O	+	+ +	+ O	+
	M.	+ +	O O	+	+ +	+ O	+
	G.	+ +	O +	+	+ +	+ +	+
Psittacosis.	S.	+ +	O O	+	+ +	+ +	+
	M.	+ +	O O	+	+ +	O O	+
	G.	+ +	O +	+	+ O	+ O	+
Black plague.	S.	O O	O O	+	O O	O O	+
	M.	+ O	O O	+	+ O	O O	+
	G.	O O	O O	O	O O	O O	+
Staphylococcus pyo. aur.	S.	+ +	O O	+	+ +	+ O	+
	M.	+ +	O O	+	+ +	O O	+
	G.	+ +	+ +	+	+ +	+ +	+
Pneumonia (Fraenkel).	S.	+ +	O O	+	+ +	O O	+
	M.	+ +	O O	+	+ O	O O	+
	G.	+ +	O O	+	+ +	O O	+
Green pus.	S.	+ +	O O	+	+ +	+ O	+
	M.	+ +	O O	+	+ +	O O	+
	G.	+ +	+ O	+	+ +	+ +	+
Streptococcus pyogenes.	S.	+ +	O O	+	+ +	+ O	+
	M.	+ +	O O	+	+ +	O O	+
	G.	+ +	+ +	+	+ +	+ O	+
Tuberculosis.							
Total positive growths.[1]		96	13	54	95	40	55
Deducting hay bacillus.		91	13	51	89	39	52

[1] See footnote to Table I.

the distillation of the ordinary forty-per-cent. solution of formalin. One hundred and fifty cubic centimeters of formalin solution (5¼ fl. oz.), containing therefore 60 grams (2 oz.) of formaldehyd, were placed in a one-and-one-half-liter flask, and ten per cent. of sodium chlorid was added to prevent polymerization. Subsequent experiments showed that the addition of the sodium chlorid was unnecessary. The flask was provided with a rubber stopper and a bent glass tube, which was inserted into the room through the keyhole. The contents of the flask were then heated to boiling by means of a Bunsen burner. In about fifty minutes the liquid was completely evaporated, and at no time was there a sign of polymerization. At the end of twenty hours, when the room was opened, the formalin vapors were intolerable.

Table III. combines the results obtained in four separate experiments. The first ten organisms were tried first in order to test the efficiency of the method. Subsequently suspensions of the other organisms were prepared and tested in a similar manner. These suspensions, as stated in the beginning, were very rich in bacteria. It should be understood that they were different from those employed in the Tables I. and II.

In the first set, 150 c.c. of formalin solution, representing 60 grams of pure formaldehyd, were distilled as rapidly as possible. In the second set double this amount was used, corresponding to 120 grams of pure formaldehyd. The distillation in this case was carried on at a slow rate, requiring about three hours to evaporate almost to dryness. It may be incidentally added that the formalin solutions employed were examined quantitatively and found to contain 39.7 per cent. of formaldehyd. The temperature in the room during the first set ranged from 17° to 24° C. (60.2° to 75° F.); whereas, in the second set, it ranged from 20° to 29° C. (67° to 80.4° F.).

As a result of the slow distillation many of the cover-glass preparations and silk threads dried out before enough formalin was present in the room, and hence acquired the resistance of dried specimens. This experiment is intended to show the importance of having the object to be disinfected in a wet condition and of rapid distillation of formalin. Although twice as much formalin was distilled as in the first set, yet the results were decidedly inferior, owing to the reason just given.

When the formalin is rapidly distilled the results are in no wise inferior to those obtained with paraform.

THIN SUSPENSIONS.

The first three tables contain the results obtained with thick suspensions prepared in the manner de-

TABLE IV.—THIN SUSPENSIONS.

Organisms tested.		Sulphur, A.		Formalin, B.		Formalin (large room), C.			Formalin, D.	
		3 pounds. 20 hours.		60 grams. 20 hours.		60 grams. per 1000 cubic feet. 20 hours.			60 grams. 10-hours exposure.	
		Dry.	Control.	Dry.	Control.	Dry.	Wet.	Control.	Dry.	Wet.
Anthrax.	S.	+ +	+	+ +	+	+ +	O O	+	O O	O O
	M.	+ +	+	+ +	+	O O	O O	+	O O	O O
	G.	O O	+	+ O	+	+ +	O O	+	+ O	O O
Symptomatic anthrax.	S.	+ +	+	+ +	+	+ +	O O	+	+ +	O O
	M.	+ +	+	+ +	+	+ O	O O	+	O O	O O
	G.	+ +	+	+ +	+	+ +	O O	+	+ +	O O
Malignant edema.	S.	+ +	+	+ +	+	+ +	O O	+	+ +	O O
	M.	+ +	+	+ +	+	O O	O O	+	O O	O O
	G.	+ +	+	+ +	+	+ +	O O	+	+ O	O O
Tetanus.	S.	+ +	+	+ +	+	+ +	O O	+	+ +	O O
	M.	+ +	+	+ +	+	O +	—	+	O O	O O
	G.	+ +	+	+ +	+	+ O	O O	+	+ O	O O
Potato bacillus.	S.	+ +	+	+ +	+	+ +	O O	+	+ +	O O
	M.	+ +	+	+ +	+	+ +	O O	+	+ +	O O
	G.	+ +	+	+ +	+	+ +	O O	+	+ +	O O
Cholera.	S.	O O	O	O O	O	O O	—	O	O O	O O
	M.	O O	O	O O	O	O O	—	O	O O	O O
	G.	O O	O	O O	O	O O	—	O	O O	O O
Diphtheria	S.	+ +	+	+ +	+	O O	O O	+	O O	O O
	M.	+ +	+	+ +	+	O O	O O	+	O O	O O
	G.	O O	+	+ O	+	O O	O O	+	O O	O O
Glanders.	S.	+ +	+	O	+	+ O	—	+	O O	O O
	M.	+ O	+	O O	+	O O	—	+	O O	O O
	G.	O O	+	O O	O	O O	—	+	O O	O O
Typhoid fever.	S.	+ +	+	+ O	+	+ +	—	+	O O	O O
	M.	+ +	+	+ +	+	O O	—	+	O O	O O
	G.	O O	+	O O	+	O O	—	+	O O	+ +
Colon bacillus.	S.	+ +	+	+ +	+	+ +	—	+	+ +	O O
	M.	+ +	+	+ +	+	+ +	—	+	+ +	O O
	G.	O O	+	+ +	+	+ +	—	+	O O	O O
Sanarelli.	S.	+ +	+	+ +	+	+ +	—	+	+ +	O O
	M.	+ +	+	+ +	+	+ +	—	+	+ O	O O
	G.	O O	+	+ +	+	+ +	—	+	O O	O O
Havelburg.	S.	+ +	+	+ +	+	+ +	—	+	+ +	O O
	M.	+ +	+	+ +	+	+ +	—	+	+ +	O O
	G.	+ O	+	+ +	+	O O	—	+	+ +	O O
Psittacosis.	S.	+ +	+	+ +	+	+ +	—	+	+ +	O O
	M.	+ +	+	+ +	+	+ +	—	+	+ +	O O
	G.	O O	+	+ O	+	+ +	—	+	+ O	O O
Black plague.	S.	O O	+	O O	+	O O	—	+	O O	O O
	M.	O O	+	+ O	+	O O	—	+	O O	O O
	G.	O O	O	O O	+	O O	—	+	O O	O O
Staphylococcus pyogenes aureus.	S.	+ +	+	+ +	+	+ +	O O	+	+ +	O O
	M.	+ +	+	+ +	+	+ +	O O	+	+ +	O O
	G.	+ O	+	+ +	+	+ +	O O	+	+ +	O O
Pneumonia (Fraenkel).	S.	+ +	+	+ +	+	+ +	—	+	O O	O O
	M.	+ +	+	+ +	+	+ O	—	+	O O	O O
	G.	O O	+	O O	+	O O	—	+	O O	O O
Green pus.	S.	+ +	+	+ +	+	+ +	—	+	+ O	O O
	M.	+ +	+	+ +	+	+ +	—	+	+ +	O O
	G.	O O	+	O O	+	O O	—	+	O O	O O
Streptococcus pyogenes.	S.	+ +	+	+ +	+	+ +	O O	+	+ +	+ O
	M.	+ +	+	+ +	+	+ +	O O	+	+ +	O O
	G.	+ +	+	+ +	+	+ +	O O	+	+ +	+ O
Positive growths out of 108 specimens and 54 controls.		75	50	81	50	67		51	50	4

scribed. The silk threads, muslin squares, or cover-glasses were coated with a mass of organisms, such as will hardly be met with in practice or in an ordinarily well-kept room. Such experiments, therefore, may be considered as very severe tests of the efficacy of the several methods studied. Ordinarily infectious material that may be scattered about in a room is in a fine state of division as dry dust. Even when infectious material as saliva or sputum in diphtheria, tuberculosis, etc., is spread over the surface of an article it dries down in a very thin layer, and it is safe to say contains but relatively few organisms in a given area, as compared with the test specimens from the thick suspensions mentioned above.

In order to obviate this objection a series of experiments were carried out, as given in Table IV., using very thin, *homogeneous* suspensions. For this purpose most of the test-organisms were grown for several generations of twelve hours each at 39° C. (102.2° F.). In this way very thin and perfectly homogeneous bouillon cultures were obtained. In one or two instances, where there was a tendency to the formation of scum, this was removed by filtration through a sterile absorbent cotton and glass-wool filter. The anthrax and potato-spore material were obtained from agar cultures. Only a portion of the surface growth was rubbed up with bouillon, and diluted to about 8 c.c, with sterile bouillon, and then filtered as above. Bouillon cultures of the anaerobic germs were employed, diluted with an equal volume of bouillon, and filtered to remove gross particles.

For each trial fresh specimens were prepared from these thin suspensions in exactly the same manner as in the preceding experiments. The same suspensions were used for all four experiments given in Table IV. In order to prevent alterations in the suspensions in the two and one-half days necessary for the four experiments, the suspensions were kept in a jar in melting ice. No change was observable in the material thus kept.

In experiments A, B, and C the exposure was continued twenty hours, as in all previous experiments. Experiment D was of only ten-hours' duration. In experiments B, C, and D the vapors of formaldehyd were distilled into the room through the key-hole by boiling formalin solution in the apparatus to be presently described. The same room has been used for all the experiments described in this paper except in Experiment C, Table IV.

Experiment A.—A comparison of the results obtained with thin suspensions will show little or no difference from the results given in Table I. Only dry specimens were exposed, as previous trials had clearly shown that three pounds of sulphur would destroy all vegetating forms in the wet condition. Omitting the hay bacillus results in Table I., inasmuch as this organism is not represented in Table IV., it will be seen that out of a total of 108 dry specimens 74 survived exposure in Table I. and 75 in Experiment A, Table IV. The temperature of the room varied from 20 to 24° C. (60.7°–70.5° F.). The odor at the end of 20 hours was tolerable.

Experiment B.—In this experiment 150 c. c. of formalin solution was distilled into the room within about thirty minutes. The temperature of the room varied from 20 to 22° C. (60.7°–70.1° F.). The odor at the end of twenty hours was tolerable. For the reason mentioned under Experiment A only dry specimens were exposed. The results were fairly satisfactory, as 81 out of 108 dried specimens survived the exposure. These results however are by no means as good as those in Experiments C and D, wherein the same method was followed. This is probably due to slower and possibly less complete distillation.

Material from a tuberculous lung cavity, very rich in tubercle bacilli, was divided into three portions and placed in wide Esmarch dishes. One of these was exposed to a temperature of 39° C. (100.2° F.) for about three hours or until dry. A second was exposed in the wet condition and the third reserved for direct use as a control. After exposure bouillon was added to each of the dishes, the material was thoroughly rubbed up and injected intraperitoneally into guinea-pigs. The control guinea-pig died within twenty-four hours as a result of diplococcus infection. The guinea-pig that received the dried material likewise died of diplococcus infection within less than three days; whereas, the guinea-pig that received the material which was exposed in a wet condition survived without the slightest illness, but when killed three weeks later it showed small tuberculous nodules in which tubercle bacilli were demonstrated. These results show that in a *dried layer* of sputum the micrococci of sputum septicemia (Fränkel's diplococcus) will survive exposure to formaldehyd and undoubtedly this is likewise true of the tubercle bacillus since it possesses in general a greater resistance than these organisms. In moist material the diplococci are killed more readily than tubercle bacilli. The latter undoubtedly escaped destruction owing to the large amount of material used (3 c. c.) and the presence of more or less solid particles.

Experiment C.—This experiment is given as a crucial test of the value of the formalin-distillation method. The large laboratory-room was employed for this purpose. The dimensions of this room are 36⅓x36⅙x12½ feet. It contains therefore 17,334 cubic feet (490.84 c.m.). The room has seven large windows and two doors; also, six or eight ventilating-shafts which unite into a main shaft in the attic. Large cracks extended around the entire edge of the ceiling. The ventilating- and cold-air shafts were plugged with bundles of old cloth. The cracks in the ceiling, about the edge of the floor, windows, and doors were caulked with strips of cloth.

On the basis of 60 grams of pure formaldehyd per 1000 cubic feet, 2600 c.c. of the 40-per-cent. formalin solution was necessary for the disinfection of this room. This amount could not be added all at once to the apparatus which was employed and will presently be described. One liter of the solution was placed in the apparatus and in about three-fourths of an hour a second liter was added, and after a like interval the remaining quantity was introduced. A little over three hours was necessary to distil this amount of formalin. Attention may be called to the great advantage of this apparatus over the so-called formalin lamps, or even the paraform apparatus. The same apparatus will do for large or small rooms. If all the formalin necessary for disinfection cannot be at once added, it can be introduced in portions during the process itself.

The specimens were placed at the further end of the room. A complete set of dry specimens and in addition wet specimens of spore material were exposed. At the end of twenty hours when the room was entered the formalin vapors were intolerable, and at no time were they noticeable in the adjoining rooms.

As shown in Table IV.,C, all the wet-spore specimens were disinfected. Of the 108 dry specimens 67 survived exposure. The fine dust taken from the floor at the farther end of the room was sterile. The dust on the top of the cases in the room had apparently lain there for a year or more. A considerable amount of this could easily be gathered by means of a sterile spatula. Portions of dust, the size of a small pea, placed in bouillon showed no sign of growth for the first couple of days, eventually however a "potato bacillus" developed. Practically therefore all surface dust in the room, and a large portion of the specimens exposed were disinfected.

Experiment D.—One hundred and fifty cubic centimeters of formalin solution was distilled as rapidly as possible (within ten minutes) into the disinfecting room of 1000 cubic feet capacity. The formalin vapors were allowed to act during ten hours. The room was then opened. The vapors were present in such amount as to be insupportable. The temperature ranged from 20 to 22° C. (60.7°–70.1° F.). Both dry and wet specimens were exposed. The control-tests given under *C* are also applicable to *D* since both tests were made at the same time and with the same material.

Of the wet specimens only four survived. Three of these were cover-glass preparations, and one a silk thread. They undoubtedly dried out before the gas had acted a sufficient length of time. Of the 108 dry specimens only fifty survived. This it will be seen is the best result obtained in this series of experiments.

By *rapid* formalin distillation it is, therefore, possible to disinfect all wet material within ten hours. Possibly one-half this time is sufficient for the accomplishment of the same result. Dried specimens of the germs of cholera, diphtheria, glanders, typhoid fever, black plague, and pneumonia, were all destroyed in the same time.

No experiments were made with less than 60 grams of formalin per 1000 cubic feet.

AVAILABILITY OF FORMALIN.

While sulphur fumigation under certain conditions (as shown in the preceding experiments) is of value, it is nevertheless evident that it is more obnoxious to persons in adjoining rooms, more injurious to fabrics, and certainly less effective than formalin. There can be no question but that formalin will eventually wholly displace sulphur fumigation. Formalin, perhaps, as yet, may not be obtained in every drugstore, but it undoubtedly will soon be as easy to obtain as sulphur.

As indicated heretofore formaldehyd vapors may be obtained in three ways: (1) By incomplete combustion of methyl alcohol. This is the basis of the so-called formaldehyd lamps in which the slow combustion and uncertain action make them of very little or no practical value. (2) By the polymerization of formalin, thus converting it into the solid form. On heating this material by means of an alcohol lamp the formaldehyd is regenerated. While this method gives excellent results and is much more certain than a formaldehyd lamp, it nevertheless possesses certain drawbacks. In the first place an additional and unnecessary expense is created in making paraform out of formalin and in regenerating the gas from this compound. Again, the apparatus for heating the paraform is placed within the room to be disinfected, and remains there until the room is opened. It is not possible to disinfect a number of rooms in the course of a day, unless a corresponding number of "disinfectors" are at hand. For the disinfection of a very large room a number of such machines must be employed. Moreover, the apparatus cannot be almost constantly watched either to prevent fire or to control the method itself. The third method of using formaldehyd consists in heating the commercial formalin or formol which is a forty-per-cent. solution of formaldehyd. Formaldehyd vapors are thus generated, and can be injected through a key-hole into a room. The statement is freely made that formaldehyd solutions cannot be heated without polymerizing and thus interfering with further evaporation. Formalin if heated slowly in an open dish may possibly polymerize, especially when concentrated to about 25 c.c., but we have never found this to take place when the formalin solution was rapidly heated in a glass flask or copper container. This fact can be utilized as the basis of a practical method for room disinfection.

Roux and Trillat devised an autoclave in which the formalin could be superheated and the resultant vapors then injected into the room. Various modifications of their apparatus have appeared from time to time. So far as our knowledge goes none of these can be said to possess the merits of cheapness, simplicity, and general usefulness. The results obtained by distillation of formalin from a glass flask (given in Table III.) were such as to justify further experimentation. The outcome was the construction of a very simple apparatus shown in the accompanying sketch. A similar apparatus, designed by Professor A. B. Stevens, has been in use in the Chemical Laboratory to produce steam for distillation purposes. The experiments with formalin described in Table IV. were made with this apparatus, and are a sufficient testimonial of its usefulness.

Fig. 1.

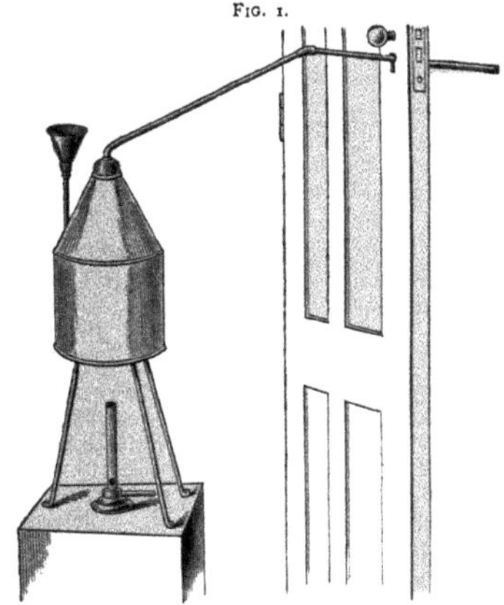

Formaldehyd Generator.

The container is six inches in diameter. The height of the cylindrical part is five inches; the total height to the top of the neck is ten inches. The capacity of the cylindrical part of the container is 2300 c.c. (approximately, 5 pints). An inclined tube twelve inches long and one-fourth inch in diameter screws into the neck. This is connected by means of a short piece of rubber tubing to a narrower tube, which is twelve inches long and three-sixteenths of an inch in diameter. A rubber connection between the tube is better than a rigid one. The end tube readily passes through an ordinary key-hole. The first tube is inclined to permit reflow of condensed water.

The funnel-tube is prolonged into the interior of the container, and extends to within one-sixteenth of an inch of the bottom. The height to the top of the funnel is eleven inches, and the diameter of the funnel-tube is five-sixteenths of an inch. The funnel-tube serves a double purpose in that it permits the introduction of the formalin solution, and serves as an indicator of the completion of the distillation. As soon as the liquid in the container has evaporated down to the level of the bottom of the funnel-tube, the formalin vapors and steam will issue from the tube. Therefore, when this tube extends down to within one-sixteenth of an inch of the bottom, practically the entire quantity of the liquid can be distilled into the room to be disinfected, not more than 10 grams of residue being left in the apparatus at the close of distillation.

The vessel is made of copper and the tubing of brass. The apparatus is placed on a tripod and heated with a Bunsen-burner. It may be placed on a gas or gasoline stove, or over a kerosene lamp. A portable heater similar to a plumber's lamp will undoubtedly be most useful.[1]

The formalin should be as rapidly boiled as possible. A good Bunsen-burner will distill 150 c.c. (5 oz.) of formalin, the amount necessary for 1000 cubic feet of space, within ten or fifteen minutes. When the room is very large, as in Experiment C., Table IV., the necessary amount of formalin may be added in several successive portions. It is perhaps desirable not to add the formalin too rapidly, inasmuch as the rapid cooling of the contents might result in the production of paraform. An increase of heat immediately after such addition will serve to promptly dissolve any paraform which might be formed. It is well to repeat, by way of emphasis, that there will be no trouble with polymerization when formalin is heated in a flask or in this disinfecting-apparatus. Should there be a tendency for the formalin to polymerize it can be prevented by the addition of 5 or 10 grams of borax. Solid paraform may be added to boiling formalin in a flask, and it will dissolve, forming an opaque white liquid. If a little borax is present the paraform will dissolve perfectly. It may be interesting to note that if 5 grams of borax and 60 grams of paraform are added to 100 c.c. of forty-per-cent. formalin and heated, perfect solution will result.

Commercial formalin, then, dissolves a considerable amount of paraform on heating, and the amount may be increased by the addition of borax. This fact may be utilized in shortening the time of distillation. Thus, to disinfect a room of 2000 cubic feet capacity, 150 c.c. of formalin, 60 grams of para-

[1] A small ordinary kerosene burner can be used to heat the formalin in the apparatus. Two hundred and fifty cubic centimeters of formalin can be raised to the boiling-pointin about ten minutes, and the distillation will be complete in about one hour. A parallel test, made with a modified plumber's gasoline lamp, especially made for us by Wm. A. Nicholas & Co., 940 North Clark street, Chicago, caused a like quantity of formalin to boil in four minutes, the distillation being complete in less than thirty minutes.

form, and a little borax can be introduced into the apparatus. This mixture could be distilled in one-half the time necessary for 300 c.c. of formalin.

Paraform when suspended in water and boiled will cause much foaming, and it cannot therefore be distilled with water in this operation. If, however, it is added to formalin, with or without borax, it can be distilled very rapidly without the slightest foaming.

At the close of a distillation it not infrequently happens that the formalin vapor present in the container condenses and polymerizes. A solid plug of paraform is thus formed. Consequently, before using the apparatus care should be taken to see that the tube is open. If this is not the case, on gentle heating the paraform will be readily volatilized, or a wire probe can be passed through the tube.

As seen from the illustration and description the apparatus is simplicity itself, and can be made by any tinsmith. It can be obtained from the Eberbach Hardware Company of Ann Arbor, or from Parke, Davis & Co. of Detroit.

The advantages possessed by this apparatus may be briefly summarized. One apparatus is sufficient regardless of the size of the room or rooms to be disinfected. The same apparatus can be used for almost any number of disinfections in the course of the day. The distillation of formalin into an ordinary room need not take more than twenty or thirty minutes. It is easily portable since it is very light, and is not voluminous. Inasmuch as it remains on the outside of the room before the eyes of the operator, there is absolutely no danger of fire or explosion. The apparatus, formalin, and fuel are inexpensive.

In conclusion, the following general directions for the disinfection of rooms may be of value:

1. All cracks or openings in the plaster or in the floor or about the door and windows should be caulked tight with cotton or with strips of cloth.

2. The linen, quilts, blankets, carpets, etc., should be stretched out on a line in order to expose as much surface to the disinfectant as possible. They should not be thrown into a heap. Books should be suspended by their covers so that the pages are all open and freely exposed.

3. The walls and floor of the room and the articles contained in it should be thoroughly sprayed with water. If masses of matter or sputum are dried down on the floor they should be soaked with water and loosened. No vessel of water, should, however, be allowed to remain in the room.

4. One hundred and fifty centimeters (5 ounces) of the commercial forty-per-cent. solution of formalin for each 1000 cubic feet of space should be placed in the distilling-apparatus and as rapidly distilled as possible. The key-hole and spaces about the door should then be packed with cotton or cloth.

5. The room thus treated should remain closed at least ten hours. If there is much leakage of gas into the surrounding rooms a second or third injection of formaldehyd at intervals of two or three hours should be made.

A CASE OF FECAL COMMUNICATION WITH THE BLADDER, WITH RESULTING CALCULUS FOLLOWING APPENDICITIS.[1]

By GEORGE RYERSON FOWLER, M.D.,
OF BROOKLYN, N. Y.;
PROFESSOR OF SURGERY IN THE NEW YORK POLYCLINIC; SURGEON-IN-CHIEF TO THE BROOKLYN HOSPITAL; SURGEON TO THE METHODIST EPISCOPAL HOSPITAL.

THE following history illustrates one of the possible sequels to appendical abscess, and is offered for the purpose of further emphasizing the importance of removing the vermiform appendix sufficiently early during an attack of inflammation of the organ and before the occurrence of suppuration, or failing in this, providing a safe exit for the suppurative collection, as well as a contribution to the literature of the complications and sequels of appendicitis:

J. B., a German, aged sixty-two years, was admitted to the Methodist Episcopal Hospital of Brooklyn March 4, 1895, with the following history: Twelve years previously, having up to this time enjoyed good health, he was suddenly seized with cramp-like abdominal pains, accompanied by nausea and vomiting. The pains were at first referred to the epigastrium, but afterward centered in the right iliac region. He was confined to bed several weeks with fever and anorexia. Finally, he passed a quantity of pus with the urine; this was followed by relief of the symptoms. Shortly afterward he began to pass fecal matter with the urine. This has continued to a greater or lesser extent ever since.

Since the first appearance of fecal matter in the urine he has suffered from chronic cystitis, with occasional acute exacerbations. One year prior to admission to the hospital these symptoms became greatly aggravated, with severe pain in the perineum and penis, together with dysuria and vesical irritability. The pain has kept him confined to his home, and most of the time to his bed, during the past few months. He has frequently suffered from obstruction to urination, due to the engagement of fecal masses in the vesico-urethral orifice, but of late, in addition to this, there has been the sudden cutting off of the outflow during the act of micturition characteristic of vesical calculus.

Upon admission the patient presented the appearance of a feeble and broken-down old man, and hav-

[1] Read at the Nineteenth Annual Meeting of the American Surgical Association, Held at New Orleans, April 19, 20, and 21, 1898.

ing been placed under the influence of an anesthetic, the sound detected the presence of a medium-sized calculus in the bladder. The bladder was at once opened with the double purpose of removing the calculus, and at the same time affording ready exit of the fecal matter which passed into it from the bowel. A phosphatic calculus the size of a horse-chestnut was removed.

The right lateral portion of the fundus of the bladder was found adherent to the structures in the neighborhood of the cecum, forming a deep pouch, from the bottom of which fecal matter in small quantities was forced during the manipulation incident to the examination. No neoplasm was present. Owing to the feeble condition of the patient the abdomen was not opened.

The patient gained rapidly in strength, but declined further operative interference. He was discharged from the hospital several weeks from the time of the operation, wearing a Bolton Bangs' suprapubic drainage-tube. His family physician has since reported to me that the suprapubic opening has healed, and that the patient is free from all traces of his former difficulty.

It would seem as if there could be no reasonable doubt that this case was originally one of appendicitis, and that the fecal communication between the bladder and intestine resulted from a rupture of an appendical abscess, either into both the bowel and the urinary viscus, or into the latter alone. In the latter case the communication occurred with the cecum as a result of the restoration of the patency of the appendix following the subsidence of the inflammatory condition.

WAR ARTICLES.

SANITARY NOTES UPON THE PROVINCES OF PINAR DEL RIO, HAVANA, MATANZAS, AND SANTA CLARA.[1]

By HENRY I. RAYMOND, M.D.,
CAPTAIN AND ASSISTANT SURGEON, UNITED STATES ARMY, STATIONED AT CAMP TAMPA HEIGHTS, FLORIDA.

THROUGH the courtesy of the Chief Surgeon of the Second Independent Division of United States troops in the field I am enabled to present to the readers of the MEDICAL NEWS a full and reliable report, submitted by S. Cueroo, M.D., a Cuban physician of many years' professional experience in that country, upon the water-supplies and the healthful or infected conditions of all important towns or localities throughout the four most westerly provinces of the Island of Cuba.

The report by Dr. Cueroo is so succinct and important for our practical guidance in the event of the occupation of Cuba by United States troops, that I present it without abridgment.

[1] The facts herein contained are based upon the personal knowledge and experience of Cuban physicians.

HAVANA PROVINCE.

Havana.—All kinds of infectious diseases. Water-supply contaminated.

Marianao.—Yellow fever, when imported; good supply of water.

Guanabacoa.—Same conditions; good water.

Guines.—Yellow fever, when imported; malaria; bad water.

Jaruco.—No yellow fever; good water.

Alquizar.—No yellow fever; malaria; good water from wells.

San Antonio de los Baños.—Yellow fever, when imported; springs and river water good.

Guanajay.—Yellow fever, when imported; malaria; good well water.

Bepical.—No yellow fever; good well-water.

Guincan.—No yellow fever; good well-water.

Santa Maria Bosano.—Very healthful city; no yellow fever; springs and good well-water.

Santiago de las Vegas.—Healthful city; deep wells; good.

Guira de Melena.—No yellow fever; malaria; well-water.

Batabano (south shore).—Very unhealthful; yellow fever, malaria, and typhoid fever; very bad water.

Aguacati.—Healthful place; well-water.

Madruga.—Very healthful locality; very good water; sulphur springs.

Nueva Par and *San Felipe.*—No yellow fever; well-water.

Guava, Castatina, Melena del Sur, Hoyo Colorado, Cannito, Guayabal, Guatao, Wajay.—No yellow fever; malaria; well-water.

Bauioa.—No yellow fever; healthful place; well-water.

MATANZAS PROVINCE.

Matanzas City.—Yellow fever and all kind of infectious diseases. Contaminated water.

Union de Reyes.—No yellow fever; well-water.

Suba Mocha.—Healthful locality; deep wells; good water.

Sabonitta.—No yellow fever; malaria; well-water.

Cardenas (Dr. Menvial).—Twenty-five thousand inhabitants; has two classes of water-supply: from wells which are almost all contaminated, and from the town's reservoir, supplied by a spring, but this spring-water is heavy and very sedimentous or incrustant, and is but slightly palatable. Many people there drink rain-water.

Malarial locality in autumn; dysenteric in summer. Yellow fever prevails there every year from June to October. Many cases of diphtheria and sore throat in dry season on account of the dust.

The soil is very permeable and the material of the macadam is very fragile. In time of grippe, this disease spreads very rapidly, because the dust forms clouds throughout the whole town.

Recreo.—Situated fifteen southeast of Cardenas; has four or five thousand inhabitants; low and red earth; paludic region; dysenteric in summer; no yellow fever except when imported; all the zone between the two places is very low, marshy, and swampy; somewhat malarial; travel almost impracticable by horses. San Anton River and what is called the "Canal of San Anton" (by which the inundation of "El Roque" empties its waters into the bay of Cardenas) are the water-channels of this district.

Hato Muevo.—Situated about fifteen miles east northeast of Recreo; has two thousand inhabitants. A range of uninterrupted mountains, fifteen miles long, divides this section of country into two zones; one in the southern part, higher, has many wells; some of them of good quality as to their water, and about ninety feet deep; without rivers in all the extension of this zone. The northern part, in which is situated Hato Muevo, is supplied from wells whose water is contaminated; these wells become filled up with water, usually in the summer season after heavy rainfalls. We have in this northern zone, malaria and dysentery, but never yellow fever. That part of the zone south of Cardenas is deprived of rivers and we have very few springs.

The Cuban physician furnishing this information on Matanzas Province has practised medicine for nine years in the zones above-mentioned and extending from Cardenas to Colon, and is therefore, well qualified to speak *ex cathedra.*

PINAR DEL RIO PROVINCE.

City of Pinar del Rio, Consolacion del Sur, Paso Real de San Diego, Palacios, San Cristobal, Candelaria.—Yellow fever only when imported; water good. All these cities are located in the southern plains of the province; more or less malarial localities.

Cabanas, Bahia Honda, and *Mariel.*—On the south shore; are very malarial; no yellow fever. All small localities in the hills are quite healthful and well supplied with good water.

SANTA CLARA PROVINCE.

The territory of "Sancti Spiritus," located in the central and southern part of Cuba, is very abundant in spring water, of excellent quality for drinking-purposes. One can rest assured that within a circumference of four miles in the greater part of this territory, a stream of water can be found. The territory forms an inclined plane that gradually rises from the southern coast with an occasional abruptness. It extends from southeast to northwest, forty-eight miles; from northeast to southwest, seventy-eight miles; from north to south, sixty miles.

The principal city, Sancti Spiritus, with fourteen thousand inhabitants, is thirty-six miles from Tunas de Laza, the port of entry, and is 570 feet above the level of the sea. A railroad runs between these two places, making four different stops on the road at as many villages.

Tunas de Laza, the port of entry, has only rain-water, but the railroad crosses one river and five streams of very good drinking-water.

The city (Sancti Spiritus) is divided by the Yayabo River, and its water is supplied to the inhabitants through iron pipes; there is also a small stream to the east of the city; one mile east and west of the same city there are found two other streams; all of these streams have very good water.

Leaving the city of Sancti Spiritus at any point of the compass, about every four miles good and abundant water can be found in all this territory.

This section of country continues rising toward the north and more so toward the west, terminating in mountains, some of which rise about 9000 feet, giving rise to many streams.

The principal rivers are: The *Laza,* navigable twenty-one miles; traverses the whole territory from north to south; its waters are good up to six miles south of the city of Sancti Spiritus.

The *Jatibonico del Norte* and *Jatibonico del Sur* have very good water; these two rivers form the eastern boundary of the territory, both rise from the same spring, one following north and the other south.

The *Tuinucu,* quite deep, rises in the mountains in the west from the same source as the Yayabo. The *Banos* rises also in the mountains and flows south into the sea, twelve miles to the west of Tunas de Laza; near the coast this river is known as the Tayabacoa. The *Higuanojo* rises also in the mountains and flows south into the sea, eighteen miles west of Tunas de Laza. This river forms the territorial boundary to Trinidad.

In the country lying between these rivers are innumerable springs, all of excellent water.

The climate is not excessively damp on account of the excellent drainage due to the gradual slope of the land. All the rivers have many good fords, except the Laza and Tuinucu, which in the rainy season are impassable for some days. To the east of this territory water is less abundant.

This territory suffers from yellow fever only when that disease is imported by Spanish troops, and at various times eight years in succession have elapsed without a case. The vegetation is luxuriant and woods are plentiful. The maximum temperature is about 95° F., and the minimum 45° F. No typhoid fever or diphtheria.

This short account of the Sancti Spiritus' waters and its excellent territorial conditions as to climate and healthfulness is very refreshing to one's mind after contemplating the plague-stricken cities along the shores of the more westerly provinces.

SANITARY SERVICE IN BATTLE.[1]

BY H. F. NICOLAI, M.D.,
MILAN, ITALY.

LOCATION OF THE FIRST DRESSING-STATION.

ON approaching the enemy, the regimental surgeons should make careful note of the ground gone over, in order to be prepared to select the best locations for the establishment of dressing-stations in case it comes to battle. Until the conflict actually begins, and it is clear in what direction it is going to develop, no dressing-stations are, however, actually instituted. The bearers assemble at the hospital wagons, and, superintended by an assistant surgeon, place their own equipment on the wagons and take their dressing-cases therefrom. Upon consultation of the senior medical officers of the battalion, regiment, and brigade, and of the regimental commander, the exact location of the dressing-stations is decided, but nothing is unpacked until the battle assumes a distinct form, the line of advance and of possible retreat become apparent, and the direction of fire and of available cover are considered. The dressing-station, once established, does not require to be removed unless the distance from it to the line of battle becomes too great for the bearers to traverse, or the station comes under fire; or, finally, the troops retreat. Under the first two conditions there is usually an abundance of time for the chief sanitary officer to select a new site for the station. But a retreat, if it occur, takes place suddenly, and in locating and conducting a dressing-station surgeons should always have this eventuality in mind. To facilitate rapid evacuation, as well as not to encumber the sanitary officers during battle, the slightly wounded should be immediately sent to the rear, and those who are not able to walk must be put in condition as soon as possible to stand transportation to the principal dressing-station, field-hospital, or some fixed point where they may receive proper care. For this purpose a number of vehicles should be kept close at hand. Surgeons in charge of advanced dressing-stations should keep in mind that only those must be treated who require immediate attention; for the medical officers at these points must be free to meet and grapple with unexpected emergencies. The choice of the site for the principal dressing-station is made in the same way. The Division Surgeon informs himself of the probable line of action and of the topography of the country; while, acting under his direction, the commander of the sanitary detachment and his subordinates select the exact site of the station, and make arrangements for the sanitary wagons and ambulances, for the erection of tents, and for cooking. Nothing is actually unpacked, however, until the conflict begins, as there will be plenty of time thereafter to prepare for even the most complicated operation. The possibility of a forward or backward movement should again be remembered, and every one should know his duties and be able to perform them rapidly and systematically in case a sudden movement is necessary. In choosing a position for a dressing-station, it is advisable to recall the three zones of battle described by Bircher: (1) The marching zone—to within about 1500 meters of the enemy; (2) from that point to the main firing position, or to within 500–600 meters of the opposing force; and (3) the zone of decisive conflict (Entscheidungszone). While gunshot injuries may occur in all three zones, at first the greatest losses will take place while the troops are deploying or in the zone of development; and both they who wish to approach in safety as near as possible to the enemy, and the sanitary officers who desire shelter for the wounded, will utilize all available cover. The flat trajectory of the modern missile has the advantage that, at short range, a relatively slight elevation will afford protection. A bullet shot from a distance of 2200 yards, if it pass over an elevation of 270 feet, will not reach its mark until it has traversed 1300 yards behind it; and a greater elevation than this cannot be shot over if aim is taken along the line of vision. An obstacle 250 feet high affords protection to a space about 2000 yards behind it; one 100 feet in height, at a distance of about 1000 yards from the enemy, shelters 1500 yards, and an elevation of 40 feet, if the enemy be distant less than 1000 yards, protects a distance of from 600 to 1000 yards in its rear. These facts are of the greatest moment in the choice of a location for a dressing-station, which must be near enough to the firing-line to afford aid to the wounded, and yet occupy a position where those already injured may be sheltered. From what has been said, the importance of adequate cover will be readily seen, and it will also be clear that withdrawal in a straight direction from the firing-line is not the way to secure necessary protection. In fact, the site chosen should be behind cover within the area of danger; which position may, however, become untenable in the event of the retreat of the enemy and necessitate an advance of the dressing-station, as was exemplified in the case of Sanitary Detachment No. 2, Eighth Army Corps, at Spicheren. Finally, the question arises, How can those who fall wounded in the fighting-line be most efficiently succored. The War Sanitary Regulations provide that one-half of the regimental surgeons and hospital assistants must remain at the dressing-station, while the other half accompanies the troops into action. It is maintained by some that a surgeon, if in line of battle, can save many lives by promptness, and that the moral effect of his presence is of great service to soldiers in danger. The author is of opinion, however, that the four bearers of a company, if properly trained, can render, on the few occasions when immediate aid is needed, far more assistance than one surgeon, however skilful and cool he may be, and that

[1] *Deutsche Mil.-Arztl. Zeitschr.*, Berl., 1897; as translated, and appearing in the *National Medical Review*, May, 1898.

the latter can do much more good at the dressing-station than with the troops. One point upon which the author lays particular stress is that it is never wise to select buildings of any kind for dressing-stations, on account of their liability to catch fire. Many instances of this lamentable accident, where it was impossible to remove the wounded, have been recorded, one in the war of 1870–71. It is far better to select positions, not *in* buildings, but *behind* them, since these can be the more readily evacuated.

MEDICAL PROGRESS.

A Sanitary Barber-shop.—According to BERGER (*Centralbl. für Bakteriol.*, March 10, 1898) the conditions existing in barber-shops are responsible for the spread of many diseases, not merely of the skin, hair, and beard, but infectious maladies as well. He suggests the following rules for practical guidance of barbers and legislators, since he considers that a barber-shop is properly subject to public control. The barber himself should be free from epilepsy, spasms of any kind, drunkenness, and infectious diseases. Persons afflicted with contagious diseases of the skin, hair, beard, or genitals, should not be allowed in a public shop, but should be attended to at their homes, where they should have all their own instruments. In the shop all brushes and combs should be made of good material, so that they may withstand frequent disinfection. Puff-balls should be replaced by balls of absorbent cotton, which should be thrown away after they have been once used. Towels, etc., should be freshly laundered for each person, unless paper napkins are employed and used only once. Combs should be cleaned and disinfected with corrosive-sublimate solution after each use. Shears, razors, and clippers should be boiled or wiped thoroughly with alcohol after each use. A barber should never wipe the razor upon his hand. Brushes to dust away the cut hair from the neck should be forbidden. A barber should pay special attention to the cleanliness of his own hands and person, and should be instructed in the appearances of diseases of the skin, scalp, beard, and genitals.

A Digestive Fever in Children.—COMBY (*Med. Moderne*, February 16, 1898) says that a light or severe fever is often observed in children from three to ten years of age, who are given improper articles of food. It shows itself at night by restlessness, redness of the cheeks, or perspiration. In the morning there is no fever, but the little one is pale and languid. These attacks may come every day, or only occasionally. The fever is moderate, usually 38 to 38.5° C. (100.5° to 101.5° F.), and lasting one, two, or three days. Anorexia, great thirst, a coated tongue, chronic constipation, and fetid stools, are the common symptoms. The treatment should correct the diet, and facilitate digestion by the administration of pepsin, magnesia, rhubarb, nux vomica, calomel, etc. Quinin and alcoholic preparations will do more harm than good.

Two Cases of Purulent Pleurisy in the Child Cured by Puncture.—VARIOT (*Rev. de Therapeut.*, April 1, 1898) succeeded in curing a certain number of cases of purulent pleurisy in children by simple puncture. Clinical observation is the best guide in determining what patients should be subjected to puncture, and what ones should be subjected to the usual operation for empyema. If the amount of pus is small, and the respiratory function is not interfered with, if the digestion is good and there is little fever, the conditions are such that one may well hope for a complete cure from a simple puncture. If on the other hand, the heart beats strongly and respiration is hampered, while there is high fever, and the amount of fluid in the pleural cavity is large, resection of a rib is indicated. Also, if after a puncture, the symptoms grow worse with high fever and putrid discharge, no time should be lost, but the chest should be opened widely and thoroughly drained.

THERAPEUTIC NOTES.

Treatment of Cutaneous Anthrax by Injections of Iodin.—ASMOUSS (*Rev. Therapeut.*, April 15, 1898), practised injections into the periphery of cutaneous nodules of anthrax of tincture of iodin, diluted with one or two parts of distilled water. Two patients so treated received from four to eight injections each, and injections were also made in the vicinity of secondarily infected glands. Treatment in one case was continued for ten days, in the other for two weeks. Both patients recovered. No symptom of iodism was at any time manifested. The author says that this treatment is especially adapted to anthrax occurring under circumstances prohibiting surgical treatment.

Tincture of Strophanthus in Cardiac Affections.—JACOBÆUS (*Klin. Ther. Wochenschr*, March 13, 1898), warns against a too hasty conclusion that strophanthus and digitalis have benefited a patient suffering from heart disease, because improvement has followed the use of these drugs. Rest in bed alone will often cause a marked improvement in such patients, and it is better to defer the administration of these precious remedies until it is manifest just how much benefit is going to follow decubitus. Strophanthus has the great advantage over digitalis in not being cumulative in its action. In grave emergencies, however, some physicians prefer not to trust to it alone. It is then best to give it alternately with digitalis and in small doses, for in this manner an effect is produced which could not be obtained by the administration of either of the drugs separately, in the same amounts. In all cases in which there are associated disturbances of digestion, as well as in all cases in which the medication will have to be administered for a long time, strophanthus ought to play the chief part. In conclusion the writer states that there are certain cases of asystole, in which small doses of strophanthus are more efficacious than large doses of digitalis. At present he is not able to recognize such cases in advance, and it is therefore advisable in all cases to begin with strophanthus, a remedy which is always more manageable and sometimes more powerful than digitalis.

THE MEDICAL NEWS.

A WEEKLY JOURNAL

OF MEDICAL SCIENCE.

COMMUNICATIONS are invited from all parts of the world. Original articles contributed *exclusively* to THE MEDICAL NEWS will after publication be liberally paid for (accounts being rendered quarterly), or 250 reprints will be furnished in place of other remuneration. When necessary to elucidate the text, illustrations will be engraved from drawings or photographs furnished by the author. Manuscripts should be typewritten.

Address the Editor: J. RIDDLE GOFFE, M.D., No. 111 FIFTH AVENUE (corner of 18th St.), NEW YORK.

Subscription Price, including postage in U. S. and Canada.

PER ANNUM IN ADVANCE	$4.00
SINGLE COPIES	.10
WITH THE AMERICAN JOURNAL OF THE MEDICAL SCIENCES, PER ANNUM	7.50

Subscriptions may begin at any date. The safest mode of remittance is by bank check or postal money order, drawn to the order of the undersigned. When neither is accessible, remittances may be made, at the risk of the publishers, by forwarding in *registered* letters.

LEA BROTHERS & CO.,
No. 111 FIFTH AVENUE (corner of 18th St.), NEW YORK, AND Nos. 706, 708 & 710 SANSOM ST., PHILADELPHIA.

SATURDAY, MAY 21, 1898.

FOOTGEAR FOR THE SOLDIER.

THE greatest English soldier and commander of modern times said that the most essential thing for a soldier is a good pair of boots, and the second most essential thing is a second pair of boots. Every one who has had any experience with marching troops will be likely to agree with this immortal. Now that 125,000 of our National Guardsmen, from all walks and stations of life, have been mustered into the regular service, it behooves the commissary department of the army and its various agencies to use supreme vigilance, precaution, and wisdom in providing suitable footwear for this vast number of practically raw recruits.

It probably does not overshoot the mark to say that eighty per cent. of the men who have enlisted are improperly shod on entering service. And if the commissary department is not in possession of properly accredited and well-advised purchasing agents, these soldiers are likely to be seriously handicapped and many of them made useless as implements of war when they come to be landed in Cuba or the Philippines, where they will be subjected to tests of unaccustomed climate and soil. The quartermasters of companies should therefore bear in mind in attending to the shoeing of their troops that they are not dealing with the normal foot in the vast majority of cases. This is the first obstacle to contend with. The second is the vanity of man concerning his feet, even though he be a soldier.

The absolute requisites in a shoe for marching are that it be comfortable and enduring; that is, that it be made on the right kind of a last from the proper material, and that it be properly and firmly put together. The essential elements of the first are that it have a straight inside line; that the sole lie flat or nearly flat upon the ground; that the arch be firmly and solidly supported; that the shoe fit snugly around the heel and the instep, and finally, in order that the pressure may be equally distributed, that there be sufficient room for the unhampered play of each pedal articulation when the weight of the body is successively thrown upon it. Unless the shoe fulfils these indications it should be discarded. The sole should project beyond the upper so as to give firm support to the foot when it is fully expanded under the combined influence of the weight of the body and the resultant muscular relaxation of fatigue; and it should be composed of solid double sole, not paper or leather packing sandwiched between two thin pieces of leather which unfortunately is often found. The uppers should be of stout, yet pliable, thoroughly seasoned hide, double stitched, and by proper dressing made impervious to moisture. If these details are insisted upon more will be done toward contributing to the capacity of the soldier than by the most elaborate system of acclimatization. It is more necessary to make Mulvaney immune to fatigue than it is to make him immune to fevers; by accomplishing the former you encompass the latter.

A properly clad, well-fed American soldier is well prepared to give battle to the Cuban germ and the Spanish parasite, but he expects his Government and its officers to provide him with the most approved implements of war and accoutrement. It is the poorest sort of economy to grudge a few cents on a pair of shoes, especially in the light of what has just been said. Yet this is what the quartermaster's department has set out to do, if we may give credence to the reports in the daily press. In response to an invitation for estimates for 25,000 pairs of shoes, Chicago manufacturers offered to furnish army footgear at prices varying from 90 cents to $2 per pair. It is not at all improbable that the latter figure embraces the cost of manufacture plus a fair profit for shoes that will meet all the requirements mentioned above, while it is just as certain that any figure very much below it does not do so. This is not the time to be cent wise and dollar foolish. A few cents extra expended on a pair of boots may mean a live, fighting soldier in time ot pressure and of need, while a 90-cent pair will be very sure to be found bound in tatters on a lamed or dying sacrifice.

A WORD TO MEDICAL GRADUATES.

THE tendency to specialization in every department of life is patent to all, but to none is it more evident than to the bright, wide-awake young medical graduate who has just finished his college work, and is about to step out into active life. He has already noticed in medicine the pressure of competition, the over-crowding in many places, and the difficulty of securing a foothold, to say nothing of a decent livelihood, much less recognition and fame. A specialist seems to have a better chance in every way. There are not so many of them, they command higher remuneration, they sooner come into public notice and become famous. It is not to be wondered at then that so many of our graduates are deciding to be specialists. In this way is most hope of a living, and perhaps fame. And, let us be fair, there is also the fact that there is so much to learn in each department of medicine, that to be able to concentrate all the thought and effort upon one subject strengthens one's confidence in himself, and kindles the hope that he surely can master that one subject. It therefore appeals to him not only as the best thing to do, but the most reasonable thing to do.

While this is all true, are there not some salient facts of the utmost importance that ought to be most carefully considered before making so serious a decision as this must necessarily be? Before one decides to become a specialist ought he not to remember that to be a specialist implies not only that he makes one subject his sole business, but also that he knows all there is to be known about that subject? To limit one's work and attention to one specialty, however, does not make one a specialist. The specialist must know more than is generally known in his line. He must have thought harder and longer, and pushed his investigations farther in that particular line than the general practitioner. He must know more than any or all the books have to say regarding it. And to do this means that he is deeply interested in his subject and most enthusiastic over it for its own sake, regardless of any remuneration or recognition. It will not do then to select any subject; but the would-be specialist must choose that subject he likes most, the one which will prove most fascinating and attractive the more it is investigated. If one would be sure of success as a specialist, he must be deeply and truly in love with his subject, and, forsaking all others, cleave only unto it, for better or for worse, for richer or poorer, in sickness and in health, till death them do part.

Nor is it enough merely to be enamored of some particular subject. The specialist must have the inherent aptitude, the natural gifts that such a subject demands. One may be passionately fond of the violin, and yet it would hardly be wise to spend much time or effort in trying to be an Ole Bull it one had only one arm. So one may be deeply interested in the eye, but if he be lacking in delicacy of touch, or have a beam in his own eye, how can he hope to remove the mote from another's? Each specialty demands certain qualifications which are absolutely essential to success. Of course the beginnings in any line are awkward and clumsy, faculties and powers are brought under control and made more efficient by use; but the point here emphasized is the presence of the faculty or power. Before deciding then upon a particular subject the candidate ought to make sure that he posseses the necessary powers of hand, eye, ear, and imagination which that subject requires. A specialist must not only know what ought to be done—he must know also how to do it. If the choice involves surgical work he must have the inventive faculty and the mechanical skill required by his subject. The specialist has by no means mastered his subject when he knows all that there is to be known about its etiology, pathology, signs, and symptoms. There is still a most extensive and fascinating region unentered—the vast realm of the instruments, appliances, and methods of work. The specialist must be able and willing to ponder over the shape of an instrument or the arrangement of a bandage, as over the effects of a drug, the healing of a wound, or the symptoms of a disease. Success in many cases turns quite as much upon the skilful use of an appliance specially contrived for that particular case, as upon a clearer insight into the real cause of the trouble. One can scarcely be too careful in this matter, and should be quite sure that he does really possess the inventive faculty and the mechanical skill likely to be necessary.

Not as essential as the considerations already mentioned, but still very important, is the opportunity for practice and personal experience in the chosen subject. A young man must go where he can have an abundance of opportunity for experiment and examination. The specialist must know the theories of his subject, and have his own, too, but far more some practical, personal experience in it. The more the better. Surely, if it is deemed right to insist on so many years preparation for the ordinary practitioner, the specialist needs more. For in proportion as the specialist is required to know more and to be more skilful in his particular field than the general practitioner, precisely will be the need of special study and preparation. If, then, one finds it impossible to go where such opportunities can be secured, or impossible to devote to it the extra time required, he should not persist in his choice.

Just one word more. Do not be overanxious to decide at once. Like taking a wife, the choice of a life-work is a most serious matter. One's taste changes. The darling of twenty may prove to be intolerable at forty years of age. A subject most attractive to you now may, on fuller investigation, develop lines of work not merely distasteful, but positively repellant. The advice once given to a young graduate, who was inquiring as to advisability of taking a hospital here and afterward going abroad, or of going first abroad, still stands the test of experience: Take the work here first by all means, and after a few years you will know better for what you need to go abroad. Yes, and after a few years you will know better for what you are best fitted. Wait patiently for the unfolding of your powers. Wait until you know your own self. Then in view of your own powers, your own tastes, and your own opportunities, choose and decide. Fidelity to such a choice, seconded by industry and conscientiousness, will win and bring its sure reward.

FEDERAL QUARANTINE AND SANITATION.

THE coming summer can hardly fail to bring yellow fever again to our shores; in fact, considering the turbulent times at, and within, our borders we can hardly expect to escape an epidemic unless early and extraordinary precautions are taken. A rigid watch must be kept on favorable points of ingress and modern sanitation must be enforced in all our Southern cities. Unfortunately civic cleanliness still depends upon local enlightenment and legislation and its importance is often realized only after many epidemics, entailing vast losses of life and property. Local ignorance, neglect, or parsimony therefore still leave wide breaches in the strongest bulwark against alien disease. The most we can do is to enact and put in operation laws looking to a prompt and efficient quarantine, and a uniform management of an epidemic should it prevail.

It evidently was with this necessity in mind that Mr. Hepburn introduced in the House of Representatives a bill "amending an act granting additional quarantine powers and imposing additional duties upon the Marine-Hospital Service." In the emergency confronting us we must have prompt and expert assistance, and that we can only get from the Marine-Hospital Service. We must have also authoritative and uniform management of affairs in case yellow fever invades our country and that is possible only by Federal interference. The bill in question endows the Treasury Department with power in times of epidemic to formulate and enforce rules which shall be of national scope and shall be preeminent over all local quarantine regulations. It is in this way alone that uniformity can be attained and uniformity is essential to justice and public safety.

It is only necessary for a measure like this to be proposed when opposition immediately crops out on the ground of the interference with State rights. The opponents of such a law on such grounds should be asked whether they carry their ideas to the extent of allowing States to become centers of infection or public nuisances from the interference with traffic.

The urgency is now too great to allow of creating a Department of Health even if it were desirable and the medical profession can do no better work in this direction than to exert its influence in favor of Mr. Hepburn's bill, known as House Bill No. 4363.

ECHOES AND NEWS.

Issuing of Marriage Licenses.—There has been a bill introduced in the Maryland Legislature regarding the prohibition of marriage licenses to any one suffering from insanity, dipsomania, syphilis, or tuberculosis.

The American Surgical Association; A Correction.—Dr. Claudius H. Masten desires to have it announced that the published report that he had been elected second vice-president of this Association for the coming year is incorrect. Dr. Solon Marx is the second vice-president.

Dainties for Dewey's Wounded.—The Surgeon-General of the Navy has sent one hundred dollars to the Navy Pay Office at San Francisco to purchase clam-juice, lemons, beef extract, and jellies to be sent to the sick and wounded of Admiral Dewey's fleet. The money was contributed by the National Relief Association of the National Society of Colonial Dames of America.

Meeting of the American Gastro-Enterological Association.—At the annual session of this Association, held at Washington, D. C., May 3, 1898, the following officers were elected: President, D. D. Stewart, Philadelphia; first vice-president, Max Einhorn, New York; second vice-president, John C. Hemmeter, Baltimore; secretary and treasurer, Charles D. Aaron, Detroit.

Meteorological Conditions of the Klondike Region.—Some interesting observations on the climate have been made in regard to the Klondike region, particularly at Dawson between August, 1895, and November, 1896. From December 1, 1895 to February 1, 1896, the temperature fell below zero every day. July was the only month in which the mercury did not sink below freezing.

The Marine Biologic Institute of the University of Pennsylvania.—This institution will be opened during the summer, after being closed for five years. It is situated on the shores of Ludlam's Bay, at Sea Isle, N. J. The laboratory will be in charge of Dr. Milton J. Greenman of the university. The intention is to build a floating house-boat of some extent for the accommodation of the students.

The Hospital-Ship "Solace."—The Surgeon-General of the Navy, Dr. Van Reypen announces that the hospital-ship "Solace" is at Key West and that her splendid equipment is ready to give every care to the wounded. Aside from the "Solace," the Navy has at Key West a temporary hospital. It is the purpose of the department, however, to use the "Solace" mainly for the wounded, and to bring them North as fast as their condition will permit, in order to get them out of the Southern climate.

The Title of Doctor in Prussia.—The German universities, with the exception of Fiessen, Leipzig, and Rostock, independently of the Staats-Examen, which alone can give the right to practise medicine, have been conferring the degree of doctor of medicine. So a man could be a doctor of medicine without being legally qualified. But the Minister of Public Instruction has recently put a stop to this practice. No university can grant a degree of doctor of medicine to any one who has not passed the Staats-Examen. This law goes into force October 1st.

New York Train to the Denver Meeting of the American Medical Association.—At the last meeting of the New York County Medical Association, the following Committee on Transportation was appointed to arrange for a Greater New York special train to the Denver meeting of the American Medical Association. Inquiries should be addressed to the chairman or secretary. J. J. A. Maher, M.D., chairman; F. H. Wiggin, M.D.; L. Fisher, M.D.; W. R. L. Dalton, M.D.; A. E. Gallant, M.D., secretary, 60 West Fifty-sixth street, New York City.

The Alphabet Only of the Nervous System Mastered in This Life.—Two veteran neurologists sat talking late into the night of the difficulties and inexplicable phenomena daily presented in their practice, and then the talk diverted to the question of the immortality of the soul. Said one of them to the other, "Do you believe the soul is immortal?" and he replied abstractedly, "I hope so. I would like to exist some time longer. I would like to know more about the nervous system." The plentitude of the ages yet to come seems to be necessary for the neurologist's line of work.

A First-Class Fraud.—A man, short, thick, well-dressed, with stick in hand, about forty years old, has been "operating" Boston for several weeks, till two weeks ago, when, with wife and baggage, he left by the Providence railroad. He presented his card as Dr. C. C. Perry, putting out his sign at 94 Compton street, corner of Tremont, and stated that he had just returned from a visit to Europe. The janitor where he stopped says about forty people have come inquiring after him, some for money borrowed, others for goods furnished on instalments, etc. He has probably transferred his operations to some other large city to the Southward. Look out for him!—*Boston Medical and Surgical Journal.*

Dr. Porro in the Milan Riot.—A cablegram gives the following story about the recent riot at Milan: "The mob did not even respect the hospitals, but wished to invade them, and the Ospedale Maggiore was particularly threatened. Behind the gate at that building stood Professor Porro, a senator and well-known doctor, the most noted conservative in Milan. The crowd was quick to see him. 'There is Porro, our oppressor!' they cried, threateningly. Insults were shouted at the professor, who, pale but calm, resolutely opened the gates and stood with arms folded, saying sternly: 'Let him who has the courage advance. He will find a good revolver ready for him, and I will show how a good physician does his duty.' Nobody accepted the invitation."

The American Gynecological Society. — The next annual meeting of this society will be held at Boston, May 24, 25, and 26, 1898. The meetings will be held at the Hall of the Boston Society of Natural History, corner of Berkeley and Boylston streets. The sessions for the presentation of papers and scientific discussions will be held daily from 9 A.M. to 12 M., and from 2 P.M. to 5 P.M.; executive session Wednesday 5 P.M. One of the following subjects for discussion will be presented each day: (1) Has Electricity Ceased to Be a Useful Therapeutic Agent in Gynecology? (2) Should Non-Absorbable Ligatures Be Discarded in Gynecological Surgery? (3) The Surgical Treatment of Sterility—How Far Is It Justifiable or Expedient? The program of papers is unusually full and varied.

The Commencement of Bellevue Hospital Medical College.—This institution held its thirty-seventh annual commencement at the Carnegie Laboratory, Monday, May 9, 1898, and sent forth into active professional life 132 graduates. In addition to the above, 160 candidates have passed three or more of their examinations in the following primary subjects: Materia medica and therapeutics, physiology, anatomy, and chemistry. The successful candidates for appointment in Bellevue Hospital are William W. Beveridge, William Martin Richards, William D. Robertson, William Ray Gladstone, Harry Neafie Taylor, Edward Henry Cary, Reginald McCreery Rawls. The graduates with honorable mention and a prize of $100 each are: Samuel Spiegel, William Martin Richards, Samuel Benjamin Yow, Peter Frederick Holm.

Niemeyer's Anecdote about the Ventilating of Vehicles.—In one of his lectures, Niemeyer tells a story of a scene in an omnibus, which hinged on the question whether the conductor should open or shut the windows. On the left was seated a corpulent lady with full face, shrill voice, and labored respiration. The lady on the right was of lean, slender dried-up figure; on entering the omnibus she had coughed; after taking her seat she held her handkerchief to her mouth and fairly changed color when the one opposite wheezing, took her place and called out for "Air, air!" exclaiming she would fairly be smothered if the window were to remain closed. "But I," objected the other, "would get my death of cold if the window were opened." The conductor, who for some time stood undecided what to do, received this piece of Solomonic advice from one of the passengers: "Open the window," said he, in a deep voice, "and then one of them will die; then close it, and the other will die, and so at last we shall have peace."

Climate in the Philippines.—The Philippine Islands are peculiar in having three seasons, a cold, a hot, and a wet. The first extends from November to February or March. The winds are northerly and woolen clothing and a fire are desirable, the sky is clear and the air bracing. The hot season lasts from March to June, the heat becomes oppressive, and thunder storms of terrific violence are frequent. During July, August, September, and October the rain comes down in torrents and large tracts of the lower country are flooded. Manilla, though low, is, broadly speaking, healthy except for smallpox, which flourishes unnoticed in the crowded houses of the lower, half-caste natives and Chinese, and malarial typhoid, which chooses the careless foreign resident for its attentions. The black plague has never reached the Philippines, but cholera used to decimate Manila's native population before a generous benefactor gave the city its present good water-supply system. Since then that dread disease has kept away, and the mortality in that center of 350,000 Malays, half-castes, Chinese, and Europeans does not probably exceed three per cent. per annum.

Diamond Cut Diamond.—The recent death of Sir Richard Quain, who had been what some Americans might call a "hustler," has brought forward the following anecdote of London high-life practice. Dr. Quain, as the *London Practitioner* states it, had in a very high degree the power of inspiring confidence, which is of vital importance in the equipment of a successful city physician. He was a past master in the art of managing patients. There is a legend, however, that he was once driven from the field by a still more consummate artist. A financial magnate of Israel had been suffering for a long time from renal trouble of a grave character, and which it was considered expedient by Quain and other physicians in attendance to conceal from the family. The wife insisted, much to Quain's annoyance, on calling in Sir William Gull, who, she said, would be sure to tell her what her husband was suffering from, which apparently none of the doctors knew. Gull, when interpolated on the subject, replied in his most oracular manner: "Madam, your husband is suffering from a cachexia." "There," said the lady, triumphantly, "I knew Sir William Gull would tell me!"

Protection of the Red-Cross Flag.—The bill passed by the United States Senate two months ago to protect the Red-Cross insignia against use by other associations having a similar purpose has now been favorably reported by the House Committee on Foreign Relations. The text of the bill is the same as that of the measure passed by Congress two years ago, but which failed to receive the President's signature. It would seem to us an advantage if the present measures were amended so as to include protection against mercantile use of the Red-Cross emblem, and we wish that such an amendment might be introduced. At all events, it is essential that the bill to protect the Red-Cross flag be passed at once. The Red Cross is no mere ordinary society; it should be a Government agency, and should receive Government recognition and protection. In other countries agreeing to the Geneva Convention we understand that it has been so recognized. The steamer "State of Texas," which sailed from the port of New York with twelve hundred tons of provisions for the suffering in Cuba, called at Key West last week, taking on board Miss Clara Barton and her assistants. It is awaiting instructions from Admiral Sampson. — *New York Times.*

Prophylactic Gargle in Scarlatina. — The frequency of otitis media as a complication of scarlatina is said to be reduced to a minimum, if several times a day the tonsils and pharyngeal vault be gently brushed with absorbent cotton, wet with the following solution:

℞ Beta-naphthol . . . . . . ʒ i
Camphoræ } aa . . . . . ʒ iv.
Glycerini }
M. Sig. For application to throat.

CORRESPONDENCE.

OUR PHILADELPHIA LETTER.

[From Our Special Correspondent.]

AN ATTEMPT TO ESTABLISH A NATIONAL FORMULARY OF POPULAR PRESCRIPTIONS—ANOTHER INSTANCE OF MILK INFECTION—A MEMORIAL TABLET DEDICATED TO TWO NEW JERSEY PHYSICIANS—TO STUDY THE POLLUTION OF THE SCHUYLKILL RIVER—JEFFERSON MEDICAL COLLEGE'S COMMENCEMENT AND ITS NEW BUILDINGS—DR. SCHWENK ELECTED SURGEON TO WILLS' EYE HOSPITAL—A WARNING AGAINST SMALLPOX BY THE STATE BOARD OF HEALTH—OPENING OF THE PENNSYLVANIA EPILEPTIC HOSPITAL AND COLONY FARM—A "DIVINE HEALER" IN THE TOILS.

PHILADELPHIA, May 14, 1898.

AT the last meeting of the Philadelphia County Medical Society, held May 11th, a report was made by a committee from the Philadelphia College of Pharmacy, advocating the establishment of what may be called a "national formulary," to be prepared by representatives of various pharmaceutical societies of the United States, and having for its purpose the substitution of the so-called "shot-gun" prescriptions marketed by the large manufacturing pharmacists by formulæ which have, by long usage, become popular with the medical profession. Briefly, the stand taken seems to be one of defense on the part of the druggist against the trade-demoralizing influences of the ubiquitous tablet-triturate and like preparations. Dr. F. W. E. Steadman, for the College of Pharmacy Committee, exhibited four preparations of a standard drug obtained from four leading drug-stores of this city, and all unlike both in value and appearance. While disavowing any intention of criticising the value of the combination put up by the wholesale manufacturer, he held that these prescriptions should contain the precise ingredients and in the exact proportion stated by the makers. That wide variations between the actual composition of these preparations and the formulæ printed on their labels does exist to a large extent was further claimed by other representatives of the college, who declared that the great variations, both in the quantity and the quality of the drugs put into these preparations, and the chemical incompatibility of many of the ingredients, was often a source of positive danger to the patient. It was stated that the employment of skilled labor by the druggist ensures to the physician a more accurate compounding of his prescription than could be promised by the wholesale manufacturers, who, it was charged, employ unskilled laborers for the work, and not registered pharmacists, like the drug-stores; the mixing and weighing of ingredients in these factories is done by boys and girls of twelve and fourteen years of age. As a result of such methods, mistakes are bound to occur, with unfortunate results to the patient, to sustain which charge a recent case in court was cited, which involved the sale of 40,000 strychnin pills, where suspicion was raised as to the amount of strychnin contained in each pill, a patient having shown signs of strychnin poisoning after the administration of some of them. Dr. H. A. Hare, in the discussion which followed, said that as modern therapeutics aims at securing the effects of single drugs, prescriptions containing the combination of a large number of different drugs are not in general demand at the present time. He also expressed the opinion that the large manufacturers, with their superior facilities for obtaining pure drugs in large quantities and with the supervision of skilled chemists during the processes of manufacture and assaying, can furnish perfect and reliable prescriptions more cheaply and more certainly than the druggist.

Of the eighty-six new cases of diphtheria reported in this city last week, a large majority were confined to a limited district in Germantown, which had hitherto been considered a healthy locality. Upon investigation of the cause of this unlooked-for outbreak, Dr. Taylor of the Health Bureau, found that the patients had been served with milk from a single dairy, the sanitary condition of which, according to the official report, must have been so bad that it surprised even the stench-proof inspectors. It was found by these gentlemen that the stables and cow-yard of the establishment (which, it should be noted, is situated within the city limits) drained through the open street, past dwellings, by an open gutter, together with, during rains, the overflow of two privy wells, all after a liquid carnival of filth, finally reaching the Schuylkill River by way of the Wissahickon Creek. Is it any wonder that our water-supply is tainted, when such menaces to health exist right under the noses of our accomplished corps of sanitary inspectors? Of course the dairy was promptly closed by the authorities, after their attention was directed to it by the outbreak of diphtheria, but this very circumstance prompts the question, How many more such foci of disease still exist undisturbed within the limits of the city, and how many more outbreaks of diphtheria must be recorded to direct, as in the present and other instances, the attention of the health officials to the condition of affairs, and to induce them to take, as the newspapers delight in saying, "active measures to stamp out the source of the infection"?

The Camden County (N. J.) Medical Society, at its fifty-second annual session, held May 10th, presented to the county authorities a brass memorial tablet in commemoration of the heroic services of Dr. John W. McCullough and Dr. Henry E. Branin during the severe epidemic of typhus fever in the Camden County Almshouse during 1880 and 1881. It may be recalled that Dr. McCullough died during the course of the scourge, and that Dr. Branin's life was shortened by many years as a result of his labors at this time. The principal addresses at the dedication of the tablet were made by Dr. E. L. B. Godfrey, who read a memoir of the deceased physicians, and by Dr. James Tyson, who related some personal experiences of the late epidemic, which he had an opportunity to study, and also spoke feelingly of the unselfish services rendered by the members of the Camden County medical profession at that time.

In order to arrive at, if possible, a final solution of the cause of the pollution of the water-supply of Philadelphia, a committee of the local and State Boards of Health this week began a special tour of investigation of the Schuylkill river, including its tributaries, drains from factories and workshops situated along its course, and other places which are liable to contribute to its infection. A steam-launch has been placed at the disposal of the committee, and they have equipped it with the necessary apparatus for chemic and bacteriologic examination of the samples of water which will be collected at various points along the river, in the hope of locating definitely points of especially serious pollution. It is the present intention to pursue the investigation as far as the city of Reading, some sixty miles up stream, but, if required, the commission will extend their labors to a still more remote point. The following prominent sanitarians constitute the commission entrusted with this work: Dr. George Woodward, of the Philadelphia Board of Health; Dr. A. C. Abbott, Director of the Bacteriologic Laboratory of the Philadelphia Board of Health; Dr. Benjamin Lee, of the Pennsylvania State Board of Health; Dr. R. L. Pittfield, Bacteriologist of the Pennsylvania State Board of Health; John W. Trautwine, Chief of the Philadelphia Water Bureau; George L. Hughes, Chief of the Philadelphia Bureau of House Drainage, and Charles F. Kennedy, Chief Inspector of Nuisances of Philadelphia. At the conclusion of their investigations this commission will report to Councils for the guidance of this body during its deliberations on the question of a new water-supply for the city.

The seventy-fourth annual commencement of the Jefferson Medical College was held in the Academy of Music on May 13th, fifty members of the graduating class receiving the degree of the doctorate from the hands of the Hon. William Potter, President of the Board of Trustees. The opening prayer was made by Archdeacon Cyrus T. Brady of Pennsylvania, and addresses were delivered by President Potter, and by the dean of the college, Professor James W. Holland.

At the conclusion of the present college year, work on the new buildings of Jefferson will be commenced. On ground immediately adjoining the present college buildings, now in the possession of the trustees, a structure extending 118 feet 6 inches on Walnut street, and 107 feet 6 inches on Tenth street, will be erected. The buildings will be of the Italian *Renaissance* style of architecture, of brick, terra cotta, and limestone, five and six stories high. In addition to offices and rooms devoted to the business needs of the institution, the plans provide for an extensive library, museum, and gymnasium, and reading- and lounging-rooms for the students. The larger lecture-rooms, of which there are to be two, have a seating-capacity, one of 400, the other of 300 students; a number of smaller rooms for section work are also provided. The clinical amphitheater seats 520 people, the seats rising from the ground floor to the second story, and the floor space of the whole measuring 76 feet by 21 feet 6 inches. Fronting on Tenth street are the students' laboratories, six in number, each occupying an area of 76 feet by 21 feet 6 inches. A number of other laboratories, for advanced workers and for the use of the members of the faculty and other instructors, are conveniently situated in this section of the building. The dissecting-room measures 64 feet by 46 feet, and is to be provided with every modern improvement as to sanitation and facility for work. The new structure will be completed early in 1899, the work of the college classes meanwhile being carried on in the present rooms of the college which may be undisturbed by the builders, and in the hospital building. As soon as the new college building is finished, the present hospital will be torn down to make way for a more modern and much larger hospital on the same site.

Dr. P. N. K. Schwenk has been unanimously elected an attending surgeon to the Wills' Eye Hospital to fill the vacancy caused by the resignation of Dr. Edward Jackson. Dr. Schwenk has been senior assistant surgeon a the hospital for eight years, and is also one of the attending surgeons on Dr. Harlan's clinic at the Pennsylvania Hospital.

All the local health boards in this State have received an official warning from the State Board of Health against the danger of smallpox, two cases of which disease have recently developed in this city, and a third in one of the western counties of the State. The board lays emphasis in their notice upon the necessity for enforcing vaccination by the local health officials, and also dwells at length upon the importance of careful inspection and supervision of cotton mills, inasmuch as it is believed that the present cases, all in mill-hands, received the contagion by handling cotton which was brought here from infected districts in the South.

The formal opening and public inspection of the Pennsylvania Epileptic Hospital and Colony Farm will take place May 19th. Addresses will be made by members of the medical staff and boards of managers, and by other prominent persons. The hospital buildings were completed last October, since which time final arrangements as to their interior furnishing and other details have been progressing.

"Father" Girand, who posed in this city as a "divine healer" a few months ago, has been arrested on the charge of criminal assault alleged to have been committed by him upon two young girls, his patients at the time of the occurrence. The evidence against this individual seems strong, and, with Archbishop Ryan as the prosecutor, Girand has been held under heavy bail for appearance at court.

For the week ending May 14th, the total number of deaths reported in this city was 430, of which number 134 were of children under five years of age. There were 161 new cases of contagious disease reported, as follows: Diphtheria, 61, with 17 deaths; scarlet fever, 50, with 6 deaths; and enteric fever, 50, with no deaths.

Treatment of Ecthyma.—BROCQ recommends the complete removal of the crusts by means of warm wet compresses or oils, and the subsequent daily application to each ulcerous base of a two-per-cent. solution of silver nitrate, or a one-half-per-cent. solution of chloral hydrate. Tincture of iodine is also of value, followed by the use of the following powder:

℞ Iodoformi . . . . . ʒ ss
Bismuthi salicyl. . . . . ʒ v.
M. Sig. Apply as a powder.

Regulation of the diet, hot salt baths, fresh air and tonics are generally indicated.

OUR FOREIGN LETTER.

[From our Special Correspondent.]

JENA AS A CENTER FOR MEDICAL EDUCATION—UNIVERSITY STUDENTS FULFIL THEIR ANCIENT USAGE OF "WELCOMING THE MAY" AT 12 P.M.—THE PROCEEDINGS OF THE THIRD SEMI-ANNUAL MEETING OF THE SOCIETY OF PSYCHIATRISTS AND NEUROLOGISTS OF MIDLLE GERMANY—BRACHIAL NEURALGIA DISCUSSED BY PROFESSOR OPPENHEIM OF BERLIN—PROFESSOR SAENGER OF HAMBURG DISCUSSES OCULAR-MUSCLE DISTURBANCES IN HYSTERIA—PROFESSOR MAYSER OF HELDBURGHAUSEN PRESENTS A PAPER ON MANIA—NERVOUS AND MENTAL DISEASES OF WORKERS IN A RUBBER-FACTORY—GOETHE AS A PSYCHIATRIST.

JENA, May 1, 1898.

THE third semi-annual meeting of the Society of Psychiatrists and Neurologists of Middle Germany was held here to-day, Sunday being chosen for the meeting day usually in order not to interfere with the regular work of the professors and privat-docents at the universities, who naturally form the majority of the members of the Society. Under the term Middle Germany is understood practically the Prussian province of Saxony and the Kingdom of Saxony, territory limited enough, but containing the three universities of Leipzig, Halle-Wittenberg, and Jena, besides the city of Dresden, in which, despite the absence of a university, some excellent and progressive scientific medical work is always being done. As the proceedings of the society are usually supplemented by papers from distinguished neurologists from other parts of Germany, they are always of considerable interest to neurologists generally.

Members who came to Jena on Saturday evening for the congress had the opportunity to see and hear the Jena University students fulfil their ancient usage of welcoming the May at 12 P.M., April 30. To the old German song, "'Tis the May," they paraded the streets in hundreds at that hour, while all the town (Jena has but about 12,000 inhabitants to 1000 students) looked interestedly on. The statue of the founder received the usual ovation, and was drenched with beer, each student carrying a mug in the procession for that purpose. Then around the monument to the Jena students who fell in defence of Germany during the Napoleonic wars and the soldier students of 1870-71, they sang *vivas* to Jena and the national hymn.

It was an inspiring moment in the midst of the seemingly utter levity of the occasion. It showed how thoroughly earnest the German character is even at moments when only superficial feelings seem to rule. One could better understand after witnessing the scene the truth of their great Roman historian Mammsen's remark, that the war of 1870-1871 was won at the universities.

But to the Congress. Professor Oppenheim of Berlin read the opening paper on "Brachalgia, or Brachial Neuralgia." In some 200 patients that had come to him during the last three years with the sole complaint of pain in *one* arm, in 15 the cause proved to be vertebral caries, spinal tumor, or tabes; in 30 cases there were the tenderness along nerve trunks, the special points of tenderness that pointed to neuritis of toxic, infectious, or traumatic origin; 6 of these cases followed influenza; 12 of the cases were not long enough under observation to decide whether they were peripheral or central in origin. In 7 cases the neuralgic pains were the so-called referred pains, due in 6 patients to heart affection; in 1 to liver disease. There were 22 cases of genuine neuralgia; that is, of nervous pain, for which no organic cause, central or peripheral in the nervous system itself, could be found. All the rest of the cases, considerably more than one-half the total number, were practically occupation neuroses developing on a hysteric or neurasthenic basis, really a psychalgia, not a local neuralgia.

The discussion, which was prolonged, brought out the generally accepted opinion as to what neuralgia is; that it is, except in a very small proportion of cases, less than one-tenth, either a neuritis or a psychic symptom in neurotic patients, having a local manifestation because of overwork or injury of the part. Genuine neuralgia constitutes a nervous manifestation as yet without a pathologic basis, but the near future and improved technic in the examination of nervous tissue it is expected will furnish this before long. The therapy of the psychalgia is mainly suggestive, and a number o striking examples of its rapid effect were given.

Another paper that was very thoroughly discussed was Professor Sanger's (Hamburg) on "Ocular Muscular Disturbances in Hysteria." Charcot's opinion that the ptosis of hysteric patients is *always* due to spasm of the lids, was considered to be too general. *Nearly all* hysteric ptosis is due to lid spasm, but there are a certain number of cases in which a real palsy exists. Sänger showed photographs of such cases, and Oppenheim, Stentzing (Jena), Bruns (Hanover), and Möbius (Leipzig) reported cases. In the spasmodic cases the symptoms noted by Charcot, *viz.*, the lower eyebrow on the affected side, and certain folds in the lower and upper lids are present; in the paralytic cases these are wanting.

When it came to the question of internal ocular muscle palsy, especially the Argyll-Robertson phenomena, all the cases of it so far reported were considered not to prove that it was ever due to hysteria alone, but that when it occurred in hysterical patients it was due to other causes, especially incipient tabes or brain syphilis. Möbius thought that tabes might exist with this for the only symptom for years. Oppenheim considered that in practically all cases it could be referred to syphilis, this single symptom sometimes remaining after an oculomotor ophthalmoplegia had receded under specific treatment.

Mayser (Heldburghausen) read a paper on "Mania." He showed from statistics how extremely rare it is to see a single attack of mania in a patient whose life is prolonged for any considerable time after the attack. His argument is that the psychic diseases even in their franker typical forms, though these are becoming ever rarer and rarer, are very seldom the acute mental diseases, episodes in life like other diseases, which they are often considered to be. The mental condition that underlies them is permanently pathologic and a single attack of mania, in a lifetime is almost as rare as a single attack of epilepsy, the last being a medical curiosity.

Laudenheimer of Leipzig reviewed the *nervous and mental diseases of workers in rubber-factories, i. e.*, among employees who, in the vulcanizing-rooms, come in contact with carbon bisulphid. The characteristic nervous symptoms are paraparesis affecting the legs and especially noticeable in the peroneal group of muscles. That the fumes of the bisulphid of carbon are often the real cause of the mental troubles noted in rubber-workers he had no doubt. He had seen some forty cases from various factories around Leipzig and only one case of mental disease in a rubber-worker had occurred in a person not employed in the vulcanizing-rooms. From one factory ten employees had been under treatment during the year, and six had exhibited psychic symptoms; all six were vulcanizers.

In nearly every case disturbances of the ventilation of the vulcanizing-rooms, by which the noxious fumes of the carbon bisulphid had been allowed to collect in the rooms in dangerous amounts, had been found. Careful ventilation, it has been discovered, furnishes almost complete protection against the toxic effects of the fumes.

Heredity plays a large rôle in the development of the psychic symptoms in people exposed to the vapors. Very seldom does a case occur without nervous heredity directly or indirectly. The personal idiosyncrasy in the matter is very marked. If employees are not affected at the beginning of the term of service they escape entirely. An individual who develops no symptoms before two months are over is reasonably safe from infection later. No case has been known to develop after two-years' employment. The personal index of mental equilibrium, so important in all mental diseases, is even more noticeable here.

Küstner of Leipzig demonstrated Nissl preparations of the nerve-cells of animals which had been poisoned by carbon bisulphid. All of the nerve-cells were affected, the sympathetic ganglion cells, the cells in the cerebral and cerebellar cortex, the large cells in the anterior horns of the cord, and in the cells of the spinal ganglia on the posterior roots. In all cases where the poisoning had been carried far enough, there was an increased pericellular space, a dislocation of the nucleus, an increase of the staining property of the intracellular substance, and an irregular distribution of the Nissl bodies within the cells.

Professor Stentzing of Jena demonstrated the nervous cells of a case of tetanus, also prepared by Nissl's method. The degenerations in this case, an extremely rapid fatal case, were much more pronounced than the only other case of tetanus in which Nissl preparations have so far been made, that of Professor Goldscheider at Berlin.

Professor Möbius of Leipzig read a paper on "Psychiatry as Goethe Had Studied It in Certain of His Famous Characters." Goethe had once refused to visit with the Grand Duke of Weimar the very insane asylum in which this Congress was being held, because he said he found plenty of fools to study in ordinary life without having to seek them out in an asylum. How much he had profited by his studies in real life, to get at the real essence of the pathologic in mental symptoms long before the profession had properly grasped them, his portrayal of the characters of Werther, Gretchen, Mignon, Benvenuto Cellini, and especially Tasso amply prove. An analysis of this last character formed the basis of the paper. The drama was really a study of paranoia long before the word had been coined or the idea of it realized. It had been grasped all unconsciously perhaps by the poet's genius and crystallized in perfect literary form for immortality.

TRANSACTIONS OF FOREIGN SOCIETIES.

London.

THE VAGUS ORIGIN OF ASTHMA AND ITS TREATMENT—OSMIC ACID INJECTED TO CURE NEURALGIA—SARCOMA TREATED BY COLEY'S FLUID—INTERSCAPULOTHORACIC AMPUTATION—ADVANTAGES OF GLEOSIGMOIDOSTOMY—DIPLOCCOCUS FOUND IN ACUTE ASCENDING MYELITIS—EXPERIMENTS WITH COBRA POISON—MENSTRUATION OF MONKEYS AND THE HUMAN FEMALE.

AT the Medical Society, March 28th, KINGSCOTE read a paper on *the vagus origin of asthma and its treatment.* It is pretty generally conceded, he said, that the origin of asthma is to be found in the irritation of one or several of the many ramifications of the vagi. Whether it be from the origin in the medulla or from Meckel's ganglion, as in hay fever, or from the superior laryngeal, from ear mischief, through Arnold's nerve, or through the recurrent laryngeal, or through pressure on the main trunk in the neck, or through irritation of the heart, lungs, stomach, liver, spleen, bowels, or sympathetic system, it is difficult to evade vagus origin. There is only one known means of artificially producing asthma. If we chloroform a dog and divide the left vagus and gently stimulate the proximal end with electricity we produce asthma in the right lung, and tonic contractions of the right half of the diaphragm. In addition to these ascertainable causes of vagus origin there still remains, however, a large class of obscure cases whose origin is not ascertainable as yet. Thus, in treating chronic heart-lesions Kingscote noticed that an accompanying asthma of unascertainable cause was frequently cured. These patients were invariably found to have a deep-seated dilatation of the heart. When this condition improved the asthma disappeared. Considering that a dilated heart when distended with blood weighs about half as much as a bucket of water it is not surprising that in the supine position the organ can make considerable pressure upon the vagi, and by its pulsations hammer their nerves against the spine.

There are two obvious criticisms of this theory which naturally occur: (1) If these things be, why are these cases not oftener diagnosed? and (2) why do not all persons with heart dilatation have asthma? They are not often diagnosed, because in asthma of long standing there is usually a large amount of emphysema, which makes accurate percussion of the heart's margin very difficult. The asthma need not occur where the dilatation is very great, for the heart flops over on either side of the bony spine and thereby assumes a hollow conformation immediately over it, by which means perhaps the vagi escape pressure.

The speaker's method of treatment in these cases of asthma, combined with cardiac dilatation, consists in a modification of the Schott treatment with the inhalation twice daily of free oxygen gas. The gas seems to relieve the paroxysms by supplying the oxygen of which the system is in need.

WILLIAMS said he was not convinced that the pathology of asthma described by the speaker was correct. He thought that the posterior pulmonary plexus was principally affected, and that this plexus contained sympathetic and spinal filaments as well as vagus fibers. Neither did he take so gloomy a view of the administration of medicine for the relief of asthma. Iodid of potash in 10-grain doses three times a day is often of great benefit.

MAGUIRE thought that the view that asthma was due to spasm of the muscles of the bronchi was a pure assumption. It was difficult to believe that such spasm could be so universal or so prolonged as it was in many attacks of asthma. In cases of spasmodic asthma there were, first, sudden dyspnea coming on early in the morning, then ineffective cough, and later expectoration of tenacious mucus often containing Curschmann's spirals. There was evidence of congestion, if not of inflammation, of the mucous membrane. Attacks similar to these were seen affecting the larynx in the "false croup" of children in which the larynx could be seen by actual inspection to be congested. The value of antispasmodic remedies could be explained by their action on the muscularis mucosa rather than on the circular muscular fibers.

MORRISON thought the vagus theory of Kingscote untenable on anatomic grounds, yet a neurotic reflex causing dyspnea might arise from various organs. As examples he mentioned the effects of gastric and intestinal catarrh, and cardiac dilatation. Groedel of Nauheim advocates the use of baths in the treatment of dyspnea primarily dependent upon the state of the heart, and that in which the heart is secondarily affected in consequence of emphysema. Cases of so-called idiopathic asthma are however not suited for the Nauheim bath treatment.

At the session of April 4th, TURNER showed a woman, aged thirty-three, who had for two years an *obstinate neuralgia of the infra-orbital nerve.* Before exploring the antrum as a preliminary, if necessary, to the removal of the Gasserian ganglion, he injected a one-per-cent. aqueous solution of osmic acid into the infra-orbital nerve by passing an ordinary hypodermic needle into the infra-orbital canal. Considerable pain and tenderness resulted, and when in the course of ten days this passed away, the patient had lost the pain, which had not since returned. He suggested that the nerve-fibers were destroyed by the acid. For this purpose an aqueous solution is preferable to one in glycerin.

RICHARDS doubted whether the acid penetrated the neurilemma and was disposed to attribute the relief to the effects of a transitory traumatism.

BATTLE showed a man, aged thirty, with a *history of syphilis six years previous.* Eight months ago he noticed a swelling under his right arm, and soon after swellings above the clavicle and near the sternum. In the axilla were numerous enlarged glands. Iodid of potash in increasing doses produced no improvement. Sections of sternal and subclavicular growths were removed and found to be fibrosarcomata containing giant cells. The patient was, therefore, given half minim doses of Coley's fluid every other day, from January 21st to March 21st, the iodid mixture being continued until March 6th. The dose was then raised to one minim every other day. The man's general health had improved and all the tumors had disappeared excepting two comparatively small ones. The temperature had been normal throughout.

At the Clinical Society, March 25th, BARLING read an account of two cases of *interscapulothoracic amputation for sarcoma of the humerus.* Both patients recovered from the operation. In one the growth recurred in six months, but in the other there was no recurrence at the end of fifteen months. In each case the axillary vein was ligatured through the anterior flap instead of being tied as was the artery in the third part of the subclavian. Otherwise the operation was performed as recommended by Bèrger. The mortality of this operation is slight. Nineteen cases have been recorded since 1890, and in all of them the operations were successfully performed.

BIDWELL related a case in which he had performed *ileosigmoidostomy* in order to close an artificial anus at the umbilicus. The colostomy was of the transverse colon and had been performed on account of a stricture in the splenic flexure. The ileum was united to the sigmoid flexure by lateral anastomosis according to Halsted's method. After the operation about one-half of the feces passed per rectum, and the remainder by the colotomy opening. Two months later, in order to drain the whole of the contents through the anastomotic opening, the abdomen was reopened and the portion of the ileum between the cecum and the anastomosis was divided transversely, and the two ends were invaginated on themselves. This procedure was completely successful.

This operation leaves the patient in a much more comfortable position than does a colostomy. It is, therefore, to be recommended in cases of irremovable tumor of the ascending or transverse colon.

BUZZARD and RUSSELL related a case of *acute ascending myelitis* in a man aged thirty-six years. Numbness and weakness commenced in the feet and spread rapidly up through the legs into the trunk, and into the arms. Control of the bladder was lost, and there was slight difficulty in swallowing. The temperature rose to 102° F., then to 103° F., respiration became feeble, edema of the lungs set in, and death followed six weeks from the time of the first symptom. At autopsy there was found a marked meningomyelitis, most intense in the lumbar region. A diplococcus was found in the exudation of the meninges, and in the substances of the cord. There were many points in common between the diplococcus and that described by Weichselbaum, but in the present state of knowledge of this subject the speakers hesitated to express an opinion as to the relation of this diplococcus to the disease.

At the Pathological Society, April 5th, MYERS described some *experiments bearing on immunity against cobra poison.* He tried to find out whether any of the organs of the guinea-pig had any antitoxic action on the poison. He used a ten-per-cent. emulsion of the organs in sterilized normal salt solution. The only organ which gave positive results was the suprarenal body. Seven animals were injected with a mixture of emulsion of this organ, and more than a lethal dose of cobra poison. Four of them survived and the remaining three lived much longer than the control animals. Positive results were also obtained by using the suprarenal body of the sheep.

At the Obstetrical Society, April 6th, HEAPE read a paper on *the menstruation and ovulation of monkeys and of the human female.* He is of the opinion that the menstrual process is practically identical in women and in female monkeys. He pointed out that although monkeys menstruate all the year round they (at least some of them) are fertile at only certain times of the year and thus occupy an intermediate position between the lower mammals and the higher primates. He believes that the histologic homology of "heat" and menstruation will be established. He combated the view that in the lower animals "heat" is brought about by ovulation or that the ovary is the seat of stimulus which induces "heat." He urged that both menstruation and ovulation are closely connected with congestion and that in the primitive condition they are both due to the same cause. His conclusions were that in women and female monkeys ovulation and menstruation are not necessarily coincident; that menstruation may take place without ovulation, and that in women ovulation may occur without menstruation.

SOCIETY PROCEEDINGS.

THE NORTHWESTERN MEDICAL AND SURGICAL SOCIETY OF NEW YORK.

Stated Meeting, Held April 20, 1898.

THE Vice-President, WILLIAM STEVENS, M.D., in the Chair.

TWO CASES OF APPENDICITIS; STONE REMOVED FROM THE JUNCTION OF THE CYSTIC AND HEPATIC DUCTS.

DR. JOHN F. ERDMANN: This appendix was removed from a medical student twenty-one years of age. The history of the attack is rather peculiar. He was taken ill on Saturday three weeks ago. I saw him at 1.30 P.M. He then had very acute pain, rather cutaneous than deep-seated, extending from the ninth costal cartilage down to Poupart's ligament. This area was so sensitive that the slightest touch caused the patient to cry out with pain. There was also deep-seated pain from the lower border of the twelfth rib to the crest of the ilium posteriorly. His temperature was 102° F., and his pulse 116. There was no rigidity of the rectus muscles on either side, no pressure point (McBurney's), and no mass could be felt anywhere. I saw the patient again at six o'clock, and found the condition the same. At eight o'clock I operated, and found an appendix with two perforations and partly gangrenous. An enterolith was found in the base of the appendix. An extensive dissection was done, the entire mass tied off, and the wound drained. On the following morning the temperature was 99.5° F., and the pulse 94. In the afternoon the temperature was 101.5° F., and the pulse 120, the symptoms pointing to a condition of profound sepsis with a grave outlook. At nine o'clock that night the condition was just the reverse, the temperature being 99.5° F., and the pulse 104. Since then the patient has made a good recovery.

The next appendix was removed two weeks ago, during the patient's fourth attack. The first three attacks were very mild, none being severe enough to cause confinement to bed. When I first saw the patient there was a slight amount of parietal rigidity, some cutaneous sensitiveness, and the usual pressure-point was present. He was removed to St. Mark's Hospital, where an operation was performed. A clean abdomen was found with no evidences of the former attacks which had occurred within a year or eighteen months. The veins and arterioles were tortuous and dilated, but the appendix otherwise appeared to be healthy. Upon grasping it, however, I felt small, hard bodies within it, which proved to be enteroliths. There were six of them, each about the size of a grain of wheat. Four points of ulceration were found inside the appendix. The patient recovered, and returned to his home at the end of ten days.

This third specimen is a stone which I removed from the junction of the cystic and hepatic ducts. In January the patient had an attack of pain in the abdomen which was relieved by mild remedies. A second attack occurred in March, the pain being just below the ensiform cartilage. The pulse was 112, and the temperature 104° F., and the patient was considerably jaundiced. The temperature and pulse soon went down, but three days later had again become elevated. A longitudinal incision was made along the border of the right rectus muscle, but as this was not large enough, I opened across to the left rectus in order to reach the duct, which was bound down on that side by adhesions which had formed at the time of the previous attack. The mass discovered resembled a new growth. Search was made for a stone, but none found until just as I was about to close the wound, when one was discovered at the junction of the cystic and hepatic ducts. It was displaced into the gall-bladder, from whence it was removed. Owing to the adhesions, suture of the gall-bladder to the parietal peritoneum was impossible, but the sac was grasped with a pair of Halsted forceps and drawn up as close to the abdominal wound as possible, and held there with gauze pads. The patient made a perfect recovery, both the longitudinal and transverse incisions healing primarily and the sinus closing within five weeks.

DISCUSSION.

DR. WILLIAM STEVENS: I would like to ask Dr. Erdmann what his experience has shown to be the average length of the normal appendix.

DR. ERDMANN: That is a rather difficult question to answer, but probably the average length is between three and a half and five inches. In the dissecting-room at

Bellevue I once saw one which measured eleven inches. I have seen but one case in which there was supposed absence of the appendix. Close examination, post-mortem, will usually show the presence of a small, rudimentary appendix in cases in which it is believed to be entirely absent.

DR J. RIDDLE GOFFE: It is interesting to note what Dr. Erdmann has said about the average length of the appendix. This seems to vary greatly. I have removed two which were about five inches long, and in performing laparotomy I have seen appendices which were so long that they reached down over the brim of the pelvis. They were not diseased, so they were not removed. I do not consider five inches an unusual length.

In regard to the case in which there were several points of ulceration, it is astonishing to what an extent ulceration will go before marked symptoms appear, as shown by the following case: Two weeks ago a young unmarried woman was seized with sharp pain in the abdomen while she was at a lunch-party. This was the first indication of appendical trouble. She promptly rallied from this attack, and although operation was considered, it was postponed for more positive indications. When the operation was performed two days later, the appendix was found gangrenous in nearly its entire length. The intestine was also involved, and there was a general septic condition of the peritoneum. The case was hopeless, of course, and the patient promptly died.

DR. J. H. FRUITNIGHT: Speaking of long appendices, I would remind the members that Dr. Grauer once presented to this Society an appendix thirteen inches long which had been removed post-mortem.

A CASE OF DIPHTHERIA.

DR. ROBERT MILBANK: I have a case to report which is interesting as showing rapid recovery from diphtheria after the use of antitoxin in spite of the fact that it was employed some days after the beginning of the disease. At the last meeting of this society I was called away to see a child, seven years of age, who had been for some days under the care of a homeopathic physician. I found the child with a temperature of 103° F., a pulse of 130, and the fauces covered with diphtheritic membrane. The larynx was not especially involved. I at once consulted our friend Dr. Dillon Brown and upon his advice administered 5500 units of antidiphtheritic serum. On the following morning the child was much better. The next day 2000 units of the serum was given, and an additional 2000 on the succeeding day, 9500 units in all being administered. The child seemed to improve after the first injection and soon recovered, the temperature not rising above 100° F. after the second day. The albumin rapidly disappeared from the urine and the membrane was all gone after the fifth day.

CATARACT.

DR. E. S. PECK: These two specimens are interesting as showing two widely different forms of cataract. The small white one is calcareous and was removed from a man twenty-seven years of age. The second is a ripe cataract and was removed from a man eighty-two years old. Both patients were in first-class hygienic environment, and both were operated upon in October, 1897, within two days of each other.

The first case is unusual as the patient was a deaf-mute and also because the lens was dislocated. He was brought to me having, as was supposed, a large drop of pus in the right eye which had suddenly appeared on the previous day. I found that the white substance was a hard body, that it was in the anterior chamber, and that it followed the movements of the patient's head. It was diagnosticated as a dislocated calcareous cataract, which must have formed a long time before. The man's history was rather interesting. He was born with all his faculties, but in his third year had a severe attack of cerebrospinal meningitis which left him a deaf-mute and with a white speck in the right pupillary field. The latter caused no symptoms except almost total loss of sight until recently when the eye became painful on account of the presence of the hard white body in the anterior chamber. It is probable that the dislocation of the lens into the anterior chamber occurred on the day mentioned, and, although the idea may be ridiculed, I think it was caused by a violent attack of coughing. Extraction was performed without difficulty and healing occurred without accident. Later the ophthalmoscope revealed two large plates in the choroid, showing that the cataract was the result of a calcereous deposit of lime, a manifestation which occasionally follows cerebrospinal fever. The case is unique on account of the unusual cause of dislocation of the cataract and because of the fact that the patient was a deaf-mute. In addition the small size, white appearance, and stony feel of the cataract are in striking contrast to the large size, brown color, and semi-solid consistency of the senile cataract.

DR. JOHN F. ERDMANN then read the paper of the evening, entitled

HEMORRHOIDS AND THEIR TREATMENT,

which will appear in a future issue of the MEDICAL NEWS.

DISCUSSION.

DR. R. C. M. PAGE: It seems to me that if we consider hemorrhoids as a symptom rather than a disease, we can more intelligently apply treatment. For instance, in nearly all cases we find that hemorrhoids are due to obstruction of the portal circulation, and if this obstruction be due to some chronic disease of the heart or to chronic atrophy of the liver, we will find the hemorrhoidal condition very difficult to manage. I doubt if anything short of operation will accomplish anything. If, however, we have an obstruction which is only temporary, the hemorrhoids will disappear under proper treatment. For example, a young man applied to me some years ago for relief of a hemorrhoidal condition which was undoubtedly due to excessive eating and drinking during the holidays by one who was usually temperate. I found him in a very bad condition, there being a tremendous projection of the bowel from the rectum. The gut was almost black and several points of ulceration were to be seen. I gave him a good dose of calomel, followed by castor oil, and sprinkled the ulcerated parts with a powder of bismuth and opium. It was impossible to replace the mass. The patient was seen by the late Dr. Sands, who advised immediate operation. The young man, however, begged not to be cut, saying that he had once before had a similar condition from which he recovered. So it was decided to wait. No operation was performed, for by alternately irrigating the parts with tepid water and keeping them dusted with the bismuth and opium powder, stopping the use of alcohol, but allowing the patient a nutritious liquid diet, I was able to replace the tumor at the end of four or five days, and within ten days the young man was perfectly well. Ever since then I have thought that I would never again be in a hurry to operate in such a case. Last January I saw a patient who had a similar condition. It was impossible to replace the tumor when first seen, but it entirely disappeared after a week of palliative treatment. Much can be done in these cases to reduce the hemorrhoidal tumor by regulating the diet.

DR. FRUITNIGHT: In regard to simple incision of the thrombotic variety of hemorrhoids, my experience confirms what the author has said about the tendency of the tumor to refill. This has happened several times in my practice, and I now invariably excise part of the skin. The old nut-gall ointment combined with extract of belladonna and opium as a local application, together with the use of Van Buren's old prescription

Lac sulphur.
Potassæ bitartrat. } aa . . . . ℥ ii
Pulv. buisi . . . . . . ʒ ii

to keep the bowels open, will generally relieve mild cases.

In regard to the skin-tab or itching pile, when the patient will not consent to removal, I have employed with good results applications of a twenty-per-cent. white precipitate (mercurial) ointment. Strict attention should be paid to the diet and the habits of life should be regulated.

DR. MILBANK: I have employed Whitehead's operation in a great many cases and with most satisfactory results. There are some objections to it, particularly the difficulty of maintaining asepsis, although this may be overcome by frequent irrigation after operation. Its advantages are that it is unnecessary for the patients to remain long in bed—not longer than three days—and there is very little pain after its performance. In young people recovery is uncomplicated. I have performed the operation upon two old patients, the first being a woman aged sixty-five years, who had suffered from hemorrhoids during many years. She remained in bed only four days. The second case was complicated by extensive prolapse of the rectum. The patient was obliged to replace the bowel several times a day. He dreaded operation, and put it off from year to year, but finally submitted to it six years before his death at the age of sixty-six years. He made a rapid recovery, being up on the second day and out of the house on the twelfth. To my mind, however, the Whitehead operation is justifiable only when the case is a very bad one. I have never seen it followed by a rise of temperature.

DR. S. N. LEO: I have seen a great deal of rectal trouble among old people in the institutions with which I am connected. I relieve most of the cases by surgical procedures, but I think that a great deal can be done by medicinal treatment and regulation of the diet and bowels. Pulna water (domestic, not the imported) gives good results in cases of this kind.

DR. S. H. DESSAU: I can add nothing to the paper except a word, perhaps, in regard to the etiology of the condition. I am convinced that a very important factor in the causation of hemorrhoids is the chronic intestinal indigestion to which adults seem to be so liable nowadays. It has been noted by a number of surgeons that hemorrhoids have been more commonly seen during the last few decades than ever before. Chronic intestinal indigestion has also been more frequently encountered during this same period.

DR. A. M. JACOBUS: From a surgical standpoint the author has covered the ground very thoroughly in his most practical paper. I desire, therefore, merely to allude to a remedy which has proved very useful in my hands in the treatment of hemorrhoids; but first I wish to emphasize the importance of teaching our patients how to defecate. A large proportion of women, as we find in gynecologic practice, go to the closet only once or twice a week, and even then never completely empty the bowel but only pass hurriedly such small scybalous masses as may be in the lower rectum. The fact must be impressed upon them that they should go to the closet every morning and at such other times as there may be the slightest desire, thus forming a habit of regularity, and at the same time they must be urged not only to empty the lower bowel but to take time enough to wait for the second desire and thus pass the feces which subsequently pass down from the upper rectum after the first discharge. To relieve straining they should pass into the anus some lubricant such as vaselin, lard, etc., on arising each morning and again just before the call to defecate. A remedy which I have found useful as a local application for hemorrhoids is an ointment consisting of 2 drams of ichthyol to an ounce of lanolin. A small mass of this, the size of a grape, passed up the anus three times daily, acts like a specific in many cases. In this connection I will add that Dr. L. D. Bulkley recently told me that for some time past he has prescribed ichthyol by the mouth, 10 to 15 drops, in capsules, three times daily, and declared that this, through its action on the liver and intestines, will cure nearly every case of hemorrhoids. In fact, he looks upon its internal use as a specific.

DR. PECK: I would like to ask the author of the paper if Krüll's method of flushing the lower bowel, which came into vogue some years ago, is not a good means of relieving pressure on the hemorrhoidal veins.

DR. GOFFE: In examining patients per rectum I do not employ the rubber finger-cots, as suggested by the author, because I find them annoying. I am in the habit of covering the examining finger, and, indeed, the whole hand, with balsam of Peru in order to protect it. It also forms an excellent lubricant.

In treating hemorrhoids we must carefully differentiate the various degrees of involvement from simple congestion to the extreme condition described by the author. The milder forms can be relieved by regulating the diet and habits. Glycerin and gluten suppositories have proved useful in my hands in relieving the constipation. Horseback riding is an old remedy which acts well in some cases, but I have been told that hemorrhoids are of frequent occurrence in men who ride a good deal. On the Western plains it is said to be a common complaint both among cowboys and cavalrymen.

In regard to the method of dilating the sphincter, I use the two thumbs instead of pushing in first one finger and then another, for I find that I can pull down and roll out the mucous membrane to a greater extent in this way, which is also Nature's method. With the hands on the tuberosities, the floor of the pelvis is readily drawn down and converted into a cone by the thumbs in the anus.

Of the various surgical procedures recommended by the author, I usually employ the Whitehead operation, which I prefer to the clamp or ligature, and I am glad to know that others are of my opinion. I frequently see cases in which the extensive involvement calls for it, and I have never known infection to follow the operation. My plan is to wash out the rectum with a bichlorid solution and to pass a tampon up into the rectum before beginning the operation. In doing this operation, however, the possibility of the bowel retracting and healing by granulation, thus producing a stricture, should be borne in mind. This happened in one of my cases, and the man was so indignant that he disappeared before I had time to ascertain how extensive the stricture was. Now, in order to avoid this, I am always careful to dissect out the rectum high up—fully two inches above where I cut it off. This removes the strain and relieves the tension upon the sutures. Primary union then follows, and a smooth orifice is the result. I have also used the clamp and cautery with satisfaction. In one or two instances I have found that in separating the blades of the clamp after using the cautery the tissues adhere to the blades and the wound is torn open, thus occasioning considerable hemorrhage. Since then I have been careful to separate the tissue from each blade of the clamp as it is opened and find that the cut edges adhere together, and thus avoid any raw surface.

DR. LEE: I have very much enjoyed the paper and the discussion. The subject has been well covered, but there is one way of treating a large hemorrhoid which has not been referred to, *i. e.*, dividing it into quarters by transfixing it with a double-threaded needle, tying off each quarter, and this without incising the skin at the base, as is usually done. I find that a large hemorrhoid can be very much better controlled in this way than by a single ligature. There is less pain and healing is rapid. I do not employ general anesthesia, but merely inject the tumor with a solution of eucain or cocain.

DR. GOFFE: There is a little maneuver which has served me well in replacing large hemorrhoids which have become strangulated. I make the patient bear down as hard as possible while I press the tumor up into the rectum. The patient's efforts will cause the sphincter to relax.

DR. ERDMANN: The point just brought out by Dr. Goffe is also true in strangulated hernia.

In answer to Dr. Page, of course if we can treat the cause we will cure the hemorrhoidal condition without operation. There is no doubt that these affections are often due to obstruction of the portal circulation. As to local applications, Goulard's extract and cherry-laurel water applied on a cloth at night will often relieve the pruritus.

I am surprised to hear Dr. Milbank say that he allows his patients out of bed on the third day after a Whitehead operation. I would not think of letting a patient up so soon. Perhaps it is because I have seen several cases of stricture follow this operation, which, by the way, I never employ unless a large area is involved.

In regard to Dr. Goffe's use of balsam of Peru on the examining finger instead of the rubber finger-cot, I have found that the balsam produces considerable smarting if there is any abrasion of the skin. Patients, too, complain that it causes smarting and burning about the anus which lasts for hours.

I have not found that any particular degree of pain follows the ligation of hemorrhoids. The method employed by Dr. Lee of quartering the mass is nothing more than a modification of Allingham's operation. Personally, I do not like it. It is better to dissect the skin off the pedicle. After this operation the patient may be allowed out of bed on the second day.

DR. R. A. MURRAY: I have found that the replacing of a hemorrhoid is much facilitated by putting the patient in the knee-chest position. I have also used the chlorid-of-ethyl spray as a local anesthetic when operating upon hemorrhoids when the patient refuses to permit me to inject a solution of eucain or administer a general anesthetic.

DR. ERDMANN: In regard to the knee-chest position, I have lately been using the Kelly proctoscope, and find that when the patient is in that position not anesthetized it is almost impossible to insert it; whereas when the patient is on the back its introduction is easy.

In ligating hemorrhoids under local anesthesia I nearly always spray them with chlorid of ethyl before inserting the needle.

REVIEWS.

THE ELEMENTS OF CLINICAL DIAGNOSIS. By PROFESSOR G. KLEMPERER, Professor of Medicine at the University of Berlin. First American, from the seventh (last), German edition. Authorized translation by NATHAN E. BRILL, A.M., M.D., Adjunct Attending Physician, Mount Sinai Hospital, New York City, and SAMUEL M. BRICKNER, A.M., M.D., Assistant Gynecologist, Mount Sinai Hospital, Out-patient Department. New York: The Macmillan Company, 1898.

THE fact that Klemperer's "Clinical Diagnosis" has in seven years reached as many editions is an excellent proof of its value and of the demand by the profession for a work of this kind. It is therefore surprising that its translation into English has so long been deferred. Drs. Brill and Brickner are to be congratulated for giving this book to the English-reading student and physician, and also for the admirable manner in which their work has been accomplished. In the translation, the original style and diction have been faithfully followed, as far as possible, and nothing has been amended, added, or omitted. The book is the best one of its kind published, and on every page the ripe and mature impress of a scientific and well-grounded clinical experience can be discovered. All the modern methods of examination necessary to a complete and scientific diagnosis are recognized, and each subject receives the consideration which its importance merits. The excellent scheme for examination of the patient which has long been in use at the Charitéin Berlin, receives the first consideration. Following this is a chapter on the general condition of the patient, which contains many valuable hints in diagnosis. Chapters II. to XIII. are devoted to the diagnosis of the acute febrile and acute infectious diseases, diseases of the nervous system, diseases of the digestive system, diseases of the upper-air passages, diseases of the respiratory tract, diseases of the circulatory system, examination of the urine, diseases of the kidney, disorders of metabolism, diseases of the blood, animal and vegetable parasites, and the Röntgen-rays as diagnostic aids. The last-named chapter is a new addition to the work. In every chapter the special symptomatology of each disease is considered, which adds greatly to the usefulness of the book. We are thoroughly in accord with the translators' plan of adhering to the original technical terms and Latin names, and this plan will be of immense service to those physicians who intend taking courses in any of the German clinics.

The book is a veritable store-house of useful methods in clinical diagnosis, and a full description of all the chemic, microscopic, and bacteriologic technic necessary in clinical medicine is clearly and concisely stated. We are amazed at the amount of practical information contained in something less than 300 printed pages. The book is of a convenient size for the pocket, is well bound and printed, and contains sixty-one illustrations and an adequate index.

We cordially commend it to all teachers and students in medicine as a thoroughly safe and valuable book on clinical diagnosis, and we also congratulate the publishers and translators for a most useful contribution to English medical literature.

INCOMPATIBILITIES IN PRESCRIPTIONS. By EDSEL A. RUDDIMAN, Ph. M., M.D., Adjunct Professor of Pharmacy and Materia Medica in Vanderbilt University. New York: John Wiley & Sons, 1897.

IN this work Dr. Ruddiman has presented, in alphabetical form, the more common incompatibilities occurring when the drugs ordinarily employed by physicians are combined. In the form in which the book is written reference to any drug is convenient and easy. The second part of the book contains a long list of prescriptions whose ingredients are wrongly combined for the training of the medical student and the student of pharmacy.

We have no doubt that Dr. Ruddiman's work will have a ready sale, since it is eminently practical, easy of reference, and because few physicians have the opportunity of practical work in pharmacy which would enable them to know as well as the pharmacist what drugs are incompatible with each other.

A SYSTEM OF MEDICINE. By many writers. Edited by THOMAS CLIFFORD ALBUTT, M.A.,M.D., LL.D., Regius Professor of Physics in the University of Cambridge, etc. Vols. I., II., and III. New York and London: The MacMillan Co., 1897.

THE tardy appearance of the review of this important work in the MEDICAL NEWS is unfortunate as it is unavoidable; for through no fault of the reviewer the readers of this journal have not been made acquainted with the virtues of this excellent system. One needs but to consider the list of contributing authors to become aware of the superior merit of the monographs comprising the work, which is at once complete and scientific. The editor, moreover, has accomplished his harmonizing work in a remarkably adroit manner, and, although external evideuces thereof do not appear, this much is clear, that the usual faults of contradiction and overlapping are absent. The work is marked by a breadth and comprehensiveness which stands in marked contrast to the ordinary medical writing, and takes this fundamental note, perhaps, from the introduction to the first volume, written by the editor. This is not only a master-piece of medical thought and of depth of knowledge, but is marked by elegance of diction and strength of purpose. It is medical, biologic, philosophic, and classic all at once, and he who reads it must of necessity have a broader view of medical science.

Vol. I. is divided into two parts. The first division, under the title prolegomena, deals with general themes related to internal medicine. The treatment of the individual articles is broad, and their contents useful. Among the subjects discussed are medical geography, climatology, aerotherapeutics, hydrotherapeutics, electricity, dietetics, massage, medical statistics, inflammation and its relations to fever, the pathology of disturbed nutrition, and the general pathology of new growths. In the second part of this volume fevers are considered. Insolation is separately described, and is followed by a chapter on the individual infectious diseases. The articles are all modern, and where new discoveries have been made since the publication of this volume they are noted in Vol. III., as is the case with the serum diagnosis of typhoid fever, the recent outbreak of the plague, and the newly discovered bacterium of yellow fever.

Volume II. deals with gynecology, and the editor has availed himelf of the services of Dr. W. S. Playfair as the co-editor of this volume. This volume offers within its 973 pages a complete treatise on the diseases of women. It is progressive, recent in its nomenclature and expression of opinion, and unhesitatingly decries obsolete and useless measures of therapeutics. In this it is unique, that it does not mention many remedial measures, leaving the choice to the confused reader; but it states emphatically what is the best recognized procedure for each particular ailment. Chief among the notable articles are the ones on the anatomy of the female pelvic organs, gynecologic diagnosis, the relation of the nervous system to the etiology of gynecologic diseases (by Playfair), displacements of the uterus, extra-uterine gestation, the diseases of the bladder and urethra. All gynecologists will not agree with the author of the chapter on electric treatment, who is something of an optimist, and here and there are to be noted other mooted points which are stated with dogmatic earnestness; but this does not vitiate the value of the book, for it is but the expression of individual opinion, and, usually, very high opinion. We may conclude the consideration of this volume by saying that it is an up-to-date, classic text-book of gynecology, replete with good things and practically with no blemish.

Volume III. deals with infective diseases of chronic course, diseases of uncertain bacteriology, subdivided into the endemic and non-endemic varieties, the infective diseases communicable from animals to men, the diseases due to protozoa, the intoxications and internal parasites. Here again, the broad comprehensiveness of treatment appears and makes what is frequently dull reading a pleasure. Under the treatment of tuberculosis, however, no recognition is given, nor is mention made, of the various serums and tuberculins which have been vaunted as curative agents. Leprosy is not deemed contagious; its communicability by contagion is, at least, not considered proven. Constitutional syphilis (Jonathan Hutchinson) and the "Co-existence of Infectious Diseases" (Dr. Calger) are significant chapters, the former, especially, being brimful of suggestion and valuable consideration. The articles on endemic diseases are written for the most part by men who have lived in the tropics, and their discussion is preceded by a chapter on the climate and some of the fevers of India.

Glanders and farcy, vaccinia, foot and mouth disease, rabies, and glandular fever are next described. Under vaccinia are considered vaccinal eruptions and complications, vaccinal injuries, alleged and real, and the appearance of syphilis after vaccination. This chapter is concluded by a discussion of the relation of vaccination to various diseases in which the writer takes the ground that direct communication of bacterial diseases is possible when the operator is careless or when the materials employed are not properly prepared. Malarial fever is discussed by Dr. Osler, and is illustrated by two beautiful plates showing the parasites of the tertian and quartan types and the organism of estivo-autumnal fever. There is little that is new in this article, but it bears the usual mark of scholarliness and of perfect writing, which we have learned to expect from this teacher.

The intoxications, vegetable and mineral, including opium, alcohol, cocain, haschisch, and ether poisoning, are fully described. Several of these articles are from the pen of the editor, and he has adduced much that is new and interesting concerning these conditions. The volume is concluded by a chapter on the internal parasites of man.

This cursory view of these superb volumes must suffice for the present. It has brought to light but few of the many excellencies of this remarkable work. As far as the writer's knowledge extends, no English system has ever been published which has an array of contributors so famous or a list of monographs so valuable. It is almost puerile to say that the work forms a decided addition to medical literature; it is medical literature; and other systems published in time to come must be modeled from it to hold an equally high place. The books are handsomely printed on heavy paper, the illustrations are numerous and apt, the indexes of authors and subjects are complete and make reference easy.

THERAPEUTIC HINTS.

Treatment of Painful Dentition.—

1. Frequent hot irrigation of the mouth with a solution of the following:

℞ Chloralis hydratis . . . grs. xlviii
Aq. menth. pip. . . . ℥ i.
M. Sig. One teaspoonful to 3 ounces of hot water for irrigation.

2. Gentle friction of the gums with the following mixture.

℞ Chloroformi . . . . . . *m*. vii
Creosoti pur. . . . . . . *m*. iii
Vini opii . . . . *m*. ii
Tinct. benzoini . . . . . . ʒ iii.
M. Sig. External use.

—*Danchez.*

Prophylactic Treatment of Hereditary Syphilis—PINARD prescribes one of the following formulæ which, according to his observation, never cause digestive disturbances and only seldom a slight coryza. The treatment is carried out during the whole course of pregnancy.

℞ Hydrarg. iodidi rubri . . . gr. i
Potass. iodidi . . . . . . ʒ iss
Syr. simpl. . . . . . . ℥ vi.
M. Sig. One tablespoonful twice a day at mealtime.

℞ Hydrarg. iodidi rubri . . . . gr. i
Potass. iodidi . . . . . ʒ iss
Aq. menth. pip. . . . . . ʒ iii
Aq. dest. . . . . . . ℥ v.
M. Sig. One tablespoonful twice a day at mealtime.

For Blepharitis.—FAGE highly recommends bathing the affected surfaces every other day with a watery solution of picric acid (5 or 10 parts to 1000), or with this solution mixed in equal parts with glycerin to render it more adherent. The action is antiseptic, analgesic, and non-irritating.

For Seborrhea of Scalp with Beginning Alopecia.—BAYET advises that the following procedure be carried out daily or once or twice weekly according to the severity of the case. (1) Wash scalp with tar soap for ten minutes. (2) After rinsing, wash scalp with one-half-per-cent. solution of corrosive sublimate in hot water. (3) Dry scalp, and rub into it a five-per-cent. naphthol pomade, removing any excess of the same.

THE MEDICAL NEWS.

A WEEKLY JOURNAL OF MEDICAL SCIENCE.

VOL. LXXII. NEW YORK, SATURDAY, MAY 28, 1898. NO. 22.

ORIGINAL ARTICLES.

THE ANATOMY AND FUNCTIONS OF THE PELVIC FLOOR IN WOMEN AND THE OPERATION FOR ITS REPAIR.

BY J. RIDDLE GOFFE, M.D.,

OF NEW YORK;

PROFESSOR OF GYNECOLOGY IN THE NEW YORK POLYCLINIC MEDICAL SCHOOL AND HOSPITAL; VISITING GYNECOLOGIST TO THE NEW YORK CITY HOSPITAL, ETC., ETC.

PROBABLY no part of the female pelvis has been the subject of so much painstaking thought as the pelvic floor, or, more particularly, that portion of the pelvic floor known as the perineum. It would therefore seem somewhat audacious to attempt to offer anything new, as the present teaching concerning the dynamics of these parts, especially of the functions of the female perineum, leaves little to be said. With the elaborate exposition of its functions and anatomy, however, students and general practitioners become confused and discouraged.

It shall therefore be my endeavor to simplify as far as possible the important points of the subject. The essential feature which distinguishes my position from that of many authorities is my belief that the essential structure in the floor of the pelvis is not the perineum, but rather the levator ani muscle. Page after page in gynecologic literature has been expended in describing the perineal body, and opinions have varied from the elaborate theory mentioned above to the more recent dictum of Emmet that "no such body as a perineal body exists save as an imaginary one." Inasmuch as there is no particular structure in the perineum which is not common to the pelvic floor, in just so much am I in accord with Dr. Emmet.

In order that the points at issue may be clearly defined, I may perhaps be permitted to state, somewhat axiomatically, (1) that the important, essential structure of the pelvic floor, and the one upon which all active functions depend, is the levator ani muscle and its fascia; (2) that the functions of the perineum are entirely passive and may be classified as follows: (*a*) Anatomically the perineum fills a certain amount of space between the outlets of the two canals, the vagina and rectum; (*b*) give it attachment to the movable end of the levator ani muscle, and (*c*) it must get out of the way of the advancing head in parturition and of fecal matter in defecation—or more correctly, to be drawn out of the way. All active movement of the pelvic floor is accomplished by the various muscles composing the muscular diaphragm of the pelvis. These muscles are all under one nervous control, all act in unison, and all of the less important ones are simply accessories of the levator ani proper.

Considering as a unit the muscles and fascia which compose the pelvic diaphragm, it may be said that

FIG. 1.

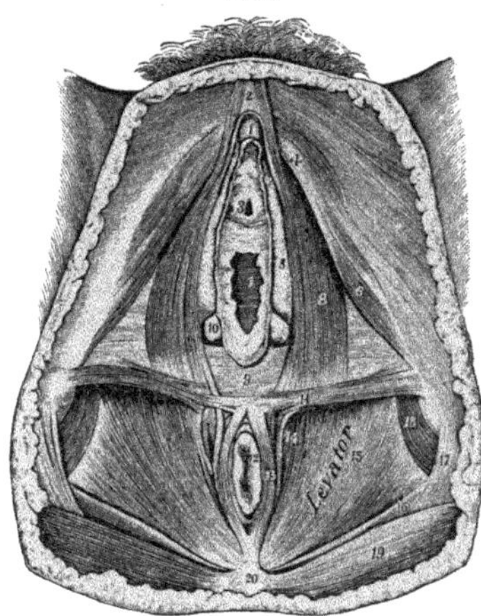

The muscles of the pelvic floor, and the relations of the sphincter and its fellows. Note the close union with the tendinous center of the perineum and the interweaving with the transversus perinei and the bulbo-cavernosus, also the lateral flattening of the anus and the tendon front and rear. 1, glans clitoridis; 2, corpus clitoridis; 3, meatus urinarius; 4, tendon of ischiocavernosus muscle; 5, bulb; 6, ischiocavernosus muscle; 7, vaginal entrance; 8, sphincter vaginæ or bulbo-cavernosus muscle; 9, fossa navicularis; 10, Bartholin's gland; 11, superficial transversus perinei muscle; 12, anus; 13, sphincter ani externus; 14, 15, levator ani muscle; 16, coccygeus muscle; 17, great sacrosciatic ligament; 18, obturator internus muscle; 19, glutæus maximus; 20, os coccygis. (Dickinson, modified from Breisky and Savage.)

together they make a cone-shaped muscle, with a bony origin and a tendinous attachment, the bony origin being the entire circumference of the pelvis, and the attachment, the tendinous center known as the perineal raphe. A vulgar illustration of the shape of this combined muscle is an ordinary meal-bag.

[1] Read at the Ninety-second Annual Meeting of the Medical Society of the State of New York, held at Albany, N. Y., January 25, 26, and 27, 1898.

with a hoop in the top to keep the mouth open and a string tied around the middle of the bag, concentrating its fibers at one point. The bag from the hoop to the string represents the levator ani muscle and its accessories. All of the divisions of this great muscular diaphragm reach directly from the bony origin of the pelvis to the tendinous raphe of the perineum, and, with the exception of the levator ani proper, terminate there. These divisions are the superficial and deep transversus perinei, the bulbocavernosi or constrictores vaginæ, and the erectores clitorides. The fibers of the levator ani, assuming a more or less oblique direction and interlacing with each other, sweep entirely across the outlet of the pelvis, and are bound together and to the fascia in the raphe of the perineum, at which point they anastomose with the internal sphincter ani. Practically, therefore, the result of its contraction is to elevate this point of attachment, and thus, to all intents and purposes, this point may be regarded as the distal point of insertion of this muscle, as well as of all others of this group. The conical shape of the muscular diaphragm is not so apparent when the parts are quiescent as when the perineum is forced down by intra abdominal pressure, as in parturition or defecation. This conical shape may be readily demonstrated in a subject who is anesthetized by hooking (through the anus), the two index-fingers above the sphincter ani muscles and then dragging down strongly.

Accepting then, the description of these muscles as I have given it, with a bony attachment above and a tendinous insertion below, we are in a position to inquire into their functions. Briefly stated they are: (1) to assist in parturition; (2) to assist in defecation, and (3) to assist in coition. The contraction of all the muscles of the pelvic floor has one important result, *viz.*: lifting the point of common insertion—the perineum. Before the muscular diaphragm can be stimulated to act, however, the point of insertion must be depressed. This is accomplished in parturition and defecation by the intra-abdominal pressure which forces down the floor of the pelvis, and in coition, by the admission of the male organ. To illustrate the action of this muscle more in detail, it may be said that as the child's head advances in parturition, the pelvic floor gradually yields and descends until the head reaches that point at which the occiput engages under the symphysis. As soon thereafter as the head in advancing to the front affords opportunity to the levator ani to contract, exerting its power along a line posterior to the point of greatest protrusion of the head, this muscle contracts, and, sweeping the perineum over the face of the child, lifts it up into its proper position. During this process the head does not necessarily advance. The intra-abdominal pressure holds it firmly while the perineum is lifted back into its normal position by the levator ani, thus leaving the child's head without the genital canal.

In defecation the levator ani muscle acts in precisely the same way, with the exception that its movable point of insertion is in front of the protruding mass instead of behind it. Its action, however, is most apparent in a condition of extreme constipation. Let us consider then, step by step, the details of this important function, *viz.*, defecation. Let us suppose the rectum to be distended by a large, solid, fecal mass. In order to force this out, the subject draws a long breath, fixes the abdominal muscles, thus increasing the intra-abdominal pressure and forcing down the rectum and its contents together with the floor of the pelvis. The sphincter ani muscle is made to open only by forcing down the pelvic floor. The structure of the levator ani in the median line between the tip of the coccyx and the anus is almost entirely fibrous in character and devoid of elasticity. As the anus descends, its posterior segment swings backward in an arc the radius of which is the distance from the tip of the coccyx to the anus. The perineum also descends and swings slightly to the front. These two movements naturally open the anal orifice, and, while the intra-abdominal pressure maintains the position of the contents of the rectum, the levator ani lifts the perineum over it and the fecal matter is extruded in a manner analogous to the mechanism of labor. While this process is more plainly demonstrable in cases of constipation, it is pursued to a greater or less degree in every act of defecation.

The process of coition need not be particularized, except to state that in this act the function of the floor of the pelvis is performed by the levator ani muscle in lifting the perineum.

It becomes apparent, therefore, that the proposition laid down in the beginning of this paper, that the essential structure of the floor of the pelvis is the levator ani muscle and its accessories, is true. It is likewise manifest that the functions of the perineum are entirely passive and may be summed up in three concise statements, as follows: (1) To fill in a certain amount of anatomic space; (2) to give attachment to the levator ani and its accessories, and (3) to get out of the way of the advancing head of the child or of the protruding fecal mass.

We are now ready to lay down the proposition that injuries to the pelvic floor are serious in proportion to the degree of impairment which they produce in the structure and functions of the levator ani. Lacerations may occur directly in the median line of the perineum, splitting the raphe and so dividing it into two equal parts. In my experience such lacerations occur in unassisted labors in which the head is forced down by unusually strong pains so rapidly that the levator ani and its fascia are not allowed time to stretch. In hasty deliveries by forceps, the median tear is also not unusual. In this injury, the muscular fibers are rarely interfered with. The two ends of the transversus perinei are separated, and the tendinous center to which all these muscles are attached or bound down is destroyed. The muscles are therefore set free, and the more powerful ones, the transversus perinei, retract, thus drawing the torn edges of the fascia with them into the tissues on either side of the pelvis. The floor of the pelvis, from the pubis back to the rectum, and the fibers of the levator ani muscles, being split along the median line, are drawn aside by the contraction of the transversus perinei as one would separate two halves of a portière. This illustration was original with Dr. Emmet, and is most apt.

In the majority of instances the laceration is very irregular in its outline, and usually passes obliquely across the perineum and follows either one or both of the sulci of the vagina. The lacerations may or may not extend into the rectum. A careful study of such injuries has been made by both Dickinson of Brooklyn and Reynolds of Boston, and it has been determined that the tendinous center escapes, but as the laceration extends across the fibers of the levator ani and the transversus perinei and their fasciæ of the side on which the injury occurs, the result is the same although not to an equal degree: the transversus perinei retract upward and outward into the deeper structures, carrying the fibers of the levator ani and the fasciæ of both muscles with them. The result of this injury is that the function of the levator ani is destroyed. The distal end no longer has a firm point of attachment. The muscle therefore can no longer assist either in defecation or in parturition. The support which it ordinarily gave to the posterior wall of the vagina and the anterior wall of the rectum is removed. The outlet of the vagina gapes and the anterior wall of the rectum with the vagina prolapses downward forming a rectocele.

Studying this condition, now, as applied to the two functions, parturition and defecation, we find that in the former, as there is no longer a perineum, it is no longer placed under the obligation of getting out of the way, and therefore there is no function to be performed by the levator ani muscle. Parturition, as far as the floor of the pelvis is concerned, is simple and easy and usually occurs without deleterious influence upon these parts. Defecation, on the contrary, is seriously interfered with. The anterior pull upon the sphincter ani no longer obtains, and the orifice dilates with difficulty. This dams back, as it were, the content of the rectum, which now tends to crowd down the anterior wall and make its exit through the vulva. It becomes apparent that this unfortunate consequence is the direct result of impairment of the function of the levator ani muscle. The effect of this laceration upon the position of the uterus is due to the fact that when the insertion of the levator ani is destroyed, the prolapse of the posterior vaginal wall gradually carries the cervix uteri downward and forward until finally the fundus retroverts, and, in aggravated cases, the entire organ is protruded through the vulva.

It remains now to consider the condition when the laceration has extended through the sphincter ani into the rectum. In these cases the function of the levator ani is destroyed and the perineum no longer offers resistance to the advancing head of the child. In defecation, the sphincter muscle being torn, it cannot offer resistance to the fecal mass; therefore, a rectocele is not developed and no malign influences are brought into play to drag down and displace the uterus. While, under these circumstances, there is no occasion for the levator ani muscle to act, the condition of the patient is even more deplorable, in that there is no longer control of the rectum and constant, fecal discharges and escape of gas annoy and vex the patient beyond endurance. It may be incidentally remarked that when the laceration results in absolute destruction of the perineum and extends through the sphincter muscle into the rectum, the uterus, as a rule, remains in normal position, thus demonstrating the fact that the perineum cannot be regarded as a support to the uterus, as was formerly taught.

The Operation.—The only active function that any muscle is called upon to perform is that of contraction, but in its contraction it can accomplish nothing unless it has a fixed point of origin and a movable point of insertion. The levator ani is no exception to this rule. Any operation for the repair of the pelvic floor in order to be effectual must aim to restore to this muscle its distal attachment. It has been seen that in lacerations of the perineum of every form the torn ends of the muscles, with their fasciæ, have retracted into the tissues on either side, and must be brought again into apposition in order that continuity may be restored. This is a simple matter in the primary operation performed immediately after delivery, but, in cases in which the injury is of long standing, before these tissues can be drawn out of their retracted positions and brought into apposition, the rectocele must be carried back out of the way so that approximation of the muscles may be effected at their original site in front of the rectum. In other words, the tissues constituting the rectocele must be carried upward and backward, and the anus must be drawn forward and upward, and, at the same time, the ruptured edges of the fasciæ and the tendinous edges of the muscles must be brought in contact. This, I find, can be accomplished by a procedure which is readily understood, extremely simple in its execution, and effectual in its results. Its advantages as compared with other operations are that it restores the perineum to a more nearly normal condition than any other operation known to me; moreover, convalescence from the operation is entirely devoid of pain, and the patient may assume any position in bed which affords her comfort, and, if she cannot af-

FIG. 2.

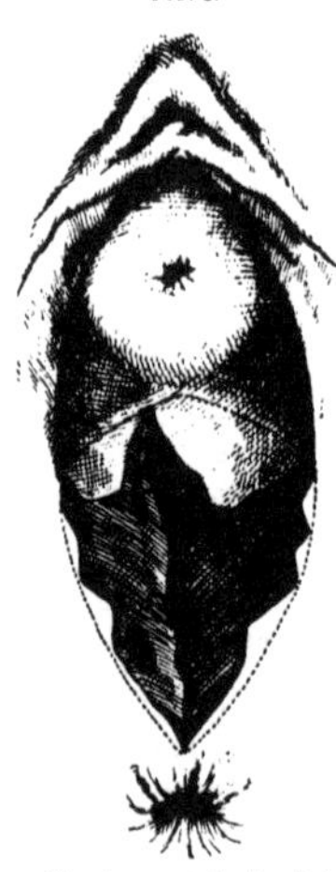

Showing area to be denuded.

ford to pay for the constant attendance of a nurse, the operation permits of her getting out of bed to attend to the calls of Nature. This commendable feature is explained by the fact that only such tissues as normally belong in apposition are brought together, and all the stitches are passed through the mucous membrane inside of the vagina instead of through the skin.

It is hardly necessary to say that the field of operation is made aseptic. By rolling out the labia on either side the remains of the hymen can be followed down from the lower border of the meatus urinarius until it finally terminates in an abrupt caruncle. This caruncle is caught by a tenaculum or artery-clamp, and snipped off with scissors, thus serving as a landmark to indicate the outer boundary of the denudation. Then the caruncle on the opposite side is sought and treated in the same way. A point is now selected which marks the highest border of the rectocele, and a bit of mucous membrane is snipped off by scissors to mark its site. This point on the rectocele is then connected with the outer landmark by an incision made by drawing a scalpel from one point to the other, and extending through the mucous membrane. A similar incision is made upon the opposite side, and then a third, connecting the two outer landmarks by following the curve of the mucocutaneous juncture, and completing the outline of the denudation. This large, triangular flap is dissected off in one piece by stripping it from the underlying tissue with the handle of a scalpel. It is best to begin the denudation near the outer landmarks, as the line of cleavage can be easily found at this location. Thus, by catching a point of the flap between the thumb and index-finger and setting it free a short distance and rolling it toward the axis of the vagina over the finger, the underlying tissue can readily be stripped off by successive short strokes with the handle of the knife, keeping constantly in mind the fact that the operator must closely hug the mucous membrane.

In cases in which the flap has been carefully outlined and the above method of removal followed, it is no unusual experience to remove the flap in one and a half to two-minutes' time. This denuded surface corresponds very closely to that described in the Hegar operation. The point of originality consists almost exclusively in the manner in which the stitches are passed. Catching the tissues at the upper part of the rectocele with an artery-clamp, which is elevated by the hand of an assistant, and with the index-finger of the left hand in the rectum, the needle is inserted about one-fourth of an inch from the angle of the denudation. Passing through the mucous membrane, the needle is swept out toward the side of the pelvis and gradually curved toward the median line until it emerges near it, and about an inch and a half down the rectocele. It is then withdrawn, and again inserted about one-eighth of an inch on the opposite side of the median line, and swept back through the tissues in a reverse direction until it emerges upon the mucous membrane at a point equally distant from the angle of denudation and corresponding with the point of insertion. A second stitch is inserted about a quarter of an inch further down the edge of the mucous membrane, and made to pursue a course corresponding to the first suture.

In inserting these sutures they should be passed

sufficiently far down the rectocele to carry it entirely up into the vagina when the sutures are tightened. The two or three succeeding sutures which are similarly passed bring together the separated edges of the muscles and faciæ in front of the rectocele. The last suture is inserted just above the position of the caruncle, which was removed on one side, swept down around the entire circumference of the denuded surface, and made to emerge above the site of the corresponding caruncle on the opposite side. To understand the action of the sutures as inserted in this method, the fact must be borne in mind that the vaginal mucous membrane and underlying fasciæ through which the two first sutures are passed afford a more resisting tissue than that which makes up the rectocele. Therefore, when these sutures are tightened, the line connecting the point of exit and insertion of each suture near the median line of the rectocele is drawn up under a line connecting the points of insertion and emergence in the mucous membrane, and thus, to that extent, lifts upward and backward the rectocele. The same principle applies to the remaining sutures, so that their combined effect is not only to unite the torn borders of the muscles and fasciæ, but at the same time to lift the anus upward and forward and so restore it to its normal position. The last suture surrounds the edges of so long an incision that these margins will usually be found to gape a little along the line from the point of insertion of the last stitch to the bottom of the fourchette. To secure primary union and prevent the secretions from entering this little gap, it becomes necessary to insert one or two superficial silk or catgut sutures at this point. The entire strain, however, is taken by the sutures which are passed through the mucous membrane of the vagina.

It will be noticed that the sutures, instead of being passed through the skin, as is the case in Hegar's operation and also in that of Emmet, are inserted in the mucous membrane of the vagina, and take their points of support from the fasciæ, thus lifting the rectocele and the anus instead of dragging them down, as is true of the operations mentioned. This method of passing the sutures seems to me not only mechanically more nearly correct than others, but also has the additional advantage of not causing pain. The suture material which I prefer is silver wire, about No. 25, which is inserted by hooking it into a carrying-thread of silk attached to a strong, straight needle.

When the laceration involves the sphincter ani and the anterior wall of the rectum, the tear in the rectal wall is first closed by interrupted catgut sutures which unite merely the mucous membrane of the rectum. In closing this tear the sutures should be continued from the upper angle down beyond the outer border of the torn ends of the sphincter muscle, which are indicated by dimples in the tissues on each side. Of course, the denudation of all the parts to be brought together in the perineal operation is made previous to the insertion of this suture. The silver-wire sutures are now passed, as previously described, with the one exception that the two final sutures are both made to include the ends of the sphincter muscle. Previous to passing any sutures, however, the sphincter muscle is grasped between the thumb and finger of both hands and stretched as much as possible in order

FIG. 3.

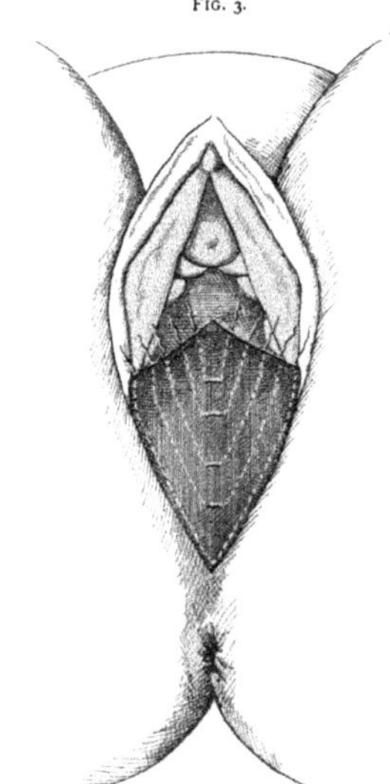

Showing method of insertion of sutures.

to secure as large an anal opening as the length of the muscle will permit.

If, after tightening the sutures, the orifice of the anus seems too small, it is my custom to insert a bistoury at the posterior edge of the muscle and divide it subcutaneously clear across its entire structure. This affords sufficient patency to the orifice and at the same time does not interfere with the function of the muscle in maintaining fecal continence after healing has occurred. The explanation of this latter fact is as follows: It is a common experience with all surgeons to find that the sphincter ani can be completely divided in cases of fistula in ano, not only in one direction, but even in two, and the function of the muscle not be interrupted after recovery provided the incision in the muscle is not made *anteriorly*. If this provisional incision is made in the median line anteriorly, the same consequences follow as in rupture of the perineum during parturition, *viz.*, the transversus perinei muscles separate, retract into the deeper structures, and so draw apart the two divided ends of the sphincter that it becomes impossible for them to unite.

After-Treatment.—The after-treatment is comparatively simple. As a rule no anodyne or sedative is required. If the patient is uncomfortable, she can be relieved by changing her position. The open bowel treatment is employed. This is accomplished on the second day after the operation by giving Seidlitz powders in divided doses every half hour until four doses have been taken. When the laceration has extended into the rectum, all rectal injections are prohibited. The patient is kept upon a liquid diet, consisting of soups, broths, hot water, etc., during the first two days, but no milk is allowed. After the bowels have been freely opened the patient is allowed a small quantity of meat, such as chops, steak, roast-beef, with toasted bread. No vegetables are permitted. Every morning a dose of Apenta water is given, and a free, watery evacuation of the bowels secured. Apenta water acts especially well in these cases.

A self-retaining catheter is usually inserted into the bladder at the close of the operation, and left there two days. Through this the urine is allowed to escape every six or eight hours. After the second day the catheter is removed and the patient is usually able to void urine naturally. The parts should be bathed after each urination. The stitches are not removed until the tenth day, and the patient is kept in bed until the seventeenth day.

TUBERCULOSIS.[1]

BY LEVI D. JOHNSON, M.D.,
OF MUSCATINE, IOWA.

WHEN it is considered that at least one-seventh of all people die of some form of tuberculosis, it is no wonder that so much earnest attention has been paid to the etiology, pathology, and treatment of this disease. All must agree that it is one of the most dreaded, and, unfortunately, most common and widely spread diseases to which mankind is subject. It is an erroneous idea to think for a moment that it is a modern disease. We know that it has persisted through the ages. For many generations before the discovery and use of the microscope tuberculosis was not always clearly differentiated from cancer. Nevertheless, there are unmistakable signs of its existence in the early literature of medicine. We not only find it described in medical works, but also know that in some of the old countries in which its ravages were great, laws were passed providing means to be taken for its radical prevention.

Men of keen insight and close observation have believed for ages that tuberculosis was of parasitic origin, and that the time would come when its true cause would be discovered, when some form of treatment would be known with which to successfully combat its terrible inroads upon human life. The first object has been undoubtedly and satisfactorily accomplished. Of the second we cannot speak so assuredly, but still we have much to be thankful for in this direction.

Many experimenters, especially Klebs, Villemin, and Conheim were on the verge of the discovery of the specific bacillus, but its successful demonstration remained for Professor Koch of Berlin, who wrote so accurate a description of the organism and the lesions which it produces that it became comparatively easy to satisfactorily isolate and study the specific bacillus of tuberculosis.

It has long been known that tuberculosis was an inoculable disease, but it is only since 1883 that Koch and his pupils were able to demonstrate that a specific organism could be separated from tuberculous tissue and cultivated outside of the body, the cultivated organisms having all the characteristics of those found in the tissues, and that when introduced into certain animals, this organism was capable of producing tuberculous disease, the organism again being demonstrable in the new tuberculous deposits.

One of the great hindrances to the study of this bacillus was for a long time the inability to color it with anilin or other nuclear stains. Baumgarten made the first real advance in this direction, but while he was working out his method Koch completed some investigations by which he proved that by the addition of a small quantity of an alkali to the anilin stain the dye was rendered capable of penetrating the resistant outer membrane of the tubercle bacillus. It has since been found that some other agents have the same property of acting as a mordant, of which thymol, turpentine, and carbolic acid may be given as the most important. The next essential step was taken when it was found that the tubercle bacillus differed from others in that it most tenaciously retained the staining reagent, even the strong mineral acids not being sufficient to at once remove it, as they do from other bacteria and nuclei. In sputum or sections a most beautiful differential staining can be obtained as a result of this fact. The stained tubercle bacilli are seen as delicate rods or

[1] Third Prize Essay, MEDICAL NEWS' Prize Contest.

threads, generally slightly curved, being in length from 1.5 m to 3.5 m, and about 2 m in thickness, although these dimensions may greatly vary. The bacilli quite commonly occur in pairs, and may be in apposition end to end, usually overlapping somewhat, but not attached to each other. At first it was claimed that they did not contain spores, but afterward Watson Cheyne taught that from two to six spores could frequently be seen in these rods. It is quite common to observe a peculiar beaded appearance in the bacilli when they are contained in pus and sputum, due to contraction of the protoplasm within the resisting capsule, at least this is the general opinion. Some have thought that these fragments were bacilli in the stage of sporulation, though at the present time it is generally believed that the bacilli do not contain spores. It has been repeatedly demonstrated that the spaces between the bacillary fragments cannot be stained as can the spores of other species of micro-organisms. It has also been shown that these degenerative forms do not stand the heat test for spores. The tubercle bacillus is not motile and does not possess flagella.

Many modes of staining the bacilli have been advised, but none are better and few as satisfactory as that known as the Koch-Ehrlich method. The formula for the staining solution used in this method is as follows:

Anilin	4 parts
Saturated alcoholic solution of gentian violet,	11 parts
Water	100 parts.

The prepared cover-glass is to be floated smeared side down, upon, or immersed smeared side up, in a small dish of the solution, and placed in an incubator and kept for twenty-four hours at about the temperature of the body. When removed from the stain it should be momentarily washed in water, and then, alternately, in a twenty-five to thirty-three per cent. solution of nitric acid and a solution containing sixty per cent. of alcohol until the blue color of the gentian violet is almost entirely lost. Ten to thirty seconds is long enough for this washing. After a final thorough washing in a solution containing sixty per cent. of alcohol, the specimen may be counter-stained in a dilute aqueous solution of vesuvin. Then wash in water, dry, and mount in balsam. The tubercle bacilli will appear a dark blue, while the other material, having been decolorized by the acid, will be colored brown by the counter-stain. To be successfully practised this method requires at least twenty-four hours.

Many physicians in active practice, and who simply desire to know as quickly as possible whether the sputum contains bacilli or not, prefer a shorter method. Under such circumstances Ziehl's Carbol-fuchsin is an excellent stain, the formula for its preparation being as follows:

Fuchsin	1 parts
Alcohol, 95 per cent.	10 parts
Five per cent. aqueous solu'n of phenol crystals,	100 parts.

After having the cover-glass spread with sputum, dried and fired, and held with a pair of cover-glass forceps, from a pipette carefully drop the staining solution on the glass until the surface is completely covered, then hold it over a Bunsen-burner or spirit lamp until vapor is seen to rise from it, and keep it at the same temperature five or six minutes, dropping on more stain from to time if necessary to keep the glass covered. Now, wash the glass in water and absorb the excess of stain with blotting-paper, and then wash in a fifteen-per-cent. solution of sulphuric acid, or a solution containing twenty-five per cent. of nitric acid for a period not to exceed thirty seconds. Some recommend stronger solutions of acid, but I have found that weaker ones act more satisfactorily, especially in the hands of beginners. The acid is washed off in water and the specimen dried and mounted in balsam. Nothing will be colored except the tubercle bacilli, which will be red. Before mounting, the specimen can be lightly stained with an aqueous solution of methyl-blue if a counter-stain is desired. This makes a very pretty picture under the microscope. There are many other methods of staining, but it is much better for the beginner to adopt some method similar to the above and use it continuously until he is perfectly familiar with it. It is also necessary to remember that the bacilli will not be found in every suspected sputum or tissue, and the examiner should not permit himself to be led to imagine that tubercle bacilli are present when they are not clearly visible.

As before indicated, the association of this organism with tuberculous disease is undoubted; it is found in the lungs and sputum in various forms of consumption, in the kidneys and urine, also in tuberculous ulcers of the intestine, around the vessels in the tuberculous inflammations of the membranes of the brain, especially in children, and also in tubercle of the liver. Briefly, no organ of the body is free from the possibility of invasion by the tubercle bacillus. The most common mode of infection is through the respiratory tract, and the most frequent seat of the disease is in the lungs, usually beginning at the apex. Most frequently the bacilli gain entrance into the body by being inhaled in air which contains dried tuberculous sputum pulverized into dust. If the invading organisms find a congenial soil in a catarrhal mucous membrane, for instance, or the vital powers of the patient are so low that phagocytosis is not active, they will rapidly multiply, and soon give evidence of their presence in the dreaded disease of which they are the cause. The alimentary canal is the next most common channel of infection. This occurs in various ways. The bacilli may be taken with the food, as in improperly cooked tuberculous meat, or they may be swallowed with sputum containing them, in either event passing through the stomach unaffected when the gastric functions are performed with diminished acttivity. It has been quite satisfactorily demonstrated that when the gastric juice is in a normal condition its action upon the bacilli will prevent their further growth or reproduction, at least to a very great degree. In children, especially, the intestinal tract is frequently invaded, either producing tuberculous ulceration of the intestine or tubercles in the neighboring glands. Many children die from obscure diseases in which the physician is greatly puzzled as to the diagnosis, when if the facts became known, tuberculous disease would be found to be at the bottom of the difficulty.

A very common medium of infection is through the use of infected milk. Much attention has been given to this subject abroad, and in some countries a very complete system of milk inspection has been instituted in order to protect the people from infection through this source.

Treatment. — All accessible tuberculous glands should be removed as soon as possible. In tuberculosis of any of the internal organs a general supportive treatment should be instituted, combined with much out-door exercise in the sunshine. I will not enter into details relative to treatment, but suffice it to say, that glycerin, wine of cod-liver oil, oleomargarin, creosote, the phosphates, guaiacol, and sometimes whisky, are among the most valuable therapeutic agents. As yet no antitoxin has fulfilled the expectations of the clinician. I believe, however, that one will eventually be found which will greatly advance the treatment of this disease.

There is an agent, however, which I think promises much, especially in tuberculosis of the lungs. I refer to formalin. I have never seen it recommended, but we all know of its wonderful germicidal powers. In a culture-tube in which tubercle bacilli are growing, a few drops of formalin placed on the cotton in the end of the tube will, through the vapor given off, cause their destruction. It is also well known that it is very important in the treatment of tuberculosis to keep the air-cells in the lungs well dilated. With any good inhaler in which hydrogen dioxid can be used as the means for suppling oxygen, a sufficient quantity of formalin may be added to make a solution of a strength of 1–1000 or 1–1500. With this apparatus the vapor of formalin, mixed with oxygen, can be deeply and slowly inhaled; thus at the same time thoroughly expanding the lungs. The treatment should be applied twice daily, and continued ten or fifteen minutes at each sitting. By these means faithfully applied in the incipiency of the disease I believe all cases of tuberculosis of the lungs may be very much relieved and the patients' lives made more comfortable, while in quite a large per cent. there will be permanent cure. I especially desire that the readers of this paper will try the formalin treatment and report their results. In conclusion, I believe that a consumptive patient will derive great benefit by sitting a few hours each day in a room in which a formaldehyd generator is in operation.

SUTURE OF THE CLAVICLE FOR SIMPLE FRACTURE.[1]

BY E. M. FOOTE, M.D.,
OF NEW YORK.

A WELL-BUILT, healthy lad, thirteen years of age, was struck by a heavy piece of machinery upon his right shoulder two months ago. The clavicle was broken by the blow slightly outside of its center. I saw the patient two days after the accident. There was not much pain, but the shoulder had dropped so far inward and downward, the body at the same time being bent toward the right, that the mother of the boy feared he would be permanently deformed. There was only a slight effusion of blood. The outer fragment of the clavicle overlapped the inner by more than an inch, and this deformity could not be wholly reduced. Under these circumstances operative treatment seemed indicated, and the mother agreeing to it, the following day ether was administered and the bone was exposed. It was interesting to note that with the patient in the dorsal position, and with the aid of full anesthesia it was impossible, by manipulation of the shoulder, to draw the fractured ends wholly apart. They still overlapped by a half-inch. The periosteum on the outer fragment was uninjured; that of the inner one had been split anteriorly for about 1½ inches. To this fact is due, I think, the presence of the slight callous which still can be felt —eight weeks after fracture. The ends of the bone were drilled, and a stout kangaroo tendon was passed through them and tied. The periosteum was closed as well as possible by a catgut suture. The wound was sutured over a silkworm-gut drain, which was removed on the second day.

The skin united primarily, but two weeks later a small sinus opened, leading to the bone. This closed again without treatment other than a protective gauze pad. Union is now firm, and the functional result is perfect. There is a minimum amount of deformity, the only noticeable sequence of accident or treatment being a linear scar two inches long which will soon be invisible. The dressing was of the simplest character. The arm was confined for ten days, and carried in a sling for another ten days.

[1] Read before the Surgical Section of the New York Academy of Medicine.

Long confinement in rigid apparatus of a fractured bone in which there is little tendency toward displacement is inexcusable.

A cursory glance at recent literature, shows that an operation of this character has seldom been reported in this country. In Germany, France, and Italy, however, several surgeons have reported cases, and one writer has collected forty-four examples of this operation, all of the patients being cured by it. Owing to its simple character, and the successful healing which now almost always follows a reasonably clean technic, it is somewhat strange that so few surgeons have resorted to this satisfactory method of treating what is universally admitted to be one of the most troublesome of fractures.

Let it be clearly understood that a bone suture is not advocated as a routine treatment for all cases of simple fracture of the clavicle. Many such fractures heal without treatment, or with a simple body bandage and sling, with little or no deformity. During the past year I have seen several patients who came to the Vanderbilt clinic from a few days to two weeks after fracture of the clavicle, not having had any treatment, and in whom union in a good position was already well begun. But there are other cases in which no apparatus will reduce the deformity, or maintain it in position when reduced. From a study of the reported cases the following reasons are given on account of which suture of the clavicle may be advisable:

1. Irreducible deformity, or one which will not stay reduced.

2. Interposition of muscle between the ends of bone.

3. Pressure upon, or injury to, a nerve.

4. Injury to a vessel, causing a large hematoma.

5. The protrusion of a sharp piece of bone to the skin.

6. Cases of compound fracture would naturally be treated by suture.

7. As a secondary operation suture is required in cases of continued pressure on the nerves, as shown by pain or paralysis; and also in cases of non-union.

The results of the late operation are not apparent as soon as when operative interference has been at once instituted, but nevertheless they are good. Most of the reported operations have been performed with silver wire, a few with silk, but none, so far as I have been able to observe, with an absorbable suture. There seems to be no good reason why the last-named material should not be employed and the patient thereby spared the possibility of future trouble with the suture material. Some writers have advised the removal of the wire within four or five weeks; others leave it permanently.

Kinnarnen recommended that both bones be bored through with an awl and a peg inserted. Postemski treated several oblique fractures by binding a wire around them as a broken spar is lashed. This method is certainly the most clumsy of all. Hassler says that only fractures of the middle third of the bone present difficulties, but as this includes two-thirds of all cases the remark is not very significant.

Those who are interested in this subject will find the following references of value:

Langenbuch (*Deut. med. Wochenschr.*, No. 5, 1882) wired a fracture with success.

Whitson (*Brit. Med. Jour.*, vol. i, 1883). Patient, a boy, aged fifteen years, who had been run over; compound fracture about the middle of the clavicle. The ends of the bone were smoothed, and one week later were wired. The wire was removed within three weeks, it being already loose, and the union was good.

Poirez (*La Sem. Méd.*, No. 2, 1891) operated upon a patient to avoid pressure upon the brachial plexus. A good result followed.

Ninni (*Gir. Internaz. d. d.*, Professor Cantani, No. 9, p. 333, 1892) operated once on account of great deformity. Result good.

Routier (*Bull. et Mem. de la Soc. Chir.*, p. 664, 1894). Operation upon a young woman to reduce deformity caused by interposed fragment; silk suture of bone; suture of periosteum; good result.

Mauclaire (*Cong. Fr. de Chir.*, p. 516, 1894) had a patient, female, aged twenty-one years, with a fracture of the outer half of the clavicle. It was dressed in a Desault bandage. Three weeks later there was a large callous and paralysis of the arm due to pressure on the brachial plexus. Incision; removal of callous and a spicule of bone; suture of bone with silver wire; of periosteum with catgut; primary union; paralysis disappeared within two months. After the operation electricity and massage were applied. Direct injury of the plexus in simple fracture has been reported by Earle, Charier, and Mercier, and in compound fractures by Gibion, Gross, Hamilton, Boone, and Chipault. Indirect injury of the plexus may be due to effusion of blood and cicatricial contraction (Hilton) or to callous (Polaillon, Chalut, Chipault, and Mauclaire).

Postempski (*Del. R. Acad. d. Rom.*, xiv, p. 46) reported six cases, all acute, and all in the outer half of the clavicle. In some of them drilling and wiring was done, and in some the fractured ends were wrapped with wire. In all treatment was successful.

Demons (*Cong. fr. de Chir.*, p. 620, 1895) advocated operation for deformity, pseudo-arthrosis, vicious callous, wound of a vessel or nerve, injury of the skin, and in comminuted or compound fractures. He reported five successful cases in which silver wire was buried, a light dressing applied, and the arm moved after a few days.

Reboul (*Cong. fr. de Chir.*, p. 620, 1895) sutured two comminuted (not compound) fractures of the clavicle in patients aged sixty and sixty-three years, respectively, with good results. Silk was used. In one case loose fragments of bone were removed.

Smits (*Centralbl. f. Chir.*, p. 566, 1896) wired a fracture of the inner half of the bone caused by direct violence in a male aged eighteen years, with perfect results.

Davis (*Ann. of Surg.*, p. 147, vol. 23, 1896) operated with entire success eight weeks after fracture for incomplete union, persistent pain, and paralysis. Silver wire was used and removed within seven weeks.

Fevrier (*La Sem. méd.*, p. 433, 1896) says that he collected forty-four cases in which operation was successfully performed. The only disadvantage of operation was the anesthesia of the front of the chest resulting from the incision. In thirteen instances troubles referable to irritation of the nerves were relieved by an immediate operation. The results after a late operation are not as prompt and the operation is more difficult, but in these cases also the results were satisfactory.

Spencer (*Am. Jour. Med. Sciences*, p. 445, 1897) reports two cases due to indirect violence, occurring in young men, in both of which wiring was successfully performed by Hearn.

The other articles to which reference has been made are:

Kinnarnen, *Jour. Am. Med. Assoc.*, p. 116, 1892.

Hassler, *Lyon. Med.*, Nos. 2 and 3, 1896.

Franklin, *Ann. of Surg.*, p. 716, vol. 25, 1897.

WAR ARTICLES.

NEWS OF THE WEEK.

AMONG the many lessons taught by the Civil War of thirty years ago, one of the most important was that showing the necessity for broad, earnest study of military medicine and surgery. At that time the entire available supply of medical literature for army use consisted of a library of less than 400 volumes in the Surgeon-General's office.

The great importance of a prompt and substantial improvement in this direction is amply evidenced by the action of Congress, which even in those days of financial depression appropriated $5000 yearly to be used for the purpose of compiling a "Medical and Surgical History of the War." This work was begun in 1865 under the personal supervision of Dr. John S. Billings, by whose wise and far-seeing management it was merged into the National Medical Library, which at this date contains 120,000 bound volumes, nearly double that number of pamphlets, and atlases, engravings, charts, and plates in almost endless array.

Our army and naval medical men now have access to what is admittedly as complete a collection of medical and surgical literature as can be found in the world.

. . . .

A most convenient and valuable addition to the soldier's equipment is the "first-aid-to-the-injured package" recently adopted by the War Department. The packages are four inches square by one and one-half inches thick, and contain antiseptic bandages, compressors, etc. The War Department has contracted for 100,000 of these packages.

. . . .

The question of an insufficient supply of pure water at Key West is one which may well be viewed with serious apprehension. We quote from *The* (New York) *Times* as follows:

> Key West's water-resources are most primitive and limited. Every one is afraid to drink water from several shallow wells in town, all being more or less brackish and under suspicious surface drainage. Two companies, at various times, have driven artesian wells 1800 and 2300 feet deep, but they have never secured fresh water. The town lives by cisterns and rain-barrels, and the latter are only a shade less unhealthful than the wells. These cisterns are filled during the rainy season, and usually run very low by the close of the dry season, which is due now.
>
> This year, in addition to the rains coming very late, the town has practically had its population doubled by the presence of troops, ships, and war vessels, and the army of newspaper correspondents and their tugs, which vessels take water by the thousand gallons for their boilers and crews. Of course, the war vessels and some of the hospital and other craft have condensers, but the drain on the town's supply is still abnormal.

The large condenser (said to have a capacity of 40,000 gallons daily) which was to have been erected by the Government and in operation by April 21st, has not, at this writing, arrived at Key West, and the situation grows more serious every day. A water famine is almost appalling to consider in connection with an army of soldiers, and the risk of impure water with its train of diseases is still more to be dreaded.

. . . .

The Medical Department U. S. A. is evidently making extraordinary preparations for the care of the Cuban invading army. The daily papers report the supply of quinin at 135,000 grains, put up in capsules of 3 grains each. Fifty-four ambulances were ready in Key West on May 10th, and on May 18th one manufacturer alone shipped seventeen carloads of new military ambulances to Mobile.

Other medical stores are ready in the same abundant proportion, and the Government appears to be using every precaution to meet what might prove the most dangerous ally of the enemy.

. . . .

In regard to some customs, it will doubtless be well for our soldiers to paraphrase the old saying, and "When in Cuba do as the Cubans do." The New York *Evening Post* says:

The War Department has given orders for 10,000 hammocks, to be delivered immediately. It is stated by experienced men that the hammock is an absolute necessity in a Cuban campaign, and it is the only way to escape the vermin and the fatal dampness of the soil. It is thought that the hammock will be finally adopted for the full army of invasion.

We have long been accustomed to associate the sailor with his hammock and the soldier with his blanket, but the innovation now suggested is supported by sound reason, and will doubtless go a long way toward preventing sickness and death in the ranks.

. . . .

The large steamer "John Englis" has been purchased by the Government from the Maine Steamship Company, and will be fitted up as a hospital ship. It will require about three weeks to put her in proper condition for this purpose, and her large size (300 feet long, 46 feet beam, and 3000 tons) will admit of a refrigerating-plant, a distilling-apparatus, and a machine for making carbonated waters, etc. The boat has a speed of fifteen knots, and it is the purpose of the War Department to use her for transporting sick soldiers to permanent hospitals as well as for regular hospital purposes. She will be in charge of Major George H. Torney as surgeon-in-chief, with five assistants. A corps of six women nurses from Johns Hopkins Hospital, Baltimore, will also be carried, not as recruits, but as civilian employees.

. . . .

The story so widely circulated in the daily papers of the arrest of three men at the Chickamauga camp with arsenic in their possession, presumably to be used for poisoning the water used for drinking-purposes by the soldiers, has been authoritatively pronounced an invention pure and simple. Such a catastrophe would be well-nigh impossible, as the wells which furnish the water-supply are constantly guarded to prevent not only pollution but waste.

YELLOW FEVER; HOW IT IS REGARDED AT CAMP TAMPA HEIGHTS.

BY HENRY I. RAYMOND, M.D.,
CAPTAIN AND ASSISTANT SURGEON, UNITED STATES ARMY.

I AM indebted to my colleague, Surgeon Samuel Q. Robinson, United States Army, who has recently arrived in camp by way of Mobile, for notes taken by him during an informal lecture given, by invitation, before a small gathering of medical men especially interested in the subject of the *practical* management of yellow fever, and being the latest words on this important subject, from the lips of Surgeon Murray of the Marine Hospital Service, in charge for many years of Southern quarantine-stations.

On the first intimation of the fever give the patient three or four improved compound cathartic pills. These are preferable to a solely calomel purge, as the latter requires six hours to act, while the compound cathartic pills will usually act within three hours, and they contain sufficient mercurial. As soon as possible give a hot-water bath; if this is impracticable have recourse to a blanket or sheet wrung out in hot water for enveloping the body, thereby inducing profuse diaphoresis. Follow this by some antiphlogistic coal-tar derivative, with soda and caffein. Caffein is the proper heart stimulant for the first stage. Sulphate of soda is preferable to the magnesium salt, as being less griping. Coal-tar products are indicated if fever is above 102° F., and for the boring pain through the temples. If the fever persists about 102° F., repeat the coal-tar products at intervals of from three to six hours.

For the first movement of the bowels, the patient may sit up; the evacuation is thought thereby to be more complete; after that, the bed-pan should be used. If the bowels are not relieved in six hours, give a saline, or castor oil if it can be borne. Lemon juice is recommended as a vehicle for the oil.

As refreshing fever drinks, employ ginger-ale, hot lemonade, or small sips of ice water, or bits of cracked ice; no spirits. Sago or mush, composed of well-cooked, boiled hominy, or corn-meal, may enter the dietary when the stomach can retain them.

For the relief of nausea, rub ice rapidly about the neck, lips, and temples, or give cocain in 0.016 gram (gr. ¼) tablet-form; wash rapidly down the throat. As a pleasant draft for this purpose, or as a fever drink, use any flavored (orange) water. It is better retained than plain water; the orange grows everywhere in the South, and anybody can prepare this flavored and much-favored drink. When giving fluids to a fever patient, administer in a glass just the quantity you wish him to take.

If albumin appears as a trace in the urine, give more liquids. If the albumin increases, especially after sixty hours, administer turpentine in 10-minim doses, every four hours. Dropping the turpentine into a spoonful of water is as good a way as any to combine it for administration.

For sleeplessness make use of sulphonal. Chloral and the bromids are useful, but sulphonal is the best hypnotic in yellow fever.

In collapse an enema of turpentine and whisky is indicated. Hypodermatic injections of strychnin sulphate are useful.

As nutrition, liquid preparations of farinaceous foods alone are best for at least five days. Milk and eggs are regarded as poison at any stage of the disease.

Always keep the patient protected by a covering. This fever is so commonly complicated with malaria that Surgeon Murray makes quite a routine practice of giving 4 grams (grs. lx) of quinin sulphate during the first twenty-four hours of the attack, and then further withholds this specific altogether. The patient ought to be back on duty at the expiration of eleven days.

The only hours during which it is at all prudent to be on the streets in a town where yellow fever is prevalent are between 9 A.M. and 3 P.M. Surgeon Murray affirms that it is practically safe for a non-immune person to visit the shops between these hours if he does not go into dwellings where yellow-fever patients are housed. On the other hand, it is his conviction that a non-immune going into town before 9 A.M., or after 3 P.M., will almost certainly contract the disease. He knows of no medicinal preventive.

Dr. John Guiteras, Professor of Pathology in the University of Pennsylvania, who has been assigned to special duty with the Chief Surgeon of the United States Forces at Tampa, as adviser on yellow fever and other tropical diseases, when seen recently at the Tampa Bay Hotel, cordially gave me his views on yellow fever, with permission to use his notes as I deemed proper. He frankly differs in some particulars with Surgeon Murray's views as expressed above, especially in regard to the supposed immunity conferred upon persons visiting the shops of an infected locality during and only during the high noon hours. He is strongly opposed to the prevailing opinion that yellow fever is contracted usually at night. During last year's epidemic he made it a point to find out in the affected Southern cities what kind of people were first affected, and he found that the disease never broke out among the night-watchmen. He did not find a single case among these. On the other hand, he has seen many outbreaks of the disease among people who moved out of the cities during epidemics and came into town only during business hours. It is not so much a question of time of day or night as it is one of duration of exposure.

If our troops are sent into Cuba his advice is to locate our forces, if possible, in the interior of the country, or if along the sea coast, then in small places or near small harbors. Probably nine-tenths of the territory of Cuba is free from yellow fever; in fact, this fever is circumscribed and confined to the populous cities of the seaboard. Small harbors are free from this pestilence, and if we can quarantine our camps against the populous cities of the coast, there is no reason why they should suffer from yellow fever.

How this fever is transmitted or admitted into the system is still unknown. The drinking-water has nothing to do with the case. The poison may possibly be conveyed in food, in air, or by insects.

The treatment is largely symptomatic. The bowels should be kept free; coal-tar products are useful for pain, distress, and sleeplessness; but not for the control of temperature. In suppression of urine, the form of treatment generally employed in such cases under other circumstances is to be recommended. There are some special advantages found in calomel as a diuretic, in doses of 0.2 gram (grs. iii). If stagnation of the circulation and tendency to hemorrhage present themselves, resort to the old tincture of the chlorid of iron. Carburated waters are very agreeable to the patient. Alcohol cannot be used in yellow fever in the large doses we employ it in typhoid fever and pneumonia. The diet should be extremely light during the first three or four days of the disease; practically, nothing at all.

There is no disease in which the mortality varies so greatly as in yellow fever. It is to be expected that the mortality in cities should be lower than among soldiers, because mortality is relatively so low in children, who constitute a large proportion of the population of cities.

With respect to serum-therapy in this disease, the experience with the serum of Sanarelli, as reported by himself in a lecture recently given in San Paulo, Brazil, is not at all encouraging.

The diagnosis can be made with great positiveness. Among a group of symptoms almost pathognomonic, there are the peculiar facies, albumin in the urine, and the discrepancy between the pulse and temperature.

Dr. Guiteras is a Cuban born, familiar with the topography and climatic conditions of his native country, and by long experience and study is peculiarly adapted for the mission in which his heart and mind are enlisted.

THE SANITARY REDEMPTION OF HAVANA; THE NEED AND THE MEANS.[1]

BY GEORGE HOMAN, M.D.,
OF ST. LOUIS.

THE Harbor of Havana, or Habana, received its distinctive name (the Haven) because of the exceptionally safe refuge it afforded the sailing craft of earlier times from the stormy seas and tempests of that latitude. It is a land-locked bay, deep, spacious, easy of access, and well sheltered on all sides. Its general direction is from

[1] Abstract of a paper read before the Medical Society of City Hospital Alumni, May 5, 1898, and published from advance sheets furnished through the courtesy of *The Medical Review*, St. Louis.

southwest to northeast, while the outlet points about northwest, this passage being less than one thousand feet wide and about four thousand feet long. With the exception of some arms, or inlets, that reach in different directions the main bay, or harbor proper, may be likened roughly to a bottle or narrow jug with the neck set on the shoulder in an oblique direction.

There are no streams of large size flowing into the bay, the Gulf tides are inconsiderable (only about two feet), the sewage and surface drainage of a large population have been poured for centuries into the almost stagnant basin, and with a temperature seldom falling below 70° F., and when it does the fall being of too brief duration to affect either soil or water, the conditions afforded for breeding and storing disease are well nigh perfect. It is, indeed, a huge cesspool festering in sub-tropical heat. To borrow the terms of house-drainage as applied in modern dwellings, Havana practically presents to the world trading in its port the conditions that would follow the continued use of sanitary conveniences in a residence where only the most scanty means of flushing were provided.

The situation, in so far as it relates to the genesis and spread of yellow fever, is the result of maladministration, for while the local configuration is peculiar in affording an especially safe refuge for shipping it has become through sanitary neglect an equally snug harbor for a particular disease, so much so, that for more than half the year it is deemed unsafe for any unacclimated or susceptible person to visit there. The danger that attends intercourse with this seaport is so great that the chief commercial nations have recognized it for many years, and special precautions are observed by their shipping in order to lessen the risks incurred.

During the centuries when the slave trade flourished Havana was the principal mart for the traffic, reputable writers stating that for many years not less than one hundred ships annually discharged their human cargoes at the wharves. Aside from other potent influences the pollution of the harbor from this source was extensive, and as no means were employed to freshen the waters of the bay it is not surprising that the place became the mother city of the most fatal infection having restricted geographical range of which our profession has present knowledge. Depots or centers of yellow fever were developed at other Cuban points and in other islands of the West Indies, and on the mainland along the Atlantic and Gulf coasts, but it is believed that these all reached back, directly or indirectly, to Havana as the principal source.

The growth of knowledge, with increased skill in sanitation as applied to seaports, shipping, and cities in the countries and colonies surrounding the Spanish islands has served to thrust back the disease toward its original habitat. Except as an occasional visitor it is now no longer known in this country. To the westward, Mexico has very nearly freed herself from the disease as an endemic, an important change having been effected at Vera Cruz in this respect, as late reports show; to the southward Jamaica and other British colonies have substantially rid themselves of it except as it may be brought in by shipping, and the same condition is reported of the Danish islands to the eastward, so that north of the equator Havana stands as the chief source of this peculiar form of danger to the trading nations of the world; and from them has gone forth the demand that an end shall be put to a state of affairs that is a perpetual menace to health and life in those waters.

Yellow fever being essentially a disease of sea level, thriving best in combined moisture, filth, and heat, clinging especially to the foreshore, wharves, docks, shipholds, etc., Havana presents special conditions for its growth and harboring, and, therefore, requires special means for its eradication. This implies one or two things, to wit., either that some method shall be found by means of which the waters of the bay will be regularly and frequently changed—flushed out thoroughly as a catch-basin should be—or else that the pollution now poured into it shall be diverted and safely disposed of elsewhere.

These propositions necessarily raise questions of engineering and finance, but there is no reason to doubt that every difficulty can be overcome, as the normal commerce of Havana is of such magnitude, and under changed administrative conditions would be so greatly increased, that the financial cost of the work necessary for the regeneration of the port, if wisely undertaken, could be easily carried and met.

As already pointed out the main sanitary problem hinges on the possibility of either keeping the waters of the bay clean by frequent changing, or by cutting off the dangerous contamination that now enters it. To effect the former it has been proposed to cut a canal leading from the bay to a point on the north coast with a view to establishing a current toward the Gulf. But I am not sufficiently informed concerning the local topography to say whether or not this would be likely to achieve the desired end. It has been claimed that a work of this kind in one of the seaports of the Danish islands has proved to be a remedy for like conditions, but still there may have been essential differences in the two situations.

It will be remembered that Milwaukee, in order to overcome the foul stagnant condition of the stream whose course traverses that municipality, several years ago installed a powerful pumping-plant on the lake shore and by this means forced fresh water across the area separating river and lake, and thus started a current in the channel of the former, and it has been suggested that such means established near the Tallapiedra Bay could be employed to force the sewage into the Gulf and thus induce an inward current through the harbor entrance. The other alternative is the diversion of the sewage now delivered into the bay and its disposal elsewhere without prejudice to public health. This would involve the construction of an intercepting sewer along the water front to receive the outfall of drains carrying domestic and manufactured waste, and is a measure so commonly resorted to that no novelty presents itself in connection with the suggestion. Generally, the adoption of such a sewerage scheme requires in connection with it the operation of receiving-basins and pumps to overcome adverse gradients, or for delivery of the sewage to its final destination whether into the open sea, or for irrigation purposes.

The construction of an intercepting sewer as suggested would probably eventually lead to a renewal of the drainage system of the entire municipal area, such as was accomplished at Memphis, whereby the sewage proper or house-drainage would be cared for apart from the rainfall, and the initial cost of the reconstructed work thus greatly reduced.

From a sanitary standpoint there would appear to be no objection to allowing the rainfall from the municipal surface to continue to flow into the harbor, if proper scavenging was regularly performed, but provision for subsoil drainage would be necessary, and, preferably, in connection with the sewerage system on the score both of economy and efficiency. Wherever the condition of the ground demanded it subsoil drains should be laid below and in the same trenches with the pipes carrying the sewage and a dry sound condition of the subsurface assured in this way.

To a progressive commercial world doing business by clean methods in clean ships, and desiring exemption from unnecessary risk in so doing, such a condition became intolerable when it was seen that problems akin to this elsewhere were successfully grappled with and solved, and the time was deemed ripe for the abatement of what in fact constituted a gigantic international nuisance. The safety of our own people is yearly put in too great jeopardy while things continue as they are, and with the present hopeful outlook for a radical change of régime in Havana and Cuba—political, racial, and economic—it may be fairly assumed that there are those now present here who will live to see the day when yellow fever will become practically a lost disease, and the deliverance of its present citadel from this form of pestilential dominion be duly chronicled as one of the victories of peace and science not less renowned than those of war.

CLINICAL MEMORANDUM.

REPORT OF AN UNUSUALLY SEVERE CASE OF DIPHTHERITIC PARALYSIS, WHICH WAS FOLLOWED BY COMPLETE RECOVERY.[1]

By WILLIAM FLITCROFT, M.D.,
OF PATERSON, N. J.

ON November 7, 1897, I was called to treat L. S., aged eight years, suffering from a malignant type of pharyngeal diphtheria. The pseudomembrane was the most extensive I have ever seen. The fauces were completely covered and the nares closed with the exudate, so that breathing was very difficult. Upon entering the sick chamber the foulness of the membrane was very plainly perceptible at the door. The boy was in great distress because of the degree of toxemia already present and the impediment to respiration, although the larynx was not involved. I immediately injected 2000 units of Mulford's extra-potent antitoxin deep into the gluteal muscles, after first scrubbing the surface with antiseptic soap.

During the early part of the following day the child was decidedly better, having passed a good night; but toward evening, finding him growing worse, I repeated the dose, injecting it into the opposite buttock. On the third day the characteristic red line of demarcation, seen wherever membrane was visible, showed that the disease was fully under control. Exfoliation of membrane soon became quite marked.

Late on the third day I was hastily summoned, to find the first of the series of sequels that greatly impeded the progress of the case. This was epistaxis. Before bleeding was arrested probably as much as one pint of blood had been lost. From this time, however, convalescence was uninterrupted save by the persistence of albumin in the urine for three weeks. Six weeks after treatment for diphtheria had been inaugurated, paralysis was first observed. This affected the left eyelid. Later, in rapid succession, the right eyelid, the muscles of deglutition, and finally both lower limbs became involved. The boy was entirely helpless as regarding swallowing of liquids, and locomotion. He became frightfully emaciated. Counsel was given that he be placed in a hospital ward, and he accordingly was brought to the Paterson General Hospital where, however, he remained but a very short time. Treatment was then given him at his home.

I administered nourishment by means of a stomach-tube introduced through the nose. This was supplemented by rectal feeding. Various efforts to use the stimulants and tonics generally employed in such cases proving futile, sole reliance was placed upon forced feeding. The results were that after about two weeks, to use the parent's words, "He was better than before he was sick." Severe neuralgic pains along the larger nerve-trunks, notably the anterior tibial, were controlled by massage and applications of alcohol.

The most interesting feature of the case aside from the complete recovery, is the fact that the only medicine employed in the case from first to last was 4000 units of antitoxin. Basing my judgment upon considerable experience with diphtheria, embracing eighty antitoxin-treated cases, I am convinced that without antitoxin this patient would not have lived to develop paralysis; and similarly had treatment been instituted earlier, recovery would have promptly followed the initial dose and paralysis would not have resulted.

[1] Read before the Passaic County District Medical Society.

MEDICAL PROGRESS.

A New Diagnostic Sign of Measles.—KOPLIK (*Medical Record*, April 9, 1898) mentions a new sign of measles which is evident some two or three days before eruption can be seen. It consists of small irregular spots of bright red color which appear on the mucous membrane lining the cheeks and lips. In the center of each spot is a minute bluish-white speck. These specks are so delicate that a strong window light is required to make them out. He has never seen them under other conditions, and when once seen their appearance will never be forgotten. This sign is of especial importance since it occurs before any of the other symptoms of the disease manifest themselves. These spots are characteristic. They never coalesce but always retain their punctate character.

Danger of Sudden Changes in the Diet of a Diabetic Patient. —O'DONOVAN (*Maryland Medical Journal*, April 23, 1898) warns against a sudden stoppage of diet containing starches and sugar in case of diabetic patients. He quotes from his own experience the notes of two cases, both of which terminated fatally within five days after the sudden change from a mixed diet to a diabetic one. Both patients were men who, as far as they knew, were in good health up to the time they came to his office for consultation. Neither presented any symptoms that would lead one to suspect impending collapse. Both were passing large quantities of water containing four or five per cent. of sugar. Both were very fond of sweets which they ate in large quantities, as well as bread and other starchy foods. These things were forbidden them and they were put on a strict diabetic diet, with the result that they became suddenly weak and passed into a semisomnolent state, and in spite of stimulants, opiates, and all sorts of concentrated foods, died in less than five days. This accident is not properly described in American text-books and its omission is a very serious fault.

The True Nature of Yellow Fever.—KLEBS (*Journal of the American Medical Association*, April 16, 1898) says that the feeling of blind terror in connection with yellow fever in our Southern States, combined with the cruel shot-gun quarantine, has been productive of much injury and fails to accomplish what it aims at, *viz.*, the prevention of the spread of the disease. It is time that our medieval notions in this respect are given up as has already been done in connection with smallpox and diphtheria, and in Europe in connection also with cholera. It is important, therefore, to understand the manner of dissemination of yellow fever.

In the first place the disease is transported by sick people, and not by goods, and not by water. No known case is reported in which it was imported by the products of the West Indies, Central and South America, and that water does not act as a propagator of the disease is shown by the fact that an epidemic never follows a river downward but spreads upward, as in the Mississippi Valley.

In the second place the personal contagion is not confined to a very near contact. While many individuals in immediate contact with the sick do not contract the disease, there are other instances which show that contagion lingers in the vicinity of a sick person for a long time. Thus, in December, 1897, long after the epidemic in Mobile was extinguished, a workman moved to a house in which there had been cases months before, and which had been cleaned and disinfected. He was there infected and died in a short time. Yellow fever often develops very slowly in certain places so that the nature of the disease is only detected later, when graver cases follow the lighter ones. This was notably true in the recent epidemics.

Klebs does not believe that the bacillus discovered by Sanarelli is the true germ of yellow fever. He could not find it in every case, which seems strange if it is so easily stained and cultivated. Furthermore, Sanarelli's is a pronounced water bacillus, while yellow fever does not seem to be conveyed by drinking-water. In years gone by different observers claimed to have discovered the bacillus of malaria and to have proved it by injecting it into animals, thereby producing swelling of the spleen, etc. The truth of the matter was that the fluids they were experimenting with contained the plasmodium as well as a bacillus. Klebs believes that yellow fever is due to protozoa which he has succeeded in staining in hepatic tissue from yellow-fever patients as well as in the mucous membrane of the duodenum. He admits, however, that these discoveries must be supported by further examinations, especially of living patients. He looks upon the disease as a gastro-duodenitis set up by these organisms, which find their way from the duodenum into the liver, producing the well-known atrophy. This theory will explain why some cases are mild and lingering, since in them the protozoa remain in the intestine; and other cases take on a virulent aspect when the protozoa reach the liver.

Rumination in Man.—SINKLER (*Journal of the American Medical Association*, April 9, 1898) mentions four cases of rumination which occurred in his practice and gives some history of the literature of this subject. Very few cases of this trouble have been reported, apparently because the habit gives individuals who practice it so little annoyance that they do not consult a physician, or because they are ashamed to say anything about it. It must not be regarded as simple regurgitation or vomiting of the food; it is a return of the food shortly after it has been swallowed, unattended by nausea, retching or disgust. In many cases only the portions of food which need remastication are returned. Regurgitated food is rejected from the mouth or is remasticated and again swallowed. Rumination in man is analogous to the chewing of the cud in certain lower animals. Hasty eating, and imperfect chewing, and drinking much liquid with meals are frequent causes. It may be the result of imitation, as seen in the cases of two children who acquired the habit from a governess and who were readily cured of it as soon as she was sent away. There is generally a neurasthenic condition, and treatment should be directed to the improvement of the general health, and especially of the digestion. Strict attention should be paid to the amount and character of food taken into the stomach and the patient should be cautioned to masticate his food thoroughly.

A Case of Echinococcus of the Breast.—VITRAC (*Centralb. für Gynakol.*, April 9, 1898) mentions a case of echinococcus of the breast occurring in his practice. A woman, aged twenty-one, noticed about the time of the birth of her first child, a tumor of the breast the size of a hazel-nut, which was movable and painless. It increased so rapidly that five months later she consulted a physician who found a tumor the size of the fist, not adherent to the skin and giving evidence of fluctuation. He assumed it to be a cystic adenofibroma and removed it without difficulty. Microscopic examination, however, showed it to be an echinococcic cyst.

Vaccination by Denudation.—HUTCHINS (*Journal of the American Medical Association*, April 23, 1898) claims that vaccination may be robbed of its terrors by the appiication of liquor potassæ to remove the superficial epidermis. Two or three minutes after the application is made the superficial epidermis may be wiped off with a bit of wet cotton, when a moist shining surface will remain without bleeding. The vaccine material is now applied and allowed to dry in the usual manner. The results obtained by this method show that the lymph will "take" as often when applied to a denuded surface as when it is applied after scarification.

Methods of Preserving Eggs.—A writer in *Food and Sanitation*, February 12. 1898, describes the results of experiments recently made by Director Strauch, of the Agricultural School, in Neisse (Germany), with various methods for keeping eggs fresh. At the beginning of July twenty fresh eggs were treated by each method and examined at the end of February. The results are given below:

Kept in brine: all unfit for use. Not decayed, but unpalatable from being saturated with salt.

	Per cent. spoiled.
Wrapped in paper	80
Kept in a solution of salicylic acid and glycerin	80
Rubbed with salt	70
Packed in bran	70
Coated with paraffin	70
Painted with a solution of salicylic acid and glycerin	70
Immersed in boiling water 12-15 seconds .	50
Treated with a solution of alum . . .	50
Kept in a solution of salicylic acid . .	50
Coated with soluble glass	40
Coated with collodion	40
Coated with varnish	40
Rubbed with bacon	30
Packed in wood ashes	20
Treated with boric acid and soluble glass .	20
Treated with potassium permanganate .	20
Coated with vaselin and kept in lime water	All good
Kept in soluble glass	All very good

Infection of Gun-shot Wounds from Clothing.—KARLINSKI (*Centralb für Chir.*, April 16, 1898) conducted a large series of experiments upon rabbits in order to determine the likelihood of infection of gun-shot wounds from clothing through which the bullets may have passed. The missiles and rifles were thoroughly disinfected as was the skin of the rabbit. The shot was made usually at a distance of one hundred meters, less often at two hundred meters. The wounds were immediately sealed with iodoform collodion. When the intervening clothing was artificially infected the result was both local abscesses and general infection in spite of immediate attempts at disinfection of the wound with solutions of corrosive sublimate. Infection also followed if old clothing was used although not artificially infected. If this cloth was light as, for instance, of linen or cotton, infection was sometimes absent. It was remarkable in all the experiments to what a distance fine bits of the cloth and single fibers were disseminated in the vicinity of the wound. Thus in one instance in which the femoral artery was injured, minute fragments from the intervening cloth were disseminated microscopically in its wall.

THERAPEUTIC NOTES.

Validol.—In the *Wiener Medizinische Blätter*, December 16, 1897, mention is made of a new remedy, validol, which is a chemically pure combination of menthol and valerianic acid, containing thirty per cent. of the former. It is a clear, colorless fluid of the consistency of glycerin, with a slight, pleasant odor, and a cooling, slightly bitter taste. Schwersenski has found it a medicine which is easily borne by nervous and feeble people. The quantity of menthol contained may be readily increased, as it dissolves menthol. It is a powerful restorative and may be used in the place of musk, camphor, ether, alcohol, etc. It is also a valuable carminative, and antihysteric. Locally it can be applied when menthol is indicated, and, as it is strongly bactericidal, it is useful for the disinfection of the skin. Internally it is given in doses of 10 to 15 drops one or more times daily, in either water or wine or with sugar. It may also be inhaled.

Nourishment of a Woman During the Puerperium.—In the *Wiener Medizinische Blätter*, December 16, 1897, attention is called to the wrong ideas which many physicians hold in regard to the amount of nourishment which a woman should receive immediately after childbirth. It is a well-known fact that after a severe surgical operation, nourishment is given to the patient as frequently as it is safe to do so, and in generous quantity. On the other hand a woman who has borne a child is often kept for days upon a little tea or zwieback or thin gruel, when in reality she should be receiving a very nutritious and abundant diet. This is a bit of ancient tradition which has come to us from the time when puerperal fever was common and when it was supposed to be dangerous to feed anything to the mother of a new-born child for several days. How unreasonable this idea is, has repeatedly been demonstrated clinically.

Use of Formaldehyd in Malignant Tumors.—BAYER (*Die Arzt. Praxis*, March 15. 1898) believes that the hardening and mortifying properties of formaldehyd will make it especially useful in malignant tumors. He applied to the surface of an inoperable cancer of the scrotal region a two-per-cent. solution of formaldehyd upon absorbent cotton, but finding this strength insufficient he increased it to eight-per-cent. With this solution it was necessary to protect the healthy parts. The application caused a dry slough, which was removed after the application of compresses soaked with acetate of aluminum. This required about fifteen days, and there was then left a clean granulating surface, with only a few nodules of tumor tissue visible in its area. In his opinion the result was better than could have been obtained by any of the topical applications heretofore recommended, and the danger of septic absorption was absent. To increase the action of the formaldehyd, it may be combined with arsenic or alcohol.

THE MEDICAL NEWS.

A WEEKLY JOURNAL

OF MEDICAL SCIENCE.

COMMUNICATIONS are invited from all parts of the world. Original articles contributed *exclusively* to THE MEDICAL NEWS will after publication be liberally paid for (accounts being rendered quarterly), or 250 reprints will be furnished in place of other remuneration. When necessary to elucidate the text, illustrations will be engraved from drawings or photographs furnished by the author. Manuscripts should be typewritten.

Address the Editor: J. RIDDLE GOFFE, M.D.,
No. 111 FIFTH AVENUE (corner of 18th St.), NEW YORK.

Subscription Price, including postage in U. S. and Canada.

PER ANNUM IN ADVANCE	$4.00
SINGLE COPIES	.10
WITH THE AMERICAN JOURNAL OF THE MEDICAL SCIENCES, PER ANNUM	7.50

Subscriptions may begin at any date. The safest mode of remittance is by bank check or postal money order, drawn to the order of the undersigned. When neither is accessible, remittances may be made, at the risk of the publishers, by forwarding in *registered* letters.

LEA BROTHERS & CO.,
No. 111 FIFTH AVENUE (corner of 18th St.), NEW YORK,
AND NOS. 706, 708 & 710 SANSOM ST., PHILADELPHIA.

SATURDAY, MAY 28, 1898.

ABSCESS OF THE THYROID GLAND.

ALTHOUGH much attention within the last few years has been called to the thyroid gland in connection with its physiologic and pathologic function, disease of this portion of the body is by no means as frequent as might be inferred from a perusal of current medical literature. Aside from goitrous swelling, as seen so commonly in certain portions of the world, and exophthalmic goiter, pathologic conditions in association with this organ are very rare, although when they do occur they are sufficiently extraordinary to attract marked attention and to be the subject of interesting study. Even more infrequently, however, than myxedema and cretinism do we meet with acute inflammation of the thyroid gland, and therefore a case which has been recently reported by Barclay in the *Australian Medical Gazette* for March, 1898, seems to us of considerable interest.

The patient was a man aged thirty-seven years, who presented himself for treatment suffering from dyspnea and high fever. The ultimate result of the case revealed the fact that he was suffering from a purulent pleurisy and that a large abscess, secondary to this purulent focus, had developed in the thyroid gland. The case was obscure because of the fact that soft lymph covering both pleuræ led to the absence of pleuritic-friction sounds and abolished almost all thoracic symptoms. The patient's dyspnea seemed to be chiefly due to a swollen thyroid which pressed on the trachea and, on one occasion, when the patient suffered from an alarming attack of exaggerated dyspnea, it was believed that the pressure on the laryngeal nerves had set up a reflex spasm. The post-mortem examination of the thyroid showed it to be greatly enlarged, one side of it being diffluent and the other being represented by an abscess-sac from which fluid and pus spurted on section. The pus contained streptococci in abundance.

As with most cases of abscess of the thyroid gland this case, it will be seen, was due to a secondary infection; for true primary strumitis is exceedingly rare. In most of the cases which have been reported by such authors as Bowlby, Havel, Erichsen, and Thornton the condition has followed some one of the infectious diseases, such as typhus, puerperal fever, pyemia, or pneumonia. It is interesting to note that in this case, apparently owing to a sudden breaking down of a portion of the gland, thereby allowing the pus to escape through its tissues, a sudden increase in the size of the thyroid occurred in the course of half an hour, causing urgent symptoms which were exceedingly puzzling to Barclay and to other clinicians who saw the case with him in consultation.

AN IMMORAL ADVERTISEMENT.

A DECISION in an action recently brought against a newspaper in England may be of interest at this time when the editors of several American medical journals are engaged in a lively discussion about the propriety of printing advertisements of certain "remedies." The owner of a "remedy for female irregularities" known as Irristum, claimed damages against the advertising agents of *Pick-Me-Up* for breach of contract in refusing to insert their advertisement. No one reading the advertisement could doubt for a moment that the intention ot the writer was to convey the meaning that the use of Irristum would bring about miscarriage. To this end the medicine was advertised in three strengths, for which different prices were charged. The official analysis did not show any material difference in the composition of these three kinds of medicine, nor was it proven that the ingredients of the so-called remedies were in any wise capable of interrupting pregnancy. It follows, therefore, that their sale is fraudulent as well as immoral, and the jury returned a verdict for the defendant. Is it not time that similar offenders in American newspapers were made to feel that they cannot with impunity vaunt their deceptive and illegal wares in the columns of the public press? The fight ought to be taken up on all sides until reference to "female irregularities" shall be legally excluded from all advertisements.

THE AMALGAMATION OF BELLEVUE HOSPITAL MEDICAL COLLEGE WITH THE NEW YORK UNIVERSITY.

A FEW weeks ago the MEDICAL NEWS devoted considerable editorial space to a discussion of the discord between the council of the New York University and the professors in its medical department, which led to the recession of the latter and their successful endeavor to establish another medical college in this city, to be known as the University Medical College of Cornell University. Thus was chronicled the second act in a drama which has interested thousands of the alumni of these two institutions. The curtain has now been rung down upon the third, and we trust the final, act of a controversy that has been waged with no little animus and acrimony during the past year.

The union of the medical department of the New York University and Bellevue Hospital Medical College, the consummation of which was announced by the chancellor of the former institution at the fifty-seventh commencement, which was held in this city last week, is obviously a gain for medical education. It might be more correct to say that Bellevue Medical College has become the medical department of the university because the university has been, practically, without a medical faculty since the decession of its professors on April first. The new institution will be called, it is said, "The University and the Bellevue Hospital Medical College," but we venture to doubt it. Thus it may be called on paper, and thus it may be inscribed on the diplomas of its alumni, but it is contrary to the traditional hurry and bustle of the American to say that he will waste so much time and breath on designating that which will be known in every day parlance as "Bellevue College." Just as to-day, three years after the consolidation of the College of Physicians and Surgeons of this city with Columbia University, no one thinks of going deliberately through the intricacies of this explanatory phrase when referring to that institution, so it will be with the one which has now been so infelicitously baptized. Bellevue Medical College serves, but when called upon we can probably call up the other in proper sequence and phraseology. Many an infant is hampered throughout life by the freakish baptismal indulgence of indiscriminating parents and sponsors. A word, particularly a wholly disinterested one, to the wise will no doubt be sufficient.

This new medical school will occupy the three large and extremely well-adapted structures which they are now in possession of in Twenty-sixth street, and which will probably be somewhat remodeled during the summer, particularly the building which has been a part of the university. It is stated that the clinical professors who did not go out with the regular faculty of the university will be given places in the amalgamated institution. To do this may require considerable diplomacy on the part of the council, and not a little self-sacrifice on the part of some of the individuals. It is not quite apparent how more than one incumbent of a chair of the highly specialized subjects can be tolerated. The opportunity for self-renunciation in the interests of the corporate whole may be offered.

The amalgamation of the two schools a year ago was hailed with joy, because in union there is strength, and because it tended materially to center medical students in large, well-equipped, and well-endowed institutions. Moreover, it separated the teaching side entirely from the financial side. Interpreted as a sign of the times it meant that medical colleges as entities distinct from the university connections were in transit. Although the present arrangement afflicts us with another and unneeded medical school, we can suggest a way by which this can be remedied, and very likely to the interests of the two institutions. Cornell University is a coeducational institution and its medical department to be opened next autumn will welcome both sexes. At the present time there is in New York a long-established, honorable, and prosperous institution, known as the Woman's Medical College, which was founded for the purpose of furnishing women opportunity to enter the portals of medicine, and less for the personal aggrandizement and glorification of its incorporators than almost any institution of the kind. As the prime necessity for its existence now ceases by the establishment of a medical school open to women in connection with one of the leading universities of this country, we suggest that the councils of these two institutions put their heads together for the purposes of propounding a plan of union. In truth, there will not be the slightest reason for the existence of the Woman's Medical College after next autumn. One of the appointees as instructor of general medicine and professor of clinical medicine in the Cornell institution has been elected recently to the chair of practice of medicine in the Woman's Medical College, and other professors in the latter institution are connected with the former. Although these gentlemen are probably quite able to discharge their dual rôle, the necessity for their so doing is not obvious. If our suggestion is adopted the buildings of the Woman's Medical College which have recently been restored and enlarged may be utilized, and this with the present laboratory and hospital facilities of the new school should be ample to train the comparatively restricted class which a beginning institution must naturally expect to have. Moreover, the adoption of such a plan would insure it a goodly number of students to start with, and would endow it with an honorable tradition, and a considerable body of alumnæ. We trust that this suggestion, made in the best faith, and in the interests of medical education, will receive due consideration. The consummation of it would be, we are sure, an important forward step in the line of recent advances in the study of medicine.

ECHOES AND NEWS.

Long Island College Hospital.—The thirty-ninth annual commencement took place on the 18th inst. There were sixty-nine graduates.

Formalin as a Disinfectant of the Skin.—It has been suggested by Professor Landerer of Stuttgart to apply bandages treated with a one-per-cent. solution of formalin to the skin, twelve to twenty-four hours before an operation.

Serum Treatment in Austria-Hungary.—According to a late report by the Bohemian National Committee serum was used during the year in 493 cases of diphtheria in 31 public hospitals; 401 patients were cured, a death-rate of 18.6 per cent.

The Study of Military Surgery. — The family of the late Professor Von Lagenbeck has endowed the German Surgical Association with 50,000 marks, to enable the German surgeons, civil and military, to study military surgery in countries which may be engaged in war.

French Medical Congress.—The French Medical Congress will hold its next meeting at Lille in August, 1899, under the presidency of Professor Grasset of Montpellier. The discussions will be on (1) "Myocarditis"; (2) "Adenitis" and "Leukemia;" (3) "Acquired Tolerance of Drugs."

Complimentary Dinner to Playfair.—Lord Lister will take the chair at a complimentary dinner to be given to Dr. W. S. Playfair, who retires from hospital work after thirty-five years of service. The dinner will be given by his colleagues, former residents, and friends at the Grand Hotel, London, on June 4th.

Association of Military Surgeons of the United States.—The eighth annual meeting of this association, which was announced to occur on June 1st, 2nd, and 3rd next, has been postponed owing to the occupation of its members in the war with Spain. A date, however, will be arranged later by the executive committee.

The Prevalent Diseases in New York City.—The Health Department of New York City announces that for the week ending May 14th there were reported 500 cases of measles, with 17 deaths; 202 cases of diphtheria, with 37 deaths; 244 cases of scarlet fever, with 26 deaths; 189 cases of tuberculosis, with 168 deaths.

Potable Water on the Army Transports Provided by Distillation.—The Quartermaster's Department at the Army Building in New York recently received orders to purchase twelve complete distilling-plants for immediate shipment South, to be installed on the transports there. The plants are to vary in price from $300 to $2800 each, and will produce about 1080 barrels of water a day.

Improper Use of a Doctor's Signature.—Dr. A. L. Benedict of Buffalo complains that a certain pharmaceutical manufacturing company is making use, without authorization, of his name in recommending eucalyptol. A private letter written eight years ago in regard to eucalyptol, manufacturer unspecified, has been used by this firm to advertise its wares through the ruse of an interpolation.

Acting Assistant Surgeon, Marine Hospital Service.—The United States Civil Service Commission announces that on June 7, 1898, examination may be taken at any city in the United States where the commission has a competent board of examiners for the grade of assistant surgeon in the Marine Hospital Service, Treasury Department. There is at present a vacancy in this grade at Chicago, Ill., at a salary of $100 per month, which it is desired to fill. In filling this vacancy preference will be given to eligibles who are legal residents of Chicago or vicinity.

Life Insurance and the War.—President Thomas H. Bowles of the National Association of Life Underwriters recently issued a letter to the Presidents of all the life-insurance companies in the United States recommending the establishment of a cooperative hospital service between the American life-insurance companies for the benefit of policy holders who are taking part in the present conflict between the United States and Spain. He suggests the organization of a hospital service for the purpose of rendering assistance to the policy-holders who may be sick or wounded, as well as serving as a bureau of information concerning those who fall in battle.

The Thirteenth International Medical Congress.—The organizing committee of the Thirteenth International Medical Congress, which is to be held in Paris in 1900, held its first meeting April 23rd. The officers of the committee are: President, Professor Brouardel; vice-presidents, Professors Bouchard and Marey; general secretary, Professor Chauffard; treasurer, M. Duflocq. The Executive Committee consists of Professor Lannalongue, chairman; M. Chauffard, general secretary, and MM. Bouchard, Bouily, Brouardel, Dieu, Gariel, Le Dentu, Malassez, Nocard, Reymond, Rendu, and Roux. The formal opening of the Congress has been provisionally fixed for August 2, 1900.

Hot Oil as a Sterilizer.—*The Hospital* extols the virtues of hot oil as more efficient than boiled water in sterilizing instruments, especially syringes. Olive oil at a temperature of 320° to 356° F. acts very quickly and with great power. To obtain complete sterilization of the instruments, it suffices to dip them for an instant into the hot oil, and in the case of syringes it is sufficient to fill them twice with oil at the temperature mentioned. The temperature of the heated oil may be determined by a thermometer, which certainly is the scientific way, but Professor Wright of the Netley Hospital in England suggests the very crude but rough and ready method of dropping a bread crumb into the oil, which becomes brown and crisp as soon as the required temperature is obtained.

The Royal Army Medical Corps.—On May 4th the Lord Mayor of London gave a banquet to the medical profession for the first time. It was an occasion long to be remembered by the medical men, not only for the brilliant manner in which the Lord Mayor extended the traditional hospitality of the city, but also for the speech of Lord Lansdowne, which marks the end of the long dispute into which the medical profession was forced on behalf of those of its members who entered the military service of the State. The compliments paid to army medical officers by Lord Lansdowne were handsome. Among his numerous remarks he said that there is no department in the public service which owes more to or depends more upon, the medical profession than the army, and that medical officers are soldiers in the fullest sense of the word, and on this account the Government was prepared to treat them with the respect to which they are entitled.

Suicide of Professor Seidel.—Professor Seidel was the chief surgeon of the Brunswick Hospital, Berlin. Through the dissatisfaction of assistants, who wrote a complaint to the Brunswick Ministry stating that the professor was careless in antiseptic precautions, and had thereby caused the death of a patient, the professor was suspended. Being a man of very sensitive and nervous temperament, he felt disgraced, and committed suicide the following day, leaving letters asking his brothers to clear his name. The brothers of the professor brought suit for libel against the assistants, which terminated in a verdict for the brothers. The great interest of this lawsuit from a medical point of view is undoubtedly the evidence of Professor v. Bergamann, which he gave in favor of the late Professor Seidel and against the assistants. Bergamann stated that it was his decided conviction that the problem of asepsis and antisepsis in surgery is as yet by no means scientifically solved; that the most distinguished surgeons are very much at variance on the subject.

President Eliot's Advice to Harvard Students Regarding the War.—At the concluding talk to students of Harvard University, on "Soldiers' and Sailors' Life," President Eliot voiced the sentiments of the faculty in the matter of enlistment for the war. He said that a student's duty lay between his personal obligations and those to this country. In times of crisis the latter are above everything, but at present the situation is not sufficiently grave to force the student to put his all behind him and rush to the front. In closing the President said that the faculty and board of overseers had decided to establish a permanent organization where students who desired it might receive military instruction, and that next year such an organization would be formed. Every man who joined would be put to the physical test required for recruits for the regular army. The President also recommended that the students avail themselves of the opportunity to become expert marksmen by practice in the new base-ball cage, which has been fitted up with targets and rifle racks for the purpose. He closed by urging every man to take part in the military drill now going forward.

Entente Cordiale.—The friendliness of the rivalry between the faculty of the old University Medical School and that of Bellevue Hospital Medical School has long been recognized. Still there are degrees of intimacy that pass the point of endurance, and when the members of these two rival faculties found themselves one year ago sitting in each other's laps in the professorial chairs of the combined institution, the limit seemed to have been reached and they flew from each other's presence like pith-balls charged with opposite electricity. Now that their distinct paths have been marked out and lie in parallel lines at a sufficiently safe distance, we find them again falling on each other's necks, after the manner of imperial personages. When the Czar of all the Russias and the Emperor of Germany meet they signalize their friendship by appearing in each other's clothes. Behold! our medical friends adopting the same custom and presenting themselves in each other's domicile. Upon the opening of the fall session of the medical schools, Bellevue will be domiciled in the old buildings of the University Faculty and the University Faculty under the designation of the Medical College of Cornell University, will have its temporary home in the old Bellevue buildings on the grounds of the Hospital.

Law Governing the Practice of Medicine in the British Possessions on the Klondike.—To those contemplating a professional residence in the gold fields of Yukon the following extracts from the official Medical Register of the Northwest Territories will be of interest: (*a*) "The Council shall admit upon the Register any person possessing a diploma from any college in Great Britain and Ireland (having power to grant such diploma), entitling him to practise medicine and surgery, and who shall produce such diploma and furnish satisfactory evidence of identification. (*b*) The Council shall admit upon the Register any member of the College of Physicians and Surgeons of the Provinces of Manitoba, Ontario, and Quebec, upon producing satisfactory evidence of the same and of identification. The fee for registration under any clause of this ordinance shall be $50. (*c*) The Council shall admit upon the Register any person who shall produce from any recognized college or school of medicine and surgery a certificate or certificates that he has taken a four-years' course of study or a diploma of qualification from such recognized college or school, provided also that the applicant shall furnish to the Council satisfactory evidence of identification and pass before the members thereof, or such examiners as may be appointed for the purpose, a satisfactory examination touching his fitness and capacity to practise as a physician and surgeon, and provided that every applicant for such examination shall pay to the Registrar of the College of Physicians and Surgeons of the Northwest Territories the sum of $50 toward defraying the expenses of the examining board. Examinations: The examination for candidates for registration will take place on the second Wednesday in January, May, and September in each year." Further information may be had by addressing Dr. Hugh U. Bain, Registrar, Prince Albert, Saskatchewan.

The Navy Will Cooperate in Preventing the Introduction of Yellow Fever.—In accordance with the request of the Secretary of the Treasury made at the suggestion of Surgeon-General Wyman of the Marine Hospital Service, the Honorable J. D. Long, Secretary of the Navy, has issued instructions to the commandant of the United States Navy Station at Key West and the Commander-in-Chief of the North Atlantic Squadron to keep a lookout for and apprehend any small vessels which it is believed intend to affect a surreptitious landing on the Florida coast and to take them immediately under guard to the nearest quarantine station for necessary detention and disinfection. In his letter to the Secretary of the Navy, Secretary Gage says: "I am informed by the Surgeon-General of the Marine Hospital Service that even under ordinary circumstances there has been danger of the introduction of yellow fever from Cuba into the State of Florida through the medium of small craft containing persons and baggage, seeking for various reasons surreptitiously to land upon the Florida coast. Under present conditions it is believed that the danger from these small crafts is greatly increased. During the active quarantine season from April 1st to November 1st it is contrary to the United States Quarantine Regulations for persons from Cuba not immune to yellow fever to be landed at any point South of the southern boundary of Maryland without detention in quarantine from three to five days and disinfection of their baggage. The importance of enforcing these regulations throughout the summer is very great, and I have to request that the officers of the fleet in Florida or Cuban waters be instructed to aid in the prevention of the introduction of yellow fever in the United States by keeping vigilant outlook for small vessels of the character above described and upon their apprehension such vessels and their personnel be taken immediately under guard, to the nearest quarantine station for necessary detention and disinfection."

National Quarantine.—Dr. H. M. Folkes of Biloxi, Miss., in a paper read before the Mississippi State Medical Association, April 8, 1898, and published in the *Virginia Semi-Monthly*, May 13th, says: "While a strong advocate of State's rights in health affairs, I must confess to a fascination with the idea of Federal handling of epidemics for the following reasons: They have the power of securing uniformity in rules and regulations, the authority in interstate questions, the likelihood of its officers not being swayed by local influences—though this has certain drawbacks—and, finally, what to my mind most recommends it is the opportunity to organize a company of immunes properly officered, equipped, and drilled, to act as a cordon around infected points. This company should be stationed constantly at some Southern place, and should be prepared to march at an hour's notice. Such an organization should be ordered to an infected point, placed on duty at once, and could lend invaluable aid in checking the spread of the disease. They should be instructed in all sanitary matters, and those not under arms as guards could be of service as sanitary inspectors, nurses, etc., in the afflicted place. Not a wheel should turn in the town, not a person be allowed to go in or out, until this force has arrived by special train. Uniformity of rules and regulations is so essential to an intelligent handling of an epidemic that it seems hardly necessary to refer to the fact; yet in our own State the recent law is so modified as to almost entirely subordinate the authority of the State Board of Health to any little town which may decline to receive persons absolutely non-dangerous. The proper intent of a law based upon modern sanitary and commercial requirements, is to afford protection and enable business to proceed. Unfortunately, our law largely nullifies the good accomplished at the recent Quarantine Conferences in New Orleans and Atlanta, where were adopted a series of rules and regulations positively accomplishing the two requirements above mentioned, safety and continued commerce. Our future laws should be based upon the lines laid down by the above-mentioned conventions."

CORRESPONDENCE.

THE GERMAN UNIVERTITY SEMESTERS.

THE special correspondent of the MEDICAL NEWS in Germany, who has been absent from Berlin for several weeks in attendance upon the German Medical Congress at Wiesbaden, and the Neurological Congress at Jena, and who has been taking extensive notes on the system of medical teaching at the smaller universities in Western and Middle Germany, Bonn, Giessen, Marburg, and Jena, requests us to publish the following note:

To the Editor of the MEDICAL NEWS.

DEAR SIR: Through your columns I beg to express my thanks to Professor George Dock of the University of Michigan, Ann Arbor, for his courteous correction, as printed in the MEDICAL NEWS of April 2d, of certain statements of mine contained in the Berlin correspondence of March 19th. I regret not having been in a position to acknowledge it before. It is the *Austrian*, not the German, universities which close about July 1st. Hence my mistake. The latter close about the 25th of July. May I add, however, that the kernel of the bit of information imparted in my letter, and which is of special interest to American medical men, remains absolutely true. The German medical course consists of nine semesters of scant three months each, on an average, of actual required attendance at clinics and lectures, etc., while the course at our best American medical colleges consists of four years of more than seven months each of actual work. May I add too, that while we lack the preliminary training in America, unfortunately, our actual medical courses compare very favorably with those given here even at the best universities. Personal observation has convinced me that our best American medical schools are at the present moment turning out, on the whole, at least as well trained, practical physicians and surgeons as the corresponding German institutions.

BERLIN CORRESPONDENT OF THE MEDICAL NEWS.

OUR PHILADELPHIA LETTER.

[From our Special Correspondent.]

THE DANGER FROM YELLOW FEVER TO THE AMERICAN ARMY IN CUBA: OPINION OF DR. JOHN GUITERAS—PENNSYLVANIA STATE MEDICAL SOCIETY MEETING—A PROTEST FROM THE HOMEOPATHS—THE PENNSYLVANIA EPILEPTIC HOSPITAL FORMALLY OPENED — COMMENCEMENT EXERCISES OF MEDICAL COLLEGES.

PHILADELPHIA, May 24, 1898.

IN view of the almost universal belief in the danger from yellow fever to unacclimated American troops sent to Cuba at this season of the year, the following remarks, expressed by Dr. John Guiteras, of the University of Pennsylvania, and now in the service of the United States Army, as a yellow-fever expert, are important and of timely interest. Concerning the geographical distribution of the infection, Dr. Guiteras has this to say: "By far the greater part of the territory of Cuba is free from the yellow-fever infection. The disease is, in fact, circumscribed to the larger and more important seaport towns, such as Havana, Matanzas, Sagua, Nuevitas, Santiago, Manzanillo, Cienfuegos, and Batabano. The interior of the island, in a general way, may be considered free from infection. This is not due, as it is generally believed, to altitude. The seacoast, outside of the centers of population, is as free from yellow fever as the highest mountains. On the other hand, it is well to know that there is no part of the territory of Cuba where yellow fever may not be carried. The experiences of the Spanish illustrate this very clearly. It has been their practice to make the city of Havana their base of supplies. They have actually had, and probably still have, a large depot of military outfits in San Ambrosia hospital. These supplies became infected, so that this yellow-fever hospital in Havana may be looked upon as a distributing center of the disease to the Spanish army. If, therefore, we should be able to keep our army outside of the yellow-fever centers, if we have our base of supplies in the United States, if these supplies are landed or kept at an uninfected port, and if we are able to prevent communication between the army and the infected location, all the forces of the United States could be held in Cuba without infection."

If the disease should be introduced by importation into one of our army camps, active measures could be taken to prevent the further spread of the disease. In the first place, preparations have been made for the prompt detention of such cases, and in the second place, isolation-tents and hospitals will be provided for their immediate segregation. By such measures the large detention-camps that have been established by the Marine Hospital Service in our late Southern epidemic have been kept from all contamination. Cases of yellow fever have broken out in these camps among the recent arrivals, but the system of segregation has made it possible to keep the camp itself in the condition of an uninfected place. As a last resort, if there be evidences of actual infection of the camp, we may appeal to the radical measures of change of site of the whole camp, after disinfection or destruction of all the possible sources of infection. The American army having occupied Havana, Dr. Guiteras recommends that the following sanitary measures should be followed: First, diagnosis of all cases of yellow fever, including the native children; second, disinfection of all premises in which yellow fever has occurred; third, a modern system of sewerage extending throughout the city; fourth, the proper paving of the streets. It is not thought that the popular belief in the contamination by the harbor rests on much foundation, for attention is drawn to the fact that it is a very rare occurrence to hear of yellow fever breaking out among the crews of merchant vessels which are kept anchored and all communication with the shore cut off. Finally, Dr. Guiteras states that the annual epidemic of yellow fever breaks out in Havana regularly during the month of June, and increases during July and August. It begins to decrease during September, and practically disappears by November.

The semicentennial meeting of the Pennsylvania State Medical Society was held in Lancaster, May 17th, 18th, and 19th. Several hundred delegates from all parts of the State were in attendance, and a most successful three-days' session resulted. Inasmuch as in Lancaster was held the first meeting and the organization of the Society, and as its first president was a native of that place, it seemed especially appropriate that the jubilee of the Society should have been held in that city. Elaborate exercises commemorative of the fiftieth anniversary of the Society were held in the Court House. The scientific business of the meeting reached a high plane, the discussions of papers were spirited and instructive, and a total absence of that sectional prejudice and personal enmity which so often mars the proceedings of State societies, contributed to ensure to the sessions most valuable results.

At the last monthly meeting of the Homeopathic Medical Society on May 16th, an animated discussion took place concerning the movement, now in progress in this city, to prevent "discrimination," as the followers of Hahnemann are pleased to term it, against the appointment of homeopaths to Government positions in the army and navy. A number of letters from indignant protesters were read, a flood of comment unfavorable to the army, navy, and militia officials was indulged in, and it was triumphantly announced that a bill has been introduced in Congress by Senator Allen of Nebraska, making it illegal to discriminate against any school of medicine in making appointments to any branch of the various services. A committee, appointed at this meeting, was introduced to the President at Washington a few days later, to present a petition embodying the main features of Senator Allen's bill. It will be amusing to follow the proceedings which are booked to develop along the lines of homeopathic agitation. The antivaccinationists and antivivisectionists have had their fling at the public, the faith-curers are many of them in jail, and it is but fair to give these other agitators their chance. The public must be amused.

The Pennsylvania Epileptic Hospital and Colony Farm at Oakbourne was formally opened, with appropriate exercises on May 19th. The number of invitations issued was large, and many well-known persons were present. The farm is an outgrowth of the original institution which occupied for many years inadequate quarters in the heart of this city, and it is a matter of much congratulation that the managers have acquired for the treatment of this unfortunate class of invalids such admirable facilities as the new hospital possesses.

The graduating exercises of the class of '98 at the Medico-Chirurgical College were held in the Academy of Music, May 21st, at which degrees were conferred upon the largest class ever graduated from this institution. Rev. Dr. Edsall Ferrier of Easton made the opening prayer, and Charles M. Swain, acting president of the college, conferred the degrees. Dr. Isaac Ott, professor of physiology, delivered the annual address to the graduating class.

The annual commencement exercises of the Woman's Medical College of Pennsylvania were held on May 18th, in the Academy of Music. The annual address to the graduates, who numbered thirty-five, was made by Dr. A. A. Stevens, professor of pathology.

TRANSACTIONS OF FOREIGN SOCIETIES.

Vienna.

THE VARIOUS REACTIONS OF THE BODY UNDER THE INFLUENCE OF INFECTIONS.

Paltauf read a paper before the Imperio-Royal Society of Physicians, March 18th, upon the "Reactions of the Organism against Infections." As most of the symptoms of disease are produced by infection the consideration of the above subject includes almost the whole of pathology. Reactions which for a long time have been known to exist are fever, degeneration of the tissues, and inflammation. Fever is produced by substances either manufactured directly by the micro-organisms or which result from their injury to the tissues. Such substances act as poisons upon the nerve-centers that regulate the temperature of the body. Fever may be produced by living bacteria, by dead bacteria, or by extracts from them. Although an increase of fever in an infectious disease accompanies the increase of bacteria and defervesence is associated with their destruction, still one dare not conclude that the fever is a process designed to oppose infection; for fever comes not only in infections, but also as a result of other poison, and its favorable effects are lost in the numerous accompanying injuries which it works.

The degenerations of tissue do not result altogether from the high temperature. They are due rather to the products of the activity of the micro-organisms. The proof of this lies in the fact that by different infections different organs are the chief sufferers, as the muscle of the heart in diphtheria, the liver in typhoid fever, or the central nervous system in tetanus and rabies. And these last two infections differ, for in tetanus the poison is absorbed and acts upon the nerve-centers, while in rabies it proceeds from the periphery to the center of the nervous system along the nerves themselves.

Inflammation has long been known to be one of the reactions of infection, although at first only suppurative inflammation was recognized as such. Now it is known that the same micro-organism, according to its virulence, may produce different kinds of inflammation, and suppuration may be produced by very different kinds of bacteria. The tissue, too, determines to a certain extent the kind of inflammation. Thus in the mucous membrane of the air-passages and in the tissue of the lungs fibrinous inflammation is most common irrespective of the kind of bacteria which excites it. The chronic inflammations which occur have peculiar characteristics, and are known as specific. Under this heading are included those of glanders, tuberculosis, syphilis, leprosy, and more recently to these have been added the inflammations of actinomycosis, scleroma, mycetoma pedis, and mycosis cutis chronica, or Aleppo evil. In all these inflammations the limited extent of the influence of the infection is noticeable. In all of them there is produced a peculiar granulation tissue which probably has other differences except the presence in it of the various bacteria, although little is known about them.

Inflammations appear to be a struggle between the organism and the invading micro-organisms. Metschnikoff's original idea was that bacteria were digested by the cells. Later researches have shown that bactericidal powers must be attributed to the fluids of the organism as well as to its cellular elements. There are certain other reactions produced in the body by infection which may well be called physiologic. Behring and Kitasato found out that the blood of an animal which had withstood diphtheria and tetanus possessed substances which, while they would not kill these bacteria, would nevertheless protect other animals from the fatal effects of these infections. Such products are known as antitoxins. It was once assumed that an antitoxin was itself a poison which counteracted the poison of the bacteria. The counteraction, however, is not a simple chemical process, as it requires the cooperation of a living animal in order to be carried out. Similar protective powers have been found in the serum of animals which have withstood the infections of typhoid fever and cholera. But in these cases the protection arises by actual destruction of the micro-organisms, for the infection of typhoid and cholera can only be produced by the bacteria themselves as the toxins of these diseases are not known.

Gruber showed that the antityphoid and anticholeraic serums could be used to make a diagnosis of these diseases, since the addition of either of these serums to a drop of a fresh culture of the corresponding bacteria caused them to gather together in clumps and to cease their motions. This phenomenon, which is known as an agglutination, is found also in the plague and in Malta fever, as well as in the infection produced by the bacteria coli, protenis, and pyocyaneus, but not in influenza or in the infection produced by the meningococcus.

In other affections the serum contains certain protective properties which are neither bactericidal nor are they to be spoken of as weakening the power of the micro-organisms. Their action is rather a stimulating one upon the cells, since they incite the leucocytes in the animal in question to a more active phagocytosis. Since normal serum possesses a certain anti-infectious power, one must be on his guard in experiments in this direction.

Berlin.

ACTINOMYCOSIS OF THE THORAX AND LUNGS—EGYPTIAN OPHTHALMIA NOT TRACHOMA—ASCENDING NEURITIS.

At the Medical Society, March 16th, KAREWSKI read a paper on actinomycosis as it appears in the thorax and lungs. This disease, which has been known only twenty-three years, is by no means an uncommon one, and the reason that it did not sooner attract attention is that it was mistaken for other diseases, usually tuberculosis. Recent communications upon it have shown that it is in many instances amenable to treatment, both surgical and medical, and that in various parts of the body it has a marked tendency to heal spontaneously. But only three cases have been recorded in which actinomycosis of the lungs was not fatal. Karewski spoke of a fourth successful case which occurred in his own practice. The patient was a strong man of middle life, who had symptoms of trouble with the right side of his chest, and a rapidly growing tumor. At operation, four months after the beginning of the trouble, it was found necessary to remove the third, fourth, fifth, sixth, and seventh ribs from the sternum to the posterior axillary line, together with a portion of the underlying pulmonary tissue as large as a small fist. Owing to collapse, the anesthetic was stopped before the operation was completed, and the lung was removed by the cautery, without pain or hemorrhage, although the patient was conscious at the time. A tedious convalescence followed. The large wound was covered with skin grafts, which adhered, except over the pulmonary tissue. A large bronchial fistula persisted, sufficiently large to permit of respiration through it, when the mouth and nose were covered. The man was also unable to raise the right arm. Otherwise the recovery was satisfactory, and is to be attributed, according to the writer, to the fact that all the diseased tissue was removed or destroyed.

Pulmonary actinomycosis may be divided into three stages, a latent one, in which the affection is confined to the lungs themselves; a florid stage, in which the growth extends into the pleural cavity, causing exudation or adhesions, or both, and attacks the chest wall; and a chronic period, in which the disease extends into the abdominal cavity, or breaks externally, or forms metastases. Naturally therapeutic efforts can avail only in the first two stages, and hence the importance of an exact diagnosis.

In the first stage, the affection greatly resembles phthisis, although the subclavicular and axillary portions of the lung are more likely to be attacked than the apex. Later the sputum becomes mucopurulent, and possibly bloody, and the characteristic organisms may be found in it, though this seldom happens. Elastic fibers are wanting. From the pleural cavity there is usually no fluid to be obtained, or at best a little serous or bloody fluid.

This fact combined with the elastic character of the swelling, explains why in the second stage, the affection is often mistaken for sarcoma. In the third stage owing to many abscesses, and metastases in various organs, the disease takes on the form of pyemia.

Without operation pulmonary actinomycosis, according to the eleven recorded cases, is absolutely fatal in from one to five years after its first appearance.

At the session of March 23d GREEFF spoke of the alarm which the recent outbreak of "Egyptian" ophthalmia had occasioned, owing to the fact that the disease was falsely assumed to be the same as trachoma. The latter shows little tendency to travel from those places in which it is endemic, and it does not exist in Berlin. For the sake of clearness, acute epidemics of ophthalmia, which are liable to occur anywhere, should be characterized by the particular agent which causes them, *e.g.*, the pneumococcus, or various bacilli, as the case may be. The distinction between the swollen follicles which accompany contagious conjunctivitis, and the granulations of true trachoma, is not a difficult one for a good observer to make. A mistake in this regard, however has led in many instances to a long and needlessly harsh treatment.

At the Union for Internal Medicine, March 21st, LEYDEN discussed a case of ascending neuritis in which the autopsy revealed in a striking manner how, in the gangrenous right leg of a paralytic (a left-sided hemiplegia), an infection of streptococci had commenced in the sciatic nerve and had proceeded, with lessening intensity, clear into the corresponding half of the spinal cord. In the popliteal space the streptococci were found to have made their way into the nerve, and were found to be lying between the very nerve fibers. A little higher up, no micrococci were to be seen, but only an infiltration of the sheath and interstitial tissue of the nerve with leucocytes. In the spinal cord, the leucocytes were crowded into the perivascular spaces of the anterior horn of the right side, thus showing plainly that this was an ascending infectious neuritis, in the strict sense of the words. The pathologic changes were the same as those which have been produced in animals by a chemic irritation of a peripheral nerve.

SOCIETY PROCEEDINGS.

SEMICENTENNIAL MEETING OF THE MEDICAL SOCIETY OF THE STATE OF PENNSYLVANIA.

Held at Lancaster, Pa., May 17, 18, and 19, 1898.

FIRST DAY.

AFTER the President, DR. MURRAY WEIDMAN, had called the society to order and the usual benediction had been given, Dr. G. W. Berntheisel, President of the Lancaster City and County Medical Society, delivered an address of welcome. Dr. H. S. McConnell of New Brighton then delivered the "Address on Medicine," laying stress on the matter of dietetics and reviewing therapeutic progress.

After an essay on "Alcohol," by Dr. J. M. Batten of Pittsburg, and one on "The Ice Treatment in Pneumonia," by Dr. Thos. J. Mays of Philadelphia, Dr. J. I. Johnson of Pittsburg read a report on "A Case of Tuberculous Cirrhosis of the Liver," which he considered an important and rarely diagnosed condition. "The Variation in Strength and Consequent Unreliability of the More Common Officinal Preparations of the Materia Medica, as Proven by Special Clinical Observations," by Dr. Henry Beates, Jr., of Philadelphia, was next on the program. He hesitated, he said, in presenting the paper, for he knew in so doing he attacked subjects never before questioned, and hinted a departure from a life-long foundation. He questioned whether the profession has an exact science in its materia medica, and were it not for many years of clinical observation he would not feel justified in his results. All drugs in the Materia Medica are classified by the *preparation* of each, a tincture, a fluid extract, etc., and not by the potentialities of the several derivatives even though they may be antagonistic. As an illustration, he took opium, which the U. S. P. directs shall contain not less than nine per cent. nor more than fourteen per cent. of morphin; from this a tincture of ten-per-cent. strength is made, and how can the tinctures be uniform? Further than this, no two roots of any plant contain the same amount of active principles, and we therefore get the physiologic effect of whichever may be present in the greater amount, and confusion is the result of the action attributed to the drug. As a specific instance he quoted digitalis, with its almost innumerable alkaloids, one of which is known to be a cardiac depressant, while the others are stimulants. This typifies the complexity of drugs, and it is not strange under the circumstances that we encounter such diversity of opinion as to the value of any drug. Aconite, he had found, will sometimes act most satisfactorily as a sensory paralyzant, while at other times its depressant action on the heart will preclude its use for this purpose, showing the ascendency of one property at one time, the other property at another.

DR. ALFRED KOENIG of Pittsburg followed with a paper on "Therapeutic Fasting in Typhoid Fever," in which he advocated a limited diet, claiming that feeding of certain prescribed quantities at certain prescribed times was often nauseous to the patient, and in excess of Nature's demands.

DR. S. SOLIS COHEN of Philadelphia read the next paper on "The Treatment of Patients with Typhoid Fever." He called attention to the fact that a physician should guide his patient through the illness, and only interfere as occasions arise. Temperature, of itself, not being a factor to be dreaded, the coal-tar products as antipyretics are abandoned, and cold water is used with reaction as its chief object. He wished, he said, to put himself on record as being against the extreme use of the Brand method; of "systems" it is the best, but "systems" are poor. In his opinion, also, to strike at one symptom, unless most urgent, is often to put the patient in his grave. Feeding, like the entire treatment, should be fitted to the case, water should be used freely internally and externally. Where sponging is employed it is necessary to see that it is properly done; the bed should be warmed for the patient's return, red wine before and after the bath should be given in place of whisky, and for severe cases the bath should be used. The "pump-handle" charts, produced by frequent bathing, and exhibited in hospital wards, he condemned, together with the practice of wakening a patient for a bath. As initial treatment he advised calomel and intestinal antiseptics.

An interesting case of "Orchitis Complicating Typhoid Fever" was reported by Dr. A. A. Eshner of Philadelphia, together with a brief review of forty-three other cases collected by the author. From his experience and from the literature on the subject, he summarized as follows: Orchitis is rare, generally a sequel, occurring during convalescence, involving one or the other testicle, and not infrequently the epididymis. It usually lasts a week or ten days, and generally ends in resolution, though suppuration or subsequent atrophy may follow. Its cause is probably an infection of the blood by the typhoid bacillus.

DR. MCCORMICK of Williamsport, in the discussion which followed, condemned the practice of locking up the bowels in hemorrhage. Dr. H. A. Hare of Philadelphia spoke of the extreme use of the Brand bath, the excess of which he condemned, recommended a more liberal diet, and spoke of the advantages of camphor as a stimulant, comparing it to strychnin, than which he thought it more lasting. He employs it in 1-grain doses, dissolved in oil, and given hypodermically. Drs. Heyl of Pittsburg, Judson Daland of Philadelphia, and McConnell of Pittsburg also joined in the discussion.

DR. WM. T. ENGLISH of Pittsburg advocated the use of "Opiates in Bronchitis," and from observation in some 200 cases drew the conclusion that they (1) reduce inflammation, (2) alter and limit secretion, and (3) relieve pain and insomnia. He explained the great benefit obtained on the ground that opium (which he uses) equalizes circulation, thus overcoming the congestion, and supports the heart.

One of the most interesting papers read was by Dr. H. A. Hare of Philadelphia on "The Treatment of Toxemia by Intravenous Injections and Hypodermoclysis; of Aneurism by Electrolysis; of Hemorrhage by Calcium Chlorid." After describing the technic of the first-named treatment, he stated that it was his custom to bleed on the opposite side of the body to which the transfusion was given, when arterial tension was high, and that unless the condition was pressing he preferred hypodermoclysis. Under the second heading he reported a case of aortic aneurism in which electrolysis was most successful. The patient, who was suffering from a large aneurism, was operated on March 3, 1898, with the assistance of Dr. D. D. Stewart of Philadelphia, to whom the credit of the introduction of electrolysis in this country is due. Nine feet of gold wire was introduced, and a current of from forty to seventy milliamperes passed through for about an hour and forty minutes. At the end of forty-eight hours there was no bruit, less thrill, and less expansion, which symptoms had been most marked. Since that time the patient has gained ten pounds in weight, and is now walking around the wards; expansion is absent, and the only symptom present is a slight impulse felt at the seat of the lesion.

He reported, also, two cases in which he had used calcium chlorid in hemorrhage with marked success, and called attention to the fact that an excessive use of the drug for any prolonged time has a deleterious effect on the coagulability of the blood.

DR. J. MADISON TAYLOR of Philadelphia read a paper on "Three Cases of Lumbar Puncture for the Relief of Symptoms of Leptomeningitis," after which Dr. A. B. Dundore of Reading delivered the "Address on Hygiene." Dr. J. V. Shoemaker of Philadelphia closed the afternoon session by exhibiting two interesting cases, one of psoriasis and the other of fibroma molloscum.

In the evening, at the Lancaster Court House, an interesting musical program was rendered, and an address of welcome was made by Hon. W. U. Hensel, President of the State Bar Association. The State Medical Society's president, Dr. Weidman, then reviewed the work of the Society, calling attention its long record and the advances made in medicine.

SECOND DAY.

The first paper, entitled "The Natural Agencies Concerned in the Purification of Polluted Waters" was read by Dr. H. Bergy of Philadelphia, and he was followed by Dr. H. S. Anders of Philadelphia with a paper on "The Individual Communion Cup and Its Critics," which was discussed by Dr. Diller of Pittsburg, who did not agree with the author as to the wisdom of agitation on the subject.

A paper, entitled "Some Points on Infant-Feeding" was read by Dr. Edwin Rosenthal, who pointed out the necessity of having a "home-made" ***modified milk*** which would be less expensive than that prepared by the laboratories. Cow's milk, next to mother's milk, he believes to be the best, and for the new-born child gives equal parts of milk and boiling water with a pinch of common salt. Bowel movements he controls to a large extent by oatmeal for constipation and barley for diarrhea. He also advised a more liberal use of salt in the diet of children and urged the necessity of modifying the diet to suit.

DR. CHARLES W. DULLES of Philadelphia read a paper on "A Simple and Satisfactory Method of Examining Urine." After twenty-years' experience he considers albumin, sugar, and sediment the objects to be examined for and to search for chlorids and indican is a waste of time. He classifies the presence of albumin and sugar as "very little" or a "great deal" and decries the importance paid to small amounts of either. For albumin he uses heat and nitric acid; for the phosphates he considers caustic potash ***par excellence***, as it is, in his opinion, a most delicate test for sugar at the same time. To a microscopic examination he gives the most attention, believing that it reveals pathologic conditions not yielded by chemic tests. Blood and pus, whenever present, are important, but a few hyaline casts or small amounts of epithelium are not of importance.

Extracts from the "Address on Surgery," read by Dr. W. L. Estes of South Bethlehem, are as follows: During the past year, among the many advances may be mentioned the removal of the entire human stomach by Schlatter of Zurich, not only as an evidence of remarkable surgical technic but also as a contribution to our knowledge of the physiology of digestion. It should be remembered however, by those who would follow, that all the conditions existing in his patient were particularly favorable to success. Another notable instance of ablation and the marvelous adaptability of the gastro-intestinal tract was the case of Shepherd. In extirpating a thirteen-pound fibromyomata of the mesentery he removed seven feet, eight inches of the small intestine, and the patient not only recovered but gained in weight. Hepatic and renal surgery have also had a great impetus—Robson, Lange, Senn, Halsted, Murphy, and Fenger in cholelithiasis, Kelly, Weir, Fenger, Gerster, and others in renal surgery. Among other advances may be mentioned Kelly (in this country) and Pawlik (on the Continent) in ureteral catheterization, and Kelly in the air-distention method for cystoscopic examination of the bladder.

Gynecology has also advanced. A further knowledge of the Röntgen-ray has narrowed down its possibilities, and Schleich's anesthesia has not received the hearty endorsement of American physicians. In the field of antiseptics, formaldehyd has found much favor.

The distinction between "gynecologic" surgery and "general" surgery is disappearing while the hitherto neglected "traumatic" surgery, as opposed to pathologic surgery and observed by the mine, railroad, or mill surgeons, is beginning to receive recognition.

By a personal practice, founded on the danger of anemia in operations, the mortality of amputations has been greatly reduced. To wait thirty or forty hours before operating, meanwhile using antiseptics, can do no harm, while it offers an opportunity to stimulate the patient, fill the blood-vessels, and greatly decrease the danger from shock and exhaustion.

A recent notice in Stephen Paget's book on John Hunter sums up the year's lesson. It says: "The lesson of Hunter's life was never more needed than to-day, when mechanical conceptions of surgery are so dominant and when technic has so largely replaced pathology."

"The Removal of Stone in the Bladder" was the title of a paper read by Dr. William S. Forbes of Philadelphia. He called attention to the advantages of litholapaxy over suprapubic cystotomy, and gave statistics of mortality showing a large difference in favor of the former. American physicians, to his regret, seem far behind English operators in this one field.

DR. EVAN O'NEILL KANE of Kane, in his paper on "Catgut," condemned its use, and was followed by Dr. Ernest Laplace of Philadelphia, whose topic was "The Pathology and Surgical Treatment of Chronic Varicose Ulcers of the Leg." Being due to a disturbance of the superficial circulation of the leg, he advises removal of the cause, the varicose veins, which he accomplishes by a circular incision around the leg, and ligation. He advises also the treatment of any diathesis the patient may suffer from, as well as the local treatment of the ulcer.

DR. J. R. CARE of Worcester reported a "Case of Unilateral Castration and Its Effect on an Enlarged Prostate Gland." This case was markedly successful, the prostate gland diminishing in size and affording great relief to the patient. He believes that bilateral castration causes a more rapid diminution in size, but that the unilateral operation is indicated in cases seen early.

"Chronic Diarrhea as a Symptom of Rectal Disease," by Dr. W. M. Beach of Pittsburg, was the next paper. After speaking of the futility of internal medication in many cases, he classified the causes of diarrhea as follows:

(1) General proctitis; (2) ulceration; (3) fecal impaction; (4) polypi and neoplasms. The treatment in general should consist in keeping the intestinal canal aseptic and clear of *débris*, in depleting the engorged mucosa, and in removing diseased areas. He also described in detail the treatment for the various causes.

DR. L. J. HAMMOND of Philadelphia read the next paper entitled "The Radical Cure of Hernia by the Method of Nelaton and Ombradin, with Report of Cases." He reviewed the methods of Halsted, Bassini, and others, and described the technic of Nelaton and Ombradin, who make a hole in the pelvis for the proximal end of the spermatic cord. Of three cases in which the speaker operated by this method, two were eminently successful, and the third, though protracted, was finally satisfactory. His experience promises few recurrences by this method.

"The Surgical Treatment of Common Deformities of the Face," by Dr. John B. Roberts of Philadelphia, was next read. His principal points were as follows: The deleterious influence on the mental aspect of persons so deformed is well known, as is also the effect on the earning capacity of the individual, particularly servants, nurses, and salesmen. In urban communities, being familiar with the safety of surgical science, persons so afflicted more often consult the surgeon, but in sparsely settled localities the sufferer is rarely relieved. The abundant blood-supply of the face, insuring against gangrene of the flaps, is an important factor, and it remains to have the operation well planned and artistically performed to insure success. It is important to insist upon the necessity for repeated operations, for very often crude restoration of the parts is all that can be accomplished at first.

DR. B. D. DETWILER of Williamsport delivered the "Address in Mental Disorders." There are 10,000 insane in Pennsylvania, and an annual increase of from 300 to 500. One cause for this unusual number is the allowance of unfit marriages. Sterility of those so afflicted is the natural cure, but so slow is this extirpation that it must be hastened and the law invoked. Two instances were quoted of families having many descendants who were mentally defective, and so great was the increasing number of insane thus descended as to confirm the opinion of the necessity of State interference. Of patients treated for insanity, those suffering from cerebral exhaustion, when treated by isolation, rest, and sleep, the prognosis is good; of those caused by syphilis and alcohol, seventy-five to eighty per cent. recover if treated early, but in those suffering from hereditary insanity, recovery is the exception. Country "homes" where the harmless, hopelessly insane can be kept was advised, while the State hospitals can keep all cases for one year under observation and keep violent cases. This system has been very successful in Wisconsin, and an appeal on the part of the society to the Legislature was asked.

"Provision for the Insane in Hospitals" was read by Dr. John Curwen of Warren. In his exhaustive paper most careful methods for treatment were presented as well as a large amount of statistical matter relative to the cost of caring for the insane.

"Hypnotism, Dominant and Relaxant," was read by Dr. George E. Brill of Harrisburg, and this closed the exercises for the afternoon. In the evening Dr. J. T. Rathrock, Commissioner of Forestry, gave an illustrated lecture on "Sanitary Relations of Our Highlands to the State." The views exhibited were beautiful and the lecture most interesting. Attention was particularly called to the necessity of protecting existing forests, and to the advantage of planting trees upon the barren mountain sides of the State, thus insuring a water-supply and adding to the general sanitary health of the State. Later the faculty of Franklin and Marshall College entertained the delegates.

It is to be regretted that the committee having in charge

the assignment of papers should have so crowded them. Many which promised to be most interesting were "read by title," presumably because their various authors had not the time at their disposal to wait from session to session in the hope of finally being able to read them. For the same lamentable lack of time, discussion was greatly limited, some papers receiving none. The papers in general were excellent, and the meeting an undoubted success.

The following officers were elected for the coming year:

President, W. B. Lohman, Cambria County; first vice-president, R. B Watson, Clinton County; second vice-president, G. W. Guthrie, Luzerne County; third vice-president, J. A. Ehler, Lancaster County; fourth vice-president, Henry Landis, Berks County; secretary, C. L. Stevans, Athens; assistant-secretary, G. W. Wagoner, Johnstown; treasurer, G. B. Dunmire, Philadelphia.

Johnstown was selected as the place for next year's meeting. Two thousand dollars was voted the Rush monument fund.

THIRD DAY.

DR. C. W. DULLES of Philadelphia opened the session with a "Report on Hydrophobia." During the past year he has been able to collect from various sources reports of but six cases of the affection in this country. Of the six, three gave negative results from inoculations and the cases generally confirmed his belief in the non-existence of rabies.

During the past twelve years in the United States, the average number of cases collected by Dr. Dulles has been fourteen. France, where Pasteur's methods have been instituted, shows no decrease, but Germany and England, without the method, do. The speaker advised against the wholesale dosing with narcotics and the forced feeding of patients, the former treatment causing some deaths in his opinion, from their depressing action.

"Corneal Ulcers, Varieties and Treatment," by Dr. Joseph E. Willitts was then read. Dr. Lautenbach of Philadelphia discussed the paper and dwelt upon the importance of early, frequent, and thorough cleansing of the eye. Dr. P. J. Kress of Allentown then read a paper, entitled "Determination of Errors of Refraction by the Skiascope During Sleep," and spoke of its value in the case of children.

The "Address in Obstetrics" was read by Dr. S. S. Fowler of Marionville. The paper, written from the standpoint of the general practitioner, said it would be a sorry day when the "family doctor" existed no more. The specialist should be the friend of the family doctor, and if called for consultation, should still leave him, the doctor, in charge. He called attention to the gynecologist who, seeing a woman who has had eight or nine children, exclaims, "Madam, you have a frightful tear, the physician who attended you last must have been most careless!" Carelessness gives rise to the calamities of obstetrics and just as long as the practitioner thinks his case "will do as well as the majority do," so long will he take risks. He decried the delay in emptying the uterus in cases of persistent vomiting until the patient becomes weak and exhausted; the undue haste to use forceps; and the excessive preparation and paraphernalia of obstetric cases.

DR. MORGAN J. WILLIAMS of Scranton, and Dr. B. S. Pollak of Pottsville, then respectively read papers, entitled "Puerperal Eclampsia" and "Eclampsia." "Extra-uterine Pregnancy, with Report of Cases" was read by Dr. G. D. Nutt of Williamsport. He said the diagnosis of this condition has advanced greatly during the past two or three years, which he thinks is as easy as that of appendicitis. Few cases are seen or recognized before rupture, hence he advises operation by the abdomen.

DR. J. M. BALDY of Philadelphia then read a paper with the title "Gynecological Reflexes." He condemned the universal custom of attributing various nervous phenomena to lacerations of the cervix and other gynecologic conditions. Such conditions have their local symptoms, but he can see no reason why the uterus should be considered a nerve-center capable of causing general nervous disturbances: on the other hand, it is quite probable that a general disturbance does affect the uterus as it does other organs. "The Conservative Treatment of Fibroid Tumors of the Uterus" was read by Dr. E. E. Montgomery of Philadelphia, who advocated enucleation of the fibroid; by the vagina when possible, by the abdomen when not. Dr. Charles P. Noble then read "The Conservative Treatment of Fibroid Tumors of the Uterus by Myomectomy," in which he said the age and desire for children relatively, and the character of the tumor absolutely, should determine the question of myomectomy or hysterectomy.

DR. M. PRICE of Philadelphia next read a paper on "The Use of the Curette," which he scathingly condemned, and Dr. Anna M. Fullerton of Philadelphia related "Some Experiences in Operative Gynecology." In "The Primary Malignant Diseases of the Corpus Uteri, and the Practical Value of the Microscope in Establishing an Early Diagnosis," Dr. H. L. Williams of Philadelphia made an earnest plea for the more liberal use of the microscope in diagnosis. Dr. W. S. Brenholtz of Lancaster read the next paper, "Nasal Catarrh and Its Relation to Diseases of the Ear." He called attention to the importance of early treatment, not local applications, but general treatment in which he was ably seconded by Dr. Lautenbach, who discussed the paper.

The last paper of the meeting was "Rupture of the Ear-Drum, Not Necessarily Incurable," by Dr. Louis J. Lautenbach. So many untruths are afloat concerning this important matter, and so many errors are accepted as truths, that he wished to call attention to this matter. In the common-school physiology the statement is made that once the ear-drum is ruptured permanent deafness results; as a matter of fact, if treated early, nearly every case is curable, and many ruptured drums heal of themselves. Under ordinary conditions the ear-drum has considerable recuperative power, and even after removal of the ossicles there may be a new membrane formed. The drum-head may be entirely absent and yet the hearing good, let alone simple perforation, and it is to be remembered that the articulation of the stapes with the oval window is *the* essential to hearing.

DR. W. B. LOHMAN, the newly elected president, was then escorted to the Chair by Drs. Fowler and Craig, and after a brief speech the Society was declared adjourned. In the evening the Lancaster County and City Medical Society entertained the delegates with a dinner, and the fiftieth anniversary of the State Medical Society ended.

FORTY-THIRD ANNUAL MEETING OF THE KENTUCKY STATE MEDICAL SOCIETY.

Held at Maysville, Ky., May 11, 12, and 13, 1898.

THE President, J. M. MATTHEWS, M.D., of Louisville, in the Chair.

FIRST DAY—MORNING SESSION.

DR. JAMES B. BULLITT of Louisville read a paper, entitled

DIAGNOSIS AND TREATMENT OF OSTEOMYELITIS.

He stated that the affection is an inflammation of bone, its medulla and its covering, the medulla being the starting-point as a rule; for anatomic reasons the bone and its fibrous covering are secondarily involved. It is caused by chemic irritants, or infections of micro-organisms. It is definitely known that no specific germ exists, the infection being by a number of pus-producing organisms. Of these the most frequent are the golden pus coccus and the staphylococcus pyogenes aureus. In fulminant cases the latter germ is the most frequent cause. It is essentially, though not exclusively, a disease of childhood, the condition of the circulation in growing bone being responsible for this. Many terminal twigs or loops of blood-vessels exist in the ends of the long bones, permitting a stagnation of foreign particles, micro-organisms and the like, starting as a rule at the diaphyseal side of the cartilage. In adults it generally follows injury to the bone. The femur is most frequently the seat of the trouble, as it grows the most rapidly. Males are more frequently affected than females. The pathologic process consists of rapid thrombosis, coagulation necrosis, and suppuration, along with the local destruction incident thereto, with possibilities of septic intoxication.

The symptoms are a feeling of great exhaustion, followed quickly by pains. Chill accompanies the pain, at first general, but rapidly becoming localized, and very severe. Fever follows, and may be high. Tenderness, swelling, and redness develop over the area affected. With this is the characteristic muscular spasm pointing to the bone affected by posture incident thereto. Edema should be regarded as pathognomonic. A scarlatinaform rash may appear upon the skin. Fat embolism may occur, and there is often albumin in the urine. It is to be diagnosed from acute rheumatism and from typhoid fever.

The treatment is essentially surgical; no drug can be of any service. In the fulminating type rapid interference is necessary for the preservation of life as well of limb. Open the bone by trephining, scrape out thoroughly with a spoon, and incise freely any neighboring joint affected.

DISCUSSION.

DR. JOHN M. FOSTER of Richmond: My experience has been limited to some dozen cases, and but one of these was seen early enough for intervention to save the limb. One patient had had a fall of about ten feet, alighting on his feet, the process developing in the ankle. The condition was not recognized at first, and when I saw it there were two large pus-sacs in the leg on its posterior surface. Finally an amputation in the middle thigh had to be done. In this case a large part of the bone was saved by scraping out the medulla for some distance up and draining. I mention this to show the rapid and extensive involvement sometimes seen in these cases, it having extended in a short time from the ankle to the middle thigh. I hope that now the subject is more thoroughly taught in the schools than was formerly the case. The treatment is surgical, and it should be prompt and thorough.

DR. W. L. RODMAN of Louisville: I arise only to emphasize a few points brought out by the essayist in his excellent paper. It is frequently impossible to differentiate between osteitis, periosteitis, and osteomyelitis, they merge so one into another, especially those of an explosive character being difficult to diagnose. The medicinal treatment avails nothing, and it was a pleasure to hear the essayist so positive on this point. Prompt and judicious surgery is the only thing. Trephine and drain the medullary canal upon the same principles that one would drain any other cavity. If this were done promptly we would see fewer cases in the chronic state. I would not agree with the essayist that the femur is most frequently involved, though only on personal experience, having seen it more frequently in the humerus and tibia.

DR. B. MERRILL RICKETTS of Cincinnati: I am convinced that operative procedures are not resorted to frequently enough. Frequent explorations should be resorted to, trephining two or three places into the bone to find out the cause of the symptoms. I use the irrigating curette, and Wyeth's method, curetting out the canal of the bone and leaving a large part of the bone, the tube being drawn out a half-inch every day until entirely removed.

DR. BULLITT, in closing: My statement that the femur is more frequently involved is not from any personal experience, but from the statistics of Tallmann, who has had more opportunity of observing a large number of cases than any other observer.

DR. R. ALEXANDER BATE of Louisville then read a paper on

THE RATIONAL THERAPEUTICS OF THE ANIMAL EXTRACTS.

He referred to the group of animal extracts, and called attention to pepsin, pancreatin, ox-gall, beef-blood, bone-marrow, spermin, nuclein, thyroid, suprarenal, thymus, orchitic, brain, renal, splenic, ovarian, uterine, cardiac, and lymphatic extracts. There are two classes of extracts—those made from secreting organs and those from non-striated muscle. The use of these extracts cannot be limited to isopathy, but when administered upon isopathic principles, as thyroid in myxedema, etc., they must be continued, just as food must be repeated to relieve recurring hunger. In all cases reported cured the subsequent history of the case has shown that withdrawal of the medicine has been followed by a recurrence of the disorder, but again controlled by its administration.

DR. R. C. MCCHORD of Lebanon read a paper, entitled

THE UTILITY OF THE BLOOD-CLOT IN THE TREATMENT OF WOUNDS.

He detailed his experience with Schede's method, and considered it a valuable agent, especially in the condition resulting from injuries to fingers made by machinery, leaving some of the bone exposed. He had seen good results follow the use of the clot in injuries where as much as one-fourth of an inch of bone was exposed.

EVENING SESSION.

The annual address of the President was delivered in the Baptist Church. In his address he paid a feeling tribute to the late Dr. J. Q. A. Stewart, an ex-president of the Society, recently deceased. He then said that when addressing the Medical Society of the State of New York he had stated that there were no "quacks" in the State of Kentucky, and the remark had evoked considerable applause, and he further stated that Kentucky was the only State in the Union that had accomplished so much. Attention was called to the fact that the law against quackery now rests with the courts and not with the Board of Health. Any person who knows of the violation of the law has only to swear out a warrant, have the person arrested and prosecuted, and the board will assist. Due credit was given to the secretary of the board for obtaining the much needed legislation during the last session of the Legislature regarding the "osteopaths," which makes them undergo an examination before the board before they can practise in the State.

Regarding the relation of the people to the profession, the speaker said he hoped that the day is not far distant when the people will learn to discriminate between the pretender who strews pamphlets at the door and the hard-working and competent physician, to know the difference between jealousy and contempt, and not ascribe envy to the family physician, when in truth he is trying to protect them. Especially he hoped the minister of the gospel would withhold his pen from endorsing that which would ruin his wife or daughter or his trusting parishioners.

Attention was called to the lack of any action of the State Society in the matter of the Rush Monument Fund, and he urged that some action be taken at once. A splendid tribute was paid to the American Medical Association, "the peer of any medical organization in the world." He urged every one that possibly could to make the sacrifice of time to attend the meeting in Denver, and congratulated the profession of the State of Colorado for its excellent preparations. He stated that the Association is the owner of a journal equal to any in the world, which, under the management of its able editor, has increased its subscription to over 10,000. He urged each member to subscribe for it, even though not a member of the American Medical Association. He stated that there was noticeable a lack of interest in the State meetings, and believed that the cause of it is the large number of local and district societies. He suggested as a remedy for this condition a reorganization of the society, making a membership in it dependent on membership in a county society. This would necessitate the formation of county societies where they do not now exist, delegates being appointed to the State society according to the membership in the county bodies, one for every five. No paper should be read at the meeting of the State society that has not already been read before the local county body, and the assessment for the use of the State society should be $1 per annum. A committee consisting of Drs. Henry E. Tuley of Louisville, John A. Lewis of Georgetown, and J. N. McCormack of Bowling Green was appointed, and reported a change of the constitution as suggested by the President, to be voted on at the next regular meeting.

(To be continued.)

REVIEWS.

THE FACULTY OF SPEECH. By JOSEPH COLLINS, M.D. Pp. 432. The Macmillan Co., New York, 1898.

THIS volume, which as an essay gained for the author the Alvarenga prize of the College of Physicians of Philadelphia in 1897, is the most thorough and comprehensive study of aphasia which has so far been published. Aphasia has always been a difficult subject to master for the general student of medicine as any subject must be when there are so many and diverse opinions concerning the exact limitations of the term, and when so many deductions are based upon theories instead of facts. Dr. Collins' work shows that he has been an indefatigable student. His style is facile yet forcible. He smoothes out the tangle of theories in which aphasia has, for so long, been embedded in a way which is both comprehensive and entertaining.

We must, however, take exception to the numerous new and often enigmatical words which grace the text from the dedication page to the end. Simplicity of expression is a great and pleasing boon to the reader and is infinitely to be preferred to terms which though they may be expressive to the initiated are often confusing and incomprehensible to others.

The work opens with an introduction on the "Disorders of Intellectual Expression."

This classification, in the main, conforms practically to that adopted by neurologists generally. The recognition of motor and sensory aphasia and the division of the latter into word-deafness and word-blindness are universally accepted. We cannot, at the present time, find fault with the author for classifying the so-called subcortical aphasia as forms of aphasia. Properly speaking, subcortical aphasia, as Dr. Collins admits in a foot-note on page 155 and elsewhere, is not aphasia at all, but it is so generally accepted as a variety of aphasia that a classification would be incomplete without a reference to it. It is probable, though, that in future works this interesting condition will not be spoken of as aphasia. The same leniency, however, cannot be extended to that part of the classification in which aphasia is made to depend upon lesions of the peripheral neural mechanisms of the visual, auditory, and articulomotor systems. Lesions of the retina and of the organ of Corti may, and often do, interfere with the transmission of impressions to the cerebral centers, but it is clearly inadmissable to consider such conditions as forms of aphasia, a term which should very properly be confined to disturbances of speech resulting from lesions of the cortical speech-centers only.

The chapter on the history of aphasia is most complete and interesting. It shows the thoroughness of the author's research and is a model of what such a chapter should be. The pages on the genesis and function of speech constitutes one of the most important and valuable parts of the work. This is a subject which is rarely touched upon by writers on aphasia except in a most superficial manner, and yet a knowledge of it is essential if one would comprehend the fundamental principle upon which the theory of aphasia is founded. The author treats his subject thoroughly and comprehensively and the student is advised that a careful perusal of this part of the work will rob aphasia of many of its difficulties.

In the chapter on the "Conception of Aphasia" the author illustrates topographically the centers concerned in aphasia. The region which embraces these centers he very appropriately terms the "zone of language." The functions of the centers are discussed; their relation to each other through the medium of association paths is pointed out, and the site of the revival of words in silent thought is carefully elaborated.

The author believes the primary revival of spoken words is in the auditory center, and of written words either in the visual or the auditory centers, and that the kinesthetic center plays no part in silent thought at all. This agrees fully with the views expressed by Bastian and should meet with no opposition by those who have carefully studied the subject.

Exner's view in regard to the existence of a distinct graphic motor center is combatted with fair criticism of the cases offered in support of such a theory and also by convincing arguments, yet there are some recent writers, of whom Mills is one, who still describe such a center. Most readers will agree with the author that the existence of such a center is, at least, decidedly improbable.

The chapters on motor and sensory aphasia contain graphic descriptions of these conditions. They are illustrated by the citation of numerous cases which materially assist in explaining and enforcing the author's opinions. He advances the doctrine that impulses from the percipient visual and auditory centers travel through the articulatory kinesthetic center in Broca's convolution in order to reach the motor centers in the Rolandic region. This differs totally from the teachings of Bramwell and Bastian both of whom believe the percipient visual center is in direct communication with the Rolandic centers for movements of the fingers. According to Collins, in spontaneous writing and writing from dictation, the impulses travel respectively from the percipient visual and auditory centers through Broca's center to the Rolandic center for movement of the fingers, while Bramwell, Bastion, Mills, and other recent writers believe visual impulses travel directly from the higher visual center through special association fibers to the motor centers for the fingers. The latter hypothesis seems more reasonable. In Appendix II. the author cites a case which seems to support his statement, but the diagnosis was not confirmed by an autopsy and there are those who might, with propriety, disagree with him in regard to the situation of the lesion.

Interesting chapters follow on the diagnosis, etiology, morbid anatomy, and treatment. They are thorough, artistic, and show deep thought and great care in their preparation. The book is one that will be read with deep interest both for the fund of information it contains and for its scholarly construction.

A Text-Book of Mental Diseases. By Dr. Theodore H. Kellogg, former Superintendent of the Willard State Hospital, New York: Wm. Wood & Co., 1897.

In this volume the main facts of modern psychiatry are set forth in readable and interesting form. Although a brief chapter is devoted to the pathology of insanity and an occasional reference to psychologic explanations is found, the work is mainly clinical in character, and it is in its value as a practical treatise that its chief claims for merit lie. Dr. Kellogg divides his theme into two parts. The first and larger part consists in discussions of the statistics, nasology, etiology, symptomatology, and pathology of insanity; the evolution, and terminations of mental diseases; their diagnosis, prognosis, and treatment.

Under the heading of etiology, heredity, environment, education, climacteric changes, shock, fear, etc., etc., the various divisions of the subject are treated at length and their relative importance estimated. Few writers on insanity can resist the temptation to offer their own nasologic arrangement and Dr. Kellogg is not one of the few. His classification is careful and comprehensive, and is defended on logical grounds.

The psychic manifestations of insanity are presented seriatim, each with a terse description. The author wisely devotes several pages to physical symptoms without, however, laying too much stress upon the so often overdone "*stigmata degenerationis*." One of the most interesting parts of the book is the chapter on treatment. It is a presentation of the deductions of modern efforts in psychiatric therapeutics, and reflects, in great degree, the writer's State hospital experience. Prophylactic, educational, psychic, hygienic, and dietetic measures, home and institutional methods, medical and surgical procedures are all discussed in detail. Medicinal remedies are suggested with, perhaps, too much enthusiasm. Recent therapeutics, organic extract feeding (especially thyroid), lumbar puncture, etc., receive due mention.

The second part of the work is devoted to concise delineations of the various types of insanity as arranged in the author's classification. It presents, among others, the following noteworthy features. An effort is made to portray the progression of each form of mental disease through *stadias cœnaestheticum, acutum, debilitatis et terminale.* Dr. Kellogg insists upon the scientific propriety of the term "partial insanity" and, with Spitzka and others, treats under the heading "primary monomania" those cases which constitute so large a number of otherwise-styled paranoiacs.

The book is carefully arranged and conveniently indexed. The illustrations are well chosen, but for a descriptive work, altogether too few.

ABOUT CHILDREN. By SAMUEL W. KELLEY, M.D. Cleveland: The Medical Gazette Publishing Co., 1897.

THIS little book is a collection of six lectures delivered to the nurses in the training School of the Cleveland General Hospital in February, 1896. As their treatment is somewhat general and in a short space they cover a wide ground, they are not primarily designed for physicians. The manner of presentation is easy, conversational, and taking, so that they make interesting reading not only for nurses but also for mothers and those interested in the practical care of children. Their scope is large enough to include information on anatomy and physiology, artificial feeding, the effects of medicinal and hygienic remedies and symptomatology. The advice given is, in the main, sensible and rational. There is a short appendix containing a few recipes of foods for sick children.

ATLAS AND ESSENTIALS OF BACTERIOLOGY. By PROFESSOR K. B. LEHMANN, Chief of the Hygienic Institute in Würzburg, and DR. RUDOLF NEUMANN, Assistant in the Hygienic Institute in Würzburg. Illustrated. New York: William Wood & Co., 1897.

BY republishing in English Lehmann's popular hand atlases the publishers have done the English reading medical public a service. This particular volume is so widely known in the original German that it need but be stated that the plates are from the original source and that the text is a good translation to render the book the highest possible praise. The extreme condensation of the reading matter is to be regretted.

A HANDBOOK OF THERAPEUTICS. By SYDNEY RINGER, M.D., F.R.S., Holme Professor of Clinical Medicine, University College, etc., and HARRINGTON SAINSBURY, M.D., F.R.C.P., Physician to the Royal Free Hospital, Victoria Park, etc. Thirteenth edition. New York: William Wood & Co., 1897.

RINGER'S "Therapeutics" has always occupied a unique place among the books on the subject, its popularity chiefly depending upon clinical aspect of the work. The present edition, the thirteenth, does not vary from former ones in this aim. Particular emphasis is laid upon the use of drugs in disease, the indications and the contraindications for their employment. No more than is essential for the comprehension of the mode of action of a drug or other remedial agent is given of physiologic action; but the influences of therapeutic measures of all kinds in disease are thoroughly considered. This is the key-note of this work and to this position must be ascribed its wide fame.

In the present edition we note, as additions, a discussion of the Schott treatment of heart disease, scarcely of the length the subject deserves. Serumtherapy and organotherapy are considered at length and the articles on these subjects contain all that is recent in their relations to the treatment of specific diseased conditions. The digestive ferments are described under "Dietary for Invalids." Among the newer drugs which have found a place here are eucain and iodol; but we find no mention, for instance, of Golde's work on the antiseptic silver salts. The edition is, of course, thoroughly modern, and will undoubtedly meet the same cordiality that has been extended to its predecessors.

THERAPEUTIC HINTS.

For Herpes Progenitalis.—If the surface be dry, apply one of the following ointments:

1. ℞ Emplast. plumbi } aa . . . ʒ v
Lanolini }
Adipis . . . . . ʒ i.
M. Ft. ungt. Sig. External use.

2. ℞ Lanolini } aa . . . ʒ iv
Ungt. hydrarg. }
Ol. olivæ . . . . . ʒ ii.
M. Ft. ungt. Sig. External use.

If the affected parts be moist with secretion, first wash with a solution of boric acid, and then employ the following powder:

℞ Bismuthi subnitratis . . . gr. xvi
Ac. tannici . . . . gr. lxxx
Pulv. amyli . . . . ℥ iii.
M. Sig. External use. Dusting-powder.

For Pityriasis of the Scalp.—

℞ Salophen . . . . . gr. xiv
Vaselini . . . . . ℥ i.
M. Ft. ungt. Sig. For inunction morning and evening.—*Fournier.*

For Pustular Acne.—

℞ Bismuthi subnitrat. }
Hydrarg. ammoniat. } aa . . gr. xxx
Ichthyol }
Vaselini . . . . . ʒ v.
M. Ft. ungt. Sig. Apply at night.—*Von Hebra and Ullmann.*

For the Bites of Vermin and Mosquitoes.—

℞ Balsam. Peruvian . . . . ♏ lxxx
Ung. styracis . . . . ʒ vi
Ol. olivæ . . . . . ʒ v.
M. Sig. External use.

Or the following ointment:

℞ Naphthol . . . . ʒ i–ʒ ii
Ætheris . . . . q. s. p. diss
Menthol . . . . gr. iv–xlvi
Vaselini . . . . ℥ iii.

THE MEDICAL NEWS.

A WEEKLY JOURNAL OF MEDICAL SCIENCE.

VOL. LXXII. NEW YORK, SATURDAY, JUNE 4, 1898. NO. 23.

ORIGINAL ARTICLES.

PREGNANCY AND FIBROID TUMORS.[1]

BY H. C. COE, M.D.,
OF NEW YORK.

THE subject assigned to me is not only quite familiar, but is one in regard to which there has been no essential change in the views of accepted authorities during the past twenty years, or since the publication of Gusserow's exhaustive monograph on uterine neoplasms. It would, therefore, seem to be a thankless task to discuss such a well-worn theme. However, with the advance of aseptic surgery, we may at least record more intelligent methods of dealing with the complication in question.

Assuming that the question of fibroids in connection with labor and the puerperium is one that more directly concerns the obstetrician, we shall confine ourselves to what may be called its gynecologic phase.

It is a curious fact that in spite of the somewhat extensive literature of this subject there exists a considerable diversity of opinion with regard to the significance of pregnancy occurring in a fibroid uterus. Thus, we read in a recent text-book that "with tumors above the internal os from 70 to 80 per cent. of the patients may be expected to go on to term;" while a well-known authority (Bland Sutton) states in a clinical lecture just published that "when a woman with a myomatous uterus conceives it is certain that her life is in jeopardy, not only so long as the fetus remains within it, but also when it is expelled, whether this occurs prematurely or at full time." It is evident that the acceptance of either of these extreme views must lead the inexperienced either to adopt an ultra-conservative policy, or to lean too strongly toward radical methods.

It is impossible to lay down general rules for the treatment of a complication in which the conditions differ so essentially in different cases. The skill, experience, and bias of the surgeon, as well as the anatomic conditions, are to be considered. One who regards the presence of a uterine fibromyoma of moderate size as a sufficient indication for a radical operation, irrespective of serious symptoms, will naturally be more indifferent to the interruption of pregnancy than the gynecologist who operates only for the relief of urgent symptoms, and prefers to save the uterus when this is possible. But, from the standpoint of the general practitioner, whose laudable desire is to avoid operative interference wherever it is compatible with the safety of the patient, it is desirable that a few definite facts should crystalize out of the mass of conflicting evidence.

The statement so frequently reiterated that conception is rare in women with fibroid uteri is doubtless correct, but with certain exceptions. That it does not apply to subserous growths is well known to those who practice among the negro race.

Unfortunately, the presence of small interstitial fibroids in the lower uterine segment, especially those which develop between the folds of the broad ligament, do not by any means offer that hindrance to conception which we are ordinarily taught to believe.

It is unsafe to assume that the presence of any uterine neoplasm is absolutely incompatible with pregnancy; so that the natural corollary is that, having an unmarried patient with a fibroid even of moderate size (unless it be of the subperitoneal variety) it is the duty of the physician to state frankly the possible risks of matrimony and to dissuade her from it.

In considering the influence of pregnancy upon fibroid tumors, and conversely, the effect of such growths upon the course of pregnancy, we shall assume that the elementary facts with regard to the genesis, mode of growth, degeneration, and usual complications of fibromyomata are sufficiently familiar to you. Without subscribing to the extreme view that every fibrous neoplasm, though innocent in itself, is to be regarded as a possible menace to life at some indefinite period in the future, we must all admit that certain changes may occur in the tumor itself, or in its environment, which may cause it to assume serious clinical importance. As is well known, the indications for surgical interference in these cases are progressive increase in the size of the tumor, hemorrhage, and pressure-symptoms—one or all. That these may develop in connection with a fibroid which has previously been quiescent under the influence of pregnancy, at once suggests the importance of the complication. That such a tumor, especially when interstitial, should rapidly enlarge under the influence of the increased blood-supply is self-evident. This enlargement is not always permanent;

[1] Read at a meeting of the New York Academy of Medicine, April 7, 1898.

it may be simply due to edema, but none the less it gives rise to marked pressure-symptoms, especially if impacted within the pelvis.

Changes in position of the tumor and uterus as the latter enlarges are not unimportant. A subserous growth at the fundus may cause retroflexion and incarceration of the gravid organ, or may press it downward upon the bladder.

The liability of pedunculated tumors when displaced by the enlarged uterus to suffer torsion of the pedicle—with all the serious results which may ensue—has been noted by several writers. Moreover, the occurrence of localized peritonitis with the subsequent fixation of the growth and uterus by adhesions has often been demonstrated at the operating-table.

Among the internal changes which may take place in the neoplasm itself in consequence of prolonged pressure, obstruction to the circulation, etc., are hemorrhage, cystic degeneration, and even necrosis.

Clinically, the site of the growth is by far the most important point. All agree that subserous tumors at the fundus, even when of large size, may be influenced but slightly, if at all, by pregnancy, which may advance to full term and be terminated in an entirely normal manner. Small interstitial growths may be equally quiescent, and many cases have been reported in which submucous polypi have been recognized only after the birth of the child. But, it is equally certain that growths of either the subserous or interstitial variety situated in the true pelvis, especially if these be impacted or adherent, may give rise to disturbances entirely out of proportion to their size, hence they always cause more or less apprehension should pregnancy occur.

Did time permit, I could report fatal cases of ureteral and intestinal obstruction, of septicemia, and of thrombosis, due to the pressure exerted by fibroid tumors of small size complicated by pregnancy. I have discussed this subject in a former paper on "Impacted Intrapelvic Tumors" (MEDICAL NEWS, October 30, 1897). Nor is this the only danger from growths so situated. If abortion occurs spontaneously or is induced, even as early as the second or third month, the cervical canal may be so encroached upon that it is impossible for the product of conception to pass, and then serious hemorrhage or sepsis may result.

Fortunately the condition of the endometrium in cases of sessile submucous fibroid is such that conception is unlikely to occur, but when it does, premature expulsion of the fetus is the rule, and with it often an alarming hemorrhage. We need not dwell upon the dangers of conception in connection with intra-uterine polypi—a somewhat rare complication. Sloughing of the growths during pregnancy or after delivery is always to be apprehended, as experience proves.

As to the influence of fibroid tumors on the course of pregnancy, it may be said in general that we cannot always predict what the outcome of an apparently unfavorable case will be. While the gravid uterus is apt to enlarge irregularly, and often to suffer displacement, as before stated, it may, as it rises out of the pelvis, carry with it a tumor which was supposed to be impacted, and thus naturally prevent the complications which were feared. Such a fortunate development could, of course, not be hoped for in the case of growths in the lower segment. The latter, however, may not affect the course of the pregnancy, which goes on to term with all the risks attending labor under such circumstances. With large interstitial fibroids, on the other hand, the probability of early detachment of the placenta is great, or if pregnancy advances there is imminent risk of accidental hemorrhage. The imperfect contractile power of the uterus in this condition is well recognized, as is also the consequent risk of hemorrhage and retention of the product of conception.

Although foreign to the present discussion, it may not be amiss to call attention to the fallacious view that while fibroids may enlarge under the influence of pregnancy, they undergo a notable diminution in size, or even disappear, during the process of involution. Under favorable conditions (as in the case of small intramural growths) such a diminution may sometimes be observed, but to hope that such a growth will entirely disappear is hardly less reasonable than to expect its total removal by electricity. One would hardly recommend pregnancy as a cure for fibroids.

The question of the diagnosis of pregnancy in a fibroid uterus is one which concerns the general practitioner quite as much as the specialist. The history may be entirely misleading, especially where the patient is unmarried or the periods are irregular. Rapid enlargement of the tumor in a woman who has previously been under observation, in the absence of evidences of degenerative changes, would cause suspicion. This sign alone led to the diagnosis of pregnancy in two cases in which I performed hysterectomy for large multiple fibroids. Both patients were unmarried, one being a young girl, the other a negress so advanced in years that she was thought to have passed the menopause.

With a retro-uterine or intraligamentous growth the diagnosis would be comparatively easy because the softer body of the uterus could be isolated from the tumor. Asymmetry of the uterus is not an infallible sign, by the way, as it has been noted in normal pregnancy. Dermoids and solid tumors of the ovary, when impacted in the cul-de-sac, and adherent to the uterus, are so often mistaken for fibriods that the error should never be a subject for criticism.

If there is any doubt as to the true condition, examination under anesthesia is not only advisable, but obligatory. It is so important to determine not only the fact of pregnancy, but the precise character, relation, and range of mobility of the tumor, that one cannot afford to neglect any means of arriving at an exact diagnosis. This is especially true if the question of the performance of a radical operation is under consideration. Any one can recognize a good-sized fibroid; this is an elementary point. There are many other things to be taken into consideration.

The reproach that gynecologists of the present day have become more careless in regard to diagnosis as they have increased in operative skill is not undeserved. We do not examine either the inside or the outside of the uterus as carefully as did our predecessors in the art, being content to wait until the abdomen is opened before trying to settle disputed points. The prompt recognition and proper appreciation of the complication which is under discussion calls for no small amount of diagnostic acumen. If skill and experience are requisite for the making of a correct and exhaustive diagnosis, certainly in the decision as to the best course of treatment to pursue there is opportunity for the display of the ripest judgment. As was stated at the outset; no fixed rules can be applied. Each case must be decided by itself, since no two are exactly alike. While the physician will naturally be somewhat influenced by the wishes of a patient who earnestly desires offspring, he cannot allow this factor to have much weight when it is evident that it is impossible for pregnancy to continue to the full term without imminent risk to the patient.

When the tumor, or tumors, is subserous and the uterus enlarges symmetrically, there will, of course, be no occasion for solicitude. A pedunculated, movable growth will bear watching, since symptoms of torsion may require a prompt resort to celiotomy; or, it may slip down into the pelvis, so that it will be necessary to push it above the brim. A fibroid of considerable size, situated in the anterior or posterior uterine wall, may also take care of itself and cause no solicitude even during labor.

It is hardly necessary to say that a woman with a large interstitial fibroid who becomes pregnant should be kept under careful observation. Doubtless such patients may go on to full term, though rarely. Few of us would care to have any member of our family take such a risk, but would prefer to terminate the pregnancy at an early stage, or to at once perform hysterectomy.

From what has been said about tumors springing from the lower uterine segment, it will be inferred that in these cases pregnancy is a serious complication. The dystocia which is present during labor is a familiar theme in all text-books on obstetrics. From a gynecologic standpoint they are equally important. While it is granted that pregnancy may often continue to full term with impacted pelvic tumors, it is certain that the patient will suffer from various disturbances, and has the almost certain prospect of a difficult labor, usually with a dead child, unless an abdominal operation is performed. There can be little question that if an intelligent effort to dislodge the tumor from the pelvis under anesthesia is unsuccessful, the uterus should be emptied, provided that the cervical canal is not so contracted that it is impossible for the fetus to pass. It will be a question in most cases in which the patient is not seen until the fifth or sixth month (or even the fourth), whether it would not be better to allow the pregnancy to advance to term, and then to perform an elective Porro-Cæsarian operation.

The possibility of enucleating *per vaginam* an extraperitoneal (or even an intraperitoneal) fibromyoma of the lower segment will naturally suggest itself to one who is familiar with such work, and this procedure if practicable would seem to be preferable to sacrificing the entire uterus. It should be borne in mind, however, that the increased vascularity of these growths during pregnancy entails some risk of hemorrhage, so that the surgeon may be obliged to ligate the uterine arteries in order to control bleeding, or perhaps to extirpate the uterus. Pregnancy is not necessarily interrupted, and if it is, abortion does not imply an untoward result for the operation, since the obstruction to the escape of the product of conception has been removed.

The persistence of pregnancy after accidental injury of the gravid organ during the course of abdominal operations shows that myomectomy by the upper route may be attempted with good prospect of success under favorable conditions. Certainly an explorative celiotomy does no harm, and may enable the surgeon to free an impacted or adherent tumor from the pelvis, so that the patient may go on to term—a far more rational procedure than to attempt enucleation of the growth *per vaginam*, with the finger, unaided by the eye. In fact, it may be better in a doubtful case to at once perform celiotomy in order to determine the exact nature and relations of the tumor. The incision may then be closed, and the growth attacked *per vaginam*, especially if pus be present, as in a successful case reported by the writer.

The indications for supravaginal amputation or total extirpation do not differ essentially from those in the case of the non-pregnant fibroid uterus. Rapid enlargement, marked pressure-symptoms, serious impairment of the general health, may lead the surgeon to adopt radical measures at the outset. He will be influened in this decision by the fact that under these conditions pregnancy can not, and should not, continne, and the inevitable abortion will diminish the chances of recovery from a subsequent operation. The operation itself is no more difficult than under ordinary circumstances, and the prognosis is equally good. The abdominal is certainly preferable to the pelvic route, in view of the more perfect control of bleeding and the diminished risk of injuring adjacent structures, especially the displaced bladder or ureter.

To summarize: Submucous polypi may be removed in the ordinary manner when they are accessible. Subperitoneal growths can be disregarded unless they are pedunculated and become impacted in the pelvis, undergo torsion of the pedicle, or contract adhesions. Liberation of the tumor under anesthesia failing, it is entirely in the line of conservatism to open the abdomen, to separate adhesions, or to remove the tumor, leaving the uterus undisturbed.

Tumors in the lower segment may be let alone if they are found to rise out of the pelvis as the uterus enlarges. Should the contrary be true and pressure-symptoms arise, abortion should be induced if the patient is seen at a sufficiently early stage to allow the fetus to pass the obstruction.

Conservative myomectomy may be performed subsequently, and the hope of a second normal pregnancy may be confidently held out. If there is any reasonable doubt as to the diagnosis, explorative celiotomy is indicated, especially in view of the frequency with which impacted ovarian tumors are mistaken for fibroids. Liberation or removal of the tumor may not interfere with the course of the pregnancy. Should the tumor not be discovered until the latter half of pregnancy, it would seem better (in the absence of serious pressure-symptoms) to wait until near full term, and then to perform Cæsarian section, followed by supravaginal amputation, subject, of course, to the wishes of the patient.

The usual indications for hysterectomy in cases of fibroid tumor become more urgent if pregnancy occurs, since an exaggeration of the symptoms may be expected. The patient cannot bear a living child, her life is imperiled, and conservatism is out of place under the circumstances. The abdominal is preferable to the vaginal route for the extirpation of the pregnant fibroid uterus.

LOCAL ANESTHESIA, WITH SPECIAL REFERENCE TO THE INFILTRATION METHOD.*

BY MARTIN W. WARE, M.D.,
OF NEW YORK;
ATTENDING SURGEON TO THE GOOD SAMARITAN DISPENSARY.

THE introduction of cocain as a local anesthetic nearly fifteen years ago marked an era in surgery greatly enlarging its limits. Mindful of the suffering that mankind has been spared by the use of this agent, an everlasting tribute can best be paid to its introducer, Dr. C. Koller,[1] by daily extending the sphere of its usefulness.

In the first decade of its employment unintelligent, reckless application claimed for it a considerable number of victims. Thus, Reclus[2] quotes one authority who, up to 1893, collected 128 deaths from cocain. In a careful analysis of sixteen cases Reclus accounts for the causes of death as follows: (1) "The use of very strong solutions in too great quantity. (2) The sudden emptying of large quantities of the drug into the general circulation, by puncture of a vein or injection into areas, vascular by virtue of the presence of an inflammation, or naturally so, as is the case with the head. (3) Operating in the erect position was a factor in all of these cases."

Untoward experiences like these called for improvements in the method of its administration, which but recently culminated in the infiltration anesthesia of Schleich. In an effort to make it clearer wherein the true advance of this latter procedure lies, I will rapidly sketch the evolution of cocain anesthesia.

At first the strength of the solution was considered most important, and it soon became a dictum that 10 to 30 minims of a four-per-cent. solution could be safely injected. On account of its concentration the small volume of cocain which could be employed limited the extent of the field of operation. When, following its very liberal use, toxic symptoms supervened, the administration of such antidotes and antagonists as caffein, whisky, and amyl nitrite was resorted to; hence, the suggestion of Gauthier[3] to add, as a prophylactic, a small quantity of nitroglycerin when using stronger solutions.

The earliest technic consisted of the subcutaneous injection of stronger solutions of from four to five-per cent. so as to form a depot from which the drug was carried by the capillary or lymph current in a more or less diluted form to the tissues and nerve filaments. After the lapse of a few minutes anesthesia occurred, most marked at the point of injection, and growing less toward the periphery of

*Read at a meeting of the Metropolitan Medical Society, January 25, 1898.

the anesthetized area. This method is referred to as regional anesthesia, and identified with it are the names of Landerer[4] and Woelffler.[5]

The next to perfect a method was Corning.[6] In his brochure, entitled "Local Anesthesia," he calls the procedure "local anesthesia by incarceration of the anesthetic in the field of operation." The steps of this method are, first, emptying the extremity of its blood up to the area intended to be operated upon, and then injecting subcutaneously the four-per-cent. solution of cocain, awaiting its diffusion by the blood still in circulation, and finally applying the Esmarch constrictor to prevent further absorption. With this method Corning performed major operations, but, rather frequently encountering toxic phenomena, he advocated the use of one-per-cent. solutions, and in his appendix says that "by heating the solution its anesthetic effect is enhanced so much that a 1-500 and even 1-1000 solution of cocain has performed good service. Thus, we shall see that the greater credit must redound to Corning for having anticipated almost all the conditions which we now regard as recent improvements.

The teachings of Corning were temporarily unheeded, and it remained to Reclus,[7] seven years later, in his able articles on the subject, to again advocate a reduction of the strength of the solutions to one and two per cent. for all purposes. In addition, he proposed the technic which consists of anesthetization of the tissues successively from the surface to the depth. This is, perhaps, the method most in vogue among us. Reclus' success in the performance of 3000 operations, a large number of capital ones being included, went far to popularize this method.

In 1894 Krogius[8] enriched the technic of local anesthesia by a procedure which might be styled peripheral anesthesia, and was dependent upon the injection of cocain into or about a nerve trunk, thus causing anesthesia in the area of peripheral distribution of the nerve. Here, again, priority for this advance must be claimed for Corning, and in 1890 Pernice[9] refers to this procedure as being practised in the Clinic of Professor Oberst of Halle. Success with this is attendant upon the most fortuitous condition of having the area operated upon solely innervated by the injected nerve; for otherwise, the free anastomosis of nerve filaments compensates for the exclusion of nerve impulses from any limited source.

This completes the first decade of cocain anesthesia, during which there was as wide a latitude in the method of its application as now characterizes the administration of general anesthetics.

Desirous of still further promoting the safety of using cocain, and thus make it a competitor of the more dangerous general anesthetics, Schleich of Berlin studied the question anew. His experiments resulted in the method, entitled "Infiltration Anesthesia," which he officially demonstrated at the German Surgical Congress in 1894. Subsequently he published a report of his successful application of the new method in 3000 cases, together with his improvements in general anesthesia under the title of "Schmerzlose Operationen." [10]

Schleich's starting-point was the anesthesia dolorosa of Liebreich. This phenomena, following the injection of indifferent fluids in animals, is characterized by a preliminary period of hyperesthesia due to the irritation of nerves, followed by anesthesia dependent upon the destruction of the nerve filaments. Of such a nature is the anesthesia produced by the injection of guaiacol dissolved in sweet almond oil, a mixture introduced by Championnière.[11]

Schleich found that the injection of water caused an anesthesia dolorosa, and that the injection of a six-tenths-per-cent. sodium chlorid solution was unattended by any disturbance of sensation. He, therefore, premised the existence of a concentration intermediate between these two which would produce anesthesia without paresthesia, and he realized it in a two-tenths-per-cent. sodium chlorid solution. This solution ought then in itself to suffice were it not that the use of anesthetics is called for in tissues rendered hyperesthetic by pathologic conditions; therefore, the necessity of adding some narcotic poison such as cocain in a strength of .02 per cent., this being the minimum concentration capable of producing anesthesia. For morphin likewise a minimum was found. It was incorporated in the solution for the purpose of allaying the paresthesia incident to the wearing off of the anesthesia. With a .2-per-cent. sodium chlorid solution as a vehicle a further reduction of the amount of cocain and morphin was practicable. This led to the construction of the following graded solutions:

(1) Cocain mur., 0.2; morph. mur., 0.025; sodium chlorid, 0.2. (2) Cocain mur., 0.1; morph. mur., 0.025; sodium chlorid, 0.2. (3) Cocain mur., 0.01; morph. mur., 0.005; sodium chlorid, 0.2.

To each of these is added 100 c.c. of distilled sterilized water. A few drops of a five-per-cent. solution of carbolic acid is added to prevent decomposition. To effect anesthesia over large areas with these weaker solutions Schleich conceived the ingenious method of rendering the tissues artificially edematous. Briefly stated, the technic is as follows: With a hypodermic syringe, while ether or ethyl chlorid spray is played upon the skin so as to render painless the first puncture with the needle, the fluid is injected merely into the skin so as to raise a wheal.

In the periphery of the latter the needle can be again inserted without pain and another wheal formed. This is repeated to the extent of the incision contemplated. The same procedure is followed in the depths of the wound.

There are a number of minor details which I will mention in recounting my experiences within the last two years, based upon the application of this method in nearly 400 cases. Not unlike others, I found my early failures dependent upon poorly constructed syringes. The Neal dental syringe I have found answers all purposes. It can be easily sterilized, being entirely of metal, and for the same reason the calibration is more perfect than when glass cylinders are used. The packing, originally of leather, now of asbestos, is in the stuffing-box at the head of the instrument into which the piston fits. If there is any leakage the packing may be compressed with the wrench. The piston and inner casing of the cylinder are made of non-corrosive metal. The power at times necessary can be developed with this syringe. Short, sharp, slender, and straight needles, to the exclusion of the curved ones, have been found adequate; a quick sharp thrust with such a needle at times causes less pain than the ether spray which we have latterly discarded.

Solutions must always be freshly prepared from powders or tablets, and with Schleich we hold that the temperature of the solution should be that of the body or below it. In the few instances in which we followed the suggestion of T. Costa[11] to raise the temperature of the solution to 100° or 105° F. much pain was caused. Our experience is confined to the use of solutions Nos. 1 and 2. In non-inflammatory conditions, where a large surface is to be exposed to operation, No. 3 is indicated.

Under all circumstances it is best to begin the infiltration in healthy tissue, and, when the conditions can be prejudged, to infiltrate every thing at once. Infiltration in the open wound is more difficult, as the fluid escapes. One should not aim, as the tendency is, to infiltrate over the surface, but should inject the fluid at right angles to the surface into the depth, forming the same succession of wheals as in the beginning. The skin incision is made larger than is necessary with general anesthesia, so as to obviate the pain incident to any strong retraction of the margins of the wound when working in the depth. Infiltration increases the thickness of the tissue layers even if much fluid escapes on cutting. The waxy appearance of the tissues and the sensation imparted to the knife will indicate to the operator whether he is working in infiltrated areas. The zone of hyperemia which surrounds the infiltrated area also affords an index of the extent of the anesthesia. To afford a guide, I colored the fluid with methyl-blue. This procedure gave satisfaction, yet on a few occasions the diffuse discoloration obscured large veins, which, on being cut unrecognized, caused annoying hemorrhage.

Infiltration renders the parts fairly bloodless, yet wherever possible the constrictor should be applied, and that, as Hofmeister[12] suggested, after the injection; for otherwise the blood still in the extremity will be displaced under stress of pain. Where hemostasis was necessary longer than five minutes I preferred digital compression by an assistant.

In the majority of instances the anesthesia continued about half an hour, and was unattended at all times by symptoms of poisoning. No regard was paid to the position of the patient. Fainting, which occured a few times with patients in the erect attitude, was due merely to psychic impressions occasioned by witnessing the operations. The patients were instantly restored to consciousness by the simple expedient of doubling them upon themselves so as to place the head between the legs. In children the method was a failure, for the reason that they became unruly upon seeing the knife. At all times delicacy of touch is necessary, and blunt dissection is to be dispensed with as much as possible; nor is sponging to be as vigorously indulged in as when general anesthetics are employed.

The exquisitely acute painful affections, furuncle, carbuncle, and whitlow require a thorough mastery of the technic. Not infrequently the difficulties obliged us to resort to the method of Reclus or nitrous oxid. Here also we had occasion to test the method recently suggested by Hackenbruch under the title of "Circular Anesthesia.[14]" From two points opposite each other he injects the fluid so as to surround the area to be operated upon. He uses a solution of cocain and eucain, of each one-half per cent. The cocain thus overcoming the pain caused by the eucain, which I found to be the case when eucain was substituted for cocain in Schleich's solutions. The advantages in favor of eucain are its stability when subjected to heat for purposes of sterilization, and, being a laboratory product, it is a surrogate for Nature's supply in time of need.

It may seem paradoxic to say that deep-seated abscesses are more amenable to operation by this method than those that are superficial; for in the the latter the skin and loose cellular tissue are as a rule already infiltrated with inflammatory products. No difficulty will be experienced if the caution of Schleich is followed: to first make a small incision into the abscess to relieve tension and then proceed with the infiltration. In the removal of growths the displacement previously alluded to is a temporary embarrassment, and it seems to me that the greater field for the extension of this method is just in this class of cases, though I recall decided failure or obstacle in the removal of friable glands. In the extirpation of an angioma, the profuse hemorrhage washed away the solutions so quickly that in spite of fifteen syringefuls of solution No. 1 the anesthesia was imperfect. Ganglions intertwining with the tendons could be removed with ease. Three ranula removed afforded difficulty only on account of the motions of the tongue, and in the removal of a growth from the tongue the hemorrhage was annoying. Foreign bodies could be quickly located; for the track made by their introduction stands out very clearly in the white edematous tissue. In the removal of ingrown toe-nails no difficulty was experienced.

Sequestra were easily removed from the bones of the hand, radius, humerus, skull, and a subperiosteal resection of a metatarsus was easily performed. In all of these the bone could be infiltrated through the cloaca which existed in each instance. Once, in the operation for hallux valgus, the bone had to be divided under nitrous oxid, the remainder of the work being completed under infiltration. Amputations and exarticulations of fingers afforded the least trouble. In the extraction of teeth, I had a personal experience of the efficiency of this method. Some dentists advocate the addition of antipyrin[15] to the solution to enhance and prolong the anesthetic effect and control the hemorrhage.

For sewing wounds the interrupted suture is best adapted, for with it one can better approximate the edges which very often lie at different levels owing to variations in the quantity of infiltrated fluid. Tenorrhaphy was successfully performed three times. In the hand a larger incision than necessary had to be made, because the fat protruded into the wound on account of the pressure of the injected fluid. For the excision of ulcers, curetting of granulations, and sinuses, and circumcision in adults the infiltration method is very suitable. My latest triumph with infiltration consisted of two successful Thiersch skin-grafts for large defects on the neck following the extirpation of carbuncles.

Following the employment of infiltration, wounds, as a rule, healed kindly, and never following the use of the method in infected areas was there any lymphangitis or dissemination of the infectious material. At all times a rigid observance of the rule to cut only in infiltrated areas will contribute to success.

The following contraindications or limitations to the infiltration method suggest themselves:

1. Whenever the limits of disease are not reasonably definable.

2. In diffuse cellulitis requiring free incisions.

3. In malignant new growths, for here there is danger, says Braatz, of forcing the *materies morbi* into the lymph-channels. The same danger is to be apprehended in conditions of diffuse tuberculosis.

4. Special attitudes long to be maintained during operation. On sentimental grounds, in operations requiring exposure, a general anesthetic may be preferable.

Reclus and Schleich, with their large experiences with their respective methods, stand for the use of cocain, as the rule, and general anesthesia as the exception.

It is perhaps too early in the career of the infiltration method to assign figures, but so much is certain, that the majority of authors consulted are of the opinion that a decided inroad has been made upon general anesthesia since the introduction of the new method.

The skepticism I first entertained as to the efficiency of infiltration anesthesia gave way with increased experience to that confidence which I feel certain will be the position of those who give this method the painstaking study its successful application calls for.

BIBLIOGRAPHY.

1 *Wien. Med. Blät.*, Jarg. vii, p. 1352.
2 *La Sem. Médicale*, p. 244, 1893.
3 *Centralbl. für Chir.*, p. 1100, 1893.
4 *Wien. Med. Wochensch.*, p. 263, 1887.
5 *Wien. Med. Wochensch.*, No. 50 and 52, 1885.
6 "Local Anesthesia," Appleton, New York, 1886.
7 *La Sem. Médicale*, pp. 33 and 434, 1893.
8 *Centralbl. für Chir.*, p. 241, 1894.
9 *Deut. Med. Wochensch.*, No. 14, 1890.
10 "Schmerzlose Operationen," Berlin; first edition, 1894.
11 *La Sem. Médicale*, p. 318, 1895.
12 *Centralbl. für Chir.*, p. 252, 1896.
13 *Beitr. zur klin. Chir.*, xv, p. 563.
14 "Oertliche Schmerzlosigkeit," Wiesbaden, 1897.
15 *Therap. Monatsch.*, p. 267, 1896.

CRANIAL DISTORTION IN THE NEWBORN AND ITS CONSEQUENCES.

BY M. A. VEEDER, M.D.,
OF LYONS, N. Y.

DR. MARION SIMS regarded distortion of the cranial bones during childbirth as a cause of trismus neonatorum, and recommended placing the child in such a position when recumbent as would tend to restore the normal shape of the head, together with the use of gentle manipulation. Other dangers beside that of trismus emphasize the necessity for the precautions suggested by Dr. Sims. For example no accident of childbirth, not even compression by the forceps, is so likely to result in permanent injury as is delivery with the head in the occipitoposterior position. Such labors are always difficult and often impossible, and yet again and again in consultation the writer has seen the source of the difficulty pass unrecognized. It seems to be the fact that the general practitioner is, as a rule, not very sharply alive to the dangers of this particular form of abnormal labor. Its mechanism, as the occiput sweeps over the perineum, is such as to crowd the bones together from before backward in a way that does not occur when the occiput is in its normal position under the symphysis. Thus originates a peculiar deformity at the back of the head readily recognized when attention has once been directed to it.

The permanent results that may follow this particular form of cranial distortion during delivery are well illustrated in two cases which recently came under the observation of the writer, and which appeared to be typical. Both the patients were women and had reached adult life. One of them, who exhibited by far the milder case, had for years been in an institution for the feeble-minded. In her case overlapping and synostosis of the occipital and parietal bones along the line of the lambdoid suture were well marked; there was a prominent ridge in that location, and the back of the head and neck were in a line with each other, and almost perpendicular when the patient was in an upright position. No other cause for this deformity is known than abnormal delivery with the head in the occipitoposterior position. The crowding together, overlapping, and distortion of the bones thus produced are specially liable to be maintained by the habit which nurses have of placing children habitually on the back. Simply to turn the child on its side tends to restore the normal shape by giving free play to the elasticity of the bones which in most cases is sufficient to this end without any manipulation whatever. If the deformity becomes permanent there will ensue more or less impairment of the functions of the brain of life-long duration. In the case just described as the result of the malformation at the back of the head, the power of muscular coordination was more affected than mentality, and the patient had been thought to have a mild form of St. Vitus' dance.

The other patient to whom reference has been made had a similar deformity of the back of the head, with even more pronounced symptoms of incoordination. Her gait was staggering and awkward, her hands writhing and twisting in an aimless way on any attempt at motion, and she was able to utter only stammering and inarticulate sounds. At first glance she would be regarded as a gibbering idiot, and yet the functions of the cerebrum were but slightly impaired as compared with those of the centers at the back and base of the brain. Memory and reasoning were fairly good for one in her helpless condition.

There are multitudes doubtless suffering from lesser degrees of impairment due to the same cause. Other forms of cranial distortion might be considered in detail. Enough has been said, however, in regard to the variety most apt to have serious consequences, and most frequently met in general practice, to indicate the importance of the subject, and the desirability of keeping it in mind at the critical period immediately following birth, during which prevention of these consequences may be possible. It is not the difficulty of management but the neglect of such cases that does the mischief. Very little mechanical ingenuity is requisite, provided that it be employed at the right time in accordance with the obvious indications in each case.

WAR ARTICLES.

NEWS OF THE WEEK.

THE following statistics recently published in a German exchange are interesting as showing the comparative heights required by the several nations in their soldiers: Germany, 1.54 meters (one meter equals 39.37 inches), 5 feet .63 inches; France, 1.54 meters, excepting the cuirassiers, who must measure from 1.70 (5 feet 7 inches) to 1.85 meters (6 feet .83 inches); Austro-Hungary, 1.55 meters (5 feet 1 inch); Russia, 1.54; Switzerland, Belgium, and Holland, 1.55; Sweden, 1.608 (5 feet 3.3 inches); United States, 1.619 (5 feet 3.74 inches), and England, which has the highest minimum standard, namely, 1.65 meters (5 feet 5 inches). As a matter of fact, the great majority of recruits in the English army actually measure 1.68 meters (5 feet 6 inches).

. . . .

The prospects for a plentiful supply of pure water at Camp Thomas are excellent. A large force of men has been put to work laying a pipe-line from Chickamauga creek, and another from Crawfish Springs, to the camp. An immense engine and pump are already in working order, and the supply of water will be ample for every need. The men at Chickamauga are in excellent condition, and improvements in the sanitary condition of the several camps are progressing favorably.

. . . .

Plenty of hard work, drilling and exercise, but good health, good spirits, and good sanitary conditions is the gist of the report from the 71st Regiment of New York Volunteers encamped at Lakeland, Florida. Several men have succumbed to the heat during drills, but all quickly recovered, and the regiment is rapidly becoming acclimated. Colonel Greene has prohibited board floors in the tents as out of consonance with serious campaigning, a regulation which opens up a question of hygiene, and the possibilities of a course of toughening to the inexperienced civilian. It seems doubtful whether in a country like Florida a man can accustom himself to sleeping on the damp earth in a heavy moist night atmosphere richly laden with an extensive and varied collection of malarial germs. Even the "crackers" who take their daily ration of "chills" or "ague" as one of the regular conditions of life do not sleep on the ground, and the risk of implanting seeds of disease in our troops to ripen and bear fruit under the climatic influence of Cuba would seem to be too great to hazard for the sake of military ethics. The adoption of the hammock is a long step in the right direction.

. . . .

Nearly ten thousand men are encamped at Falls Church, Va. This is known as Camp Alger, and the conditions here are not so favorable as at any of the other camps. We quote from the daily press:

> It is doubtful if clearer grounds for complaint could be afforded than those which exist at this camp, whose natural facilities are not sufficient to meet the wants of one regiment, let alone a full army corps. The volunteer officers, all of whom have had experience in camp life and in the selection of camps, cannot understand why this particular site was selected when there are other points where the two great needs of a camp—water and fuel—are in abundance, and where transportation is not a matter of mule-killing over muddy country roads. The commissary arrangements have been inadequate, and the volunteers are being subjected to a rigorous hunger drill. It is suggested that they will be prepared for any hardship that Cuba or the Philippines may offer after a tour of duty on the desert plains near Falls Church.
>
> Owing to the inadequate water-supply, some alarm is felt that typhoid fever may gain a foothold. Two cases, one fatal, already have made their appearance, and strenuous efforts are being put forth to avoid its spread.

. . . .

At the suggestion of General Wesley Merritt the War Department has detailed the following officers of the Medical Department to duty in the Philippines: Colonel Henry Lippincott, who has been on duty at Fort Sheridan, Ill.; Captains William O. Owen, who has been on duty at Fort Bayard, N. M., and E. R. Morris, who has been on duty at Fort Spokane, Wash., and Lieutenant Henry Page, who has been on duty in Washington.

. . . .

A meeting of Cuban physicians was held at the Red Cross Hospital, New York City, on May 22d, to discuss the effects of climatic diseases in Cuba. Those who took active part in the discussion were Dr. Morrill of the Hospital of the Holy Virgin, Havana, Dr. Riviere of Havana, Dr. Munoz, recently chief of the Civil Hospital in Havana, Dr. Sollosso, until recently surgeon in the Spanish army, and Drs. Carvona and Lesser. The points determined were that men from the United States suffer more from disease in Cuba than men from Southern countries. Of the Spanish soldiers who have gone to Cuba seventy-five per cent. have suffered from malaria and twenty-five per cent. from yellow fever. Deaths have occurred in about twenty-five per cent. of the cases. The seriousness of the diseases in Cuba has depended on the seasons and location; malaria has prevailed during the entire year, and yellow fever only during the months of August, September, October, and November. Yellow fever prevails mostly on the coast and in the cities. At a distance of eight to ten miles from the coast and in the mountains the island is healthy during the entire year. The physicians came to the conclusion from their observations that diseases do not spread as rapidly, nor are they as severe, as on the southern coast of Florida.

. . . .

Actual experience and statistical records show beyond question that disease is more disastrous to an army than the enemy's bullets, and hygienic rules and conditions, and medical and surgical equipment, are quite as essential as ammunition, arms, forts, and tactics. During the recent Greek war, Turkey lost about 1000 men in battle, 19,000 died of disease, and 22,000 were sent home invalided. Of the latter 8000 subsequently died.

. . . .

Although it was positively announced at the beginning of the war that women nurses would not be enlisted in either the army or the navy, the plans have been changed, and for the first time in the history of this country women are being enlisted into military service as nurses. Dr. Anita Newcomb McGee of Washington has just been charged with the selection of all of the women nurses for the Government during the present conflict. There were women nurses during the Civil War, but they were not enlisted, being paid by the Sanitary Commission. By the present plan, applicants must be between the ages of thirty and fifty; they must be graduates of reputable training-schools, and preferably with practical experience and without family ties. They must be strong and healthy; surgical nurses are in much the greater demand. They will receive $30 per month, wear a uniform consisting of white dress, cap and apron, and a badge in the form of a red cross of enamel, surrounded by a circle of blue enamel. In addition to their pay, each nurse will receive her rations daily, and lodging when practicable. There is a great demand for nurses who are immune to yellow fever, but so far not one has applied. No women nurses will be sent to Cuba, neither will any be permitted aboard the naval vessels.

. . . .

Dr. Walter Wyman, Supervising Surgeon-General of the Marine Hospital Service, has notified the medical officers of the service that the United States Marine Hospitals are available for the reception of the sick and wounded of either the army or the navy, and that they are directed, upon a written request of the proper military or naval authority, to receive and care for said patients, the Marine Hospital Service to be reimbursed the actual cost of maintenance.

THE EFFECT OF THE EXPLOSION OF A SHELL.

By RAYMOND SPEAR, M.D.,
ASSISTANT SURGEON, UNITED STATES NAVY, ON BOARD FLAGSHIP "NEW YORK."

DURING the bombardment of San Juan de Puerto Rico on May 12th, the U. S. S. "New York" was struck once by a 14 cm. shell at a distance of about 5500 yards. The shell came over the stern of the ship and struck an iron stanchion three inches in thickness which was broken short off at the point of contact. The shell went on for a distance of about fifteen feet and exploded in a wooden boat which was covered with canvas. The boat was demolished, the lighter planking being badly splintered and driven downward and forward against an iron steam-winch. The oars in the boat were broken and one piece was driven forward along the spar deck but did no damage. The canvas covering the boat was torn and rent into shreds by the force of the explosion and by splinters passing through it and then caught fire, showing that canvas under such conditions will not stop splinters.

The shell itself burst into many pieces varying from the size of a pea to large pieces weighing about five pounds. The direction these fragments took was forward, downward, upward, and to both sides, many of them going over the ship's side, others passing through the copper ventilators and smoke-pipes and doing but little damage.

The fragments that went downward and forward struck about the port 8-inch waist gun, where there were twelve men stationed, killing one man and injuring several others. The man killed, Wiedemark, was struck by a piece of shell about two inches square by one inch thick. It entered the left side of his neck near the angle of the jaw, severed the blood-vessels, proceeded upward and backward into his brain, probably injuring the medulla, and lodged under the skin just beneath the occipital protuberance. The man fell forward, losing consciousness immediately. His respiration ceased as soon as he was struck, but his heart continued to beat feebly for about five minutes, when all signs of life disappeared.

Another fragment of shell of about the same size struck a man named Fettman on the anterior inner surface of the left thigh about three inches above the knee and went through the limb, taking a backward and downward course. The femur was shattered into numerous fragments and the muscles were torn considerably in the track of the wound. The effect of the missile on the bone was peculiar in that the bone was not only splintered for about three inches of its length but it was also pulverized, hundreds of minute pieces of bone being embedded in the muscles. The wound of entrance was smaller than the wound of exit, the piece of shell probably entering the thigh edgewise, turning and presenting a flat surface at the point of exit. At this point there were shreds of tissue protruding from the wound showing that the ragged piece of steel drew muscular fibers and fascia along with it. The leg was operated on and a portion of the femur resected, the splinters and crumbs of bone were removed, the fragments were trimmed off and wired together, and through-and-through drainage established, the limb being put up in a fenestrated plaster-dressing. The man was transferred to the Hospital Ship "Solace" two days after the operation and is now in the hospital at Key West. The wound at last accounts was healing by primary union and there is every reason to believe that the leg will be saved.

Another man was struck in the left leg by a piece of shell about 1 in. x ½ in. x ½ in. It entered the leg about its middle on the outer side, went inward and forward, grooving the anterior surface of the tibia. The fragments of bone were taken out of the leg by the piece of shell.

There were several other minor injuries. Pieces of shell struck several men but did no damage. One man felt something hot on his breast and investigating found a small piece of shell that had burned its way through his clothing and reached his skin. There were a few contusions due to flying splinters, but no serious injury from this source. The fragments of the shell were all hot, as was shown by burnt wood and canvas. The men injured by the shell all said they felt a burning, stinging sensation about their wounds, and in some cases the clothing was scorched.

The shell receives a great deal of heat from the friction it incurs in leaving the gun; some of this heat is lost through radiation in its flight through the air, more heat is developed on the impact of the shell, and still more energy takes the form of heat when the missile explodes, making the fragments hot enough to set fire to wood. All of the wounds made by the pieces of shell were aseptic, but they all were sluggish in healing, due to the lowered vitality and burning of the injured parts.

EXTRACT FROM THE LOG OF THE AMBULANCE SHIP "SOLACE."

[From our Special Correspondent.]

WE left Norfolk early in May and after touching at Key West, joined Admiral Sampson's fleet and accompanied it in its cruise to Puerto Rico. The "Solace" was in attendance upon the fleet at the bombardment of San Juan where, directly after the engagement, we took on board the wounded and cared for them. The casualties in the bombardment consisted of one man killed and five wounded. The injuries received were all produced by the fragments of bursting shells, except in the case of one man who received a lacerated and contused wound of the back produced by a splinter from one of the steel girders. The fatal injury was caused by a fragment of shell which passed directly through the sailor's head from side to side, producing almost instant death. Another fragment of the same shell struck another man producing a compound comminuted fracture of the femur; the third man received a flesh wound only. These casualties happened on board the flag-ship "New York."

The "Iowa" was the only other ship that was struck during the engagement. The fourth man was wounded by a fragment of a shell which entered the ship's superstructure and burst. It carried away the bones entering into the formation of the right elbow-joint. The fifth man received a slight wound of the foot. The wounded were all attended by the surgeons of their respective ships, the effort being made in all instances to save the parts.

At the present time, May 20th, the patients are all doing well, with the prospect of a successful outcome of the treatment. The "Solace" returned with the fleet to Key West and transferred the patients to the well-equipped hospital on shore, which is conducted by the Medical Department of the army.

SANITARY ORGANIZATION, REPORT OF SICK AND WOUNDED, AND ROSTER OF MEDICAL OFFICERS IN THE VICINITY OF CAMP TAMPA HEIGHTS.

[Special Correspondence of THE MEDICAL NEWS.]

CAMP TAMPA HEIGHTS, TAMPA, FLORIDA, May 26, 1898.

THE following circular has been issued from the office of the chief surgeon in reference to our medical organization in the field:

"For the purpose of efficient administration of the medical department of this division the senior surgeon of each brigade will be considered its chief surgeon. Except under conditions of urgency, he will be the usual medium of communication of orders to the regimental medical officers, and he will have a general supervision of the enforcement of the orders of the chief surgeon of division which pertain to the medical department. Under direction of the chief surgeon of the division, the brigade surgeons will act as medical inspectors and will advise him upon all matters which pertain to the health of the commands or the efficiency of the department.

"All monthly or special sanitary reports will be transmitted through brigade surgeons, and will receive their consideration before they are sent to the chief surgeon."

Regimental surgeons are required to submit semi-weekly reports of sick and wounded promptly after sick call on Wednesday and Sunday mornings, covering the following points: Numerical summary of cases under treatment at last report; admitted to sick report; returned to duty; died; discharged, and those remaining at date of report; also, general character of diseases and condition of camp sanitation, with remarks.

There are now thirty-one medical officers, commissioned and contract, in the field with the United States forces at this point and quite an additional number are expected to join soon. The following is a roster of commissioned medical officers and acting assistant-surgeons attached to the United States forces in the vicinity of Tampa, and their respective assignments:

Major B. F. Pope, chief surgeon, United States forces; Major H. S. Kilbourne, chief surgeon, Infantry Division; Major L. A. LaGarde, chief surgeon, Cavalry and Artillery Division; Major A. H. Appel, commanding division field hospital, Infantry Division; Major S. Q. Robinson, brigade surgeon, 1st Brigade, Infantry Division; Major R. J. Ebert, brigade surgeon, 2d Brigade, Infantry Division; Captain Wm. Stephenson, assistant surgeon, in charge 4th U. S. Infantry; Captain C. M. Gaudy, assistant surgeon, in charge 1st U. S. Infantry; Captain Jas. E. Pilcher, assistant surgeon, in charge 22d U. S. Infantry; Captain W. D. McCaw, assistant surgeon, in charge 6th U. S. Infantry, and division ambulance surgeon; Captain Henry I. Raymond, assistant surgeon, in charge 13th U. S. Infantry; Captain H. T. S. Harris, assistant surgeon, in charge 9th U. S. Cavalry; Captain Paul Shillock, assistant surgeon, in charge 25th U. S. Infantry; Captain E. B. Frick, assistant surgeon, in charge Lt. Bat. "F," 3d U. S. Artillery; Captain A. M. Smith, assistant surgeon, in charge Lt. Bat. "D," 5th U. S. Artillery; Captain M. W. Ireland, assistant surgeon, in charge Lt. Bat. "C," 3d U. S. Artillery; Captain Henry C. Fisher, assistant surgeon, in charge 21st U. S. Infantry; Captain Henry A. Shaw, assistant to division field-hospital surgeon, Artillery and Cavalry Division; Captain Robert S. Woodson, assistant to division field-hospital surgeon, Infantry Division; 1st Lieut. Edw. L. Munson, assistant surgeon, in charge Lt. Bat. "F," 2nd U. S. Artillery; 1st Lieut. J. M. Kennedy, assistant surgeon, in charge, Lt. Bat. "E," 1st U. S. Artillery; 1st Lieut. Guy C. M. Godfrey, assistant surgeon, in charge Lt. Bat. "K," 5th U. S. Artillery; 1st Lieut. W. W. Quinton, assistant surgeon, in charge Lt. Bat. "A," 2nd U. S. Artillery; 1st Lieut. Doane C. Howard, assistant surgeon, in charge 9th U. S. Infantry; 1st Lieut. Wm. H. Wilson, assistant surgeon, in charge 1st U. S. Artillery; 1st Lieut. Thos. J. Kirkpatrick, Jr., assistant surgeon, in charge 24th U. S. Infantry; Dr. John Guiteras, acting assistant surgeon, on special duty with chief surgeon, U. S. forces; Dr. W. E. Parker, acting assistant surgeon, assistant to division field-hospital surgeon, Infantry division; Dr. H. W. Danforth, acting assistant surgeon, on duty with 9th U. S. Cavalry; Dr. W. W. Calhoun, acting assistant surgeon, on duty with 4th U. S Infantry; Dr. B. C. Leonarde, acting assisting surgeon, on duty with 17th Infantry; Dr. J. Lawrence, acting assistant surgeon, on duty with Lt. Bat. "B," 4th U. S. Artillery.

I have tabulated a consolidated report of sick and wounded of the United States forces near Tampa, *i. e.*, at Camp Tampa Heights, Picnic Island, and Port Tampa, for the last ten days of April, being the first ten days that the troops were in camp, and I find that disorders of the gastro-intestinal tract largely predominate. Assistant-Surgeon Fisher reports thirty-seven cases of acute diarrhea in the 21st Regiment, and as to their causation he justly remarks: "The prevalence of diarrhea is attributed to the great difference in temperature between the days and nights. The days were excessively hot, while some nights the thermometer fell below 50° F., and the men became chilled; also, to the use of iced drinks while heated, and to indiscretions in dietary."

Only seven cases of heat exhaustion were reported from all the regiments. Some of these cases occurred during noon (1 P.M.) drills, which were prudently discontinued after a short trial, and active work of all kinds largely suspended between ten and four in the day. One case of croupous pneumonia occurred in my own regiment. The local health physician tells me that this disease is so infrequent in this locality that he has seen but three or four cases in eight-years' practice. The patient did admirably in a hospital tent with free ventilation, and very little medication was required.

One case of measles has broken out in camp, but the patient was promptly isolated, and no second case has occurred. Should the infection spread it might work havoc among the young recruits, as was the case in the Sixties. Only four cases of acute alcoholism are recorded. It would appear that the men already begin to realize that alcohol must be avoided if effective campaigning is to be carried on under a tropical sun.

Four cases of vaccinia are reported. Several hundred vaccinations have been performed in the field, aside from many that were practised upon the troops before leaving their respective posts. The virus, contained in hermetically-sealed tubes (Sternberg's), has given such a large percentage of successes in persons not vaccinated for five years previously, that I feel confident a person in whom it does not "take" is already immune.

Three gunshot wounds and one saber thrust are reported, all probably accidental and without fatality. The first semiweekly medical returns show fifty-four cases of sickness among nearly 5000 men; only a little more than one per cent. non-effective, a very gratifying condition of affairs.

Since the publication of my letter on "The Medical Organization of the United States Forces at Tampa," some modifications in the general plan therein outlined have been made leaning toward the fuller equipment of the regimental hospital organization, so as to allow each regimental surgeon a personnel consisting of at least three privates and one acting hospital steward, and an allotment of one red-cross ambulance with two horses, one hospital tent, and one wall-tent.

In view, also, of our immediate embarkation for Cuba, there has been issued to each regimental surgeon one field surgical box containing the following named articles, specially selected and packed under lock and key for this campaign: Schering's sterilizer, lamp, etc., 1; rubber gloves, 4 pairs; rubber envelopes, 2; finger-cots, assorted sizes, 2 dozen; rubber aprons, 2; green soap, 2 pounds; Halsted's rubber cylinders, 4; gauze bandages, three sizes, 300; gauze sublimated bandages, one meter long, 300; absorbent cotton, in one-ounce packages, 150; iodoform gauze, one-half meter length, 50; catgut ligatures, three sizes, 150; silk ligatures, strands, 150; rubber irrigation-bags, 2; compressed sponges, cotton, 24 dozen. Each box, with its contents, weighs 140 pounds.

HENRY I. RAYMOND,
Captain and Assistant Surgeon, United States Army.

ARMY LIFE IN 1861-1865.[1]

BY PROFESSOR HENRY P. BOWDITCH, M.D.,
OF HARVARD UNIVERSITY.

THOSE of us who, in 1861, saw how the sons of Harvard sprang to arms at their country's call little thought that they would live to witness a repetition of the call and the response. For months we had watched the heavy war cloud gather on the Southern horizon as one State after another strove to pluck its star from our Nation's banner. Gloom and doubt filled every breast. The condition of the country was of course the one theme of conversation in every group of students, and many men who afterward fought well for their country did not at this time hesitate to express their conviction that "if the whole South wanted to secede we should have to let them go." This condition of uncertainty grew daily more and more intolerable, till at last, in the words of the Phi Beta Kappa poet of that year,

" . . . a red flash like lightning across the darkness broke
And with a voice that shook the land the guns of Sumter spoke."

How the men of Harvard replied to that voice this stately building rose to bear witness.

And now Harvard may be called upon to arm herself again for battle, but under very different conditions. There has been no insult to our flag demanding instant atonement in blood. We are engaged in a war in which our part may perhaps be best described as that of ministers of fate charged with the duty of exacting from Spain the penalty of her four centuries of misrule, oppression, and cruelty. Let us see to it that we perform this function with dignity and self-restraint. Though the call for troops is not yet so urgent as to make every Harvard man feel, as he felt in 1861, that he must be able to show good cause if he fails to don the uniform, yet it may well happen that in the progress of hostilities complications with other Powers may arise, and that the war power of the Nation may be taxed to the utmost. In view of the possibility that our country may require the services of all her loyal sons, it is well for the present generation of Harvard men to take counsel with their older brethren to see if perchance the experience of a former generation may contain useful lessons for those who are about to undertake the unfamiliar duties of the soldier.

The class which will graduate next month stands in the same relation to the war with Spain as the class to which I belong stood to the War of Secession. That is, the members of the class who enter the service of the country will pass directly from academic to military occupations, and the figures of the student and the warrior decorating the window of the class of 1861 in the neighboring hall will seem to be as appropriate for the class of 1898 as for the class which placed the window in position.

Since those of you who pass at once from the college to the camp will have no preparation for army life except that which the university affords, it seems to me important to inquire how far an academic training may fit a student for a military life. In other words, what advantages, if any, does a college-bred man, entering the army or navy, have over a man who has not been trained in college halls? In the first place we like to think that Harvard men are so much in the habit of striving for high ideals that their conduct in the field will be guided by the noblest of motives; that they will not take up the calling of the soldier from a mere love of adventure, or from a restless desire for a change, but from a profound conviction that war, while it should always be the last argument to which nations resort, must, in order that it may not fail to carry conviction, be urged with all the power which the contestants have at their disposal.

In the second place, it seems to me that a very obvious advantage possessed by the college man is the power of rapidly acquiring and practically utilizing the information contained in books. It was a matter of common observation in the army that men of considerable intelligence, but without a liberal education, often had a good deal of difficulty in understanding a military movement from a printed description of it, although, when it had once been shown on the field, it was grasped and retained in all its details. It was this power, in the early days of the war when officers and men were alike ignorant of their duties, which enabled the young college-bred lieutenants to read up their tactics in the morning and drill their men in the afternoon. This, of course, is not to be regarded as the most desirable way of securing a well-drilled army, but when an army had to be improvised in the shortest possible time, the faculties of students trained in cramming for examinations served an excellent purpose.

There is one other inestimable advantage which you young men will have in entering upon a military career, and that is the advantage of youth. Youth is not troubled with misgivings. Doubts come with age. You will not shrink from any responsibility which you are ordered to assume from a doubt about your ability to perform the task. I have often thought that if I had been asked at any time during the last twenty years to take command of troops or execute military orders, as I did unhesitatingly before I was twenty-five years old, I should have felt and perhaps said, "This is no work for me. I have had no experience which will justify me in assuming such a responsibility."

Fortunately for the country no such feelings entered the minds of the young men who fought in the war of 1861. If they had stopped to think whether they were fitted for their task the war would never have been fought. You too, if you enter your country's service will assume your new duties with the same feeling of confidence that the end will justify your efforts, thus furnishing an illustration of a lesson which, if I mistake not, you have all learned from your professor in psychology, *viz.*, that an absolute faith in one's own power to accomplish a given result is an important, perhaps the most important, factor in determining the result itself. Let us trust that your individual experiences will conclusively demonstrate this principle.

[1] Professor Bowditch, who was a cavalry officer during the Civil War, recently gave a "war talk" at Sander's Theater, Cambridge, before the students of Harvard University. Through his courtesy the MEDICAL NEWS is enabled to publish the accompanying short abstract of his remarks.

MEDICAL PROGRESS.

The Incubation Period of Malaria Experimentally Lengthened.—CELLI and SANTORINI (*Fortschrt. der Med.*, January 15, 1898), by rendering animals somewhat immune with malarial parasites, and by taking their serum and injecting it into patients before inoculation, have been able to delay the period of incubation of the parasites from an average of thirteen days to an average of twenty-five days; that is to say, the incubation period has been doubled. In autumnal fever the incubation period has been found to range from two to five days, the mean being three days. Men who were treated with serum of immunized animals, and afterward infected with malarial poison, were found to have an incubation period ranging from six to seventeen days, but the investigators were not able to prevent altogether the infection by this method of treatment, even in a single case.

Advantage of Previous Castration in the Diagnosis of Stone in the Bladder.—HORWITZ (*Therap. Gaz.*, February 15, 1898) mentions four cases in which he was unable to make a diagnosis of stone in the bladder until the atrophy of the prostate gland which followed double castration enabled him to pass a stone-searcher and establish the diagnosis. The youngest of these four patients was sixty-two years old. All presented symptoms of cystitis, and in the most of them the existence of stone was strongly suspected. In every case the atrophy of the prostate was sufficient in from ten to fourteen days after castration to allow the passage of the stone-searcher. One of the stones was small and soft, and was crushed and washed out. In the other three patients a suprapubic cystotomy was performed, with complete success. It is interesting to note that an attempt was made in two of these cases by means of the Röntgen-rays to determine the presence of the stone, but without success. Horwitz has no hesitation in recommending this method of procedure to patients of advanced age with enlarged prostate glands where the symptoms point to the presence of a stone if the diagnosis cannot be determined by instrumentation.

Suture of an Artery.—BRIAU (*Echo Medical, Lyon*, March 15, 1898) succeeded in making a complete circular suture of the carotid artery in an animal. The wound healed and the continuity of the vessel was not interrupted. The wall of the vessel showed only small traces of the suture, and at the points where pressure had been applied so as to control the flow of blood there were slight white thrombi. The inner coats of the artery were approximated with great care, and the thread was kept out of its lumen in order not to form a starting-point for a thrombus.

Dangers of Ligating the Axillary Artery.—SOUPART (*Belgique Médicale*, March 24, 1898), in commenting upon an instance of gangrene of the arm following ligation of the axillary artery, says that the ligation of this vessel between the subscapular branch and deep humeral ought to be proscribed in surgery, except in those cases in which an irregular arrangement of its branches allows the radial pulse to be felt after compression of the axillary at the point at which it is proposed to apply a ligature. Thus for axillary aneurism the vessel has been successfully tied in the situation referred to. However, for all such troubles, it is both easier and safer, and equally successful, to tie the subclavian rather than the axillary artery.

THERAPEUTIC NOTES.

A Simple Method of Curing an Ingrowing Nail.—TARDIF (*Anjou Médicale*, February 1, 1898) says that he has been able to cure all cases of ingrowing nail, without recourse to the knife. He proceeds as follows: With a flat probe, or a match, he slips a bit of cotton between the edge of the nail and the inflamed flesh. Another strip of cotton is put along the outer margin of the ulcerated area, and the space between these two strips of cotton, and which is occupied by the ulcer, is thickly powdered with nitrate of lead. The whole is covered with cotton, and the toe is bandaged. The dressings are repeated the following day, and every day until the incarcerated edge of the nail is plainly visible. Usually four or five dressings suffice. Then with patience the edge of the nail is lifted away from the flesh and a bit of cotton is introduced under it, to keep it up. As it grows it will gradually take its proper position above the flesh, this having in the meantime shrunk and shriveled by reason of the applications of lead nitrate. The lead is to be discontinued as soon as it appears that the exuberance of the fleshy bed of the nail has been overcome. The difficulty seldom recurs. If this does happen it is necessary to repeat the treatment from the beginning.

Treatment of Diarrhea in Children by Sterilized Water.—MONGOUR (*Correspondenz-Blatt f. Schweiz Aerzte*, April, 1898) says that the intestines of infants suffering from gastro-enteritis contain in great numbers, and in a high degree of virulence, those bacteria which produce abnormal fermentations in the articles of food which they ingest. There are therefore two indications for treatment; first, to free the intestines as quickly as possible from the products of fermentation, and second, either to frequently change the contents, in which the bacteria develop, or else to keep these fluids in an aseptic condition. The first indication is secured by laxatives, but these cannot be many times repeated in the case of a weakened child. Asepsis of the intestine cannot with certainty be obtained. It is easy, however, to frequently renew the nourishment, although such children suffer more from lack of water than from lack of food. Moreover, water is one of the poorest media for the development of bacteria which it is safe to introduce into the stomach. The clinical results are in accord with this theory, and if a child is given from ten to twelve ounces of sterilized water daily vomiting will cease at once, diarrhea will soon disappear, and the temperature will fall so that in a relatively short time milk can again be given. Absolutely no medicine will be required. Mongour has obtained most brilliant results from this simple treatment.

THE MEDICAL NEWS.

A WEEKLY JOURNAL

OF MEDICAL SCIENCE.

COMMUNICATIONS are invited from all parts of the world. Original articles contributed *exclusively* to THE MEDICAL NEWS will after publication be liberally paid for (accounts being rendered quarterly), or 250 reprints will be furnished in place of other remuneration. When necessary to elucidate the text, illustrations will be engraved from drawings or photographs furnished by the author. Manuscripts should be typewritten.

Address the Editor: J. RIDDLE GOFFE, M.D.,
No. 111 FIFTH AVENUE (corner of 18th St.), NEW YORK.

Subscription Price, including postage in U. S. and Canada.

PER ANNUM IN ADVANCE $4.00
SINGLE COPIES 10
WITH THE AMERICAN JOURNAL OF THE MEDICAL SCIENCES, PER ANNUM 7.50

Subscriptions may begin at any date. The safest mode of remittance is by bank check or postal money order, drawn to the order of the undersigned. When neither is accessible, remittances may be made, at the risk of the publishers, by forwarding in *registered* letters.

LEA BROTHERS & CO.,
No. 111 FIFTH AVENUE (corner of 18th St.), NEW YORK, AND NOS. 706, 708 & 710 SANSOM ST., PHILADELPHIA.

SATURDAY, JUNE 4, 1898.

THE DENVER MEETING OF THE AMERICAN MEDICAL ASSOCIATON.

THE annual pilgrimage of the faithful has already begun, and the numerous pilgrims are now centering at Denver preparatory to laying their contributions upon the sacred altar of Science at that Sanitary Mecca of so many of the afflicted ones of this world. Not all of these pilgrims, however, are burdened with offerings; indeed, it is quite safe to say that a goodly proportion have left such burdens behind them, and are journeying thence in search of recreation, rest, and enjoyment. This, however, should be no reflection upon the character of the assembly, for the serious concerns of the doctor's life are so constantly with him that an annual excursion in which the chief motive is a change of air or social fellowship with his professional brethren, even though it has only the mildest flavor of scientific and professional work, is good for the doctor, and indirectly beneficial to the patients whom he has left at home.

There is every assurance that the Denver gathering will be strong in all the features that make up a successful meeting. Some fears have been expressed lest the president of the Association would be detained and unable to be present, but General Sternberg has made provision for a brief absence from his pressing official duties, and announces that he will certainly be present for at least a part of the meeting. The programs of the various sections give promise of most instructive discussions, and the number and character of the men who will take part insure to the scientific features of the meeting a full measure of success.

The profession of Denver has been wide awake to the opportunity this meeting affords of giving the medical men from the various parts of the country who will assemble there, not only a bird's-eye view, but a quasi initiation into the elements of, the climate and soil that make Colorado the Mecca of health-resorts.

The Greater New York excursion train started on Thursday evening last, and by the time this notice reaches our readers will be approaching the end of its journey. A similar train has gone from Philadelphia, and the Chicago train, known as the Journal Train, is expected to leave Saturday night, June 4th.

The entertainment that has been provided at Denver by the local profession is most attractive, and the excursions into the mountains and to Colorado Springs and its vicinage will afford interesting diversion and prove restful to tired brains and nerves. No band of men and women can be happier or more jovial than doctors and their wives when thrown together in these annual outings. With the stimulus of Colorado air and scenes the customary exuberance will doubtless be overflowing.

The MEDICAL NEWS has made arrangements for a prompt and complete report of this meeting, which will appear in the next issue.

THE RECENT MEETING OF THE AMERICAN NEUROLOGICAL ASSOCIATION.

THE twenty-fifth annual meeting of the American Neurological Association, held at New York last week, was, both in point of attendance and in the scientific efforts that it called forth, the most successful in the annals of this important and vigorous society. Altogether forty-three communications were presented, many of which were of great practical importance, while others were genuinely scientific in the highest sense of the term.

Dr. Wm. Osler's paper on the combined symptoms of myxedema and Graves' disease, occurring without discernible cause in a young man, and leading quickly to a fatal issue, was one of the most interesting clinical contributions. The fact that symptoms of myxedema develop in patients who have suffered for a considerable time with Graves' disease is universally recognized, a number of such cases having been recorded; but the simultaneous development of these two diseases, which in causation, course, and pathogenesis seem to be antithetical, must be extremely rare. The report of such a case prompts one to think anew of the functions of the thyroid gland, which seems to stand in such important genetic relation to both of these diseases.

A disease whose clinical course and morbid anatomy received satisfactory explanation is one that is now known, perhaps temporarily, as amaurotic family idiocy. At the present time about thirty cases of this remarkable disease are on record, although but a few years have elapsed since it was first described. All writers on the disease are in accord concerning its occurrence solely in the Jewish race, its onset after birth, its progressive course characterized by idiocy and bodily decay, and its fatal termination in from a few months to a year or two after its onset. Heretofore the lesions constituting the basis of the disease have not been satisfactorily understood, but the communications on this subject by Drs. Hirsch and Holden go far toward filling this gap in our knowledge. The former demonstrated a large number of sections taken from different parts of the central nervous system, which showed very clearly that there was a slowly progressive widespread degeneration of the cerebrospinal system, like unto that caused by toxic agencies; a gradual destruction of the ganglion cells or parenchyma of the various components of the central nervous system. The latter investigator showed that changes exactly analogous occurred in an extra-cranial part of the brain: the retina. Dr. Holden's communication served also to emphasize the necessity of studying the retina in cases of nervous disease and of employing the same histological technic as that which had been of such signal service in unraveling the intricacies of neuropathology.

Of the purely scientific contributions one presented by Drs. B. Onuf and Joseph Collins, on the localization of the sympathetic nerves in the cerebrospinal system, deserves especial mention. These investigators showed from experiments on cats, consisting of extirpation of different segments and ganglia of the sympathetic system, that the mesal and lateral portions of the gray matter of the spinal cord and corresponding parts of the oblongata are the seat of the sympathetic nerves. By using the Marchi and Nissl methods of staining they were able to follow the degenerations resulting from the extirpation of ganglia to certain groups of cells in the spinal cord, especially to one situated mesad and ventrad of the central canal, which they call the paracentral group, and to a lateral marginal group, and in the oblongata to the dorsal vagus nucleus. The importance of these researches bearing on many obscure questions in pathogenesis and symptomatology of nervous diseases, such as the occurrence of visceral symptoms and crises in tabes, pupillary, ocular, and trophic symptoms in syringomyelia, and in injuries of the spinal cord, as well as in clearing up many mooted points in connection with the physiology and symptomatology of the pneumogastric, was brought out in the paper and in the discussion which followed.

A paper on the morbid anatomy and the surgical treatment of the tic-douloureux by Drs. W. W. Keen and W. G. Spiller goes far toward answering the questions, How much can be expected from surgical treatment in this most intolerable of all diseases, and when should such treatment be resorted to. After Hartley, Krause, and other surgeons showed that the Gasserian ganglion could be successfully removed there was a decided tendency on the part of neurologists, both here and abroad, to recommend this measure to patients whose suffering resisted all other therapy, but the frightful mortality attending the operation, and the comparatively transient relief that it gave soon deterred them save in those few instances in which it was absolutely incumbent to adopt the most heroic measures to stay the sufferer from suicide.

Since then surgeons have been assiduously at work to perfect the details of the operation so that to-day the percentage of mortality is less than one-fourth, while the certainty with which all of the ganglion can be removed, and without great laceration, insures a large percentage of cures or protracted and acceptable amelioration. The authors concluded that the operation of extirpation of the ganglion should never be resorted to until every form of therapy, including peripheral operations of resection and exsection the fifth nerve, had failed. In this conclusion we heartily concur.

Many other noteworthy and most suggestive papers were read. Taking it altogether the neurologists have every reason to feel satisfied with this year's convocation.

NURSES FOR THE ARMY AND NAVY.

THE question of nurses for the wounded and sick of the Army and Navy is an extremely important one. At the present writing, when thousands of enlisted recruits and soldiers of the regular army have gone to the Philippines, and when we are apparently on the eve of throwing all our available forces into Cuba, the need for thoroughly trained and disciplined nurses subservient to the orders of the Surgeon-General is a pressing one. It is a matter of history, as well as of common experience, that death claims more victims through sickness, pestilence, and neglect, which always hover around an army, and particularly when in the tropics, than it does through the missiles of the enemy. Despite this, scarcely any provision has yet been made to combat the mortality arising from insufficient care and nursing of the sick and those not mortally wounded in the present conflict. We have been informed that the Surgeon-General of the Army purposed not to employ any female trained nurses during the campaign, yet we note that four female nurses have recently been engaged and sent to the Army Hospital at Key West. This is probably the beginning of a movement very propitious for the soldier and the sailor which will be looked upon with favor. There is no dearth of trained, graduate nurses in this country—in fact the supply during the past few years has been enormously in excess of the demand—who would willingly enter the service if given adequate remuneration. Their presence in the bays of hospital ships and in hospital camps would prove a most desirable addition.

It is regrettable that no provision exists for the training of nurses for our Army similar to that in vogue in England. Years ago, the English Government, recognizing how necessary it is to have the assistance of capable women in caring for sick and wounded troops, established a training-school for female nurses in connection with the army hospitals and medical school at Netley. The work which these women have since done with Robert's soldiers in India and with Wolseley's in Egypt has received the highest praise and commendation and has more than justified their professional existence. In this country we have hospitals at Washington, West Point, and other places in connection with the Army where nurses could be properly trained and fitted to meet such emergencies as the one now upon us. Moreover, the Marine Hospital Service, which is to-day one of the most efficient departments of the Government, would be an ideal place for the preparation of such nurses. True it is that the Red Cross Society has for one of the purposes of its existence the furnishing of nurses both for the side of the friend and of the enemy, and no one can fail to appreciate the immense amount of good which this organization may encompass, but it would be ludicrous, if it were not so sad, to read the accounts in the daily papers of the young women who are volunteering to enter the society as nurses from all over the country, and who come to New York, and we presume to other cities, to receive a course of training of a week's duration, which they are deluded enough to believe will fit them for caring for the sick.

In many instances the instruction is given by physicians who have never seen a battle-field nor a hospital ship; and whose knowledge of many of the tropical diseases which the nurses are expected to combat, have been gained solely from text-books. Many of these volunteers are women of the finest spirit, animated by a desire to make the misery and suffering of their brothers who are defending the honor of their country less poignant, and whose patriotic sentiment is akin to a touch of the Divine wand. Others, however, are emotional and notoriety-seeking, who see in this an opportunity to add a new stimulus to their sentient souls and who enjoy the hysterical exaltation and enthusiasm of it all. In their imagery and highly colored dreams they see themselves clad in the robes of a sister of the Red Cross moving about a battle-field strewn with bleeding, dying, and agonized men, giving a word of comfort and solace to him whose life is ebbing, binding up the wounds and staunching the blood of him whose spirit is struggling to open the golden gate, receiving a message of love for those at home from another who is already en route across the Stygian River; in short, they picture a realization of the inspiring, if conventional, picture of the ministering angel on the battle-field after the smoke has cleared away. But how different the realization. The nurse never sees the battle-field, except in rare instances. Her duty calls her to the hospital ward, at camp or on shipboard; there she is the physician's left hand, and oftentimes his right. To be the one, or both, cool-headed, non-emotional, properly trained, mature women are needed, and the surest way of getting them is to train them as every other Army servant is trained.

ECHOES AND NEWS.

The Problems of Charity.—The recent National Conference on Charities by one passing incident, served to punctuate the essential difficulty that attends all attempts at giving. Bishop Henry C. Potter did this in reminding his audience of the old-time epigram of Henry Ward Beecher that "The next worst thing to not helping a man is helping him."

Position of Women Physicians in Russia.—A decree has just been issued in Russia permitting women physicians to enter the Government service. By this fact women in Russia have won an important privilege. The Government service carries with it extremely liberal pensions. It is expected that this will be the forerunner of other extensions of privilege to women.

The Anatomy of the Drawing-Room.—Not long ago an officer died at a certain British military station. At an afternoon "at home" of one of the leading ladies on the station, the captain's death was mentioned, and the hostess who knew all about it, volunteered the information that he had died of disease of the kidneys, adding, with some unction and a little bashfulness, "how thankful we women ought to be that we have no kidneys."

The Medical College Laboratory Sues the University of the City of New York.—The Medical College Laboratory of the City of New York, which is in fact the former Medical Department of the University, has brought an action in the Supreme Court against the University to recover property which it recently conveyed to that Institution. The brief also attempts to enjoin the defendant, pending the suit, from disposing of the property or collecting the rents.

Army Surgeons Detailed as Delegates to the Denver Meeting.—The following named officers are detailed to represent the Medical Department of the Army at the annual meeting of the American Medical Association to be held in the City of Denver, Colorado, June 7 to 10, 1898: Lieutenant-Colonel Alfred A. Woodhull, deputy surgeon-general; Major Curtis E. Munn, surgeon.

Summer Recreation for New York Children.—Two of the large recreation-piers, extending about one-eighth of a mile into the moving currents of water and air on either side of the city have been opened to the public for the season. These piers are two stories in height, and each will afford spacious accommodations for from 10,000 to 12,000 women and children. The Association for Improving the Condition of the Poor will undertake this summer to pay all the expenses of managing fifteen public-school playgrounds as small parks for the people. The plan contemplates the use of the roof and basement playgrounds, the presence of kindergartners to direct the games of the children, and an adequate supply of clean sand in which the children may frolic.

Advance in Oral Instruction of the Deaf in Illinois.—Dr. J. C. Gordon, Superintendent of the Illinois Deaf and Dumb Institute at Jacksonville, reports progress in respect to the instruction for deaf and dumb in the State, and says: "A notable development in the past few years has been the advancement made in both the quality and the extent of oral instruction. The attitude of the State school toward the instruction of the deaf in speech and lip reading has always been liberal and progressive. Ten years ago nearly thirty-five per cent. of the pupils were receiving oral instruction. At present fifty-five per cent. are in the oral department, in which speech and lip reading are the ordinary means of communication, or are receiving special instruction in this art every school day."

Christian-Science Healing Invades England.—The Christian-Science lunacy is just now invading England. Investigators are taking it in hand, but find difficulty in making much out of it as a real curative factor. There, as here, it is found to offend common sense, contravene human experience, and run counter to Infallible Writ. An English investigator of the States, in the *Westminster Gazette*, says that he "could extract no coherent scheme of teaching from the mystical negation of matter," and that the thing "certain about it" is that "fees are charged for the treatment, and persons initiated into the arena of scientific healing are required to pay $100 for the same." If its money-making features were removed it would soon lose its charm and attraction for its professional advocates.

Dangerous Odors.—Berzelius, who discovered the element called "selenium," once tried the experiment of permitting a bubble of pure hydrogen selenide gas to enter his nostrils. For days afterward he was not able to smell strong ammonia, the olfactory nerves being temporarily paralyzed. Selenium gas has the odor of putrid horse-radish. Tellurium is even worse. There is a story of a physician whose patient, a lady, refused to take an absolutely necessary rest because she was so fond of being always on the go in society. He gave her a pill containing a small quantity of tellurium, and her breath was affected by it to such an extent that she was not able to appear in public for a month. She never guessed what the trouble was. The volatilized essential oil of roses is supposed to cause "rose cold." This peculiar complaint is so far nervous in its character that paper roses sometimes excite it.

Official List of Changes in the Stations and Duties of Officers Serving in the Medical Department, United States Army, from May 17, 1898, to May 23, 1898. *Washington, D. C., May 26, 1898.*—The following named officers of the Medical Department will proceed to San Francisco, Cal., and report for duty with the expedition to the Philippine Islands: Lieutenant-Colonel Henry Lippincott, deputy surgeon-general; Captain William O. Owen, assistant-surgeon; Captain Edward R. Morris, assistant-surgeon; 1st Lieutenant Henry Page, assistant surgeon. Acting Assistant-Surgeon Douglas F. Duval, U. S. Army, will proceed from this city to West Point, N. Y., and report for duty at the U. S. Military Academy. Acting Assistant-Surgeon S. Melville Waterhouse, U. S. Army, will proceed from this city to Fort Hamilton, N. Y., and report for duty at that station. Major William B. Davis, surgeon, is assigned to duty in charge of the general hospital at Fort Myer, Va., in addition to his duties as surgeon at that post. Acting Assistant-Surgeon David Baker, U. S. Army, will proceed from Waltonville, Ill., to Fort Thomas, Ky., and report for duty in the general hospital at that place. Acting Assistant-Surgeon George H. Richardson, U. S. Army, will proceed from this city to San Francisco, Cal., and report in person to the Commanding General of the expedition to the Philippine Islands for duty. Acting Assistant-Surgeon Arthur Jordan, U. S. Army, will proceed from Richmond, Va., to Mobile, Ala., and report for duty with troops in the field at that place. Major William H. Corbusier, surgeon, is relieved from duty at Angel Island, Cal., and assigned to duty as acting medical-purveyor of the expedition to the Philippine Islands. Captain Charles B. Ewing, assistant-surgeon, will proceed at once to New Orleans, La., and report to the commanding officer, 5th Cavalry, for duty. Acting Assistant-Surgeon Frederick J. Combe, U. S. Army, will proceed from Brownsville, Tex., to Tampa, Fla., and report for duty with troops in the field at that place. Acting Assistant-Surgeon Clarence J. Manly, U. S. Army, will proceed from this city to Fort Thomas, Ky., and report for duty in the general hospital at that place. Acting Assistant-Surgeon Ira A. Shimer, U. S. Army, will proceed from this city to Fort Myer, Va., and report for duty in the general hospital at that place. A contract having been made with Dr. A. D. McArthur of Littleton, Col., for duty as acting assistant-surgeon at Fort Logan, Col., he will proceed to that post and report to the commanding officer for duty to relieve Acting Assistant-Surgeon Carroll E. Edson, whose contract is about to terminate.

CORRESPONDENCE.

AN IMPROVED METHOD OF TREATING IVY POISONING.

To the Editor of the MEDICAL NEWS.

DEAR SIR: With the advent of summer that very annoying skin irritation resulting from exposure to the poison-ivy will make its appearance. Having been annoyed at the persistence of the dermatitis caused by it in spite of the use of medicated oils, ointments, and lotions, I was led during the summer of 1897 to use collodion (contractile) freely in such cases, with very gratifying results. The benefits derived from its use are the relief of itching, the cessation of the extension of the dermatitis, and the rapid subsidence of that which is already present.

The collodion should be freely applied when the diagnosis is first made and every inflamed patch and any isolated vesicles entirely covered, also to a slight extent the surrounding healthy skin. The result is that the inflamed parts are no longer exposed to the air and the itching and burning usually cease. The collodion contracting slightly, exerts some pressure on the inflammatory area and seems to squeeze the vesicles out of existence.

The patient should be directed to reapply the collodion whenever any cracking occurs in that already applied, and, indeed, to paint it over all the affected parts once or twice a day; also, to immediately cover any new patches that may appear. Used in this way without other treatment I have been enabled to cure this disease in from two to four days, the usual duration being from one to two weeks.

W. F. MARTIN, M.D.

COLORADO SPRINGS, COL., May 25, 1898.

THE LIFE-INSURANCE COMPANY AND ITS ENCROACHMENT UPON PERSONAL RIGHTS.

To the Editor of the MEDICAL NEWS.

DEAR SIR: A number of idealists and enthusiasts designate the Life-Insurance Company a public benefactor, totally ignoring the important fact that it is a purely mercantile enterprise founded on business principles and intended to yield lucrative results. As a mercantile institution it has the right, nay, even the obligation, to protect itself and those already insured against possible loss. To accomplish this it adopts, as is perfectly right and proper, more or less stringent tests for those seeking admittance. Based on the same ground as that on which the business man refuses credit to a customer of doubtful standing, the Life-Insurance Company, considering it a financial undertaking, may exert its right to reject habitually those applicants whose family records from a medical standpoint are deficient, whose renal excretions present so-called abnormal constituents (even if they be without specific significance), and may debar from admittance those who are laboring under certain systemic conditions, inherited or acquired, or are afflicted with well-defined diseases, no matter of how comparatively innocent a nature these affections may be. In short, the Life-Insurance Company may be justified in adopting such conservative methods as will secure profitable results, and in regard to the rules it has laid down, though they may seem ever so preposterous, there is no contention.

If a life-insurance institution demands a rigid physical

examination of the applicant it is the duty of the examiner to make it as thorough and complete as possible, both in justice to the applicant and to the company, and the benefit of a reasonable doubt should be extended to the latter.

But is the examination as to the physical condition of the applicant a thorough and trustworthy one in every case? Does it not frequently decree against the applicant in an arbitrary manner? A number of instances have been brought to my notice in which the company's physician caused the rejection of the applicant on account of the apparent occurrence of dextrose in the urine. Now it seems to me that an experienced and careful examiner cannot possibly mistake the presence of a certain urinary constituent for glucose; if he does, he is either a novice in the profession or else extremely careless, and such a physician is in no way qualified to be an examiner of life-insurance applicants.

A competent and careful examiner is acquainted with and guards against the inaccuracies and insufficiencies of certain methods in the detection of dextrose. He knows that other bodies may occur in the urine besides glucose which possess the power of reducing copper compounds. He is aware of the fact when applying one of the copper tests (still the most common tests in vogue) that a number of normal urinary constituents, especially when they occur in excessive amounts as uric acid, the urates, creatinine, hippuric acid, and hypoxanthin may bring about a similar reduction of the copper solutions as does dextrose, and that a variety of abnormal urinary bodies as indican and alkaptone, and some alkaloids, and tannin, gallic acid, pyrogallo, camphor, copaiba, cubebs, and also some other carbohydrates possess analogous copper-reducing properties. Moreover, the painstaking and conscientious examiner will never omit to apply control-tests when he makes use of one or the other copper solution, and he will never fail to employ two or more testing methods when the presence of glucose or any other abnormal constituent is suspected.

A colleague, aged forty-five years, of good physique, good family history, and good habits, applied for life insurance in one of our companies. He was rejected on account of "diabetes." Numerous examinations of his urine did not reveal to me any glucose, nor does his general condition warrant the assumption of a glycosuric or diabetic state. The applicant himself was and still is in the habit of examining his urine from time to time, and as yet has never detected any grape sugar or any other abnormal constituent. The "inefficient examiner" was evidently mistaken and negligent. Possibly his Fehling's solution had deteriorated; possibly the few pieces of chemical apparatus used were not previously thoroughly cleaned. No matter what caused the apparent copper reduction, it was this official's duty to apply at least one control-test to ascertain the presence of glucose. Had he done so, the rejection of the applicant on account of "diabetes" could not have occurred. I have selected this case from a number of others which I have in mind as it occurred recently, and as the applicant is a well-informed, conscientious and trustworthy physician.

The insurance companies—among themselves—have established some kind of a bureau of information for mutual protection. The data as to the physical condition of a rejected applicant are cheerfully transmitted from the medical director of one company to that of another, who, when called upon, will return this favor. In other words, *the insurance companies have combined to form a trust* —if I may so term it—*to effect the exclusion of certain applicants.*

The cited case will illustrate how unreliable the data as to the state of health of an applicant may occasionally be. Thus a reasonably healthy man may be debarred from obtaining *any* life insurance. The companies will ostracize him because at some possibly remote period an incompetent examiner alleged to have found diabetic sugar or another abnormal urinary constituent. True, the company may grant a subsequent examination to the applicant after some months have elapsed, and the applicant may present himself for such an examination at the "home office," but is it not remarkable that in the rarest instances the second examination reverses the unfavorable verdict of the first?

Furthermore, it may even occur at times that the medical director of one company will ignore the report of the same officer of another institution as to the bodily condition of an applicant, but how often will the medical chief of the average company be unbiased enough to overlook a previous examination made for another association which proved disadvantageous to the applicant?

Under these existing conditions there seems to be an urgent necessity of reform. Is it not the duty of the governments of the different States in which the life-insurance companies are transacting business to ameliorate this unjust state of affairs? Is it not the duty of the government of the State to protect the individual interests of the inhabitants? While one company has a perfect right to reject a candidate who is unsound, it has no authority whatsoever to communicate and circulate the information privately obtained under the supposed seal of professional secrecy. Do the physicians who are connected with the insurance companies deem themselves not subject to the laws of propriety observed by the other members of the medical profession?

Most States, if not all, have a department of insurance. The Superintendent of Insurance of the State of New York acts as a general public overseer of the whole insurance system. But while the Insurance Department thus protects the *insured*, it does not protect the *insurable* public from the encroachments of the companies. In this connection the people may demand: (1) That the Insurance Department of every State create a special medical board to supervise the medical departments of the life-insurance companies, and to examine and license physicians who wish to devote themselves to life-insurance work. (2) That the medical departments of the insurance companies shall be forbidden to communicate to each other any knowledge as to the physical condition of an applicant obtained by and from an examination of the same; that such a communication shall be considered a breach of a privileged communication; that it shall be deemed a conspiracy between the insurance companies in thus imparting and receiving such communication, and be punishable as such.

The following propositions, were they constitutionally authorized, would still more assist the advocated cause: (*a*) That each and every insurance company file an authoritative statement with the State Department of Insurance setting forth its classes of insurance, its standards and limits for the acceptance of an applicant. (*b*) That the State Department of Insurance may deputize one or more physicians to inquire into the state of health of a rejected applicant, provided the same applies to the department on a prescribed formula, signed by two reputable practitioners of medicine, who state why an official examination should be made. (*c*) That the insurance companies be compelled to insure the applicant if the medical examination ordered by the Department of Insurance pronounce the same elegible, and that he shall enter that class of insurance for which he is conditionally (*a*) qualified.

HEINRICH STERN, M.D.

NEW YORK, May 16, 1898.

OUR FOREIGN LETTER.

[From our Special Correspondent.]

BEHRING AND THE TUBERCLE TOXIN—BEHRING'S NEW LABORATORY—DIPHTHERIA SERUM AT HOCHST—TETANUS AND THE TETANO-ANTITOXIN IN NERVOUS TISSUE—THE UNIVERSITY CLINICS AT MARBURG.

MARBURG, Germany, May 21, 1898.

THE political press had said so much of Behring's communication to the Congress of Hygiene in Madrid as to a cure for tuberculosis that I was naturally anxious to hear definitely what there was in it. That there was a great deal of exaggeration in the popular reports I felt sure. Daily newspapers are all very well in their way, but when it comes to war news and medical, especially therapeutic, discoveries, it is advisable to wait to hear what they say next day or next week before putting too much faith in to-day's announcements.

Professor Behring himself proved ready to say what the drift of his recent communication had been. Its first formal appearance in print will be in French, the manuscript immediately after translation to be given to the *Deutsche Medicinische Wochenschrift*. He is, of course, not at all pleased that the political press has given the idea publicity that he has discovered a new antitoxic serum or tuberculin for tuberculosis. He has even thought it advisable to make a formal public correction of such reports in the *Temps*, one of the most prominent of the Parisian newspapers.

His paper at Madrid merely discussed the results of the experiments that he has been carrying on at Marburg for some time with the toxins of tuberculosis. He has found that there is a series of toxic substances produced by the growth of tubercle bacilli in cultures. One of these at least he has been able to segregate, and he finds that it possesses a toxic power at least one hundred times as great as that of Koch's old tuberculin. Observations with this on the smaller animals are almost hopelessly unsatisfactory owing to the fact that a fatal issue so often enters into the experiments. On the larger animals, however, Behring has found that the reaction so faithfully sought for by Koch in his experiments with the old and the new tuberculin is produced by this new and powerful agent. In the blood of cattle infected with tuberculosis and then injected with this tubercle toxin a very striking therapeutic effect is produced. Whether this effect consists in the production of certain sozalbumins, an antitoxin for the animal itself, or whether it is a cell-stimulus that arouses tissues to new resistive vitality is not clear. It is sure, however, that cattle seemingly hopelessly infected with tuberculosis have been cured by careful injections of the remedy. Further experiments are to be made on cattle at the Veterinary School in Berlin and the remedy will be thoroughly tested before its use is commended even to veterinarians. There is no question as yet of its application to human therapeutics. So much says Professor Behring himself, who is extremely modest and states absolutely only the results of actual observations. Professor Loeffler, who was at Madrid and took part in the discussion of the subject, expresses his sincere conviction that there is in these experiments with tubercle toxin the germ of even a greater discovery for therapeutics than diphtheria serum has proved to be. Koch and Behring have both been so fascinated by therapeutic results in animals that their results must be undisputed. Both are too acute observers, too well disciplined in the school of control-experiments to be deceived by a series of mere coincidences. Professor Loeffler expresses the opinion, too, that the return of Professor Koch will see a revulsion of opinion with regard to the new tuberculin R., the manufacture of which, despite reports to that effect, has not been given up.

As to the question of an antitoxin for tuberculosis on the principle of the diphtheria antitoxin Professor Behring expressed himself as very doubtful of any such thing being possible last year during a visit to Paris. Further experiments have confirmed this view. All of the mammalia practically have been experimented upon for the purpose and none produce antitoxic substances in quantities that would make their serum available therapeutically for others affected by the disease. The therapeutic reaction must, it would seem, take place in the circulation of the tuberculous themselves; no part of this reaction can be accomplished by proxy. This opinion is not absolute because it is possible that birds may yet furnish some surprises in the matter. Their reaction to their own form of the disease—aviary tuberculosis—has been carefully observed. Whether future observers will find the identity of the infections, human and aviary tuberculosis, at present a matter of dispute, and then avail themselves of the fact for human therapeutics, remains to be seen.

At Marburg, where everything is magnificently arranged for scientific work of the most exact kind, it is easy to see how much the study of tuberculosis is occupying the attention of the head of the department. The brooding chambers are filled with thousands of cultures of tubercle bacilli and other rooms contain a number of evaporating apparatuses where at a low temperature under decreased air-pressure a comparatively rapid concentration of the liquid of the cultures is secured. Not everything is given up to the study of tuberculosis, however. The observations for the still further perfection of the diphtheria antitoxin are continued and not without result.

The serum prepared under Behring's direction is put on the market by the Farbwerke (dye works, a stock company), formerly Meister, Lucius & Brenning, the well-known dye and drug manufacturers, to whom the antipyrin patent belongs. The members of the Congress for Internal Medicine at Wiesbaden were invited out to see the works at Höchst, not far from Frankfort, just after the close of the Congress. Besides seeing the preparation of the serum, they were shown the product as it is now put on the market. By a careful mixture of serums of different strengths the possibility of the most exact dosage has been secured. One may inject but 5 c.c. of serum, and in that have any number of antitoxic units required—100, 200, 300, 500, 750, etc.

An interesting fact that came out in the discussion of Behring's paper at Madrid is the observation that adults afflicted with tuberculosis do not stand injections of blood-serum well. That is to say, simple blood-serum injected into such patients produces an increased activity of bacterial growth, or else lessens tissue resistance, and so leads to a further invasion of the tuberculous process. This seems to be true, too, even of diphtheria antitoxic serum, the presence of the antitoxins not lessening this liability to undesirable and at times serious reaction in tuberculous patients.

The work on tetanus is, of course, continued under Professor Behring's direction. The discovery made in his laboratory some time ago that the central nervous substance possesses qualities that make it antitoxic for tetanus, has been confirmed by a number of observers in France and Germany. So far, however, it has been found to exist in but very small quantities, and in a practically insoluble state. None of the ordinary chemic solvents or any liquid as yet tried has taken up any of the substance from the tissues, so that its sphere of activity, and observations with it, are extremely limited. It is hoped that further experiments will make it more amenable to experimentation.

To an ardent medical devotee who wishes to make a medical pilgrimage I should certainly commend the road to Marburg. The town itself is most picturesquely situated in the prettiest valley imaginable. The clinics and laboratories are all magnificent new buildings, most of them having been erected within the last few years. No expense has been spared to make them thoroughly modern in every scientific appointment. Owing to the peculiar relations of the Prussian Government to the province of Hesse, in which the university is situated, money seems to be no object. The medical faculty is one of the best in Germany. If one wishes to study German student life in its most characteristic form, here is the place to carry out the observations. Professor Behring has a private laboratory of his own on the hill above the town. It is a pretty little stone building situated at the very summit, and the view from the windows over the picturesque valley of Marburg is beautiful almost beyond description. Some time the ardent worshipers at the shrine of the new medicine will found a pilgrimage to the spot where, surrounded by all that is prettiest in Nature, the master studied out the hidden secrets for suffering humanity.

TRANSACTIONS OF FOREIGN SOCIETIES.

Paris.

HYPERCHLORHYDRIA PRODUCED BY ALKALIES—RESULTS OF THE SERUM-TREATMENT OF DIPHTHERIA IN THE PARIS HOSPITALS—BULLETS ARE NOT STERILIZED BY THEIR DISCHARGE FROM A GUN—CONTINENCE IN GASTRIC FISTULÆ—POSTERIOR VAGINAL OPENINGS FOR HIGH PELVIC ABSCESSES—MEASURES ADVOCATED BY THE ACADEMY OF MEDICINE TO LIMIT THE SPREAD OF TUBERCULOSIS.

AT the Medical Society of the Hospitals, April 15th, HAYEN spoke of hyperchlorhydria as produced by alkalies, and the habitual use of laxatives, such as rhubarb, podophyllum, and cascara. Thus, bicarbonate of soda, if given for a considerable length of time, will strongly increase the acidity of the stomach. This is due apparently more to the elimination of the alkalin salt than to any local effect upon the gastric mucous membrane. Hyperchlorhydria only follows the administration of alkalies in case there are numerous active glands in the stomach. If the gastric mucous membrane is degenerated so that the gastric juice is hypopeptic, the use of alkalies instead of producing hyperchlorhydria will depress the stomach and produce a condition almost of apepsia. In other words, alkalies exaggerate when given continuously whatever abnormal chemic state may exist in the stomach.

MATHIEU expressed himself as in substantial accord with these views. He is not in the habit of prescribing long-continued doses of an alkali. It is better that a patient should take at the moment when pains from hyperacidity are coming on, a sufficiently large dose to afford relief. Alkalies and alkalin waters are, nevertheless, of benefit to patients suffering from a diminished secretion of gastric juice.

RICHARDIERE gave results obtained in the treatment of diphtheritic children at the Trousseau Hospital in 1897. Six hundred and ninety-six children were brought to the hospital for treatment of diphtheria during that year. Upon entrance, each once received an injection of antitoxin serum. The dose varied from 10 to 20 c.c. according to the age of the child. Of these 696 children, 125 died, a mortality of 17.9 per cent. If one leaves out of calculation 31 cases in which death occurred within twenty-four hours of entrance to the hospital, and before any serum was given, the percentage of mortality of the remainder is 14.1.

BARBIER said that the size of the dose of antitoxic serum ought not to be determined simply by the age of the child. More reliable guides are, first, evidences of diphtheritic intoxication, such as rapid anemia, prostration, rapid pulse; and second, the occurrence with the diphtheria, or before it, of another bacteriologic inflammation.

At the session of April 29th, SEVESTRE said that 580

patients were treated during 1897 for diphtheria in the Children's Hospital; 101 died, giving a mortality of 17.41 per cent.; or, excluding forty-three cases in which death occurred during the first twenty-four hours, the mortality was 10.80 per cent. It was interesting also to divide the cases according to the nature of the infection; thus, those children in whom streptococcic as well as diphtheritic inflammation existed had a mortality of 32.32 per cent., while all the others taken together had a mortality of 13.34 per cent. All the children received an injection of serum upon entrance. The dose was 20 c.c. or more, for those two years old and upward.

At the Surgical Society, April 20th, BROCA explained that while by the discharge of a gun its barrel is rendered sterile, the ball itself is not sterilized, and even if it were, it would make little difference since the probability of infection of the wound from bits of clothing, etc., is so great. Absolute asepsis of a gunshot wound is rarely possible. Experiments upon animals have shown that attempts at disinfection are almost useless; the indications for operation are due to injuries of the bones, viscera, or blood-vessels. If these do not exist a simple dry dressing which can be easily removed and watched is the best treatment unless septic complications arise.

At the session of April 27th, RICARD spoke of the favorable action of the valvular gastrostomy of Fontan. By this method the stomach is attached to the anterior abdominal wall, around a little circle an inch or two in diameter. The mucous membrane in the center of this circle sinks inward, so that a cone is formed with its apex in the cavity of the stomach. At this apex a minute opening is made. The effect of this position of the stomach wall is that no gastric contents escape through the fistula.

TUFFIER said that the continence or incontinence of a gastric fistula depends chiefly on its situation in the gastric wall. An opening which is near the cardiac end will give little trouble; but there often is great difficulty in raising the cardiac portion to the surface. Routier said that the simplest operation is usually the best; and that even incontinent fistulæ will not be found inconvenient if a catheter is passed several times a day. The opening, whatever method is employed, should be made very small.

SCHWARTZ rejected the operation performed in two stages, since he had the misfortune to make an opening on the sixth day, not into the cavity of the stomach, but into that of the lesser peritoneum, and the accident was not discovered until a considerable quantity of food had been poured into that cavity.

MONOD stated that a similar accident had occurred in his hospital.

At the session of May 4th, MONOD said that he had forty times employed an opening into the posterior cul-de-sac of the vagina for the removal of purulent collections high up in the pelvis. It is necessary in this treatment to be on guard against neglecting a second abscess. Four times he had found such to exist after he had opened a perisalpyngeal pouch containing only serous fluid. In seventeen cases there was a double purulent focus on one side. One of these patients died. Four times there was a double purulent focus on both sides, two of these patients dying. Hence the necessity in these cases of making a bimanual examination, after one focus has been opened, to discover if others are palpable.

At the Academy of Medicine, May 3d, GRANCHER read the report of the commission appointed to consider the best means of preventing the occurrence of tuberculosis. The report which was confirmed by the whole body contained the following recommendations:

1. Collect sputum in pocket bottles containing a colored solution of carbolic acid, five per cent., or at least a little water; to substitute for sweeping, wiping with a moist cloth; and to boil milk before it is drunk.

2. As far as family life is concerned, physicians were urged to control as far as possible the spread of the disease, both by the enforcement of hygienic regulations, and by the early diagnosis and treatment of phthisical patients, so that they may not become sources of infection.

3. In the army the temporary subjection of those persons who have a commencing phthisis to the regulations of Section 1, was advocated, as well as the permanent subjection to them of all persons in whose sputum tubercle bacilli are present.

4. The attention of those in charge of schools, stores, and work-shops should be called to the simplicity of preventive measures, and the necessity of their observance, in order that every family in the land may be free from this scourge.

5. In hospitals, tuberculous patients should be separately treated and separate hospitals for them should be provided in high altitudes.

6. Stock-raisers were to be advised to use the tuberculin test to keep their stock free from the disease, and all meat should be inspected, and if found to be infected, should be destroyed at the slaughter-house.

A new and permanent commission was appointed whose object shall be to further all efforts to prevent the spread of tuberculosis.

SOCIETY PROCEEDINGS.

FORTY-THIRD ANNUAL MEETING OF THE KENTUCKY STATE MEDICAL SOCIETY.

Held at Maysville, Ky., May 11, 12, and 13, 1898.

(Continued from page 701.)

THE President, J. M. MATTHEWS, M.D., of Louisville, in the Chair.

SECOND DAY—MORNING SESSION.

The resignation of Dr. W. L. Rodman as a member of the Society was read, as he will move to Philadelphia in the fall. It was stated that Dr. Rodman had attended eleven meetings of the Society without missing one, and had read eleven papers. He was elected an honorary member by a rising vote. A committee was appointed to canvass the Society for funds to be added to the Rush Monument Fund.

A number of papers on diphtheria were then read, the first by DR. C. W. AITKEN of Flemmingsburg, entitled

PATHOLOGY AND DIAGNOSIS OF DIPHTHERIA.

The author stated that the diphtheria bacillus is capable of being grown through several generations, which, after an interval of several months, is capable of producing the disease. This is not true of the non-pathogenic bacteria which resemble this germ. Nasal, pharyngeal, laryngeal, and faucial mucous membranes are most frequently affected. The first macroscopic change at the site of the disease is a passive hyperemia, an increase of secretion of mucus and necrosis of superficial epithelium. An important point is to be able to differentiate at the bedside. The throat of every sick child should be examined, as they so infrequently complain of the throat. There are no pathognomonic bedside means of diagnosis but there are many helps. Diffuse redness of the pharynx and high temperature indicate scarlatina, but the diagnosis is more difficult from follicular tonsillitis. In the latter, sudden onset is the rule, high temperature during the first twenty-four hours, no asthenia, rapid but full pulse, absent glandular swellings, reaches its height in twenty-four to thirty-six hours, no albumin in the urine unless very high temperature, membrane superficial and easy to remove unless accompanied by bleeding, it does not reform, appears on the first day and is nearly always bilateral. Microscopy is a great help, but both the microscopic and macroscopic findings must be taken into consideration. As to the microscopic technic, the use of the one-twelfth oil immersion lens is to be recommended, Lœffler's culture-medium and stain giving the best results. Animal inoculation is a final valuable confirmatory test.

TREATMENT OF DIPHTHERIA

was the title of the paper presented by DR. S. G. DABNEY.

The author considered the prophylaxis and treatment of nasal, pharyngeal, and laryngeal diphtheria. He considered the withdrawal of cases from quarantine too early was a frequent cause; a number of examinations of the throat should be made microscopically of scrapings from it and no antiseptic used at this time. Well-ventilated rooms and sunlight are valuable agents. Removal of enlarged tonsils and adenoids should be considered under this head, also prevention of public funerals. Antitoxin as a preventive was extolled on the weight of accumulated statistics. It gives an immunity of three weeks. Antitoxin should be used in all suspicious cases, the earlier the better the result. In laryngeal cases its use, even if late, is of great efficacy when assisted by the use of the intubation-tube. Comparatively little can be accomplished by the use of antitoxin after the third day; it should be given during the first twenty-four hours. Any practitioner who has read the report of the collective investigation of the American Pediatric Society and fails to use antitoxin should not be allowed to care for a case of diphtheria. Statistics were quoted showing the result of the use of antitoxin, both in private and hospital practice, and its use urged most emphatically. A concentrated dose is recommended, 600 units in mild cases to a child of two years; in severe cases, 1000 units. In laryngeal cases the prognosis is grave. Hypodermic injections should be made in the thigh, back, or abdominal wall. In rare cases an eruption and pain in the joints may be caused, but nephritis is certainly not caused by it, and the frequency of this complication has been diminished since its use was begun. Stimulation is next in importance to the use of antitoxin, strychnin and whisky being of the most value. One ounce of whisky should be given to a child of four years when the pulse and depression indicate it. Muriated tincture of iron should be given when there is streptococcic infection. Local applications should consist of cleanliness rather than of antiseptics, using no force in applying them at any time. The author did not recommend the use of hydrogen dioxid. The proportion of the cases in which intubation is indicated has been much smaller since the use of antitoxin. Practice in intubation on the larynx of a dog was recommended to those who were unfamiliar with the technic of the procedure. Inhalations of steam was considered of valuable assistance. When the breathing becomes labored, as shown by drawing in of the clavicular spaces, insufficient expansion of the chest, great restlessness and evident distress, the tube should be inserted at once. In rare cases the membrane is pushed down in front of the tube. The tube should be left in four or five days.

A paper, entitled

MEMBRANOUS CROUP AND INTUBATION,

was read by DR. G. G. THORNTON of Gravel Switch.

The writer took the position that membranous croup and diphtheria are two distinct diseases, and based his opinion on the cases he has seen in which membranous croup has existed in patients who have not been exposed, and others who had been exposed and were not attacked by the disease. He never isolates a case of croup, and none had any trace of infection or exposure; others had been exposed to these and had not contracted the disease. It is often influenced by heredity. Antitoxin is not advised, as this disease is distinct from diphtheria. He has failed to find any remedy of avail among the host recommended. Intubation and tracheotomy are to be employed when indicated, preference being given to the former.

DISCUSSION.

DR. J. A. STUCKY of Lexington: I believe that I can hazard the statement that diphtheria is practically a stranger in Lexington, not more than fifty cases having occurred in the town during the last ten years. I believe there is a difference between diphtheria and membranous croup, the former a blood poison, a treacherous disease, contagious and infectious, leaves sequelæ, while in pseudo-diphtheria or membranous croup, the opposite is the condition. An early diagnosis is essential, and sun and fresh air are valuable prophylactics. I doubt the efficacy of treating the throats of other members of a family who have been exposed to infection. We should not tamper with the natural filtering properties of the nose. I believe there is some benefit to be had from the use of protonuclein.

DR. J. H. SHOEMAKER of Morganfield: Diphtheria is a rare disease in my neighborhood, I having seen but few cases in the last thirty-three years of practice. I am inclined to the belief that it is a filth disease and a constitutional disease. Antitoxin has taken the fear of the disease which we formerly had away, and it should be used more often.

DR. J. H. LETCHER of Henderson: I wish to emphasize the importance of making an early diagnosis, for we are on the safe side when we suppose a case to be one of diphtheria and begin work early. I believe a good many more cases occur than are recognized.

DR. F. L. LAPSLEY of Paris: I believe that there is some difficulty in determining whether a given bacillus is the true bacillus of diphtheria or a pseudo one, as they closely resemble each other. I consider the use of ice-cloths to the neck a valuable remedy, soothing and allaying lymphatic engorgement. Cases should be examined early and thoroughly, and antitoxin should be employed early, for I believe it is criminal to fail in its use.

DR. AITKEN, in closing: Only by animal inoculation can the differentiation be made in many cases between the pseudo and true bacillus. I would be most emphatic in the statement that croup and diphtheria are one and the same disease. The physical structure of the larynx and pharynx is not the same. When the larynx is affected the patients die from suffocation, and when the pharynx is the seat of trouble the death is from sepsis. It is a local disease from the beginning. I do not believe in the use of steam, as it favors the growth of the bacillus by supplying heat and moisture.

DR. S. G. DABNEY, in closing: My statement that steam is a good remedy was made from personal experience, as it certainly aids in the separation of the membranes. Those cases in which great glandular swelling of the neck occurs are cases of streptococcic infection, and ice applications certainly do a great deal of good. Diphtheria is certainly more common in cities, and there should be no question as to the diagnosis when a laryngeal case occurs after a follicular or membranous condition in the throat. Antitoxin has certainly caused us to see less of the complications in these troubles than formerly.

DR. W. L. RODMAN of Louisville read a paper, entitled

THE INFLUENCE OF AGE, RACE, AND SEX IN SURGICAL DISEASES.

It treated in an interesting way of the most common surgical conditions in the various races, especially the white, negro, and American Indian, and of the points of difference in each.

DR. T. C. EVANS of Louisville read a paper on

DEFLECTIONS OF THE NASAL SEPTUM.

Among the difficulties due to this trouble are deformity of the nose, distortion of the face, contraction of the alveolar arch, and dental irregularities. The complications and sequelæ are mouth-breathing, disturbance of speech, chronic deafness, hay fever, frontal headache, hypersecretion of the nasal cavities, defective drainage, diseases of the accessory sinuses, pharyngitis, laryngitis, and asthma.

The operation described by the writer for the relief of the condition is practically that of Dr. Morris J. Asch. A general anesthetic is recommended, and as hemorrhage is usually profuse, precautions should be taken as to the position of the head. The instruments necessary are the Asch septal scissors, Adams septal forceps, two vulcanite tubes and a probe-pointed septal knife. Digital exploration of the stenosed side is first carried out, and if adhesions are present they are dissected up. The first incision is made in the septum in a line of the greatest convexity and parallel with the floor of the nose, and a second incision at right angles to the first, intersecting it near its center. These incisions are extended to the limit of the cartilaginous septum, which divides the septum into four irregular and unequal triangles. An Adams forceps is now introduced, one blade in either nostril, and each triangle caught separately and twisted on its base to loosen its articulation and destroy its resiliency. The thoroughness with which this is done will insure the result. After irrigation of the nasal cavities the nasal tubes should be introduced, the hemorrage ceasing at once. Irrigation should be practised every few hours at first, then every two days, and after the first week the patient can do it himself. The results of this operation are most excellent.

DISCUSSION.

DR. J. A. STUCKY of Lexington: I have not been very enthusiastic over the Asch operation for some time. In the majority of cases it is better to use the beak or bayonet-pointed knife than the scissors, as they are liable to injure the inferior turbinated bones when there is marked stenosis. The Asch tube has too large an external and too small an internal opening. When the patient is under an anesthetic and there is much bleeding it is easy to push the tube through the wrong place. I use a longer and narrower tube. Cocain should be used cautiously and never alone. Combine it with a one-per-cent. solution of resorcin and no ill effects will be noticed.

DR. S. G. DABNEY of Louisville: Many cases of nasal deflection do not require operation. The Asch operation is the best in older patients. I generally make the incision first, before the anesthetic is given, the use of the Asch forceps requiring general anesthesia later. The nasal septum is very tolerant of work done upon it. The bistoury makes the best and most accurate incisions. The Asch tube is open to many criticisms; the side openings are entirely unnecessary. I never use the cocain spray, and believe the reason I have never seen any toxic effect is due to the fact that I never use it except with an applicator to the place which it is desired to anesthetize.

DR. T. C. EVANS, in closing: I rarely use cocain in a spray except when the first cleansing is done after the operation and think it is needed then, as there is so much injured surface that it would be impossible to make the application by means of a cotton swab. I think the scissors is a valuable instrument to make the first incision with, using the bistoury afterward.

DR. HENRY E. TULEY of Louisville exhibited an obstetric outfit. This had been made for his personal use by a drug company, but because of the demand for them had been prepared for general sale. The speaker referred to the fact that there have been a number of outfits or kits suggested from time to time, and they have not proven practical because they have not been selected with the best interests of the patient, nurse, and accoucheur in mind, and have been too expensive. The one exhibited can be purchased for three dollars, and is within the reach of patients of all classes. The following articles are enclosed in a hermetically sealed box, after thorough sterilization, and instructions are printed on it that it must not be opened except by the physician or nurse in attendance. It contains the following articles: Lochial pads, an obstetrical bed, five yards of plain sterilized gauze, one-half pound of absorbent cotton, two dozen safety-pins, fountain-syringe, nail-brush, nail-file, antiseptic soap, antiseptic tablets (mercuric bichlorid), six ounces of a saturated solution of boracic acid, a tube of white vaselin, plain vaselin, one ounce of Squibb's chloroform, sterilized tape for the cord, cord dressing (made of balsam of Peru, m. xx, to ol. ricini ½ ounce, which causes the cord to separate more quickly, and makes it more easy to care for, and minimizes the chances of infection), Credé eye solution, pipette, and fluid extract of ergot.

DISCUSSION.

DR. F. L. LAPELEY of Paris: These are useful articles but cannot be utilized in country practice as a rule. I use a strong cord for tying the funis, never using silk for this purpose, and use a dry dressing which is not changed until the cord falls off, which is between the third and fifth days as a rule.

DR. T. A. REAMY of Cincinnati: Looking toward asepsis, the outfit is a good one. I do not recommend douches either before or after labor, and only after labor when there has been manual or instrumental interference. In cases of prolonged labor there are conditions present which are favorable to the development of sepsis, and ergot should be given then only. Ergot can be injected, if deeply, and not cause an abscess.

DR. TULEY: I do not use the cord dressing exactly as recommended by Dr. A. E. Gallant, who first called my attention to it. He advises that only a slit be made in the gauze, the cord drawn through enough layers of it to cover it, the oil dressing applied, and the whole confined to the abdominal wall by adhesive strips, which are not removed or disturbed until the cord separates. I do not advise the use of the bichlorid as a routine practice for I think it unnecessary if thorough application of soap and nail-brush is carried out. The outfit is a most acceptable adjunct to the equipment of a lying-in chamber.

DR. F. F. BRYAN of Georgetown read a paper on

EXTRA-UTERINE PREGNANCY.

As a cause that is reasonable, it was suggested that mechanical conditions such as offered by obstructions to the passage of the ovum to the uterine cavity is a prominent one. Gravity, muscular action, and vibratile cilia are the best-demonstrated factors to this end. The causes that interfere are gonococci, strepto- and staphylococci, and all of the other members of the family of pus-producing organisms. Traumatism plays an important part. It is a fairly frequent condition, occurring as often as once in every 500 pregnancies. The usual signs of pregnancy are modified, menses cease for three months, as a rule, and then reappear irregularly as to time, quantity, and quality. The expectant plan of treatment should be condemned. Medicinal treatment, consisting in the administration, of morphin, strychnin, atropin, or electricity, should not be resorted to. Thorough surgical intervention is indicated in all cases.

MALIGNANT DISEASES OF THE UTERUS

was the title of a paper read by DR. LOUIS FRANK of Louisville.

He stated that the uterus is among the organs most frequently attacked by malignant processes. Malignant disease occurs between the ages of thirty-five and forty, and from fifty to sixty, although it may be found in the very young. The early symptoms are often obscure; the least irregularity during the climacteric period should arouse suspicion; suspicious cases should be subjected to microscopic examination; early operation is the only hope for cure; extirpation of the uterus after the disease is evident, after the appearance of cachexia, is harmful rather than beneficial; women should be taught to consult physicians for any irregularities of menstrual flow.

A paper, entitled

THE MIDWIFE AND MIDWIFERY,

was read by DR. L. C. WADSWORTH of Newport.

The writer stated that while Nature does in a majority of instances care for cases of labor, interference is often indicated and intelligent interference or assistance makes midwifery a science. The midwife attends the labor for a small fee and returns daily for nine days, washing the patient and baby and doing all the household work. In Kentucky midwives are especially exempt from State laws governing the practice of medicine. He felt that while they could not be entirely gotten rid of it would be a good plan if their education could be brought up to a standard and suggested that the way to accomplish this is to have laws enacted compelling them to procure a license and pass an examination for fitness. An ordinance governing this, as in effect at Newport, was read in substance.

DISCUSSION.

DR. EDWIN RICKETTS of Cincinnati: I have recently seen a family in which there were six cases of delivery and six cases of sepsis, all attended by midwives. I wish to go on record as being opposed to the midwife. I believe they should go. They are the cause of more puerperal peritonitis than any other being and the physician has to shoulder the blame, or at least cover up their mistakes, and I think the time has come when we, as intelligent physicians, should demand their getting out.

DR. REAMY: I believe because a woman is a midwife she should not be charged with every case of puerperal sepsis, procidentia, and other complications. Abroad the midwives are encouraged and recognized by the profession. Restrictions should be placed on these women, when they desire to practise midwifery, until they are thoroughly prepared. If they are trained in aseptic principles, and in the anatomy and physiology of the parts, they should be allowed to practise in proper quarters.

DR. BULLITT: I believe the view of Dr. Reamy the better one and the proper one. The midwives we have here now should go but good midwives should be welcomed. Many women prefer to be served by women if they are capable in occasions of this kind. Midwives should be educated to recognize abnormalities and to care for the normal cases.

A paper was read by DR. GEORGE E. DAVIS of Lawrenceburg, entitled

THE PHYSIOLOGY OF THE LIVER AND THE ROLE IT PLAYS IN DIGESTION AND NUTRITION.

DR. ISAAC A. SHIRLEY of Winchester read a paper, entitled

A CASE OF HEMATOMA OF THE VULVA FOLLOWING LABOR; OPERATION; RECOVERY.

Hematoma occurs but once in 1600 deliveries, according to one observer, and one in 14,000, according to another. The case reported was that of a primipara, nineteen years of age, the labor a dry one four hours long. Twenty minutes after labor there was a slight prolapsus of the uterus, and a tumor appeared in the left labium. Three days later the pulse was 130 and temperature 104° F., with a gangrenous odor from the pent-up lochial discharges. The clot was turned out and the cavity packed and thorough drainage obtained, without hemorrhage. Generally speaking varicose veins, a large head and severe expulsive pains are given as causes of this trouble. If occurring during labor immediate interference may be necessary.

THIRD DAY—MORNING SESSION.

The nominating committee made the following report: President, Dr. David Barrow of Lexington; first vice-president, Dr. H. K. Adamson of Maysville; second vice-president, Dr. James B. Bullitt of Louisville; secretary, Dr. Steele Bailey of Stanford; treasurer, Dr. C. W. Aitken of Flemmingsburg; librarian, Dr. B. W. Smock of Louisville; chairman, committee of arrangements, next meeting, Dr. John G. Cecil of Louisville; place of next meeting, Louisville, May, 1899. Dr. B. L. Coleman was elected chairman of the board of censors and of the committee on topics for the next meeting, and Dr. Henry E. Tuley chairman on publication.

DR. TULEY offered the following resolutions, which were unanimously adopted:

WHEREAS, Strenuous efforts are being made by the Marine Hospital Service to have the Caffrey bill passed by the House of Representatives and Senate of the United States, which practically gives the Marine Hospital Service complete control if this bill is passed to create a National Bureau of Public Health;

Resolved, That this society condemns the Caffrey bill and endorses the bill drafted by the American Medical Association and endorsed by the American Public Health Association, and urges the Kentucky senators and representatives to earnestly support the Association bill.

WHEREAS, It has been brought to the attention of the Kentucky State Medical Society in session at Maysville, Ky., May 11, 1898, that there is a bill now pending before the Congress of the United States relative to the suppression of vivisection in all its forms, be it

Resolved, That we, the Kentucky State Medical Society, fully realizing and deeply appreciating the great achievements in the domain of medicine and surgery which may be directly attributable to a practice of legitimate vivisection in the past, and feeling that its suppression as called for by the said pending bill would be a most serious blow to research in the future, do most heartily condemn the passing of such a bill; and be it further

Resolved, That a copy of these resolutions be spread upon the minutes of this society and that a copy be sent to each representative and senator from Kentucky, with an autograph letter from the secretary of this society, urging them to use their influence to defeat the passage of this bill.

After the reading of a number of papers by title, in the absence of the authors, the society was declared adjourned.

TWENTIETH ANNUAL MEETING OF THE AMERICAN LARYNGOLOGICAL ASSOCIATION.

Held at Brooklyn, N. Y., May 16, 17, and 18, 1898.

FIRST DAY.

THE President, DR. THOMAS R. FRENCH, of Brooklyn, in the Chair.

In his opening address the president said:

"As the result of the work of Pasteur, Lister, and Koch a new pathology has been created. The foundation of medical education is to-day normal histology and pathology. The searchlight of biology and bacteriology is only beginning to reveal the fields for study, which doubtless contain many truths that the future will disclose. Our dependence on the microscope in diagnosticating disease is growing with each year, but a proper conservatism in regard to its findings must be observed. The useless removal of important structures due to the not infrequent simulation by inflammatory tissue of conditions requiring thorough eradication demands serious consideration.

"Three classes of workers are needed in scientific work; the first is the original investigator who seeks for truth for its own sake; the second, the teacher who diffuses the knowledge acquired by the original investigator; the third is he who applies knowledge to its practical uses. Tyndall, in an address delivered in New York twenty-five years ago, said that in no other country would science, in its highest forms, exert a more benign influence than in ours. At that time those who confined themselves to work in one line were few; now their number is legion and the tendency toward a special field for practice is growing stronger each year. In no department of medicine have the workers increased so rapidly as in ours. Years of practice together with natural aptitude are absolutely necessary in order to acquire skill in the surgical treatment of diseases of the larynx, but much less practice is required to permit of intranasal surgical work, and this fact is unquestionably accountable for the large amount of indifferent or mischievous surgery which is yearly growing more noticeable. The advice of Sir Morrell Mackenzie that a man should practise medicine and surgery during the first ten years of his career is of greater value to-day than ever before. It is wise to remind a student of the advice given by Dr. William Osler, 'as a man values his future life let him not get early entangled in specialism.' To a certain extent it is true that many workers in various departments of medicine are becoming too narrow in their studies, devoting themselves to the acquisition of a limited field at the expense of general medical and surgical information. The charge is also made that specialism is doing great harm because of the charlatans who live and thrive under its influence, yet it is a fact that there are fewer of them to-day than ever before; this condition is due, not to specialism, but to the weakness and selfishness of mankind. Despite the evils that are growing out of specialism, the fact that men are centering their thoughts on special lines of work more than ever will result in the largest amount of good to mankind, for we are beginning to realize that concentration is the price we must pay for efficiency. It behooves us to think well on these things and to secure to specialism the minimum of harm and the maximum of good."

DR. J. N. MACKENZIE of Baltimore then read a paper on

THE LARYNGOTRACHEAL NEOPLASMS OF TUBERCULOSIS.

The larynx and the trachea are the seat of various forms of neoplasms which may be divided into three groups. To the first group belong that variety which may be termed granular hyperplasia (ordinary granuloma). Anatomically this variety is allied to granulation tissue and may be regarded as a conservative effort to promote cicatrization. If a section be made through the tubercular ulcer more or less clearly defined hyperplastic granulation is found, which is the effort on the part of Nature to isolate the tubercular process from the adjacent tissue. In the second group may be placed that variety of growth termed papillomata; this is less common than the preceding and may be found in any part of the larynx, especially in the posterior wall. The gross appearance shows nothing by which to differentiate it from simple papillomata, and the microscope reveals nothing of a tuberculous nature. Stürk long ago insisted that these growths are one of the earliest signs of tuberculosis, and since his time they have often been found to be the precursors of trouble in the lungs.

The third variety is the true tubercular tumor which is found in the windpipe. By tubercular tumor is meant an isolated, well-defined growth occurring independently of ulceration or tubercular infiltration and covered by normal mucous membrane, with little or no tendency to ulcerate. These tumors are of great rarity, the experience of the essayist having yielded but three cases. These growths are probably due to secondary deposits from the lungs or to metastasis. They have little tendency to ulceration, which, if it occurs at all, takes place at a late stage. The only sure way of reaching a correct diagnosis is by means of the microscope. The color, situation, presence of tuberculosis in the body, etc., are of some value.

DR. W. F. CHAPPELL of New York read a paper, entitled

LARYNGEAL TUBERCULOSIS AT THE LOOMIS SANATORIUM.

This sanatorium is 2300 feet above the level of the sea, and the surrounding country is hilly and undulating. The temperature varies from 0° F. in the winter to from 70° 80° F. in the summer. The prevailing winds are northwest and southwest and there is but little humidity in the air. The institution is conducted on the cottage plan. In tubercular laryngitis the local treatment consists in applications of lactic acid, creosote, ichthyol, nitrate of silver, etc. Clothing, exercise, and food play an important rôle in the systemic treatment. Hypodermic injections of horse serum are largely used and the effect on temperature and cough is far in advance of any other agent yet used. The history of the cases shows improved command of the voice, greater clearness, lessening of pain, better general condition, increase of weight, and absence of bacilli.

DR. W. K. SIMPSON of New York demonstrated

THE USE OF THE BERNAY SPONGE IN THE NOSE AND NASOPHARYNX, WITH SPECIAL REFERENCE TO ITS USE AS A HEMOSTATIC.

The Bernay sponge consists of cotton fiber which has been subjected to many hundred pounds of pressure and compressed to a disc of one-sixtieth of an inch in thickness. By the absorption of liquids it will attain fifteen times its size and twelve times its weight. Its great absorbing power makes it useful both as a cleansing agent and afterward to pack the wound. For the purpose of tamponing the anterior and posterior nares they are far more efficient than cotton or gauze, which have to be frequently inserted; this inconvenience is done away with by the use of the Bernay sponge. The slow absorbing power of cotton or gauze is no guarantee against hemorrhage. In case of epistaxis the sponge should be cut in semicircular size and introduced into the nostrils with the convexity upward.

DR. BEVERLY ROBINSON of New York read a paper on

ENLARGEMENT OF THE LINGUAL TONSIL AS A CAUSE OF COUGH.

For many years it has been a recognized fact that enlargement of the lingual tonsil may be the cause of cough, although few appreciate the condition. It is apt to occur in persons of a lymphatic or sluggish temperament. The beginning of this trouble is insidious, particularly in young adults. If the cough lasts for a few hours only, the general practitioner, after obtaining negative results from a chest examination, thinks that it is either a stomach or a reflex cough. Possibly he may think of laryngeal inflammation. An enlarged tonsil may be inspected with the laryngeal mirror, but this examination is often difficult and sometimes impossible. In children of from two to three years of age a laryngeal cough without reasonable cause is usually due to pressure upon an enlarged tonsil. This condition is often treated as an irritable cough for a long time without obtaining satisfactory results. In small children an irritative cough may be nothing more than the initial stage of whooping-cough. Impaired condition of the general health or the continuance of a catarrhal relaxation are predisposing causes. Anemia, constipation, and habitually irregular habits as regards food and rest are also responsible for this condition. In children overfeeding may cause congestion of the lingual tonsil. Rheumatic dyscrasiæ frequently found in adults are causative factors which should be attended to.

DR. JOHN O. ROE of Rochester read a

REPORT OF A CASE OF FRACTURE AND DEPRESSION OF THE ANTERIOR WALL OF THE MAXILLARY ANTRUM, WITH RESTORATION OF THE DEPRESSED WALL.

On February 15th, X., aged thirty-five years, received a severe blow with the fist which broke in the anterior wall of the antrum. Three days afterward, when the speaker first saw him, the face presented a one-sided appearance on account of the cavity situated in the cheek. In operating, the upper lip was raised, the dissection being carried high; by keeping close to the bone there was but little hemorrhage. A hole was drilled into the antrum through the canine fossa. By means of a curved sound the crushed wall of the antrum was raised to its proper position. The cavity was cleansed and iodoform gauze introduced. On the sixth day the dressing was removed and the cavity cleansed. The hole in the antrum no longer existed and the contour of the face was entirely normal.

DR. ROE then read a paper, entitled

THE TREATMENT OF FRACTURES OF THE NOSE.

These fractures are infrequent on account of the yielding character of the cartilaginous septum. They are usually accompaniments of fracture of the superior maxilla, and are usually attended by severe hemorrhages. Fractures of the nose are usually bilateral, and may be classified as simple, compound, and comminuted. Injury to the lacrimal apparatus affects the resonance of the voice, and therefore one should be careful in examining these parts.

DR. HENRY L. WAGNER of San Francisco read a paper on

EARLY DIAGNOSIS IN WHOOPING-COUGH.

He said that the duration of this disease can be shortened and its spread prevented by the adoption of proper measures. A diagnosis can be made at once by a bacteriologic examination of the secretions. The nose is the primary seat of infection. The secretions from a normal mucous membrane contain but few bacteria, while in whooping-cough a large number of characteristic bacteria are present. The bacterium of whooping-cough when full grown is two or three times as long as broad, is rounded, and somewhat thickened at the ends and is divided apparently in the middle. It is surrounded by a capsule not unlike Friedlander's pneumococcus. A one-per-cent. acetic-acid solution is used in staining, followed by Loeffler's solution, which consists of fuchsin, 1 part; carbolic acid, 5; glycerin, 50, and water 100 parts.

Dr. Wagner also read a paper on

LEPROUS ULCER OF THE LIP.

This condition is rare, only one case having been reported. At the International Congress it was held that the primary seat of this contagious disease is the mucous membrane of the upper respiratory tract.

DR. EMIL MAYER of New York read a paper on

THE USE OF THE SCHLEICH'S SOLUTIONS FOR ANESTHESIA IN NOSE AND THROAT OPERATIONS.

In summing up he said that Schleich's theory that the boiling-point of the anesthetic has an adaptability to the temperature of the body has been amply proven. The Schleich mixtures are safe for short operations. There is no stage of excitement. The tension of the pulse is increased. The patient becomes rapidly conscious.

SECOND DAY.

DR. S. W. LANGMAID of Boston read a paper, entitled

THE HOARSENESS OF SINGERS.

The symptoms of the condition are swelling of the nasal mucous membrane, enlarged turbinates and congested larynx. Occasionally there is absence of catarrhal affection, but there is disability resulting from impaired muscular power of the glottis. The acute catarrhal condition may be superimposed upon long-existing infection of the cavity by catarrh of the nose. The predisposing factors of this affection are neuroses, constitutional defects, anemia, rheumatism, atmospheric conditions, etc. Weakness of the intrinsic muscles—the tensors, the adductors, and the sphincters—always exist. The bending inward of one or both cords, the divulgence of the posterior portion of the cord, and what is more constant, deflection of one or both cords are conditions often noted.

DR. J. EDWIN RHODES of CHICAGO read a paper, entitled

SPASM OF THE TENSORS OF THE VOCAL CORDS.

Dr. Mackenzie was the first to describe this condition. Dysphonia spastica is a very rare condition, Dr. Mackenzie having seen only thirteen cases. The causes of this affection are an abnormal use of the voice, and possibly a neurotic condition not yet understood. It is present in incipient multiple sclerosis and is usually connected with some nasal affection. The symptoms appear on attempted phonation. The voice jerks when an attempt is made to pass from a low note to a high one and there is difficulty in getting started. There is an involuntary breaking in the speech. One of the peculiarities of the disease is that cocain used in the nose relieves the spasm for some time.

The prognosis is very unfavorable. In the treatment local applications, strychnin, sprays, etc., are of no benefit. The best treatment is long rest for the voice, general tonics, such as iron, arsenic, iodid of potassium, electrical treatment, etc., which may give some relief. Astringent applications are occasionally of some value. The use of cocain in the nose cannot be recommended.

DR. F. W. HINKEL of Buffalo read a

REPORT OF A CASE OF LIPOMA OF THE LARYNX.

In 1883, a patient, now aged fifty-five years, was conscious of a tumor at the back of her tongue and consulted

Dr. Park, who removed it. After some years there was a gradual return of the symptoms and Dr. Park again removed a tumor smaller than the first. In 1894 he again removed one similar to the one removed the previous year. In 1895 the patient consulted the essayist for cough and difficulty in swallowing. She stated that her father had died of cancer of the face. From the left epiglottis a pinkish body was growing which was soft or doughy in consistence and there were varicosities at the root of the tongue. Having difficulty in drawing the loop through the snare it was necessary to remove the growth in three pieces. It was dense and hard and no bleeding accompanied the operation. Behind was left some fulness of the epiglottis. In 1898 she again consulted him for discomfort, and a tumor was found at the free edge of the epiglottis and bending toward the right. The left aryepiglottic fold was thickened. There was no involvement of the ventricular band. The growth resembled a polyp. It was readily removed with forceps and scissors and was found to be three-quarters of an inch in length. The epiglottis presented a curious appearance, the epiglottic fossa being filled with tissue similar to that removed The persistent occurrence of the tumors suggested the advisability of a microscopic examination. Dr. Wright reported the case to be one of lipoma of the larynx.

Dr. Hinkel also read a paper reporting

DEATH IMMEDIATELY FOLLOWING AN OPERATION FOR NASOPHARYNGEAL ADENOIDS UNDER CHLOROFORM ANESTHESIA.

A boy, six years of age, never a mouth-breather or snorer, complained of ear trouble and deafness. Examination of his throat revealed a moderate amount of lymphoid tissue in the vault of the pharynx. He continued to be troubled with deafness and when eight years of age it was decided to operate. Chloroform was used, the mask being applied dry and the chloroform dropped on it by an experienced anesthetist, who was prepared for any emergency. The boy had a systolic murmur which was probably not due to organic lesions. Vomiting and spasm of the glottis occurred. One ounce of chloroform in all was used. The lymphoid tissue was found to be quite firm. Careful watch of the respiration and pulse was kept. A temporal pulse was noted. The operation had been finished when suddenly respiration ceased; no pulse could be felt and there were no heart sounds noted. Digitalis, strychnin, and other drugs were given, and also hypodermics of ether, atropin, and digitalis. Cold effusions were also tried. Artificial respiration was kept up for two hours. No post-mortem was permitted.

DR. ARTHUR AMES BLISS of Philadelphia read a paper, entitled

THE RECURRENCE OF ADENOIDS AFTER EXCISION.

In three of his cases in which there had been recurrence the operation had been performed in two instances from the region of the vomer. The prevent the return of the tumors the best method is complete and thorough removal. Incomplete removal often results in their return.

DR. D. BRYSON DELEVAN of New York read a paper, entitled

PRESENT METHODS FOR THE OPERATIVE TREATMENT OF PHARYNGEAL ADENOIDS.

Attention had not been called to this subject for twenty years. In the surgical treatment of these adenoids two points should be kept in mind, thoroughness and humanity. Thoroughness means the complete removal of the condition, as any tissue left behind is certainly unhealthy, and half-way measures are useless. As to the humanitarian side one should choose as far as possible those methods which inflict the smallest amount of pain, shock, and injury. The statement that this operation is not painful is incorrect. The patients questioned in regard to the pain during a long period of years invariably replied that the removal of the adenoids had been accompanied by sharp pain.

The paper was discussed by Drs. Gleitsmann, Casselberry, Wagner, Thrasher, Logan, Swain, Bryan, Rice, and Hinkel.

THIRD DAY.

The discussion of Dr. Delevan's paper was continued. In his closing remarks the essayist said that during the first two years he used chloroform, and in operating upon more than two hundred patients he had had two accidents, neither of them fatal. Unfavorable reports that came from abroad, together with these accidents, caused him to discontinue the use of chloroform. Ether often is not given properly and produces complete relaxation of the pharynx, while only partial relaxation is wanted. People in this country are more familiar with the administration of ether than with that of chloroform. Adults do not require a general anesthetic; the paper read referred only to children. In operating about the orifices of the Eustachian tubes the finger should be used, and with great care. Any nasal obstruction may give rise to failure of the adenoid operation. He did not think that ether had anything to do with the amount of hemorrhage present. Certain anomalies, such as stammering, had been removed after adenoid operations.

DR. J. C. MULHALL of St. Louis read a paper, entitled

THE UPPER RESPIRATORY ORGANS AND THE GENERAL HEALTH.

The national triad of affections is catarrh, dyspepsia, and nervous prostration, all due to our bad habits of living. Diseases of the upper air-passages may produce disturbances of the general health and it is equally true that if the general health suffers there may result diseases of the upper air-passages.

Prophylaxis should begin in childhood. There should be as near an approach to outdoor life as possible. The head covering should permit of free ventilation; the same should be true of foot covering. But three meals a day should be eaten. Hot bread should be eschewed. Rubber shoes and mufflers should be done away with. Careful diet does as much for the outside skin as it does for the inside. Nasal affection cannot be properly treated until the ptomains are swept from the system. The Salsbury method, consisting of beef diet, hot water, and plenty of exercise is very beneficial in properly selected cases.

DR. HENRY L. WAGNER of San Francisco read a paper, entitled

NATURAL IMMUNITY; A BIOLOGICAL RESEARCH,

and was followed by DR. J. W. FARLOW of Boston, who reported

A CASE OF DISEASE OF THE ACCESSORY SINUSES.

This case was of particular interest from the fact that it followed scarlet fever. There was a thickening of the superior maxilla and absence of discharge from the nose. The eye was pushed outward, downward, and forward, and there was possibly a secondary involvement of the antrum of Highmore.

DR. HENRY L. SWAIN of New Haven read a paper, entitled

SOME OBSERVATIONS ON THE USE OF AQUEOUS EXTRACT OF SUPRARENAL GLANDS, LOCALLY, IN THE UPPER AIR-PASSAGES.

He concluded his paper as follows:

1. We have in the aqueous extract of suprarenal glands a powerful, local, nasoconstrictor agent, and a contractor of erectile tissue, which it is safe to use in very considerable amounts without any dangerous or deleterious effects locally or to the general constitution of the individual.

2. These local effects can be reproduced in the same individual, apparently, any number of times without entailing any vicious habits to either the tissue or the individual.

3. The use of the extract seems rather to heighten the effects which may be expected from any given drug which may be used locally after it.

4. In acute congestions it has its widest application and greatest opportunity for good, but in certain chronic conditions of the hay-fever type where redundant tissue seems prone to develop it can be relied upon as one of the most helpful adjuvants which we have at command.

5. The only difficulty seems to be the production of it in quantities and preventing its decomposition on standing.

DR. CLARENCE C. RICE of New York read a paper on

ACUTE INFLAMMATORY CONDITIONS OF THE UPPER AIR-PASSAGES ACCOMPANIED BY LARYNGEAL EDEMA.

In the classification of this disease he wished to have it understood that laryngeal edemas due to diphtheritic infection were to be carefully excluded, which had not been done in many of the cases published. He thought it was also well to leave out of consideration cases of non-inflammatory edema, or so-called "passive edema," which are only a symptom of general disturbance and due to cardiac, renal, and hepatic disease. Another line of cases which properly should be excluded are those which might well be termed "chronic" edema of the larynx, where the swelling is occasioned by a chronic local disease, such as tuberculosis, syphilis, and malignant disease. The late Sir Morrell Mackenzie stated that in nearly all the instances of so-called idiopathic edematous laryngitis, the disease is due to blood-poisoning, and that he had met with it among hospital physicians, medical students, and nurses. He stated, also, that in every case that had come under his notice ample opportunity for acquiring septicemia had been present.

Dr. Rice tabulated for his paper 41 cases reported by journals from the year 1887 to date, exclusive of 14 cases by Semon. He found that but 4 or 5 cases were reported annually and that the prevalence of *grippe* since 1890 has not materially increased the number of reported cases. In about fifty per cent. of all the cases the cause is put down as "catarrhal," that is, as due to exposure to cold. The author cited 3 cases of moderate laryngeal edema of his own following peritonsillar inflammation; 2 cases of edema of the larynx due to traumatism, that is, one following the use of the galvanocautery applied to the lateral wall of the pharynx, and the other to a foreign body which lodged in the pyriform sinus; and 2 cases of edema due to constitutional causes. These 2 cases seemed both to be preceded by inflammation at the base of the tongue, possibly due to inflammation of the lingual tonsil. There was no indication of diphtheritic exudation. Exactly what the infection was in these cases it was difficult to determine, but in neither was there pre-existing inflammation of the respiratory tract unless of the tongue. The author thought the cases very rare in which there is an acute primary edematous laryngitis which exists without relationship to any other inflammation in this location. He thought the possible existence of diphtheritic poisoning in many of these cases should be more carefully considered, and that it is likely that in some which are put down as primary and acute are really secondary to renal disease. Extraordinary exposure to cold, together with the effects of alcohol and tobacco, are potent etiologic factors.

At the executive session the following were elected to active fellowship: Dr. J. W. Goodale of Boston, Mass., thesis, "A Contribution to the Histopathology of Acute Tonsillitis;" Dr. D. Braden Kyle of Philadelphia, thesis, "The Position of the Orifice of the Eustachian Tube and the Possibility of Catheterizing It through the Mouth;" Dr. G. Hudson Makuen of Philadelphia, thesis, "Artistic Breathing."

The officers elected for the ensuing year are as follows: President, William E. Casselberry of Chicago; first vice-president, J. W. Gleitsmann of New York; second vice-president, F. Whitehill Hinkel of Buffalo; secretary and treasurer, Henry L. Swain of New Haven; librarian, Jonathan Wright of Brooklyn; delegate to the Council, Thomas R. French of Brooklyn; representative to the Congress of Physicians and Surgeons, W. K. Simpson of New York; members of the Council, Thomas R. French of Brooklyn, John O. Roe of Rochester, W. H. Daly of Pittsburg, and Charles H. Knight of New York.

Chicago was chosen as the next place of meeting, the time to be at the discretion of the Council.

To Remove the Odor of Iodoform.—Ordinary mustard flour has been recommended for the removal of the extremely clinging and disagreeable odor of iodoform from the hands. Orange-flower water also is said to accomplish a like result.

REVIEWS.

INTERNATIONAL CLINICS. Edited by JUDSON DALAND, M.D., Instructor of Clinical Medicine and Lecturer on Physical Diagnosis in the University of Pennsylvania, J. MITCHELL BRUCE, M.D., Physician to and Lecturer on the Principles and Practice of Medicine in the Charing Cross Hospital, London, England, and DAVID W. FINLEY, M.D. Professor of the Practice of Medicine in the University of Aberdeen. Vol. IV., Seventh series. Philadelphia: J. B. Lippincott Co., 1898.

THE present volume of the "International Clinics" contains some excellent lectures. Among the more notable ones are: "A New Department in Therapeutics," by Dr. Roberts Bartholow; "The Value of Venesection in Certain Cases of Heart Failure," by Dr. Francis Warner of London; "The Treatment of Secondary Syphilis," by Dr. John E. Hays; a striking article on the "Treatment of Emergency Cases in Common Practice," by Dr. James F. Rinehart. Professor Klemperer of Berlin contributes an instructive lecture on diabetes mellitus, and Dr. Boas furnishes a contribution on the present diagnosis of gastric diseases by chemic investigations. An instructive lecture is that of Dr. Charles L. Greene on the differential diagnosis of typhoid fever. The departments of neurology, surgery, gynecology and obstetrics, ophthalmology, laryngology and rhinoscopy, and dermatology are well covered as usual.

A SYSTEM OF MEDICINE BY MANY WRITERS. Edited by THOMAS CLIFFORD ALLBUTT, M.A., M.D., LL.D., Regius Professor of Physic in the University of Cambridge. Vol. IV. New York: The Macmillan Co., 1897.

THE standing of this classical system of medicine is not impaired by the present volume. Its contributors, as well as its articles, combine to furnish a volume of unusual merit and interest. The volume opens with a discussion of diseases of obscure causation, including rheumatism in its various forms, rickets, gout, diabetes, and lardaceous disease. Dr. Garrod writes of rheumatism, and Dr. Saundby of diabetes. The next division is devoted to diseases of alimentation and excretion, including articles on the general pathology of digestion, by Drs. Ralfe and Soltan Fenwicks; the general pathology of secretion by Dr. Rose Bradford; shock and collapse by Dr. Cobbett, and closes with diseases of the mouth and esophagus by Drs. Wills and Rolleston. The diseases of the stomach follow, and contain articles by the editor, by Drs. Lauder Brunton, Leith, Stocker, Dreschfeld, and Hale White. Dr. Lee Dickinson considers subphrenic abscesses and diaphragmatic hernia. Dr. Playfair has an admirable article on abdominal diagnosis from a gynecologic standpoint. Mr. Treves contributes a classical paper on peritonitis. We know of nothing better than Mr. Treves' conception of acute peritonitis as described by him in this volume. It must be read to be thoroughly appreciated. Other diseases of the peritoneum are discussed by Allchin. The diseases of the intestines ("diseases of the bowels") are thoroughly considered. Dr. Lauder Brunton writes of fecal evacuation and on diarrhea, and Mr. Treves on intestinal obstruction. The diseases of the colon are described by Dr. Hale White. Dr. Herbert Allingham considers the differential diagnosis of diseases of the anus and rectum. The diarrheas of children are considered by Dr. Eustace Smith.

This volume is illustrated with the same profuseness and generosity that have characterized its predecessors. The book is handsomely made, and forms a valuable and splendid accompaniment to the volumes that have gone before. We have previously stated that Allbutt's System of Medicine would long be considered among the classics of distinctly modern medical literature. We have nothing to detract from this assertion, and feel more thoroughly convinced of it than before after perusal of the present volume.

THERAPEUTIC HINTS.

For Chancroid. — Daily applications of guaiacol are highly recommended as effecting an early cure. A small quantity is first employed to anesthetize the part, which is then thoroughly swabbed with the guaiacol to produce a caustic action.

Abortive Treatment of Acute Rhinitis.—COURTADE recommends hot nasal douches (122° F.), with a mildly antiseptic solution. RABOW claims equally good results from the use of fine common salt as a snuff.

For Soft Corns.—

℞	Iodi	gr. ii
	Collodii flex.	℥ iii
	Spiritus	℥ i
	Potass. iodi	gr. ii.

M. Sig. Apply at night.

For Stye.—The following combination is very efficacious in the treatment of styes:

℞	Tinct. camphoræ	m. xv
	Sulphuris precip.	gr. xv
	Aq. calcis } aa Aq. rosæ }	℥ iiss
	Pulv. acaciæ	gr. iii.

M. Sig. External use.

Hemostatic Action of Calcium Salts. —SILVESTRI has obtained excellent results from the use of the hypophosphite of calcium in cases of metrorrhagia, epistaxis, and gastric and intestinal hemorrhage. He prescribes it in the form of cachets of 15 grains each, one to be administered every two hours, until from eight to ten doses have been taken.

For Acne and Furunculosis.—

℞	Syr. calcis lactophos.	℥ iii
	Ol. morrhuæ	℥ iv
	Ol. amyg. amaræ	gtt. iii
	Aquæ	℥ i
	Pulv. acaciæ	q. s.

M. Ft. emulsion. Sig. One tablespoonful three times a day.—*Purdon.*

THE MEDICAL NEWS.

A WEEKLY JOURNAL OF MEDICAL SCIENCE.

VOL. LXXII. NEW YORK, SATURDAY, JUNE 11, 1898. NO. 24.

ORIGINAL ARTICLES.

FORTY-NINTH ANNUAL MEETING OF THE AMERICAN MEDICAL ASSOCIATION, HELD AT DENVER, COLORADO, JUNE 7, 8, AND 9, 1898.

PRESIDENT'S ADDRESS.[1]

BY GEORGE M. STERNBERG, M.D.,
SURGEON-GENERAL, UNITED STATES ARMY.

I DESIRE at the outset of my presidential address to express to you my high appreciation of the honor conferred upon me and my thanks for the same. I esteem it a special honor to have been elected president of the American Medical Association at the semicentennial meeting in Philadelphia.

Our association, as the representative body of American physicians, will no doubt continue to increase in membership and in influence. The day is perhaps not far distant when no reputable physician will be willing to confess that he does not belong to the American Medical Association, and when no progressive physician can afford to do without our journal. I would not exclude a reputable physician from membership because the State, county, or district medical society to which he belongs declines to adopt our code of ethics. If he, individually, is willing to be governed by the regulations made by this representative body, I see no good reason for rejecting his application for membership.

A liberal and progressive spirit will do much toward promoting the growth and influence of the Association. The medical profession in this country has suffered more from the ignorance of some of its members who hold diplomas from regular schools of medicine than from the attacks of those whom we call irregulars, or quacks. To maintain our standing in the estimation of the educated classes we must not rely upon our diplomas or upon our membership in medical societies, but must show ourselves superior in knowledge and in professional resources to the ignorant pretender or to the graduate of a medical school which is bound in its teachings by an untenable creed, adopted before the light of science had taught physicians to reject theories and the dicta of authorities in favor of truths demonstrated by modern methods of research. There are those who still speak of us as "old-school physicians," ignorant, apparently, of the fact that scientific medicine is, to a great extent, of very recent origin, and that all of the great discoveries in relation to the etiology, prevention, and specific treatment of infectious diseases, and nearly all the improved methods and instrumental appliances for clinical diagnosis and surgical treatment, have their origin within the ranks of the regular profession. While, therefore, we still have with us some "old-school doctors," who have fallen behind the procession, the profession, as a whole, has been moving forward with incredible activity upon the substantial basis of scientific research, and if we are to be characterized by any distinctive name, the only one applicable would be "*the new school of scientific medicine.*" Not that our science is complete, for we have still many things to learn and many problems which have thus far resisted all efforts at their solution. But we have learned how to attack these problems, and no one any longer expects that they can be solved by the exercise of the reasoning powers and the facile use of the pen. The old saying has it that "the pen is mightier than the sword." This is no doubt true in politics, but in science the pen is a feeble instrument compared with the test-tube, the microscope, the chemical balance, etc. Nevertheless, I am about to advise well-informed physicians to make greater use of the pen, not for the elucidation of those problems which remain to be solved, but for the purpose of calling the attention of the non-medical portion of the community to the recent achievements of scientific medicine. It is a remarkable and lamentable fact that many persons belonging to the so-called educated classes, are grossly ignorant as regards the present status of medical science. They not only speak of us as "old-school doctors," but they entrust their lives and those of their children to pseudo-scientists who, taking advantage of the popular interest in the great discoveries of the day, make extravagant claims as to the curative power of electricity, the X-ray, oxygen, ozone, or some wonderful microbe destroyer. It seems to me that those familiar with the truths of scientific medicine would do well to give to the public concise and comprehensive statements suitable for publication in newspapers and popular magazines, setting forth the facts and the evidence upon which these facts are accepted by well-informed physicians. If we had an association organized for the purpose

[1] Abstract.

of answering such false statements as have circulation in public print much good might result. Certainly it seems to me that the profession has a duty to perform in this direction, and I hope some steps will be taken to bring about such an organization.

Whenever any new discovery in medicine is announced, some conservative physicians, and often men of reputation in the profession, are sure to commit themselves to a positive denial of the alleged fact. This occurred when the discovery of the tubercle bacillus was announced by Koch, it has occurred with reference to the treatment of diphtheria by antitoxin, and to the preventive treatment of hydrophobia by Pasteur's method. Yet these discoveries are based upon experimental evidence of the most unimpeachable character. To deny their reliability at the present day is simply to show ignorance of the nature of this evidence or a failure to appreciate its scientific value. Often the positive and premature statements of a physician relating to new discoveries in medicine are corrected, or at least regretted at a later date, but sometimes the pride of opinion prevents a retraction in the face of the most conclusive evidence. The result is that such opinions, although they may have been given years ago, are always available to controvert the statements of those who maintain the value of vaccination, of experiments on the lower animals, of the diphtheria antitoxin, etc., and the non-medical public often accept the opinions which coincide with their preconceived views, or arrive at the conclusion that there is nothing settled in our so-called medical science. It should be our aim to remedy this evil by elevating the standard of medical education, as we are doing in many parts of the country; by impressing upon the rising generation of physicians the importance of laboratory work not only as a means of instruction, but for the purpose of cultivating a scientific spirit of inquiry and just appreciation of the value of experimental evidence, and finally, by instructing the public with reference to the present status of scientific medicine, the difference between fact and fancy, between the vagaries of the imagination and the demonstrable results of scientific investigation.

With the progress of scientific medicine we have improved methods of teaching, and it is now generally recognized that reading medical books and listening to lectures is not a sufficient preparation for the practice of medicine any more than the reading of books on navigation would be for the responsible position of captain of an ocean steamer. It is for this reason that we insist upon the study of anatomy in the dissecting-room, the teaching of methods of diagnosis and treatment at the bedside, and of chemistry, physiology, and pathology in the laboratory. It is only within the past few years that our leading medical colleges have provided suitable facilities for practical laboratory work, and even at the present day, as I understand, the laboratory courses are not compulsory in some institutions which provide for a four-years' course of study as a requisite for receiving the degree of doctor of medicine. From my point of view these laboratory courses are a most essential part of the medical curriculum, not only because the student becomes familiar with the use of instruments and methods which will be of inestimable value to him in the practice of his profession, but especially because of the effect of the kind of training he there receives in enabling him to judge of the imperfections of our unaided senses and the small value of opinions in comparison with that of facts capable of demonstration; as also the relative importance of many things which to the superficial observer might appear to be insignificant and unworthy of attention. He learns not to accept the assertion of the professor in the lecture-room or the dictum of any authority if this is in conflict with experimental evidence which he is able to verify for himself. On the other hand, he learns not to have an overweening confidence in his own judgment and powers of observation. He may fail to demonstrate the flagella on the typhoid bacillus or the presence of the plasmodium in the blood of a malarial-fever patient, or of a trace of arsenic in the tissues of one who died with symptoms of arsenical poisoning; but having learned by repeated investigation that the failure was due to his want of expert skill in the use of the microscope or in the application of delicate methods of investigation, he learns that it is unscientific and injudicious to give a premature opinion in regard to any subject under investigation, and especially so when this opinion is based upon negative evidence. Failure to find the tubercle bacillus in a given specimen of sputum has little value unless the examination has been repeatedly made by an expert. It unfortunately too often happens that physicians, after a very perfunctory investigation, give a positive opinion based upon negative evidence. I have investigated, I have not found, consequently it does not exist. This is the attitude of the unscientific but self-satisfied man, and it often leads to mistakes which are not only discreditable to the individual, but damaging to the profession of medicine, for the mistakes of the doctors, as a rule, attract much more attention than their successes. The painstaking work and attention to details required of students engaged in chemical, physiological, bacteriological, or histological studies, and the failure in their attempts to repeat an experiment or demonstration, if through haste or carelessness they neglect any step in the necessary technical processes, constitute an invaluable lesson. Indeed, the scientific medicine of the present day can only be taught by such methods, and the scientific physician of the future must make his way to fame and fortune by traveling this somewhat difficult and time-consuming road.

Having referred to the injurious consequences of premature and unfounded opinions, especially when given by men of prominence in the profession, I desire to call attention to the best method of counteracting such mischief. This is undoubtedly by united action on the part of the more enlightened members of the profession in behalf of truth and progress. This assistance we have had in combatting the antivivisection bill introduced into the United States Senate and vigorously pressed by the members of the Washington Humane Society, supported by their misguided friends in various parts of the country. The result has been eminently satisfactory, and shows that when exercised in a just cause the influence of the medical profession is a factor which will not be ignored even by the Senate of the United States.

The principle involved in the construction of the compound microscope was discovered as long ago as the Sixteenth Century, but it is only within the present century, and principally during the last half of the century, that those improvements have been made which have made it available for etiological and histological studies. There is, however, a growing disposition to suspect that our microscopes, notwithstanding the great degree of perfection attained in their construction, are still inadequate to the task of revealing to us the specific infectious agents of certain diseases, because of their minute size.

In a late number of the *Centralblatt für Bakteriologie*, Löffler and Frosch have published their official report of investigations made for the German Government, relating to the etiology of foot and mouth disease of cattle, the results of which are very interesting in this connection. As in smallpox, rabies, scarlet fever, typhus fever, and certain other infectious diseases, the efforts heretofore made to demonstrate the specific etiological agent in foot and mouth disease have been unsuccessful. The carefully conducted investigations of Löffler and Frosch also failed to demonstrate the presence of any specific microorganism in the lymph drawn with proper precautions from about the mouths or udders of infected cows. Cultures in various media inoculated with this lymph remained sterile and no micro-organism could be demonstrated by the use of the microscope in stained preparations. Nevertheless, experiments showed that this lymph was infectious material, and that calves inoculated with a very small amount of it invariably developed the disease in two or three days. Very much to the surprise of the investigators named, they found that lymph which had been filtered through a porcelain cylinder, which was proved by experiment to arrest the passage of bacteria, retained its full infecting power. That the result was due to the multiplication of the infectious agent in the body of the infected animal and not merely to the introduction of a very toxic non-living substance present in the lymph, was shown by the small dose required to produce the disease ($\frac{1}{10}$ to $\frac{1}{40}$ c.c. of filtered lymph), and also by the fact that the disease could be transmitted to other animals by inoculating them with like amounts of lymph taken from the vesicles which developed in the calves inoculated with filtrated lymph. The authors conclude their report as follows:

"It seems difficult to escape the conclusion that the action of filtered lymph does not depend upon a soluble constituent, but upon an agent capable of self-multiplication. This must be so small that it can pass through a filter which retains the smallest known bacteria. The smallest hitherto known bacterium is the influenza bacillus of Pfeiffer."

In the department of etiology the most brilliant and farreaching discoveries of the century are the discovery of the anthrax bacillus (1850) and demonstration of its etiological relation to the disease with which it is associated—by Davaine, Pasteur, Koch, and others (1863–1875); the discovery of the tubercle bacillus by Koch (1882) and the discovery of the malarial parasite by Laveran (1879). These discoveries, so essential to the progress of scientific medicine, would evidently have been impossible without the aid of the compound microscope. But just here I wish to insist upon another point, which is, that for the untrained eye the microscope is little better than a toy, and it may even be regarded as a dangerous instrument because of the inevitable mistakes which the novice will make if he undertakes to decide questions of diagnosis by the use of high power oil-immersion objectives without having had the necessary training for such delicate work.

For the illiterate, and even for many of the so-called educated class, the whole of medicine consists in the cure of disease by medicines, or by some agency, natural or supernatural, and a failure to cure is evidence that medicine is not a science. We readily admit that the cure of disease is one of the principal objects which medical science has in view, and that from a scientific standpoint therapeutics is very much behind some of the other branches of medicine. This is shown by the diversity of remedies prescribed for certain diseases and the failure of any one of these remedies to effect a cure in many cases. But, on the other hand, therapeutics has made great advances during recent years, and by the application of scientific methods of research the exact value of alleged remedies and of various methods of treatment is now determined with far greater precision than formerly. Recently several additions have been made to the list of specific therapeutic agents, and there is good reason to believe that further discoveries in this direction will be made as a result of investigations now being conducted in pathological laboratories in various parts of the world. Among the most important recent discoveries in this department of scientific medicine I may mention the use of thyroid extract for the cure of myxedema and the antitoxin of diphtheria. The discovery of the diphtheria antitoxin promises to be as important for therapeutics as the discovery of the anthrax bacillus was for bacteriology, and will no doubt henceforth be regarded as one of the most notable achievements of the century. It resulted directly from laboratory experiments relating to the production of immunity. While the practical results of this discovery have been most notable in the case of diphtheria, some success has been attained in the specific treatment of tetanus, streptococcus infection, pneumonia, and even in tuberculosis. These results give encouragement to the hope that future investigations may develop methods of obtaining these antitoxic substances in such form and amount as will enable us to successfully use them in the treatment of those infectious diseases for which we have not heretofore had a specific remedy. Another recent discovery of considerable importance from several points of view, is the so-called Widal-reaction.

Where thousands have been saved by the timely administration of suitable medicines or by the skilfully performed operation of the surgeon, tens of thousands have been saved by preventive medicine. And preventive medicine is to day established upon a strictly scientific foundation. If our practice was *pari passu* with our knowledge, infectious disease should be almost unknown in civilized countries, and those degenerative changes of vital organs which result from excesses of various kinds would cease to play a leading part in our mortuary statistics. But while our knowledge is still incomplete in some directions, and while individuals and communities constantly fail to act in accordance with the well-established laws of health and the scientific data which furnish the basis of preventive medicine, the saving of life directly traceable to this knowledge is enormous.

The time at my disposal is entirely inadequate for the purpose of setting forth the present status of scientific medicine, but I trust enough has been said to justify the claim that we are not "old-school doctors" and to show that medicine has not been behind other branches of science in taking advantage of improved methods of research and in establishing itself upon the sound basis of facts, demonstrated by experiment and observation with instruments of precision.

What has been said will also prove that there is no room for creeds and pathies in medicine, any more than in astronomy, geology, or botany. Every man is entitled to his own opinion upon any unsettled problem, but if he entertains an opinion in conflict with ascertained facts, he simply shows his ignorance. There is no restriction placed upon any physician who graduates from our regular schools as to the mode of treatment he should pursue in any given case. If he sees fit to prescribe a bread pill or a hundredth trituration of carbo vegitabilis, there is no professional rule of ethics to prevent him from doing so. But if his patient dies from diphtheria because of his failure to administer a proper remedy, or if he recklessly infects a wound with dirty fingers or instruments, or transfers pathogenic streptococci from a case of phlegmonous erysipelas to the interior of the uterus of a puerperal woman, it would appear that the courts should have something to say as to his fitness to practise medicine. There is, however, nothing in the code of ethics which will prevent him from associating with reputable practitioners. But no matter where or when he obtained his medical degree, he can scarcely be said to belong to the modern school of scientific medicine. We must not fail to recognize, however, that the progress of knowledge has been so rapid that it is impossible for the busy practitioner to keep pace with it, and that even the requirement now generally adopted by our leading medical sohools for a four-years' course of study, is inadequate for the attainment of such a degree of professional knowledge and practical skill in diagnosis and therapeutics as is desirable for one who intends to practise scientific medicine.

THE DIFFERENTIAL DIAGNOSIS BETWEEN DENGUE AND YELLOW FEVER, WITH SOME ACCOUNT OF THE EPIDEMIC OF 1897 IN TEXAS.[1]

BY H. A. WEST, M.D.,
OF GALVESTON, TEX.

THE diagnosis of disease is universally and justly regarded as the foundation-stone upon which rests the entire superstructure of practical medicine. The question, however, is in most instances a personal one only; it concerns the health, life, or death of

[1] Abstract of a paper read at the Forty-ninth Annual Meeting of the American Medical Association, Denver, Col., June 7, 8, and 9, 1898.

the individual affected, his family and friends, the public in so far as he may be a useful and influential member of society, and the physician as affording a basis for his prognosis and treatment. But there are occasions when far more momentous interests are implicated in the correct diagnosis of prevailing diseases. A complete paralysis of commerce, arrest of the wheels of industry, enforced idleness with the consequent poverty and suffering of thousands, enormous depreciation in property values of every kind, universal fear and panic, and the possibility of widespread death and desolation may be involved. To the physician himself an error in diagnosis ordinarily implies results which are comparatively inconsequential. On the other hand, there are times when such an error means public denunciation or disapprobation. A correct diagnosis, even when opposed to commercial interests, may subject him to loss of reputation and business which may last for a lifetime.

This was the state of affairs in Texas during the summer and autumn of 1897. So long as yellow fever was supposed to prevail east of the Mississippi only, and that dengue was the epidemic disease in Texas, peace reigned, but when the trouble came to our own doors by the announcement of yellow fever in Galveston and Houston, there arose a contest over the subject of diagnosis. With visits of local experts from city to city, and the gradual passing of the epidemic with no record of deaths from yellow fever, there was a popular conviction that a stupendous error had been committed by those who believed in the presence of that disease. These are matters of such recent history it is only necessary to mention them. The majority both of physicians and laymen in the State are firm in the conviction that dengue alone was the disease which was prevalent in Texas during the past summer. A minority believe that yellow fever alone prevailed, but that owing to its mild form, indisposition to spread, exceptionally small mortality, and resemblance to dengue, it was usually unrecognized. Confusion has arisen in the minds of many. They naturally ask themselves, "Are the landmarks all swept away? Have the authorities led us astray? Has a new disease, *anomalous dengue*, made its appearance? Is there no such thing as dengue? Is the so-called dengue a mild form of yellow fever, and does the latter arise *de novo*?"

The important issues dependent upon a knowledge and recognition of the truth relative to these points render it not only pertinent, but imperative, upon the part of those who are familiar with the facts to study them in concert. Now that the obscuring mists due to commercialism, prejudice, and passion have for the most part passed away, we approach the subject from a scientific standpoint. It is with this end in view, and in no spirit of dogmatism or self-assertion, that I introduce the matter for consideration.

The following hypotheses have been assumed in relation to the recent epidemic: (1) The disease was dengue only. There was no yellow fever in Galveston, Houston, or the State of Texas in 1897. (2) There were anomalous cases of dengue presenting all the symptoms of yellow fever, but proven not to be that disease by the indisposition to spread from numerous foci, and the low mortality-rate. (3) During the progress of an intense epidemic of dengue throughout the State, in Galveston, Houston, and possibly other places, yellow fever made its appearance, and in consequence of its mild form and resemblance to the prevalent disease was generally unrecognized. (4) An imputed hypothesis that the epidemic of 1897 in Texas was yellow fever only. (5) A few cases terminating fatally and others attended by marked jaundice and albuminuria were denominated acute infectious jaundice (Weil's disease).

In order to obtain definite information upon the subject a circular of inquiry was distributed to a limited extent. I regret very much that replies could not have been obtained from every infected place in the State so as to have made the report exhaustive. Summarizing reports obtained from twenty observers in eighteen places we find as follows:

The epidemic of dengue of 1897 prevailed chiefly in Southern Central Texas within a radius of 200 miles from Houston, but was prevalent to a limited degree 300 miles to the north. San Antonio, Houston, and Galveston, followed by Schulenberg and Navasota, appear to have been most intensely infected, the proportion of population in these places affected varying from seventy-five to ninety per cent. Belton, Palestine, and Huntsville followed closely with a percentage of sixty to sixty-five. In the extreme northern and eastern portions of the State, as in Gainesville, Sherman, Bonham, Terrell, and Tyler, there were but a few sporadic cases. At Dallas and Paris a very mild epidemic affected not more than six per cent. of the population. San Antonio, Galveston, and Houston seem to have been the centers of infection, as appears from the following statement: In Palestine, a railroad center about 150 miles north of Houston and 200 miles northeast of San Antonio, with double daily train service, Dr. Link states the probable origin was from these two cities. Dr. Tabor reports from Bryan, which is about 100 miles from Houston, with direct rail connection, that both the first and second cases were in persons who had been exposed in Houston. Dr.

Thomason reports from Huntsville, about seventy miles north of Houston, with direct train service with the latter place and Galveston, that the first case was that of a young lady from Galveston, and that other foci of infection were developed by persons from Houston and Galveston. Austin's first case was in a hotel clerk recently returned from San Antonio. Dr. Lee reports from Galveston that his first case, seen July 29th, was from San Antonio. The first two cases seen by the writer, August 11th, were in the persons of young men who had returned to Galveston from the Interstate Military Drill at San Antonio. Schulenberg is about equidistant from Houston and San Antonio, and may have been infected from either. Navasota is only about seventy miles from Houston.

The intensity of the disease at San Antonio, the presence there of companies of militia not only from numerous points in the State, but from States east of the Mississippi, the coincidence in time (latter part of July) of the return of the militia to their homes with the outbreak of the disease, and the positive identification of the first cases in several places in persons who had returned from the encampment, is evidence going to prove that San Antonio was the initial point of infection in the State. As to the origin of the disease in the latter city, I have no means of tracing it, but can only say that ample opportunity for conveyance of dengue was afforded by the collection there from July 19th to 26th of troops and visitors from points east of the Mississippi where the disease had already made its appearance.

Further confirmation is also afforded by the facts above cited that dengue is an infectious, a portable, and contagious disease, *i. e.*, the specific micro-organism which produces it may escape from the body of an infected individual and be transmitted by persons and fomites to other persons, thus speedily multiplying foci of infection and accounting for the rapidity of its dissemination. The fact previously observed that the progress of the disease is arrested by the advent of cold weather or frost, has also been confirmed by the consensus of the statements received. As to the effect of meteorological and hygienic conditions, the majority of observers describe the existing weather as excessively hot and dry. The mean daily temperature in Galveston during the month of October, 1897, was nearly eight degrees higher than during the corresponding month of the three previous years, and the continuance of unusually hot weather during November and December was the subject of general comment. Local sanitary conditions do not appear to have played any important part in the propagation of the disease. Dr. Paschal, however, calls attention to the excessively unsanitary condition of San Antonio at the time of the outbreak, and Dr. Tabor ascribes the comparative immunity in Bryan (only 100 cases out of a population of 4000) to the extraordinary precautions to better the sanitary condition of the town.

In regard to the symptomatology, I have not attempted to obtain information as to the complete clinical history of the cases under consideration, but rather to determine the distinctive value of those symptoms which have heretofore been regarded as of great importance in the differentiation between dengue and yellow fever, *viz.:* the presence of an eruption, hemorrhages, nausea, and vomiting, evidence of an acute nephritis, as albuminuria, scantiness of urine, presence of casts, uremia, etc., divergent pulse and temperature, jaundice and mortality.

There is almost perfect unanimity upon the part of observers as to the presence of an eruption, the proportion with this symptom varying from twenty-five to ninety per cent.; seventy-five per cent. would be a fair average. It is variously described as miliary, scarlatiniform, rubeloid, erythematous, reddish papules, macular dermatitis, urticarial, desquamative, as localized upon the face and neck, upon the face and upper part of the body, with profuse perspiration, irregular as to time of appearance, coming on the second or fourth day or end of fever, hyperemia appearing on the first day. Dr. Peeples notes the fact that while frequently absent in adults, an eruption was almost invariably present in children. The consensus of opinion is that glandular involvement occurred to a very limited extent in this epidemic, the majority of observers not noting this symptom at all, but one observer mentioning enlargement of the cervical glands and tonsils in twenty-five per cent. of the cases; another the connection between enlargement of the glands and the rash; another observed swelling of parotid and sublingual, inguinal, and suboccipital glands, especially in children; one observer noted enlargement of the submaxillary glands in twenty per cent. of his cases. With but three exceptions every observer noted the occurrence of hemorrhages. The nose, throat, stomach, intestines, uterus, and kidneys were the chief sources mentioned. The proportion in which this symptom was present varied from one to ten per cent. Three or four observed black vomit. Nausea and vomiting were notable symptoms, and occurred in a large number of the cases, varying from eighty to ninety per cent. With but few exceptions it was described as severe, excessive, incessant, almost universal, etc.

Unfortunately, observations pertaining to the urine were made so infrequently and imperfectly as to render them of but little value. Most of the observers made no examination at all; a few examined for albumin only in the worst cases. Dr. Wilkinson of Galveston, out of 500 cases, says he tested for albumin in many and found it absent, but the specific gravity was generally high. Dr. Lee of Galveston states he examined for albumin in 50 cases out of 490. Eight of these had previous kidney trouble; of the remaining 42, 20 showed slight albuminuria on the third and fourth days, and in six albumin was present in large amounts. Dr. J. M. Coble, Dallas, examined the urine in twenty-five per cent. of his cases, and found slight albuminuria in ten per cent. of them. Drs. Wilson and Harris of Navasota only made urinary examinations toward the end of the epidemic in about fifty cases. In forty of these albumin was found in considerable quantity. The urine was diminished in quantity and highly colored; casts and blood-cells occurred in three cases, and uremic symptoms in four. Dr. Taylor Hudson of Belton tested the urine only in a few suspicious cases, and found albumin in several; the urine was usually dark and diminished in quantity, uremic symptoms pronounced in several patients. Dr. D. L. Peeples, Navasota, found albumin from slight traces to abundance; in some cases there was almost total suppression, color varying from a deep straw to the color of blood. Dr. R. R. Walker, Paris, found albumin in twenty-five per cent. of his cases. Dr. W. W. Walker, Schulenberg, only tested for albumin in worst cases, found it in ten; in some in large amounts. The remainder of the reporters fail to note condition of the urine. If dengue was the only disease prevalent, albuminuria is not a rare symptom in that disease, which is contrary to the opinion heretofore entertained.

Ten out of 16 observers mention that the pulse was abnormally slow and not in proportion to the pyrexia; 3 state the ratio was normal, and 3 made no note of the symptom. Our reporters mention jaundice as present in about seven per cent. One, Dr. Wilkinson of Galveston, mentions jaundice as being of frequent occurrence, and of severe grade after October 1st. One notes it as generally present of a mild grade; another states that it was mild in ten per cent., and severe in two to five per cent. One found it more or less present, and seven failed to note icterus at all. There is almost perfect unanimity as to want of mortality in the recent epidemic. The few deaths occurring were usually ascribed to some complication. As regards progressive severity, a majority state there was no marked difference; a few assert aggravation in the beginning and in the midst of the epidemic. Dr. Wilkinson notes mildness in August, increased severity in September, progressing to violence in October. Only two or three out of the twenty suspected the presence of yellow fever.

The onset was usually sudden, attended by slight rigors or chilly sensations, with more or less severe headache, and pains in the back, limbs, and joints. As regards the paroxysm, there is a remarkable discrepancy in the statements of Drs. Lee and Wilkinson, each of whom treated about 500 cases. Dr. W. (I quote his exact language) states: "The fever in all my observations contained but the one single paroxysm; there was no secondary fever from first to last; it departed by lysis after three or four days' duration, and never returned except in cases of relapse several weeks later." Dr. Lee, on the contrary, says: "In a large proportion of the above mentioned cases two paroxysms were noticeable, the first coming on usually without positive chill or chilliness; temperature usually high in the beginning became, after slight remission, high again toward end of the attack." It is difficult to reconcile such contradictions. The probabilities are that there is no invariable rule in regard to the paroxysm. In ten cases at the Sealy Hospital, where careful thermometric observations were made, there was only one paroxysm in seven. In one there was an exacerbation in the afternoon of the day following the return to normal temperature; in one the fever was of remittent type, rising at mid-day for three successive days; in one there was a slight return of fever on the evening of the first day after the temperature reached normal.

Before proceeding to make any deductions from the foregoing, I beg leave to show what has been the accepted teaching by referring my readers to the following authorities upon the differential diagnosis of the two diseases under consideration. H. D. Schmidt, on Dengue, "Pepper's System of Med.," pp. 884–885. Matas, Keating's "Cyclopedia," vol. i, p. 894, quotes Holliday, who makes a comparison of the symptoms as follows:

YELLOW FEVER.	DENGUE.
Temperature rising regularly.	Temperature rising irregularly.
Tongue, white center, red edges, pointed.	Tongue, broad, white, indented edges, rarely red.
Stomach irritable, vomiting frequent.	Vomiting rare.
Conjunctivæ congested, jaundice appearing early.	Conjunctivæ rarely red, jaundice never observed.
Secretions all suffering, urine scanty, often albuminous, suppression frequent.	Secretions natural, urine *usually* normal, sometimes (exceptionally) traces of albumin.
Hemorrhages frequent and alarming, black vomit an urgent symptom.	Hemorrhages slight, black vomit very rare.

In regard to the condition of the urine in dengue, Matas observes (see footnote p. 889, Keating) that "in tropical pyrexiæ it is always a matter of great importance, both from the diagnostic and prognostic standpoint.'' Eugene Foster (''Ref. Handbook Med. Sciences,'' vol. ii, p. 397) gives the following summary of the points of similarity and dissimilarity in dengue and yellow fever:

In time of appearance, and generally in geographical distribution, they seem related to one another. Dengue has, however, prevailed in Asia and Egypt where yellow fever is unknown. Both diseases are arrested by severe frosts. Both dengue and yellow fever are diseases characterized by one febrile paroxysm. In order to show contrast, the symptoms will be arranged in parallel columns:

YELLOW FEVER.	DENGUE.
	The fever regular until the acme is reached, when a short stadium of a few hours occurs, followed by a remission, when a second rise of temperature takes place, but not reaching the former height.
The pulse becomes slower, while the temperature rises.	The pulse increases in frequency with the rise of temperature.
Fever lasts seventy-two hours.	Fever lasts five to eight days.
Vomiting frequent.	Vomiting rare.
Eruption rare.	Eruption common.
Jaundice almost invariably present.	Jaundice extremely rare.
Urine scanty, frequently albuminous, and often suppressed.	Urine generally high-colored, normal in quantity, free from albumin, and never suppressed.
Hemorrhages frequent, alarming, and often fatal.	Tendency to hemorrhage from nose, gums, bowels, lungs, and womb, with occasional black vomit, but hemorrhages as a rule insignificant.
Often fatal.	Proverbially non-fatal.
One attack protects from another; not protective against dengue.	One attack not protective against another; not protective against yellow fever.

Sternberg (Buck's ''Ref. Handbook, vol. viii, p. 60) says: ''Of the three prominent features making up the clinical tableau of yellow fever, *viz.*, a yellow skin, highly albuminous urine, and black vomit, only one is a constant character which can serve in establishing the diagnosis in mild cases; this is the presence of albumin in the urine. At some period in the disease, even in the mildest cases, there will be a distinct trace of albumin in the urine as shown by the usual test, and this will usually be sufficiently abundant to leave no doubt in the mind of the observer as to the nature of the precipitate. The value of this test in the differential diagnosis is indisputable. The second stage of the disease is commonly, however, well-marked in non-fatal cases, and is its most characteristic feature; the remarkably slow and soft pulse, the evident prostration of the vital powers, although the patient may be comfortable and even cheerful and desirous of getting up and taking food; the yellow tinge of conjunctivæ and skin (not always present); the tenderness on pressure in the epigastric region, and often a feeling of weight and distress, attended with intense thirst and vomiting of a transparent acid fluid, or of the characteristic black vomit; the tendency to passive hemorrhages from the mucous surface of the mouth or nose, oozing of dark blood from the gums, or lips or sides of the red and fissured tongue; the scanty urinary secretion, and the presence of albumin, usually in considerable amount, constitute an unmistakable ensemble of symptoms.''

It appears from the above quotations that the symptoms which have heretofore been relied upon to differentiate between yellow fever and dengue, are the occurrence in the former of albuminuria, the characteristic facies (inclusive of jaundice), the divergent pulse and temperature, excessive irritability of the stomach, and increased disposition to hemorrhages. The absence of such symptoms in the main, the presence of an eruption in a large proportion of cases, and a want of mortality are characteristic of dengue. In the epidemic herein described we have an apparently inextricable confusion. A widespread epidemic of fever presented the symptomatology of yellow fever in many instances, but with the eruption of dengue and practically with no mortality. One of two deductions is irresistible; either the two diseases approximate more intimately in their symptomatology than has heretofore been taught, or else yellow fever of remarkably mild type has been associated to a greater or less degree with dengue. Granting the reliability of the testimony herein presented both conclusions are warrantable. I shall not attempt here to solve this problem so far as the epidemic of the interior is concerned, but will present the evidence which is convincing to my mind that the latter proposition is true as to the coast cities of Galveston and Houston.

Before doing so, however, let me refer briefly to certain facts in regard to the epidemic east of the Mississippi, taken chiefly from the report of the Louisiana State Board of Health, dated December 6, 1897. The first death from yellow fever was reported by Dr. J. M. Holloway of Louisville, Ky., about August 18th, the patient having gone to that city from New Orleans *via* Ocean Springs, where the disease was supposed to have been contracted. Subsequent to this four official investigations were made as to the nature of the epidemic at Ocean Springs, resulting as follows: (1) The visit of Dr. S. R. Oliphant, President of the Louisiana Board of Health, August 22d, 1897, who reports finding an epidemic had been prevailing the previous six weeks, that 400 cases had occurred in the practice of two physicians without a single resultant death, and that it was considered to be dengue of mild type. (2) On August 23d a commission of experts from the New Orleans Board, from the Mississippi State Board, and others, signed a report which concludes as follows: ''After a careful inspection and examination of the aforesaid cases we are positive in our opinion that the disease is dengue and that in no case is there, or has there been, any symptom which would lead to even a suspicion of a more serious disease." (3) On August 27th we have a report of another commission to which the name of the health-officer of Alabama is added, stating "in reply to your request we have again investigated the fever at Ocean Springs, which is abating and is absolutely without fatality. The conclusion arrived at is that *it is not yellow fever*." (4) On September 6th we have the following statement: "The patient died Sunday night, and early Monday morning the expected autopsy was performed by the bacteriologist of the board in the presence of the medical gentlemen assembled. Unmistakable evidence of yellow fever having been revealed, we arrived at a unanimous verdict."

According to Dr. Oliphant the grand total of cases in New Orleans did not reach 2000 nor the deaths 300, a mortality-rate of fifteen per cent. based upon reported cases which would doubtless be much smaller if founded upon the actual number. Another significant fact noted by Dr. Oliphant in the epidemic, which verifies the history of previous ones in New Orleans and elsewhere, is that yellow fever does not burst forth suddenly, but gathers volume and force after smouldering for a time, *e. g.*, it was introduced into Edwards, Miss., August 8th, but gained no headway until the middle of September. Confirmatory as to the remarkable mildness of the last epidemic[1] Dr. L. Sexton writes from New Orleans, September 20th, "*Our present death-rate is lower than in any epidemic of yellow fever.* If the present death-rate prevails throughout this visitation we will have to send around a subscription-list for our undertakers."

What bearing have these facts upon conditions as they existed in Texas? In my opinion they are convincing, when taken in connection with the clinical history of certain cases, that the epidemic upon the Texas Gulf coast was similar to that in Louisiana, Mississippi, and Alabama, the results being modified by the late introduction of yellow-fever infection and by the presence of unfavorable conditions for its dissemination. It should be remembered that the declaration of quarantine at Galveston was made on September 10th, nearly a month after the recognition of yellow fever at Ocean Springs, that the latter place is directly upon a common route of travel between Eastern and Texas points, and that a month subsequently the diagnosis of yellow fever in Galveston and Houston was made by Dr. Guiteras. Under such circumstances it is not surprising that yellow-fever infection should have been introduced into Texas; nor should it be a matter of wonderment that it should not have been generally recognized, when we take into consideration that it came in the guise of dengue, was introduced late in the season into localities where the conditions were unfavorable for its spread, and that according to all testimony it was the mildest epidemic of yellow fever ever known in the history of the country.

Admitting that there is greater similarity in the symptomatology of the two diseases than has heretofore been acknowledged, the question arises How can they be differentiated? In my opinion chiefly by the occurrence of a complicating acute nephritis in yellow fever and its absence in dengue. In the latter simple parenchymatous changes may occur in the kidneys and be manifested by an evanescent and mild albuminuria, while in the former, in a series of cases, many will afford incontestable evidence of the occurrence of a severe nephritis, *viz.*, scanty urine of high color and specific gravity, intense and persistent albuminuria, hematuria, casts, decided tendency to suppression and the accompanying uremia.

One of the arguments which has been repeatedly used against the existence of yellow fever in Texas during the past season, was the want of mortality. Upon this point let me quote Dr. Morris.[1] "From October 1 to November 18, 1897, the death-rate in Houston was $33\frac{1}{3}$ per cent. greater than in the corresponding period of 1896." The causes given in death-certificates are as follows: Senility 11 (four of whom were not over sixty); dengue 5; enteritis and gastritis 11; fever 10; meningitis 1; kidney disease 5. The record of Galveston does not show any increase of deaths during the months of August, September, and October over the three previous years. There were five deaths, however, preceded by symptoms of yellow fever. It is a significant circumstance that in four of these uremia was given in the certificate as the cause of death. In the other congestion of the lungs was mentioned as the primary, and bilious fever as the remote, cause.

Those who deny the existence of yellow fever in Texas during the past season rely chiefly upon the apparent indisposition of the disease to spread from numerous foci. In other words, they contend that the presence of the infection necessarily involves its dissemination. No extended argument is requisite to demonstrate the fallacy of such conclusions. The pathogenic micro-organism of yellow fever is a facultative parasite, but its ordinary mode of life is saprophytic. It grows and develops outside of the body when the conditions are favorable for its repro-

[1] *American Medico-Surgical Bulletin*, page 903, October 10, 1897.

[1] *S. W. Med. Record*, pp. 413-414, January, 1898.

duction. The fact that the soil of Texas was an unfavorable one for the multiplication of the yellow-fever germ last season is an adequate explanation of the history of the recent epidemic. It is not contended that the hygienic condition in our cities was perfect, but that the combination of circumstances was antagonistic to the extensive dispersion of the infection. Instead of being a blot upon the sanitary escutcheon of Houston and Galveston, it is another demonstration of the fact, which has previously been observed, that yellow fever may be brought to these places without necessarily involving an extensive epidemic or serious mortality.

Two important lessons should be emphasized: (1) the urgency of promptly recognizing the early cases, and calling them by their proper name, for by this means only may subsequent disaster in many instances be averted; (2) we should put our houses in order, in other words, adopt every possible method of domiciliary and municipal cleanliness. Napoleon is said to have remarked that "Providence was on the side with the strongest artillery." When yellow fever is around, Providence is on the side of the town with the best sewers. Again has it been demonstrated that yellow fever may masquerade in the garb of dengue, and that the latter is a portable disease. Leaving out of the case the probable association with yellow fever, it becomes a serious question whether dengue should not be considered a quarantinable disease. The suffering and expense incident to an extensive epidemic like the one of last season would certainly appear to justify measures of prevention.

ELECTRICITY IN GYNECOLOGY.[1]

BY HENRY J. GARRIGUES, M.D., OF NEW YORK.

WE shall, perhaps, arrive at an answer to the question propounded by the Society in the easiest and clearest way by passing in review the different kinds of electricity—franklinism, faradism, and galvanism.

Franklinism, or static electricity, has never played a great rôle in gynecology. Few gynecologists own the expensive Holtz machine. It belongs rather to the domain of the neurologist, and the general practitioner. Those who have it will, however, probably find its current of value as a general nerve tonic, and capable of subduing local pain, when chiefly of a neuralgic origin.

Faradism, or the interrupted induced electric current, has widened its therapeutic field considerably of late years. The old-time little machine with its short, coarse wire has given way to the modern apparatus with a secondary coil composed of three wires of different gage, measuring together 1½ miles in length. By improved mechanical contrivances the pain incident to the application of this current may be greatly reduced or abolished altogether. By using a thicker, shorter wire we obtain a stimulating effect which may be utilized to the greatest advantage in gynecological disturbances, such as subinvolution, infantile uterus, amenorrhea, sterility, or uterine hemorrhage. For subinvolution I take it to be the best of all known remedies. It works in two ways, partly by disintegrating and eliminating diseased tissues, partly by causing the muscle-fibers, composing the bulk of the uterine walls, to contract. A similar effect may be expected in cases of chronic metritis which do not originate in childbirth.

For infantile uterus this remedy is likewise the best known, but here the prognosis is less favorable, as the condition in most cases is incurable.

In amenorrhea I have been so successful with galvanism that I have not had occasion to test the value of inductional electricity, but it is highly praised by those who use it.

For uterine hemorrhage, if only caused by laxity of tissue and lack of proper innervation, the bipolar electrode, applied either in the vagina, or in the uterus, is a powerful therapeutic agent. In this connection I may also recall the peerless value of faradization in securing uterine contraction in cases of post-partum hemorrhage.

In the long, thin wire, on the other hand, we have of late years obtained a most valuable addition to our therapeutic armamentarium. This high-tension current has great analgesic power. It answers, therefore, an excellent purpose in cases of dysmenorrhea, pelvic pain, dyspareunia, coccygodynia, and such cases of salpingo-oophoritis, and local peritonitis, in which the nervous elements predominate over the inflammatory.

Galvanism.—Of still greater importance is the galvanic current in gynecological treatment, and it is serviceable in a variety of ways. By using a large, wet electrode on the abdomen, and a large, wet electrode in the vagina, we can send a strong current through the uterus, or the appendages, where it exercises its interpolar, electrolytic action. Thus it becomes a valuable therapeutic agent in the treatment of chronic metritis, and chronic or subacute forms of inflammation of the adnexa, with or without pelvic exudation, or deposits of organized lymph. By this means I have saved many an ovary which otherwise would have been sacrificed. This treatment is effective in many cases in which tincture of iodin, ichthyol-glycerin, and hot douches, fail to give the desired results; but, if there is cystic degeneration, one helps

[1] Read at the Twenty-third Annual Meeting of the American Gynecological Society, Boston, Mass., May 24, 25, and 26, 1898, in discussion of the topic, "Has Electricity Ceased To Be a Useful Therapeutic Agent in Gynecology?"

as little as the other, and surgical interference becomes necessary.

It often happens that there is produced a painful swelling around the stumps, left by salpingo-oophorectomy, or supravaginal amputation of the uterus. This condition is easily cured by the galvanic current.

By connecting an intra-uterine platinum electrode with the negative pole of the battery we have the best remedy for functional amenorrhea I know of. A similar electrode made of copper and connected with the positive pole destroys the gonococcus, and has, therefore, been used in gonorrhea of the cervix. It is, however, apt to produce stenosis of the cervical canal, and must be used cautiously.

In extra-uterine pregnancy electricity is used much less now than some years ago, but if this condition were found in an early stage, say during the first two months of pregnancy, in a woman personally dear to me, I would prefer it to surgical interference. Facts remain facts, even if lost sight of for a time, and numerous cases observed by men whose diagnostic skill is unimpeachable have been recorded in which this method has killed the fetus and has not had any bad influence on the mother. Either galvanism or faradism may be used, preferably the former.

The other chief form of galvanism is galvanocauterization, and in this form, electricity, far from being obsolete, has constantly enlarged its field of usefulness. A mild degree of cauterization used without an anesthetic is one of the best remedies for ectropion. Cervical membranes that have resisted all sorts of applications, douches, and suppositories sometimes become healthy by a few applications of a nearly dry gas-carbon electrode connected with the positive pole and applied to the everted part or through the whole length of the canal. A similar treatment carried out with the intra-uterine platinum electrode has often allowed me to cure a menorrhagia which had resisted thorough curetting by my own hand.

In the Apostoli treatment for uterine fibroids we have a combination of galvanocauterization of the mucous membrane of the uterus and of interpolar electrolysis. It is not an infallible remedy; I have seen cases in which it had no effect; but the worst cases are the most grateful. In the majority of cases, pain ceases very soon, menstruation becomes normal, the patient regains general health, and the tumor is reduced in size and becomes stationary. In one patient whose uterus reached an inch above the umbilicus there was no diminution, but when I saw her six years later, the uterus had not grown, and she had been well in the meantime. In some cases I have seen tumors pushed out of the wall so as to form prominences in the peritoneal cavity. Only in one case have I seen the myoma disappear altogether, but this is so marked a case that I take this opportunity of publishing its chief features. Mrs. K., from New Orleans, forty-two years old, had a myoma in the posterior wall of the uterus as large as a medium-sized orange. She suffered great pain, had fearful hemorrhages, which only could be controlled by tamponade, and she led the life of an invalid. She had thirty eight applications in nine months, all pain disappeared, menstruation became normal, and she became a healthy woman, so that treatment was discontinued. When seen a year later, there was not a trace of the tumor to be felt; and she was in perfect health. One such case is enough for me nearly always to recommend a trial of electricity before resorting to operative procedures as did Thomas Heith, the most successful operator for fibroids in his time.

In operations for carcinoma the galvanocautery is of great value, whether used with the dome-shaped cautery to sear a cavity left by the curette, or with a wire to extirpate the cervix, or with a knife with which we either can cut off a portion of the uterus or remove the whole uterus with its appendages. The last-named method is recognized as the best of all methods of vaginal hysterectomy for carcinoma, because it avoids wound infection and perhaps even destroys the germs of the disease at some distance beyond the place where it is applied.

In closing I will only recall the value of the electric lamp in abdominal or vaginal operations.

Far from having ceased to be a useful therapeutic agent in gynecology, electricity not only holds its own, but has of late years enlarged its territory in different directions and deserves the closest study from every gynecologist.

HAS ELECTRICITY CEASED TO BE A USEFUL THERAPEUTIC AGENT IN GYNECOLOGY?[1]

BY EGBERT H. GRANDIN, M.D.,
OF NEW YORK.

IN taking the affirmative of this question, it seems fitting that I should glance back ten years in order to suitably account for the faith that is in me to-day. From 1884 to 1892 I delved deep into the mysteries of electricity and fully equipped myself for the formation of an unbiased opinion in reference to its sphere of utility in the treatment of the diseases of women. The outcome of my study and of my practical experience was the publication of a monograph on the subject, the keynote of which was a

[1] Read at the Twenty-third Annual Meeting of the American Gynecological Society, Boston, May 24, 25, and 26, 1898.

protest against the ultra enthusiasm which pervaded other workers in a similar field. As I read that monograph in the light of views held by me to-day I regret little that I wrote then, with the single exception of the opinion I advanced in regard to the treatment of ectopic gestation; an opinion founded on what was then the weight of distinguished authority, controlled by a limited amount of personal experience. The doctrine preached by me in this monograph was simply this: Electricity constitutes a valuable adjuvant to other routine methods of treatment; its rôle is palliative, pure and simple. To-day, even as I have rejected certain other routine methods of treatment because experience has taught me their futility, even so have I shelved electricity, because experience has taught me that cure is possible through resort to surgery and that this is better than palliation through electricity. Five years ago my electrical outfit was an elaborate one; to-day I possess no outfit, having given it away to a colleague whose credulity was born as mine died. And yet I would not have you think that I was not as honest in intention in the days when I used electricity as a remedial palliative agent as I am to-day when I discard it. My change in belief has been due to causes of a two-fold nature; in the first place I gradually emerged from a pathology which held sway for years over the minds of the leaders in the profession into the clearer and truer which rules to-day; and, in the second place, I found out practically that there were speedier ways of accomplishing the cure of certain conditions than through electrical treatment, and that in other conditions electricity was an absolute failure on account of the different pathology underlying them than that which I formerly had in mind. In short I had been taught badly, although my teachers were unquestionably honest in belief, and I emerged from under their influence a little later than some of my colleagues, but with the decided advantage over them that I declined to condemn absolutely an agent until after I had tested it and found it wanting. My policy was and still is: Test all things and after the test hold fast to that which proves good.

It appears to me that I can best exemplify the reasons which actuated me in shelving electricity by taking up in turn the affections peculiar to women wherein I formerly contended it was of value and stating succinctly my reasons for preferring the methods of treatment—surgical and non-surgical, to which I resort to-day.

Among the minor affections formerly treated by me by electricity may be noted uterine flexions with stenosis and endometritis (uncomplicated by tubal or ovarian disease). As I look backward it appears to me that I selected electricity in the spirit of protest against other methods then current, such as gradual dilatation and intra-uterine medication. I became satisfied that by means of the negative pole of the battery and low milliamperage I could overcome stenosis more quickly than by graduated dilators, aside from the fact that asepsis was thus better secured than was possible with dilators in routine office work. One method was certainly as rational as the other. The complicating endometritis, furthermore, or this condition aside from stenosis, it was fully as rational to treat by the intra-uterine electrode as by the highly problematical application of drugs carried on cotton-wrapped sticks And, again, asepsis in office work was more thorough. My success was fair as regards the abatement of discharges and relief of dysmenorrhea, but relapses were frequent. I therefore discarded electricity even as I had previously the intra-uterine applicator, and at one sitting under anesthesia, with the dilator and the curette, I accomplished with greater certainty and more speedily the cure of the symptoms due to the stenosis and to the endometritis.

Passing to the inflammatory affections of the uterine adnexa, my reason for advocating their treatment by electricity was simply because I was steeped in the then prevailing doctrine of cellulitis. It seemed as rational to treat cellulitis by electricity (and I still believe it was) as it did by the painting of the vaginal vault with iodin and the insertion of tampons *ad infinitum*, methods which, at the time I am considering, were in high favor, and, indeed, as I speak to-day, I wish to go on record as believing that the one method is as safe, as effective, as rational as the other. With the disappearance of the cellulitic-cobwebs from my eyelids, with the acceptance of what is now the general teaching that, with rare exceptions, cellulitis is a myth and that we are dealing with diseased tubes and ovaries and with peritonitis, I perforce rejected electricity and at one and the same time iodin and tampons. I would still claim that by means of the one or the other, in selected cases, symptomatic cure for a variable period is possible, but anatomical cure never. The careful reader of my writings will find that the latter I never claimed. To-day I am satisfied that there is but one way to secure cure and that this is through surgery. The mortality-rate in my hands in non-selected cases is held at two per cent. Attempts at palliation by electricity or iodin and tampons simply postpone the surgical day and then many a case is in more desperate straits and the mortality-rate inevitably rises.

Passing to the treatment of fibroids by electricity, it was tested by me in about fifty cases, and I may say that I never saw one disappear except where the menopause entered as a factor. In fully thirty per cent. of the cases I could check the discharges, but only temporarily. The latter effect I found I could secure more speedily and for a longer interval by curettage, and, therefore, from the standpoint of the discharges I found no use for electricity. Be it understood that I never resorted to electropuncture, but that my experience was limited to the Apostoli method. Puncture I always feared on account of the probability of producing local necrosis of the tumor. Fibroid tumors carrying pain as a symptom practical experience soon taught me were unsuitable for any treatment short of the knife because the pain was due (in my experience) to the association of diseased appendages. Thus I have record of a number of instances where complicating pyosalpinx, ovarian abscess, suppurating ovarian cyst (thick-walled) were the causal factors of the pain and not the fibroid, and in some of these cases these factors were only certified to after opening the abdomen. Instances of this type it would be dangerous to treat by electricity, while surgery gives me a mortality-rate in unselected cases of two and one-half per cent., this mortality rate not being traceable to the operation but to the complicating factor making the operation one of urgency, such as suppurating ovarian cyst, peritonitis consecutive to rupture of a pus-sac, etc. Subjects of this type would assuredly die also under any other form of treatment. Patients with uncomplicated uterine fibroids operated on by me have up to date uniformly recovered. Little wonder then that I prefer the certainty of surgery to the uncertainty and protracted delay entailed by electricity.

The last subject I touch upon is ectopic gestation. The first patient I saw treated by electricity went into deep collapse and although, if my memory serves me, the woman recovered, I now realize that this was due more to good luck than to good management. This experience should have been an eye-opener to me but I was easily swerved by the weight of distinguished authority and at this date the leading gynecologists of America favored electricity, being under the subtle influence of this agent to a blinding degree. I treated four to six patients personally by electricity and they all recovered. Of course it was open to doubt if any one case was an instance of ectopic gestation, since the abdomen was never opened for absolute certification. The customary symptomatology was present however. Finally a woman thus treated by me lay in collapse for hours; she had a consecutive hematoma and hematocele. The latter eventually suppurated and was incised per vaginam. The woman recovered. About eighteen months thereafter I again saw this woman in collapse with precedent symptomatology of ectopic. I opened the abdomen at once, found free intraperitoneal hemorrhage from a ruptured tube and the other tube was distended with pus, agglutinated and utterly useless to the woman except as a source of pain and of danger. In short, the tube I had treated electrically for ectopic had become a pyosalpinx and here I had a *demonstratio ad absurdum* of the electrical treatment of ectopic gestation. The woman recovered and so did I from the effects of erroneous belief. At the first opportunity which offered I told the Fellows of the New York Obstetrical Society that I had permanently discarded electricity and why.

Since that date I have operated on fourteen cases of ectopic gestation, inclusive of two cases in collapse from free intraperitoneal hemorrhage. One of my patients died suddenly thirty-six hours after operation and the certified cause of death (without autopsy) was fatty heart. In fully half my series disease of the adnexa of the other side has been a complicating factor. In none of the patients operated on by me would electricity have availed aught unless to expedite a fatal issue. To-day I take the ground that in the presence of a presumptive history of ectopic gestation a clean cut is preferable to and safer than expectancy.

Thus, briefly, have I outlined my views in regard to electricity. Whatever weight they have must be due purely to the fact that they emanate from a man who has had ample experience with the agent and did not condemn it untried. Surely such views should carry greater conviction than hysterical claims in favor of the agent advanced by men who have never operated or but rarely; and, furthermore, I would contend that the position I have assumed in this controversial matter is more befitting the scientific man than that of colleagues who decried electricity without trial and abused those who used it even though by chance it has eventuated that the views they expressed were the sound ones. There is little room for dogmatism in this science of ours where views change almost daily. Electricity had as much warrant for existence in the therapy of gynecology as many another method equally obsolete so far as I am concerned, and yet practised and taught still by a no means insignificant school. Need I state that I refer to tamponade and iodin to the vaginal vault for months and years until you or I operate on the patient and cure her? It is in the spirit of charity toward all that I view these false prophets—and yet earnest workers and honest in belief. I would like all to do as I have attempted: Admit error as soon as convinced.

WAR ARTICLES.

NEWS OF THE WEEK.

IN all probability during the present war disease will be the element of danger rather than Spanish bullets, and the physician will be more in demand than the surgeon; nevertheless, the effect of the small balls used in the modern rifles, projected with almost inconceivable velocity, will prove a most interesting study. The force with which these bullets travel is said to be sufficient to cause one to perforate eight men in succession standing directly behind each other with a space of three feet separating them, the shot being fired from a point twenty feet distant from the first man. In an experiment with one of these modern military rifles recently, the writer, from a distance of five yards, drove a bullet completely through a maple log twelve inches in diameter. In another test, firing at the end of the log, the bullet penetrated to a depth of forty-six inches.

. . . .

The great progress of late years in surgery, especially abdominal surgery, will doubtless result in the saving of many lives during the present conflict. Until quite recently, and notably during the Civil War, and all prior wars, an abdominal wound was regarded as inevitably fatal, but now, provided surgical aid can be rendered promptly, as will be the case under nearly all circumstances, the probability of saving life is very great. During the Civil War it was not unusual for two or more days to elapse before even the most dangerously wounded men could receive surgical attention. The awful aftermath of death following the battle of Gettysburg will be recalled with horror, but thanks to the systematic and thorough preparations being made by the Medical and Surgical Departments, and the achievements and advances in the science and art of surgery the proportion of deaths to wounds will be greatly lessened.

. . . .

If there is such a thing as an optimistic view of a bullet wound perhaps it will arise from the fact that the bullet of a modern rifle strikes and penetrates its victim with such velocity that there is practically no danger of shreds of cloth being carried into the flesh, and the prospect of infection from this source is thus reduced in very great degree. The Spanish troops are mostly armed with Mauser rifles, which carry with tremendous velocity. Wounds made with these weapons are rarely infected as above described, and unless a bone is struck heal rapidly under favorable conditions.

. . . .

The Daughters of the Revolution have taken upon themselves a grand work and one which reaches far beyond the actual care of the soldier in the field. The Government has accepted their offer as embodied in the following resolutions, which were unanimously adopted at the recent meeting of the Society in Washington:

Resolved, That the members of the society be requested to unite in a general effort to succor needy families of men who have gone to the front, and to furnish comforts for soldiers and sailors, whether regular or volunteer. That a large sum of money to be used in emergency and exigency calls of every kind, such as are attendant upon the condition of a nation engaged in warfare. That a war committee, composed of the members of the National Board of Management, with the addition of Mrs. George M. Sternberg and Mrs. Charles L. Alden, be formed. That the treasurer-general, National Society of the Daughters of the American Revolution, be elected treasurer of the war fund, and that the moneys be under authority and direction of a sub committee.

. . . .

Plans are well under way to prevent the introduction of yellow fever into this country by troops returning from Cuba. Rigid quarantine regulations will be enforced at every point along the Atlantic and Gulf coasts. Surgeon-General Wyman of the Marine Hospital Service has the supervision of this far-sighted and most important matter.

. . . .

The number of rejections of candidates for the volunteer service from the militia of the several States because of failure to pass the required physical examinations, has occasioned much and reasonable surprise. We say reasonable surprise, because although it has always been necessary for a man to pass a physical examination before enlisting in the militia it now appears that the physical requirements in time of war are quite different from those in times of peace. Perhaps it does not require a very high physical condition to enable a man to parade for a few hours through a fine street lined with admiring citizens, but if our State militia is intended to be capable of military service in time of need should not the physical standard required be just as high as that necessary for volunteers in the regular army?

. . . .

As affording striking evidence of the fitness of college men for the life and duties of a soldier the report of the condition of the Yale men in the State camp at Niantic is interesting. Out of more than sixty undergraduates from Yale who went into camp not one failed to pass the required physical examination.

. . . .

The best record made by any company of militiamen in the matter of physical condition is held by the Second Separate Company, Third Regiment, of Auburn, N. Y. There were but two rejections from the entire company.

REQUISITES FOR AN ARMY CAMP; EXISTING CONDITIONS IN THE VICINITY OF TAMPA.

By H. S. KILBOURNE, M.D.,
MAJOR AND SURGEON, UNITED STATES ARMY, WITH THE 5TH ARMY CORPS AT TAMPA, FLORIDA.

APART from purely military considerations the first three requisites for an encampment are good water, good wood (fuel), and good grass. The first two are closely related to the health and efficiency of the troops, while the first and last involves the well-being of horses, the constant auxillaries of men engaged in war. To these three must be added a fourth of little less importance, *viz.:* a dry, well-drained soil. The vicinity of Tampa meets all these requirements save the third. The water-supply is abundant and pure and fuel is plentiful and readily obtained. The soil on Tampa heights is sandy and dry, with natural surface drainage into the adjoining tidal river (Hillsboro), but grass for the horses and train animals is lacking, a deficiency for which an arid soil and a prolonged period of drouth are sufficient causes.

The above-mentioned sanitary advantages are combined with the military features of a practicable harbor and railway facilities for the movement of troops and supplies. The water source is a large spring situated within the city limits, independent of local rainfall, unfailing, and yielding water having a small percentage of organic mattei and of a moderate degree of hardness, and shown by analysis to contain less than ten grains per gallon of dry solids in suspension or solution. The spring is protected by a retaining wall of brick, the water being pumped directly into the mains for distribution to the city and outlying camps by service pipes laid down by the water company according to requirements. A three-inch main or its equivalent in pipes of smaller caliber, will supply sufficient water for the troops and trains of a division for all purposes excepting bathing, facilities for which are found in the tide-water of the river and bay. About two gallons per diem is a minimum allowance per man, eight gallons being allotted to each horse or train animal, but as there is no scarcity of the supply the water is more freely expended. The outflow of the spring is estimated at three million gallons per diem, more than sufficient for the needs of the town consumers and an army corps.

In addition to this natural source of water-supply, there are a number of shallow driven wells scattered in and about the town from which the poorer sort of the citizens obtain a precarious supply derived from the ground and surface waters and which, owing to the absence of sewers and the general use of privy vaults in many localities, are subject to contamination and infection. The sanitary regulations of the camps require that all water excepting that from the spring be boiled for use, preliminary boiling of the authorized supply not being required. Ice produced from distilled water by ice-machines in the city and neighboring towns is procurable at fair rates and finds a ready market among the troops, the hospitals being supplied by expenditure of the hospital funds.

METEOROLOGIC SUMMARY, TAMPA, FLA., FOR THE YEAR ENDING DECEMBER 31, 1897.
(Compiled from record of United States Weather Bureau.)

	January.	February.	March.	April.	May.	June.	July.	August.	September.	October.	November.	December.
Highest temperature	78	82	88	86	90	94	94	94	90	88	82	82
Lowest temperature	29	39	50	47	55	68	70	70	54	56	50	40
Range, absolute	49	43	38	39	35	26	24	24	36	32	32	42
Precipitation	1.42	5.40	1.44	4.65	.33	8.46	6.23	7.84	10.73	4.78	.63	2.50
Number of clear days	10	10	11	10	22	13	8	12	8	17	16	14
Number of partly cloudy days	14	15	16	13	8	15	19	14	15	11	12	11
Number of cloudy days	7	3	4	7	1	2	4	5	7	3	2	6
Average humidity, per cent	78	86	81	73	70	78	79	82	86	80	81	81

The climatic conditions of Tampa are subtropical with modification due to proximity to the coast. A rainy season, delayed this year, usually begins in May or June, continuing for nearly one-half the year and is followed by a dry season during which a scanty rainfall occurs. The humidity is variable according to the direction of air currents from or toward the sea, ranging between an average percentage of 70 to 90. The month of May was hot and dry and the air in and about the camp exceedingly dusty and irritating to sensitive throats. A meteorological summary for the year 1897 is appended for the information of any of the statistic-tolerant readers of the MEDICAL NEWS. It will be noted that the summer heats are not extreme but continuous and that the difference between summer and winter maxima is less than 20°.

The City of Tampa, with a population of about 25,000, exhibits for the year 1897 a mortality-rate of 13.30 per 1000.[1] Out of a total of 346 deaths for the year phthisis heads the table with 47 deaths, followed by enteritis and enterocolitis with 25; malarial (?) fever with 16; pneumonia, 14; trismus nascentium, 12; hepatitis, 11, and Bright's disease, 10; typhoid fever is charged with only 6 deaths, all other diseases and injuries having a lower rate. The high death-rate from phthisis is accounted for by the fact that Tampa is a winter-resort for invalid Americans with narrow chests and long purses who come here in the vain hope of recovering from pulmonary tuberculosis in the later destructive stages of that disorder. The city is favored with one hotel of the first-class, heretofore open only to winter visitors, but now having its wide corridors and ample grounds thronged with the gathering military, war correspondents, and the adventurous and curious from all quarters of the world.

[1] "Annual Statement of Vital Statistics," J. W. Douglas, M.D., 1897.

MEDICAL AID DURING AN ACTION.

BY RAYMOND SPEAR, M.D.,
ASSISTANT SURGEON, UNITED STATES NAVY, ON BOARD FLAGSHIP "NEW YORK."

WHEN "general quarters" is sounded aboard the U. S. S. "New York," the sick-bay is immediately converted into an operating-room, an operating-table is placed in the center, the ordinary instruments for amputating limbs are arranged in trays, and immediately disinfected by steam, aseptic dressings are laid out, and antiseptic solutions prepared for immediate use. In former times during an action the doctors remained in the sick-bay and the wounded were brought to them, but conditions have changed, and now on a ship like the "New York," where there is practically no protected place during an action, this is impossible. The injuries on the old ships were spread out probably over several hours, and the doctors could perform many of the necessary operations during the fight. The engagements between modern ships do not last long, and operations during the period of action is not to be considered on an unprotected ship.

The question which confronts the medical officers is how to save the most lives. It is a known fact that the majority of lives lost during a war are due to the loss of blood. Some authorities estimate the loss of life from hemorrhage alone as seventy-five per cent. of the total. It becomes the duty of the medical officers to take measures to stop all bleeding from wounds. To do this the crew of each gun receives instruction in First Aid to the Wounded by the medical officers. Each gun has its own outfit of rubber tubing and packages of aseptic dressings. The men are instructed how to apply the rubber tubing to the limbs in order to arrest hemorrhage, how to apply aseptic dressings, being especially cautioned against touching wounds, and finally how to support limbs when broken, and how to carry the wounded and where to place them.

Each deck of the "New York" is divided up into several compartments, separated by watertight bulkheads. During an action these bulkheads are closed. Under these conditions the medical officers cannot reach all of the wounded if they are in different compartments; therefore, if a man be injured sufficiently to be disabled, he is attended to by some of his companions. If an extremity be badly injured, a piece of rubber-tubing is applied so as to arrest hemorrhage, an aseptic dressing is applied, the leg is bound to the other one for support, or the arm is bound to the body if fractured, the man is placed in a hammock, and dragged to the best protected place nearby where he will not be in the way, and here he waits for the surgeon. The wounded are placed athwart ships if possible, thus offering the smallest possible target for the shells that come through the ship's side.

The doctors take their stations in the most protected parts of the ship, *viz.*, behind the turrets, and here establish dressing-stations and attend to all the wounded in the immediate vicinity. The surgeons have received orders to expose themselves as little as possible during action, as their real work begins when the fight is over. Each surgeon carries a haversack in which are pieces of rubber-tubing for controlling hemorrhage from the extremities, hemostats, a pocket-case, hypodermic syringe, and solutions of strychnin and morphin ready for hypodermic use, and some first-aid packages. Stationed with each doctor is a nurse, who carries in a knapsack surgical dressings, antiseptic solutions, whisky, etc. When the action is over, the surgeons will take a hasty survey of the wounded and give such attention as is absolutely necessary to each. When the wounded have been attended to, those cases needing immediate operation will be looked after, three operating-tables being established if necessary. The wounded will not be disturbed, but will await the arrival of the hospital ship "Solace," and will then be transferred to her, where they will receive medical attention during their transportation to the hospitals in Key West.

BAKING OF BREAD IN THE FIELD.

[Special Correspondence of THE MEDICAL NEWS.]

CAMP TAMPA HEIGHTS,
TAMPA, FLA., May, 30, 1898.

IN my last semiweekly medical report to the surgeon of division, through the brigade surgeon, the following note was entered under "remarks": "The bread was sodden and heavy, not sufficiently baked." Before the ink was dry, Brigade Surgeon Ebert and myself investigated the causes of the failure to provide good bread for the regiment, and sought to find means for insuring a wholesome, well-baked loaf under all circumstances hereafter.

Inquiry elicited the fact that the companies of the regiment had arranged to turn in their flour rations to a civilian baker near the camp, and to receive bread from him, in return, pound for pound. The terms were fairer than the bread, for a second regiment was turning in to another bakery 196 pounds of flour, and drawing out therefor only 160 pounds of bread, but the fact of the case is that the bakeries of Tampa have not sufficient capacity to supply the present large demand made upon them by the resident community and by the large increment of floating population incident to the encampment of nearly 5000 troops in the vicinity, consequently to compass as large an output of bread as possible, the proper duration of the baking process is cut short, and the bread loaves are underdone.

But (and this is the gist of the whole matter), if the thriving town of Tampa cannot fully provide us with well-baked bread with all its bakeries in force, how is the army to be provided with this desirable and very necessary article of diet when our troops are landed in Cuba? The answer is simple—the *portable ovens*. We have all heard of them, and can read of them in the "Manual for Army Cooks," published by the War Department, but so accustomed are we to make use of the Dutch oven for small detachments, and so seldom are we thrown on our own resources for large field bakings, that I dare say but few of the regiments are provided with portable field ovens.

Our brigade commissary officer, 1st Lieut. Arthur Johnson, 17th Infantry, finding that his regiment was taxed 100 pounds of bread for the baking of 196 pounds of flour by a civilian baker, purchased and put into operation two small portable field ovens of a capacity of ninety-six loaves for each oven, and sufficient, when operated by two enlisted men as bakers, to furnish a regiment with its bread ration. These ovens were manufactured in Tampa on twenty-four-hour's notice, at a cost of $17.50 each, and were readily "set up" underground in the field. They are provided with removable sheet-iron bottoms, which are taken out before the fire is started and replaced when the dough in pans is introduced. The arched body of each oven is made of sheets of steel in preference to sheet-iron.

It is a common practice when encamped on a clayey soil for troops to construct a bake-oven by baking a clay body; for instance, by placing a barrel filled with combustibles in an excavation, covering with sand and clay, and after combustion has ceased, removing the sand and débris, leaving a clay oven. But in this locality there is no clay, only a deep, sandy soil, and in Cuba, a rich red loam, hence the body of an oven in these localities must be constructed from metal.

So important does this subject appear to medical officers with large bodies of troops in the field, and in the hope that these small portable ovens will be more generally adopted by regiments already mobilized or about to be mobilized, that I venture to quote somewhat in extenso from the manual above referred to: "The body of each oven is made of two pieces of $\frac{1}{16}$ of an inch sheet-iron (sheet steel). These sheets are 5 feet long by 2 feet 6 inches wide, and so curved that, when their upper edges are connected and the lower edges fixed in the ground, they form an arch, the span of which is 3 feet 9 inches, and the rise 1 foot 4 inches. The lower edge of each sheet is bent outward into a flange, so as to secure a firm rest on the ground. On the inside of each sheet are riveted 3 longitudinal bars, 1 inch wide and $\frac{3}{8}$ of an inch thick, and on the outside 5 transverse ribs, $1\frac{1}{4}$ inches wide by $\frac{3}{8}$ of an inch thick. The upper ends of the transverse ribs on one of the sheets are formed into hooks, and those of the other sheet into eyes, by means of which the sheets are securely attached to each other along the ridge of the oven when erected. (The front of the oven is closed by a sheet-iron or steel door with a handle.) When the soil is of clay or of other favorable quality, the rear end of the oven may be closed by the natural earth, but if it is sandy or loose a sheet-iron plate will be required to close it. No chimney is necessary. When set up, the whole, excepting the door, is covered with a mass of earth eight inches in thickness.

"The depth of the earth is named for the reason that a larger quantity would be liable, from its weight, to bend the iron when heated, and a smaller quantity would allow too much heat to escape. An excavation three or four feet in depth should be made a foot or two from the door for the convenience of the baker. Two hours are required for heating the oven at first starting, but for each heating immediately following one hour will be sufficient.

"A small quantity of wood is placed in the oven at

the extreme rear and ignited, the door being kept open to afford a draft and a vent for the smoke. Small quantities of wood should then be added as combustion progresses. In this way the fuel will burn more freely and the oven be heated quicker than if all the fuel necessary for the heating were put in at once. As soon as the oven is at a white heat the ashes should be raked out, the floor swept clean (or the sheet-iron floor put in), and the dough in pans introduced. The time required for each baking is about forty-five minutes.

"The oven can be erected and prepared for use in fifteen minutes, and if kept in constant operation for twenty-four hours can bake sufficient bread for 1000 men. By the use of two of these ovens, therefore, a regiment of 1000 men, if it make a halt of fourteen hours each day, can be supplied with fresh bread daily on the line of march. Ordinary kneading troughs can be made and placed on trestles, or they may be fixed on the ground and trenches excavated near them for the kneaders to stand in."

Compressed yeast may be used under ordinary circumstances, but it should be kept on ice. The rising with this yeast will take from four to six hours. It is more practicable, however, for troops going into Cuba to make use of a dry yeast (yeast foam, yeast powder) that is guaranteed not to deteriorate for three months from time of manufacture. The rising process with the dry yeast will consume eight or ten hours.

A hospital tent should be allowed for a bakery, and two men from the fighting force can well be spared as bakers, for a supply of wholesome bread is not only a comfort to soldiers in the field but virtually strengthens the effective force numerically as well as physiologically through avoidance of dietetic errors.

If these ovens do not turn out sweet, wholesome, and delicious bread it is no fault of their own, as attested by the character of the bread issued from the ovens already in operation in this brigade.

HENRY I. RAYMOND, M.D.,
Captain and Assistant-Surgeon, United States Army.

THE ADVISIBILITY OF A SUMMER CAMPAIGN IN CUBA.[1]

To the Editor of the MEDICAL NEWS.

DEAR SIR: About four weeks ago I wrote an article, which was published in one of the daily papers, in which I took the ground that an immediate invasion of Cuba at that time of the year (May 1st) by a small body of men, 10,000 to 15,000 well-drilled veteran troops, would be followed by no more danger of sickness than an active campaign in the State of Florida under the same conditions; and I also made the statement that I believed that there would be little or no danger from yellow fever to such troops so long as they were kept out in the country and not permitted to enter the cities, making use of the insurgent forces for such purposes. But I must confess, that as matters stand now, I cannot help but take a different view.

The unpreparedness of the military branch of the government has become so apparent, and from all accounts the necessity of a much larger body of troops to invade the island so evident, that I can well understand the hesitation on the part of the Washington authorities to land troops at this season of the year around Havana and Matanzas. In fact, I am about convinced that unless Havana in the meanwhile capitulates from lack of food, no troops will be landed in that province before the month of October or November.

Around Santiago the conditions are different. The country all about is hilly and much healthier, and by utilizing the several thousand insurgents in the neighborhood for the purposes of garrisoning the city after its capitulation, the American troops could be safely encamped all summer under decidedly more advantageous conditions than either at Chickamauga or Tampa.

From the point of view of a Cuban, this pacific blockade, especially if kept up all summer means the practical extermination of all the people in these three provinces, Pinar de Rio, Havana, and Matanzas, and as this war, we are told was undertaken for the very purpose of saving these people, why should American troops not be immediately landed on the island, even if they do run the risk of a high death-rate from climatic conditions, etc.?

On the other hand, as Americans we are justified in reasoning in this manner: We are certainly not prepared for such an undertaking. Our soldiers, mostly men who were only yesterday clerks and mill-hands, are not even supplied with one of the most essential and vital things for a summer campaign in the tropics, and that is suitable clothing. In such an undertaking we know that climate does not influence mortality as much as deficient preparation and lack of organization, therefore, let us take into consideration the lives of 20,000 or 30,000 Americans, as against these unfortunates, who perhaps are already beyond any human aid. This pacific blockade will certainly force Havana to capitulate long before October, and by that time we shall have a thoroughly trained and properly equipped body of troops. There are many sides to this Cuban question, and the position of the men at the head of affairs in Washington, who must decide these questions, is certainly not one to be envied.

The sinking of the "Maine" will bring about the ultimate freedom of Cuba, but she will have many more victims to count than those who went down with her.

Yours very truly,
D. T. LAINE, M.D.

218 SOUTH FIFTEENTH STREET, PHILADELPHIA,
June 6, 1898.

[1] Dr. Lainé's papers on the Cuban question have received wide attention of late and the readers of the MEDICAL NEWS will be interested in the opinion of a Cuban-American of such extensive experience regarding the proposed invasion of Cuba at this time by the United States forces.—ED.

MEDICAL PROGRESS.

Intralaryngeal Hemorrhage. — GEYER (*Münch. Med. Wochenschr.*, April 12, 1898), in speaking of hemorrhage into the larynx, mentions a case in which a hematoma resulted, the appearance of which some time afterward suggested a malignant tumor, and was most puzzling. The difference in appearance between a shriveled hematoma and a malignant growth may be very slight, so that the differential diagnosis may rest in a large measure upon the fact that in the latter trouble infiltration of the cords produces at an early stage some interference with their normal action.

The Direction of the Ciliary Motion in the Uterus.—MANDL (*Münch. Med. Wochenschr.*, April 12, 1898) has demonstrated the truth of the assertion made by some histologists, Hofmeier among them, that the ciliary motion in the uterine canal is from above downward. He examined eleven uteri immediately after extirpation. In seven of them no ciliary motion was detected. In four it was shown to exist, and in all of these the direction was from above downward; that is to say, in the same direction as the motion in the Fallopian tubes. This clinical demonstration clears up this disputed point, for histologists have not been in agreement upon it, Wyder, for example, having claimed that the motion was from below upward.

Purpura an Infectious Disease.—LAPIN (*Med. Moderne*, April 9, 1898) mentions two cases of purpura, one of which ended fatally, and in both of which micrococci were found in the blood. In the fatal case streptococci were present. He states that our present knowledge regarding infectious purpura is as follows:

1. It is not always accompanied by fever, so that one ought never to say that a given case of purpura is non-bacterial until a microscopic examination has been made.
2. Even in septic cases bacteriologic examination ought to be made in the early hours after the appearance of ecchymosis.
3. Individual predisposition exerts a decided influence.
4. Werbol's disease is not a simple purpura confined to hemophiliacs, but is a disease by itself.
5. Purpura frequently enters by the mouth, the pharynx, etc.
6. Predisposing factors other than hemophilia are excesses at table, the use of alcohol, nephritic and hepatic lesions, and such cardiac troubles as cause venous congestion.

Spontaneous Disappearance of Pigmented Keloids.—GOTTHEIL (*Amer Jour. Surg. and Gyn.*, April, 1898) mentions a case of the disappearance of numerous deeply pigmented keloids which had developed in the scars following burns from potash solution. The burns were upon the backs o' the hands of a girl aged nineteen, and healed with difficulty. Proud flesh appeared, and was several times burned away, and it was not until four months had elapsed that cicatrization was complete. The following year, without known cause, the scars began in places to increase in size and to grow dark in color, until there were some forty sharply circumscribed elevations of a dark, bluish purple, varying from a quarter of an inch to an inch in diameter. Some of them were treated by electrolysis without marked success, and after six or eight sittings the patient disappeared from view. Eight months later she reappeared, and showed with delight that all the keloid growths had disappeared. As only a half a dozen of the smaller tumors upon one hand had been subjected to electrolysis, the conclusion was inevitable that the involution was spontaneous.

The Use of the Bone-Clamp in Difficult Fractures.—PARKHILL (*Annals of Surgery*, May, 1898) gives numerous illustrations of the advantage of bone-clamps in the treatment of ununited fractures, of fractures with malunion, and of recent fractures with tendency to displacement. The method of application is as follows: Four holes are drilled in the broken bone in such a manner that when the deformity is reduced they shall all be in the same straight line, and in the long axis of the bone. They are an inch or two apart, and about the same distance from the broken ends of the bone. Into each one a slender pin is screwed. These pins are of steel, heavily plated with silver. To their upper ends bent strips of steel are fastened by nuts. These strips overlap, and are held together by a small clamp. The fractured bone is reduced, the ends brought together, and the clamp is tightened. It is then impossible for the ends of the bone to become separated, or for the angle between them to vary. As the pins stand up a considerable distance from the surface of the leg, it is easy to apply a sterilized dressing which will remain for some weeks in an aseptic condition. The claims for this instrument have been well established by its use. They are that it is easily and accurately adjusted, that it prevents longitudinal and lateral motion between the fragments, that the presence of the pins in the bone stimulates the production of osseous tissue, and that no secondary operation is necessitated. Union has resulted in every case in which they have been used, as against fifty-six per cent. of successes which, according to the statistics of Bruns and Gurlt, follow the use of other mechanical appliances.

A Simple and Safe Method of Locating Intestinal Obstruction.—REED (*Jour. Amer. Med. Assoc.*, April 30, 1898) says that the old method of finding collapsed bowel and following it upward in order to locate a point of obstruction in the intestines is often unreliable, for the reason that collapsed bowel may be found above the obstruction as well as below it. When the sense of touch is depended upon to locate the stricture it is advisable to pass the hand first into the left inguinal region in order to exclude hernia and see if the sigmoid flexure is collapsed. If so, the hand is next passed into the right inguinal region, and if the cecum is collapsed the difficulty must be in the small intestine. This may be turned out and the obstruction found, but a simpler and a safer method is what may be properly termed a "color-guide." At the seat of strangulation congestion exists, which deepens and extends further along the bowel the longer the exciting cause continues. If one loop after another of distended intestine is brought into view at the bottom of the abdominal incision and their appearance carefully noted, a clue will shortly be found to the point of obstruction by following in the direction in which the color grows deeper.

A Retroperitoneal Chyle Cyst.—SARWEY (*Centralb. f. Gynakologie*, April, 1898) removed a retroperitoneal cyst from a girl of eleven years. The cyst, which was very large, had its origin apparently in the pancreas, and as it grew it forced its way through the gastro-colic omentum so that the greater portion of it was in front of the transverse colon. According to the chemic examination of the fluid contents of the cyst, its origin was not in the pancreas but in the lymph vessels. This fluid had the appearance of milk, both macroscopically and microscopically, but was absolutely lacking in pancreatic ferments. The operation showed, also, that the total removal of a cyst in this situation presents by no means insurmountable difficulties. No accident occurred during the operation, and the patient made a speedy recovery.

The Primary Essential Lesion of Typhoid Fever.—MALLORY (*Jour. Boston Soc. Med. Sciences*, April, 1898) has made histologic examinations of the intestinal lesions in nineteen cases of typhoid fever in order to determine which lesions are primary and which secondary. As a result of his investigations he denies that the inflammatory theory of the disease is the correct one. This ancient theory, which has recently been revived by Ribbert, supposes an acute inflammation with exudation to occur, followed by enormous proliferation of the endothelial cell of the lymph sinuses (a reparative process), necrosis, and sloughing, and finally repair by granulation. Mallory finds, however, that the essential lesions of typhoid are proliferative, and may very well be compared with those of tuberculosis. In the former they are diffuse, however, while in the latter they are focal. We have to do in typhoid fever with a mild toxic agent, which in part is absorbed from the intestinal tract, and in part is produced within the body in the various organs and in the blood. The intestinal lesions depend on absorption mainly through the lymphatic apparatus, but in part through the capillaries. The toxin is diffusible, as is shown by the extension of the lesions in the submucosa, serosa, and muscular coats to a varying distance outside of the path of absorption. The lesions in the mesenteric lymph nodes depends on absorption through the lymphatics.

The lesions in the rest of the body depend primarily on the toxin in the general circulation. These lesions are not peculiar to typhoid fever except in rotation, sequence, and degree.

THERAPEUTIC NOTES.

Quinin Instead of Ergot in Midwifery.—MACKNESS (*Edinburgh Medical Journal*, May, 1898) thinks that ergot is often administered in labor when better results might be obtained from the use of quinin. All preparations of ergot are unreliable. The liquid preparations are nauseating, and ergotin keeps badly and is not suited for hypodermic use. Moreover, ergot causes tetanic contraction of the uterine muscles, and while it sometimes produces spasms of uterine contraction there is not complete relaxation between the pains. This tetanic contraction is dangerous to the mother and even more so to the child, so that if delivery is not accomplished within half an hour after the administration of the drug, other means have to be resorted to.

The advantages of quinin are numerous. It keeps indefinitely and can be administered in tasteless form. It has no tendency to produce vomiting. Its action is certain and is manifest within twenty minutes after its administration. It increases the strength of the labor pains while relaxation occurs in the intervals just as in normal labor. This fact can be verified by any one who chooses to keep his hand upon the abdominal wall after the drug has been administered. It is therefore of especial use in cases where inertia is caused by the general exhaustion of the patient or by actual lack of power in the uterine muscles themselves. If delay is caused by obstruction in the passages no drug, of course, can avail. In normally formed primiparæ where slow dilatation of the passages causes exhaustion of the uterine muscles, quinin will often stimulate them anew so that delivery can be accomplished without instrumental interference. Two four-grain pills of the sulphate are given and if the pains do not increase sufficiently another is given in an hour, and yet another an hour later. The third dose is, however, rarely required. Toxic symptoms need not be feared. Ergot should be administered after labor to control hemorrhage. It is useful in threatened abortion where hemorrhage occurs without pains, the os uteri being closed. Given in small doses it is beneficial in subinvolution of the uterus.

Duration of Life of Thiersch Grafts.—LJUNGGREN (*Deut. Zeitschr. f. Chir.*, vol. lxvii. p. 608), by the microscopical examination of Thiersch grafts which had been kept for three months in sterile ascitic fluid, found that the epithelial cells were well preserved, and their nuclei took stain well. The epithelial layer was for the most part separated from the underlying fibrous and fat tissue, but in grafts which had been kept for several weeks these structures were still firmly united. To determine whether grafts of such an age were really composed of living cells a number of them which had been kept for varying periods of time were planted upon fresh and ulcerated surfaces, every precaution being taken to insure the accuracy of subsequent observation, so that a growth from the edge of the wound, for instance, should not be mistaken for an increase in size of the grafts. The oldest grafts which the writer was able to make adhere and grow had been kept for a month at the room temperature, the ascitic fluid not being changed. This is certainly a remarkable result, and the question at once presents itself whether at a lower temperature, or with some nutrient fluid, or by changing the fluid from time to time, it might not be possible for a still longer time to preserve alive epithelial grafts. Ljunggren, in fact, suggests that it may be found practicable for surgeons to keep on hand among their surgical supplies a number of grafts for future use.

THE MEDICAL NEWS.

A WEEKLY JOURNAL

OF MEDICAL SCIENCE.

COMMUNICATIONS are invited from all parts of the world. Original articles contributed *exclusively* to THE MEDICAL NEWS will after publication be liberally paid for (accounts being rendered quarterly), or 250 reprints will be furnished in place of other remuneration. When necessary to elucidate the text, illustrations will be engraved from drawings or photographs furnished by the author. Manuscripts should be typewritten.

Address the Editor: J. RIDDLE GOFFE, M.D.,
No. 111 FIFTH AVENUE (corner of 18th St.), NEW YORK.

Subscription Price, including postage in U. S. and Canada.

PER ANNUM IN ADVANCE $4.00
SINGLE COPIES 10
WITH THE AMERICAN JOURNAL OF THE MEDICAL SCIENCES, PER ANNUM 7.50

Subscriptions may begin at any date. The safest mode of remittance is by bank check or postal money order, drawn to the order of the undersigned. When neither is accessible, remittances may be made, at the risk of the publishers, by forwarding in *registered* letters.

LEA BROTHERS & CO.,
No. 111 FIFTH AVENUE (corner of 18th St.), NEW YORK,
AND NOS. 706, 708 & 710 SANSOM ST., PHILADELPHIA.

SATURDAY, JUNE 11, 1898.

THE RED CROSS.

THE present time would seem to be opportune for saying a few words concerning the Red Cross Society, which is now attracting such widespread attention. The fact that our Government was rather late in officially recognizing it, having entered the compact in 1882, may explain why so few fully comprehend the origin and functions of the society, or the Geneva Society of Public Utility, as it is properly called. The Red Cross is an organization which owes its existence to the initiative of Henri Dunant, who, after witnessing the terrible and preventable suffering of the wounded at the battle of Solferino, June 24, 1859, addressed a petition to the Swiss Government that it should foster an international conference whose object should be to devise a plan for the amelioration of the suffering of the sick and wounded in war. As a result of M. Dunant's agitation the Swiss Government appointed a committee in February, 1863, which invited the nations of the world to send delegates to an international conference in Geneva during October of the same year for the formulation of such a plan. This conference adopted regulations for the establishment and government of civil organizations in each country to supplement the work of the medical department of the army and navy on the battle-fields and in hospitals, and for the international legal existence of such organizations.

The conference having laid the foundation for the international work of relief, the Swiss Government then invited the nations to send delegates who would convene in congress endowed with authority to ratify its action. This convention, held in August, 1864, resulted in the adoption of nine articles of international treaty known as the Convention of Geneva. The pith of the articles is that all sick or wounded persons shall in time of war be regarded as neutral and that the Red Cross shall care for the enemy's disabled as for their own. A sick or wounded soldier is a Red Cross subject, it matters not to which army he may belong or into what hands he may fall. The red cross upon a white field was agreed upon as the distinctive badge of neutrality. This insignia must be displayed at all times, and the badge or brassard must bear the viseé of the duly authorized military or naval officer under whom the member of the Red Cross serves, as a guarantee of its right of recognition. In every country which signed the Red Cross Treaty originally, or which has since signed it, there is a civil Red Cross organization whose duty it is to cooperate in time of war with the sanitary services of the army and navy when called upon. The civil arm of the Red Cross can extend unmolested through the lines of battle to reach the suffering, it matters not who they are, or where they are. Members of the Civil Red Cross Corps whose services are accepted by the military authorities become as subservient to the medical department of the army as duly enlisted members of the army. Their badge gives them the protection of neutrality.

Many are unable to understand why the ambulance-ship, "Solace," which was equipped and is supported by the United States Government, and which is under the direction of the Medical Department of the Navy, is flying the Red Cross alongside the Stars and Stripes, and they naturally ask if the former flag gives the protection of neutrality despite the fact that the ship is a part of our armamentarium of warfare. If it does, many interesting questions arise, some of which it would seem quite impossible to answer. Sailing under the Red Cross flag, the "Solace" is bound to give succor to wounded and ailing friend and foe alike, and she forfeits her right to be considered neutral by favoring the one or the other. If an American ship and a Spanish ship were put *hors de combat* during an engagement and both stood in most urgent need of an ambulance ship, to which would the "Solace" turn her attention? It is beyond the belief of the most divinely generous and altruistic that the enemy's wounded should be cared for before those of our own flesh and blood; and still it would seem to be incumbent for the ship to do this if she happened to be nearer that of the enemy than her own.

Another question that suggests itself is, Why should our Government fit out ships which may dispense their aid entirely to the sick and wounded enemy? Spain was one of the first to see the eternal fitness of the Red Cross, but she has not despatched a ship flying the red cross with Cevera's fleet, nor do we hear of any such making ready to accompany the Cadiz fleet. It would seem to us that ships flying the Red Cross should be those fitted out with the funds that flow into the exchequers of that Society, and that the Government of this country should expend its moneys for the relief of the sick and wounded at sea only upon ships that will care for her own soldiers and sailors.

THE VACCINE VIRUS FURNISHED BY THE NEW YORK CITY DEPARTMENT OF HEALTH.

NEW YORK CITY does not have a system of compulsory vaccination, yet the fact that no child is allowed to enter a public school until it has been successfully vaccinated makes it probable that more than ninety per cent. of all children within the city limits are vaccinated before the age of eight years. Since the majority of these children are vaccinated with virus obtained from the Laboratory of the Department of Health, either by inspectors appointed for the purpose, or by private physicians, who obtain it from the various drug-stores, it is pertinent to consider whether the department is furnishing to the profession and community a safe and reliable virus.

The physician should have confidence that the vaccination will not only be successful but will pursue a regular course without dangerous complications, and he should be able to give this assurance to the family of his patient. It may therefore be of interest to call attention to the work which is being done by the Department of Health in regard to these points. In the first place it may be stated that only bovine virus is employed. The calves are carefully selected and after the virus is collected from a calf, the animal is killed and a thorough examination of all the organs made. A sample of the collected virus is then given to the bacteriologist, who makes tests upon culture-media for the presence of extraneous germs. A second sample is sent to an inspector, who is required to vaccinate five children, making three scarifications on each.

In case the calf shows disease of any organ or the bacteriologist discovers organisms which would render the virus dangerous, or if fifteen perfect vesicles are not obtained from the clinical test all of the virus collected is destroyed. In other words, unless the vaccine matter is clearly proved to be safe and one-hundred-per-cent. efficient it is not sent out of the laboratory for distribution. Should it respond to all these tests it is put up in sealed capillary tubes, each containing sufficient for one vaccination, or in small vials of a capacity sufficient for ten or fifty vaccinations.

The results of this careful work are shown in the statistics of the Health Board for 1897, when over 20,000 primary vaccinations were performed by the inspectors with a percentage of success greater than 99. All authorities on this subject agree that in a very small percentage of cases considerable inflammation may arise from a skilfully performed vaccination with sterile virus; but in the vast majority of cases this results from an improper method of vaccinating or from a mixed infection due to rupture of the vesicle.

The virus furnished by the Department of Health is very concentrated and only a small quantity is necessary for a successful "take." Caution is also to be observed in making the scarification, which should be small (not more than one-eighth of an inch in diameter) and exceedingly shallow, so as to remove only the outer layers of skin, scarcely drawing blood. The instrument recommended for this purpose is an ordinary sewing-needle, which causes very little pain and after being used can be thrown away. The virus should be taken upon the broad end of a sterile, smooth, wooden toothpick and gently but thoroughly rubbed into the scarified area.

Various methods of protection have been devised, but all are open to the objection that they are liable to crush and macerate the vesicle. As the result of experience the department has found that a loose sleeve lined with a piece of soft linen affords the best protection. If this method is carefully followed it may safely be said that very few failures or serious complications will occur.

THE BRITISH PHARMACOPŒIA OF 1898.

THE new volume is printed but is not quite ready for public distribution. It follows quite closely the edition of 1885 as to arrangement and size. The accessions to the list are seventy-seven in number, while the omissions are one hundred and eighty-three. Among the latter are several of the older decoctions, infusions, tinctures, and unguents which are at the present time little used. Among the additions we find that comparatively few of the newer preparations find place, the principal ones being salol, salicylate of bismuth, hyoscin hydrobromid, hyoscyamin sulphate, terebene, naphthol, and two preparations of thyroid. Most of the other additions consist of pharmaceutical preparations, and of these a series of concentrated solutions are perhaps those which will be most acceptable to the medical profession, inasmuch as this innovation appears to constitute an attempt to keep pace with the dispensing practice of late years and to establish a standard of purity for many preparations which have hitherto been much employed with no certainty of their composition. Considering the small number of additions it is somewhat curious to find that there are no less than seven new syrups, most of which appear to be intended to render medicines more palatable.

Some of the alterations affect drugs which are in every-day use; at the head of the list stands aqua chloroformi, which is so extensively used as a vehicle. This preparation in the new volume is reduced to one-half of its former strength, so that it no longer affords an indication of the degree of solubility. The alcoholic extract of belladonna now contains one-third the proportion of the alkaloids present in average samples of the former extract and is prepared from the new liquid extract, instead of directly from the root. The extract of nux vomica now contains five per cent. of strychnin, which is two-thirds of the alkaloidal strength of the extract of nux vomica of the edition of 1885, and this also is prepared from a liquid extract, instead of being obtained as formerly from the seeds. In this case the dose is the same as before, but the dose of the alcoholic extract of belladonna has been increased. The phosphorus pill of the last edition contained about one grain in ninety of phosphorus of the mass. The new pill is made so that it may contain two per cent. of phosphorus and the whole method of preparation has been completely altered, carbon bisulphid being now employed as a solvent. The strength of the morphin suppositories has been reduced, each containing now a quarter instead of half a grain.

ECHOES AND NEWS.

Vaccination in the Orient.—In Japan the law not only makes vaccination compulsory but directs that revaccination be practised every five years.

Another Hospital Ship.—The "John Englis" of the Maine Steamship Company has been purchased by the Government to be used as a hospital ship for the army.

Holidays in the University of Paris.—The future doctors, lawyers, and politicians of France devote but 149 days out of 365 to their education, the remaining 216 being holidays.

First Use of the Term "Microbe."—The word "microbe" was introduced to the scientific world by M. Sedillot in a communication presented to the Académie des Science of Paris, in 1878.

Foreign Practitioners in Italy.—Foreign medical men are permitted to practise among people of their own nationality in Italy, but are forbidden under pain of prosecution and fine to give first aid to an Italian in a street accident.

Degree for Medicine-Mixers.—Following the lead of the Philadelphia College of Pharmacy the Paris Society of Pharmacy has decided to grant the degree of "Doctor of Pharmacy" to those who excel in the mixing of medicine.

Telephone Service and London Physicians.—It is said that in London not more than twenty or thirty physicians have telephones in their offices. This seems strange to the American physician who finds the telephone service indispensable.

Society of Infantile Medicine and Surgery.—At a recent meeting of the physicians and surgeons of the various hospitals for children in Paris, held under the presidency of M. Cadet de Gassicourt, it was decided to form a society with the above name.

A Phonetic Reporter.—The *Times* (London), in speaking of the condition of Mr. Gladstone shortly before his death, makes his physician say that his patient had "change-stroke in his breathing." Presumably the illustrious patient was suffering from Cheyne-Stokes' respiration.

New University Degree.—According to the *Medical Press and Circular* (London) a new degree has been created by the Council of the University of Paris, to-wit, that of "Doctor of the University of Paris." It will be granted to students of science or of medicine on conditions similar to those required for the German Ph.D., namely, the preparation of a thesis embodying original research.

Corns and a Learned Judge.—According to the ruling of a German law court "corns on the feet are not a disease" and, consequently, remedies for this condition cannot be considered as coming under the head of medical treatment. The contemporary which makes this statement expresses the hope that the millions of mortals who are afflicted with corns will find comfort in the decision of this learned judge.

Felons May Not Practise Medicine.—The Supreme Court of the State of New York recently upheld the constitutionality of the law which forbids a physician who has been convicted of a felony to practise his profession after his liberation from prison. An appeal had been taken on the ground that the law was unjust and unconstitutional in that it added a new punishment to the sentence already served.

L'Amende Honorable.—The resident medical officer of the West Ham Infirmary, Leytonstone, England, who was inexcusably attacked by the *Twentieth Century Press* in an article headed "How They Treat Poor Children in the Workhouse," has had the satisfaction of forcing the editors to publish an apology in three newspapers, to bear all costs of the suit, and to pay over to the Infirmary the sum of ten pounds and ten shillings.

Sudden Resignations.—There is good authority for stating that Professors Austin Flint, Frederic S. Dennis, and Samuel Alexander have resigned their respective chairs in the faculty of the Bellevue Hospital Medical College. It is inferred from this action that these gentlemen will not become members of the faculty of the combination of Bellevue College with the Medical Department of the New York University. It would seem that they do not find the prospects in the new school as inviting as its friends have anticipated.

An Ancient Pocket Code of Ethics for Surgeons.—The Master in Chirurgie, Guy de Chauliac, who flourished between 1300 and 1370 was the author of the first surgical treatise of importance after the Middle Ages, a work that had full sway for two centuries. He grouped together a few precepts for his own and his pupils' guidance, which might be taken as the nucleus of a code for surgeons of the present day. "In dangers cautious. Be bold when sure. Friendly with fellow-workers. Not greedy of gain. Constant in duty."

Gift to the Kings County Medical Society.—The late Dr. Cornelius Olcott of Brooklyn, through his heirs, has given to that society copies in oil of the three best known medical paintings in Europe; namely, first, "The Lesson in Anatomy," the Rembrandt masterpiece at The Hague; second, "Harvey Demonstrating the Circulation before Charles I.," and third, "The Anatomist," by Gabriel Max. These paintaings will be cared for privately until the proposed new building for the society shall have been erected.

Anthrax Contracted in a London Post-Office.—A case of anthrax contracted under peculiar circumstances is reported in a recent number of the *British Medical Journal.* The patient was a man employed in the Parcels Post-Office of the London post-office whose duty it was to repair wooden boxes and baskets broken in transit. Strips of leather cut from untanned hides were used for this purpose. The man had a pimple on his neck and had scratched it, and anthrax appeared as a result of handling raw hides. It was stated that nine years ago a case of blood poisoning occurred in the same department from a similar cause.

Medical Education Gratis.—At the Faculty of Medicine in Cairo, Egypt, a man may study medicine at the expense of the government. There are no fees for the examinations, or any other expenses, and each student is allowed $10 a month for pocket money. Furthermore, there are restaurants near the college buildings where students may take their meals at the expense of the government. The reason for this strange state of affairs is stated by the *Lyon Médical* to be due to the fact that all the Egyptian students deserted the college when Englishmen took possession of it, and it then became necessary to replace them at any cost.

Return of the "Solace" from Key West.—The United States Hospital Ship "Solace" returned to New York on June 5th from Key West, bringing fifty-four men belonging to the various warships, who have been invalided either on account of illness or from wounds received in the bombardments, in which the vessels have recently been engaged. Four of the men were suffering from tuberculosis. Four surgeons, eight trained nurses, and three apothecaries looked after the welfare of the sick and wounded during the trip. Ambulances from the Naval Hospital were awaiting the arrival of the vessel to transfer the patients. The men have improved very rapidly since leaving the enervating climate of Key West.

Indictment against Dr. Cleaveland Dismissed.—It is a pleasure to announce that Dr. Turnbull W. Cleaveland, a Fellow of the New York Academy of Medicine and of the New York Obstetrical Society, and a highly esteemed member of the profession, who for nearly three months has been under bail on a criminal charge, has been honorably discharged by Judge Cowing in Part II. of the Court of General Sessions. The indictment was found in March by two members of the Grand Jury on the uncontradicted statement of the defendant, James L. Carhart, a theatrical manager, who alleged that the death of his infant daughter was due to the criminal negligence of Dr. Cleaveland. Previous to the criminal charge a civil suit for damages had been unsuccessfully brought against the physician by the parents of the child.

Electric Anesthesia.—In a brief communication to *Science* Professor E. W. Scripture of Yale University states "that while making some experiments on the sensations derived from sinusoidal currents he noticed that anesthesia of the tissues resulted from currents of high frequency, the condition lasting for some time after the removal of the electrodes. While in this condition the fingers could be pricked with a pin without any resulting sensation except that of dull contact. Sensitiveness to cold was also removed. The investigation has been continued and has shown the possibility of employing a sinusoidal current of high frequency as an anesthetic." The observations of Professor Scripture, which evidently led him to more than suspect that in especially adapted electric currents there exists a local anesthetic power of practical value, should excite the interests of surgeons, and we are glad to record his promise to publish at an early day the details necessary for the application of his discovery.

Unexpected Demands.—The unpreparedness of our nation to go immediately to war is just now becoming painfully manifest on every hand and carries a telling rebuke for those critical jingoes who have liberally abused the conservatism of our central authorities. The appeal of the American Bible Society through its Treasurer, Mr. William Foulke of the Bible House, New York City, for contributions required for its work among our soldiers only presents another phase of the situation. To supply the Army and Navy of the United States now expanded to a war footing, very large demands are being made on the American Bible Society for pocket testaments. Tens of thousands of copies have been called for by the chaplains of regiments, Young Men's Christian Association officers, and other responsible parties who are at work in the camps all over the country and at the front. Care is used to insure the wisest distribution accompanied by a friendly word with each man. Deprived as they are of reading matter, the soldiers gladly accept the books, and will treasure them as a souvenir of the war.

An Eastern Branch of the Battle Creek Sanitarium.—New York City is to have a branch of the famous Battle Creek Sanitarium. Dr. J. H. Kellog, the well-known Superintendent at Battle Creek, has engaged the Park Hotel, at Prohibition Park, Staten Island, for this purpose, and he and his helpers open the doors of the hotel for guests this week. It is not generally known that the Battle Creek Sanitarium is a huge benevolent enterprise of the Seventh-Day Adventists, and that this sanitarium has now fifteen branches under its charge in various countries, almost encircling the globe. None of the profits from these sanitariums go to individuals, but all are turned into what is known as the Medical Missionary Work. It is a cardinal principle of these Adventists that the human body, as well as the soul, is sacred to God, and that it should be religiously cared for. A more delightful and profitable place to spend a summer vacation it would be difficult to find than one of these sanitariums or health-resorts.

CORRESPONDENCE.

OUR PHILADELPHIA LETTER.

[From Our Special Correspondent.]

RESULTS OF THE SCHUYLKILL INVESTIGATION—PHYSICIANS WHO WILL REPRESENT PHILADELPHIA AT THE AMERICAN MEDICAL ASSOCIATION CONVENTION—PATHOLOGICAL SOCIETY—RED CROSS SOCIETY IN PHILADELPHIA—THE EVANS' WILL CONTEST—ANOTHER INSTANCE OF INSUFFICIENT MARRIAGE LAWS—HEALTH-BOARD STATISTICS.

PHILADELPHIA, June 8, 1898.

THE local health authorities completed their investigation of the pollution of the Schuylkill River on last Wednesday. This river, furnishing as it does the water-supply of this city, has long been a menace to health and the investigation promises to reveal some facts which will astound the authorities. A trip was made as far as Reading, photographs and samples of water being procured at various points along the course, and while the report will not be made public until the views are developed and the samples analyzed, it has become public property that causes exist which may at any time give rise to an epidemic of fever or dysentery.

The secretary of the State Board of Health, Dr. Benjamin Lee, who was a member of the investigating party, said that the Commission hopes to produce such evidence of impure water that legislative action will be taken to protect not only the Schuylkill but all streams of the State. Such action has been taken by New York and many other States and in time it is hoped all towns will arrange some satisfactory method of disposing of sewage or at least of rendering it innocuous.

Camden, across the Delaware, is also in the depths, for after suffering for years from an insufficient and unwholesome supply of water the city contracted for an artesian well capable of furnishing 2,000,000 gallons of water every twenty-four hours. After relishing this welcome change for ten days the residents have been compelled to return to the old source of supply, for the contractor, claiming to have been unfairly treated by the city officials, cut the new one off. In all probability the matter will be settled in the courts next week.

Philadelphia will be well represented at the convention of the American Medical association in Denver, about two hundred physicians having gone. Among the number were Drs. J. H. Musser, Hobart A. Hare, W. W. Keen, Crozier Griffith, B. Alexander Randall, W. B. Atkinson, Edward Jackson, Judson Daland, L. F. Flick, George M. Gould, J. V. Shoemaker, James Tyson, and J. C. Wilson.

At the National Education Association Convention to be held in Washington, July 7-12, Dr. D. H. Bergy of the University of Pennsylvania is to read a paper on "Heating, Lighting, Ventilation, and Sanitary Arrangements of School Buildings."

Among the specimens presented at the last meeting of the Pathological Society were a spleen weighing 5600 grams (nearly 15 pounds), and a liver weighing 6300 grams (nearly 17 pounds). These were shown by Dr.

H. A. Hare, who reported the case, one of splenomedullary leukemia.

The local Red Cross Society in its desire to interest and receive support from the public, recently conceived the idea of holding a mass-meeting. Many prominent men were to take part and it was hoped to raise sufficient money to maintain an ambulance and field-hospital at the front, but the idea did not receive sufficient encouragement and has therefore been abandoned, much to the regret of many who are interested.

At a recent examination of applicants for the position of Assistant Surgeon in the Navy Dr. T. L. Rhoads, a graduate in 1893 of Jefferson, and lately pathologist to the Surgical Department of Jefferson Hospital, scored a percentage of 841 points, beating the previous record of 826 points.

The first hearing in the will case of the celebrated Dr. Evans, the American dentist who accumulated an immense fortune in Paris, was held on Friday, Clara Davis, a niece, objecting to the probating of the will. The city will defend the will inasmuch as the municipality is to receive $8,000,000 if the will is proved. Under its terms this sum is left in trust for the founding of "The Thomas W. Evans' Museum and Dental institute." In the event of success no doubt the interests of the city will be incorporated in one of the existing dental schools, of which there is already an overabundance.

Samuel Henderson, the fifteen-year-old murderer, was sentenced this week to twenty-years' imprisonment. The case, which was detailed in the MEDICAL NEWS of April 9th last, attracted much attention because of the expert testimony and the endeavor of the defense to prove insanity. A similar case having occurred during the present week attention is brought to the necessity for legislation prohibiting the marriage of defectives; in the Henderson family there is a history of a homicidal heredity.

The total number of deaths reported at the Health Bureau for the week ending June 4th was 406, of which 120 occurred in children under five years of age. There were 155 new cases of contagious diseases reported as follows: Diphtheria, 57, with 15 deaths; scarlet fever, 47, with 2 deaths; typhoid fever, 51, with 7 deaths. It is interesting to note that the mortality from typhoid in Philadelphia has been decreasing each year for the past decade. In 1888 it was 21 per cent. of the number of cases reported and a steady decrease has brought it down to 13 plus per cent. for 1897. A lower rate is probable this year. A similar fall in the number of cases has occurred also, though it is not so marked. From 1887 to 1892 the average number was from 3400 to 3700, and from 1891 to 1897 from 2300 to 2600.

Liniment for Myalgia.—

℞		
	Aq. ammoniæ	ℨ iiss
	Ext. hyoscyami } aa Ext. opii }	ℨ ss
	Ol. thymi	gtt. v
	Ol. camphorat.	℥ iii.

M. Sig. Rub painful parts morning and evening.

OUR FOREIGN LETTER.

[From our Special Correspondent.]

A GREAT SURGEON'S VIEWS AS TO MEDICINE AND SURGERY IN WAR—THE IMPORTANCE OF THE CARE OF THE SICK AS WELL AS THE WOUNDED—THE DISINCLINATION BILLROTH NOTED AMONG PHYSICIANS REGARDING THE CARE OF THE SICK—VENESECTION AND THE USE OF LEECHES IN CHILDREN—A NEW HOSPITAL FOR BERLIN.

BERLIN, May 28, 1898.

As everything in America breathes a martial air and war and its affairs occupy all attention an expression of expert opinion as to the German medical arrangements during the Franco-Prussian war of 1870-'71 may not be untimely. Most of the medical men who volunteer for actual service go with the idea, of course, of having to treat wounded soldiers, firmly persuaded that they are to have extensive practice in surgery, especially the surgery of gunshot wounds and with very little prospect that most of their duty will be to treat purely medical cases. Yet in the campaign about to be inaugurated in Cuba, their aid as medical men will, beyond doubt, be much more often invoked than their skill as surgeons.

Billroth, in a series of surgical letters written from the war hospitals of Weissenburg and Mannheim in 1870, expressed himself very forcibly on this subject. (The letters contain other interesting observations of the great surgeon that may be of interest to military medical men at this time.—*Briefe aus den Kriegslazaretten in W. and M.* Berlin, 1872, August Hirschwald.)

"The thanks of the poor jaded sick soldiers," says Billroth, "for the care taken of them are not less hearty than those of the wounded. The disinclination among the physicians to treat sick *unwounded* soldiers was formally epidemic, though most of them were certainly better prepared to treat medical than surgical cases. At the beginning of the campaign the number of wounded was naturally in excess of that of the sick, but after the first month, despite the fact that this war has been especially favorable to the health of the troops, the number of sick and wounded was equalized. After two months the number of sick was always greater than that of the wounded and remained so.

"This fact, which has been noted in all wars, was not sufficiently taken into account. The number of lazarettos in the immediate neighborhood of the scene of operations seems to have been too small, otherwise they would not have had to materially reduce the number of men in the ranks by sending to distant hospitals for treatment men afflicted with but slight diarrheas, who might have gone back to service again in a couple of days. It seems to me that in this I can see the absence of a sure, level-headed, experienced clinician, who at the same time understands military matters, as the guiding-head of each military medical department.

"It is certain that men with light cases of dysentery transported for nights and days on the scarcely even straw-covered floors of freight-cars, often without medical attendance, were frequently made much worse, though it is certain too that the newspaper reports as to inadequate and crude hospital and transport conditions were greatly exaggerated.

"Had I time personally," the war was then practically over, "after the transfer of the lazaretto from Mannheim, I should have traveled as far as possible into France itself and would have devoted my attention in conjunction with the Red Cross Society and the various aid organizations to the care of the sick.

"What I missed in the field hospitals and military medical department generally, was the presence of young, strong medical men, whose youth and health fitted them for the arduous duties, and whose experience in internal medicine made them eminently suitable for that thoroughgoing care of the sick that was so much needed. They would have reaped, besides the consciousness of duty to Fatherland in efforts that were of the most humane and practical character, a rich reward in the most varied experience in internal medicine. I saw practically none such. I hope that I shall meet them in the next campaign. The authority which a distinguished well-known surgeon or physician brings into a lazaretto is enough not only to assure its proper scientific conduct, but also assures the proper subordination in various ranks of the physicians in charge, without which I need not say that things will not be carried on properly in such large institutions."

These words of the greatest of modern surgeons as to the necessity for physicians in time of war cannot but be precious at a time like this. Most of the medical volunteers for the war look, as we have said, for surgical practice. Billroth's experience in the war in which sickness played the least rôle of any war in history is important to consider. The disinclination to attend the sick must not be found among American physicians, though of course the privilege of tending the brave fellows who are wounded in action will be an enviable one. The condition of things in Cuba is such that sickness will inevitably be one of the most serious factors to deal with during the campaign.

The eyes of Europe are turned with deepest interest to watch how the well-known inventive and organizing genius of Americans will deal with the problems presented in this war. The medical army organization during our last war, from '60 to '65, was the source of many a suggestion that was eagerly adopted over here and the invention of the barrack or pavilion-hospital plan revolutionized military medicine. Patriotic medical men will not be wanting now, any more than thirty years ago, and will be as satisfied to take obscure, hard-working positions in the care of the sick, because their duty and the really greatest benefit to the army and the country in the care of soldiers is thus secured. Out of it all will come, we feel sure, some organization of the military medical service that will not leave it any longer liable to the objections which the great surgeon Billroth found some twenty years ago. This much one can confidently say medical Europe expects to see result from practical American methods.

The extent to which the reaction in favor of venesection as a therapeutic measure has set in may be gathered from the fact that at the last meeting of the Berlin Medical Society Professor Baginsky, on the strength of recent personal experience with it, recommends it even for children. Up to this it has always been considered, at least since venesection went out of fashion at the beginning of the century, that for children, who bear loss of blood very badly, it was an absolutely unsuitable measure. In severe cases of convulsions in children Baginsky has found it most efficient. He has felt himself practically forced into its use by finding at the autopsy of eclamptic children in several instances intense cerebral hyperemia. Actual venesection he reserves for extremely bad cases. In ordinary cases of children's convulsions he uses leeches—one leech for each year of the child's age. He applies them over the mastoid so as to be able to easily control the bleeding afterward by pressure. He considers it imprudent to allow any after-bleeding. Where the leeching is not followed by immediate relief he opens a vein and takes away 60 to 100 c.c. (2½ to 3½ ounces) of blood.

I said some time ago, in describing the improvements that were to be made in the near future in the Charité Hospital here, that Berlin was alive to the fact that to retain her place as the great medical center advance and improvement in modern clinical facilities must be the watchwords. Another evidence of the determination that the city shall retain its place at the head of medical education is the announcement that a new hospital is about to be erected in the extreme northern part of the city. The plans have already been adopted and give some idea of how extensive the new institution is to be. It is to cost 13,200,000 marks, more than three and one-fourth millions of dollars. Its grounds will contain over 116 acres, more than sixty-six of which will be covered by buildings. Professor Koch's department, the Institute for Infectious Diseases, which at present occupies an extremely unsuitable place in connection with the Charité in the heart of a populous part of the city is to have its quarters transferred to the new hospital, which is to be finished in 1903. No expense is to be spared to make it eminently suitable at once for the care or patients and the investigation of disease. Its hospital wards are to be on the pavillon plan, though the administration and some of the other buildings not connected with the hospital proper are to be ambitious architectual structures.

TRANSACTIONS OF FOREIGN SOCIETIES.

London.

PRECIPITATED ALBUMOSE IN THE URINE—INTRA-PLEURAL TENSION—CENTRAL GALVANIZATION IN CARDIAC AND OTHER NEUROSES—TREATMENT OF TUBERCULOUS DISEASE OF THE BLADDER—A CASE OF COMPLETE HEPATOPTOSIS—RENAL CALCULUS DISCOVERED BY THE ROENTGEN-RAY—TRANSPLANTATION OF TENDON TO CORRECT THE DEFORMITIES OF PARALYSIS.

AT the Royal Medical and Chirurgical Society, April 26th, BRADSHAW read a paper on "A Case of Albumose-Uria, in Which the Albumose Was Spontaneously Precipitated." The patient, an old man, who had enjoyed good health, passed two or three times a week a milky urine which deposited a copious white sediment, giving the reactions of a proteid. At other times the clear urine contained a proteid substance in solution. Cases have been reported in which albumose in solution has existed in the urine, but this is the first case on record in which it has been passed in a precipitated form. In the cases recorded there has usually been some disease of bone, and this patient also showed a certain degree of kyphosis and rigidity of the lower vertebræ.

MARTIN reported a case in which the urine contained precipitated-albumose. The patient was a woman from whom an ordinary multilocular ovarian tumor had been removed. There was no evidenee of bone disease but there was chronic renal inflammation and hypertrophy of the heart. The substance met with in the urine in such cases is usually spoken of as hetero-albumose, but it differs from true peptic hetero-albumose in not being dialysable. It differs from deutro-albumose in being redissolved after coagulation in a 0.2-per-cent. solution of caustic soda. Further observations are necessary to show whether the body more closely resembles proto-albumose or peptone. In cases associated with multiple new growths, rapid cell degeneration leads to the formation of proteids which cannot be used within the body and are excreted.

DICKINSON said he had met with both proto- and deutro-albumose in the urine of patients suffering from pneumonia, in some cases as much as one per cent. The cases were always marked by severe symptoms, depression-pulse of low tension and hemorrhagic tendency, symptoms similar to those which are observed on injection of mixed albumoses into the blood of animals.

At the session of May 10th WEST read a paper on "Intrapleural Tension." During normal quiet breathing intrapleural tension is always negative. During forced inspiration its negative value is increased, but during forced expiration tension may become positive. In pneumothrorax during inspiration the pressure cannot exceed that of the atmosphere or very slightly so, but the expiratory pressure is always positive and may be high, hence the lung will be compressed and the mediastinum may be displaced. These statements are based upon observations made in eleven cases of pneumothorax. In two of them the inspiratory pressure was zero, but in the rest it was positive, and in those in which effusion was associated it was high. The pressure when serous effusion exists alone varies greatly. There seems to be no definite relation between the size of the effusion and the amount of pressure, and the pressure may not be affected at all by inspiratory and expiratory movements. Inasmuch as the normal pleura is probably kept dry by the "lymphatic pump," *viz.*, respiration acting upon the stomata and the valved lymphatics into which they lead, it is evident that when the respiratory oscillation is absent the mechanism for the removal of food is at a standstill. When the respiratory oscillation has been found absent at the commencement of paracentesis it often returns at the end. This explains why the removal of a small amount of fluid often determines the rapid disappearance of the rest. In all cases of empyemia the pressure is considerably increased, though here, too, small effusions are quite as likely to have high pressure as large ones. Respiratory oscillation is likewise practically absent.

At the Medical Society, April 26th, ARMSTRONG read a paper on "The Therapeutic Value of Central Galvanization in Cardiac and Other Neuroses." The want of judgment in the selection of cases, and of precision in its application, together with the extravagant claims made for it, have brought this excellent method of treatment into disrepute. Its physiological effects are three-fold: stimulating, sedative, and tonic. The stimulating effect is immediate, the sedative quickly follows, and the tonic comes on more slowly. The most important effect is upon nutrition. During the passage of the current through the body heat is generated, substances are passed from one pole to the other, endosmosis and exosmosis are modified, and there is a marked acceleration of the process of oxidation. Secretion is largely influenced, as is excretion, especially in those gouty cases where there is deficient excretion, especially urea and uric acid. The structures mainly influenced by this method are the medulla, the pneumogastric nerves, and the sympathetic system. The applications should be neither too long nor too strong, and if headache, insomnia, nausea, or over-excited pulse, or a prolonged reaction of the nerves of special sense follows the treatment, its continuance should be watched with more than special care. Cases suitable for galvanization are: (1) cardiac and gastric neurosis; (2) neurasthenia and hypochondriasis; (3) cerebral exhaustion; (4) migraine; (5) exophthalmic goiter; (6) Raynaud's disease, and (7) spasmodic asthma. The therapeutic effects noted in the patients treated were a feeling of better health, an increase in brightness and clearness of thought, an improvement in appetite and digestion, and a marked decrease in the formation of indican, skatol, cresol, and oxalates. Sleep was markedly increased and was more calm and peaceful. The action of the heart became more regular, anginoid pains were relieved, the rapid pulse became slower, and the unstable nerve-centers were steadied so that they were not so readily acted upon by reflex causes, such as flatulence, absorption of toxins, etc.

At the session of May 9th MOULLIN read a paper on "The Treatment of Tuberculous Disease of the Bladder." He intimated that the local treatment of the tubercular bladder has fallen into its present state of disrepute because it has been too feeble and too late. Suprapubic cystotomy is an operation almost devoid of risk in the early stage of the disease, when excision or erasion is perfectly justifiable. The mucous membrane of the bladder rarely becomes affected through its epithelium. The bacilli invade it from some neighboring organ or through the blood-vessels or lymphatics. In the case of tuberculous pyelitis this is easy as there is a free communication between the lymphatics of the pelvis of the kidney and those of the mucous membrane of the bladder. When the disease begins around one of the ureters it is almost without doubt secondary. When it begins in the trigone this is not so certain. The success of surgical treatment depends upon early diagnosis and with the means now at hand this ought not to be difficult. In his hands operation was thrice performed with good results. In two other cases it might have been performed with equal advantage.

FREYER said that primary tuberculous disease of the bladder is very rare. He opened the bladder in six cases for tuberculous cystitis and afterward regretted it in every case but one. The trouble appeared to increase after erasion. Constitutional medical treatment does more for the patient.

BATTLE observed that it is worth while trying to benefit these patients as their lives otherwise are so miserable. He operated upon five cases; three of the patients were benefited, but in two no improvement was observed.

MACNAUGHTON-JONES described a case of "Complete Hepatoptosis in a Woman Aged Tbirty-eight." As a child she had been delicate. After marriage she bore seven children. For obstinate vomiting and occasional hematemesis laparotomy was performed and what had been taken for a tumor in the right loin was found to be the displaced liver. It extended from the costal cartilages to the iliac fossa and rested upon the right kidney. The stomach was lifted out for examination but only congestion was found. The organs were carefully restored to their normal position but were not sutured. The patient made an entire recovery, with the help of an abdominal support and a carefully selected dietary.

BATTLE said that a woman, aged forty-five, with lax-pendulous abdomen had recently consulted him on account of severe pain in the right side. There was a mass believed to be the liver lying transversely just below the umbilicus. When the patient stood up this mass sank to the level of Poupart's ligament. A flannel bandage gave relief.

At the Clinical Society, April 22nd, TAYLOR and FRITT related a case in which a renal calculus was detected by the Röntgen-ray and successfully removed. The patient gave a history of renal calculus on the right side. Through a lumbar-incision the kidney was opened but no calculus was found. A few days later the Röntgen-ray showed the existence of a calculus high up in the pelvis of the kidney, and at a second operation the stone was found and removed.

At the session of April 29th EVE showed three cases of transplantation of tendon to correct the deformities of paralysis. His operation consists in making a longitudinal incision into the tendon of a paralyzed muscle and inserting and fixing into it the cut end of the tendon of a muscle which is normal. In many cases no doubt this acts merely as a support to a lax tendon, as if the normal muscle whose tendon is cut belongs to a different group it is scarcely likely that the patient will learn to use it otherwise.

ROLLESTON showed a man, aged thirty, suffering from left hemiplegia which occurred on the twenty-fourth day of an attack of typhoid fever. The fever ran a natural course and the hemiplegia gradually improved. In all the recorded cases of this lesion which were verified by autopsy there was embolism. It is a common occurrence in cases of typhoid fever to find minute thrombi in the renal vessels.

SOCIETY PROCEEDINGS.

AMERICAN ACADEMY OF MEDICINE.

Twenty-third Annual Meeting, Held at Denver, Col., June 4-6, 1898.

[By telegraph to the MEDICAL NEWS.]

THERE was more than the ordinary amount of interest manifested in the attendance upon the twenty-third annual meeting of the American Academy of Medicine which was convened Saturday, June 4th. There was the usually attractive program provided by the Committee of Arrangements as a proof of the growing popularity and usefulness of the organization which has labored long and faithfully upon its self-imposed task of elevating the moral, literary, and ethical standard of the medical profession. The treasurer, Dr. Charles McIntire of Easton, Pa., stated that there was a net balance of over $250 in the treasury at the close of the fiscal year. It is a noteworthy fact that the influence of the Academy is now to be felt in almost every portion of the United States, its membership including men of standing from thirty-nine of the States and Territories, the Army and the Navy, as well as from England, Burmah, and other foreign countries. Not only is this true, but the good work that is being accomplished is felt in college circles, and during the year just closing twenty-one of the leading collegiate institutions of the land have extended their hearty support and cooperation to the Academy. In this roll of honor may be found the names of Yale, Harvard, Pennsylvania, Williams, Columbia, Brown, Princeton, Lafayette, and Union.

The committee which had been appointed last year in Philadelphia to consider the advisability of selecting a permanent place of meeting for the Academy failed to make any recommendation, the different members offering suggestions *pro* and *con*.

A nominating committee appointed by the retiring president, Dr. L. Duncan Bulkley of New York, presented the following report:

For President, Edward Jackson of Denver, Col.; first vice-president, W. L. Estes of South Bethlehem, Pa.; second vice-president, J. T. Searcy of Tuscaloosa, Ala.; third vice-president, William Elmer of Trenton, N. J.; fourth vice-president, Robert Hall Babcock of Chicago; secretary and treasurer, Charles McIntire of Easton; assistant secretary, Walter L. Pyle of Philadelphia.

The scientific material presented was of excellent quality, and included the following articles:

"The Prevention of Diseases Now Preying upon the Medical Profession," by Dr. Leartus Connor of Detroit; "The Esthetic Relations of Medicine and Life," by Dr. George M. Gould of Philadelphia; "The Beginnings of Disease," by Dr. H. J. Herrick of Cleveland; "The Modern Sanitarium and Its Relation to the General Medical Profession," by Dr. J. C. Lichty of Clifton Springs, N. Y.; "The Child's Brain as Illustrated by Recent Neurologic Studies," by Dr. Rupert Norton of Washington; "The Interdependence of Healthy Bodies and Healthy Brains," by Dr. Elmer Lee of New York; "The

Ethical Advertiser," by Dr. F. T. Rogers of Providence; "Snags in the Course of the Medical Examining Boards," by Dr. Charles McIntire of Easton, Pa., and a series of papers on the general subject of "The Physiologic Aspect of the Education of Youth," participated in by Drs. Rupert Norton of Washington. Elmer Lee of New York, J. T. Searcy of Tuscaloosa, Ala., Charles Denison of Denver, Thomas C. Ely of Philadelphia, G. Hudson Makuen of Philadelphia, Charles G. Stockton of Buffalo, and Edward Jackson of Denver.

Dr. Connor, in dealing with "The Prevention of Diseases Now Preying upon the Medical Profession," remarked that all disease springs from either misplaced matter or misdirected force, singly or confined. Force acting in the wrong direction is destructive; in the right direction, constructive. Among the diseases (so-called) of the medical profession now definitely recognized and fully described are the following: Over-crowding, a vast horde of incompetents, large numbers of moral degenerates, crowds of pure tradesmen, blatant demagogues, hospitals organized and conducted to the damage of the profession, patients, and people, dispensaries and public clinics of the same character, medical colleges organized for the advantage of the few at the expense of the many and unmindful of advantage to students, medical societies so conducted as to be a bye-word among honest persons and yet continued to advance the financial profits of their leaders, domination by commercial interests of drug manufacturers and promoters of secret and proprietary medicines, the prey of money-making corporations as railways, accident-insurance companies and sanitariums, and the tool of lodges, secret and other social societies. The list, he claimed, was incomplete, but sufficed to indicate the existence of morbid action in almost every portion of the profession. It conceded that these diseases result from too many doctors, and the defective quality of a large number of these. The cure consists in an elevation of the standard of education from the public schools up to the medical college, where the standard of entrance as well as of exit should be of the very highest.

Dr. Gould presented a very able and witty paper upon the "Esthetic Relations of Medicine and Life," and enlarged upon the practical importance that is to be derived in almost every walk of life from the correction of physical defects and deformities, such as astigmatism, defective refraction, cutaneous diseases and blemishes, nevi and congenital or acquired nasal or facial deformities, as hare-lip, and sunken nasal bridge.

By far the most attractive and important feature of the meeting was the discussion of the subject of "The Physiologic Aspect of the Education of Youth," a public session being held in response to an invitation from the Women's Club of Denver. The various aspects of the subjects presented and considered were as follows: "How Education Fails—Physiologically Considered," by Dr. J. T. Searcy of Tuscaloosa, Ala.; "The Child's Brain as Illustrated by Recent Neurologic Studies," by Dr. Rupert Norton of Washington; "The Interdependence of Healthy Bodies and Healthy Brains," by Dr. Elmer Lee of New York; "The Advantage of Physical Education as a Prevention of Disease," by Dr. Charles Deniso[n] of Denver; "The Importance of Training the Specia[l] Senses in the Education of Youth," by Dr. Thomas C[.] Ely of Philadelphia; "The Training of Speech as a Fac[-]tor in Mental Development," by Dr. G. Hudson Makue[n] of Philadelphia; "The Kindergarten," by Dr. Charle[s] G. Stockton of Buffalo; "The Care of the Eyes Durin[g] School Life," by Dr. Edward Jackson of Denver; "Kin[-]dergarten and Primary Grade Work in the Public Schools and Its Influence upon the Eyesight," by Dr. Casey A[.] Wood of Chicago; "The Amount of Work a Growin[g] Brain Ought to Undertake," by Dr. James L. Taylor [of] Wheelersburg, Ohio; and "The Importance of Early an[d] Scientific Training of Children with Defective Speech," by Dr. W. Scheppegrell of New Orleans.

The essential features of the discussion as summed u[p] by Dr. Connor were that the brain will not act properl[y] unless there is a sound body; it will not properly develo[p] without healthy avenues communicating with the extern[al] world, as a sound eye, and thorough ability of speech[;] the importance of good physical development to bring ou[t] the best action of the mind; all of the faculties should b[e] developed in order to secure the best results; every cell i[n] the brain and body should be brought into healthy actio[n] in order to secure a thoroughly educated child. Th[e] public schools of this country fail to accomplish this en[d] and in fact are not designed for this end at all.

The annual address of the retiring President, Dr. I[.] Duncan Bulkley of New York, was upon the subject [of] the "Dangers of Specialism in Medicine." He enlarge[d] upon the disadvantages accruing both to the speciali[st] and to the laity from this division of labor; the danger [of] narrowness of views and dogmatism; and the overloo[k-]ing of concurrent and associated diseases dependent up[on] a primary condition coming under the attention of t[he] specialist.

THE ASSOCIATION OF MEDICAL EDITORS.

The meeting was remarkably well attended and a v[...] of unusual seriousness regarding the ethics of advertisi[ng] was exhibited. The expression of this took the form [of] the following resolution which was unanimously adopt[ed]:

RESOLVED, That matter which, in the judgment [of] the editor, is clearly in the nature of an advertisement, [or] reading notice, shall be excluded from the regularly pag[ed] parts of the journal and placed exclusively in the adv[er-]tising pages.

Upon adjournment the members and their guests [re-]paired to the banquet-hall where plates were laid for [...] hundred and fifty.

A meeting of the Association of American Med[ical] Colleges was held June 6, 1898, in connection with [the] proceedings of the American Academy of Medicine. [The] address of the President, Professor J. W. Holland w[as a] very able effort. An excellent paper was also read [by] Dr. Montgomery S. Crockett of Buffalo upon the sub[ject] "Medical Education Needs Better Pedagogic Metho[ds]."

At the Executive Session the following officers w[ere] elected for the ensuing term: Dr. H. O. Walker, of troit, president; Dr. Ellis of Los Angeles, first vice-president; Dr. Woody, second vice-president; Dr. Bayard Holmes of Chicago, secretary and treasurer.

AMERICAN MEDICAL ASSOCIATION.

The Forty-ninth Annual Meeting, Held at Denver, Col., June 7, 8, 9, and 10, 1898.

[Special Telegraphic Report for the MEDICAL NEWS.]

GENERAL SESSION.

FIRST DAY—JUNE 7TH.

THE Association met in the Broadway Theatre, and in the absence of the President, SURGEON-GENERAL STERNBERG, it was called to order by First Vice-President JOSEPH M. MATHEWS of Louisville, Ky. Prayer was offered by Chancellor W. F. McDowell. Eloquent addresses of welcome were delivered by DR. J. W. GRAHAM of Denver, in behalf of local profession; by Hon. Alva Adams, Governor of Colorado, in behalf of State, and by Hon. W. S. McMurray, Mayor, in behalf of the City of Denver. The address of the President of the Association, by Surgeon-General Sternberg was read by Colonel A. W. Woodhull of Denver. (See page 737.) On motion Secretary Atkinson was instructed to telegraph the thanks of the Association to Surgeon-General Sternberg for his instructive and able address. The report of the Rush monument fund was read by DR. A. L. GIHON, showing that of the amounts pledged last year by the various State societies at the Philadelphia meeting, only $162 had been paid during the past twelve months. Colorado had announced that it has $2000 to add to the fund; New York State Medical Association $2000; and trustees of Medical Society of State of Pennsylvania, to whom was referred the report of the Rush Monument Committee, recommended to make good the pledge made at Philadelphia that the sum of $2000 be appropriated to the fund, and that amount be held in trust by the Board of Trustees of that society until a contract for erection of said monument is accepted. When these sums shall have been paid the fund will amount to $10,424.44, and there are still over forty States and Territories to be heard from. The Committee nominated for the position of treasurer, Dr. Holton of Vermont. Report closed with a resolution asking that necessary traveling expenses incurred by the Treasurer of the Rush Monument Committee, and those of Chairman or Secretary of the Committee, be paid by the Treasurer of the Association.

After the reading of the report DR. GORDON of Maine said the Maine Medical Association had appropriated $100 toward the fund; Dr Porter of Indiana had secured $500 from the Indiana State Medical Society; Dr. Cole of California, for that State $110, after which the report of the Committee was accepted.

Report of the Treasurer was read by HENRY P. NEWMAN of Chicago. He congratulated the Association upon its constantly increasing growth and prosperity. The year which closed January 1, 1898, added fifteen hundred new members and during the same time the Association had dropped for non-payment of dues only seventy-five members. Receipts during the time which he had the honor of being its treasurer had increased from $12,695.58 in 1894 to $32,200 in 1897. Balance on hand January 1, 1898, was $14,092.85, with a sinking fund of $3000. Report was accepted.

Report of the Secretary was read by DR. W. B. ATKINSON of Philadelphia. He stated that in accordance with a resolution adopted at the last meeting, he issued a circular letter to each State and Territorial Medical Society, notifying them of the action taken relative to the fund for the Rush monument and the desire to raise $100,000 for that purpose. Replies were received from several States that a special committee had been appointed to take charge of the matter and it was expected that such committees would report at this meeting.

In accordance with the by-laws the Secretary notified all in arrears for three years and in many instances these arrears were paid. On motion the report was accepted.

The general session then adjourned for the day.

SECTION ON SURGERY.

FIRST DAY—JUNE 7TH.

The committee on the Senn Medal, which was appointed last year, reported that the medal had been awarded to Dr. G. W. Grile of Cleveland, Ohio, for his paper, entitled "Experimental Research into the Effects of Temporary Closing of the Carotid Arteries; Report of the Case; Exhibition of a New Instrument," and it was arranged that this paper should be read before the Section on Thursday afternoon.

The Chairman, DR. W. L. RODMAN of Louisville, Ky., read an address, entitled

INFLUENCE OF AGE, SEX, AND RACE IN SURGICAL AFFECTIONS.

The susceptibility of the negro to disease three hundred years ago still exists, especially to local tuberculosis of the glands, skin, and bones. The negro is still obnoxious to fibroids, neoplasms, keloids, tetanus, etc., but it is believed by many that the African will at some time become as extinct in this country as has the buffalo. Cancer was rare in this race up to fifty years ago, but malignant disease has increased among them of late much more than among the whites. Cancer of the uterus is very frequent in negroes. The most common tumors of childhood are sarcomata, although the earliest case on record is that of a cylindroma occurring in a child aged eleven weeks. Tuberculosis is fast becoming the deadliest foe to the negro race, and is twice as common as in the white, while the Indians frequently develop this disease upon giving up their outdoor life to attend school. Gall-stones and chololithiasis are rare conditions before the age of thirty, but grow more common in advancing years, and are more frequent in women than in men, an explanation for which is the wearing of corsets and their sedentary habits. Several times more prominent in men than in women is aneurism, due to the greater tendency of the former to arterial degeneration. Speaking geographically, aneurism is very frequent in England, but rare in China, which freedom is due to the rice diet and habits of the people.

DR. A. D. BEVAN of Chicago read a paper, entitled

SURGICAL ANATOMY OF THE BILE-TRACTS.

He said a mental picture of the anatomy of the parts is necessary for the surgeon to do good work in this region. The surgeons of the present day are better pathologists, but poorer anatomists than in the past. For performing cholecystotomy a vertical incision along the outer border of the rectus muscle does very well, but the "T"-shaped incision is most objectionable as it is so difficult to suture, besides leaving a weak abdominal wall. The incision preferred at the present time is divided into the primary and extended, the primary being employed for exploration and other similar work, and is shaped like the letter "S," about three or four inches in length, and passes along and through the outer border of the rectus muscle. The extended portion of the incision is added when necessary, and may run from one to three inches in length, but the upper portion of the extension should not completely divide the entire thickness of the rectus muscle. This incision when complete furnishes free access to the bladder and the bile-ducts, and should always be made with a very sharp knife. In its performance a minimum amount of nerve-supply is injured as the incision runs almost entirely parallel with the nerves supplying the abdominal walls. Its relation to the costal arch makes hernia very improbable, but it should not be brought nearer than three-quarters of an inch to the costal border. In closing it is well to use silk sutures, passed through the entire abdominal wall, the skin being approximated with a continuous horse-hair suture."

DR. JOHN B. HAMILTON of Chicago, in locating the gall-bladder, first draws a line from the ensiform appendix to the superior spine of the ilium, a second from the umbilicus to the tenth costal junction, and a third transversely to these; the incision is made from one-half to three-quarters of an inch from the intersection of these lines. The gall-bladder is almost invariably found at this spot. However, the gall-bladder has a varying position influenced by atrophy or hypertrophy of the liver. Many cases of obstruction are due to the twisted or "S"-shaped condition of the cystic duct which, as pointed out by Fenger, can often be straightened and the symptoms relieved.

DR. HARRIS of Chicago entirely agreed with Dr. Bevan as to the relations existing between the ducts and the portal vein, and to the excellent advantage of the incision described by the author of the paper. Great care is necessary in suturing the extension of the lower end of the incision in order to avoid gaping.

DR. J. P. LORD of Omaha read a paper, entitled

INTESTINAL OBSTRUCTIONS FROM GALL-STONES.

After relating at length the history of the case reported and the operation performed for its relief, he said upon the third day after the operation evidence of peritonitis presented itself, lasting for two days, when convalescence began and continued uninterruptedly. The specimen removed, which was a portion of the bowel containing a mass of material about the size and shape of a small hand-bag, presented the appearance of having sustained loss of its substance by fracture of its apex. The body was for the most part smooth, with the exception of a small, irregular elevation on its side, which was believed to have been the cause of the perforation and peritonitis. Section of the specimen showed it to have a gall-stone for a nucleus. Eighty per cent. of cases of intestinal obstruction due to gall-stones occur in women, the great majority being well advanced in years. As gall-stones may exist for years without giving any evidence of their presence, it could not be any reflection upon the surgeon if the diagnosis was not made without operation. Spontaneous relief by the passage of the stone occurs in from thirty to fifty per cent. of the cases, the remainder dying unrelieved.

DR. P. S. CONNOR of Cincinnati read a paper, entitled

REMOVAL OF THE STOMACH.

After referring to the recent announcement that this operation had been successfully performed, the author claimed to have performed it fifteen years ago, the patient dying on the table. There being no physiologic, anatomic, or surgical contraindication to such an operation, he sees no reason why in cases where the stomach is functionally extinct, as in general infiltration of the gastric walls, it should not be performed, the objection being that by the time the condition is realized the patient is ordinarily in no general condition to withstand such an operation. The operation is not warranted except when the stomach has practically ceased to exist so far as its usefulness is concerned. As to removal of the stomach for other conditions than carcinoma, there certainly is no reason why it should not be done if it is simply acting as a receiving organ only, as the lower end of the esophagus can be readily attached to the duodenum or jejunum with the least amount of tension, and with the preservation of the intestinal function.

DR. D. W. GRAHAM of Chicago asked if the author anticipated much difficulty in securing the end of esophagus in cases where the entire stomach had been removed.

DR. KEEFER of St. Louis referred to the connection through the pneumogastric nerve between the floor of the fourth ventricle and the liver, and asked if it was possible to remove the entire stomach without severing some of the fibers of this nerve, and if not, what the result of such an operation would be upon the liver.

DR. HARRIS of Chicago reported having removed the entire stomach for carcinoma a year ago in the case of a man seventy-two years old, in whom the esophagus was attached to the duodenum without difficulty, and believed this would often be possible on account of the extreme mobility of the duodenum in cases of carcinoma of the pylorus. As to the pneumogastric nerve the right one need not be interfered with in this operation since it passes into the liver high up.

DR. W. J. MAYO of Rochester, Minn., read a paper, entitled

THE DIAGNOSIS AND SURGICAL TREATMENT OF MALIGNANT OBSTRUCTION OF THE PYLORUS, WITH REPORT OF THREE PYLORECTOMIES AND FOUR GASTRO-ENTEROSTOMIES.

After referring to the writings of a number of men upon

the subject of the paper, and the different views as to the etiology of the disease, the author said the diagnosis of obstruction of the pylorus and the resulting dilation of the stomach is not a difficult matter, but the differential diagnosis as to the malignant or non-malignant character of the obstruction is often very difficult and occasionally impossible without incision of the abdominal walls. The history of the case provides an important means of diagnosis, combined with results of careful inspection of the patient and examination of the gastric contents. The X-ray is of very little assistance in diagnosing this condition. The routine use of the stomach-tube, and the employment of a carefully regulated diet, bismuth, salol, and methyl blue, with three grains of powdered nutmeg after eating, promise good results. Two operations only are worthy of serious consideration, pylorectomy, which is a radical operation based on the hope of a cure, and gastroenterostomy for palliative purposes. The great mortality of the former, renders it a most unpopular operation, but improvements in the technic will soon overcome this objection. The method usually employed by the author, he divides into five steps, the first being the median incision above the umbilicus, to which, if necessary, a cross cut of the rectus is made; the second, a double ligation, and division of the necessary amount of gastrohepatic omentum; the third, the isolation of the diseased part by a piece of gauze drawn under it and the subsequent removal of this part; the fourth, the slipping to the right of the end of the stomach, and the suturing to each other the ends of the tied omentum, and the fifth, the amputation of the duodenum at a healthy point, to be followed by the insertion of the Murphy button. The author concluded his paper by giving a detailed description of the seven cases on which he had performed this operation.

DR. J. B. MURPHY of Chicago entirely agreed with Dr. Mayo as to the importance of early exploratory operation in these cases, believing that the risk of such a procedure is less than one per cent. Usually the surgeon does not see these cases until they have passed beyond the line where the preservation of life is possible under any circumstances.

DR. JOHN B. HAMILTON referred to a case of a woman, thirty years of age, upon whom an exploratory incision was done three years ago, and whose weight has since increased more than fifty pounds.

DR. WM. F. METCALF of Detroit, Mich., read a paper, entitled

INTESTINAL ANASTOMOSIS BY A NEW METHOD.

He said if any device is used in intestinal anastomosis it should be rigid, so as to hold the parts firmly in apposition, should pass away quickly, to leave the lumen of the gut free, so soon as its function is performed and the suturing is done and it should be easy of introduction. With these objects in view he experimented upon the use of sugar in the form of cylinders of hard candy and the results obtained were very satisfactory. After referring to the method of preparation and use of this device, showing diagrams and specimens illustrative of its employment, he claimed that the advantages were the quick disappearance of the approximator, the accurate adjustment of the mesentery before suturing, the ease and rapidity with which union is effected, the cheapness of manufacture, the tendency to prevent accumulation of fluid, and the formation of abscess beneath the mucous coat.

DR. H. H. GRANT of Louisville, Ky., opposes the employment of any mechanical device in performing these operations, considering them entirely unnecessary with the possible exception of the occasional use of the Murphy button. He believed that in lack of skill on the part of the operator generally arises the necessity for the use of devices and considers that they take time and add to the risk of hemorrhage.

DR. METCALF stated that it is possible to perform these operations in much less time by the aid of this device than is otherwise the case.

DR. ERNEST LAPLACE of Philadelphia read a paper, entitled

A NEW METHOD OF PERFORMING INTESTINAL ANASTOMOSIS AND ENTERORRHAPHY.

He said that the necessity for rapid and accurate suturing in performing intestinal anastomosis as well as other considerations have led him to devise a forceps which presents special characteristics as well as the advantages of being rapid and accurate, easily adjusted, and susceptible to construction in various sizes. He described the instrument at some length and demonstrated the method of its employment in cases of lateral and end-to-end anastomoses and invagination, and showed a number of illustrations.

DR. MCRAE of Atlanta, Ga., believed the instrument was a very useful one and would have a wide field for employment in the future.

DR. B. MERRILL RICKETS of Cincinnati, O., read a paper, entitled

ANEURISM OF THE AORTIC ARCH, SURGICAL TREATMENT BY LIGATION OF THE RIGHT CAROTID AND SUBCLAVIAN ARTERIES.

The author stated that he desired to call special attention to aneurism of the aortic arch, the successful treatment of which at the present time is practically nil in all ways other than surgical, even the latter having been of little consequence until in recent years. He referred to the results of ligation performed by Christopher Heath in 1865 and the nine additional operations devised since that time. He believes that recumbency and diet are advisable in all cases of aneurism, and in some cases the addition of mercury and the iodid before and after surgical intervention. Referring to the introduction of gold wire with the addition of galvanism, he thinks this the most rational method of dealing with many of these cases, although attended with great risk and mortality. As to the diagnosis of aneurism of the arch this is very uncertain and its existence may be entirely unknown until after death. The author concluded his paper with a detailed history of a case in which the subclavian and common carotid arteries of the right side were ligated and recovery followed. The patient has gained twelve pounds since the operation.

The following conclusions were submitted: First, the remedy lies within the domain of surgery. Second, there are but two methods at the present time to be considered—obstruction of the right subclavian and common carotid arteries and the introduction of wire or needles into the sac with or without galvanism. Third, either one or both of the operations should be applied in all cases after a thorough saturation with the iodid. Fourth, ligation is attended by less danger, less mortality, greater and more permanent and universal benefit. Fifth, ligation of the subclavian and common carotid arteries is less dangerous than ligation of the innominate. In fact the latter should not be done.

SECTION ON MEDICINE.

FIRST DAY—JUNE 7TH.

The Chairman, DR SAMUEL A. FISK of Denver, opened the meeting with a brief address outlining the work of the session. He expressed the hope that the ends of true scientific medicine would be served by the work of the Section.

DR. J. C. WILSON of Philadelphia read a paper upon

PERFORATING PERITONITIS.

The cause, he stated, might be the perforation of any hollow viscus, most often the stomach or intestines, notably the latter in typhoid fever. Though the discovery of a cause is to be sought, still the important point is the diagnosis of the condition from the symptoms, but it is often necessary to leave the closer diagnosis for the operator. The symptoms of most importance are pain, rigidity of the muscles of the abdominal wall, and increase in pulse-rate. Tympanitis is often too late a symptom to be of importance. The general demeanor of the patient is a valuable guide. The object of this paper is to urge the importance of early diagnosis and the immediate resort to operative interference. Delay means death in nearly every instance.

DR. W. W. KEEN of Philadelphia remarked that these cases are frequent in medical practice, and operations should be undertaken during the first hours of the attack. The incision should be large, and frequently incisions on both sides of the abdomen are advisable. The results are good in cases treated early.

DR. J. H. MUSSER of Philadelphia suggested that the difficulty of diagnosis is great, and the exploratory incision is frequently a valuable resource.

DR. L. F. BISHOP of New York said the importance of avoiding the use of opium in all suspected cases cannot be too much emphasized. The value of ice in relieving pain when applied freely by ice-bags should not be forgotten.

DR. H. A. HARE of Philadelphia claimed that pain is not a reliable symptom. When he himself had typhoid he had an attack of pain that was of the character supposed to indicate perforation, but it proved to be due to distension of the intestines by gas.

DR. WILSON, in closing, said many patients are brought to the hospital narcotized by opium, with the abdomen hard and distended by gas, the pulse rapid and feeble, and the whole condition hopeless. The use of opium certainly leads to a high mortality by obscuring symptoms until it is too late to save the patient.

DR. H. A. WEST of Galveston read a paper, entitled

DIFFERENTIAL DIAGNOSIS BETWEEN YELLOW FEVER AND DENGUE, WITH SOME ACCOUNT OF THE EPIDEMIC OF 1897 IN TEXAS. (See MEDICAL NEWS, page 740.)

SECTION ON MATERIA MEDICA, PHARMACY AND THERAPEUTICS.

FIRST DAY—JUNE 7TH.

The Chairman, JOHN V. SHOEMAKER, M.D., of Philadelphia, delivered an address upon

CHEMICAL RELATIONS OF REMEDIES IN SCIENTIFIC THERAPEUTICS.

He said a great advance has begun in the introduction of animal extracts, serums, and antitoxins into medicine. It will be worth while to make trial of suprarenal extracts and experiment with extracts of the brain and spinal cord in the treatment of neurasthenia, locomotor ataxia, and senile debility. The toxins which have been proven of value should be made officinal and adopted into the pharmacopœia, since it is in this line that future progress is to be made.

EDWIN KLEBS of Chicago read a paper, entitled

AIMS OF MODERN TREATMENT OF TUBERCULOSIS,

which was referred to a committee. A synopsis of this paper will be given before the Section to-morrow.

DR. CHARLES DENISON of Denver read a paper upon

THEORIES AND CONCLUSIONS ON THE MODERN TREATMENT OF TUBERCULOSIS.

He takes the stand that there is no settled treatment for tuberculosis as there are no two cases just alike in their several phases. Representing the benefit to patients suffering from tuberculosis as 100 per cent., 45 per cent. are affected by climate and changes involving mental influence, exercise, and out-of-door life; 30 per cent. are due to good feeling, local supervision, and medical treatment; 25 per cent. to inhaling, local medication, surgical interference, specific medication, and antitoxin treatment. So saturating the blood with creosote, for instance, that the bacillus will be stopped in its growth and the patient not be injured thereby, is, I think, a mere speculation. I doubt whether inhaled substances ever reach the air-vesicles and terminal bronchioles where the disease is located. The more a lung is diseased with tuberculosis and the accompanying infiltrating and shrinking process, the less is the possibility that inhaled medicaments can reach the affected parts. The reciprocal relation of diseased and healthy lung in the same thorax, and of the heart and blood within a given chest with reference to respiration, does not seem to me to have been sufficiently recognized by any one. I would like to demonstrate more clearly than has been done heretofore the fact that (1) correct inhaling, or, more properly, exhaling, (2) altitude above sea level, (3) rightly directed gymnastic training, all work on the same principle of mechanical distension of the air-cells. We have failed to recognize the mechanical conditions within the chest which govern respiration and blood circulation. The blood does not flow alone because the heart pumps it, but because the lung mechanism draws it in and forces it out again. Any system of training to be of use must depend upon the mechanical distension of the air-cells. I wish to make my protest against the surgeon's hasty interference in operating upon anal fistula while tuberculosis is in the lungs; it may be considered a means of elimination, and unless such elimination is provided for an operation should not be performed. If the disease is due to a special toxin working in the system it must be only through the development in that system of the proper antitoxin, or the appropriation of it from outside the body, that the disease may be opposed. The opposers of antitoxin are inconsistent in that, while they admit the existence of a toxin, they deny the possibility of an antitoxin. I firmly believe a considerable percentage of cases of tuberculosis could be held in check, if not cured, if with the present advanced technic in the manufacture of the tuberculin preparations, the physicians using them had the required knowledge to determine what patients could be treated by this method and how far the treatment should be pushed. The serum treatment of tuberculosis is as yet a beautiful dream, which I hope may be realized. My conclusions are that combined methods are superior to any given branch of treatment; that seasonable change of residence to a well-selected, high-altitude climate with its possibilities of out-door life is the best possible method for retarding the advance of consumption; that exercise is necessary to promote cell activity and distension of the cells; that it is a mistake to overwhelm the body with frequent injections of undetermined animal serums producing a cumulative toxemia; that the key to the direct method of specific treatment comes through the skilful determination of the proportion of infection, the balance between vital resistance and the disease.

Dr. Sherman G. Bonney of Denver read a paper upon

THE TREATMENT OF TUBERCOLOSIS.

He contends that climate, in conjunction with painstaking attention to details of management, offers to the pulmonary invalid greater assurance of improvement than can be otherwise attained. In many patients who come to Colorado the duration of several years of illness is disclosed with ample opportunity for earlier climatic change. Colorado is especially adapted for the early cases and contraindicated for late stages. It is a mistake to order patients away from home with directions not to see the doctor in the new location. One-third of the patients who seek a physician in Colorado present a history of several months already spent here, their medical supervision having been carried on by the home physician from a distance of two or three thousand miles. For the use of tuberculin in Colorado I see but little justification. Its use should be limited to early cases, and these cases are they which submit most easily to the favorable climate of this State. I am convinced that the moral effect of this treatment is distinctly bad. The patient should be out in the sunshine and fresh air, and removed from the depressing influence of the physician's office.

Dr. A. E. Waxham of Denver read a paper, entitled

CLIMATE VERSUS SERUM TREATMENT OF TUBERCULOSIS.

Because a patient has tuberculosis is no reason, he said, why he should be sent two thousand miles away from home, comfort, and friends, only to find perhaps his malady increased, and to die among strangers. We should prescribe climate with as much discretion and judgment as any other remedy. Whether a patient should be sent from home in search of health will depend upon several conditions. The stage of the disease, the vigor, vitality, and disposition of the patient, and the means with which to live comfortably, are all to be considered. Tuberculosis in the last stage is only aggravated, and the condition made worse by residence in this altitude. Climatic treatment should be applied early. In selecting cases for this treatment, select the early ones instead of waiting until the golden opportunity is lost in the hope of warding off the disease by less effective means. Financial factors must be considered. Many a case is aggravated as a result of anxiety and forced economy. If the patient's circumstances are such that he cannot live a year in idleness it is folly to send bim here. A contented mind, abundant food, and cheerful surroundings are essential factors. Early cases of tuberculosis, with no heart lesions, are best adapted to the high altitudes, and the invigorating, stimulating atmosphere of Colorado. More advanced cases need a warmer climate, such as Arizona or New Mexico. Many cases do well in Colorado in the summer and fall, but do not bear our cold weather. Many do well in Arizona in winter who cannot endure the heat of its summer. The success of climatic treatment will depend on the proper selection of the climate, and the proper selection of the cases as well. The effects of tuberculin in tuberculosis are disappointing. Altitude, pure air, sunshine, uniformity of climate are essential factors in treating tuberculosis because these conditions invigorate the system and stimulate the production of the normal antitoxins of the body.

Dr. E. Fletcher Ingalls of Chicago, in discussing these papers, said I think it true that patients should not be sent away for a change of climate who are not able to take care of themselves properly when they get there. I do not send advanced patients to Colorado. I think inhalations have some effect, not from the remedy used but from the fact that the air-cells are dilated. The surgical treatment of tuberculosis seems to me entirely unscientific. There is no more chance of relieving a patient in that way than of disinfecting a large sponge by injecting it with an antiseptic needle. It appears to me that the result of treatment of tuberculosis by the serum methods demonstrates that the smaller the quantity used the greater the benefit, in other words the smaller the quantity used the less harm done.

Dr. R. H. Babcock of Chicago considers the incipient stage as a pure and unmixed infection; the later stage as a mixed infection, tubercles have sunk into the background, and pus infection is in the ascendency. The former is easily curable; the latter is capable of arrest. I have used all forms of antitoxin treatment of tuberculosis, the various derivatives of tuberculin, and the various sera, and my experience is that the earlier we begin the greater the prospect of arrest. I do not believe any of these means will bring immunity.

DR. ANNAS contended that we make a mistake in discussing tuberculosis as if it were one distinct disease. We have simply a set of symptoms. I think the patient should be protected against himself, he must not swallow the sputa, must not scatter the poison about him. Confined in the house he is infecting himself; out of doors he is being protected against himself.

DR. CHAS. LYMAN GREEN plead for better statistics relative to the therapy of tuberculosis. Conclusions should not be based on less than five years of use of a treatment on an individual. I do not believe such powerful remedies as the antitoxins should be in general use.

DR. ALBERT E. MILLER of Boston thought more depends upon the nutrition than upon anything else. Climate nor tuberculin will cure unless the patient is properly nourished.

SECTION ON NEUROLOGY AND MEDICAL JURISPRUDENCE.

FIRST DAY—JUNE 7TH.

The address of the Chairman, entitled

PROGRESS IN NEUROLOGY,

was read by DR. CHARLES H. HUGHES of St. Louis, Mo., who spoke of the various advances made along neurological lines within the last twelve months. Removal of the ovaries formerly proposed for insanity among women, is now considered unjustifiable except where the generative organs are diseased, as the neuropathic diathesis is not removable by the knife. The surgical treatment of exophthalmic goiter should be condemned. It is too destructive and is unnecessary, since this disease is almost invariably curable without operation. Excellent results are obtained from arseniated and phosphorated bromid and blood reconstruction treatment, with adequate nerve and brain rest and changed mental environment for the patient. The neuron is now a proven unit in physiologic and pathologic processes.

DR. W. J. HERDMAN of Ann Arbor, Mich., presented a paper upon

NEURAL DYNAMICS.

The relations of associated neurons to each other are similar to charged electric condensers, disturbance of the potential in one producing correlated changes in the associated ones. A theory might be proposed to account for the generation of nerve force, and its conduction in the neuron and transmission from neuron to neuron. To do this it is necessary to reduce to their simplest conceptions physical and physiologic conditions present in the structure of the essential elements of the nervous system and to state what appear to be the most probable physical results of such conditions consistent with the phenomena observed.

DR. SEARCY of Tuscoloosa, Ala., said the unit of life is the cell of the nervous system, the nerve-cell. Most philosophic theories would be simplified if vital motion was described by simpler vital motion; as in the extremely complex nervous system of man by studying the movements of the lower organisms, as amebæ and protozoa.

DR. HENRY GRADLE of Chicago read an article upon

DIAGNOSTIC CHARACTERISTICS OF HEADACHES ACCORDING TO THEIR ORIGIN.

He especially referred to headaches dependent upon affections of the special senses, and said the peripheral lesion, and also the condition of the nervous system must be considered. The most important question concerning the site of a headache is whether it is wholly or predominantly one-sided. One-sided headache is always due to a lesion on the same side of the bead, intracranial, or in one of the organs of sense. As to their time relations, headaches can be classified as: (1) paroxysms recurring at (*a*) irregular or (*b*) regular intervals; (2) attacks following some specific act, and (3) more or less continuous pain. The cases classified under (1) (*a*) constitute the form called migraine. As to headaches following specific acts the most characteristic is the pain induced by use of the eyes for near work.

DR. C. M. HOBBY of Iowa City read a paper, entitled

SOME CAUSES OF WRYNECK.

Torticollis has recovered after removal of ocular conditions unlikely to have exerted a causative influence in its production. The first case was in a boy aged fifteen years. Deformity had existed several years and the muscular contraction was apparently structural. No spasmodic element was detected and the abnormal position was constant, the head being drawn well toward the right shoulder. Forcible correction was attended by diplopia, and it was found that paresis of the left inferior rectus existed. Subsequent tenotomy of superior rectus led to gradual but complete recovery from the torticollis. Second case was that of a boy aged twelve years. There was a history of impaired vision and asthenopic symptoms for more than a year. Three weeks after examination the patient had had severe headaches, nausea, and vomiting, coincidentally with diplopia. The head became twisted down toward the right shoulder. Examination showed 80° of esophoria in each eye, accompanied by low grade of hypermetropic astigmatism. Correction of refraction and "ocular gymnastics" induced recovery in two months.

DR. CASEY A. WOOD of Chicago read a paper upon

THE METHODS EMPLOYED IN EXAMINING THE EYES FOR THE DETECTION OF HYSTERIA.

The commonest ocular signs of hysteria are defects in the focusing power of eye—anomalies of accommodation. Other conditions are hysterical insufficiency of accommodation, ciliary hyperesthesia, ciliary paresis or paralysis, painful accommodation, nervous asthenopia, and are rarely permanently relieved by glasses or exclusively local treatment of the eye. This so-called paresis of accommodation is generally in the form of a true hysterical contracture of the ciliary muscle.

DR. HOWELL T. PERSHING of Denver exhibited two patients, one a young man, suffering from aneurism of the internal carotid. The prominent symptoms were diplopia, which was relieved by treatment, and occasional blowing sound in the ear. When present, the latter was readily distinguishable by the observer. Second patient, a man advanced in years, had syringomyelia with Charcot's disease of shoulder, and marked hemiplegia.

SECTION ON DISEASES OF CHILDREN.

FIRST DAY—JUNE 7TH.

The address of the Chairman, DR. J. P. CROZER GRIFFITH of Philadelphia, was read:

RISE OF PEDIATRICS AS A SPECIALTY.

This was followed by a paper from DR. LOUIS J. LAUTENBACH of Philadelphia upon "Prompt Attention to Earache in Infancy and Early Childhood." No discussion.

DR. R. B. GILBERT of Louisville read an article upon

WHOOPING-COUGH.

In this he stated that four-fifths of the deaths occurred in children under two years of age. The disease is most fatal in extremely hot or cold weather. Tincture of belladonna in increasing doses as soon as disease is recognized was advised, to which bromid of potassium and phenacetin could be added.

DR. LOUIS FISCHER of New York agreed that antipyrin in some cases does good. Bromoform properly given is also useful, but one must be sure to procure a good product. Poisoning from bromoform settling to bottom of the bottle should be avoided. The best treatment consists in sending the child into the park to receive pure air, and in sleeping with the windows open at night. Dr. W. A. Fankboner of Marion, Ind., secures good results in some cases with quinin, 10 grains three times daily. Dr. H. M. McClanahan of Omaha emphasized the importance of nourishment, and advises feeding immediately after the paroxysms. He considers antipyrin the best drug.

DR. J. M. POSTLE spoke of the pathology. Ptomains seem to affect chiefly nerve cells governing expiration, inducing a condition of depression. The peculiar inspiration results from stimulation of nerve cells governing this act by an excess of carbonic acid gas in the blood. It is believed that carbonic acid gas in blood destroys the ptomains. Strychnia is advised to overcome the depression and prevent destruction of the ptomains by excess of carbonic acid gas in blood, thus securing the immunizing effect of ptomains.

DR. I. N. LOVE of St. Louis contended that all such diseases should be treated on the principle of elimination. Improve the assimilation to build up the patient. Purge thoroughly and saturate with quinin. Acetanelin, bicarbonate of soda, and caffein are useful; also bromoform three or four times a day in increasing doses.

DR. GREEN of Michigan considered three things as important in the treatment: Warm clothing, fresh air, and nutritious food. In the last five years he has used no medicine.

DR. GILBERT, in closing, said purgation was uncalled for when there is a diarrhea. He has had bad results from antipyrin, and prefers phenacetin. The effect of bromoform is no better than from bromids. Sanitary measures contribute to the cure, but therapeutics are valuable. The theory of germ-producing toxins which act on the nervous system is attractive, but not easy to demonstrate. Strychnia is a dangerous remedy. Care should be exercised in sending children to the parks lest the disease be disseminate.

DR. A. E. GALLANT of New York read a paper upon

FRACTURE OF THE CLAVICLE IN CHILDREN,

based upon a study of 200 cases treated by Sayre's method. In a surgical service, including 18,042 children of ten years and under, there occurred 343 fractures, and of these 172 were of the clavicle. Most frequent point of fracture was in outer portion of the middle third, the shoulder dropping downward, inward, and forward, dragging on acromial fragment in such a way as to make an angle at the seat of fracture. The inner fragment has not been found displaced above the outer one, as described by Sayre and Gray.

DR. A. C. COTTON of Chicago observed that continued use of plaster may be impracticable because of irritation. Sometimes he uses a stocking over the arm, which is firmly bandaged.

DR. R. B. GILBERT, in one patient, overcame the irritation by using a moleskin bandage, perforated. Adjustment of the plaster should be accomplished undechloroform, but often only partial anesthesia is necessary.

DR. GALLANT, in closing, emphasized difficulty of preventing movement, although movement does not always prevent healing. Infants' clavicles broken during delivery may be united before the accident is recognized. He prefers the use of laughing-gas for short operations.

DR. J. A. WORK of Elkhart, Indiana, read an article, entitled

SOME THOUGHTS ON THE CARE OF INFANTS AND CHILDREN.

He referred to injury of the brain with forceps, and the cervical portion of spinal cord during delivery. After delivery, fresh aseptic lard is best for cleansing the infant. No soap or water is required. Children should not be weaned from natural food too soon without reasonable cause. When insufficiency of natural food is noticed, gradually add the artificial, and the child will usually wean itself. Next to mothers' milk cows' milk is to be preferred. If milked into sterilized containers and used soon there is no more necessity of sterilization than it would be to sterilize the mother's milk.

GENERAL SESSION.

SECOND DAY—JUNE 8TH.

The Association was promptly called to order by Second Vice-President THOMPSON. Dr. Dudley S. Reynolds of Louisville presented a resolution to the effect that after January 1, 1899, any college professor or other teacher who shall confer any degree upon any person not complying with the standards of American Medical Association regarding educational requirements, shall hereafter be excluded from meetings of the Association. This was referred to the Executive Committee.

A resolution by DR. W. W. KEEN of Philadelphia was introduced favoring vivisection for purposes of experimental research. Referred to the Executive Committee.

DR. H. A. HARE of Philadelphia offered a resolution relative to the State and County Medical Societies of the State of New York, asking that they be allowed to send regularly recognized delegates to the National Association. Referred to the Executive Committee.

DR. GEO. M. GOULD of Philadelphia presented a resolution, the purpose of which was to encourage the establishment of medical libraries throughout the United States.

DR. WILLIAM BAILEY of Louisville introduced an important matter in the form of a resolution to the effect that an office of general secretary be created with a salary not to exceed $2500 or $3000 per annum. He said that the association had grown to such proportions that the services of at least one salaried man were required, who would devote his entire time to its interests. By this resolution the present Secretary, Dr. Atkinson, would be retained as an honorary officer. Resolution was referred to the Executive Committee.

DR. SANDERS of Alabama recommended in a resolution that the Association take steps leading to the establishment of a public health bureau, having its representative in every city and town in the land and an executive head in the National Government.

DR. HUMISTON of Ohio read a report, adopted by the Ohio State Medical Society regarding the Antivivisection bill and recommended that in addition to other committees being named, one should be composed of residents of Washington, Philadelphia, and Baltimore. Under this arrangement there would be the assurance of prompt attendance of committeemen whenever the bill referred to came up.

DR. J. H. MUSSER of Philadelphia then read the General Address on Medicine, entitled

AN ESSENTIAL OF THE ART OF MEDICINE.

He said the closing years of the Eighteenth Century and the early years of the Nineteenth marked an epoch in medicine as transcendent for its welfare as the events of the past decades bespeak for the glory of the medicine of the future. The state of medicine in the Eighteenth Century was the result of deductive methods of reasoning, made possible because of the want of instruments of precision. Elaborate classification of disease and refinements of symptomatology which serve only to amuse and appal were the results. The sway of the imagination and the rule of theory were all powerful. Speculative modes of treatment grew out of the specious pathology. Venesection, polypharmacy, and stimulation were followed by expectant treatment and ninilism. Diagnosis was an intuition and an art. Cullen said theory could control observation, but medicine as a science was no higher nor lower than its cognate departments of knowledge. Science was not applied to industrial arts at this time, and so they were carried on by rule-of-thumb methods. Medicine ceased to be deductive; its practice began to be scientific.

Medicine has grown to be a science—a department of the science of biology. The history is the history of the application of scientific habits of thought to experiment, observation, and analysis. Medicine grew to a science by the labors of physicians who were naturalists. Clinical medicine, as a science, embraces diagnosis and therapeutics. Methods of diagnosis of the present day require a scientific habit of mind and skill in the use of instruments of precision. The scope and positiveness of diagnosis has greatly increased, as fifteen diseases can now be positively recognized, without any possibility of error. Diagnosis has grown to be scientific, precise, and positive. Error in method leads to error in diagnosis. Therapeutics grew to a science by the influence of various forces, all the outcome of the mode of thought of the naturalist. The science of statistics shows the fallacy of determining the value of a drug from a small number of cases in which it is tried. Analysis of 12,000 prescriptions has shown that various drugs were called for about 31,000 times, and preparations of nux vomica, iron, opium, mineral acids, cinchona and its salts, mercury, ipecac, bismuth, belladonna, arsenic, squills, hyoscyamus, and digitalis, were called for in one-third of the total, and if external remedies and excipients are excluded, in one half.

Skepticism arose because too much was claimed. The more incurable the disease the greater the number of drugs claimed to cure it. The more virtues a drug is said to have, the less its probable value. Polypharmacy was assaulted in the past, but still holds sway. Drugs no doubt have an action in health and disease. There use may be of advantage but usually is not necessary. We need not be skeptical about the power of the drug, but about its necessity. Expectancy and hypnotism, for therapeutic purposes, can be secured by an honest examination of the patient. The "lie" is not required in medicine any more than in religion, as Zola points out.

Application of science to industrial art at the present time shows that in every department scientific methods are necessary. Brewing, iron-making, leather-making are no longer an art but a science. Art is gone; science holds sway. The large amounts of capital involved and great competition have forced out the element of chance as in art and instituted the element of certainty that approaches science. Since the science of medicine is essential to the art we must educate our students to a scientific habit of thought.

Adjourned to the following day.

SECTION ON MEDICINE.

SECOND DAY—JUNE 8TH.

The first paper upon

DIABETIC GANGRENE,

was read by DR. N. S. DAVIS, JR., of Chicago. In the discussion Dr. Warren remarked that in forty per cent. of diabetic cases which live long enough tuberculosis develops. When a case is going badly it is useless to amputate, because the gangrene is only a local exhibition of a general condition which affects every cell of the body. It, however, may do to amputate in a case going well. One cannot set rules while in such ignorance regarding the disease. Dr. Davis contended that it is not necessarily objectionable to amputate a second time if the first is unsuccessful. There should be thorough antiseptic treatment of gangrenous wounds in cases of diabetes. Sudden disappearance of sugar from the urine has been observed where there was tuberculosis of the lungs. We cannot judge of arterial sclerosis entirely by the arteries we can easily handle, for it is often circumscribed within small areas. A fact brought out by study of diabetes is the very early development of arterial sclerosis, in many cases between twenty and thirty years of age, at a period of life when we rarely expect to find it.

DR. L. F. BISHOP of New York presented a paper, entitled

THE COURSE AND MANAGEMENT OF CHRONIC COMPLICATING MYOCARDITIS.

Complicating myocarditis, he said, is an important factor in many conditions. The heart muscle should be studied carefully in acute and wasting diseases of whatever nature. Arrhythmia occurring where this symptom has not been previously shown is suggestive of a complicating myocarditis. Jacobi asserts that after every case of typhoid, scarlatina, diphtheria, or smallpox we must prepare ourselves to be overtaken by some cardiac disease. Too often cases diagnosed general debility are due to disease of the heart muscle. Light, systematic exercise should be employed in treatment, with concentrated foods, but alcohol, tobacco, tea, and coffee should be eschewed.

DR. FRANK BILLINGS of Chicago read a paper upon

DIFFERENTIATION OF THE CARDIAC INCOMPETENCY OF INTRINSIC HEART DISEASE AND CHRONIC NEPHRITIS.

In all inflammatory diseases of the kidneys he said there are cardiovascular changes. In chronic nephritis while the cardiovascular changes are less marked, dropsy may occur with all the phenomena of an incompetent heart. The incompetent heart of arteriosclerosis may present phenomena so nearly like the clinical findings of inflammatory condition of the kidneys as to be differentiated with difficulty. There are some special signs valuable in differential diagnosis. If the urine shows relatively low specific gravity, with diminished total solids, lessened urea, much albumen, casts of all varieties, the pulse full and sustained, dropsical effusion poor in albumen and containing urea in a considerable amount, tendency to persistent morning nausea, vomiting of stringy mucus, frontal or occipital pain, tendency to alternating mental excitement, somnolence and coma, epigastric pain, eye ground showing changes of albuminuria, and patient possesses waxy face and general anemia, the diagnosis is favorable to nephritis. If heart action is irregular, pulse weak and not sustained, with or without arterial sclerosis, dyspnea of exertion attended with cyanosis, only moderate degree of anemia, dropsical effusion relatively rich in albumen but containing little or no urea, considerable enlargement of liver and tenderness of left lobe, urine scant, high specific gravity, but few casts, little headache, no eye-ground changes, and if thrombosis or embolism occur, the diagnosis is in favor of intrinsic heart disease.

DR. H. A. WEST of Galveston said, in discussing the paper, that if the renal symptoms are due alone to circulatory disturbance of the kidney, placing the patient upon digitalis and strychnin and freely stimulating the emunctories will in many cases clear up the diagnosis.

DR. BROWN of Illinois had made a diagnosis not upon the presence of albumen and casts, but upon symptoms which are referred to organs external to the kidneys, the forcible pulsation of the heart, palpable pulsation of the systematic arteries, etc.

DR. R. H. BABCOCK of Chicago: I would like to emphasize the point of pulse tension in this differentiation. If the pulse be carefully studied by the sphygmograph and auscultation of the aortic second sound be performed, much valuable information will be derived.

DR. ANDERS of Philadelphia: In cases of so-called chronic interstitial nephritis with lesions of the heart associated, as a rule, there is one fundamental cause, general arterial sclerosis. For a time the left ventricle meets the demands of the heart for increased work, but a time comes when the heart can no longer compensate, and the left ventricle begins to weaken and the urinary symptoms appear.

DRS. R. H. FITZ and E. P. JOSLIN of Boston, Mass., presented a paper, read by Dr. Joslin, entitled

DIABETES MELLITUS AT THE MASSACHUSETTS GENERAL HOSPITAL FROM 1821–1897; A STUDY OF RECORDS.

They found the total number of cases treated in its medical wards to be 172. The percentage in the last thirteen years has increased four fold over that of the first fifteen. Of these cases 74 per cent. were males, 26 per cent. females; the oldest was 73 years, youngest 5; average 33 years; only one was a negro. The question of hereditary tendency was considered in 42 cases, present in 10 patients, absent in 32. It is an erroneous idea that diabetics pass more liquid than they take. One case lasted twelve years; three suffered only twelve weeks; average duration was one year and a half. Cases of grave diabetes ended fatally in nearly three-fourths of the instances, and a large percentage died comatose. The average mortality of saccharine diabetes has not materially changed in these seventy-four years. Diet restrictions have undergone no marked alterations during this time, and opium is the only drug which has been persistently used throughout the period.

DR. H. A. West, in his Southern hospital, had not seen a case in the negro race. He had noticed its occurrence in very obese persons.

DR. JAS. TYSON of Philadelphia had three negro cases brought to his notice within ten days. It is especially common among Hebrews.

The next paper on

THE INFLUENCE OF SUNLIGHT ON TUBERCULAR SPUTUM IN DENVER; A STUDY AS TO THE CAUSE OF THE GREAT DEGREE OF IMMUNITY AGAINST TUBERCULOSIS ENJOYED BY THOSE LIVING IN HIGH ALTITUDES,

was presented by DRS. MITCHELL and CROUCH of Denver. They discovered, by experiments carefully performed in their bacteriological laboratory, that sputum offers very little virulence after twenty-hours exposure to solar rays. The sputum of consumptives in this altitude has ample opportunity to be blown into the atmosphere before it has been robbed of its virulence. So immunity of our population must be explained on other grounds than non-exposure. The battle for moisture, especially as it occurs in the lungs, we believe to be one of the factors of immunization. The alveoli are too dry to offer a nidus for the bacilli, so the conditions are extremely unfavorable for their development. Also this absence of moisture in the atmosphere acts favorably on the animal organism as a whole, giving increased vitality. Lessened atmospheric pressure is another factor in our immunization. When the organism is subject to increased atmospheric pressure the blood recedes from the skin, capillaries, and mucous membranes producing anemia of these parts. The reverse is true with diminished pressure. Diminished surface pressure also allows the body-heat to be easily and continuously equalized. Appetite is better; metabolism more complete; red blood-cells more abundant; percentage of hemoglobin greater. All of which is favorable to immunization.

DR. JAMES TYSON of Philadelphia presented a paper upon

OPIUM AND IRON IN BRIGHT'S DISEASE.

Contrary to the opinion he once held, much mischief is done by iron in Bright's disease. If the gallons of Basham's mixture had been poured into the gutter instead of the patients' stomachs it would have been a good thing. It is harmful in locking up secretions. It is not indicated and should not be prescribed in cases of acute Bright's disease. It is contraindicated also in chronic interstitial nephritis but is best borne in chronic parenchymatous nephritis, but even here the doses given are needlessly large. When iron barely tinges the stools it is proof that enough has been given; if they are rendered black the iron given is excessive. Death has not infrequently been precipitated by opium in uremic conditions in which opium is positively contraindicated. Under no circumstances in chronic interstitial nephritis should opium be used. It may be used in the uremic convulsions of puerpural fever.

DR. H. A. WEST expressed the belief that iron is beneficial and indicated in many cases of acute Bright's disease. It had been his experience that hypodermic injections of morphia and atropia were the only means possible after other remedies had utterly failed to control convulsions, especially of the puerpural kind.

DR. VAN HORN of Illinois remarked that if the gentlemen would use the lancet they would have no use for opium, morphin, or the bromids.

RARE CASES OF ARRHYTHMIA

was the subject of a paper read by DR. J. M. ANDERS of Philadelphia. He reported a case of tobacco poisoning in which on ausculation four sounds could be distinguished in each cardiac rhythm and both first and second sounds were duplicated, the pulse-wave being synchronous with the second element of the systole. The pulse even showed a modified double beat when moderate pressure was made upon the radial, dependent on double ventricular contraction. Also double reduplication was noted in a female with exophthalmic goiter, this being a case of asynchronous contraction of the two ventricles. The third case was complicated by marked obesity. The pulse was irregular in volume and rhythm, and 96 while patient was at rest. The systole occasionally failed to send a pulse-wave to the radial artery. Valvular affection was not demonstrable, but there was feeble, muffled first sounds, with *pulsus alternans*. On holding the breath the heart-rhythm became at times almost regular.

DR. C. S. BOND of Indiana read a paper, entitled

CONSIDERATION OF FOUR CASES OF EPILEPSY, WITH A REFERENCE TO THE CAUSE.

His first case was that of a child three months of age, of good family history, no injuries. Petit mal and convulsions represented cortical explosions caused by toxic influence of fermentation of food in the alimentary canal. Second case was in a boy of six years, whose father has developed locomotor ataxia, and the mother had uremic convulsions at the child's birth. Strict adherence to limited diet, chiefly of milk, and no bromid, has brought about long intervals between attacks. Third patient was a girl seventeen years of age, who habitually had three or four attacks a day. She was the victim of lowered power of digestion, attended by fermentation in the alimentary canal. A diet limited to a half pint of milk every six hours induced a passive condition for three years. When the diet was extended a relapse occurred. If bromids were given the stomach was disturbed and attacks increased. Fourth patient was a man, twenty-seven years of age, with a good family history, who suffered pain after eating. As a result of a restricted diet and the use of magnesia once a day he went five months without an attack. The author emphasized the fact that with the use of bromid we often ward off attacks in children, but the condition is still present, and becomes chronic.

The Section elected Dr. Frank Billings of Chicago, chairman; Dr. C. E. Edson of Denver, secretary, for the ensuing year.

Adjourned to the following day.

GENERAL SESSION.

THIRD DAY—JUNE 9TH.

The following named gentlemen were elected officers of the Association for the ensuing year.

President, J. M. Matthews, M.D., of Louisville, Ky.; vice-president, W. W. Keen, M.D., of Philadelphia; second vice-president, J. W. Graham, M.D., of Denver, Col.; third vice-president, H. A. West, M.D., of Galveston, Tex.; fourth vice-president, J. B. Minning, M.D., of Kansas; treasurer, H. P. Newman, M.D., of Chicago; librarian, G. W. Webster, M.D., of Chicago.

THE MEDICAL NEWS.

A WEEKLY JOURNAL OF MEDICAL SCIENCE.

VOL. LXXII. NEW YORK, SATURDAY, JUNE 18, 1898. NO. 25.

ORIGINAL ARTICLES.

A FURTHER PLEA FOR INTRAGASTRIC ELECTRIZATION.

BY MAX EINHORN, M.D.,
OF NEW YORK.

IN a previous paper[1] I have stated the reasons for using direct electrization of the stomach (intragastric electrization) in preference to the percutaneous method of applying electricity to the organ. In two consecutive papers[2] I have published the therapeutic results obtainable by this method of treatment in diseases of the digestive organs. Meanwhile, many writers here and abroad have also written on the value of intragastric electrization. Thus Stockton,[3] Jones,[4] and D. D. Stewart[5] in this country, Rosenheim,[6] Brock,[7] Wegele,[8] and Goldschmidt[9] in Germany, Ravé[10] and Caron[11] in France, and Goldbaum[12] in Russia have all published valuable articles on the subject. While there seems to be perfect harmony among the various writers as to the beneficial effect of direct electrization of the stomach in diseases of this organ, some difference of opinion exists with regard to the physiologic effect of the electric current on this viscus. In this connection I simply mention the papers of Meltzer,[13] Goldschmidt, and myself.[14] As the therapeutic value of the efficacy of the electric current cannot be gaged by physiologic experiments, but must be judged from clinical data empirically obtained, I will not enter into a discussion of the different views on the physiologic action of the electric current on the stomach, but will rather give my new experiences with intragastric electrization. They cover a period of five years, and contain reports of all the cases I have treated in this way since my last publication, entitled "Further Experiences with Direct Electrization of the Stomach." The great number of patients treated by me with intragastric electrization will, I trust, be of aid in deciding whether this mode of treatment is of real value or not.

The current was applied by means of the deglutable electrode, and the mode of procedure was as described by me in my book on "Diseases of the Stomach."[15]

As the number of cases treated by intragastric electrization is very large, I submit them without minute description in the accompanying tables.

These tables contain all the cases in my private practice which I have treated by intragastric electrization during the years from 1893 to 1897, inclusive.

In reviewing Table I. we find that of 118 patients treated with direct faradization of the stomach, 79 were cured (all the subjective morbid symptoms having disappeared), 32 were greatly ameliorated, 5 slightly improved, and in 2 the condition remained unchanged. Table II. contains the cases which were first treated by direct faradization, and later by galvanization of the stomach. The reason for the change from the faradic to the galvanic current was that these patients did not sufficiently respond to the faradic current (*i. e.*, the symptoms did not abate to any great extent), and that the pains within the gastric region preponderated over the other symptoms. In this table there are reports of 21 cases treated; 14 patients were cured, 6 greatly improved, and the condition of 1 was unchanged. Table III. shows the cases treated by intragastric galvanization alone. They were 38 in number. Of these, 27 patients were cured, 6 greatly improved, 4 slightly improved, and 1 unchanged.

I should like to remark again that by "cured" I mean the entire disappearance of all the symptoms of which the patients complained, and objectively the appearance of well-being. The condition of the gastric contents did not always necessarily return to the normal. In some instances there was a change in the desired direction, in some no change whatever, and in some perhaps rather an increase or decrease of the gastric juice in the opposite direction, *i. e.*, in cases of hyperchlorhydria, although rarely, it was found that the degree of acidity was higher than before the treatment; and again in cases of hypochlorhydria, occasionally, a still lower degree of acidity was found. Notwithstanding this, even in these rare instances, the subjective symptoms entirely disappeared, the patients could eat everything with impunity, and must be considered as perfectly well. The term dilatation of the stomach used in the tables simply signifies a larger size of the organ without ischochymia.

In addition to the application of electricity most of the patients were also given the usual remedies. Some patients, however, were given no medicaments whatever. The diet was a liberal one, and great stress was laid on having the patients take rather more than sufficient quantities of food. Un-

TABLE I.—CASES TREATED BY DIRECT GASTROFARADIZATION.

(From January, 1893, to December, 1897.)

No.	Name.	Age.	Disease.	Principal complaint.	How long sick before electrization.	How long treated.	Result of treatment.	Remarks.
1.	Emil R.	32 years.	Dilatation of the stomach and hyperchlorhydria.	Fulness, pains, constipation, occasionally vomiting.	3 years.	2 months.	Slight improvement.	
2.	Mrs. L. L.	35 years.	Atony of the stomach.	Anorexia, belching, constipation.	2 years.	2 months.	Greatly improved.	
3.	Mrs. A. S.	45 years.	Hyperchlorhydria.	Pains, frequent belching, constipation.	4 years.	3 months.	Disappearance of symptoms.	Patient got entirely well and has remained so ever since 1893. She can eat everything with impunity.
4.	William C.	30 years.	Dilatation of the stomach.	Anorexia, belching, weakness, frequent headaches, constipation.	3 years.	2 months.	Disappearance of symptoms.	
5.	Jacob S.	50 years.	Hyperchlorhydria.	Bloated feeling, frequent pains.	2 years.	2 months.	Slight improvement.	
6.	Charles E.	33 years.	Dilatation of the stomach and hyperchlorhydria.	Frequent belching, pains, constipation.	3 years.	3 months.	Disappearance of symptoms.	
7.	Walter C.	30 years.	Enteroptosis (ren. mob. dex.) and hyperchlorhydria.	Anorexia, feeling of fulness, and frequent pains.	4 years.	3 months.	Disappearance of symptoms.	
8.	Mrs. Amanda B.	40 years.	Enteroptosis and atony of the stomach.	Anorexia, dragging pains, constipation.	5 years.	2 months.	Greatly improved.	
9.	William D. D.	40 years.	Dilatation of the stomach and hyperchlorhydria.	Feeling of oppression after meals, pains, constipation.	7 years.	1 month.	Greatly improved.	
10.	Mrs. H. O. W.	35 years.	Enteroptosis.	Dizziness, pains, weakness, constipation.	4 years.	2 months.	Disappearance of symptoms.	Has remained well ever since (1893).
11.	Mrs. C. M.	36 years.	Neurasthenia gastrica; chlorosis.	Pains, weakness, dizziness, constipation.	2 years.	1 month.	Slightly improved.	
12.	Mrs. Julia R.	40 years.	Enteroptosis; hyperchlorhydria.	Belching, pains, occasionally nausea.	3 years.	5 months.	Disappearance of symptoms.	
13.	Mrs. F. A. R.	50 years.	Atony of the stomach.	Feeling of fulness and belching, slight pains, constipation.	3 years.	2 months.	Disappearance of symptoms.	
14.	Douglas H. C.,	19 years.	Dilatation of the stomach, hyperchlorhydria.	Pains, dizzy spells, frequent hunger, constipation, despondent feeling.	2 years.	2 months.	Condition remained the same.	
15.	Edward B.	29 years.	Dilatation of the stomach, hyperchlorhydria.	Frequent belching, dizziness, pains, constipation.	2 years.	3 months.	Slightly improved.	
16.	Mrs. B. S.	52 years.	Gastritis gland. chr.	Feeling of pressure, very frequent belching.	1½ years.	2 months.	Disappearance of symptoms.	
17.	Alexander H.	25 years.	Dilatation of the stomach, hyperchlorhydria; general neurasthenia.	Despondent feeling, pains and weakness.	2 years.	2 weeks.	No change.	
18.	George S.	40 years.	Dilatation of the stomach and hyperchlorhydria.	Feeling of fulness, burning sensation, occasionally diarrhea.	1 year.	2 months.	Disappearance of symptoms.	
19.	Edward R.	62 years.	Dilatation of the stomach and hyperchlorhydria.	Pains, occasionally vomiting, constipation.	8 years.	1 month.	Greatly improved.	
20.	William H.	43 years.	Gastritis gland. chr.	Nausea, frequent attacks of vomiting, anorexia.	7 years.	2 months.	Greatly improved.	
21.	Miss Hannah R.	26 years.	Gastritis gland. chr.	Constant belching, anorexia, constipation.	2 years.	2 months.	Disappearance of symptoms.	
22.	Mrs. Antonia R.	37 years.	Enteroptosis and atony of the stomach.	Feeling of pressure, frequent headache, poor appetite, constipation.	3 years.	2 months.	Disappearance of symptoms.	
23.[1]	William N. J.	50 years.	Gastritis gland. chr.	Nausea, poor appetite, frequent belching.	1 year.	1 month.	Disappearance of symptoms.	

[1] Cases 24 to 118 have been omitted on account of scarcity of space.

TABLE II.—CASES FIRST TREATED BY DIRECT GASTROFARADIZATION, THEREAFTER BY DIRECT GASTROGALVANIZATION.
(From January, 1893, to December, 1897.)

No.	Name.	Age.	Disease.	Principal complaint.	How long sick before electrization.	How long treated.	Result of treatment.	Remarks.
1.	Max D.	46 years.	Hyperchlorhydria.	Pains, feeling of pressure, dizziness.	3 years.	Gastrofarad., 10 days; galvaniz., 2 mos.	Greatly improved.	
2.	Henry S.	48 years.	Rumination.	Belching and rumination.	28 years.	Gastrofarad., 2 weeks; galvaniz., 1 mo.	No change.	
3.	Mrs. F. D.	35 years.	Atony of the stomach.	Pains, frequent vomiting, constipation alternating with diarrhea.	8 years.	Gastrofarad., 1 mo.; galvaniz., 3 mos.	Disappearance of symptoms.	Patient gained 20 pounds in weight and felt very well.
4.	David G.	46 years.	Dilatation of the stomach and hyperchlorhydria.	Burning sensation, nausea, dizziness, constipation.	5 years.	Gastrofarad., 2 weeks; galvaniz., 2 mos.	Disappearance of symptoms.	
5.	Lowndes T.	40 years.	Dilatation of the stomach and slight hyperchlorhydria.	Pains, despondent feeling, dizziness, constipation.	4 years.	Gastrofarad., 2 weeks; galvaniz., 2 mos.	Disappearance of symptoms.	
6.	Herman R.	30 years.	Atony of the stomach.	Frequent belching, dragging feeling, constipation.	3 years.	Farad., 2 weeks; galvaniz., 2 mos.	Disappearance of symptoms.	
7.	Herrman H.	25 years.	Dilatation of the stomach (right movable kidney) and hyperchlorhydria.	Pains, headaches, frequent diarrhea.	2 years.	Farad., 1 week; galvaniz., 1 month.	Greatly improved.	
8.	Mrs. Clara B.	40 years.	Enteroptosis and gastralgia nervosa.	Poor appetite, pains, weakness, constipation.	10 years.	Faradized, 2 weeks; galvaniz., 6 weeks	Greatly improved.	
9.	Miss Clara E.	26 years.	Enteroptosis (right movable kidney) and hyperchlorhydria.	Nausea, pains, despondent feeling, constipation.	5 years.	Faradized, 2 weeks; galvaniz., 2 mos.	Disappearance of symptoms.	
10.	George C.	42 years.	Neurasthenia gastrica, tormina ventriculi nervosa.	Burning sensation, dizziness, sleeplessness, despondent feeling, costiveness.	5 years.	Faradized, 2 weeks; galvanized, 3 mos.	Greatly improved.	
11.	Mrs. J. A. M.	43 years.	Enteroptosis (right movable kidney) and hyperchlorhydria.	Pains, occasionally vomiting, weakness, constipation.	7 years.	Faradized, 2 weeks; galvanized, 2 mos.	Disappearance of symptoms.	Patient gained 18 pounds while under treatment.
12.	Edgar C.	42 years.	Atony of the stomach, gastrosuccorrhea cont. chronica.	Pains, headache, dizziness, despondent feeling, constipation.	14 years.	Faradized, 2 weeks; galvanized, 3 mos.	Disappearance of symptoms.	Patient gained 27 pounds.
13.	Isador W.	46 years.	Dilatation of the stomach (r. movable kidney), gastralgia.	Severe pains, frequent belching, constipation.	3 years.	Faradized, 2 weeks; galvanized, 2 mos.	Disappearance of symptoms.	Patient gained 16 pounds while under treatment.
14.	Edward G.	32 years.	Hyperchlorhydria.	Pains, dizziness, despondent feeling, constipation.	4 years.	Faradized, 2 weeks; galvanized, 3 mos.	Disappearance of symptoms.	Patient has gained considerably in weight.
15.	Alfred H.	40 years.	Dilatation of the stomach, gastralgia.	Pains, headache, despondent feeling, weakness.	3 years.	Faradized, 1 week; galvanized, 2 mos.	Disappearance of symptoms.	
16.	Alfred M.	38 years.	Dilatation of the stomach, gastralgia.	Pains, constant belching, despondent feeling, irregularity of bowels.	7 years.	Faradized, 1 week; galvanized, 6 weeks.	Greatly improved.	
17.	James B.	27 years.	Atony of the stomach and hyperchlorhydria.	Frequent belching, slight pains, dizziness.	5 years.	Faradized, 2 weeks; galvanized, 3 mos.	Disappearance of symptoms.	
18.	Miss Mary W.	23 years.	Vomitus nervosus, gastralgia.	Severe pains, frequent Vomiting, weakness, obstinate constipation.	7 years.	Faradized, 2 weeks; galvanized, 2 mos.	Disappearance of symptoms.	Patient gained 8 pounds in weight.
19.	Miss Henrietta S.	26 years.	Dilatation of the stomach and hyperchlorhydria.	Pains, frequent belching, bad taste in the mouth, constipation.	6 years.	Faradized, 2 weeks; galvanized, 2 mos.	Disappearance of symptoms.	Patient has gained 15 pounds in weight.
20.	Aaron N.	36 years.	Hyperchlorhydria.	Pains, feeling of oppression, belching, constipation.	5 years.	Faradized, 2 weeks; galvanized, 2 mos.	Disappearance of symptoms.	
21.	Miss Jessie D.	24 years.	Dilatation of the stomach (right movable kidney).	Constant belching, frequent pains, constipation.	8 years.	Faradized, 2 weeks; galvanized, 2 mos.	Greatly improved.	

TABLE III.—CASES TREATED WITH INTRAGASTRIC GALVANIZATION.
(From January, 1893, to December, 1897.)

No.	Name.	Age.	Disease.	Principal complaints.	How long sick before electrization.	How long treated.	Result of treatment.	Remarks.
1.	Margaretta L.	40 years.	Ulcus duodenale, stenosis pylori.	Constant pains, frequent vomiting, obstinate constipation.	15 years.	10 days.	The pains grew less severe, but the symptoms remained.	Patient was operated (pyloroplasty of Heineke-Mikulicz) and got well.
2.	Henry S.	38 years.	Erosions of the stomach.	Slight pains, weakness, constipation.	5 years.	6 weeks.	Disappearance of symptoms.	Patient was treated besides with the intragastric spray.
3.	Siegmund F.	40 years.	Hyperchlorhydria.	Pains, occasionally vomiting, bowels irregular.	5 years.	3 months.	Disappearance of symptoms.	
4.	Samuel H. C.	34 years.	Gastralgia nervosa.	Severe pains.	2 years.	1 month.	Disappearance of symptoms.	
5.	Mrs. M. F.	38 years.	Hyperchlorhydria, gastralgia.	Severe pains, despondent feeling, constipation.	12 years.	2 months.	Disappearance of symptoms.	
6.	Mrs. Juliètte R.	35 years.	Gastrosuccorrhea continua, periodica; enteroptosis (right movable kidney).	Pains, vomiting, constipation.	8 years.	2 months.	Greatly improved.	
7.	Mrs. F. L.	54 years.	Gastralgia nervosa.	Severe pains, dizziness, constipation.	3 years.	2 months.	Disappearance of symptoms.	
8.	Gustav W.	30 years.	Ulcus ventriculi; gastralgia.	Severe pains, dizziness.	2 years.	1 month.	Disappearance of symptoms.	
9.	Samuel L.	33 years.	Hyperchlorhydria, gastralgia.	Severe pains, weakness, constipation.	5 years.	2 months.	Disappearance of symptoms.	Patient first treated in 1894; he remained well until 1896, when he had a return of his pains; galvanization relieved him again.
10.	Richard L.	30 years.	Gastralgia, hyperchlorhydria.	Severe pains, oppression after meals.	6 months.	1 month.	Disappearance of symptoms.	
11.	Arthur B.	26 years.	Hyperchlorhydria, gastralgia.	Pains, slight constipation.	2 years.	2 months.	Pains less severe, but persist.	
12.	Sam. W.	40 years.	Erosions of the stomach; hyperchlorhydria.	Slight pains, constipation, despondent feeling.	7 years.	3 months.	Disappearance of symptoms.	Patient was treated alternately with the intragastric spray and with galvanization; he has remained perfectly well since 1894 in which year he had been treated.
13.	Edward C. A.	52 years.	Dilatation of the stomach; hyperchlorhydria.	Pains, weakness, nausea, constipation.	3 years.	3 months.	Disappearance of symptoms.	Patient gained 40 pounds after treatment and remained perfectly well.
14.	Edwin N. D.	35 years.	Dilatation of the stomach, beginning ischochymia.	Pains, occasionally vomiting, attacks of shortness of breath, and tachycardia.	6 years.	2 months.	Disappearance of symptoms.	
15.	Solomon H. S.	62 years.	Atony of the stomach and hyperchlorhydria.	Pains, feeling of oppression, constipation.	3 years.	1 week.	Somewhat improved.	
16.	Miss Ruth L.	24 years.	Slight hyperchlorhydria, gastralgia.	Pains, nausea, constipation.	3 years.	2 months.	Disappearance of symptoms.	
17.	Morton R.	31 years.	Atony of the stomach, hyperchlorhydria; vitium cordis.	Pains, loss of appetite, dizziness.	4 years.	2 months.	Disappearance of symptoms.	
18.	Eugene T.	34 years.	Hyperchlorhydria.	Pains, attacks of vertigo, constipation.	8 years.	3 months.	Slightly improved; the pains disappeared, but the attacks persisted.	
19.	Frederick B.	52 years.	Dilatation of the stomach and chronic gastric catarrh.	Nausea, poor appetite, dizziness.	10 years.	2 months.	Disappearance of symptoms.	
20.[1]	Max P.	34 years.	Dilatation of the stomach and hyperchlorhydria.	Pains, despondent feeling, constipation.	5 years.	2 months.	Greatly improved.	

[1] Cases 21 to 28 have been omitted on account of lack of space.

der the heading "Remarks," a considerable increase in weight is often noted in the respective cases, but even when nothing is mentioned about weight there was very often an increase; the figures, however, were not given, as the patients did not keep track of their weight.

As mentioned above, the deglutable electrode was used in all the cases. I must again assert that I had no trouble whatever in introducing the electrode. It was rarely necessary to give the patients some bread or candy in order to facilitate the swallowing of the electrode. I may also be permitted to state that I have never as yet met with any accident resuiting from the direct faradization or galvanization of the stomach, although the number of electric applications I have performed during the last eight or nine years amounts to several thousand. It is, therefore, fair to conclude that there is no danger whatever in the direct faradization or galvanization of the stomach, provided it is done in the right manner. By this I mean to say that the current should not be too strong, and the strength required should be attained gradually. Another point is, never to employ a current so strong that it causes pain. When it does, its strength must be diminished.

The results obtained in the above cases are in harmony with those reported in my previous papers, and should serve to enhance the value of direct electrization of the stomach in most functional and neurotic disturbances of this organ.

BIBLIOGRAPHY.

[1] Max Einhorn, "A New Method for Direct Electrization of the Stomach," *Medical Record*, May 9, 1891.

[2] Max Einhorn, "Therapeutic Results of Direct Electrization of the Stomach," *Medical Record*, January 30 and February 6, 1892. "Further Experiences with Direct Electrization of the Stomach," *New York Medical Journal*, July 8, 1893.

[3] Chas. G. Stockton, "Clinical Results of Gastric Faradization," *American Journal of the Medical Sciences*, p. 20, 1890.

[4] Allen A. Jones, *Medical Record*, June 13, 1891.

[5] D. D. Stewart, *Therap. Gazette*, p. 744, 1893.

[6] Th. Rosenheim, *Berliner Klinik*, May, 1894.

[7] Brock, *Therap. Monatshefte*, p. 275, 1895.

[8] Wegele, *Therap. Monatshefte*, p. 195, 1895.

[9] Goldschmidt, "Ueber den Einfluss der Electricitat auf den gesunden und Kranken menschlichen Magen," *Deutsch. Arch. f. Klin. Med.*, vol. xv, p. 295.

[10] J. Ravé, "Contribution à l'étude du traitment des dyspepsies par l'éléctricité," Paris, 1893.

[11] Caron, "Essai sur la faradization intra-stomacale dans la médication des certains vomissements rebelles," Paris, 1891.

[12] J. Goldbaum, "Beitrag zur Electrotherapie bei Magenaffectionen," *Arch. f. Verdaunngskr.*, Bd. iii, p. 70.

[13] S. J. Meltzer, "An Experimental Study of Direct and Indirect Faradization of the Digestive Canal in Dogs, Cats, and Rabbits," *New York Medical Journal*, June 15, 1895.

[14] Max Einhorn, "Experiments upon the Effects of Direct Electrization of the Stomach," *New York Medical Journal*, December 12, 1896.

[15] Max Einhorn, "Diseases of the Stomach," p. 143, New York, 1896.

THE NOCTURNAL MANIFESTATIONS OF DISEASE IN CHILDREN.

By LAMBERT OTT, M.D.,
OF PHILADELPHIA.

By the foregoing title I do not mean to convey the impression that the ills herein considered occur only at night; on the contrary they are in some respects more prevalent during the day, therefore more evident and detectable. But such evidences of ill health occurring during sleep, and usually when the physician is seldom present, his attention is misled by other factors visible during the day, and the mother fails to detect the cause of the child's restlessness and ill health. Usually the history runs thus: The parents notice that their little boy is pale, somewhat irritable, with a capricious appetite, and restless during sleep; he rises in the morning heavy and cheerless, mopes about instead of dressing, and must be coerced by threats in order to have him make progress. Later in the day his general demeanor improves; he manifests more ambition, but remains pale and easily vexed. The physician is called, and usually, after a superficial examination, prescribes tonics, and that is the end of it until the mother by some fortuitous circumstance discovers the true cause of his restless sleep and informs the physician of it.

1. *Thread- or Pin-worms.*—Often these are overlooked unless you direct the mother to examine the child's anus or vagina under a good light. These parasites are the most prolific cause of restless sleep in children, as they migrate when the body is at rest, and, creeping over the sensitive mucocutaneous junction of the anus, cause the little one to toss about as if in great agony. I have found a single worm at the base of clitoris causing the most violent agitation during sleep, and, when removed, the child lapsed into sound slumber for the remainder of the night. So simple a cause of restless sleep is easily overlooked in our search for some complicated conditions. I hold that in most cases of night restlessness in little children who otherwise manifest no perversion of function this is the only cause. The remedy is cold salt-water injections repeated several times in the same evening, as the first injection opens the bowels and the succeeding ones kill the worms. This treatment should be continued during a period of ten days or more or the parasites will again appear. Internal medication, such as santonin and calomel three times daily act well with the injections.

2. *Nocturnal Hives.*—How few physicians think of this condition as a cause of restless nights in children. My attention was called thereto in a child in my own family. A little boy, five years of age,

about midnight began tossing and moaning in his sleep, which I at first attributed to late eating of indigestible food. Despite correction of this the restlessness continued, and not finding any of the usual causes, during one of his most severe attacks, I removed all of his clothing, when to my amazement I discovered three large nodular hives on different parts of his body to which he carried his hand in his sleep in an effort to scratch them, at the same time groaning, thus showing a distinct cause of his distress. By restricting him to milk and farinacious food, saline laxatives, tonics, and sponging with alcohol he gradually improved. There has been no recurrence of the trouble. This incident was a valnable suggestion to me and since then I have used this experience in practice with happy results. When a child is restless and moans during sleep hives is a possible cause. More than one or two blotches may not be found, and at no time the multitude observed in adults when suffering with an acute attack of urticaria. I have been surprised to find how often this is the cause of disturbed sleep in children, and, what is peculiar, the eruption does not appear during the day. The treatment consists in removing the cause, if ascertained, and the use of gentle laxatives, careful dietary, and sponging with alcohol.

3. *Night terrors* in children is another peculiar manifestation especially in those of the neurotic type. The attack is preceded by some restlessness; suddenly the child sits up in bed and screams, even shrieks, in a state of terror and no matter who approaches the bedside, even the mother, is not recognized, nor does the child recover from the fright until several minutes elapse, or until violently shaken out of the terrified sleep. When subdued and comforted by the presence of his mother he offers no explanation nor can he give one when requested, but falls back quickly into sleep. If questioned the next morning he cannot recall the event, nor does he remember having repulsive dreams. The condition is mostly caused by reciting to nervous children exciting stories especially such as pertain to midnight plundering, weird tales of spirits, and hobgoblins. I have also found an elongated prepuce distinctly causal of the attacks by creating a nerve-tension which invites all manner of frightful dreams. In these cases, retract the prepuce, clean away the smegma, give a light meal for supper, avoid all excitement, remove seat-worms if present, although male children do not complain of them as often as female children, and above all, have the child sleep in a cold room with sufficient covering so fastened that he does not lie uncovered, if restless. Have him spend as much time out doors as possible, and with the addition of an evening bath a cure will soon be effected. Aside from tonics avoid the use of all depressant medicines, such as bromids and antispasmodics I know the latter are highly recommended, but with the hygienic regimen above mentioned I have invariably succeeded in preventing the attacks.

4. *Nocturnal or Unconscious Masturbation.*—However strange this condition may seem it is not an uncommon occurrence, and my attention was first attracted to it under the following circumstances: While attending a woman in labor she spoke of her boy, seven years of age, who was pale, had a poor appetite, was rather forgetful, and easily irritated, and she asked me to go into the next room where he was sleeping. I found him lying on his abdomen in apparently sound slumber but moving his body to and fro. Raising the cover I discovered his penis erect and rubbing on the sheet. I called him by name, but this did not awaken him, so I gently touched him with the same effect, and while observing him the movements to produce friction on the end of the penis increased and there soon followed a distinct clonic spasm as the culmination of the sexual erethism occurred. Then all motion ceased, sleep continued, and by repeated calling he did not awaken, showing absolute unconsciousness during the act. Detailing my discovery to the mother as the undoubted cause of his ill health she spoke of having noticed this condition of affairs for some time but attributed it to natural causes such as indigestion, etc. We could not discover that he masturbated during the day, but on further examination I found an elongated prepuce and an irritated corona covered with malodorous smegma. This was at once remedied and I instituted careful dietary and compelled him to sleep on his side or back. In spite of all precautions he relapsed and only by forcing him to get up at midnight to void his urine did I finally succeed in preventing a recurrence of this habit. I have since claimed that when a child has penile erections from cystic distention, and incidentally friction is applied to the sensitive organ nocturnal conscious or unconscious masturbation is sure to follow. In this case, as soon as the practice was eradicated the child rapidly improved in health. This observation occurred several years ago and since then the same practice has been discovered by mothers whose attention I have directed to the matter. The ordinary form of nocturnal masturbation in young children is by pulling at an elongated prepuce prior to falling to sleep and during the early morning. My practice in cases of pallor, lassitude, and irritability in boys is to compel them to sleep on the back or side, retract the prepuce and cleanse the corona, avoid constipation,

and, if erections accompany cystic distention, have the bladder emptied several times during the night.

5. *Nocturnal Enuresis.*—Incontinence of urine during sleep has been ascribed to a multitude of causes, but in my experience the most prevalent cause is found in an elongated prepuce and a smegma-covered corona, coupled with unnaturally deep slumber. Ask the parent of a child with nocturnal incontinence as to the nature of its sleep and they invariably describe it as heavy and profound. A light sleeper is awakened by a distended bladder, while a heavy sleeper possessing a bladder rendered sensitive by preputial elongation and the consequent irritation, does not awaken, but involuntarily passes the urine. Remedying the condition of the penis does not always cure the incontinence, for a cystic habit has been established of a limited retaining capacity and when this has been reached immediate evacuation of the contents of the bladder is the result, unconsciously, if the child be in deep and heavy slumber. The only remedies I have found useful are: (1) removal of the coronal irritation; (2) have the child pass water before going to bed and again at midnight, and at the same time looking after the general health by insisting upon as much out-door life as possible, a cool bath each night and the avoidance of late and heavy eating. With medicines, such as nux vomica and belladonna, I have never obtained any good results. If the bladder has formed a habit of expelling its contents after a certain quantity of urine has accumulated, apart from the consciousness of the individual, so a counter-habit may be instituted by awakening the child at a certain midnight hour and forcing him to get out of bed and void his urine. This treatment has been repeatedly instituted with satisfactory results.

6. *Nocturnal Functional Spasm or Jerks.*—I may be wrong in naming the following condition "spasm" but there exists a nervous jerking, one clonic spasm involving the whole body in younger children and infants, occurring just as they are about to loose consciousness in sleep, when suddenly the violent single jerk of the muscular system awakens the child, who cries a moment, then sleeps and is again startled by the same contraction. They are for the most part reflex and due to some disturbance in the alimentary tract. Small doses of paregoric often repeated subdue them, but if fever occurs and no antispasmodic is given, decided general convulsions soon follow.

7. *Nocturnal Driveling.*—Driveling during sleep usually occurs in neurotic children during very sound slumber. I consider it a pathologic condition due to an abnormal relaxation and unhealthy slumber. In some who slobbered to that extent as to alarm the parents the history developed a peculiar diminished quantity of urine secreted during sleep even when liberal libations of water were taken before bed-time. Teething infants drivel profusely, less in sleep than when awake. This condition is probably physiologic and due to a superstimulated condition of the salivary glands. In older children who have all their temporary teeth and some of the permanent ones, also having no abnormal condition of the oral mucous membrane, such as stomatitis and the like, nocturnal driveling is probably associated with the condition known as renal inadequacy, when, too little urine being secreted, urinary salts are retained in the blood, producing abnormally heavy sleep and a consequent relaxation by reason of which the salivary driveling follows. There is a casual relationship between the quantity of urine secreted and the unnaturally heavy sleep, but why, one cannot easily explain. The treatment consists in toning up the general health, liberal administration of lemon-juice and sweet spirits of niter and in encouraging the child to drink large quantities of water.

8. *Nocturnal Pains.*—Pains occurring during sleep and having such causes as an affection of the teeth or ears, create, in addition to restlessness, all manner of audible expressions, such as groaning, crying, or even shrieking. The causes of simply restless sleep are usually irritative, without pain, while causes producing restlessness with sleep broken by spells of crying out are most always due to pain. A child suffering with toothache or earache cries out in exacerbations and during remission of the pain again sleeps until disturbed by a recurrence of the pain. An earache sufferer during sleep will bore the head in the pillow, carry the hand to the affected ear, and unconsciously lie on the healthy ear in order to relieve pressure. Older children are able to state the location of their pains, but in younger children we have to depend upon objective symptoms entirely. I have never yet seen a child suffer with essential neuralgia or with an attack simulating neuralgia so common in adolescence and adults, therefore the pains of childhood, apart from those of syphilis, hydrocephalus, acute inflammations, headache prodromic of the exanthemata, and local pains, as above cited, are not common even during the waking periods; therefore they are less common during sleep. Some pains in children while awake are annulled by the intense diversion at play, but as soon as they lapse into the calm quietude of sleep a subdued pain is more forcibly impressed upon the sensorium. Occasionally the joint pains of scurvy are nocturnal and only discovered during sleep. A bottle-fed baby manifested restless nights, groaning in semi-slumber, and while awake seemed cheerful and well. I happened in one afternoon while the

baby was asleep and seeing one leg flexed in an unnatural position I made an effort to straighten it when the child awakened with a scream. On closer examination I discovered spongy and reddened gums and in some places indistinct spots, purpuric in character, presenting the characteristics of scurvy, all of which disappeared like magic by the addition of fruit-juices to the dietary of the child.

SYMPATHETIC OPHTHALMIA.[1]

BY W. K. BUTLER, M.D.,
OF WASHINGTON, D. C.;
PROFESSOR OF OPHTHALMOLOGY IN THE MEDICAL DEPARTMENT OF COLUMBIAN UNIVERSITY; SURGEON IN CHARGE, LUTHERAN EYE, EAR, AND THROAT INFIRMARY.

THE subject of sympathetic ophthalmia is one of great interest and importance, both from the standpoint of the physician and of the political economist. The reputation of the one as well as the resources of the other are taxed in caring for these unfortunates, and as the condition is one for which we can do more by prophylaxis than by treatment, it is well worth the consideration of the Society during the brief time in which I would ask your attention.

It has doubtless been within the experience of most, if not of all, of the members present to have seen cases of irremediable blindness which might well have been otherwise had the proper precautions been taken. I am here reminded of a little child seen some years since who had ruined its eye by running a fork into it, and notwithstanding urgent importunity for its removal the advice was unheeded. Sympathetic ophthalmia developed, and the child is doubtless blind to-day and a probable charge on the community by reason of the obstinacy of its parents.

Sympathetic ophthalmia is a disease due to a specific cause. We often speak of sympathetic affections due to some remote cause without being able to trace the connection or to understand the mode of transmission, but the field of ophthalmology offers peculiar advantages in studying the pathology of such diseases. All diseases of the eye do not cause this sympathetic trouble, but we find that wounds of certain regions and diseases of certain kinds are among the predisposing causes.

We see sympathetic trouble in the eye so frequently on account of the intimate relation between the two eyes through the optic chiasm and their rich supply of nerves. No other special sense receives such a variety or so great a number of the cranial nerves as the sense of sight. It is only necessary to remind you that the first, third, fourth, fifth, sixth, and seventh, in addition to branches from the sympathetic, all contribute to its functions.

[1] Read before the Medical Society of the District of Columbia.

Various theories have been advanced to explain the method by which the disease travels. The two principal ones are the germ theory, supported by Deutschman and others, and that which attributes to the ciliary nerves the channel through which the irritation is conveyed. Deutschman thinks that he has proved that germs have traveled from the injured eye backward along the optic nerve, have reversed their course at the optic chiasm, and ascended in the lymph-channels along the optic nerve of the opposite eye and thus infected it. It seemed very plausible, but in numerous cases examined with the greatest care no germs could be found, and in suppuration of the eyeball where there is a wealth of bacteria, sympathetic disease is not at all frequent. Certain other symptoms fail to be explained by this theory, as the existence of the disease without alteration of the optic nerve and the failure of experiments by injecting the staphylococcus aureus into the vitreous, resulting in a panophthalmitis in the attacked eye, while the inflammation extends only a short distance backward through the optic nerve.

In my opinion the latter theory, which attributes to the ciliary nerves the path through which the irritation travels, more fully explains the progress of symptoms. Clinical facts which are unexplainable by the former theory are met by this, as in those cases in which atrophy or excision of the optic nerve appears to offer no protection. Also the rapid transfer of symptoms of irritation from one eye to the other, and the identical location, at times, of the disease in the sympathizing eye to the point of irritation in the exciting eye and the great variability in the period of incubation.

As has been stated, certain affections of the eye are more prone to cause the disease than others, but one or the other of the following conditions is usually the exciting one:

1. Punctured wounds of the ciliary region, or, as called by Nettleship, "the dangerous zone," extending about one fourth of an inch in diameter around the corneal margin. Such injuries account for probably eighty per cent. of the cases of this disease.

2. Foreign bodies within the eye.

3. Perforations of the cornea, either from wounds or ulcers in which the iris becomes incarcerated.

4. Operations on the eye resulting in one of the above conditions, as prolapse of the iris following cataract extraction.

5. Intra-ocular tumors.

6. Ossification of the choroid and ciliary body.

Sometimes, also, the pressure of an artificial eye may cause symptoms of this disease. In short, any disease or traumatism affecting the uveal tract may cause it.

The period of incubation varies from a few weeks to a number of years. Rarely is it seen as early as one week, while on the other hand, it may not develop until as late as fifty years. One patient in whom I enucleated the exciting eye was injured twenty seven years before. Alt reports one occurring as late as sixty years after the exciting cause.

The symptoms are divided between those of the *exciting* eye and the *sympathizing* eye, and usually begin as a *sympathetic irritation* rather than an inflammation.

In the *exciting* eye we usually find congestion in the ciliary region, photophobia, tenderness on pressure, lachrimation, and neuralgic pain; while in the *sympathizing* eye the symptoms are functional, *viz.*, impaired accommodation, decrease in visual acuity, contraction of the field of vision, pain, photophobia, lachrimation; in brief, all those symptoms pointing to an irritated condition of the eye. I mention these points in such detail because this is the period when we can usually prevent further trouble. When the disease has advanced to the inflammatory stage treatment is of little avail, and the best that we can hope for is to save some sight after the general conflagration has subsided. As has been intimated, more can be done for this disease by prophylaxis than by actual treatment. This consists in the enucleation of the exciting eye. Such radical treatment necessarily requires the greatest confidence of the patient as well as the most deliberate judgment of the physician, and as the result of the large experience of the best authors the following rules for performing this operation may serve as a guide:

1. Wounds of the ciliary region causing the immediate loss of sight, or its ultimate loss from inflammation reasonably certain. To this rule I would make the exception of children who can be kept under observation and the eye removed if necessary when any symptoms of irritation arise. Enucleation in children may interfere with the development of the orbit and seriously interfere with the future wearing of an artificial eye.

2. Wounds in the dangerous zone already complicated by a *severe* iritis or cyclitis, even if the sight is not *entirely* destroyed.

3. An eye containing a foreign body which is not removable, in which a severe iritis is present.

4. An eye which has been destroyed by plastic iridocyclitis, or a shrunken globe, with irritation in the ciliary region.

5. A *lost* eye with beginning sympathetic irritation in its fellow.

6. A wounded eye with repeated relapses of sympathetic irritation.

If so unfortunate as not to prevent the disease, operative interference is of doubtful propriety. It must be treated on general principles applicable to the nature of the disease, *viz.*, darkened room, complete rest, leeches, and atropin if not contraindicated. The prognosis is bad.

I do not mean to take the time of the Society by giving the history of cases, but have here a few specimens showing the nature of some of the lesions which lead to this disease. These are embedded in glycerin jelly. No. 1 was seen with Dr. Marmion and enucleated by him on account of sympathetic trouble. The eye was lost from fever about thirty years before, and had recently affected the good eye. This was due to the calcareous deposit which is shown in the specimen, forming almost a complete bony cast of the interior of the eye. The second eye was enucleated on account of an intra-ocular growth, which is seen filling almost the entire globe. The third was removed on September 29, 1896, on account of chronic absolute glaucoma, which was aggravating the other eye. On account of the loss of support from section the specimen does not show as clearly as we might wish the shallowness of the anterior chamber characteristic of this disease. The fourth case was seen with Dr. Marmion and enucleated on account of purulent iridocyclitis, supposed to be due to a foreign body having entered the eye twelve years ago. The specimen shows the purulent infection of the vitreous and the plastic exudate and cicatrix where the wound was received. The foreign body was not found.

The slides presented speak for themselves, showing the varied conditions endangering sympathetic affections. They all illustrate irritation of the uveal tract.

No. 1 shows a large anterior staphyloma with entanglement of the iris. No. 2, granuloma of the iris following perforating ulcer. No. 3, hernia of the lens resulting from perforating ulcer. No. 4, glioma of the retina. No. 5, ulceration of the cornea, followed by perforation and anterior synechia.

I cannot close this brief contribution without reference to one case recently brought to my clinic.

On September 18, 1896, Sarah T., eight years of age, was brought by her father with the following statement: About fifteen months ago she was cut in the left eye with a piece of glass. At the time of application she was totally blind in both eyes from phthisis bulbi. The eyes were then quiescent, and nothing could be done. If the injured eye had been enucleated at the time sympathetic irritation first occurred the other eye would doubtless have been saved. Such cases are sad beyond description, and impress most forcibly the necessity for early interference when sympathetic inflammation is threatened.

WAR ARTICLES.

NEWS OF THE WEEK.

PASSED Assistant-Surgeon Wood, who used to be President McKinley's physician, having been appointed colonel of the cavalry regiment popularly known as "Roosevelt's Rough Riders," Surgeon-General Sternberg has been chosen as Attending Physician at the White House.

. . . .

An innovation of the present war is the hospital train for the transportation of wounded and otherwise invalided soldiers from the coast to permanent hospitals. Arrangements for this train are practically completed; it will consist of ten tourist sleepers and one dining-car, and is to be in charge of a corps of medical officers and attendants. By using all the berths available there will be accommodations for four hundred men. Four general hospitals are ready for the reception of the sick—Key West, Fort McPherson, Ga., Fort Thomas, Ky., and Fort Myer, Va. They are capable at the present time of caring for two thousand men. The hospital-ship "Relief" will accompany the troops embarked for the West Indies, ready to return at any time with sick and wounded to the United States.

. . . .

Advices from San Francisco report the large field hospital for Camp Richmond open and in complete working order. The tents occupy an entire block and the ground on which they stand is well drained and fairly shaded.

. . . .

News of an alarming nature regarding Admiral Dewey's fleet is constantly appearing in the London papers. His men are said to be dying daily of smallpox and dysentery, but happily there is nothing direct from the fleet to confirm any rumor of the kind, and we are prone to believe that even in London "yellow journalism" has taken a hold. Although Manila itself is anything but a health-resort during the wet season just commencing there, and its climate at this time of the year together with its inferior drainage and unhygienic conditions are particularly disastrous to the white race, yet the bay where our vessels lie is breezy, salubrious, and enjoyable, and a healthier spot for a camp than Corregidor Island would be dificult to find.

. . . .

An ordinary stretcher for carrying wounded men to a place of safety on shipboard is almost impracticable, as during action hatches are battened down, water-tight compartments are closed and passages and stairways are so narrow that even an unburdened sound man must move slowly and with caution. It has remained for a woman, the wife of Commander Chadwick of the Flagship "New York," to invent a carrier suited to ship usage. Mrs. Chadwick's invention consists of an ordinary sail-cloth stretcher, at each end of which are hooks which engage in a collar with side-straps which is worn on the neck of each of the two men who are to carry the stretcher and its wounded occupant. Thus it will be seen the arms of each bearer are free to assist in holding the wounded man, or to steady himself when passing through narrow passages. The carrier can be adjusted in such a way that the patient can easily be carried down a steep stairway, such as are usual on war-ships, without danger or discomfort.

. . . .

A comparison of the medical and surgical methods and results of the present war with those of the Civil War will prove interesting to every student of statistics as well as to every medical man. The surgeon of the Civil War, for instance, would have been intensely surprised to learn that his hands, carelessly washed perhaps, or possibly not washed since the last hasty operation, were distributing almost certain infection throughout his impromptu wards. The idea of an amputation without suppuration was hardly dreamed of. The great majority of deaths from the effect of wounds, was caused by "hospital gangrene," "hospital fever," and erysipelas, and although the surgeon of that day knew the symptoms perfectly well, the field of causation was as yet unexplored. In the Northern Army during that time the proportion of deaths following wounds to instant deaths on the field of battle was very nearly as seven to eleven. Under like conditions of fighting, but with the surgical ability of to-day, and aseptic and antiseptic methods, it is confidently expected that not more than one-half of this proportion of wounded men would die.

. . . .

There would seem to be little to prevent the carrying out of the War Department's plan for sending only men who are immune to yellow fever and fully acclimated as the Cuban Army of Invasion. The climatic conditions of our most Southern States are much like those of Cuba, and thousands of men can be found in those States who either from long residence in the tropics or from an actual siege of yellow fever could safely reside in Cuba or Porto Rico indefinitely. The plans for the first invading army are as follows: The men composing the "immunes" are expected to be recruited largely from the South. They are to be organized into ten regiments, five of which will be composed of whites, and the others of colored persons. They will be made up as far as practicable of officers and men who, owing to their origin, the places of their residence and other circumstances affecting their physical characteristics, possess immunity, or are likely to be exempt from diseases incident to tropical climates. The enlisted strength of each company of the regiment will not exceed eighty-two, while the minimum enlisted strength is fixed at seventy-five. For each regiment the total commissioned officers is fixed at forty-six and the total enlisted men at 992.

. . . .

At the suggestion of Surgeon-General Senn the Illinois Volunteers will go into the field equipped with emergency supplies. Each man will carry in his cartridge belt a package containing a yard of sterilized gauze, a half ounce of absorbent cotton, and a small package each of salicylic and boric acid in powder. If as is probable, each man will receive practical instruction in the use of these materials, temporary dressings can be made on the field, the advantage of which is obvious.

. . . .

About 180 medical officers, 60 surgeons and 120 assistant surgeons, will accompany the invading army, the ratio being one medical officer to about 400 soldiers of the line. The medical service will also include 160 hospital stewards and acting stewards and 1200 private soldiers. In addition to the usual equipment of stretchers, 150 ambulances of the most modern design will be used. Not more than one-third of the entire sanitary organization will accompany the first force of regulars that lands in Cuba, the remainder following with the volunteers.

LITTER-BEARERS; MEDICAL AUTONOMY; GENERAL FIELD HOSPITAL AT TAMPA, FLORIDA.

BY HENRY I. RAYMOND, M.D.,
CAPTAIN AND ASSISTANT SURGEON, UNITED STATES ARMY.

UPON recommendation of the Chief Surgeon, an order has been issued by the Assistant Adjutant-General, United States Forces, to the effect that all members of regimental bands will be instructed in Hospital Drill and as much of First Aid to the Injured as is practicable under existing circumstances. To this end all musicians will hereafter report to a medical officer attached to the regiment to which the band belongs for one hour each day for instructions until they are pronounced qualified bearers by the medical officer who instructs them. This arrangement will add largely to the numerical force and efficiency of first-aid bearers upon the battle-field. Men will be needed who know how to handle a wounded man so as to place him with care and expedition upon a litter and transport him smoothly and without jolt to the first-dressing station or to the ambulance. Practically, therefore, the instruction that band members are receiving consists of exercises in the manual of the litter, *viz.*, marchings with the litter, as litter squads composing a detachment so as to mobilize at a given point; searching for the wounded by scattering the several squads under charge of their respective squad leaders; the proper loading of the litters with the wounded, and their easy convoy to some designated spot, and the placing of loaded litters in ambulances.

As a precious heirloom handed down to us from the Civil War, and arising out of the experience of that conflict, it is the purpose of the War Department to place under the command and immediate control of the Medical Department everything pertaining to its personnel, its equipment, and its transportation. To this end a General Order has been issued from the Headquarters of the United States Forces at Tampa, comprising the following paragraphs:

1. The Chief Surgeon of the United States Forces, Tampa, Fla., will assign for division hospitals and ambulance-train service such members of the hospital corps detachments, tentage, ambulances and wagons, animals and their equipments, hospital and medical supplies, and field equipments, as may be required, and designate the officers to receipt for the same.

2. The members of the hospital corps so assigned will be borne upon their detachment muster rolls and morning reports as on detached service with the division hospital or ambulance train, as the case may be. A *minimum* allowance to be retained with each regiment will be as follows: One acting hospital steward and three privates; one hospital and one common tent; one ambulance and necessary animals fully equipped, in order to preserve the regimental medical organization. Officers detached for duty at division hospital are authorized to take with them their allowance of tentage, each giving a receipt for same.

3. Whenever necessary, the Chief Surgeon of the United States Forces is authorized to take any or all ambulances assigned to regiments, for temporary use of the field hospital.

It is very instructive to witness the gradual development and growth of the division field hospital and ambulance-train service. They are correlated but separate organizations, inasmuch as the officer in charge of the latter is not under the direct orders of the Division Hospital Surgeon, but in like manner with him receives his orders direct from the Chief Surgeon of Division. Again, as officers outside of the Quartermaster Department can carry quartermaster property on memorandum receipt only, it is contemplated to have the surgeon in charge of the ambulance-train service assigned in orders as Acting Assistant-Quartermaster so that he may exchange invoices and receipts, and become not only responsible but accountable for all property in his hands.

Another feature worthy of remark as showing the easy and ready expansion and contraction of the regimental medical unit in its relation to the division hospital is that when the full regimental organization is in a large measure depleted in its personnel and material by contribution to the division hospital, the members of the hospital corps so assigned are still borne upon their detachment muster-rolls and morning reports, and all regiment hospital property so transferred is marked for identification, in order that if the regiment becomes detached from the command, its medical organization can be at once brought up to its full complement by retransfer of its detached personnel and reexchange of memorandum receipt for material held in custody by the division hospital. Regulations provide that on the march and in battle each medical officer will habitually be attended by a mounted orderly. To secure these mounts usually the brigade surgeons, through their respective brigade commanders and the Chief Surgeon, make application to the Chief Quartermaster for the requisite number of animals, which will be turned over to the brigade quartermasters and by them to the several regimental quartermasters who will on memorandum receipt transfer them to medical officers for use by their stewards and orderlies. Mules, harness, and ambulances complete—generally eight or twelve animals and two or three ambulances to the regiment—have been transferred to medical officers in the same manner, *i.e.*, on memorandum receipt, and are being cared for by ambulance drivers assigned from members of the hospital corps. One or more of the ambulances in full equipment attends such formations as regimental or brigade drills to pick up any men overcome by the heat or by any accident.

Not long since three men overcome by the heat were brought in by the ambulance from the field maneuvers of two regiments between the hours of 7.30 and 9 A.M.

Aside from the usual assignment of veterinary surgeons to large commands we have in this division one or two members of the hospital corps who are graduates of reputable veterinary schools, and if attached to the ambulance-train service their special knowledge may be usefully called into requisition.

A circular order from the Chief Surgeon's office requires that the following-named articles shall be regularly carried on each ambulance, secured for emergency service: 12 cans of beef extract; 12 cans of condensed milk; 1 pound of tea; 1 pound of coffee or extract of coffee; 5 pounds of hard bread; 2 guidons; 1 lantern; 1 galvanized iron bucket, in addition to litters, etc., required.

THE ADVANTAGES OF CAMP TAMPA.

[Special Correspondence of the MEDICAL NEWS.]

TAMPA, FLORIDA, June 13, 1898.

WHILE Tampa is farther South than any other place at which any considerable number of troops is encamped there has probably been less sickness among them than at any other depot. Many of the incoming regiments left Northern stations during a snow storm, and within a few days found themselves marching in a cloud of fine sand and a temperature ranging in the nineties. A few cases of heat exhaustion occurred, none of which proved fatal, and at the close of the past month but two deaths had been reported from the troops in the vicinity, one of which was accidental. This gratifying record is, I think, mainly due to two favoring conditions, *viz.*, the excellence of the water-supply and the dryness of the soil. Another contributory cause to good sanitation doubtless is to be found in the strict enforcement of orders, especially in the regular divisions, regulating the police of the camps. These are briefly as follows: The avoidance of unnecessary labor during the hottest hours of the day; the immediate construction of privy-pits and kitchen-trenches as soon as a camp is established, the contents being sprinkled with dry earth every morning and evening; the removal or burning daily of all other camp refuse from whatever source. No disinfecting chemicals are used except in the divisional hospitals. The use of water from other sources than the main supply is forbidden except after boiling. The results of the operation of these orders are clean company streets and outlying areas, a notable absence of flies and of bad odors.

Fire is the great purifier about the camp. On the heights many camps are among a sparse growth of the long-leafed Florida pine and the post-oak, both flourishing in the light sandy soil. On the lower ground and slopes the saw-palmetto take the place of a loftier vegetation. The long needle-like leaf of the pine and the fronds of the palmetto strewn inside the tents of the troops and covered with a poncho and a blanket make a bed good enough for both health and comfort.

The sudden change of climate and habit to which the troops have been subjected causes considerable disorder of the digestive organs, which, in the large majority of cases, is transitory and amenable to treatment by a little corrective medicine and a regulated diet. The men brought Northern appetites along and those who indulged freely in fruits and mixed fluids paid the usual tribute. One effect of a high temperature is to diminish digestive capacity and this is still further weakened by the ingestion of large quantities of fluids, diluting the digestive juices and distending the lumen of the *prima via*. One notable effect of the foregoing conditions and the free action of the skin is a general loss of weight among the troops, ranging from a few ounces to twenty or more pounds. On the contrary, among the Florida Volunteers examined, a gain in weight appeared; these men being acclimated and of spare habit began to take on fat on the soldier's ration from the date of going into camp when they found a regular and sufficient diet and less work than they had been accustomed to in their home surroundings.

After a prolonged drouth of many weeks the rainy season began by a heavy rainfall last week. The effect of the downpour has been to harden the sand which takes up the water like a sponge and to impart a refreshing coolness to the air. Wet blankets and clothing recovered their tone in the warm sunshine following the downpour. Few cases of infectious diseases, other than venereal cases, have been sent to the division hospital (of which more later) for treatment. Among these appears measles and typhoid fever, which have been subjected to a strict isolation and quarantine, the whole number of both being less than a dozen, all traceable to importation. New conditions will confront an expeditionary force on board transports and on the shores of the Antilles should the movement of the military forces be turned in other directions.

KAPPA.

OBITUARY.

DR. JOHN BLAIR GIBBS.

THE first member of the medical profession to offer up his life for his country in the present conflict with Spain was Dr. John Blair Gibbs of 60 West Forty-seventh Street, New York City, who was killed in the night attack on Guantanamo, June 11th. Dr. Gibbs was born in Richmond, Va., in 1859. He was a descendant from ancestry whose names are written in the honorable annals of his country. After graduating from Rutgers College he studied medicine in the University of Pennsylvania, and graduated in 1881. In the autumn of that year he entered Bellevue Hospital as an interne, taking the first surgical service. At the same time he matriculated in the College of Physicians and Surgeons, and graduated in 1882. After completing his hospital service he studied in Europe for a year, then returned to begin the practice of medicine here in 1886. He was attending surgeon to the out-door department of Roosevelt Hospital and the Demilt Dispensary for a number of years, and at the time of entering the service of his country he was an instructor of special surgery in the Post-Graduate Medical School, and assistant attending surgeon to the Lebanon Hospital. Before the war was officially declared he offered his services to the Government, and was one of the first volunteer surgeons accepted. After passing the examination he was appointed acting assistant-surgeon, was ordered to Key West, and assigned to the transport "Panther," on which were the marines who made the first landing of American troops in Cuba. The story of the attack in which the patriotic young surgeon lost his life is already well known.

Dr. Gibbs was a man with many friends and no enemies, of a modest, retiring disposition and a sensitive nature. He endeared himself to those with whom he came in contact socially and professionally, being without pretense, and in possession of those qualities that ever command success in his profession. His character was cast in the mold of patriotism and heroism. All honor to his memory!

CLINICAL MEMORANDA.

A PRELIMINARY REPORT ON CASES OF CONGENITAL DISLOCATION OF THE HIP-JOINT TREATED BY THE LORENZ METHOD.[1]

BY ROYAL WHITMAN, M.D.,
OF NEW YORK;
INSTRUCTOR IN ORTHOPEDIC SURGERY IN THE COLLEGE OF PHYSICIANS AND SURGEONS.

I PRESENT four patients before you to illustrate the stages of treatment of congenital dislocation of the hip by the Lorenz method of forcible reduction with immediate use of the limb (*functionelle belastungs methode*), and another patient in whom a cure has been attained by the treatment.

It is interesting to note the changes in the method of treatment since 1890, when Hoffa performed the first operation on the rational principle of replacing the displaced bone in its normal position by dividing resistant parts and enlarging the rudimentary acetabulum. Two years later, Hoffa's operation, which was unnecessarily severe, was modified by Lorenz, who opened the joint by an anterolateral incision, and replaced the bone without injury to the muscles. After more than a hundred successful operations in this manner Lorenz, perceiving that a well-marked ridge of bone, representing the posterior border of the acetabulum, was nearly always present, and that the acetabulum itself was often of considerable size and depth, concluded that, if the head of the bone might be forced over this ridge, and if the capsule might be sufficiently stretched to allow the head to come into direct contact with the yielding cartilage and other tissue partly filling the acetabulum, then the weight of the body thrown on the limb in standing and walking

[1] Remarks at the December meeting of the Surgical Section of the New York Academy of Medicine.

might gradually enlarge it to its normal size. Thus the disadvantages of the open operation might be avoided.

This operation was first performed by him in 1895; it has since been repeated many times, and according to his reports, with almost unvarying success in properly selected cases. The steps of the operation are as follows:

1. *Elongation.*—By preliminary traction or by manual or instrumental force applied to the limb. After the patient has been anesthetized the trochanter must be drawn down until it occupies its normal relation to Nélaton's line; in other words, one leg must be as long as the other before reposition is attempted.

2. *Reposition.*—The thigh is then flexed upon the body and the pelvis being firmly held by the assistant, the thigh is abducted to the extreme limit—practically to a right angle with the body, and at the same time it is rotated slightly inward. With one hand traction is maintained, and with the other a lifting, pushing force is exerted on the trochanter with the aim of forcing the head over the ridge of bone representing the rim of the acetabulum. When this occurs, one feels and hears a well-marked jar and thud, and the limb retains its attitude of extreme abduction.

3. *Stretching the Capsule.*—When the head has been forced over the rim of the acetabulum one must endeavor to stretch the capsule and to increase the stability of the new joint by rotating the bone vigorously from side to side, and by forcing it further forward until its head shows as a rounded projection in the groin.

4. *Reconstruction of the Acetabulum by Functional Use.*—While the leg is held in the attitude of extreme abduction and slight inward rotation, a short spica plaster bandage is applied and as soon as possible the child is induced to stand upon and to use the leg, a high sole (one inch or more) being placed on the opposite shoe. The first bandage is removed at the end of a month or more, when the new joint will have become sufficiently secure to allow a reduction of the abduction; from month to month the degree of abduction is reduced, and in successful cases the leg may be allowed to assume its normal position, and treatment may be discontinued, in from six to eight months.

The great advantages of such a bloodless operation are obvious: (1) Hospital treatment or even confinement to bed is unnecessary. (2) As the patients are using the limb during the progress of the treatment the displaced and atrophied muscles gradually take on normal function; thus the necessity for massage and special exercises, so essential after the open operation, may be dispensed with, and the dangers of limitation of motion and deformity of the limb may be avoided. (3) The consent of the parents may be obtained for an operation of this character, which is free from danger at a very early age when all the conditions are favorable to rapid cure, while it is, as a rule, not until the deformity has become an eye-sore that the "cutting" operation is permitted.

The disadvantages of the operation are sufficiently evident. Its field is comparatively limited, since children of more than six years of age are not favorable subjects. There is also an element of uncertainty in the treatment as compared to the open operation.

During the past year I have operated on eleven patients by this method. The eldest was seven and one-half years, the youngest nineteen months of age. After the first attempts no particular difficulty has been experienced in reducing the deformity (the first stage of treatment). Although considerable force has been exerted in some instances no mishaps of any kind have been encountered, and the discomfort following the operation has been insignificant. In other words, I have been able in every instance to change a dorsal dislocation into an anterior dislocation. This is in itself a great improvement, since the position of the head of the bone beneath the anterior superior spine is nearly normal in its relation to the pelvis, so that the secondary deformity of the body is corrected and the shortening is very much reduced. The actual replacement of the head and the reformation of the acetabulum has been more difficult; it has necessitated repeated operations and in several instances the entire leg has been enclosed in the bandage in order that it might be rotated far inward to force the head into its normal position as illustrated by one of the patients presented. Of the eleven cases eight are still under active treatment (in the plaster-of-Paris stage). Of the remaining three, one has been operated upon with success by the open method after failure by the bloodless operation.

One, the eldest, has been presented this evening to illustrate a partial cure, in that a posterior displacement has been converted into an anterior. A shortening of two inches has thus been reduced to one-half an inch, so that the high shoe worn before the operation has been discarded. At present the parents are so well satisfied with the result that further treatment has been discontinued. The third case is now shown to illustrate a cure. The reposition was made last April and the plaster bandage was finally removed on the 16th of October. Since this time the child has been on its feet all day without other support than an ordinary bandage about the hip.

You will notice that the child walks without limp; that the attitude of the limb is normal, and that the contour of the two sides is alike. There is no shortening and the trochanter occupies its normal relation to Nélaton's line. The success in this case is undoubtedly due to the early age (nineteen months) at which treatment was begun, and there seems every reason to hope that it will be permanent.

It would seem that this method should be the treatment of selection for the younger class of patients. If it fails the open operation can be all the more easily performed because of the previous manipulation. For the older patients and for many of those in whom the displacement is of both sides the open operation will be necessary. Three of this class have come under my care during the past summer and have been operated on with success as far as the immediate result is concerned.

Osteopathic Bill Vetoed in Illinois.—Governor Tanner of Illinois has set a good example by vetoing the osteopathic bill after it had passed both branches of the Legislature.

UNUSUAL SYMPTOMS FOLLOWING THE ADMINISTRATION OF ANTIFEBRIN.

BY P. V. BALLOU, M.D.,
OF ROWENA, KY.

ON September 13, 1897, about noon, I was called to see Mr. B. C., aged forty-five, weight 160 pounds, laborer, with a previous history of no practical interest, he having suffered only from the diseases peculiar to children.

Four days previous, on awakening in the morning, he complained of being uncomfortable and uneasy, with slight nausea, and slight headache; his breath was fetid, and he was noticed to yawn a number of times. This state of affairs continued about one hour, when his bones began aching, the pain gradually growing more severe. This was finally followed by chilly sensations up the back, and a little later the whole body felt cold. This continued for about 1½ hours, and was followed by fever lasting four or five hours, and ending in a rather copious sweat, which gave great relief. During the remainder of the day the patient felt reasonably comfortable. This condition of affairs was repeated the three following days, with scarcely any change as to time or severity, save that during the afternoon of each succeeding day the patient felt weaker.

When I saw the man, on the fourth day, the cold stage had passed and he was suffering from the effects of fever. An examination revealed a slight bronzing of the skin, an enlarged, flabby, whitish-coated tongue, with edges indented from pressure against the teeth; the pulse, 120; respirations, 23; temperature, 104.8° F. The patient complained of an almost unbearable headache and was beginning to sweat, as evidenced by slight moisture of the skin and a few drops standing on the forehead.

Cold applications being refused, 10 grains of antifebrin was given. About twenty minutes after the drug was given the patient said that his headache was relieved and that he felt easier than at any time since the previous evening. About forty-five minutes after the drug was administered, all sweating ceased and a peculiar sensation of warmth under the skin was complained of. To this, in twelve or fifteen minutes, was added intense itching, while in three or four more minutes the whole body presented a general erythematous condition. The entire surface was of a brighter red than that of a typical case of scarlet fever, and like the scarlatinal rash it disappeared on pressure, to return as soon as pressure was removed. No part of the body was exempt from this rash, the conjunctivæ, palms of the hands, and soles of the feet being as red as any part of the body. The temperature of the surface seemed elevated, but the thermometer in the mouth showed that it was gradually falling. The body appeared as if every superficial capillary was dilated, and an increased quantity of blood was rapidly flowing through each.

With the appearance of the rash the itching became more intense, the patient assuming all positions possible while scratching. Within the external ear the itching was especially intense, but there was no disturbance of hearing. This condition of affairs, so far as the rash was concerned, lasted for six hours without any apparent change. It then rapidly disappeared simultaneously from all parts of the body, requiring about one-half hour in fading away. As the rash faded, the itching abated, and when entirely gone the itching ceased. The sensation of subcutaneous warmth persisted about forty minutes after these had ceased, and then gradually disappeared. Nothing remained on the surface after the rash had disappeared but a few scratch marks to show that it had so recently been the seat of so great a change.

The pupils were unaffected. Respirations were uninfluenced save by the exertion required in scratching. The heart's action was uninfluenced until about thirty minutes before the rash disappeared, when it became irregular and slightly weaker than normal, but not increased in frequency. About this time an enlargement of the veins of the feet and legs was noticed. This cardiac irregularity continued four days, gradually improving each day; and along with this irregularity was a sense of impending danger. Nothing whatever was given to combat these symptoms, for the patient refused to take anything but quinin. It is also well to state that the only drug taken before the antifebrin was a dose of calomel (about 5 grains).

A careful examination of the urine after the rash disappeared showed only a typical febrile urine, which later was normal. The case was diagnosed as one of intermittent fever, and the patient put on quinin in full doses, with the result that he resumed work on the fifth day. No unpleasant symptoms have occurred at any time since.

MEDICAL PROGRESS.

Intestinal Auto-Intoxication.—MUELLER (*Centralbl. f. inner. Med.*, May 7, 1898) discussed in the Congress for Internal Medicine the subject of auto-infection from the intestinal tract. According to the new auto-intoxication theories of disease championed by Bouchard, Charrin, and Albu, uremia, eclampsia, diabetic coma, gout, and the conditions resulting from diseases of the thyroid gland, suprarenal body, etc., are properly called auto-intoxications, since they result from a poison found in the body. Intestinal intoxications are of another class, since they are due to products formed in the contents of stomach or intestines by saprophytic bacteria. They are rather to be classed with poisoning by meat or milk. Poisoning by meat takes one of three forms, either that of an acute gastro-enteritis, or a typhoidal form, or a form similar to poisoning with homatropin. This last form, called also botulismus, is produced by diseased meat in which is to be found the bacillus botulicus. The second form is also due to the ingestion of the flesh of diseased animals. Similarly, milk-poisoning may be due to the use of milk from diseased animals, or to the fact that the milk has spoiled. Many cases of auto-intoxication (ptomain poisoning?) are improperly so called. It is at least questionable whether putrefaction of albuminous substances in the intestine can produce symptoms of poisoning. The indol, phenol, skatol, and sulphureted hydrogen produced by the ordinary bacteria of the intestines, are comparatively harmless in their action, or perhaps it is more accurate to say that the body is accustomed to them, and so has a degree of immunity. The subject is an interesting one, but needs further investigation.

The opinion is now universal that it is not possible to destroy bacteria in the intestine. In order to accomplish this a medicine would have to be very slowly soluble in the stomach, so that it might reach the intestine unchanged. The claims of the various manufacturers of intestinal antiseptics have no foundation outside of the minds of those who write the advertisements. Calomel acts probably solely as a laxative. The best treatment lies in the washing out of the stomach and the use of laxatives. A change in diet is also beneficial.

In the discussion of this paper STERN said that he had disproved by experiment the possibility of intestinal asepsis as secured by the giving of drugs, according to the claim set forth by Bouchard. Nevertheless, there is a certain amount of prevention of bacterial action to be obtained by the administration of antiseptics, notably of calomel. Calomel stools will sometimes contain so much of the drug that after standing several hours there is a great diminution of the number of bacteria in them, or there may, indeed, be destruction of all the bacteria contained in them. It is, therefore, going too far to say that the disinfection of the intestine is absolutely impossible.

Dilatation of the Stomach Artificially Produced.—WEINTRAUD (*Centralbl. f. inner. Med.*, May 7, 1898) spoke in the Congress for Internal Medicine, held in April last, of gastric dilatations which he had produced in dogs by the application to the pylorus of thin elastic bands. If a dog so operated upon was given abundant nourishment there developed in a short time a great dilatation of the stomach, so that an organ which had held only two liters (quarts) before the artificial pyloric stenosis, would in six or eight weeks hold double that amount. There were, also, all the usual concomitants of this condition seen in man, *viz.*, hyperacidity, abnormal fermentation, etc. Hyperacidity was absent if there was a great secretion of mucus, and yeast and sarcinæ were present in large amounts only when the stomach was still full of food, twenty-four hours after the meal had been taken. In one dog, whose gastrectasia had lasted ten months, the capacity of the stomach was reduced in four weeks after the removal of the ligature from four liters to three liters, an observation which certainly gives strong support to the pyloroplastic operations for the cure of the gastric dilatation which results from benign stricture of the pylorus.

The Syphilis Bacillus.—NIESSEN (*Centralbl. f. inner. Med.*, May 7, 1898) reported to the Congress for Internal Medicine, held last April, the results of his investigation in the bacterial field of syphilis. He has obtained from syphilitic tissues, and especially from the blood, by pure culture micro-organisms which he inoculated into animals which present a reaction to human syphilis. When these cultures were injected into the veins of pigs, or inserted subcutaneously, there developed at the point of injection a hard inactive sore, and eight or ten days after the injection there appeared on the skin of the animal numerous bright red spots which disappeared after about a week. Rabbits developed at the site of injection similar hard sores. Two of these rabbits were paired, and the female gave birth to a litter of seven, all dead, and two of them, being macerated, greatly resembled in this respect syphilitic human embryos.

Neissen obtained his cultures especially from the marrow and epiphysial lines of the bones of children who had died from hereditary syphilis. The material was preserved in bouillon, and then grown in various media. He found in almost every instance a variety of streptobacilli or streptococci which he had previously obtained from the blood of patients suffering from dementia paralytica and tabes syphilitica. The bacilli can best be obtained from the blood, after the administration of mercury for a short time during the tertiary period. In the secondary period he had less success in obtaining germs from the blood, which he thought was due to the fact that at this period they lie chiefly in the skin.

THERAPEUTIC NOTES.

A Good Point in the Treatment of Hemorrhoids.—SIMS (*Maryland Medical Journal*, May 7, 1898) says that the patient upon whom operation for internal hemorrhoids is to be performed should have a gentle mercurial purgative on the second evening previous to the day of the operation, and a saline each morning before breakfast. After shaving and washing externally and within the rectum with warm soap-suds, the patient is etherized and the sphincters divulsed completely. The piles should then be everted and the whole region irrigated with a weak antiseptic solution. The individual piles are caught with the forceps, pulled out, and the mucous membrane of the neck of each one is cut through all around with a sharp scalpel, so that the silk ligature may include only blood-vessels and connective tissue. The pile is cut off close to the ligature. The cut edges of the mucosa are then sewed together with catgut over the stump, so that the raw surface is entirely covered. By this means the risk of suppuration and the suffering are reduced to a minimum. An antiseptic dressing is applied. The bowels are moved four days later by salines and an enema. The results of an operation thus carried out are most satisfactory.

Are Tablets Prepared from Digitalis Effective?—HOUGHTON (*Ther. Gazette*, April 15, 1898) has tested by experiments upon animals the question whether tablets made from fluid preparations of digitalis retain their efficacy in the dry form. The result showed that the question must be answered in the affirmative, for a fatal dose as well as the effect upon blood-pressure was found in dry preparations to be essentially the same as in the fluids from which they were formed. He therefore concludes that active fluid preparations of digitalis do not lose any activity by being manufactured into tablets, nor do the tablets become less active by keeping than do the other preparations of this drug.

THE MEDICAL NEWS.

A *WEEKLY JOURNAL*

OF MEDICAL SCIENCE.

COMMUNICATIONS are invited from all parts of the world. Original articles contributed *exclusively* to THE MEDICAL NEWS will after publication be liberally paid for (accounts being rendered quarterly), or 250 reprints will be furnished in place of other remuneration. When necessary to elucidate the text, illustrations will be engraved from drawings or photographs furnished by the author. Manuscripts should be typewritten.

Address the Editor: J. RIDDLE GOFFE, M.D.,
No. 111 FIFTH AVENUE (corner of 18th St.), NEW YORK.

Subscription Price, including postage in U. S. and Canada.

PER ANNUM IN ADVANCE $4.00
SINGLE COPIES 10
WITH THE AMERICAN JOURNAL OF THE MEDICAL SCIENCES, PER ANNUM 7.50

Subscriptions may begin at any date. The safest mode of remittance is by bank check or postal money order, drawn to the order of the undersigned. When neither is accessible, remittances may be made, at the risk of the publishers, by forwarding in *registered* letters.

LEA BROTHERS & CO.,
No. 111 FIFTH AVENUE (corner of 18th St.), NEW YORK,
AND NOS. 706, 708 & 710 SANSOM ST., PHILADELPHIA.

SATURDAY, JUNE 18, 1898.

THE DENVER MEETING.

THE meeting of the American Medical Association held at Denver during last week cannot be regarded as other than most successful. The fact that many of the local medical men originally came from the East led to the renewal of many old acquaintanceships, and this, combined with the hospitable welcome extended by the citizens of Denver, increased the feeling among the visitors that they were indeed at home. Then, too, the situation of the "City of the Plains," surrounded as it is by many features of peculiar interest to medical men, served to stimulate the activity of body and mind and to give the proceedings, scientific and social, a zest not to be found at less favorable meeting-places.

The railroad and hotel accommodations were unusually good, and thus one of the most common sources of dissatisfaction was avoided, while the good will of the visitors was obtained at the start by the efficient methods instituted for the registration of members. The meeting halls were conveniently situated, unusually large and well ventilated, and with few exceptions their acoustic properties were good.

The meeting was also very representative of the Association as a whole, for all sections of the country sent delegates to represent their views, with the result that the proceedings really represented the national profession as a whole. This general representative meeting, therefore, far surpassed in importance to the profession some of its predecessors which have had a local color, and emphasizes the fact that the American Medical Association is becoming more powerful for good in the medical affairs of the country. Sectional differences are disappearing, and politics, while active, is gradually decreasing in importance as scientific pursuits become more popular. An innovation of importance was that of asking most of the members in Denver on Monday night to the dinner tendered to the Medical Editors' Association. By this means the whole assembly started with a swing which carried it through the meeting, and friendships were formed which did much toward increasing the good feeling which was so apparent on every hand.

The work of the general sections was good and the papers in many instances were discussed in a manner which showed that their hearers had ideas worth expression and worthy of respectful attention. This was particularly true of the sections on medicine, surgery, and gynecology, in which animated and spirited debates were constantly going on. Aside from the general educational effects of the meeting there can be no doubt that it will exercise a good effect by informing many physicians of the exact therapeutic properties of the Colorado climate; for the program prepared for the entertainment of visitors was designed by the railroads and hotels to advance one's views of the possibilities of the consumptive's paradise. Low rates and personally conducted tours brought every one in contact with the sanitary side of the region, even if at times knowing the penchant for speculation characteristic of physicians, mining stocks were urged upon the credulous. As a rule, however, too many had been bitten at home to be hurt. In this connection, one trip was widely advertised with the additional information that visitors would not be importuned to buy stock if they accepted. It is only fair to state that this was not one of the official tours, but that the latter were conducted with the greatest regard for the comfort and safety of the members, and their bank accounts as well.

THE NUMBER OF PHYSICIANS IN FRANCE.

NOT long since Rouxel wrote in the *Journal des Economistes* upon what he was pleased to term the "medical crisis," and which he said was due to the "protection" in the practise of their profession afforded by the State to doctors. He assumed, as do many other writers, that the number of physicians in proportion to the population had much increased of late years. The *Journal de Medicine* disputes this assumption, and shows by official figures that the number of practising physicians in France has not sensibly increased in the last twenty years, and that it is less than it was in 1854. At that time the total number for France and Algiers was 18,438; whereas at present in the same territory there are, according to the official returns for the current year, only 17,626. Both of these figures include medical officers of the army and navy, as well as those in civil life. That is to say, in 1854 there was one practising physician for 1940 inhabitants, whereas there is one now for 2564. Leaving out of consideration these ancient figures, which may not be absolutely reliable, and taking account of the years 1876, 1886, and 1896, the doctors in France proper numbered 14,376, 14,789, and 15,017. This increase is very slight, not as great as that of the population, and so it follows that the ratio of physicians to the whole population was 2564 in 1896 as compared to 2535 in 1886 and 2511 in 1876. In different districts the figures vary considerably. Thus the number of inhabitants to one physician in Paris is only 1033, while in some of the country districts it is as high as 7000.

The most striking thing about all this to an American is the scarcity of physicians in France. The number in New York City in proportion to the population must be three times as great as that in Paris, and while in the country there are relatively fewer, still if any one should point out a locality where there was a population of 7000 persons who had only one physician to call in case of illness, scarcely would night fall before several new signs would be flung to the breeze. There is a small city not far from New York where a population of about 14,000, in the corporation and its immediate vicinity, is medically ministered unto by eleven physiciaus, and so conscious are these eleven of their unusual good fortune, that one of their number in telling the story begged that no mention of it be made in the shadow of a medical school.

And yet the French writer laments the fact that the income of some of his professional brethren is not sufficient to sustain them. The sufferers must certainly be in the cities, where practice is so unevenly distributed, rather than country physicians, where small fees and long hours of hard work come alike to all. At any rate, one must not look for an explanation of the hard times of which French physicians complain, to an increase in numbers, for such does not exist in France. Here, as has already been said, the proportion is so very different that it seems impossible that all of those licensed to practise medicine should be able to gain a livelihood. The directory of the County Medical Society contains more than 3000 names for New York County, that is, one to every 600 inhabitants or fewer; and when to this number there are added the hundreds of homeopathists and eclectics and others whose activity the State either sanctions or allows, it is certainly well within the truth to say that there is a practitioner to every 400 inhabitants in New York City.

OUR DEADLIEST FOES.

A CONSIDERATION of the events of the war so far shows that no one can forecast the conduct and plan of hostilities. For weeks past we have been on the eve of landing large numbers of troops in Cuba and of sending a formidable force to the Philippines, but the days go by and little is accomplished in this direction. We are of the opinion that we should be thankful for this inactivity. Delays are proverbially dangerous, but in this instance delay will prevent the unnecessary and unwarranted sacrifice of life. It is unquestionably a fact that the great peril of troops sent to either one of the Spanish colonies does not consist, even in small part, in overcoming the engines of war which the enemy has set up. The danger is encompassed in resisting climatic and atmospheric conditions which are hazardous, even to those thoroughly seasoned and acclimated. That this is recognized by the chief of the army and navy and his advisers there can be no doubt. Nevertheless the importance of keeping continually in mind the awful mortality of our troops were a large number of them to be landed in Cuba and the Philippines at the present time, or within the next few weeks, cannot be overestimated. There are certain parts of Cuba and of Porto Rico in which troops can be stationed that are not less salubrious than Tampa, and not much less so than Chattanooga. If a portion of our regular and volunteer armies must occupy these islands they should be confined to these less deadly localities, and they should be used for the purposes of maintaining advantages and conquests of the fleets and not for active invasion. Until the present rainy season is at an end, troops should not be sent to Cuba except to the mountainous region about Santiago and the east where they will be, with proper sanitary precautions and medical aid, comparatively safe from the depredations of miasma and infection.

Scarcely any one is so sanguine as to forecast the termination of hostilities with Spain in a few weeks. At the present time the key of the situation would seem to be to wait without forcing the enemy to expose all its vulnerabilities. With one fleet destroyed, another bottled up, and a third so crippled that it cannot slip its moorings, Spain has very little chance of landing troops in the Philippines or in Cuba. Her troops already there will be hopelessly incapacitated during the next few months through the combined activity of the insurgents and the powers that direct the forces of the microbe. This is by no means an idle statement. It is substantiated by experience and by statistics. In 1896 Spain sent 30,000 soldiers to the Philippines to quell the insurrection of that year. In twelve months about 7000 had perished from disease and exposure. Although the mortality of the Spanish army in Cuba has not been so high as this, it has, nevertheless, been very great.

Although fully alive to the righteousness of the present war we are decidely of the opinion that no justification exists for calling upon the patriotic youth of this country, who have turned from shop, counting-house, and mill to support their chief executive in giving succor to a people suffering outrages akin to those of the Inquisition, and hurling them into countries which are for the time seething with inherent potentialities of death. To require them to submit to such exposures, save in the rarest and most exceptional instances, involves the assumption by our administration of a stupendous responsibility. The inadequacy of the commissary department in caring for portions of the volunteer army has been shown during the past few weeks. It is not at all likely that it could cope more successfully with the needs of the troops if they were in Cuba or the Philippines. We have fullest confidence that these facts are fully appreciated by the commander of the martial forces in this country, and by his council and generals, and that they will show such appreciation by delaying the sending of more troops than are absolutely necessary to either of these countries at the present time.

The adoption of certain sanitary measures by the medical departments of the army and the navy, such as vaccination of every soldier destined for the Philippines, and instruction against drinking water unless it has been boiled or filtered is no doubt being effected. It is quite possible that a pocket filter might be devised that would form part of the accontrement of every soldier. Medical science has never had greater opportunities to reveal its resourcefulness than in the present conflict, and more depends upon the vigilance and skill of its votaries than can easily be estimated. The revelations of bacteriology and the strides made in the knowledge of the causation of disease will be hollow indeed if they cannot be utilized for the preservation of the health of our soldiers in such an exigency as the present. Let us pause and prepare, and in so doing prevent much wasteful slaughter.

ECHOES AND NEWS.

The Woman's Hospital, New York.—Owing to the fact that this institution is threatened with a deficiency of more than $27,000, an appeal for funds has been issued.

No "Doctored" Meats Admitted into France.—The French Minister of Agriculture has issued a notice forbidding the importation into France of meats containing borax or boracic acid.

The Next Marine Hospital Service Examination.—A board of officers will be convened at Washington, July 6, 1898, for the purpose of examining candidates for admission to the grade of assistant-surgeon in the United States Marine Hospital Service.

Scurvy-stricken Sailors.—The Norwegian bark "Elida" recently arrived at the port of New York with six of the crew ill with scurvy. During the voyage one man died of the disease and was buried at sea. It is claimed that the food was of poor quality and insufficient in quantity.

Increase of Suicide in Italy.—The official statistics of suicide in Italy for the year 1896 show an increase of fifty per cent. during the preceding ten years. This is attributed to the heavy taxation which causes a greater struggle for existence, and, to some extent, to the spread of education.

Medical Practice in India.—It is said that uneducated and unqualified persons have as much right to practice medicine in India as fully qualified practitioners, and that in the present condition of that country it is impossible to prevent the people from employing the uneducated native practitioners.

Death of Dr. Anton Krassowski.—Dr. Anton Krassowski, the leading gynecologist of Russia, professor of midwifery in the Military Medical Academy of St. Petersburg, and author of a number of text-books on obstetrics and diseases of women, recently died at the age of seventy-seven.

Rubber Operating-Gloves to the Front.—Each surgeon's chest which has gone to the front contains a package of rubber operating-gloves, which are now so much used. The surgeons who prefer those made of silk or lisle thread will presumably have to supply their own needs in this direction.

Epidemic of Skin Disease in Hungary.—Transylvania, Hungary, is suffering from at outbreak of skin disease which resembles the *pellagra* of northern Italy. It is supposed to spring from the same cause as the latter disease, *viz.*, insufficient nourishment, due to bad harvests and an exclusive diet of mildewed cornmeal.

Return of Professor Koch.—Professor Robert Koch has returned to Berlin after having spent a year and a half in Africa and India, where he has been making a study of infectious diseases. His home coming has been hailed with many expressions of delight by European bacteriologists, who esteem him as their recognized leader.

Leiter Hospital Opened.—The Leiter Hospital at Chickamauga, the gift of Mrs. Leiter of Chicago, was opened for the reception of patients on June 9. It is to be used for soldiers not seriously ill, and is in charge of Captain T. W. Carter of the surgeon-general's staff. Eighteen patients, some suffering from pneumonia, have been sent there from field hospitals.

American Pediatric Society.—At the annual meeting of this Society, recently held in Cincinnati, the following officers were elected for the ensuing year: W. P. Northrup of New York, president; G. N. Acker of Washington, first vice-president; Irving M. Snow of Buffalo, second vice-president; S. S. Adams of Washington, secretary; Edward M. Buckingham of Boston, treasurer.

Distinguished Nurses.—Miss Margaret Long, daughter of the Secretary of the Navy, and three young women who, like Miss Long, have been students at the Johns Hopkins University, Baltimore, are setting a mighty good example to all the young women of the country. They are nursing the sick and wounded men which the hospital ship "Solace" brought from Admiral Sampson's fleet to the Brooklyn Navy Yard.

Adjournment of the American Medical Association.—Dr. F. W. McRae of Georgia was selected by the American Medical Association to deliver the address on surgery at its next meeting; Dr. J. C. Wilson of Pennsylvania, the address on medicine, and Dr. Brauer of Colorado, the address on forensic medicine. The Association adjourned on June 10th to meet at Columbus, Ohio, during the first week in June, 1899.

Red Cross Army Ambulance.—The first ambulance for the New York Ambulance and Red Cross Equipment Society has been placed on view at No. 180 West One Hundred and First Street. The body is painted blue-gray, and has the letters "U. S." in gilt on each side, and also a red cross on a white ground. The top is made of canvas, as are the curtains at the sides. Inside are leather-quilted berths for four patients. It is fully equipped in every way, and has a large water-can placed under the driver's seat. The cost of such an ambulance is $1500.

Causes of Fatigue in Reading.—In continuing investigations upon this subject begun by Professor Cattell, Messrs. Griffling and Franz of Columbia University have determined that the inferior size of the type more than any other is the causative element in eye-weariness from reading, and suggest that no type smaller than eleven-point should be employed. [The type used in this column is nine-point, and the larger type in the fore part of this number is ten-point.] The amount of daylight unless reduced below the limit of distinct vision, is of less importance, as is also the variation, spacing, or style of type.

National Society for the Study of Epilepsy.—Forty-four members of the medical profession, representing eight States, recently met at the New York Academy of Medicine for the purpose of organizing a society for the study of epilepsy and the care and treatment of epileptics. The following were elected officers of the new Society: Hon. William Pryor Letchworth, LL.D., of New York, president; Dr. William Peterson of New York, first vice-president; Dr. William Osler of Maryland, second vice-president; Dr. William P. Spratling of New York, secretary; Dr. H. C. Rutter of Ohio, treasurer. Applications for membership may be addressed to the secretary, Craig Colony for Epileptics, Sonyea, N. Y.

Recent Additions to the Line of Hospital Ships.—The hospital department of the United States Army has purchased two steam launches which which will probably be carried upon davits of the "John Englis," and used as ambulance-boats. The American National Red Cross Society has ordered a forty-two-foot cabin launch, to be thoroughly equipped for use in Cuban waters. Furthermore, we learn that the British steamship "Marmion," which has been purchased from the Boston Fruit Company by the Massachusetts Volunteer Aid Association to carry supplies and medicine to the troops engaged in the Cuban campaign, and also to transfer sick and wounded sailors and soldiers to Northern hospitals, arrived in Boston last week, and is now undergoing the changes necessary for her new mission.

Long Island to Have a New Medical Association.—The physicians of Long Island are to have a new general organization under the title of the Associated Physicians of Long Island. On June 8th there was a largely attended meeting for organization held at Garden City. In addition to the preliminary and parliamentary work of such a meeting, there were presented scientific discussions in the shape of a paper by Dr. H. A. Fairbairn on the "Prognosis of Chronic Nephritis," a discourse on "Immunity from the Standpoint of the Bacteriologist," by Dr. E. H. Wilson, and "A Reported Case of Leprosy with Microscopic and Photographic Demonstrations," by Dr. J. F. Whitfield. All three authors are from Brooklyn. The officers of the association elected for the current year are: W. Browning of Brooklyn, president; L. N. Lanehart of Hempstead, William A. Hulse of Bay Shore, and Charles Jewett of Brooklyn, vice-presidents; Arthur H. Terry of Patchogue, treasurer; R. J. Morrison of Brooklyn, secretary, and Joseph H. Hunt of Brooklyn, historian. The members of the three existing county societies of Long Island are eligible to this new association, and meetings will be held quarterly in different parts of the Island.

CORRESPONDENCE.

A DROPSICAL PATIENT TAPPED FORTY-EIGHT TIMES.

To the Editor of the MEDICAL NEWS.

DEAR SIR: The following report of a case of ascites is of interest, I think, because of the number of times the patient has been tapped, the length of time the condition has existed and the fact that during the intervals between the evacuation periods she enjoys remarkably good health and does not complain of a single symptom pointing to the existence of the primary disease.

Matilda W., aged forty-seven years, married twenty-seven years, has never been pregnant. She menstruated regularly until about two years ago. In 1878 she noticed that her abdomen was gradually becoming distended, and one year later, a diagnosis of ascites having been made, she was tapped, twelve gallons of fluid being withdrawn from the abdominal cavity. One year later, the water having again accumulated, she was tapped a second time and from that date up to three weeks ago the operation has been repeated no less than forty-six times. An average of ten gallons of fluid has been removed each time, or approximately 480 gallons in all. During the last three years it has been necessary to resort to tapping once every three months.

Except during four or five days subsequent to evacuation the woman performs her household duties without discomfort. Her appetite is good, she takes plenty of exercise, and is not in the least inconvenienced until a short time before it becomes necessary to again relieve her. Her principal trouble then is shortness of breath, which is immediately relieved when the pressure exerted by the accumulation of fluid on the diaphragm is removed. Her lungs, heart, and kidneys are perfectly healthy. Diuretics have frequently been administered in the hope that the kidneys would assist in throwing off the fluid, but in each instance the accumulation has been too rapid for this method to be successful. Her feet and legs swell only when the abdominal cavity has become distended by the water.

When removing the fluid I make use of a trocar of moderate size, puncturing the abdominal wall at a point about midway between the umbilicus and pubes. The fluid is allowed to escape very gradually, firm pressure being made by means of an abdominal binder. It is necessary to employ a binder ten feet in length for this purpose. After the evacuation I am in the habit of placing six or eight folded towels on the abdomen, surmounting these with a large, heavy book, and including all in a snug binder one and one-half feet in width. The blood-pressure is thus equalized and the removal of such a quantity of fluid from the abdominal cavity is not followed by discomfort. The binder is removed on the third or fourth day.

All in all, I think this case is unique. My patient bids fair to live yet for many years and complains only of the inconvenience accompanying the periodical tapping, which deters her from social pleasures and the daily routine of household duties.

J. C. LIGHTFOOT, M.D.

ALVATON, KY., June 5, 1898.

THE OUTBREAK OF YELLOW FEVER.

IN reply to a telegram to Surgeon-General Wyman of the Marine Hospital Service, asking if he could furnish the MEDICAL NEWS with additional details of the outbreak of yellow fever in the South, the following despatch has been received as the journal goes to press:

"*To the Editor of the* MEDICAL NEWS:

"On June 9th Surgeon Murray reported that State Health-Officer Haralson had discovered seven cases of yellow fever at Ft. McHenry, Miss. Murray verified diagnosis. Notified Mobile and New Orleans. Town surrounded by guards and each infected house specially guarded. Passenger traffic stopped. On June 13th Murray wired that fifteen cases have occurred since May 20th. Nine cases now on hand. Foci of infection reduced from eight to six. Haralson is cleaning town. Examination of neighboring towns and of houses along railroad, though not yet completed, has developed no new cases or foci. Surgeon Carter and Dr. Haralson are engaged in this work. Camp Fontainebleau open for refugees. Train-inspection service begun between New Orleans and Mobile. State Board of Health has ordered that people entering other portions of the State from Jackson, Harrison, and Hancock Counties must have certificates from Camp Fontainebleau. McHenry is a small village, containing 323 white and 67 colored; on the Gulf Port and Ship Island Railroad.

[SIGNED] "WYMAN,
"Surgeon-General."

OUR FOREIGN LETTER.

[From our Special Correspondent.]

ALBUMIN AS A FOOD-STUFF DURING MUSCULAR EXERTION AND THE QUESTION OF CONCENTRATED FOOD FOR WAR USE—THE BIOLOGY OF THE TUBERCLE BACILLUS—PROFESSOR KOCH'S RETURN TO BERLIN AND SOME EXPERT VIEWS ON TUBERCULIN—PROFESSOR SCHENCK'S BOOK AND GERMAN OPINIONS—A CONTAGIOUS GENITAL AFFECTION AMONG CATTLE.

BERLIN, June 5, 1898.

A RECENT discussion in the Berlin Medical Society again brought up the question of the value of albumin as a food-product, especially its value as a supplier of muscle energy. Once more the whole subject of the energy-supplying food-stuffs would seem to be brought into question. Liebig and his school in physiologic chemistry insisted strongly on the importance of albumin as really the almost exclusive supporters of muscle energy. Then came the inevitable reaction to what seemed an exaggerated opinion and physiologists came to look upon the fats and carbohydrates as capable of replacing albumin even as regards the production of muscular energy. In general it came to be finally considered, that a food-stuff was worth in absolute value just as much as it would supply in caloric energy; that an article of diet was worth in food units, whether it did or did not contain nitrogen, as much as its heat value expressed in calories. At least this was considered true for comparative purposes.

Professor Pflüger of Bonn expressed an opinion some time ago, in opposition to this, that while muscular energy could be produced in the absence of fat and carbohydrates no muscular work could be done without albuminous metabolism. This doctrine of albumin as the immediate source of all muscular energy has been gaining a great many adherents of late, and one consequence has been the putting on the market of a series of albumin preparations by various manufacturers, each of which has claimed to be the *ne plus ultra* in the matter of a food-stuff rich in albumin for the delicate and for convalescents.

At the International Congress for Hygiene, held in Madrid in April, Professor Finkler of Bonn presented a new food-product, a very pure albumin without coloring matter, smell, or taste, which he thinks will answer the requirements of a concentrated food-stuff very fully. His product, called "tropon" by its inventor, is under investigation by the German military authorities at present with the object of determining its usefulness for campaign purposes.

It was this phase of the value of the albumin question, the preparation of artificial food-products, that was touched on at the Berlin Medical Society. The general impression seems to be gaining ground among the profession in Germany that such artificial food-stuffs may be of great value and that the fats and carbohydrates have been overvalued as articles of diet in the immediate past. The questions involved in the discussion, together with the other question, that of concentrated foods, will be of special interest to Americans in view of the campaign about to begin in Cuba, where the transportation of provisions for the troops in suitable quantity and quality, and the question of concentrated nourishment in case of forced marches will be most important problems to deal with.

Dr. Aronson, at a recent meeting of the Berlin Medical Society, demonstrated a brownish-red, thick, viscid mass which he had extracted from tubercle bacilli. This would seem to be the same (or a similar substance to that obtained by Klebs in America) though somehow it has been understood, I think, that the culture-medium used by Klebs had rendered the product suspicious. Dr. Aronson has succeeded in obtaining it even with artificial culture-media containing no animal products. The material resembles beeswax in smell and has many other of the physical peculiarities of that substance. It is true wax and Dr. Aronson has succeeded in extracting from it a higher alcohol, the properties of which he is engaged in studying. He has found a similar substance in diphtheria bacilli but in much less quantity. The wax from diphtheria bacilli reacts very differently to carbolfuchsin from that extracted from tubercle bacilli. It would seem that it is the presence of this wax in tubercle bacilli which gives it its staining properties, especially its resistance to decolorizing agents. The wax in its pure state takes carbolfuchsin well, but only after considerable time, but then it does not part easily with it.

Unable to study the life history of the single bacillus these studies in their biology by chemical investigation of large numbers of them at once have of late given some interesting results besides this wax in tubercle bacilli. Not long ago it was demonstrated in Behring's laboratory that tubercle bacilli contain a notable proportion of fat in their constitution. It thus became clear why culture-media to which glycerin was added, were so favorable to its growth, and why the bacillus would not grow where it could not obtain the fat elements.

Professor Koch has just returned to Berlin after being absent in South Africa for more than a year. Just as he returns appears Behring's article at the Madrid Congress in the *Deutsche Med. Wochenschrift* in which "the master's" work with tuberculin is considered to be the greatest work in the study of tuberculosis after the discovery of the tubercle bacillus itself. The world will, however, only appreciate it when finally the biologic cure for tuberculosis is found. Behring speaks rather sarcastically of the chance wanderers into the field of bacteriology who have of late criticized the new tuberculin. Professor Loeffler, in a private conversation not long ago, said that after Koch's return he had not the slightest doubt that this matter of the new tuberculin would be set in quite a different light from what it has been.

After the blare of trumpets that announced Professor Schenck's theory of the determination of sex it is surprising with what little interest the actual appearance of his book, "Theorie Schenck," has been greeted. The fairy godmother who presided at its birth and allowed the prophecy, so long beforehand, of how interesting the new scientific youngster was to be was evidently not properly propitiated. Like many a prophecy that may be founded on the new theory it has proven not to come up to expectations. Instead of a virile contribution to medical science we have at most a hermaphroditic conglomeration of a few scientific observations and any number of exploited theories on the determination of sex in which Schenck's own ideas are of very little weight. They are playing at one of the Berlin theaters a farce, entitled "der gefesselte Storch" ("the Stork in Irons" I suppose it must be translated since the Germans have translated our "Puss in Boots" into "der gestiefelte Kater") the reference being to the well-known office attributed to the stork in children's stories in bringing children. The farce has attracted a good deal more attention than Schenck's book. Most of the German medical journals have had references, but only of the most passing kind, to the book and German medical men seem to be agreed in the opinion, rather forcibly expressed by one of his colleagues, that its author has "bartered the birthright of his scientific reputation for the mess of potage of newspaper notoriety," but then there was something more for there was money in it.

A contagious genital affection among the cattle of northern Germany is attracting a good deal of attention. For some years it has been noticed by certain herders that a very large proportion of abortions and miscarriages were occurring in their herds. Examination disclosed the fact that animals affected with this tendency to abort were also affected by a persistent discharge from the genitals. Further observation has shown that this is contagious and that the veterinarians are in the presence of a disease that is communicated with extreme ease. So far only segregation has done good and that only in preventing the further spread of the disease. Recently irrigations with permanganate of potash have been said to be effective in producing a radical cure though this is not fully substantiated. The disease is of interest because of certain analogies with human affections, and the bacteriological and experimental therapeutic study of the disease, it is hoped, will throw more light on the process of invasion of mucous membranes by bacteria and the best means to prevent their penetration or inhibit their growth in situ.

OUR PHILADELPHIA LETTER.

[From Our Special Correspondent.]

COMMENCEMENT EXERCISES OF THE UNIVERSITY OF PENNSYLVANIA—HOMEOPATHS ENDEAVOR TO SECURE RECOGNITION—DAILY MEDICAL INSPECTION OF THE PUBLIC SCHOOLS—THE NATHAN LEWIS HATFIELD PRIZE FOR ORIGINAL RESEARCH IN MEDICINE—HEALTH-BOARD STATISTICS FOR THE WEEK.

PHILADELPHIA, June 14, 1898.

THE commencement exercises of the University of Pennsylvania were held on Thursday, June 9th, 183 graduates receiving the degree of Doctor of Medicine. Judge John B. McPherson of the Dauphin County Court delivered the address, in which he urged the profession to take more interest in municipal affairs, and spoke feelingly of the war. An interesting feature was the presentation of an oil portrait of the late Professor Theodore Wormley to the Medical School. The Society of the Alumni of the Medical Department of the University of Pennsylvania held its annual reunion on June 7. Provost C. C. Harrison announced that plans were completed for the erection of new physiologic, pathologic, and histologic laboratories, and a new laboratory of pharmacodynamics is to be established with Dr. H. C. Wood, Jr., in charge. Dr. Meredith Clymer was elected president of the society, with Drs. Claudius H. Mastin, John H. Packard, James Tyson, and S. D. Risley vice-presidents, and Dr. Joseph P. Tunis secretary and treasurer.

At the last meeting of the Homeopathic County Medical Society, held in Philadelphia, June 9th, it was determined to make an effort to have the city authorities recognize homeopaths at the Philadelphia Hospital. For this purpose a committee was appointed to confer with the authorities and to secure influence for this movement. With the valuable amount of material which this hospital has, it has always been considered the most desirable of the hospitals of the city, to secure appointments there being the aim of the several medical colleges, and it would indeed be a rich prize for the homeopaths to secure.

The Philadelphia County Medical Society held a meeting June 8th, but owing to the absence of many of its members and the pressure of business matters there was but little scientific business.

The Sanitary Committee of the Board of Health and a committee from the Public Education Association held a conference on Monday relative to establishing a daily medical inspection of the public schools similar to those made in Boston and New York. The labor involved is considerable, as there are 400 schools in this city, covering a large amount of territory. It was resolved, therefore, to have the assistant medical inspectors of the Board of Health inspect one school daily in their respective districts.

As the result of an investigation by the officials of the Coroner's office into the sudden death of a colored child eighteen months old, some startling facts were developed. Another infant had died about two weeks before under similar circumstances, without proper medical attendance, and when the last case was reported, Dr. Cattell, the coroner's physician, was assigned to investigate the case. The result of the investigation was the disclosure of a "baby farm," in which another infant and two adults were suffering from diphtheria, which, the autopsy disclosed, had caused the death of the infant in question. The place was immediately closed and the patients removed to a hospital.

Dr. Samuel G. Dixon, who has been appointed a member of the Board of Education, is a member of the bar as well as a graduate in medicine, and president of the Academy of Natural Sciences. Such recognition of medical men, it is to be regretted, is rare in this city.

The College of Physicians of Philadelphia announces that the sum of $500 will be awarded the author of the best essay in competition for the first Nathan Lewis Hatfield Prize for Original Research in Medicine. The subject selected is "A Pathological and Clinical Study of the Thymus Gland and Its Relations." The essays must be submitted on or before January 1, 1900. They must be typewritten, designated by a motto or device, and accompanied by a sealed envelope containing the motto or device, and the name and address of the author. No envelope will be opened except that which accompanies the successful essay, and all unsuccessful essays will be returned if reclaimed by their respective writers within one year. The committee reserves the right to make no award if no essay submitted is considered worthy of the prize, and the treatment of the subject must, in accordance with the conditions of the trust, be based upon original observations or researches, or original deductions. The competition is open to members of the medical profession and men of science in the United States. The original of the successful essay will become the property of the college, and the trustees will have full control of its publication. It will be published in the *Transactions* of the college, and also, when expedient, as a separate issue. The chairman of the committee having the matter in charge is Dr. James C. Wilson.

Dr. Hatfield, in whose memory his sons, Walter and Henry Reed Hatfield have founded the trust, has been dead ten years. For forty-five years he was in various capacities identified with the College of Physicians, was at the time of his death its oldest member, and was president of the Alumni Association of Jefferson Medical College.

The total number of deaths in this city as reported at the health office for the week ending June 11th, was 363, of which number 138 were of children under five years of age. There were 162 new cases of contagious diseases reported, as follows: Diphtheria, 65, with 17 deaths; scarlet fever, 35 cases, with 2 deaths; typhoid fever, 62 cases, with 7 deaths.

SOCIETY PROCEEDINGS.

AMERICAN MEDICAL ASSOCIATION.

Forty-ninth Annual Meeting, Held at Denver, Col., June 7, 8, 9, and 10, 1898.

[Specially Reported for the MEDICAL NEWS.]

(Continued from page 776.)

SECTION ON SURGERY.

SECOND DAY—JUNE 8TH.

DR. G. W. MIEL of Denver read a paper, entitled

PENETRATING WOUNDS OF THE POPLITEAL ARTERY.

He said double ligation and extirpation of the part between in all cases of incised wound of more than one-eight of an inch is recommended. One of the most difficult problems for a surgeon to solve is what to do in the case of a complicated wound of the popliteal artery. The preservation of the patient's life should be the first consideration and amputation the last resort. The external wound should be loosely closed in all cases. A mortality in complicated injury of the popliteal artery of ten per cent. may be expected. An amputation of necessity seems to be more serious than an amputation of expediency.

DR. B. MERRILL RICKETTS of Cincinnati remarked that Dr. Crile of Cleveland has proved that the common carotid can be obstructed for from twelve to twenty-four hours in a human being without injurious effects. "A case has occurred in my own practice of successful ligation of the external iliac vein, which had been torn loose in removing a tumor from the iliac fossa. My brother fourteen years ago had a case in which the deep profunda was shot off close to the femur, and the patient died forty-eight hours after the performance of amputation at the hip-joint."

DR. OLIVER of Cincinnati related the history of a case of compound fracture of the femur at the epiphyseal line in a boy twelve years of age in whom symptoms of obstructive circulation appeared on the second day after the reduction of the fracture necessitating amputation on the ninth day. Subsequent dissection of the leg showed the obstruction to be due to an effusion in the deep fascia, and it was found that two inches of the popliteal artery had been destroyed.

DR. M. B. TINKER of Philadelphia referred to an experiment made upon an ass in which the descending aorta had been ligated, firm union resulting.

DR. RICKETTS observed that anastomosis seems to be more successful in the larger arteries, which probably accounts for the success of the experiment.

DR. MIEL, in closing, said it is especially desirable to only temporarily close the vessels in wounds about the mouth. He related a case of compound fracture of the knee with injury to the popliteal artery where amputation was objected to.

DR. D. W. GRAHAM of Chicago read a paper, entitled

PRIMARY CARCINOMA OF THE AXILLA.

He said primary carcinoma of the breast often first manifests itself clinically by an enlargement of the glands in the axilla. The sweat-glands are very important from a pathologic standpoint, as cases of carcinoma had been proved to originate in these glands, which it should be remembered are situated under the skin and not in it. Although many cases of primary carcinoma of the axilla have been reported only eighteen are really reliable reports. He related in full two cases of this condition operated upon by himself.

DR. CHARLES A. POWERS of Denver said great stress should be laid upon the importance of this subject and the necessity of always removing everything at all suspicious when performing these operations. Early recognition and early extirpation are most essential to success. He referred to a patient from whom he had recently removed a nodule which upon examination proved to be a supernumerary mammary gland, the seat of a fibroid adenoma.

DR. OCHSNER of Chicago mentioned three cases of carcinomatous growth at the lower edge of the pectoralis major muscle, and the inner limit of the axilla, which doubtless originated from glandular tissue, a portion of the mammary gland.

DR. A. J. BEVAN of Chicago remarked that two possibilities should always be borne in mind in these cases, first, that the condition may be one of a small primary focus overshadowed by the secondary mass, or second, that the condition is due to encapsulation of a piece of epiblastic tissue. The primary growth may be in the mammary gland, and the secondary mass in the axilla.

DR. J. B. MURPHY of Chicago asked if the tumors in the cases reported by the author of the paper were primarily superficial or deep, and whether the skin was freely moveable in the early stages.

DR. WILLIAM L. RODMAN of Louisville, Ky., reported a case, similar to the one referred to by the author, occurring in a ship's carpenter, about sixty years of age. The case was doubtless one of carcinoma of the axilla. He thought more stress should be laid upon the fact that a very small lump in the breast may be overlooked and the growth in the axilla considered as primary when it is really secondary, and emphasized the necessity of the complete removal of the glands in these cases.

DR. GRAHAM insisted that tissue exists in the axilla which is perfectly capable of giving rise to primary carcinoma. In reply to Dr. Murphy, he stated that in one of his cases the integument was moveable over the tumor while in the other the skin was tense. It is perfectly possible to have a supernumerary mammary nodule in the male, as well as in the female.

DR. M. L. HARRIS of Chicago read a paper upon

CLINICAL RESULTS OBTAINED BY THE USE OF MY INSTRUMENT FOR OBTAINING THE URINE SEPARATELY FROM THE TWO KIDNEYS.

He said there is a great difference between chemic and microscopic examination of the urine from the two kidneys, and frequently that from one kidney is acid in reaction while from the other it is neutral. A purulent cystitis does not prevent the collection of the urine from the two kidneys when this instrument is used. Four cases were reported in detail in which it had been employed, and the results given.

DR. MCARTHUR of Chicago spoke very favorably of the instrument and of the excellent results he had obtained from its use. In certain conditions the knowledge obtained is invaluable.

SECTION ON NEUROLOGY AND MEDICAL JURISPRUDENCE.

SECOND DAY—JUNE 8TH.

DR. HUGH T. PATRICK of Chicago was in the Chair.

DR. JOHN PUNTON of Kansas City, Mo., presented the first paper, entitled

THE RELATION OF NEURASTHENIA TO INSANITY.

He said that the consensus of opinion to-day is that neurasthenia in its quintessence is a true fatigue neurosis, characterized by increased morbid reaction of the ganglionic nerve-centers to all kinds of impressions, both mental and physical, whether slight or profound; producing an excessive nervous weakness and irritability which constitute its chief cardinal symptoms. There may be nervous involvement of the motor, sensory, reflex, trophic, secretory, visceral, and psychic mechanisms furnishing a wide and varied range of clinical phenomena. All authorities agree that incipient insanity is attended by physical and mental changes that are indicative of nervous exhaustion, and clinically are expressed by a diminution of vigor in all the bodily processes. The relation of neurasthenia to insanity cannot be overestimated, the relation one bears to the other in a large number of cases being so close as to almost establish a true equivalency. Neurasthenia is an actual morbific entity with certain well-defined clinical phenomena.

DR. MEYER of New York thought the attempt should be made to single out those forms of neurasthenia which we know are initial stages of certain forms of disease, keeping these separate from neurasthenia which remained neurasthenia, without ever going over into insanity.

DR. H. S. DRAYTON of New York thought it was to Dr. Beard, late of New York, that we owe the term neurasthenia. He referred to Spitzka's elaborate opinion with regard to the difference between neurasthenia and melancholia, holding that most neurasthenic troubles were traceable to specific causes. The speaker thought that a very fine line of demarcation could be drawn between neurasthenia and melancholia.

DR. TOMLINSON said that the attempt to establish a relation between neurasthenia and melancholia only leads to confusion, and while the insane person may in the earlier stages, in fact all through the outbreak of mental disturbance, manifest neurasthenic symptoms, still the neurasthenic symptoms have nothing to do with the insanity, nor has the insanity anything to do with the neurasthenia. It was a matter of relation rather than of causation.

DR. H. H. HOPPE of Cincinnati thought that one's view was influenced by the source from which he obtained his experience, whether from the insane asylum or the clinic or office. He believed in a sharp line of demarcation between neurasthenia and melancholia.

DR. J. T. ESKRIDGE of Denver said he had seen a number of cases of neurasthenia pass into melancholia, and thought that there was a very close relation between neurasthenia and insanity. A great many cases of melancholia began with neurasthenic symptoms. Whether this passes into insanity or not depends upon several causes, but two of the principal are the hereditary condition of the patient, that is to say, the nerve stamina of the patient; and secondly, the personality of his physician, a medical attendant blessed with personal magnetism being much more likely to achieve favorable results.

UREMIC APHASIA AND HEMIPLEGIA

was the title of an article by DR. H. H. HOPPE of Cincinnati, dealing with localized lesions of the central nervous system occurring as a result of uremic attacks, and giving four interesting cases illustrative thereof. In the first case of uremia the primary symptom was aphasia, which continued for half an hour, followed by a convulsion and hemiplegia of the right side, with complete recovery in twenty-four hours. In the second case there was sudden loss of consciousness, the face being drawn to the left side, and the right arm and leg paralyzed, without convulsions or twitching of any kind. The tongue was protruded to the left. On the following morning the paralysis entirely disappeared, and the patient, being treated by alkalies and a non-nitrogenous diet, now considers himself well. In the third case there was sudden loss of power in the right arm. The attending physician diagnosed right-sided hemiplegia with involvement of the face. In twelve hours recovery was complete. The urine showed two per cent. of albumin and large numbers of hyalin and granular casts. The fourth case seemed to bear out the theory that some local predisposition is necessary for the development of the paralytic attacks; that some cause is present in the center or area of the cortex which renders this center more liable to be attacked by the poisons circulating in the blood during the uremic attack rather than other parts of the surface. The patient, a married woman of sixty-four, presented a typical fatty heart with well-marked arteriosclerosis. In August, 1897, she had a sudden attack of apoplexy, involving the external recti muscles of both eyes, especially the right. The right side of the face and tongue was involved. There was complete loss of power in the right arm and right leg, partial paresis of left leg. Diagnosis, acute bulbar paralysis due to thrombosis of a branch of basilar artery in the upper part of pons. There was gradual improvement, although the right side of the face and tongue, as well as the right external rectus did not recover. On February 12th, 1898 the patient had another attack. On examination she was found to be in a stuporous condition, with constant twitching of the left side of the face. The left arm and left leg were in a constant state of clonic spasm. When treated by purgatives, profuse perspiration was induced by the application of hot water in rubber bags, consciousness returned in about an hour. The paralysis of the arm and leg disappeared in four or five hours. On April 16, 1898, patient again had an attack of uremic coma with left-sided hemiplegia, and again recovered as in the previous attack. The real cause of these attacks is the uremic condition. As to the proximate cause, this may be either due to capillary hemorrhages (no trace of which can be found on autopsy, however), or, more probably, to toxemia or localized cortical edema. The author, however, believes that the attacks are due to intoxication and that poisons may affect circumscribed areas of the cortex of the brain.

DR. SEXTON said it was not quite clear to him how we could have a condition which must necessarily depend upon a local lesion in the brain without local lesion ever being demonstrable. He could scarcely see what the mechanism of the poison would be in producing hemiplegia. A great majority of these cases really depend upon a local hemorrhage from rupture of a minute vessel, in which the absorption of the clot was so perfect that after death autopsies do not give any evidence of its existence.

DR. CHARLES H. LODOR of Chicago said he had seen a great many cases of hemiplegia which he believed to be uremic in their origin. He did not agree with Dr. Sexton that there is necessarily an organic basis for the origin of them.

DR. TOMLINSON, in adding his testimony to Dr. Hoppe's, called attention to three cases published by Dr. Burr of Philadelphia, in which the histories were the same as Dr. Hoppe's cases, which appeared to be true hemiplegias, yet in which the autopsies showed nothing. Dr. Tomlinson related four cases of a like character which had come to autopsy within the last year, all being cases of interstitial nephritis.

DR. ESKRIDGE spoke of the differential diagnosis between Jacksonian epilepsy, due to organic lesion, and those spasms due to presumed functional disturbance of the cortex. He said that when we have an organic spasm of the cortex the muscles involved in the spasm are the last to be affected; the temperature is always high on the affected side and the patient loses consciousness. There is great difficulty in differentiating a spasm due to uremic poison from that due to a limited cortical lesion. As a rule, in organic lesions of the cortex, only those muscles affected in the initial spasm will be paralyzed after the convulsion is over.

DR. C. EUGENE RIGGS of St. Paul, Minn., said that when miliary aneurisms in the brain break, the first influence is insult to the brain, causing certain phenomena described by Dr. Hoppe.

DR. C. C. HERSMAN of Pittsburg did not think that these paralyses are caused by hemorrhage.

DR. HOPPE, in closing the discussion, referred to the autopsies made by Jurgens and Israel in Berlin, including not only gross pathologic examinations, but histologic examinations as well, in which no trace was found in the cortex of any change.

DR. FREDERICK S. THOMAS of Council Bluffs, Iowa, read a paper, entitled

THE STRESS OF MODERN CIVILIZATION AS A FACTOR IN THE CAUSATION OF INSANITY.

The higher the scale of intelligence and the more exacting the demands upon a people, the more likelihood there is, apparently, of brain disease. Civilization itself is a departure from man's primitive condition. It has made new and exhaustive demands upon his energies. Overstraining and stimulation of the nervous organism cannot fail to cause harmful effects during childhood, and frequently produce neurasthenic and nervous temperaments in later life.

DR. DAVID INGLIS of Detroit, Mich., differed with the reader's premises and conclusions, and referred to the fact that the great bulk of the men and women who constitute the inmates of our insane asylums are not people in whom the higher psychical life has had an opportunity for development.

DR. JOHN PUNTON of Kansas City, Mo., thought there was no doubt that the present methods of public-school education is largely the cause of nervous diseases among children.

DR. HAROLD N. MOYER of Chicago, in taking issue with the paper, called attention to the fact that there is no statistical warrant for the assertion that insanity is rare or infrequent among primitive races. He also referred to the fact that civilization conserves and preserves the degenerates, who would be quickly disposed of with a club among savages.

DR. SEXTON thought that the stress of civilization has

a tendency toward the degeneration of the race, the development of stable nervous organizations not being so good under this stress.

NEURALGIA AND NERVE-CRIES

was the title of an article by DR. C. H. LODOR of Chicago. Dr. Lodor said that for purposes of classification, the source of such pain may lie within the nerve itself or its environment, or may be found in irritants carried to the nerve through the medium of the circulatory fluids or in defects in said fluids. In the first class were grouped chronic inflammatory processes recognizable as neuritis, old adhesions, changes in the perineurilemma from chronic rheumatism and arthritis deformans, pressure from cicatrices and new growths, reflex pain, fatigue pain, hyperesthesia, etc. In the second class are arranged the diathetic causes, including the accumulation of gouty acids in the perineurilemma and sheath; anemia, cholemia, malaria, autotoxins, and poisons, as lead, copper, and mercury; diabetes, syphilis. Nerve-cries are also the result of change in blood-pressure, change in atmospheric-pressure, change in lymph-pressure, and in lymph constituents. The paper dwelt especially upon (*a*) the effect produced by inflammatory adhesions and by the products of, and exudates remaining after, inflammation as modifying or restricting the function of nerves so hampered; (*b*) lymph stasis, and (*c*) the autonerve poisons.

DR. C. C. HERSMAN of Pittsburg, Pa., presented a communication upon

NERVOUSNESS AS AN ELEMENT IN HYPERPYREXIA.

He detailed two cases of remarkably high temperature. In the first case the temperature on the seventh day reached 118° F. At times the temperature would drop from 110° F. to normal in twenty minutes without interference, but usually the sponge bath was resorted to with very prompt effect. There were marked hysterical symptoms. The diagnosis was that of an exaggerated nervous condition attended by hyperpyrexia and hysterical symptoms. Antipyretics had little effect. A visit from friends would provoke an attack. At the end of fifteen days the patient was sent home. The second patient, an Irish domestic aged twenty-nine, whose disease was diagnosed as articular rheumatism, had on admission a temperature of 99° F., pulse 102, respiration 24. On the second day the temperature became normal. On the fourth day it was 104° F., and on the fourteenth, it rose to 106.2° F., pulse 80. On the eighteenth day it reached 110.9° F.; on the twenty-third day at 11.30 A.M. it was 110° F., but at 2.30 P.M. had dropped to 99° F. On the thirty-fifth day her temperature was 116° F., and on the forty-second day 118.4° F. When agitated her temperature was highest. One nurse she disliked and her presence would aggravate the fever. In the first case there were tender joints, and in the latter a tender spine, but Dr. Hersman regarded these as hysterical symptoms, rather than rheumatic or meningitic.

DR. HAROLD N. MOYER said there had been a number of cases reported of extraordinary temperature, and alluded to a case he saw in 1883 in which the thermometer registered 130° F. Every precaution had been taken to eliminate the possibility of malingering.

DR. PETERSON of New York suspected that such cases as Dr. Hersman's were malingering in character.

DR. HERSMAN said that the second case was 101 days in the hospital, there being little or no emaciation during the whole time. He said the patients were not allowed to handle the thermometer at all, and there was no possibility of malingering.

SECTION ON PRACTICE OF MEDICINE.

THIRD DAY—JUNE 9TH.

DR. NORMAN BRIDGES of Los Angeles, Cal., presented a paper upon

SOME USUALLY OVERLOOKED PHYSICAL SIGNS AND SYMPTOMS IN CHEST DISEASES.

He said we look for classical symptoms and pass over the symptoms the patients coming to us actually have. It is important to make an early diagnosis in tuberculosis, before the classical physical signs are completely developed. We must learn to appreciate the signs which will eventually develop into the classical ones. We see fourfold more cases showing these slight symptoms than those with the classical signs.

DR. E. FLETCHER INGALS of Chicago said it is important to remember that in early stages of phthisis the disease is localized and even a slight change from the normal condition, if limited to a small portion of the lung, is a grave sign. It must, however, be remembered that these things may remain from a former pneumonia or pleurisy. Extreme expiration is of great value. In nine cases out of ten we get better results by examining anteriorly. More mistakes have been made in diagnosing cases as tuberculosis than the reverse. When there is a pulse of 115 or 120 and the individual seems well otherwise, I look very carefully for tuberculosis.

DR. JAMES TYSON of Philadelphia said bronchial breathing with diminished vocal fremitus means almost always a pleurisy with effusion.

DR. C. E. EDSON of Denver remarked that especially in the incipient stage the rapidity of the pulse is a sign which makes one suspect many cases. The pulse is not only quick but indescribably nervous, irritable, and of small caliber.

DR. W. N. BEGGS of Denver quoted Glasgow of St. Louis, who said that "No man was able to diagnose a case of incipient phthisis until he had examined a thousand cases more pronounced." Dr. Beggs wished to emphasize the inconstancy in the character of vocal fremitus, which with vocal resonance differs in patients from time to time and in different patients so as to cause doubt. We can emphasize not only in young but also in older children the lack of bulging, and also to a marked extent the lack of restricted movement on the affected side. Muscle tones are likely to be confused with intrathoracic sounds if we are not careful.

DR. BRIDGES, in closing the discussion, said errors are likely to occur on account of muscular action; care should be taken to put every muscular fiber at as complete rest as possible.

DR. ALLEN A. JONES of Buffalo read a paper upon

THE ASSOCIATION OF CHRONIC DIARRHEA WITH ACHYLIA GASTRICA.

In achylia gastrica there exists suspension of the secretions of the stomach. Probably all cases of this affection do not arise from glandular atrophy. Stockton thinks it may begin and continue as a neurosis and has found ocular error associated with it. Remarkable absence of fermentation is observed in the stomach in this condition. The point it is desired to emphasize is that symptoms of disturbance of intestinal digestion seems more troublesome in achylia gastrica than direct symptoms of disordered gastric condition. One of the most important factors in diarrhea from gastric disorders is the precipitancy with which the stomach sends its contents into the intestine. The diarrhea differs in different cases; sometimes there are several evacuations after the morning meal, sometimes several after each meal, sometimes they are periodic, coming on suddenly and lasting a week or two and then constipation ensues. Appetite in some cases is voracious; character of stools varies, the discharges being frequently watery and containing undigested food. In some cases constipation has been observed rather than diarrhea in this connection. A few drugs are sometimes most efficacious. Dilute hydrochloric acid, 20 to 30 drops, after the meal and repeated in the same dose in an hour, may be mentioned first. Some clinicians give it well diluted before meals. Another remedy which has proven useful and may be given with this acid, is tinct. ferri chlorid, five drops being usually quite effective. Sometimes it is better to add two drops to every glass of water taken. It is advisable to give pepsin in addition to the hydrochloric acid. This is one of the few cases which call for its exhibition. Sometimes small doses of Fowler's solution given immediately before meals are efficacious. Sometimes small doses of arsenic, gold, and red iodid of mercury do good. Gastric faradization has proven beneficial.

DR. J. M. ANDERS of Philadelphia had met with this condition in association with lienteric diarrhea. Diarrhea is more frequently dependent on a catarrhal state of the small intestine than any other single factor. This condition of achylia gastrica has been found to be associated with a tuberculous process. In a majority of cases, there is a grave general underlying condition coexistant, tuberculosis, amyloid degeneration, a marked neurosis general in character, etc., which should not be overlooked.

DR. C. G. STOCKTON of Buffalo regarded the advent of diarrhea as an unfortunate factor in persons suffering from achylia gastrica. While diarrhea does not exist there is retention of the food-products for a sufficient length of time for assimilation to be carried on. The diarrhea is largely a nervous expression, and some cases of achylia gastrica depend on a nervous condition alone.

DR. E. P. JOSLIN of Boston had observed constipation in a large portion of cases of achylia gastrica. In any nervous affection the variety of symptoms is characteristic. The benefit of hydrochloric acid is doubtful. It often happens that a test breakfast with which hydrochloric had been given, shows no hydrochloric acid present, as it has combined with the food in the stomach. Add to two or three eggs two or three pints of 2-per-cent. hydrochloric acid, normal stomach acid, let it stand a short time, and you will find no trace of the acid there at all, it having all combined with the albumen. There is no use in giving hydrochloric acid unless there is pepsin, and in achylia there is no pepsin in the stomach. If we could give two or three pints of the acid we would have the albumen saturated and in that case pepsin will act to a certain extent but then only slightly. We must get the food out of the stomach as soon as possible and that is fortunately the method Nature adopts. To avoid the diarrhea, one should eat slowly, mince the meat finely, and prepare the food as much as possible before it gets to the intestines. We must be sure these patients have enough food. From resection we learn that a person can get along without a stomach, but not without food, so in restricting the diet, be sure there is enough of it, if not proteids, then cream, fat, butter, something that can easily be digested. Pineapple juice can be given as a ferment which will act in a neutral medium.

A paper upon

SPONTANEOUS CURE OF TUBERCULOSIS AND THE IMITATIONS OF ITS METHODS,

was presented by DR. JAMES T. WHITTAKER of Cincinnati. In it he said no pathologist will dispute that tuberculosis is present in two-thirds of mankind. Two sevenths succumb tot uberculosis of the lungs alone; include intestinal, bone- and joint-infection and the fraction is brought up to two-sixths. What cures the patients who do not succumb? Those having the benefit of altitude recover. Something in altitude gives immunity and arrests the progress of the disease. Also some individuals recover under all conditions. Creasote does affect the steptococcus. The various tuberculins are antitoxic so long as the disease remains pure, and the preparations contain no impurities. Surgery fails in the lungs because of the mixed infection and because the knife cannot lay bare the mother colonies in the bronchial glands. Is there anything that will act in all cases? Universal testimony is to the effect that altitude effectually cures phthisis. It acts by dryness; by cold, which favors dryness, is a stimulus and increases the tendency to sleep; by sunshine, the germicidal action of which is due to increased oxidation; by purity, as air becomes freer of bacteria as we ascend; by rarefaction, the most important of all, because it leads to increased exercise of heart and lungs and to continuous though unconscious gymnastics. Blood-corpuscles take up oxygen only at a certain degree of pressure; they will not take up enough with greatly diminished pressure, therefore, in low-pressure climate the number and size of the red blood-corpuscles are increased. This clue should be followed up. It has occurred to many to imitate altitude in increasing red-blood corpuscles. Transfusion is one of the things which keeps coming up. Bactericidal power resides in the white corpuscles, hence defibrinated blood will not answer, and five grains of sodium oxylate will prevent the coagulation of a quart of blood. Put a teaspoonful of salt, a tablespoonful of soda and a tablespoonful of sugar of milk into a pint of water and into that a pint of ox's blood (calve's is better) and introduce, a pint at a time, into the blood by rectal enema. No rectal enema ever devised contains the same amount of nutritive. The benefit of this treatment to anemic patients is remarkable. Some gain twenty pounds in three weeks. It has not, however, the best results in fever, and the bactericidal effect is disappointing.

REST; A NEGLECTED FACTOR IN THE THERAPEUTICS OF GASTRO-ENTERIC DISEASES,

was the title of a paper read by DR. C. D SPIVAK of Denver. He defined rest as Nature's prophylactic. The surgeon was the first to recognize its value; later the neurologist took it up; they have monopolized rest, while the medical man says, Which of the thousand and one drugs of the Pharmacopeia shall I use? Rest is the greatest foe against diseases of the gastro-intestinal tract. It may be secured (1) by rest in bed, keeping the bowels regulated, and sponging the body every morning; (2) by diet; and in many cases the best diet is abstinence, for three-days' fasting will do no harm in cases of ulcers, dyspepsia, and diarrhea of all kinds and varieties. Nutritive enemata may be employed when longer fasting is required. Food must be given in small quantities and at regular intervals. (3) Poultices which make the patient feel comfortable. This treatment has been of great benefit to cases which were types of hyperacidity upon a nervous basis; neurasthenia with hyperacidity; in tubercular patients suffering from vomiting and diarrhea; and in erosions of the stomach. This rest-cure is indicated in all cases of dyspepsia, the underlying cause of which is the nervous system; where abdominal pain is present; in all cases of acute diarrhea, hemorrhage from stomach or intestines, disturbed digestion with vacillating temperature, and in many cases of dyspepsia associated with tuberculosis.

DR. O'CONNELL of Pennsylvania, did not agree to the poulticing. Applying a cold pack to the stomach twenty minutes before meals and keeping it on for an hour was more beneficial.

DR. TYSON said the author has lighted on the one thing which is likely to do more or less good in every case of gastro-intestinal disturbance. The application of our therapeutic methods is more or less haphazard. By this means we will always do some good; by other means the good accomplished is doubtful. Rest to the stomach is mainly accomplished by the ingestion of the minimum amount of food compatible with life. Food is not such a necessary thing as many imagine, out a patient may go several days without the ingestion of any food if he is in a position not to demand force.

DR. H. A. WEST of Galveston, Texas, thought the paper might be made more comprehensive. In acute infectious diseases the processes of digestion are seriously involved, and in these cases the rest-treatment is of supreme value. In acute rheumatism rest of the digestive function and rest in bed are necessary. Subsequent cardiac complications can be averted to a considerable extent by a plan of rest. Exercise is more important in tuberculosis than rest in bed, the only stomach-rest being limited to proper regulation of diet.

In closing, DR. SPAVIK said that of 100 cases of this kind, not only has the treatment done no harm, but it has in nearly every one of the cases done good. A patient with tuberculosis and fever should be in bed.

REPORT OF CASE OF ANEURISM OF THE CONCAVITY OF THE TRANSVERSE ARCH, APPEARING EXTERNALLY AS A LARGE TUMOR IN THE REGION OF THE HEART,

by DRS. H. W. MCLAUTHLIN and Wm. N. BEGGS of Denver, was read by Dr. McLauthlin.

A paper upon

THE VALUE OF SALIVA IN THE BABE AS A FACTOR IN DIGESTING MILK AND THE WAY IN WHICH IT IS TO BE OBTAINED BY USE OF AN ARTIFICIAL NIPPLE,

was read by DR. W. G. A. BONWILL of Philadelphia. He stated that the babe takes the long nipple of the nursing-bottle under its tongue and draws the milk without any effort of the buccinator muscles. The hole in the nipple is very large so the milk comes through too fast. Held under the tongue the nipple collapses. It cannot be made thoroughly aseptic. A short nipple was prepared the length of the mother's, and an external secondary one, drilling a small hole with a dental engine, so that twenty minutes was required for the child to draw four ounces of milk. The infant's parotid glands act simultaneously, which is not true in adult life, as mastication can only take place on one side at a time.

DR. ELMER LEE of New York City read a paper, entitled

THE MEDICAL TREATMENT OF APPENDICITIS.

He said the treatment of appendicitis is sometimes surgical, but more frequently medical. General measures first and local ones afterward is a broad plan. In appendicitis there is a complete clogging of the vessels of the appendix. The first determinable effect is congestion, followed by the accumulation of mucus in the appendix; swelling of the mucosa and other structures of the organ succeed. Whatever fecal matter is within the appendix is pressed into the cecum or dammed into this structure and retained there to undergo chemic action. Pain is likely to be prominent at the point affected, but in some cases it is absent. Probably vasomotor control is depressed and there is too much or too little blood in the affected part. Inflammation ensues, destructive changes take place rapidly under the influence of increased heat and chemic decomposition of fluids and tissues. When the physician first sees the patient and suspects a possibility of appendicitis he should treat the patient rather than the disease, with a view to preventing that which is suspected, or if too late for that to give him the best chance for recovery with least damage. Food should be withheld from the patient for one to four days, and the presence of temperature warrants the withholding of all food while the elevation remains. Moderate feeding is permissible at regular and long intervals where there is keen hunger. The diet should consist of sweet fruits and well-cooked vegetables. Eight ounces of pure water administered with the regularity of doses of medicine every hour for the first and second days of treatment, and if the case improves every two hours, is a therapeutic resource of striking simplicity and has a scientific value, and its only contraindication is when the patient sleeps. Heidelberg has elevated internal hydropathic therapy into a special chair. Employ an enema of hot soapy water which will free the colon and small intestines, for fermentation is to be looked for in the ascending and mesocolon. Use two or three quarts of water, half the quantity in a child, knee-chest position. The water can be made to open the appendix if perseverance is used. Intestinal antiseptics cannot stand the test of scientific experiment. Cold water applied to the affected area of the abdomen is helpful. A small napkin saturated with ice-water is useful. Generally massage of the abdominal wall contiguous to the appendix is beneficial. Rub along the spine with the hands dipped in ice-water. If fever runs high, water externally and internally in large quantities affords better means of allaying it than chemicals. A clean colon is likely to be accompanied by a healthy appendix.

DR. E. J. ROGERS of Denver doubted if an absolutely medicinal treatment could be relied upon in appendicitis, though that which Dr. Lee had outlined is certainly the best. If these lines of simple cleansing and purification were followed it would not be necessary to operate in so many cases. The cause of the difficulty is principally a mechanical one. We find a little cul-de-sac where this normal cleansing process of the intestines does not go on. Until we can determine the true nature of infection we have to treat it in the dark. It is impossible in the early stage of the disease to tell whether the patient is going to die from suppurative peritonitis in twenty-four hours or the case is going to clear up and recovery take place. The inability of determining this has led to the adoption of the rule by radical surgeons that in the early stage every case should be operated upon. If there is any disease which should be treated by the co-operation of the surgeon and physician, this is the one. The medical man should let the surgeon see the patient in the beginning, and he should continue in the case from its inception. The true surgeon is the man who avoids the knife.

DR. HENRY SEWALL of Denver agreed heartily with much Dr. Lee had said, but if the observer believes pus has formed or the inflammation leading to pus-formation is going on, there is no medical treatment. The common practice of to-day is to eliminate functional disturbance which may give rise to those symptoms. If they do not disappear when mechanical obstruction is relieved then comes a field for the exercise of judgment. The average physician should take a place midway between those who urge that every case presenting symptoms of appendicitis should be operated on and those who never allow their cases to be operated upon until the signs of death are imminent. No one can instruct another as to the use of judgment. There is no better means for keeping our patients in a condition which will act as a prophylactic measure than those the reader of the paper had advised.

DR. H. J. HERRICK of Cleveland contended that the physician deals with phenomena, the surgeon with facts. The relief of the condition by natural means is most desirable. Appendicitis is due to defective secretions which we must control.

DR. BAILEY of Louisville said that diagnosis is most difficult at the time it is most important to make it. As soon as the disease is suspected the aid of a conscientious and intelligent surgeon will never be regretted.

DR. TYSON remarked that many cases of appendicitis are extremely difficult to diagnose, and he believes that many of the cases which get well under medical treatment are not cases of appendicitis at all. When there is a just suspicion of appendicitis, one wants a skilled and accomplished surgeon, not for an operation always, but for his judgment.

DR. J. B. WALKER of Philadelphia had a case of appendicitis three years ago which recovered without operation. The young man was apparently perfectly well, but was advised that there might be a reoccurrence of the attack when he was away from where a skilled surgeon could be obtained, and the operation was done before he left Philadelphia. At the operation a pint of pus was found back of the colon; of this there was not a sign before the operation. The appendix had sloughed and was perforated.

DR. JAMES of Missouri liked hot-water applications, and let his patients get along without food for three or four days.

DR. H. A. WEST wanted to array himself beside Drs. Bailey, Tyson, Rogers, and Walker in combating the idea that there is any antagonism between the physician and surgeon so far as appendicitis is concerned. Medical treatment in these cases amounts to very little, and the cases which recover under the medical treatment without operation, would get well anyway.

A paper on

SOME CONSIDERATIONS OF UREMIA AND ITS TREATMENT,

was read by DR. E. W. MITCHELL of Cincinati, who said, that in normal urine there are seven toxic principles, two of which produce convulsions, one coma, one ptyalism, one lower temperature, and so on. We are justified in assuming that in uremia we have a state of toxemia, an intoxication which depends on the retention within the tissues of substances which should have been eliminated with the urine. The failure of the liver to properly dispose of the poisonous materials brought to it make it an important factor in the condition. Serious cases should adopt a milk diet. Elimination by the skin is to be maintained by baths of hot-air vapor, or packs selected according to the tolerance of the patient The prophylactic value of veratrum viride is not sufficiently appreciated. Alkaline mineral waters are useful, The great principle of rest is as applicable for these organs as for others. For immediate control of convulsions opium may be effective, and is not usually unsafe. Bleeding is especially to be used when combined with transfusion of normal salt solution; but not when blood-pressure is low. By transfusion poisonous matters in the blood are diluted and opportunity given to the patient to recover if the lesion in the kidney is not so far advanced that continuation of life is impossible.

(To be continued.)

REVIEWS.

PRACTICAL DIAGNOSIS; THE USE OF SYMPTOMS IN THE DIAGNOSIS OF DISEASE. By HOBART AMORY HARE, M.D., B.SC. Illustrated with 201 engravings and thirteen colored plates. Second edition, revised and enlarged. Philadelphia and New York: Lea Bros. & Co., 1898.

TO assist those not in possession of thorough medical training, and to supply the facts and statistics to others with treacherous memories are certainly praiseworthy tasks. No one could bring to them previous reputation in this particular line of work more than Dr. Hare.

To write such a book requires at the same time a broad mind and a genius for details. In it one necessarily recognizes the impress of older books. Throughout the book there is the shadow of the very ancient books on physiognomy and of the vast amount of literature of the older writers concerning posture in disease, the character of the tongue, and all those other points in diagnosis which have attracted too little notice since the causes of disease have been more clearly known and its course better understood. It would seem that in an attempt at completeness a good deal that was not of practical importance had been accumulated in so short a book.

The index, which, according to the preface, has been improved in this second edition, still leaves a good deal to be desired. Indexing is a modern development, and the first thing which one does in examining a new work is to test the indices. It is like winding up a clock to see if it will go. This index goes, but might be improved by expansion.

The real value of such a book to the profession involves the question of the value of compendiums in general. The tendency of the times to short cuts has led to an attempt to make it possible to apply the experience of one person to the direction and conduct of another; that is, to make knowledge so accessible as to supply a lack of training. Perhaps the only harm, if any, of the attempt is that persons without training may be led to believe themselves capable of working by the direction of such books. The failure of this author to produce a book that in the hands of the badly trained will enable them to make a diagnosis is not a criticism upon the author himself, because he has done well and artistically a task set him, but is dependent upon the truth that medicine has not yet been sufficiently well systematized, and that no one has yet shown a complete degree in the faculty of conveying mature medical knowledge to others.

When the book is taken for what it is intended, an index of the symptoms rather than a complete description of disease, it is of much value. It brings together as nearly as possible all the symptoms that may occur in various parts of the body, and as a careful attempt to do this the book is unique and valuable. Indeed, no one could peruse the book from cover to cover without having the memory jogged as to the unusual symptoms in familiar diseases, or increasing his stock of names of those symptoms to which unfortunately some non-descriptive proper name has been attached. The sections referring to nervous diseases are an unusually good résumé of a department of medicine in which diagnosis forms not only the chief difficulty but the chief function of the specialist. We find here in an exaggerated degree, however, that vice which is common to neurologists of making their descriptions of disease more clearly defined than the diseases themselves are ever seen actually in practice. The charts and diagrams of the nervous system, though more definite than Nature, still indicate in a general way the geography of the physiology of the nervous system. Diagrams are valuable, but in neurology they are sometimes abused to the detriment of truth.

The book will be specially valuable to the young graduate whose experience does not cover the whole field of medicine, and who is unable to correlate particular symptoms. The tendency is very marked for a student to associate a particular symptom with some particular disease, and to be surprised when the same symptom turns up in other directions; hence, a work in which symptoms are treated systematically and disease incidentally, will be of special value in the earlier and incomplete stage of education. The book will also be useful to any old practitioner whose memory is not infallible.

The book is to be commended, also, in that it does not exaggerate, as so many works do, the difficulties of such special examinations of blood, sputum, etc., as have only recently come into general use. Such examinations made by an intelligent practitioner, when admitted as evidence and not as absolute proof, are of as much value as the signs elicited by percussion and auscultation by a person of average skill.

The book is certainly one worth purchasing, and is bound to have a wide circulation.

NOTES ON MICRO-ORGANISMS PATHOGENIC TO MAN. By SURGEON-CAPTAIN B. H. S. LEUMANN, I. M. S., M. B. (London), D. P. H. (Cambridge), etc., etc. New York and Bombay: Longmans, Green & Co., 1897.

IN a preface the author states that the object of this book is to afford to those students and physicians who have no time or opportunity of working in bacteriology or of reading larger works on the subject, a clear and concise description of the commoner forms of bacteria. It would have been far better if this book had never been published, for in its ninety-six pages are errors in the greatest abundance and statements without the least foundation in fact. The proof-reading has also been accomplished with an amount of carelessness which is unique. Let us cite only a few of the errors. In discussing enteric fever, the author says, in regard to staining the bacillus,

"Loeffler's blue will clearly define both the cilia and flagella," and later on, that the Widal reaction is always seen by the fifth or sixth day. In fixing material on cover-slips the latter are to be held in the *fingers* while passing them through the flame. In Germany the intestines are frequently complicated in diphtheria, while in England this lesion is seldom if ever seen. In staining by Gram's method, the specimen is to be washed in alcohol until no more iodin comes away. We are surprised at the frequent use of "preventitive" and of "Petrier's" dishes, and amazed at the "Pasturian" inoculation for rabies. The directions for preparing nutrient agar-agar are stated in less than five lines. Although the book contains a few pages of value, it cannot fulfil its mission in its present form.

A SYSTEM OF PRACTICAL MEDICINE BY AMERICAN AUTHORS. Edited by ALFRED LEE LOOMIS, M.D., LL.D., late Professor of Pathology and Practical Medicine in the New York University; and WILLIAM GILMAN THOMPSON, M.D., Professor of Medicine in the New York University, Physician to the Presbyterian and Bellevue Hospitals, New York. Vol. III. Illustrated. New York and Philadelphia: Lea Brothers & Co., 1898.

THE third volume of this excellent system, already favorably noticed in these columns, is in keeping with the worth of the work already established by the preceding volumes. It opens with the diseases of the mouth, tongue, tonsils, pharynx, and salivary glands from the pen of Dr. Richard C. Cabot. Dr. Allen A. Jones discusses the diseases of the esophagus, and he and Dr. Charles G. Stockton treat of the diseases of the stomach in an elaborate monograph. The diseases of the intestines are taken up by Drs. William W. Johnston and Henry M. Lyman, and appendicitis is thoughtfully considered by Dr. W. F. McNutt. Dr. George Dock describes intestinal parasites and trichinosis, and Dr. Victor C. Vaughan contributes a valuable article on bromatotoxismus.

The diseases of the peritoneum are discussed by Dr. H. A. Hare, those of the liver and gall-bladder by Dr. J. G. Graham. Dr. George Roe Lockwood contributes an article on the diseases of the spleen and Dr. Stockton one on those of the pancreas. The diseases of the thyroid gland are taken up in detail by Drs. Kinnicutt and Starr, and chronic metal-poisoning, alcoholism, and morphinism by Drs. Frederick G. Finley and James Stewart, respectively. The infectious diseases common to man and animals are discussed by Dr. James Law. A series of monographs on purpura (Dr. Lockwood), beri-beri (Dr. Stewart), hemophilia and filaria sanguinis hominis (Dr. James), diabetes (Dr. Coleman), and isolation (Dr. A. Lambert), complete the volume.

We have purposely in this instance given the names of authors and their subjects that it may be seen how well the choice of the editors has fallen in the selection of appropriate men for the discussion of the various topics. The names of most of them are familiarly associated with the subjects here assigned to them, a sufficient guarantee of their uniform excellence. Here and there there may be slight differences of professional opinion, but the practitioner will find everything he can need stated in a scientific manner and thoroughly up-to-date. A pleasing feature of the work is that the reader is not left to choose between several therapeutic methods of procedure, but has stated for him the most approved forms of treatment. The present volume is not so profusely illustrated as the preceding ones, but what illustrations are given are fine examples. Volume III. can only enhance the opinion previously expressed concerning this work—that it is one of the most modern, scientific, and useful publications of its kind ever issued in this country.

ARCHIVES OF THE ROENTGEN-RAY. Vol. II. Nos. 1 and 2. Edited by W. S. HEDLEY, M.D., M. R. C. S., and SYDNEY ROWLAND, M.A., M. R. C. S., etc., London: The Rebman Publishing Company, Limited, 1897.

RADIOGRAPHY IN MARINE ZOOLOGY. *The British Echinodermata*. By R. NORRIS WOLFENDEN, M.D., Cantab. With thirty-six illustrations in fifteen plates.

THIS successor to the "Archives of Skiagraphy" appears in a somewhat modified form and increased size. The artistic merit of the illustrations and their apparent fidelity are fully up to the previous level. The editors announce their intention of retaining this feature, and of adding a certain amount of useful letterpress. This will record the proceedings of the recently formed Röntgen Society, and will consist of original communications, notes, and correspondence. The new radiation will be considered from the standpoint of practical usefulness, as well as in view of its scientific bearings. The supplement on "British Echinodermata" is exceedingly instructive, each plate showing the natural animal beside the skiagraph.

THERAPEUTIC HINTS.

For Laryngitis and Bronchial Catarrh.—KAFEMANN of Königsberg recommends the following mixture as particularly efficacious:

℞ Menthol	ʒ i
Eucalyptol	♏. xl
Terpineol	ʒ ss
Ol. picis liq.	♏. xv.

M. Sig. For inhalation.

A few drops are poured into a bottle with a convex bottom and warmed over a spirit-lamp. The patient inhales the balsamic vapors, which soon fill the bottle, by means of a glass tube with a nasal bulb.

Preparation of Yellow-Oxid Ointment.—SCHANZ recommends the use of the freshly precipitated yellow oxid of mercury, in a humid state. This can be rubbed into a very fine powder giving a perfectly smooth ointment, which is difficult to prepare from the oxid in its customary dried commercial form. It is incorporated with wool-fat and distilled water (1–10 or 1–5 of each), and is kept in a dark bottle. This ointment is said not to become rancid.

THE MEDICAL NEWS.

A WEEKLY JOURNAL OF MEDICAL SCIENCE.

VOL. LXXII. NEW YORK, SATURDAY, JUNE 25, 1898. NO. 26.

ORIGINAL ARTICLES.

ENLARGEMENT OF THE LYMPH-NODES; THEIR PATHOLOGY AND TREATMENT.[1]

BY CARL WEIDNER, M.D.,
OF LOUISVILLE, KY.;
ASSOCIATE PROFESSOR OF THE PRACTICE OF MEDICINE AND DIRECTOR IN THE LABORATORY OF HISTOLOGY AND PATHOLOGY IN THE KENTUCKY SCHOOL OF MEDICINE, ETC.

BEFORE entering upon the subject proper allow me to make a short reference to the anatomy and physiology of the lymphatic or absorbent system of spaces and vessels. The fluid contained within this system is the lymph, a colorless fluid in which leucocytes (lymph-corpuscles) are suspended, and a varying amount of very small granules of fat, giving it a more or less milky appearance, the latter most marked in the lymphatics of the intestine. Beginning as minute spaces between the elements of the tissues everywhere, without any special wall, they soon form a large, complex system of sinuous capillaries, then larger lymphatic vessels with well defined coats very much like the blood-vessels. Frequently interrupting the onward flow of the lymph are valves and a system of special filters, the lymphatic glands, which are more correctly called lymph-nodes. The lymph is finally collected principally into the thoracic duct and thence emptied into the venous blood current, the thoracic duct emptying into the left subclavian vein, and a smaller lymph-duct, collecting the lymph from the right side of the head and chest, into the right subclavian vein.

The lymph constitutes the surplus, the overflow of the nutritive fluids of the body, the tissue-juices; acts as a medium of nutrition and interchange between the fluids and solid elements, helps to rejuvenate the blood, and helps to carry on the process of metabolism. The lymph-system in addition acts as a safety-valve and safety reservoir to the blood-vessels whenever there is an increased amount of fluid and increased intravascular pressure from any cause, thus serving to prevent injury to the vascular wall as well as to permit a direct return of fluid to the blood vessels in conditions of severe depletion as well as dilatation. It, and particularly the lymph-nodes, acts as a great purifier, a filter or a depository, and in many instances as a destroyer of foreign noxious substances circulating in the blood and lymph, such as pigment, broken-down cell elements, bacteria, etc.

As I lay great stress upon the function as a filter, permit a short descriptive review of the anatomy of the lymph-nodes. The node is surrounded by a rather dense fibrous capsule containing some unstriped muscular fibers; from this capsule a system of fibrous processes—trabeculæ—run into its substance, giving off minute branches again and again, so as to form a most minute, delicate network of connective-tissue framework—the stroma. Lying within this stroma we find masses of lymphoid cells, forming in the outer or cortical portion of the gland the larger secondary nodules or follicles, in the deeper medullary portion a closer system of cord-like masses of cells, the medullary cords. Each of these is surrounded, however, by a looser meshwork containing but few cells in its meshes, lined with endothelial cells, the so-called lymph-sinuses. The lymphatic vessels enter into the gland at all points of the periphery by the afferent vessels, pour the lymph into these extensive lymph-sinuses, hence to the central gland pulp of lymph-cells, and after being acted upon by these it reenters the lymph-sinuses in the deeper part of the gland, to pass out by the efferent vessels at the indented portion of the gland known as the hilum. The blood-vessels enter at the periphery and at the hilum, and are distributed partly for nutrition of the stroma, but principally as a fine capillary plexus to the gland pulp. The flow of lymph is considerably retarded by its passage through the meshwork of the lymph-sinuses, therefore foreign substances, such as coal pigment, or noxious substances of any kind, especially also bacteria, are liable to be arrested and deposited or destroyed in the sinuses. This is a matter of considerable pathologic importance, because by this barrier pathogenic organisms or floating foreign particles may be arrested here and prevented from entering as such, unaltered, into the general circulation. We may, therefore, truly call the lymphatic glands the great filter-beds of the tissue-juices of the body, without detracting from their other physiologic function, the possible destruction of, as well as regeneration of, the leucocytes.

Disease of the lymph and lymph vessels occurs, as we may surmise from their anatomy, more or less in disease of any tissue or organ, just as the blood must be more or less affected and altered by all dis-

[1] Read before the Louisville Clinical Society.

eases. But we still confine our subject only to those cases accompanied by distinct enlargements of the lymph-nodes. As to causation in general we may classify them as: (1) Enlargements of lymph-nodes due to infection and intoxication; (2) enlargements of lymph-nodes, about the cause of which we are still in the dark, and which until our knowledge increases we may call idiopathic; (3) enlargements of lymph-nodes due to new formations or tumors. The first named, due to infection and intoxication, form the largest and most frequent examples in general medicine and surgery, and occur principally in the form of inflammations of different intensity and duration, and are, therefore, spoken of as adenitis, or as hyperplasias following adenitis.

Irritants, possibly always bacteria or their toxic products, entering into certain areas of the tissues, will cause more or less trouble in the nearest lymph-node receiving the lymph or blood from the infected distal area. Examples of this kind are the adenitides following poisoned, *i. e.*, infected wounds, the inflammatory dermatoses, catarrhal or other inflammations of the mucous membranes, as tonsillitis, otitis, diphtheria, in fact all infective diseases, particularly those with mixed infection; typhoid fever, actinomycosis, glanders, leprosy, and those of a usually more chronic character, syphilitic adenitis and tubercular adenitis, either in the local form formerly described as scrofulous, or in the form of general tubercular adenitis. The effect, the violence of the inflammation, and the result upon the tissues of the gland will depend upon the quantity of the irritant and its virulence, upon the vital resistance of the individual infected, or both. Swelling, due to increased cell formation, is, however, present very soon in all cases. Lymphatic tissue is histologically constructed more like unripe embryonic tissue, and therefore responds very promptly to comparatively slight irritation by developing considerable hyperplasia. In severer forms we have the picture of active exudative inflammation, swelling, hyperemia, sometimes hemorrhage, increase of the cells of the pulp-tissue, the lymphoid cells and proliferation of larger cells most probably derived from the endothelium of the lymph-sinuses; many of the sinuses may be entirely clogged by new cells leading to a good deal of edema. Resolution may occur if Nature's forces and particularly the cells of the gland are able to conquer the enemy. In that case there will be more or less degeneration of the exudate, or the cells reenter the general circulation of the lymph. We may have, however, as in infections by virulent pyogenic bacteria, rapid destruction of the cells, suppuration, either local or general, in one or many foci of the gland infected, usually accompanied by a periadenitis, which latter is to be looked upon as an attempt at protection on the part of Nature—an attempt to limit the disease. These suppurating glands or buboes may break, or the contents may become inspissated, dried, cheesy, or later on infiltrated by calcareous salts and enclosed by a dense fibrous tissue.

The more chronic forms are characterized mainly by proliferation of connective tissue with a comparative and proportionate destruction of the cells, leading to considerable induration, frequently with a great deal of pigmentation derived either from the blood, or substances derived from without, such as coal, iron, etc., as so well illustrated in the diseased bronchial glands. Cheesy substance most commonly occurs in tubercular adenitis, but may occur as the product of any other inflammation, or in tumors of the glands. It is most common in the bronchial, mesenteric, mediastinal, retroperitoneal, and the cervical glands. Here also we may have single or multiple foci, and single glands or many at one time affected; we may have rupture, ulceration, or a most remarkable hyperplastic periadenitis and a gradual inspissation and calcification of the entire mass. Histologic tubercles may be found in the earlier stages, before the conglomeration and transformation into cheesy masses. So also may tubercle bacilli be found by careful examination, or they may not be found. This apparently paradoxical condition may be accounted for in two ways: either the bacilli originally infecting the gland have been destroyed, or the toxins of the bacilli alone had been absorbed and caused the glandular disease. Tubercular disease of other organs is most frequently found, except in the glandular tuberculosis of young children. Syphilitic adenitis is found early near the seat of the primary infection, and resembles the mild inflammatory type, or later on as general hyperplasia in different parts of the body, or in the tertiary stage as gummata.

As idiopathic lymphadenoid swellings of unknown origin we have the enlargements of the lymph-nodes in lymphatic leucemia and those of pseudoleucemia or Hodgkin's disease; the latter are, however, enlisted among the lymphosarcomata. The blood examination of the fresh and the stained cover-glass preparations enables us without any difficulty to make a differential diagnosis between these two. In the case of leucemia the large increase of the leucocytes, particularly the mononuclear forms, is at once apparent, while in pseudoleucemia the blood examination shows a more or less advanced oligocythemia and no numerical increase of the leucocytes. The diagnosis from tubercular adenitis is usually rendered possible by the existence of other foci of tubercular disease; again, tubercular adenitis usually involves the cervical as well as submaxillary glands, whereas in Hodgkin's disease the glands along the borders of the sternomastoid muscle are the first to be involved. Softening and suppuration with caseation is very common in tubercular glands, soon matting the different glands together by periadenitis, while in Hodgkin's disease there is but little tendency to suppuration, and the glands remain isolated and movable for a long time, and furthermore, there exists in the latter disease a marked tendency to rapid involvement of other glands, the axillary, cubital, inguinal, mediastinal, and retroperitoneal, accompanied by a rapidly increasing anemia.

Of the tumors found in the lymph-nodes are to be mentioned the occasional occurrence of myxoma, fibroma and chondroma; sarcoma occurring primarily as well as secondarily in the form of alveolar sarcoma, round-celled, spindle-celled and melanotic sarcoma. The most frequent secondary tumors are the carcinomata. The type of the cell and the general character will of course depend upon the primary tumor.

The treatment of lymphangitis would of course be to treat the cause, to overcome the bad effects of the cause as far as possible. That holds true of all diseases. Unfortunately, we find the same difficulty here as we do in the treatment of other diseases. First if we can remove the cause, as can be done in many instances where there is an infected wound, and thereby prevent the disease, that would be most desirable; if we cannot prevent, then we must try to remore the caure as far as we can. I believe in many instances we can remove the cause if we see the inflammatory condition very early. Such cases as we find in the dissecting-room teach us a valuable lesson, where the infecting material might have been removed by suction, cauterization, etc., or where the surgeon might have exercised precaution as far as possible in removing infectious material entering into the tissues. However, if we have an inflammation affecting directly the lymphatic channels, with enlarged lymph-nodes, etc., what are we to do? There is hardly a subject in the domain of medicine which will stimulate us to think more over the interesting methods of Nature to combat and overcome disease and especially the warring against micro-organisms than the one being considered, and we have a good opportunity to discuss the subject to-night.

If we sum up shortly the views entertained about the methods which Nature employs to protect the body against infection and to overcome the bad effects after infection has taken place, we may classify them as mechanical and chemical mechanism. As instances of mechanical mechanism against the entrance and development of bacteria we have the healthy mucous membranes, often endowed with specially favorable protective faculties, such as the ciliated epithelium, active glands whose secretion may act both mechanically and chemically, and the healthy skin. These two we may call the superficial filters or barriers. After the entrance and possible multiplication of bacteria within some focus in the body, such as a wound, etc., we must rely upon the deep filters, the tissues, particularly the blood, and the lymphatic system, to localize the infected material, to prevent their passage into the blood and to other parts of the body, and to destroy them. The lymph-nodes and the lymphatic system answer this purpose most admirably and in many instances successfully. While the exact methods of Nature are far from being clearly understood, experiments tend, more and more, to prove, that there are, in addition to these mechanical barriers, others, dependent upon active chemical substances which either are normally and constantly present in the body, or others, which are formed and given off by the tissue-cells whenever a noxious agent irritates them or endangers their life. As instances of the first variety we mention the protective albuminoid bodies found by Buchner in the blood, and called by him "alexins," identical with the "mycosozins" of Hankin. As to their source we know nothing definitely; Hankin thinks that they are products of the leucocytes. Others, as Kossel, Vaughan, and McClintock attribute to the nucleins or nucleinic acid present in large amount in the leucocytes an antibacterial action. Metschnikoff's phagocytosis may eventually prove to be mainly an attempt of Nature to send a highly vitalized movable enemy to the front, to attack, and if possible, to destroy, the invader. And the same holds true of the motile and the stationary leucocytes, such as we find in large quantity and constantly multiplying in the lymphatic system.

As an instance of newly formed chemical substances possessing bactericidal and antitoxic action we have the "antibodies" or "antitoxins" hitherto mainly gained from the blood. Where these antibodies are manufactured is still an open question. We may not go wrong, however, to propose that all the active cells of the body help to form them, and furthermore, that possibly different cells will be found to possess specific reaction against different bacteria. Recent and most highly interesting experiments by Ehrlich, R. Pfeiffer, Wassermann, and Takaki seem to throw new light upon the subject. Wassermann and Takaki found that extracts of normal brain and spinal cord possess a certain degree of protective power against tetanus infection, also that this protective power was greatly increased if the extract was prepared from brain and cord of animals some time after artificial infection by the tetanus poison, so much so that animals were immunized as well as cured. This immunizing substance must have been furnished by the nerve-cells, as extracts from other tissues of the same animals proved not to possess the same power against tetanus. So also in another series of experiments, extracts of the lymphatic tissue seemed to possess antagonistic properties against other infections, *i.e.*, typhoid.

Now to turn back to our subject of the evening: We see that the lymph system answers most admirably several of the above methods of Nature's protective mechanisms by furnishing a most excellent filter to arrest the bacteria, and secondly to furnish a large amount of highly vitalized cells which furnish a large quantity of specific antibodies. The higher the vitality of the organism in general the greater the natural resistance to disease.

In our treatment we should support the system, the vitality of the tissues, enabling Nature to employ her natural protective forces which we know must exist, else we would die from infective diseases. Support the system in the widest sense of the word, for we have all seen cases in which we thought the patient would succumb to the disease, and where Nature has made a gallant fight and won the victory. *Rest* is one of the most important features in connection with the treatment of inflammation of the lymphatics. We do not want to encourage dissemination of the poison by moving the limb or other part of the body, we want to keep it at rest. We furthermore must do what we can to destroy the poison at the point of entrance into the body. I believe here is the indication for the application of antiseptics. Outside of incision and removal of the infectious products, I believe antiseptics have a proper place. I have frequently employed injection into the tissues of antiseptics, mainly carbolic acid, with a view of lessening the active effect of the bacteria, or lessening their active reproduction. I am of the opinion that we get benefits by this method, not only by injection into the place locally, but secondarily into the lymph-nodes themselves. The main point, however, will be to support the system. We must use every means possible to sustain the vital forces; we want to stimulate and support glandular action to assist in getting rid of the poisonous products; we want to support the vital forces in order to develop healthy blood, healthy liquids; we must feed our patients well, attend to the functions of the skin, attend to the excretions of the body, keep the bowels open, see that the urine is passed properly, place the patient in the most favorable hygienic conditions, etc. All these we know are necessary to the elimination of poisonous products which have entered the body. I believe we have in the lymphatic system, however, the best natural barrier to all infective material. Nature has no better friend than these little gland nodes which interpose between the current of the juices of the body. Aside from constituting a most excellent filter, favoring the prolonged retention or arrest of infectious materal, they contain and regenerate constantly a large number of highly vitalized cells, which are possibly the greatest factors in destroying harmful substances which have entered the body, whatever may be the exact method of action of the gland and its cells, and for that reason we have in the lymph-nodes the very best possible means for Nature to help arrest them, not only to confine these noxious substances to a certain locality, but also directly locally to destroy them and counteract their poisonous products. We must agree that this occurs in many instances.

The treatment of lymphadenitis is practically the same as that just mentioned for lymphangitis. We treat the case as much as possible by preventing infection, and if infection has taken place we try to lessen the development of the poison at the primary site; and if it has entered into the lymph-nodes either in the form of living bacteria or of their poisonous products, which is frequently the case, and which are liable to cause similar results, we use remedies to lessen its virulence in the locality where we find it. I believe here, also, particularly in case of infection by pyogenic bacteria, antiseptic injections of a three-per-cent. solution of carbolic acid into the tissues is of benefit. Then we must wait to see whether suppuration takes place, or whether Nature has gained the fight. If abscesses occur, open them, and in many cases we might incise the gland, if we find even a small focus of suppuration, and use local antiseptic measures, still leaving the rest of the healthy gland undisturbed, giving Nature a chance to throw off as much of the enemy as possible.

Syphilitic enlargements are best treated by specific treatment, as we know. They may disappear spontaneously and recover without treatment; they will often rapidly disappear, especially the earlier enlargements, by antisyphilitic medication.

In the scrofulous or tuberculous glands, I think the most important consideration is the general management, general hygiene, attention in the widest sense of the word to the hygiene, to the feeding of the patient, to his sanitary surroundings and habits, next to that climate, medicine, etc., coming into play. As far as medication is concerned, the iodin preparations are still in vogue and are used to a great extent. Injections of various agents have also been advised, and in addition we have iron, arsenic, etc.; but it is questionable how much they will act, and whether we do not gain more by strengthening and supporting the system by other measures, hygienic as well as dietetic and climatic. As to specific medication, I would suggest the use of a reliable tubercle-serum. What we shall do with tuberculous glands is a question that has probably been considered by every one present. I must say that up to a comparatively recent date I have simply removed them early and thoroughly. I am now in doubt, from reports of operations within the last few years, whether this is the correct plan, and whether we ought not to wait and delay the removal of these glands until we see that Nature has lost the fight. By that I mean the breaking down of the gland tissue into a secondary mass of caseous substance. When that occurs I think it is proper to incise the gland and remove all the diseased tissue by curetting, but not to excise the gland unless we find upon examination that the entire gland has been destroyed. In the latter case, the gland has become a totally useless organ of the body, and a possible source ot further infection. Whether we remove all the glands in the immediate locality, granting that we have made a proper diagnosis, or only that which has broken down, is another question. I have seen rather discouraging results in the last few years from the removal of tuberculous glands. After the removal of the glands, some of which were softened, others which were not, I have seen rapid spread of the tuberculous process. I would suggest, therefore, as a good rule, to remove only those glands which are softened, leaving the others which are not markedly enlarged as a protective barrier to the inroad of the disease. If, in removing these glands, we are liable to invade structures not already diseased, as all surgeons know, there is a certain danger of causing a rapid dissemination ot the poison. There is danger of infecting other lymphatics which are deeper seated and out of reach.

As to tumors I shall have little to say. As to the lymphomata of leucocythemia, we are at a loss to explain the pathology, and in consequence little can be said of the etiologic treatment. We are still dependent upon internal remedies to build up the blood, improve aeration, etc. The same may be said of all the anemias, in which we give the patients iron, arsenic, etc. The same treatment applies to pseudoleucemia, or Hodgkin's disease. I have seen several cases of this kind in my experience, which were beautifully illustrative; the rule is that all these patients die; the case is really hopeless, because we know nothing about the etiology and consequently cannot apply intelligent treatment. If we adopt the more modern view and grant that these cases are malignant lymphomata, or, if we want to draw the line sharply between lymphoma and sarcoma, we have to agree with the surgeon that all these enlargements should be removed early, provided the diagnosis can be made early. This is not always possible. Later on we may have general dissemination of the disease, and although we might remove all the superficial lymphatic glands of the body, we could not cure our patient, because there would be glands affected beyond our reach.

As to the remedies which have been recommended: I have in some cases seen temporary benefit from arsenic, which, given in doses as large as can be tolerated by the patient, seems to have considerable effect upon not only the condition of the patient but the tumors themselves. It ought to be given both by the mouth and in gradually increasing doses injected directly into the tumors, beginning with two drops of Fowler's solution daily repeated. In the cases of simple tumors where the diagnosis can be made early, they had best be removed thoroughly by surgical means.

As regards carcinomata which are always secondary, histologically considered, the treatment is a surgical one entirely. The tumor should be thoroughly removed as early as possible, together with all the glands that are enlarged, and all others within the infected zone, because we have here to deal with a disease that Nature seems entirely unable to combat.

HEMATURIA.

BY L. J. HARVEY, M.D.,
OF GRIGGSVILLE, ILL.

BLOOD appears in the urine in a variety of conditions and is always of pathologic significance. Its source is the kidneys, bladder, or urethra, and may be the result of internal disease or external violence. For practical information it is necessary to know the source of the hematuria. In hemorrhage from the kidneys the urine is usually of a reddish-brown color, of acid reaction, of lowered specific gravity, and after standing, if the hemorrhage has been sufficient, there will be a "coffee-ground" deposit. Clots are usually absent, but if present, are of the long, slender rod-like variety, showing that they have been molded in passing through the ureters, but when the hemorrhage has been profuse clots may form after the blood reaches the bladder and appear in the urine irregular in shape. The recognition of blood-casts in the urine forms the most conclusive proof of the renal origin of hematuria, and the most frequent cause of this variety of hemorrhage is the class of diseases grouped under the term "Bright's disease," and in these cases it is usually slight. In malignant growth of the kidney the hematuria is often very pronounced and its appearance frequent, as in the following case:

Mr. B., a farmer, aged sixty years, had complained of a pain in the left lumbar region for several years, but of no great severity, and during these years had repeated attacks of polyuria. In May, 1891, after a hard day's work, he passed urine several times during the night, and in the morning was surprised and alarmed to find the contents of the night-vessel to consist largely of blood. During the two succeeding days the hematuria was profuse and the pain very severe, being well-marked renal colic. These attacks continued at irregular intervals for the succeeding year and a half. Shortly after the first appearance of the hematuria a well-marked tumor was discovered in the left lumbar region, which continued to grow as long as he lived. During all this time the hematuria was frequent and profuse, the clots often being so large as to cause great pain in their passage through the urethra; he also passed several small renal stones. These attacks would be followed by polyuria without pain or hemorrhage. Microscopic examination revealed only the presence of blood-corpuscles, and at no time was albumin or pus discovered. He became greatly emaciated and died from exhaustion two and a half years after the first appearance of the hematuria. An autopsy showed a large cancerous tumor involving the left kidney. The right kidney was normal.

A renal calculus will nearly always cause hematuria most marked on exercise, and in these cases pus is usually found also in the urine. Renal hematuria may also be caused by the use of certain drugs and toxic substances. In vesical hematuria the urine is usually alkaline in reaction and if cystitis of a chronic nature be present, we will find in the urine mucopus and triple phosphates. Stone in the bladder is probably a most frequent cause of vesical hematuria and the same condition is found in cases of cystitis affecting the neck of the bladder. In these cases the flow of blood usually follows the flow of urine, and in urethral hematuria the blood precedes the flow of urine, and also occurs between the acts of micturition.

As illustrative of vesical hematuria, I cite the following cases:

Mr. A., laborer, aged twenty-four years, twelve years ago had a stone removed from the bladder and since that time has been able to hold urine only two hours during the day or night. Three years ago he had retention of urine and hemorrhage of short duration. On the morning of April 30th, he complained of great pain in the bladder and tenderness over the prostate. He had passed some blood in the early morning. I gave him the usual remedies and ordered complete rest; in two hours I was again called and found him suffering greatly from complete retention, and on passing a catheter, under an anesthetic, withdrew a small quantity of urine in which the proportion of blood was large, with several small irregular clots. Blood followed the withdrawal of the catheter, and the subsequent passage of the catheter through the prostatic portion of the urethra caused great pain. The hematuria continued for about ten days, at times slight and again profuse. I suspected the presence of a stone, but before I had an opportunity to make an examination he passed from under my observation.

Another patient, a farmer, aged fifty years, suffered similarly. In this case the hematuria was well marked, but was preceded only by slight irritation at the base of the bladder and some tenderness of the prostate; there was no fever, but the patient was much agitated by the hematuria; no marked pain; no retention; small clots frequently passed. This condition continued for about two weeks. The patient is now well.

In both these last-mentioned cases, the clear blood followed the flow of urine, which, with other symptoms pointed to the neck of the bladder as the source of the hematuria.

WAR ARTICLES.

NEWS OF THE WEEK.

THE past week has been perhaps less remarkable for events than any week since the beginning of the war. Even the "yellow journals" have been unable to hatch out of their prolific news incubators an item of sufficient importance to warrant its announcement in the customary four-inch block letters, even though it were contradicted or pronounced "a rumor" in an obscure corner of the same paper in small pica. Perhaps one of the "lessons of the war" will bear very directly upon the science of manufacturing startling war news and the business that may be done in selling the consequent "extras."

. . . .

However, if battles have not been fought on land or sea, movements of great importance have taken place, and doubtless by the time this number of the MEDICAL NEWS is in the reader's hands, some decisive results will have been attained by the detachment of the regular army now landing on Cuban soil, in time let us hope, to succor the brave little band of marines, which with such grim determination is holding the ground against Spanish guerrillas under a fierce tropical sun. Probably there was some good and tangible reason for sending this band of 600 brave marines ashore to face such odds of foe and such dangers of climate, and yet the unsophisticated non-military man is prone to wonder whether or not a delay of a few days until the reinforcements *en route* were at least in sight would have interfered with the tacticians' plans to the value of the lives of the brave lads who have already fallen under the Spanish balls.

. . . .

Two weeks ago we called attention in this column to the great velocity of the projectiles of modern rifles, and remarked that an interesting study would be that of the wounds produced by these weapons. It is of interest to note in this connection that Major Goode, who was killed by a bullet from a Mauser rifle near Guantanamo Bay, evidently did not know when he was hit, for he walked several steps before he fell dead. His immediate comrades were also unaware of his receiving any wound.

. . . .

Medical and surgical preparations having been made on such a large scale for the preventive and curative treatment of yellow fever, dysentery, and similar tropical ailments, it seems like a bit of grim jesting on the part of disease that it should manifest itself in an outbreak of measles such as has occurred at Camp Merritt. The epidemic is growing at the rate of about twenty new cases daily, but no fatal cases nor complications beyond one or two instances of mumps have been reported.

. . . .

It is not a difficult matter to compile a set of rules for protection against yellow fever, malarial fever, dysentery, etc., but when it comes to enforcing upon an army the carrying out of these rules in a measure sufficiently great to be effective the task is by no means easy or simple. The result of the climate and general unhygienic conditions upon General Shafter's army, provided as it is with Surgeon-General Sternberg's excellent and far-reaching preventive directions, will be watched with more anxiety and interest than the movements of the Spanish soldiery.

. . . .

It would seem reasonable to suppose that the officers of every grade should be required to assist in the task of compelling a continued, regular, and thorough carrying-out of the very practical regulations which have been adopted for the preservation of the health of the men, and it certainly will be a task. The soldiers will suffer more from their own carelessness and imprudence than from any other causes, and the authorities must be prepared to enforce the most exact and scrupulous attention to every detail in sanitary and preventive measures.

. . . .

Fortunately and intentionally the Cuban army of invasion is almost entirely made up of regular troops, men who are accustomed to campaign life and military discipline, and who will from experience more readily appreciate the dangers of disease in the ranks and the necessity for every hygienic and sanitary precaution. Had General Shafter's army been composed of volunteers or of National Guardsmen the difficulties and dangers would have been increased many fold. These branches of the army must follow later into Cuba, Puerto Rico, or the Philippines, but during their delay they are rapidly being disciplined and coached in these matters which are decidedly more important that an ability to cope with Spanish maneuvers and Spanish troops.

. . . .

Dr. Benjamin Lee has contributed to *Outlook* the following: "There is one phase of the Spanish iniquity in Cuba which is rarely touched upon. Nine years ago, visiting Florida with a few other sanitarians, I ran over to Havana in order to study the health conditions of that fair but insufferably filthy city. So deeply impressed was I by the truth that so long as the Spaniard ruled in Cuba Havana would continue to be a plague-spot, that, at the meeting of the American Public Health Association in Brooklyn the following autumn, I maintained the thesis that the sanitary interests of the United States demanded the annexation of Cuba. No so-called civilized government has a right to maintain a pestiferous nuisance at her neighbor's doors. Our Government will be false to its duty and its traditions if it does not abate this nuisance effectively and permanently in both regards. In this connection I call to your notice the resolutions unanimously adopted by the Associated Health Authorities and Sanitarians of Pennsylvania, at the annual meeting held recently at the City of Lancaster. The chief points in these resolves are the following:

"'WHEREAS, in consequence of the entire neglect of Spanish authorities on the island of Cuba to inaugurate and enforce such sanitary laws and regulations as exist in civilized countries, the diseases of smallpox, yellow fever, typhus fever, and leprosy constantly prevail unchecked in that island; and, as the proximity of Cuba to the United State, and the intimate commercial relations of the two countries, the conditions referred to constitute a constant menace to the public health of this country, involving anxiety, pecuniary loss, and, in repeated instances, serious loss of life. Therefore, be it

"'*Resolved*, That no settlement of the pending difference between the United States and Spain will be satisfactory to the sanitarians of this country which does not insure to the United States the absolute control of the sanitary conditions of the island of Cuba.'"

THE FIELD-HOSPITAL SYSTEM.

[Special Correspondence of the MEDICAL NEWS.]

PORT TAMPA, FLA., June 15, 1898.

THE field-hospital system put in operation by the troops mobilized at Tampa has in part been evolved by the exigencies of the situation. The regulars took the field with a complete, though small, hospital equipment for each regiment, *i. e.*, a medical officer, a detachment of the hospital corps, including a hospital steward, one or two ambulance wagons, with their outfit of medical and surgical chests, litters, and tents, field cots, bedding, and other requisites for the regimental hospital. This system, adequate for the need of a small force, was tried during the Civil War and proved inadequate for efficient service of an army. It lacked the power of combination and concentration for dealing with large numbers of disabled combatants in the radius of action of a single brigade or division.

In order to meet the requirements of field service and battle, expansion has been provided for as follows: The regimental hospitals were ordered to be skeletonized, a minimum number of their *personnel* and a minimum quantity of *matériel* being retained. The major parts were ordered turned over to chief surgeons of divisions for organization into divisional field hospitals under a surgeon in charge. In addition, the men thus collected became the companies of the hospital corps under the command of another medical officer, and the ambulance wagons thus concentrated, with the addition of other transportation, became the ambulance train under the command of another medical officer. These divisional officers are under the immediate direction of the chief surgeon of the corps, on a plan similar to the organization of an artillery corps. By this arrangement the regiments are largely relieved of the care of their sick and wounded, emergency patients only being treated in the reduced regimental hospitals, from which in case of serious disability they are promptly sent to the divisional field hospital by detachments from the ambulance-train and hospital-corps companies.

The advantages inherent in this system are apparent. It was readily put into operation by the division of regulars. More difficulty attends its development among the volunteers; the lack of provision in their organization for the creation of a hospital corps of trained men and the want of uniformity in their hastily collected medical supplies obstructing it. These organic difficulties are, however, being rapidly overcome by various expedients. With an impending movement of the troops the field hospitals are now being rapidly relieved of their accumulated disabled men by transfer by rail or steamer to the general hospitals improvised to receive them at various points in the interior.

In order to deal with the casualties of battle regimental surgeons will direct the operations of collecting wounded at the first-aid stations in the immediate vicinity of the combatants and the application of temporary dressings. From these points they will be moved to the field hospitals by litters or ambulances, according to the prevailing conditions, or as the field-hospital appliances for the immediate surgical operations demanded are available, with food, drink, and restoratives. From the field hospitals the movement of the wounded will be begun and continued according to the urgency of the situation in each case.

What amount of first-aid service can there be rendered in battle on the firing-line? This question involves the personal equation of both the wounded and first-aided. Generally when a man is struck by a missile, if he be conscious of his injury, and he often is not, his first impulse is to reach a place of comparative safety in the rear, where he can obtain succor. He will as a rule be unwilling to have his wound bound up under fire. On the part of the surgeon it is evident that there is neither time nor facilities for deliberate work and that even for the effective use of a first-aid packet it would be well to provide that the wounded man be not killed by a second shot while the wreckage of the first is on hand. But there are cases, fewer perhaps than many suppose, where the immediate arrest of bleeding from a large blood-vessel will decide the fate of some whose only hope lies in prompt assistance given without regard to surrounding conditions.

KAPPA.

TROPICAL DISEASES AND INJURIES; MOUNTS; WHEEL TRANSPORTATION; TENTAGE.

[Special Correspondence of the MEDICAL NEWS.]

TAMPA, FLA., June 12, 1898.

THROUGH the agency of reprints and oral instruction in the field by men who have had a wide observation and large experience with tropical diseases, the medical officers of the United States forces are becoming thoroughly informed upon the character, prevention, and therapy of those diseases which they will be forced to confront upon Cuban soil. Quite recently Professor John Guitéras and Dr. Moreno de la Torre have lectured to us in the open air, the former on yellow fever, regarding which I have already sent you notes, and the latter more particularly on other common diseases prevalent in Cuba. Dr. de la Torre has contracted to go with us. He formerly practised in the city of Havana and was clinical assistant at the Havana Hospital, having been appointed by the faculty of the University. He has also practised his profession at Cardenas in the Province of Matanzas.

In a very earnest manner, but with quite a foreign accent and somewhat characteristic gesticulations, Dr. de la Torre discussed the subjects of tetanus, malignant pustule, dysentery, diphtheria, etc. In Cuba tetanus is a very common disease. He said he felt very much pained in having to assure us that this disease is likely to be as terrible in its ravages among troops campaigning actively in Cuba and exposed to so many sources of vulnerability as is yellow fever, the source of infection in the latter being in a large measure avoidable by proper precautions, while the bacillus of tetanus finds its way into many unavoidably infected wounds and not infrequently attacks wounds hardly macroscopic in size. Malignant pustule or anthrax is another disease not infrequently met with, the specific bacillus finding entrance through fissures of the lips or other common abrasions or more palpable wounds.

The treatment advised in tetanus and anthrax is practically one and the same. If the wound can be found, practise deep incision into the tissues, laying them well open; then cauterize with the actual cautery and pack with powdered corrosive sublimate. It is said there is no danger of poisoning from the mercuric salt on account of absorption being prevented through its cauterizing effect on the raw tissues.

Another very common and fatal disease in Cuba is dysentery. Its morbidity and mortality greatly exceed those of yellow fever. Give plenty of Seidlitz powder and use rectal injections of hydrogen peroxid, with a most abstemious diet.

Among the insects to be dreaded stands preeminently the pulex penetrans or "nigua." Its trauma often leads to tetanus. As soon as one begins to feel the itching or stinging sensation from penetration of this insect and can detect a black speck upon the skin, extract it at once and treat the wound with kerosene oil or carbolic acid. If allowed to remain for two days one must be careful in attempting to extract the insect lest its body be torn and the ova escape, which after maturing will migrate into the tissues and set up cellulitis.

The mosquito is a fruitful source of discomfort and is regarded by Dr. de la Torre as the chief caravansary of the malarial plasmodium to the human organism. Mosquito bars, to be effective against this intruder and other smaller but hardly less annoying insectivora, must be very close-meshed, but this likewise obstructs free egress and ingress of the air. To obviate the use of netting at night when occupying a tent Dr. de la Torre has found the slow combustion of a small quantity of powdered pyretheum or Persian insect powder to be most effective.

Colonel Charles R. Greenleaf, Assistant Surgeon-General, U. S. A., and Chief Surgeon, Army in the Field, has perfected a plan of sanitary organization for the troops in the field, which I give in tabular form below. The tables "represent numerically the distribution of the personnel of the medical department and the relative proportion of the necessary wheel transportation and tentage of the combatant force." These tables are computed for a volunteer army corps of about 25,000 men, while the sanitary organization of a corps of the regular establishment, or one differing in the combatant strength, should be based upon this ratio.

Sanitary subdivisions of a volunteer army corps (about 25,000 combatant strength based upon present organization), *viz.*, twenty-four regiments of infantry, 3 light batteries, and 1 regiment of cavalry.

	Medical Officers.	Hospital Stewards.	Acting Hospital Stewards.	Privates.	Total for Corps. M.D.	H.S.	A.H.S.	Privates.
Each regiment of Infantry ..	1	1	0	1	24	24	0	24
Each Artillery Battalion (3 Lt. Bat.)	1	0	3	1	1	0	3	1
Each regiment of Cavalry ...	2	1	0	2	2	1	0	2
Total with Troops					27	25	3	27
Administration.								
1 Corps	2	1	0	2	2	1	0	2
3 Divisions	1	1	0	1	3	3	0	3
9 Brigades	1	0	0	1	9	0	0	9
Total with Administration					14	4	0	14
3 Division Ambulance Corps and 1 Corps Reserve Company, each ..	6	7	3	104	24	28	12	416
3 Division Field Hospitals (of 200 beds, each) and 1 Corps Reserve Hospital, each ...	6	6	3	90	24	24	12	360
					48	52	24	776
Unassigned ...	0	2	2	0	0	2	2	0
Grand Total					89	83	29	817

Relative proportion of the necessary wheel transportation and tentage to the combatant force of an army corps:

For wheel transportation: One ambulance to 400 men, 1 army wagon to 600 men, and 1 escort wagon to each brigade.

For tentage: One hospital tent to 300 men, and 1 common tent to 1200 men.

To illustrate the utility of the table for personnel it might be asked how many medical officers are allowed to a division of nine regiments of infantry. One medical officer for each regiment of infantry makes 9, 1 to the division adds 1, 1 to each brigade adds 3, while 6 each for the division field ambulance corps, and division field hospital adds 12, making a total of 25. According to the above schedule, the medical department in its various lines of activity will be represented by 1015 men in an army corps of 25,000 combatant strength, or about 4 per cent.. The wheel transportation, tentage, and animals pertaining to the medical department of an army corps under its own care and direction will be approximately, 62 ambulances, 41 army wagons, 9 escort wagons, 82 hospital tents, 20 common tents, 448 mules, and 201 mounts for hospital stewards, acting hospital stewards, and medical-officers' orderlies.

HENRY I. RAYMOND, M.D.,
Captain and Assistant Surgeon, U. S. A.

MEDICAL PROGRESS.

Sudden Death from an Immunizing Dose of Antitoxin.—NIFONG (*Med. Review*, May 7, 1898) mentions a death following injection of an immunizing dose of diphtheria antitoxin. The patient, a lad aged fifteen, of slight build and poor circulation, after an exposure to diphtheria, complained of sore throat. The tonsils were slightly enlarged and the throat was red. He was given an injection of between three and four cubic centimeters of antitoxin, strength 1500 units. Two girls were given similar injections from the same bottle without any bad results whatever. Within ten minutes of the time of the injection the boy became pale and complained of numbness of the extremities. Later he became cyanosed, his face swelled, and he vomited freely. An injection of nitroglycerin was given and artificial respiration was resorted to, but death followed thirty-five minutes after the antitoxin was given. The fluid used was furnished by the city chemist of St. Louis.

THERAPEUTIC NOTES.

Koplik's New Sign of Measles.—SLAWYK (*Deut. Med. Wochenschr.*, April 28, 1898) is astonished that no one should have noticed until recently the early eruption which occurs on the mucous membrane of the lips and cheeks in measles, as described by Koplik of New York, and which is said to be absolutely characteristic of the disease. The sign is of especial importance in asylums and hospitals for children, where, as is well known, the mortality in epidemics of measles is far higher than is seen in private practice, often reaching thirty per cent. or higher, and where children not unfrequently suffer from repeated attacks of the disease.

During the past winter there were brought into the Charité Hospital in Berlin fifty-two cases of measles, and the sign referred to was found to be present in forty-five of them. There developed in the hospital itself thirty-two cases, and in all but one of these the characteristic spots were found. Slawyk thus describes the eruption: The Koplik spots are round, slightly raised, bluish-white efflorescences, having minute red centers. They measure from 0.2–0.6 mm. (.01–.03 inch), and are situated upon the inner surfaces of the cheeks, less often upon the mucous membrane of the lips, and rarely (in one instance) upon the tongue. They may occur on one or both sides, most often in the vicinity of the back teeth, and the usual number is from six to twenty, though hundreds may be present. They may be seen in daylight, or by a strong incandescent light. These spots never run together, and cannot be rubbed off. They are not to be mistaken for any other eruption in the mouth.

Treatment of Anemia with Hot Baths.—ROSIN (*Centralbl. f. inner. Med.*, April 30, 1898) has used hot baths in more than fifty cases of anemia in patients who for the most part had been under medical treatment without benefit. A bath at 104° F. is given three times a week. Its duration should not exceed fifteen minutes, and at its close the patient should be douched with cool water. The immediate effect of such a bath is a feeling of lightness in the individual, and in four weeks or a less time there is a noticeable improvement in the general condition. Hot baths are taken daily by a large part of the people of Japan, as is well known.

Chronic Affections of the Heart Muscle.—At the Congress for Internal Medicine, held at Wiesbaden in April last, SCHOTT of Nauheim read a paper upon the condition of the muscle of the heart in chronic diseases of the organ. Myocarditis and fat metamorphoses are far more frequently found in cardiac diseases than is generally supposed. The latter especially is found as a result of mental and physical exhaustion, the use of alcohol, tobacco, etc.

Treatment has in the very first instance to meet this muscular insufficiency. Of drugs directed to this end there is none that surpasses digitalis. Schott then took up the diatetic-balneologic-mechanical treatment, and explained the differences between Oertel's hill-climbing, Zander's machine gymnastics, and the Schott method of treatment by graduated exercises. The exactness with which the latter can be regulated and the ease of its application are decided points in its favor. There are contraindications to any mechanical treatment, *viz.*, aneurism of the heart or great vessels, advanced arteriosclerosis, and conditions in which there is danger of cerebral hemorrhage or embolism. By means of a great number of radiograms it was clearly shown that in not too advanced cases gymnastics are capable of bringing about stronger cardiac contractions, and also a diminution in the size of the organ, even in cases of valvular disease with secondary muscular changes. In one case of advanced myocarditis with an aortic aneurism it was shown that the gymnastic exercises had greatly dilated the aneurismal sac.

THE MEDICAL NEWS.

A WEEKLY JOURNAL OF MEDICAL SCIENCE.

COMMUNICATIONS are invited from all parts of the world. Original articles contributed *exclusively* to THE MEDICAL NEWS will after publication be liberally paid for (accounts being rendered quarterly), or 250 reprints will be furnished in place of other remuneration. When necessary to elucidate the text, illustrations will be engraved from drawings or photographs furnished by the author. Manuscripts should be typewritten.

Address the Editor: J. RIDDLE GOFFE, M.D.,
No. 111 FIFTH AVENUE (corner of 18th St.), NEW YORK.

Subscription Price, including postage in U. S. and Canada.

PER ANNUM IN ADVANCE	$4.00
SINGLE COPIES	.10
WITH THE AMERICAN JOURNAL OF THE MEDICAL SCIENCES, PER ANNUM	7.50

Subscriptions may begin at any date. The safest mode of remittance is by bank check or postal money order, drawn to the order of the undersigned. When neither is accessible, remittances may be made, at the risk of the publishers, by forwarding in *registered* letters.

LEA BROTHERS & CO.,
No. 111 FIFTH AVENUE (corner of 18th St.), NEW YORK, AND NOS. 706, 708 & 710 SANSOM ST., PHILADELPHIA.

SATURDAY, JUNE 25, 1898.

A MEDICAL DUTY.

IN May, 1900, will occur in the city of Washington, the eighth decennial convention to direct the revision of the United States Pharmacopœia. All medical colleges and State medical societies will be invited to send delegates. It is rather to the discredit of the medical profession that the pharmacal delegates to the convention of 1890 outnumbered the medical, whereas the Pharmacopœia was originated by, and for some years revised entirely under the direction of, the medical profession. A very noticeable feature in the convention of 1890 was the large number of pharmaceutical societies represented by delegates in contrast to the comparatively small number of medical societies so represented. The colleges of medicine were only fairly represented, being exceeded by colleges of pharmacy.

The advantage of a large pharmacal influence in the revision of the book is apparent in the great improvements made in the last two editions; but, in view of the tendency to delegate its issue more and more to the pharmacist, it may be proper now to remind the medical profession that it is a book that we cannot afford to neglect. No book in the physician's library represents more of careful effort in preparation and no other is issued from motives so entirely disinterested. And when we reflect that it furnishes the standard for purity and strength of our drugs and preparations and that it is the basis for all our text-books on materia medica, the wonder is that the physician's library so seldom contains it. But our attitude in this respect corresponds to the present reprehensible tendency in our therapeutics to use whatever is brought to us in shape for easy administration, without much regard to purity or reliability.

It may be said that, with the tablet triturate in such a variety of combinations and the "elegant" pharmaceuticals with which we are daily sampled, many physicians do not need the Pharmacopœia. The manufacturing chemist (?) supplies all their wants. But unless we are to lose entirely the art of prescribing, it is imperative that a better appreciation of the aims, the standard character, and the resources of the Pharmacopœia be cultivated. The colleges are lax in their obligation to this book. It is not commonly found among their text-books and it must be confessed that some teachers of therapeutics do not know the difference between the United States Pharmacopœia and the United States Dispensatory.

There is need of greater independence, on the part of the rising generation of physicians, in the knowledge of drugs and how to combine and use them. A closer acquaintance with the Pharmacopœia will beget such independence.

But while our profession may be thus justly arraigned there is another side to the discussion. It is claimed, and very properly claimed by some, that the Pharmacopœia is of insufficient practical value to command the attention of the practitioner. To some extent this must be true of any book possessing the unyielding character of a standard. But is not the apathy of the profession largely responsible for the book remaining deficient in practical value? Reasonable demands for modification in the direction of the practical daily needs of the physician will certainly receive proper consideration in the coming pharmacopœial convention and there is still time for full discussion of any suggestions that may be made.

We are pleased to note that the Medical Society of the State of New York, through a committee on United States Pharmacopoeia, is doing work along needed lines and it is hoped that other State societies will follow its example. In the first annual report of this committee several items were presented for discussion during the year. Among them we note the following which appears to us to be particularly worthy of consideration: "That a section (of the Pharmacopœia) be devoted to giving reliable information concerning new remedies, without making them in any sense official; and that an annual supplement be issued for the purpose of continuing the same kind of information."

We sympathize with those who say that the Pharmacopœia ought to contain someting more practical. We are to-day simply deluged with new substances of uncertain value. All we know about them is what their manufacturers tell us. Where are we to obtain reliable information upon which to base our opinions as to their probable value? There is no disinterested source of such information.

The Committee of Revision of the United States Pharmacopœia, with an extension of its powers, would be just the body to direct the research necessary to furnish us information concerning new remedies, which need not thereby be made in any sense "official." Indeed, in case of certain substances the information might be condemnatory. If the committee were to issue a small annual supplement of that character it would, in our opinion, lead to a speedy recognition by many more physicians of the place and value of the Pharmacopœia; and if the supplements could not be obtained except by purchasing the book, we predict that there would be a great increase in the sale of the latter, which in turn would furnish means for carrying on the necessary research work.

ECHOES AND NEWS.

Suicide in a Hospital.—A patient at a Brooklyn hospital, recovering from a serious operation, recently committed suicide by jumping out of a window while delirious. He was terribly injured and died within half an hour.

The Pasteur Monument.—M. Falguière has recently completed the monument of Pasteur and it is soon to be erected opposite the Pantheon in Paris. The cost was met by an international subscription which reached $80,000.

Portrait of Dr. McLane.—The Faculty of the College of Physicians and Surgeons, the medical department of Columbia University, New York, presented to that university a portrait of Dr. James W. McLane, Dean of the College, on the occasion of his retirement from the chair of obstetrics which he held for twenty-five years.

Emergency Kits for the Army.—Among the field supplies recently shipped to Tampa are 60,000 emergency kits, consisting of two compresses, one roller bandage, and one triangular bandage, done up in a waterproof package. They cost 13 cents each. It is expected that the triangular bandage in particular will be useful in caring for a wounded soldier on the field at a distance from the surgeon.

A Generous Offer.—Mr. David H. King, Jr., of New York, has offered to the Government the use of his residence and estate on Jekyl Island, off Brunswick, Ga., without cost or restriction, as a military hospital until the close of the war. Jekyl Island is owned by a club and is rarely visited by any but its members. Half a million of dollars have been expended upon it and it has been transformed, from dreary sand and rioting foliage, into a beautiful pleasure ground. The residence is a new and handsome one and would form an ideal convalescent hospital for wounded soldiers and sailors.

A New Army Biscuit.—Dr. Barré has recently had manufactured a new biscuit for the French Army. It is made by adding thirty-three parts of gluten to one hundred parts of wheat flour and a small quantity of fat. The bread is baked in the oven, then broken, and the crumbs made in the shape of a small biscuit by means of a hydraulic press, a small quantity of sugar syrup being added to make the biscuit of the proper consistency. This new army ration is intended to be used only in time of war, but the Academy of Medicine believes that it should also be a regular article of consumption for the reserve forces.

Court Martial for a Naval Surgeon.—The news comes from Washington that Assistant-Surgeon D. H. Morgan, now at the Norfolk Navy Yard, is to be tried on charges of culpable inefficiency in the performance of duty and disrespect to his superior officer. Dr. Morgan was attached to the cruiser "Cincinnati" and is accused of having allowed three sick men to remain for an hour upon the wharf, to the detriment of their health, awaiting their transfer to the "Cincinnati." Upon being informed by his superior that he had been reported for neglect of duty, he was most disrespectful to him, hence the additional charge.

Memorial Service to Dr. Gibbs.—A service in memory of Dr. John Blair Gibbs, Assistant-Surgeon, United States Navy, who was killed in battle at Guantanamo Bay, Cuba, June 12th, was held at Trinity Church, New York City, Thursday, June 23d, at one o'clock. Many resolutions expressive of the deep sorrow experienced upon the news of Dr. Gibbs' death have been engrossed by the various clubs and hospitals with which he was connected, and the service at Trinity Church, which was largely attended by his former friends both in the profession and in other walks of life, gave expression to the high esteem and honor in which Dr. Gibbs was held by all who knew him.

OBITUARY.

R. C. M. PAGE, M.D.

DR. RICHARD CHANNING MOORE PAGE of New York died early Sunday morning, June 19th, at Philadelphia, from a stroke of apoplexy. He had been ill for some weeks and was returning home from a brief outing which he had allowed himself.

Dr. Page was descended from one of the most distinguished families of Virginia. The pioneer of the family, John Page, who settled in Virginia in 1689, was a son of Francis Page of Bedfont, Middlesex County, England, and was a member of the Royal Colonial Council of the Province of Virginia. His descendants occupied prominent positions in the government of the Province, and later took up arms against the mother country and did valiant work during the War of Independence—both in the councils of the colony and in the field.

At the outbreak of the Civil War Dr. Page was a student in the University of Virginia. He abandoned his books and enlisted as a private in Pendleton's Rockbridge Battery, attached to Stonewall Jackson's Brigade. He showed such devotion to duty and courage in action that he was promptly promoted to Lieutenant, Captain, and finally Major of Artillery. He was present at many of the important battles which were fought on Virginian soil, and commanded all the artillery at the famous Bloody Angle at Spottsylvania. A severe wound received at the battle of Gettysburg incapacitated him for a brief period.

At the close of the war Page came to New York and entered the New York University Medical School, and later served on the staff of Bellevue Hospital and the Woman's Hospital.

At the organization of the New York Polyclinic Medical School and Hospital, Dr. Page, with the late Dr. Hudson, became an assistant to Professor Leaming. In 1889 he was elected Professor of General Medicine at this school, which position he held at the time of his death.

Dr. Page has left his impress upon the minds of the medical profession more especially as a teacher of medicine. He had the happy faculty, not only of presenting a subject with clearness and comprehension, but also of impressing it upon the minds of his students in so forceful a manner that it was never forgotten. In the capacity of a teacher he won the personal gratitude and regard of all who came within the sphere of his influence, and in his association with his fellow-practitioners was the soul of honor and rectitude.

He was a member of the County Medical Society, the State Medical Society, the Southern Society, Society of Medical Jurisprudence, Sons of the Revolution, New York Pathological Society, Medical and Surgical Society, American Historical Society, Women's Hospital Society, Bellevue Hospital Alumni Association, and the New York Academy of Medicine, in the latter institution serving recently as First Vice-President. He was the author of the well-known text-book on "Practice" and a work on "Physical Diagnosis."

He married Mrs. Mary Fitch Winslow of Bridgeport, Conn., who survives him. He leaves no children.

CORRESPONDENCE.

OUR PHILADELPHIA LETTER.

[From our Special Correspondent.]

MEETING OF THE PHILADELPHIA CHAPTER OF JEFFERSON COLLEGE ALUMNI—MEETING OF THE PEDIATRIC SOCIETY—MEETING OF THE SECTION OF GENERAL MEDICINE, COLLEGE OF PHYSICIANS—OHIO'S NEW STATE CHEMIST—STATE BOARD EXAMINATIONS—HEALTH-BOARD STATISTICS FOR THE WEEK.

PHILADELPHIA, June 21, 1898.

THE Philadelphia Chapter of the Alumni Association of Jefferson Medical College held a scientific meeting Thursday evening, June 16th, at which Dr. John B. Roberts read a paper, entitled "Surgical Treatment of Deformities of the Eyelids, Nose, and Mouth." He illustrated his subject with blackboard sketches which were remarkable for the dexterity with which they were executed and for the clear outline they gave of the speaker's conception of the various procedures. He called attention to the simplicity of operations of this character and to the gratitude of patients to whom relief is afforded. A particularly grateful class are those suffering from strabismus; in this operation bulging of the eye often results from pressure by the severed rectus muscle and this bulging forces the lids apart giving one eye the appearance of being larger than its fellow. For the relief of this condition or for the protrusion seen in exophthalmic goiter, he denudes the lids at the external canthus and by means of vertical sutures "pinches in" the eye or eyes. When one eye is smaller than the other from atrophy, congenital blindness or other causes, severing the recti will bulge the eye out, force the lids apart and thus make it appear larger, or the same result may be accomplished by a double convex lens to magnify the small eye.

He illustrated also various operations for burns, the restoration of lids, etc., by means of flaps, and spoke of tattooing for leucoma. For protruding lips seen in many persons, notably "mouth-breathers," he removes a V-shaped wedge, taking care to go deep into the muscles, the neglect of which is responsible for many failures. The method for restoring the alveolar process of the superior maxilla in cases of hare-lip is as follows: Saw through the alveolar process on either side including one tooth, bring the pieces together in the median line by wire and thus obliterate the cleft; the newly formed spaces in time and with the growth of the jaw, fill in with new tissue, and if the teeth are permanently destroyed, which happens sometimes in adult life, the defect is remedied by artificial ones.

Dr. George E. de Schweinitz endorsed the speaker's method of treating "bulging" eyes, but said with modern operations for strabismus, this should never occur. As to tattooing he spoke of the washing-out of dyes and to avoid this he soaks a piece of India ink in water until it forms a soapy mass, and after spreading this upon the cornea he tattooes, the result proving entirely satisfactory.

In operating about the eye for burns he uses the already unsightly cicatricial tissue and thus avoids scars; for ectropion and trichiasis no external scars are apparent and for lotions he uses warm physiologic salt solution.

Dr. Joseph W. Hearn said he uses no dressings about the mouth as saliva lodges under them. He incidently called attention to the resistance to infection which the face enjoys as compared to the rest of the body, explaining it on the ground that the muscles of the face run transversely to the connective tissue. He uses silver wire sutures and a subcuticular stitch when possible, and in operating for hare-lip in children allowance must be made for the fact that scar-tissue does not grow. For flat or "saddle" noses a gold plate is most satisfactory, and in a case recently operated upon he dissected up the lip and soft tissues of the nose thus inserting the plate without leaving any external scar, and the result proved very satisfactory.

Dr. D. Braden Kyle believes that the thick lip seen in "mouth-breathers" will disappear when the obstruction to nasal breathing is removed. Dr. Roberts closed the discussion after endorsing the use of salt solution.

The following officers were elected for the ensuing year: President, Dr. A. Hewson; vice-presidents, Drs. Carrol, Woolf, Buckley, Davidson, Skillern, Webb, Carrell, and Hoskins; corresponding secretary, Dr. J. Salinger; recording secretary, Dr. W. M. Sweet; treasurer, Dr. J. A. Cantrell. The Association then adjourned to become the guests of Dr. Joseph S. Neff.

A meeting of the Pediatric Society was held Tuesday evening, June 14th. Dr. Meyer presented for Dr. Alfred Stengel, a case of "Chronic Lead-poisoning." The subject, a boy four and one-half years old, exhibited well-marked signs of emaciation, pallor, loss of knee-jerk, and a blue line around the gums.

Dr. Alfred Hand, Jr., followed with a case of "Essential Tremor" occurring in a negro child thirteen months old. Malnutrition probably caused the lateral to and fro movement of the head from which the child suffered, and it is interesting to note that these cases, in contrast to congenital idiopathic tremors, recover.

Dr. A. F. Witmer exhibited a case of "Hemiparesis Following Epileptic Convulsions" and a photograph showing a large subcutaneous hemorrhage of the face following a single epileptic attack in a woman.

Dr. S. M. Hamill reported a case of Dr. Faries, "Sarcoma of the Kidney of Unusual Size." The tumor which weighed 6580 grams (about 14 pounds) occurred in a child five years of age, the condition having been diagnosed as sarcoma of the retroperitoneal glands.

Dr. B. K. Chance read for Dr. W. H. Price, "Two Cases of Simultaneous Triple Infection." Both children were members of the same family and exhibited the phenomena of pertussis, varicella, and parotiditis, while a third child in the family escaped the parotiditis but had varicella and pertussis.

Dr. E. E. Graham followed with a "Report of Two Cases of Intussusception and a Case of General Peritonitis Following Appendicitis; Operation and Recovery." In the first case no blood or mucus was found in the stools nor could any tumor be felt; the child died after operation from a general sepsis induced by continuously picking at a self-inflicted wound of the mouth. The second was an ileocolic intussusception, a rare variety; although the bowel was resected and a Murphy button inserted the child died. The third case, operated upon by Dr. Joseph W. Hearn, was notable for the recovery of the patient. No trace of the appendix could be found and contrary to his usual custom Dr. Hearn flushed out the abdomen.

Dr. Alfred Hand, Jr., in his "Rapid Method for Ridding the Throat of Diphtheria Bacilli after Disappearance of the Membrane" recommended the use of silver nitrate, sixty grains to the ounce, to be applied to the mucous membrane.

A meeting of the Section on General Medicine, College of Physicians, was held Monday, June 13th. A case of "Nasal Diphtheria Complicated with Broncopneumonia" reported by Dr. Hamill was interesting because of the mild general symptoms, the location of the infection, the severe gastro-intestinal disturbances, and the ultimate recovery of the patient. Dr. M. H. Fussell in the discussion which followed mentioned several similar cases and spoke of a number of errors in bacteriologic diagnosis made by those supposed by the public and the profession to be competent.

Dr. Frederick Packard reported a case of "Intrathoracic Growth Secondary to Carcinoma of the Breast with Destruction of the Left Phrenic Nerve." The case occurred in a woman about forty years of age and, aside from the absence of cough, dyspnea, and emaciation, the case was interesting because the pancreas alone, of the abdominal viscera, was involved.

A "Case of Pyloroplasty" was reported by Dr. Fussell in which operation afforded relief.

The Ohio State Board of Health has honored Philadelphia by electing Dr. Elmer G. Horton, assistant demonstrator of bacteriology in the University of Pennsylvania, State Chemist.

The Examining Board of the State Medical Society met in this city and Pittsburg, June 14th to 17th, to examine applicants for licenses to practise medicine. The questions, on the whole, while possibly more difficult than those of previous years, were more practical and covered the subjects examined in a much better way.

The total number of deaths in this city as reported at the health office for the week ending June 18th, was 499, of which number 189 were of children under five years of age. There were 168 new cases of contagious diseases reported, as follows: Diphtheria, 49 with 9 deaths; scarlet fever, 40 with 2 deaths; typhoid fever, 79 with 7 deaths.

OUR FOREIGN LETTER.

[From our Special Correspondent.]

AN AUTOPSY IN AN ASTHMA CASE—A NEW TUMOR OF THE SPINAL CORD AND PRESENT INTEREST IN DISPLACED ORGANIC MATERIAL AS THE BASIS FOR TUMOR GROWTH—TWO CASES OF MAJOR HYSTERIA—TEN CASES OF SYPHILIS INSONTIUM IN PHYSICIANS—DOCTOR'S DAY AT WIESBADEN.

BERLIN, June 12, 1898.

PROFESSOR FRAENKEL, from whom the diplococcus of pneumonia has its name, presented two very interesting sets of pathologic specimens at the last meeting of the Society for Internal Medicine. The first were from an asthmatic patient dying during an attack. There are only three other such autopsies recorded in literature. As there is no set of pathologic changes common to all of the cases, Professor Fränkel could only conclude that asthma as we know it is not even in its immediate etiology, that is in the lung condition underlying it, a definite pathologic entity, but a clinical combination of symptoms occurring from various causes. In the discussion Professor Von Leyden took part. He himself had reported one of the three other autopsies on asthma patients, and his discovery of asthma crystals promised at one time to lead to some explanation of the attacks. He, too, considers that the bronchitis found in so many asthma cases is not specific, and that the disease is not necessarily primary in the lungs, but is a reflex neurosis, the primum movens of which may be situated almost anywhere in the body. While asthma is almost always accompanied by a fibrinous bronchiolitis, fibrinous bronchiolitis may be, and often is, uncomplicated by asthmatic attacks.

At the same meeting, Professor Frankel presented microscopic specimens of a tumor of the spinal cord, of which this is but a second example that has so far been described, though it is probable that the tumors are not so infrequent, since this second tumor turns up within a couple months after the publication of the description and plates of the first one. The tumor consists of a series of cystic cavities microscopic in dimensions, but all lined with epithelial cells, and evidently morphologically connected with the central canal of the cord, a series, as it were, of central canals grouped together irregularly. Dr. Rosenthal, in an article in *Ziegler's Beiträge* some months ago (Vol. 23, No. 1), under the name "Neuroepithelioma Medullæ Spinalis," described a similar tumor from the Pathological Institute at Erlangen. Some of Rosenthal's specimens were shown by Professor Frankel, and there is evidently identity of morphologic elements. The epithelial cells lining the cysts are cylindrical in character, and the ends situated away from the cavities of the cyst branch out into fibrillary terminals, which join the glia fibers surrounding the spaces. This is the most important distinctive peculiarity of the epithelial cells lining the canal of the cord, so that there is evidently question of an analogous combination of cellular elements.

Professor Fránkel considers that in such cases there is question of the later growth of displaced elements which probably in an embryonal stage found this abnormal situation in the cord. The term for these displaced elements in German, *Versprengte Keime*, misplaced germinal elements, is a most expressive one. The idea that it conveys is coming more and more into prominence in pathology in recent years. Grawitz's tumors of the kidney, the formerly so-called adenomata of the kidney, are now almost universally admitted to be due to misplaced suprarenal *germinals*. The last number of *Zeigler's Beiträge* contains a magnificent review of the whole subject (a much discussed one it has been), and a personal contribution of distinct scientific value, that would seem to leave no further room for doubt, from the pen of Dr. Kelly, the pathologist at the German Hospital, Philadelphia. Another phase of misplaced germinal elements, the occurrence of striped muscular tumors in the kidney, since its description at Recklinghausen's laboratory, is occupying a good deal of attention in pathologic circles, and was the subject of a most interesting discussion by Professor Grawitz recently in the Medical Society at Greifswald.

Two very interesting cases of major hysteria were presented at the last meeting of the Charité Arzte (association of physicians and surgeons connected with the charité hospital). The first, presented by Dr. Strauss, Professor Senator's assistant, was that of a young man of twenty-eight, who, ten years ago, while making his military service, was thrown from his horse and the animal fell on him. The only injury he seemed to have suffered at the time was the fracture of two ribs, and this was the only thing for which he was treated, though other internal injuries were looked for carefully at the time. Shortly after, in fact careful inquiry shows that it began while he was in the hospital for the injury, he began to suffer from most obstinate constipation. He never had a stool without some means being taken to procure one. Then began a series of attacks resembling ileus, but which ordinary medical measures sufficed to relieve. Finally, however, these attacks became so frequent and so severe that an operation was proposed and agreed to. It was thought that a stenosis of the intestine would be found, due to cicatrical adhesions from injuries produced at the time of his accident. Absolutely nothing abnormal was found.

For nearly a year after the operation, however, there were no further attacks of intestinal obstruction. Then they began again, and after awhile became again very severe. Nothing could be done for him in Berlin, so he was sent to a hospital in a distant city, where, during the course of a typical attack, he was operated on once more. This surgeon also found nothing pathologic. For more than six months after the operation he was once more free from attacks. Then they began again. He was admitted to the Charité, and from Professor Leyden's clinic referred to the surgical clinic for operation because of most exquisite ileus symptoms. In view of the patient's history, Professor Koenig refused to operate. This was more than a year ago. He is back in the Charité once more with the old complaint, but this time he has had a series of hysterical attacks, laughing and crying, and his symptoms, especially the tense distended abdomen, so characteristic of the case at its worst, has been observed to come and go without any regard to the condition of his bowels or the extent of the constipation.

The second case was presented by Dr. Westphal, Professor Jolly's assistant at the Clinic for Mental and Nervous Diseases. The patient was a young woman, who, while under treatment in Professor Leyden's clinic for pneumonia, and just at the end of her convalescence (she was to have left the hospital next day), developed during the night great tympanites, some temperature, and a rapid pulse. The condition was thought to be a fulminant perforative peritonitis, and a very bad prognosis was given. A few days later all the symptoms had disappeared. She was kept under observation for awhile longer, and the same train of symptoms developed once more. She was then referred to the nervous department, where she was discovered by an attendant swallowing air for the purpose of producing the tympanites, which she seems to be able to bring about at will. In this second case a surgical operation would undoubtedly have been suggested on the first occurrence of the symptoms, only that the fact that they pointed to an intense generalized peritonitis seemed to make surgical interference of no avail. The cases illustrate the exaggerated phases of the constitutional neurosis which is becoming more and more frequent here on the Continent.

Dr. Brandis, in a recent number of the *Deutsche Medicinische Wochenschrift* (May 21) gives an account of ten cases of syphilis from extragenital chancres in physicians. He has had the rare opportunity to watch this many cases, and gives some interesting details. In very few of the cases, practically none, was the nature of the primary sore recognized until secondaries developed, as physicians are so liable to have infected or dissecting wounds on the hands which heal slowly and become indurated. In nearly all of them the treatment was not begun till late, and the symptomatic course was severe. Most of the patients died young, though of course the mortality among physicians is always high. Dr. Brandis insists on the use of gloves in all suspicious examinations, and also during all operations on syphilitic patients, especially on suspected *buboes*. The serious sequelæ and the bad prognosis of the Doctor's cases came, he thinks, from not following the mercurial treatment exactly, a characteristic medical failing.

On June 29th the German doctors assemble for Doctor's Day at Wiesbaden. This is an annual assemblage of German doctors, in which subjects of general interest to the profession are handled. This year the subjects for discussion are "The Relations of Physicians to Insurance Companies," and the question of "Medical Studies for Women." Professor Penzoldt of Erlangen is the referee on this last question, and the drift of German sentiment in the matter is evident since it is considered worthy of a place at the discussions on *Aerztetag*.

TRANSACTIONS OF FOREIGN SOCIETIES.

Paris.

SYPHILITIC ULCER OF THE STOMACH—PROPOSED COMPULSORY DISINFECTION OF HOUSES IN WHICH PHTHISICAL PATIENTS HAVE DIED—AN INSTANCE OF THE INCREASE IN SIZE OF THICK GRAFTS—ADVANTAGES OF PERISCOPIC GLASSES — POST-OPERATIVE PSYCHOSES—VAGINAL HYSTERECTOMY WITHOUT CLAMPS OR LIGATURES—SECONDARY INFECTION WITH THE BACILLUS PYOCYANEUS—AN EPIDEMIC IN PARIS OF CEREBROSPINAL MENINGITIS.

AT the Academy of Medicine, May 17th, DIEULAFOY mentioned a case of syphilitic ulcer of the stomach. The patient was known to have had syphilis, from which he was supposed to have recovered. When a diagnosis was made of ulcer of the stomach it was assumed that this was a simple ulcer, and the patient was so treated for many months without cure. With the subsequent administration of mixed treatment the ulcer quickly healed. The writer called attention to the fact that syphilitic ulcerations of the stomach are not so rare as is supposed. They may occur in the form of ecchymoses, circumscribed or diffuse gummata, or cicatricial ulcerations. The symptoms are similar to those of simple ulcer of the stomach. Since the history in syphilitic cases is proverbially unreliable, and if for any reason it is suspected that the ulcer is not a simple one, it is advisable to put the patient at once under treatment with mercury and potassium iodid.

At the session of May 24th GIBERT proposed that every dwelling inhabited by a patient suffering from pulmonary tuberculosis, should after the death of such a person, be disinfected by the authorities. His idea was to make this a compulsory act, applicable alike to rich and poor whether dwelling in the city or in the country.

At the Academy of Sciences, May 2d, OLLIER mentioned an instance in which thick grafts were applied to cover defects in the skin of a patient whose knee had been severely burned. These grafts were taken from the patient's own skin, and after they had become adherent instead of undergoing atrophy to a certain extent their longitudinal diameters increased. He explained this by their position, for they were not only subjected to constant stretching when the knee was flexed, but they were so stimulated by the irritation thus produced, that their thickness was not diminished though their length was increased. A similar condition is sometimes found in the skin over a tumor. In support of this observation it may be mentioned that the hairs upon the grafts were further apart than those upon the skin which surrounded the spots from which the grafts were taken.

At the session of May 2d, OSTWALT spoke of the distortion of images which always occurs to a greater or less degree, with eye-glasses as usually made, since most objects are not looked at directly through the center of the lenses, but more or less obliquely. To avoid this Wollaston advocated nearly a century ago, a *periscopic* lens, that is, one in the form of a meniscus, with the convex surface toward the light, and the concave surface toward the eye. Every number of glasses is however represented by an infinite number of meniscuses, growing more and more curved. The question, therefore, arises which one is the most advantageous for the patient? Neither Wollaston nor any other person has been able to answer this question accurately, and the choice has been left to the optician. From a study of the images formed through different shaped glasses, but objects situated at an infinite distance, and twenty-five degrees to one side of the axis of vision Oswalt found that meniscoid glasses possess great advantages over planoconvex or double convex lenses. Whenever it is practicable, therefore, glasses of this form ought to be prescribed.

At the Society of Surgery, May 11th, LE DENTU said that he had studied post-operative psychoses since 1890. This state of delirium springs from several causes, but it has nothing in common with alcoholic delirium. He had himself observed twenty-three instances of post-operative psychosis. Eight times the psychosis followed an operation upon the skeleton, three times an operation upon the digestive tract, once a radical cure of umbilical hernia, and once an operation upon the urinary tract, twice an operation upon the male genitals, and three operations upon the female genitals. Of sixty-eight cases collected from literature more than half occurred after gynecologic operations. The frequency of this association is beyond doubt. In general the delirium is of two types, either of agitation or of depression. The immediate causes are numerous. Leaving aside delirium of toxic origin produced by anesthetics or antiseptics employed, as well as delirium of an infectious character, or that due to bad action of the kidneys, there remains the true post-operative delirium of purely cerebral origin. These cases may be divided into maniacal delirium, hysterical delirium, and senile delirium. The latter appears especially in atheromatous subjects, and is of a mild, tranquil form. Undoubtedly a nervous predisposition plays a considerable rôle in the production of true delirium although many cases occur in which it is impossible to determine a nervous predisposition either hereditary or acquired.

At the session of May 18th TUFFIER gave the results he has obtained by a method of vaginal hysterectomy without ligatures or clamps, bleeding being stopped by an instrument called an "angiotribe." He has employed this method twenty-three times. Operation was performed twelve times for pelvic abscess; twice for abscess complicated with hematocele; eight times for uterine fibroids; and once for carcinoma of the cervix. One patient died of septic peritonitis, the diagnosis being confirmed by autopsy; one other died in a few days of pulmonary congestion. All the rest recovered. The technic of the method is simple. The ordinary vaginal operation is performed but instead of ligating the broad ligaments or leaving clamps on them for a couple of days; they are simply grasped and crushed by the "angiotribe." If bleeding comes on rapidly or the operation is a prolonged one the ligaments are caught up in simple clamps until the operator is ready to crush them. There are two precautions to be observed, one is to close the "angiotribe" well and the other is to keep its point in the axis of the vagina. Only two incidents were noted in these twenty-three operations. Once the patient showed symptoms of collapse and the house surgeon performed laparotomy, thinking of internal hemorrhage. None was present. In another case the vaginal tampons became saturated with blood and were removed. The bleeding was found to come not from the broad ligament but from a tear in the vagina.

POIRIER showed a patient from whom he had removed the tibial diaphesis, grafting into its place the fibula by two operations. It firmly united and the functional result three years later was excellent, there being only about one inch of shortening. The fibula had considerably increased in size, thus showing the tendency of an organ to adapt itself to the demands made upon it.

At the Medical Society of the Hospitals, May 13th, VINCENT said that no disease predisposes more to secondary infections than typhoid fever. The streptococcus is very likely to attack the patient and reduce his chances of recovery. A rarer complication observed by him in one case is a general infection by the bacillus pyocyaneus. The patient was a man already weakened by malaria and his typhoid fever was complicated with a myocarditis. The symptoms lessened somewhat until on the 10th day there appeared a very painful double mastitis and then a double parotiditis, and finally a bullous eruption upon the trunk and limbs, the fluid in the bullæ being tinted. There was also a severe sore throat with high fever. The patient died three days later. In the intestine were the usual lesions of typhoid fever. There were also many foci of pulmonary gangrene of the size of a walnut, and in these foci were innumerable myriads of the bacillus pyocyaneus. This was also true of the cutaneous bullæ. This bacillus was found to be associated with the typhoid bacillus in the blood of the heart and in the spleen. This case is of interest as showing the gravity of a secondary infection by the bacillus pyocyaneus in typhoid fever. It shows further that this bacillus is capable of producing pulmonary gangrene and the other lesions above mentioned.

NETTER called attention to the existence in Paris of a small epidemic of cerebrospinal meningitis of which he had seen in a period of two months no less than five fatal cases in the Trousseau Hospital. There were three other fatal cases of tuberculous meningitis in which the meningococcus was associated with the tubercle bacillus. Most of the cases entered the hospital from different parts of the city and the suburbs. Since the prognosis in cerebrospinal meningitis is less gloomy than in tuberculous meningitis it is important to recognize it. In doubtful cases puncture of the lumbar column may give fluid enough to clear up the diagnosis. The question of isolation of a person suffering from cerebrospinal meningitis is of no importance since direct contagion is very rarely observed.

At the meeting of May 20th NETTER further reported that he had found the pneumococcus in five new cases of cerebrospinal meningitis. Four of these were primary and one complicated cerebral tuberculosis. Four of the patients were children. Twice the diagnosis was made bacteriologically from fluid obtained by lumbar puncture, and one of these patients was recovering.

SOCIETY PROCEEDINGS.

AMERICAN MEDICAL ASSOCIATION.

Forty-ninth Annual Meeting, Held at Denver, Col., June 7, 8, 9, and 10, 1898.

[Specially Reported for the MEDICAL NEWS.]

(Continued from page 807.)

SECTION ON OBSTETRICS AND DISEASES OF WOMEN.

FIRST DAY—JUNE 7TH.

THE Chairman of this Section, DR. JOSEPH PRICE of Philadelphia, delivered an address, entitled

RECENT ADVANCES IN OBSTETRICS AND GYNECOLOGY.

Several suggestions were offered in regard to improvements in methods of work. He pointed out that all troubles to which women are subject, medical and surgical, are found in the field of the general practitioner. He should be a skilled diagnostician, and be competent to deal directly with many minor gynecologic troubles. The vital question pertaining to plastic work has largely dropped out of the discussions in medical societies. All who have had to deal with vesicovaginal fistula and lacerations through the sphincter muscle and up the vaginal septum know the beautiful results following careful and successful work, and fully recognize that it is not work to be done by a mere apprentice. Failures are explainable from the certain premises that the patients had not been thoroughly prepared for operation. To do good plastic work there should be an apprenticeship of many months under a good operator. Careful training in plastic work is of more importance than in abdominal surgery. Of late years the preparation of the patient has not been sufficiently thorough and prolonged to favor the best results.

Uterine displacements are quite generally neglected. Women with uterine posterior displacements should be put to bed, the uterus replaced, all lacerations repaired, and a well-fitting pessary introduced. Large, round, soft rubber rings are useless and harmful, and much too commonly used. Stem-pessaries are of but little value. Rest-treatment for the correction of displacements is the shortest, surest, and most satisfactory. An anterior dressing for a few days, with the patient remaining in bed at rest in the Sims position, favors speedy recovery. It should not be assumed that there are no risks associated with these mechanical appliances. Early in the history of the pessary there were numerous accidents. Men familiar with placing them obtained good results and rarely had accidents. Among the accidents recorded were the following: Perforation of the rectum, perforation of the bladder, perforation of both rectum and bladder, ureteral fistula, vesicovaginal fistula, perforation of Douglas' cul-de-sac, and perforation of the vaginal wall and escape of the pessary into the peritoneal cavity. Neurasthenia is a subject that concerns all medical men. A Hodge pessary has cured many such cases. The connection of the vagina, the uterus, and the ovaries through their nervous supply with the splanchnic nerves, and with the spinal cord in the sacral and lumbar regions through the pelvic and hypogastric plexus may anatomically explain many of the reflex phenomena which follow upon stimulation or irritation of the ovarian and uterine nerves consequent upon diseases of the ovaries and uterus. Many of these nervous conditions can be averted or cured by early and careful attention to uterine and ovarian troubles.

DR. J. RIDDLE GOFFE of New York followed with an interesting paper on

ANTERIOR COLPOTOMY AND SHORTENING OF THE ROUND LIGAMENTS THROUGH THE VAGINA FOR THE RELIEF OF ALL CASES OF RETROVERSION OF THE UTERUS, SIMPLE OR COMPLICATED.

At the outset Dr. Goffe said that Dr. Kelly had collected a list of forty-five different operations which had been suggested for the relief of uterine posterior displacement. This was a proof of the general interest in the subject. The uterus rests in an unstable position, which varies with the position of the woman, so that its normal position can only be determined by a large number of investigations with the subjects in the erect posture. When the body is in the upright position the uterus nominally rests on its anterior surface, and is suspended by the uterovesical and uterosacral ligaments, while it is steadied in this position by the broad and round ligaments. It must be concluded, therefore, that the uterus is supported by its ligaments and subject to intra-abdominal pressure. In the normal position this pressure falls upon the posterior surface of the organ, and the fundus is driven still further forward and held in its normal anteverted position. If the ligaments became overstretched, that is, the uterosacral or uterovesical ligaments are relaxed, the uterus becomes displaced posteriorly. All of the ligaments then gradually become loose and lose their tone, and the organ becomes hopelessly displaced. The round and broad ligaments may be relaxed, and the uterus will remain in the normal position; but once let the uterosacral ligaments become stretched, and the uterus will sooner or later be displaced on account of the forward dropping of the cervix and backward tilting of the fundus.

The most popular operation to-day, designed to correct retrodisplacement of the uterus, is the modified or original Alexander operation. The objections to Alexander's operation are several, including hemorrhage, the making of two scars, and the difficulty in finding the ligaments and breaking of these structures. The speaker suggested the value of anterior colpotomy in all cases of retrodisplacement, whether simple or complicated. The patient is placed in the lithotomy position, and an incision made across the anterior vaginal wall in front of the cervix. The bladder is stripped from the uterus. The anterior vaginal wall is put upon the stretch and divided throughout its extent from the cervix to the internal orifice of the urethra. The finger is now passed over the uterus through the incision, hooked over the cornu, the adhesions broken up, and the fundus brought forward into the vagina and out as far as the vulva. The appendages can also be brought down and removed or treated conservatively. The round ligaments are then drawn down one after the other and shortened, the loop thus made on each side being stitched to the anterior surface of the uterus near the fundus. The uterus is then returned to its normal position. The bladder is adjusted and the vaginal incision closed by catgut, and a piece of iodoform gauze introduced into the vagina. This operation is valuable because of its wide application. The essayist had treated thirty-one cases in this way, and in all of those of simple retroversion (six in number) the results had been perfect. Some cases were complicated, requiring resection of the tube and ovary. In a number of these the patients became pregnant, but had not suffered from a return of the displacement. Attempts at loosening the round ligaments from the connective tissue were followed by profuse bleeding, in one case requiring hysterectomy.

DR. ALBERT GOLDSPOHN of Chicago, in opening the discussion, stated that he had performed this operation a number of times. In his opinion, it is not difficult, it is very feasible, and is much to be preferred to ventrofixation, vesicofixation, and ventrosuspension.

DR. HENRY P. NEWMAN of Chicago expressed his gratification at the position taken by the essayist. If the incision in Alexander's operation, however, is made over the external ring, the abdominal portion of the round ligament will be secure, and not the divided portion of the inguinal canal. This makes a much better support than the latter. The part that must be shortened is the intra-abdominal portion and not that within the inguinal canal.

DR. HOWARD A. KELLY of Baltimore believed that all of these operations should be supplemented by restoration of the floor of the pelvis. He did not believe that the round ligaments support the uterus. They are always found kinked in abdominal operations, and hence could not be supporting. With the uterus retrodisplaced the abdominal force increases the trouble, while if the uterus is anterior it increases the anterior displacement. A thread applied to the fundus holds it in this normal position, and the pressure then falls upon the posterior surface. The floor should then be restored. He had operated through an inch and a half incision more than 400 times, and only about two per cent. of the cases have relapsed. About twenty of the women have become pregnant. All are doing well but one, and in her case agglutination occurred. Fixation is not the proper procedure; it is suspension that is desired. None of the cases terminated fatally. Severe pain has not been noted in any case. He never includes the fascia or muscle in his stitch, but only the peritoneum and supraperitoneal tissues.

DR. GOFFE, in closing the discussion, stated that all gynecologists are agreed that simple retroversion of the uterus is not a condition severe enough to require a grave operation. The indications for operation are to be found in the diseased appendages, and to reach these the pelvic cavity must be opened. The question is, By which route shall this cavity be entered? The answer will be fought out in the coming years, and, in his opinion, it will be decided in favor of the vaginal operation. His rule is not to perform an abdominal operation if he can avoid it. As regards the priority of the operation, he does not claim it. Wertheim of Germany had suggested it, but he himself was the first to perform it. The operation is not simple; it takes time and patience, but the results are excellent.

SECOND DAY—JUNE 8TH.

DR. A. P. CLARKE of Cambridge, Mass., read a paper, entitled

FURTHER EXPERIENCES IN THE MANAGEMENT OF UTERINE DISPLACEMENTS,

in which he stated that in most cases of displacement of the adnexa there is also displacement of the uterus. If the latter is corrected the ovarian condition also is corrected. He had seen many cases in which ventral suspension had been performed, the results being so bad that he had become afraid of the operation. He had been interested in the Alexander operation and believed that if it is performed in suitable cases, and the perineum is made intact and existing subinvolution is corrected, the patient will be cured. If the operator fails to correct the effects of subinvolution, the operation will fail. Only in the cases in which the tubes and ovaries are involved in the morbid process and are adherent will their extirpation become necessary.

DESCENSUS OVARIORUM.

This paper was contributed by DR. ALBERT GOLDSPOHN of Chicago. The author stated that descensus of the ovary is responsible for many of the distressing symptoms of which women complain. The normal location of the ovary, as ascertained by Schultze, is against the lateral wall of the true pelvis, a little below the brim and protected by a projecting fold of its mesentery. Its free border is directed in an inverted and posterior direction. It is suspended in the true pelvis nearly as high and as far removed from the median line as possible. It is subject to the action of abdominal pressure. There are two degrees of descensus. In the first degree the ovary lies on the retro-ovarian shelf and can be felt in the posterior fornix of the vagina by bimanual palpation. In the second degree it passes over the retrosacral fold and sinks into Douglas' cul-de-sac. The left ovary descends by far the more frequently in both degrees, and in the severe cases of double ovarian prolapse it is the most displaced.

The causes of prolapse are: (1) Anything causing an abnormal or disproportionate increase in the weight of the organ, or inflammatory conditions, and in the exauthemata; (2) a multiformation of corpora lutea and unruptured, heavy, Graafian follicles. A second group of cases includes the condition in which the ovarian ligaments become elongated, as in subinvolution, or when vicious traction is made upon them in minor gynecologic operations. Especially is this common in vaginal celiotomy, which is useful for extirpation of the adnexa but not for the conservative treatment of these organs. (3) The chief cause of descensus is retroversion and retroflexion of the uterus. Harmful factors incident to descensus are: (1) Venous stasis; (2) traumata from the uterus and the rectum. During coughing, sneezing, and other acts of straining the pelvic viscera are displaced downward, owing to the action of the intra-abdominal pressure. If the ovary leaves its sheltered nook and approaches the median line of the pelvis, the intra-abdominal pressure falls upon it and painful traumata results. In complete descensus the ovary lies in a vise and is pressed upon by the retroverted uterus and overloaded bowel, while coitus is impossible. In the first degree of descent, when the ovary lies in the sulcus under the fold of ligament, the pressure from above will sooner or later produce descent of the second degree unless some operative procedure be resorted to. Hematomata, edema, connective-tissue hyperplasia, chronic oophoritis, leading to multiple cystic degeneration in one part of the ovary and cirrhosis in other portions, and peri-oophoritis are the pathologic changes in prolapsed ovaries.

The so-called medical treatment of this condition is effective in cases in which descent is associated with retroversion and uterine subinvolution subsequent to parturition. A properly fitting pessary and a vagino-abdominal faradic current, with massage and tonic medicinal treatment will do good in a few cases. Non puerperal cases, however, are not benefited by this course. Wool tampons impregnated with glycerin and renewed daily will reduce the tenderness, and manual massage may then correct the displacement, when a pessary must be introduced and be worn for life. The best treatment for these cases, however, must be surgical. The displacement of the uterus must be corrected at the outset. Vaginal fixation, vaginosuspension, and ventrosuspension are not eligible as curative procedures in women subject to conception. The round ligaments of the uterus are proper structures to act upon. They may be shortened by vaginal section, but this route is only of service in some cases in which a conservative operation on the appendages is not needed. Ventral celiotomy is the proper route in all cases complicated by adhesions and lingering septic action. Intra-abdominal shortening of the round ligaments then acts admirably. The ovarian fimbriæ are caught by a thread and secured to the inner free margin of the spermatic or main suspensory ligament of the ovary near the iliopectineal line. Thus, the ovary and fimbriated extremity of the tube are suspended in normal relation to each other and with a proper degree of mobility. Alexander's operation is not an ideal method for the treatment of ovarian prolapse. Only skin and fat should be cut, all other tissues being separated bluntly and the internal inguinal ring stretched. In this way hernia will be prevented. A small opening, large enough to introduce the index-finger is thus obtained, and any degree of fixation can be loosened and the tube and ovary brought up and out of the ring, when incision or conservative treatment of the appendages may be practised.

DR. GOLDSPOHN, in closing the discussion which followed the reading of his paper, condemned what he designated as the surgical monstrosities of ventrosuspension, ventrofixation, and vesicofixation. Fixation is so serious a thing that soon it will be malpractice to perform it. Suspension exposes the patient to the risks of intestinal obstruction. If the bands made by these operations are the result of traumatism the operators themselves will open the abdomen to remove them. Two-thirds of the women so operated upon have troubles in gestation or labor, or both. Ileus becomes a common sequence after these operations. Ligaments are merely guy-ropes; intra-abdominal pressure is the fixing force that condemns the retrodisplaced uterus to remain in a permanent position. The best route to correct displacements is through the inguinal canal. The cardinal point in the technic of the Alexander operation is that the way into the abdomen is not cut, but the tissues so split that they fall together. Each layer must also be closed individually. At least ninety-five per cent. of the cases of descent of the ovaries are associated with uterine retroversion; hence, the treatment is to be directed to both conditions. The gynecologist who knows no middle ground between excising an ovary and doing nothing stands in the same position as the surgeon who would amputate every diseased leg.

DR. W. D. HAGGARD, JR., of Nashville, Tenh., contributed a paper, entitled

A PLEA FOR THE MORE CORRECT APPLICATION OF EMMET'S METHOD IN PLASTIC SURGERY,

in which he dilated upon the importance of removing from the cervix all cicatricial tissue in suturing a laceration, at the same time retaining, as far as possible, the original conical shape of the cervix. The incision should be conoidal. Emmet's operation on the vaginal wall was of more gradual evolution than his trachelorrhaphy. It includes the rectocele as well as destroyed muscle. The perineal body is of no consequence. As Emmet said, it is the body which does not exist. The sense of bearing down in injury of the pelvic fascia is due to the pelvic congestion that is present. Women who have a true laceration of the floor, a complete tear through the sphincter and up the posterior vaginal wall, do not have prolapse. The fascia is not torn, and hence support is not lost. The proper treatment of the torn floor is to catch up the retracted fascia, so as to take up the slack, as it were, and thus restore its function. The denudation is all effected on the posterior vaginal wall, and does not involve the bladder or the labia.

The afternoon session of this Section was devoted to a joint discussion with the Section on Neurology on

THE RELATION OF PELVIC DISEASES TO NERVOUS AND MENTAL AFFECTIONS.

The first paper was by DR. FREDERICK PETERSON of New York, entitled

IS PELVIC DISEASE A CAUSE OF NERVOUS AND MENTAL AFFECTIONS?

The author stated that specialists should first of all equal the general practitioner in ability. The specialist is likely to attribute hysteria, neurasthenia, chorea, and other neuroses to the viscus that is most prominent in his intellectual sphere. The specialist who is broad enough to look upon man as a biologic unit will not fall into this narrow rut. He had looked recently into five books on gynecology to see what was said upon the subject under discussion. Three said nothing about it; the others attributed the nervous conditions of women to disorders of their sexual organs. The pelvic organs play but a small part in nervous complications which have to deal with the entire organism of woman. Pelvic disease in women attended by exhausting pain may give rise to neurasthenia or hysteria, but exhausting pelvic pain is no more deleterious than exhausting pain elsewhere. Profuse hemorrhage may cause serious trouble, no matter what its source. The pelvic organs have little if any effect upon psychic conditions. The field of the gynecologist, in the opinion of the essayist, is very limited in the nervous domain, and there is but little opportunity for gynecologic operations on insane patients.

ARE NERVOUS AND MENTAL DISEASES CURED BY PELVIC OPERATIONS?

This paper was contributed by DR. F. X. DERCUM of Philadelphia, but, in the absence of the author, was read by Dr. Patrick of Chicago. The author pointed out that the most important neuroses encountered by the gynecologist are neurasthenia and hysteria. Neurasthenia is marked by chronic fatigue; hence, he terms it the "fatigue neurosis." There are nervous irritability and nervous weakness or tire. Hyperesthesia is often marked in these cases, as over the coccyx, the iliac spines and in the eye. The resistance to fatigue is diminished; hence, symptoms of tire become marked, as headache and nervous irritability. A woman with some morbid pelvic condition, as laceration of the cervix or perineum, or displaced uterus, may not complain until neurasthenia develops, when she commences to suffer from the symptoms of the pelvic complaint. Hysteria is often said to be a disease without a syndrome, but this is untrue. It has as marked a syndrome as any disease known. Its symptoms are sensory, motor, and psychic. In hysteria anasthesia may be present. This sensory loss never occurs in neurasthesia. Hemianesthesia of the left side is a common symptom of hysteria, and it may also be limited to areas, as the foot, the hand, or a segment of the body. The anesthesia is not referred to any nerve area, or to any territory governed by a spinal center. Hyperesthesia is occasionally found in hysteria, and usually under the breast or above the groin, where it is grossly miscalled ovarian tenderness. This also is more common on the left side. Areas of hyperesthesia may become areas of hyperalgesia, for example, the clavus hystericus. So-called ovarian tenderness may be found in men, and also in women without ovaries. This is in reality an inguinal or groin pain. It is always associated with other well-marked hysterical stigmata. It is superficial, in the skin of the groin, and not deep in the body, as true ovarian pain would be. Pressure between two fingers, one on the spot and the other in the vagina, will differentiate this pain from ovarian pain.

The psychic symptoms of hysteria are important to the gynecologist. The patient is, as a rule, exceedingly impressionable. She is open to suggestion, especially as regards her pelvic condition. Hysteria is a psychoneurosis because of the prominence of these psychic manifestations. Neuresthenia may exist without pelvic disease. If both coexist they have no relation with each other. If pelvic disease exists with neurasthenia the pelvic symptoms become more marked because of increased irritability. Hysteria may exist without pelvic disease. The possibility is denied of nervous and mental disease arising from pelvic operations. The pelvic condition should be operated on for the local condition only, and not to relieve the nervous condition. In cases of profound hysteria an operation should never be undertaken unless the surgical condition is very urgent. The hysteria should first be cured in order to prevent the disastrous effects of the operation upon the nervous condition. The insanities are not due to local organic disease, but to disease of the neurons as a result of various derangements of tissue metabolism. Pelvic operations will not cure insanity.

DR. B. SHERWOOD DUNN of Boston discussed

THE PATHOLOGICAL RELATIONS OF UTERINE AND NERVOUS DISEASES,

saying that neurasthenia is undoubtedly the result of tire, as from a repeated reflex action that gives no time for the neuron to recuperate. As a result, chronic fatigue symptoms appear, and these may be referred to different parts of the system, the muscles, special senses, etc. The generative organs of woman are most closely allied to her nervous organism. Disease of the pelvic organs probably furnishes the most frequent cause of irritability of the nervous system. The rest cure, diet, electricity, and massage may cure temporarily the symptoms of neurasthenia, but if they be stopped the nervous symptoms return. Gynecologists are in the front rank of conservatism and do not operate on all nervous cases that come to them. Pelvic operations occasionally do cure nervous conditions. Nymphomania may be cured by local pelvic operations. There are certain microbic pathologic conditions of the ovary that give rise to persistent and troublesome neuroses. These are often relieved by operation.

DR. HAROLD N. MOYER of Chicago dwelt upon

NERVOUS AND MENTAL DISEASES FOLLOWING PELVIC OPERATIONS.

He propounded the question as to whether there is any difference between operations on the pelvic organs of women and operations in general. Investigation has shown that a large number of cases of neurasthenia and insanity follow pelvic operations, and one was led to believe that the nervous condition is the result of the operation. However, if one looks into the patient's condition he will find that she is run down and the subject of a long-continued infection. Dr. Moyer took fifty cases of operation on the prostrate, excluding all cases in which there was marked disease of the kidneys, and found that a larger number of males suffered from nervous symptoms than a similar number of women operated on for pelvic disease. He concludes, therefore, that pelvic operations are not more likely to be followed by nervous disorders than are general operations. Neurasthenia and mental debility are the common forms noted. Does the removal of an ovary exert any profound effect upon the body similar to that produced by the removal of the thyroid gland? He believed that when possible the ovary had better be left, or at least a part of it, and that resection is better than excision.

DR. JOSEPH EASTMAN of Indianapolis, Ind., spoke on

THE ASSOCIATION OF UTERINE AND NERVOUS DISTURBANCES,

stating that it is often difficult to determine whether the local condition is the result of neurasthenia or *vice versa*. A simple laceration of the perineum may result in profound neurasthenia that will disappear when the perineum is restored. Impaired sexual gratification in both male and female may result from laceration of the perineum, and therefrom result unhappiness and neurasthenia. In some cases the nervous condition is the result of irritation from the vermiform appendix. Coccygodynia is a condition that may give rise to nervous symptoms on account of the intimate relationship that exists between the coccyx and the ganglion impar. The fear of bearing children, with the resulting efforts to induce sterility, he thought is a frequent cause of neurasthenia.

DR. W. H. HUMISTON of Cleveland, O., dwelt upon the

INDICATIONS AND CONTRAINDICATIONS FOR SURGICAL INTERFERENCE.

He believed that the indications for operative interference are numerous, but doubts if there are any gynecologists who are operating on healthy structures to relieve nervous conditions. In all patients operated on there will be found marked deviations from the normal in the genital organs, as a tear of the cervix or of the perineum, a conical cervix, areolar hyperplasia of the uterus, endometritis with prolapse of the uterus, displacements of the uterus, dysmenorrhea, thickening of the tunica albuginea of the ovary, fissure of the rectum, fissure of the urethra, urethral caruncle, adherent glans clitoridis, etc. The pelvis should not be examined until the body has been carefully gone over. Auto-intoxication from the intestinal canal is a common cause of nervous phenomena. The contraindications to operation are to be found in the family history, the length of time the insanity has existed, and the independence of the symptoms of menstruation.

DR. HENRY P. NEWMAN of Chicago read a paper on

THE INDICATIONS FOR PLASTIC SURGERY UPON THE CERVIX UTERI, TRACHELOPLASTY, WITH A NEW METHOD OF OPERATING.

He said that the operation known as Emmet's operation has been in vogue for thirty-five years, but there is a wave of interest abroad concerning improved methods, and many reports of admirable work are being made in foreign journals. For some years he had sought to do operative work of such a character that as much as possible might be accomplished at one sitting, and the patient led to expect prompt recovery and encouraged to consider herself well and free from bondage to the gynecologic chair. His results have been, so far, satisfactory, and it was to call attention to a method of cervical operation which meets these requirements that he had selected this subject. The essayist then went into the technic of his method at great length, after which he summarized its advantages as follows:

1. The quickness and ease of operating by the knife; the manner of making the flaps transcending in certainty and safety of execution the ordinary methods of excision.

2. Clean, smooth cut surfaces which are obtained without haggling of tissues, always most desirable in plastic surgery.

3. The easy approximation of flaps and the avoidance of all hemorrhage beneath them by deep placing of sutures and compression of the flaps.

4. The accurate approximation of mucous membrane to mucous membrane, thus avoiding granulating surfaces, formation of cicatrix, and constricting of the canal. This feature, which obtains also in Schroeder's operation and modifications of it, is of great importance and a decided advantage over trachelorrhaphy, especially where the entire cervical mucous membrane is removed.

5. The certainty of obtaining a permanently patulous canal and well-formed cervix with pronounced reduction of the hyperplastic uterus.

6. The simplicity of the after-treatment.

THE TREATMENT OF AMBULATORY GYNECOLOGICAL CASES.

DR. DENSLOW LEWIS of Chicago read a paper on this subject, in which he referred to the gynecologic cases he had seen at the Chicago Polyclinic during the past four years. He directed attention exclusively to those cases, very properly designated as ambulatory, in which the women, although often seriously diseased or suffering from a condition which seems to demand some surgical treatment, are unable to submit to any radical measures which would necessitate a sojourn in a hospital or cause them to give up their daily work.

The officers elected for this section next year are: Chairman, Dr. A. H. Cordier of Kansas City, Mo.; Secretary, Dr. W. D. Haggard, Jr., of Nashville, Tenn.

THERAPEUTIC HINTS.

To Prevent Adenitis in Cases of Seborrheal Eczema.—The cervical adenitis due to auto-infection, especially by scratching, may be avoided in large measure, according to STEINHARDT, by scrupulous cleanliness and by relief of the pruritus. The infant is to be bathed frequently, its hands and nails cleansed at least every two hours, body and bed linen changed often, and the playthings washed.

Compresses wet with pure fresh water frequently renewed for one hour, will relieve the pruritus, after which the following ointment is applied:

℞ Ac. salicyl. . . . . gr. viii
Menthol . . . . . gr. xv
Ol. lini, Aq. calcis } aa . . . . ℥ iss.

M. Sig. External use.

Ichthyol in Acute Larnygeal Catarrh.—CIEGLEWICZ claims remarkable results in both adults and children from inspiration of a cold two-per-cent. ichthyol solution. The treatment is carried out once or twice daily for a period of three to five minutes by means of a Richardson atomizer, and causes rapid decrease of the cough and hoarseness.

For Chronic Eczema of the Fingers Due to Occupation.—For this affection, seen in various trades, such as masonry, and in women whose hands are much in contact with water, EDLEFSON recommends the following application:

℞ Iodi pur. . . . . . gr. iss
Potass. iodi . . . . . gr. iv
Glycerini . . . . . ʒ iii

M. Sig. Paint affected parts morning and evening and cover with linen or gloves.

Under this treatment the itching rapidly subsides and improvement of the eczema soon takes place. It may sometimes be well to use a twenty-per-cent. boric-acid ointment in the morning, painting at night only.

INDEX.

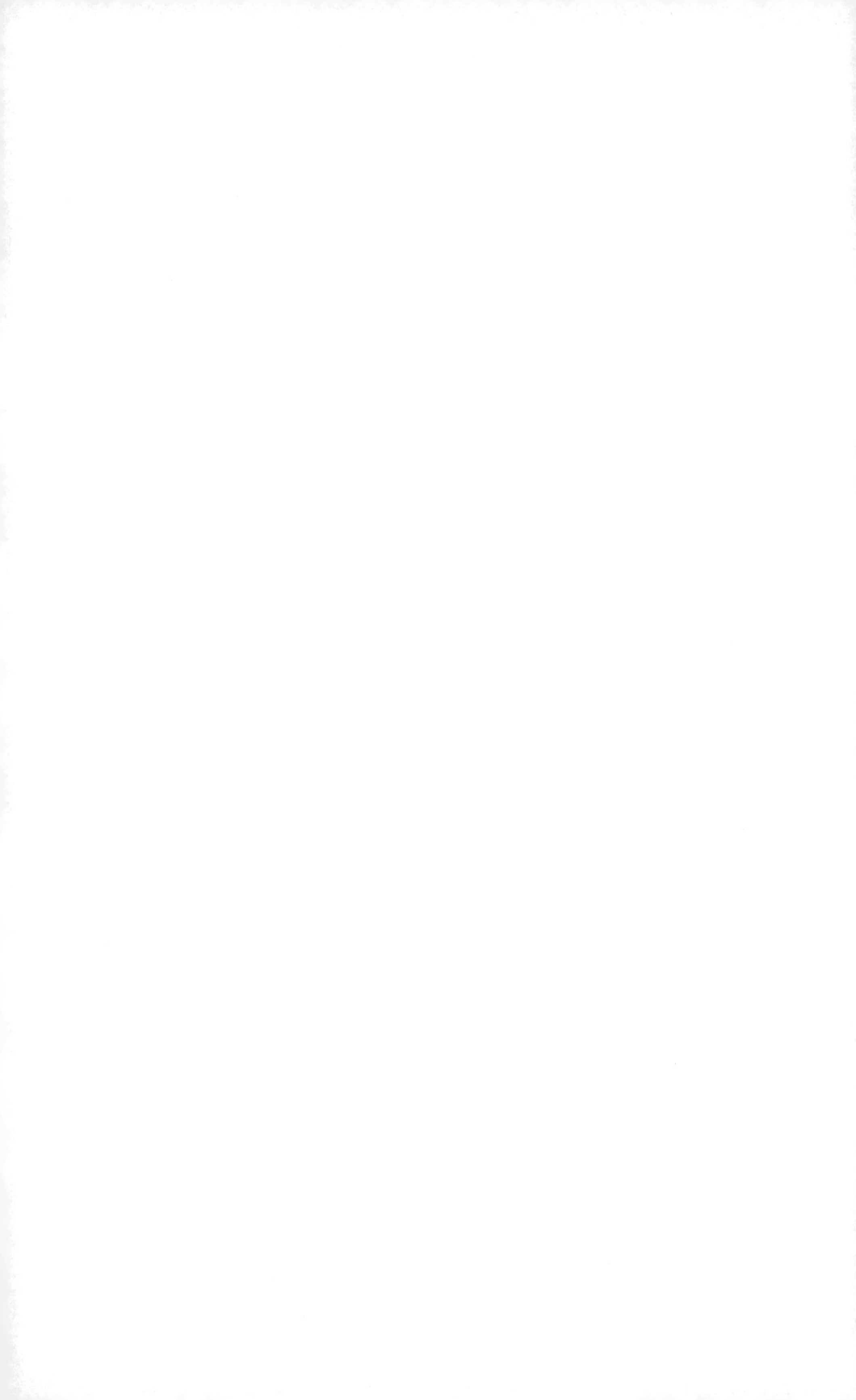

Lightning Source UK Ltd.
Milton Keynes UK
UKHW021108160119
335572UK00008B/289/P

9 780484 074605